Vaccine Design

The Subunit and Adjuvant
Approach

Pharmaceutical Biotechnology

Series Editor: Ronald T. Borchardt
The University of Kansas
Lawrence, Kansas

Vaccine Design
The Subunit and Adjuvant Approach

Edited by

Michael F. Powell
Genentech, Inc.
South San Francisco, California

and

Mark J. Newman
Vaxcel, Inc.
Norcross, Georgia

Assistant Editor
Jessica R. Burdman
Genentech, Inc.
South San Francisco, California

With a Foreword by Jonas Salk

Plenum Press • New York and London

Library of Congress Cataloging-in-Publication Data

Vaccine design : the subunit and adjuvant approach / edited by Michael
F. Powell and Mark J. Newman.
      p.   cm. -- (Pharmaceutical biotechnology ; v. 6)
   Includes bibliographical references and index.
   ISBN 0-306-44867-X
   1. Vaccines.   2. Immunological adjuvants.   I. Powell, Michael F.
II. Newman, Mark J.   III. Series.
QR189.V24   1995
615'.372--dc20   95-16401
                                                                      CIP

ISBN 0-306-44867-X

© 1995 Plenum Press, New York
A Division of Plenum Publishing Corporation
233 Spring Street, New York, N. Y. 10013

10 9 8 7 6 5 4 3 2 1

Printed in the United States of America

To those people who have supported us with this effort and also throughout our careers. Mike gives special thanks to his parents, Frank and Terri, in-laws, Sam and Joan, and especially to his wife Tana. Similarly, Mark thanks Joe, Adair, Kim, and his wife Gale.

Contributors

Sally E. Adams • British Bio-technology Ltd., Oxford OX4 5LY, United Kingdom

Jeff Alexander • Cytel Corporation, San Diego, California 92121

Alexander Andrianov • Virus Research Institute, Inc., Cambridge, Massachusetts 02138

Gail L. Barchfeld • Chiron Corporation, Emeryville, California 94608

Robert A. Baughman • Emisphere Technologies, Inc., Hawthorne, New York 10532

John W. Boslego • Walter Reed Army Institute of Research, Washington, D.C. 20307

Robert N. Brey • Vaxcel, Inc., Norcross, Georgia 30071

Carsten Brunn • Department of Pharmaceutics, University of Washington, School of Pharmacy, Seattle, Washington 98195

Jeanine L. Bussiere • Department of Pathobiology and Toxicology, Genentech, Inc., South San Francisco, California 94080

Noelene E. Byars • Syntex Research, Palo Alto, California 94304

Esteban Celis • Cytel Corporation, San Diego, California 92121

Donna K.F. Chandler • Division of Vaccines and Related Products Applications, Center for Biologics Evaluation and Research, Food and Drug Administration, Rockville, Maryland 20852

David Chernoff • Chiron Corporation, Emeryville, California 94608

Robert W. Chesnut • Cytel Corporation, San Diego, California 92121

Masatoshi Chiba • Department of Chemical Engineering, Massachusetts Institute of Technology, Cambridge, Massachusetts 02139; *present address:* Pharmaceutical Development Laboratory, Mitsubishi Kasei Corporation, Kashimi-gun, Ibaraki 314-02, Japan

Silas Chikunguwo • Department of Tropical Public Health, Harvard School of Public Health, Boston, Massachusetts 02115

Jeffrey L. Cleland • Pharmaceutical Research & Development, Genentech, Inc., South San Francisco, California 94080

Peter D. Cooper • Division of Cell Biology, John Curtin School of Medical Research, Australian National University, Canberra, ACT 2601, Australia

Richard T. Coughlin • Cambridge Biotech Corporation, Worcester, Massachusetts 01605

Daniel E. Cox • Cambridge Biotech Corporation, Worcester, Massachusetts 01605

Charles Dahl • Department of Biological Chemistry and Molecular Pharmacology, Harvard Medical School, Boston, Massachusetts 02115

Lawrence W. Davenport • Genentech, Inc., South San Francisco, California 94080

Penny Dong • Department of Pharmaceutics, University of Washington, School of Pharmacy, Seattle, Washington 98195

Ronald Eby • Lederle–Praxis Biologicals, West Henrietta, New York 14586-9728

Ronald W. Ellis • Virus and Cell Biology, Merck Research Laboratories, West Point, Pennsylvania 19486

Patricia E. Fast • Vaccine and Prevention Research Program, Division of AIDS, National Institute of Allergy and Infectious Diseases, National Institutes of Health, Bethesda, Maryland 20892

Donald P. Francis • Genentech, Inc., South San Francisco, California 94080

Glenn R. Frank • Paravax, Inc., Fort Collins, Colorado 80526

Steve Furlong • Department of Rheumatology and Immunology, Harvard Medical School, Boston, Massachusetts 02115

Reinhard Glück • Department of Virology, Swiss Serum and Vaccine Institute Bern, CH-3001 Bern, Switzerland

Karen L. Goldenthal • Division of Vaccines and Related Products Applications, Center for Biologics Evaluation and Research, Food and Drug Administration, Rockville, Maryland 20852

Michael G. Goodman • Department of Immunology, The Scripps Research Institute, La Jolla, California 92037

Susan Gould-Fogerite • Department of Laboratory Medicine and Pathology, University of Medicine and Dentistry of New Jersey, New Jersey Medical School, Newark, New Jersey 07103

James D. Green • Department of Pathobiology and Toxicology, Genentech, Inc., South San Francisco, California 94080

Howard M. Grey • Cytel Corporation, San Diego, California 92121

Robert B. Grieve • Paravax, Inc., Fort Collins, Colorado 80526

Rajesh K. Gupta • Massachusetts Public Health Biologic Laboratories, State Laboratory Institute, Boston, Massachusetts 02130

Susan Haas • Emisphere Technologies, Inc., Hawthorne, New York 10532

Justin Hanes • Department of Chemical Engineering, Massachusetts Institute of Technology, Cambridge, Massachusetts 02139

Donald A. Harn • Department of Tropical Public Health, Harvard School of Public Health, and Department of Rheumatology and Immunology, Harvard Medical School, Boston, Massachusetts 02115

Mary Kate Hart • Division of Virology, U.S. Army Medical Research Institute for Infectious Diseases, Fort Detrick, Frederick, Maryland 21702

Barton F. Haynes • Department of Rheumatology and Immunology and the Duke Center for AIDS Research, Duke University Medical Center, Durham, North Carolina 27710

Andrew W. Heath • Department of Medical Microbiology, University of Sheffield Medical School, Sheffield S10 2RX, United Kingdom

Stanley L. Hem • Department of Industrial and Physical Pharmacy, Purdue University, West Lafayette, Indiana 47907

Rodney J.Y. Ho • Department of Pharmaceutics, University of Washington, School of Pharmacy, Seattle, Washington 98195

Stephen L. Hoffman • Malaria Program, Naval Medical Research Institute, Bethesda, Maryland 20889-5055

Glenn Ishioka • Cytel Corporation, San Diego, California 92121

Sharon A. Jenkins • Virus Research Institute, Inc., Cambridge, Massachusetts 02138

Charlotte Read Kensil • Cambridge Biotech Corporation, Worcester, Massachusetts 01605

Alan J. Kingsman • British Bio-technology Ltd., Oxford OX4 5LY, and Department of Biochemistry, Oxford University, Oxford OX1 3QU, United Kingdom

Peter J. Kniskern • Virus and Cell Biology, Merck Research Laboratories, West Point, Pennsylvania 19486

Jörg Kreuter • Institut fur Pharmazeutische Technologie, Johann Wolfgang Goethe-Universitat, D-60439 Frankfurt am Main, Germany

Ralph T. Kubo • Cytel Corporation, San Diego, California 92121

Lawrence B. Lachman • Department of Cell Biology, University of Texas M.D. Anderson Cancer Center, Houston, Texas 77030

John R. La Montagne • Division of Microbiology and Infectious Diseases, National Institute of Allergy and Infectious Diseases, National Institutes of Health, Bethesda, Maryland 20892

Robert Langer • Department of Chemical Engineering, Massachusetts Institute of Technology, Cambridge, Massachusetts 02139

Dale N. Lawrence • Division of AIDS, National Institute of Allergy and Infectious Diseases, National Institutes of Health, Bethesda, Maryland 20892

Deborah M. Lidgate • Syntex Research, Palo Alto, California 94304

B. Michael Longenecker • Department of Immunology, Faculty of Medicine, University of Alberta, Edmonton, and Biomira Inc., Edmonton, Alberta T6N 1H1, Canada

Jianneng Ma • Cambridge Biotech Corporation, Worcester, Massachusetts 01605

Raphael J. Mannino • Department of Laboratory Medicine and Pathology, University of Medicine and Dentistry of New Jersey, New Jersey Medical School, Newark, New Jersey 07103

Stephen Marburg • Synthetic Chemical Research, Merck Research Laboratories, Rahway, New Jersey 07065

George C. McCormick • Department of Pathobiology and Toxicology, Genentech, Inc., South San Francisco, California 94080

Kent R. Myers • Ribi ImmunoChem Research, Inc., Hamilton, Montana 59840

Bernardetta Nardelli • Medicine Department, Infectious Diseases Division, New York University Medical Center, New York, New York 10016

Mark J. Newman • Vaxcel, Inc., Norcross, Georgia 30071

A. D. M. E. Osterhaus • Department of Virology, Erasmus University Rotterdam, 3000 DR Rotterdam, The Netherlands

Gary Ott • Chiron Corporation, Emeryville, California 94608

Thomas J. Palker • Department of Rheumatology and Immunology and the Duke Center for AIDS Research, Duke University Medical Center, Durham, North Carolina 27710

Lendon G. Payne • Virus Research Institute, Inc., Cambridge, Massachusetts 02138

Christopher Penney • Immunomodulator Research Project, BioChem Therapeutic, Inc., Laval, Quebec H7V 4A7, Canada

Patricia J. Freda Pietrobon • Connaught Laboratories, Inc., Swiftwater, Pennsylvania 18370

Michael F. Powell • Genentech, Inc., South San Francisco, California 94080

Ramachandran Radhakrishnan • Chiron Corporation, Emeryville, California 94608

Xiao-Mei Rao • Department of Cell Biology, University of Texas M.D. Anderson Cancer Center, Houston, Texas 77030

Edgar Relyveld • Office d'Etudes en Vaccinologie, Paris, France

Sandra R. Reynolds • Department of Tropical Public Health, Harvard School of Public Health, Boston, Massachusetts 02115

G. F. Rimmelzwaan • Department of Virology, Erasmus University Rotterdam, 3000 DR Rotterdam, The Netherlands

Bryan E. Roberts • Virus Research Institute, Inc., Cambridge, Massachusetts 02138

Bradford E. Rost • Massachusetts Public Health Biologic Laboratories, State Laboratory Institute, Boston, Massachusetts 02130

John B. Sacci, Jr. • Malaria Program, Naval Medical Research Institute, Bethesda, and Department of Microbiology and Immunology, University of Maryland School of Medicine, Baltimore, Maryland 21201

John Samuel • Faculty of Pharmacy and Pharmaceutical Sciences, University of Alberta, Edmonton, Alberta T6G 2N8, Canada

Noemi Santiago • Emisphere Technologies, Inc., Hawthorne, New York 10532

Leigh A. Sawyer • Vaccine and Prevention Research Program, Division of AIDS, National Institute of Allergy and Infectious Diseases, National Institutes of Health, Bethesda, Maryland 20892

Alessandro Sette • Cytel Corporation, San Diego, California 92121

Li-Chen N. Shih • Department of Cell Biology, University of Texas M.D. Anderson Cancer Center, Houston, Texas 77030

George R. Siber • Massachusetts Public Health Biologic Laboratories, State Laboratory Institute, Boston, Massachusetts 02130

Laura L. Snyder • ImmunoTherapy Corporation, 14262 Franklin Avenue, Tustin, California 92680

Sean Soltysik • Cambridge Biotech Corporation, Worcester, Massachusetts 01605

Vernon C. Stevens • Department of Obstetrics and Gynecology, The Ohio State University, Columbus, Ohio 43210

James P. Tam • Microbiology and Immunology Department, Vanderbilt University, Nashville, Tennessee 37232

Pierre L. Triozzi • The Ohio State University Comprehensive Cancer Center, The Arthur G. James Cancer Hospital and Research Institute, Columbus, Ohio 43210

Cynthia A. Tripp • Paravax, Inc., Fort Collins, Colorado 80526

Stephen E. Ullrich • Department of Immunology, University of Texas M.D. Anderson Cancer Center, Houston, Texas 77030

J. Terry Ulrich • Ribi ImmunoChem Research, Inc., Hamilton, Montana 59840

Peter van Hoogevest • Ciba Geigy Ltd., Basel, Switzerland

Gary Van Nest • Chiron Corporation, Emeryville, California 94608

Antonella Vitiello • Cytel Corporation, San Diego, California 92121
Frederick R. Vogel • Division of AIDS, National Institute of Allergy and Infectious Diseases, National Institutes of Health, Bethesda, Maryland 20892
Peggy Wentworth • Cytel Corporation, San Diego, California 92121
Susan L. Wescott • Vaccine and Prevention Research Program, Division of AIDS, National Institute of Allergy and Infectious Diseases, National Institutes of Health, Bethesda, Maryland 20892
Joe L. White • Department of Agronomy, Purdue University, West Lafayette, Indiana 47907
Nancy Wisnewski • Paravax, Inc., Fort Collins, Colorado 80526
David V. Woo • ImmunoTherapy Corporation, Tustin, California 92680
Jia-Yan Wu • Cambridge Biotech Corporation, Worcester, Massachusetts 01605

Foreword

When my interest was first drawn to the phenomenon of vaccination for virus diseases in the late 1930s, the state of the art and the science of vaccine design was not far advanced beyond the time of Jenner at the end of the 18th century and of Pasteur a century later. In the 1930s it was still believed that for the induction of immunity to a virus-caused disease the experience of infection was required, but not for a toxin-caused disease such as diphtheria or tetanus, for which a chemically detoxified antigen was effective for immunization. This prompted the question as to whether it might be possible to produce a similar effect for virus diseases using nonreplicating antigens.

When in the 1930s and 1940s it was found possible to propagate influenza viruses in the chick embryo, protective effects could be induced without the need to experience infection by the use of a sufficient dose of a noninfectious influenza virus preparation. Later in the 1940s, it became possible to propagate polio and other viruses in cultures of human and monkey tissue and to immunize against other virus diseases in the same way. Later, with the advent of the era of molecular biology and genetic engineering, antigens and vaccines could be produced in new and creative ways, using either replicating or nonreplicating forms of the appropriate antigens for inducing a dose-related protective state.

Influenza virus vaccine effectiveness was observed to correlate with levels of serum antibody acting to block infection at the portal of entry. The need for antibody at the portal of entry in influenza virus infection is necessitated by the short incubation period (1 to 2 days), too short for an anamnestic antibody response to have a protective effect as in the prevention of paralysis following effective poliomyelitis vaccination. In poliomyelitis, the incubation period is sufficiently prolonged for the anamnestic response in a vaccinated individual to precede invasion of the central nervous system and prevent paralysis, and to prevent pharyngeal infection and spread of virus by that route.

The role and importance of the length of the incubation period and of the presence and persistence of immunological memory for long-term immunity to paralytic polio revealed that the presence of serum antibody at the time of exposure was not a necessary prerequisite for the prevention of paralysis; thus, the presence of immunological memory alone is the necessary and sufficient requirement for effectively preventing paralysis. To produce a persistent memory state a single dose of a sufficient concentration of antigen in saline can be uniformly effective when administered at any time after loss of maternal antibody. When incorporated in a mineral oil adjuvant as previously used for an influenza virus vaccine, much smaller doses of antigen are effective even in the presence of maternal antibody.

It now appears that for the control of cell-associated or cell-free pathogens by immunoprophylaxis a Th1-type or Th2-type memory pattern, respectively, is required. This is now evident for the immunological control of HIV, as for other cell-associated pathogens, for which a Th1-type memory state is required, and for which many more adjuvants, as well as antigen preparations, are now available for enhancing the induction of either cell-mediated or antibody-mediated immunological memory, required to protect against either cell-associated or cell-free pathogens, respectively.

Thus, for the design of vaccines and vaccine strategies for the control of viruses and other microbial pathogens, consideration must be given to the requirements appropriate to influence the immunodynamics and pathodynamics for each pathogen for which a specific immunizing agent is intended. Since infectious agents for which humans are the only reservoir may be eradicated from the human population through the phenomenon of the herd effect, it is also necessary to consider the epidemio-dynamics as well.

Through the availability of an extensive armamentarium of reagents and the science to guide their use it will now be possible to design safe and effective vaccines and vaccine strategies, for use with a greater economy of means in suitable combinations to produce the desired effect for many more pathogens than can now be controlled by vaccination.

This comprehensive volume considers and elaborates on all the relevant considerations for vaccine design, revealing the many possibilities that now exist to meet the multiple challenges for the control of infection and disease that the science and technology of vaccinology now make possible.

JONAS SALK

San Diego

Preface

Most of the more traditional types of vaccines developed for use in humans are based on replicating pathogens that have been attenuated. Vaccination with these agents results in a limited infection but with little or no disease pathogenesis and the resultant immune responses protect against the fully virulent pathogens. Attenuated vaccines are still widely used and efforts to develop the next generation continue. Subunit vaccines differ since they are based on only one or a few proteins or polysaccharides from the target pathogen. They can readily be designed for safety but their failure to induce the appropriate types of immune responses has plagued their development. Novel biotechnology techniques are now providing ways of producing better subunit vaccines and with these advances, we may soon be able to protect the population against many more diseases.

The purpose of this book is to provide descriptions of scientific theories, product development strategies, and results from preclinical studies for many of the newest subunit vaccines or components designed for use in subunit vaccine formulation, such as adjuvants and vaccine delivery systems. We have selected topics that we feel highlight many promising technologies and novel products rather than focusing on disease states or individual pathogens. Most of these products are still considered "experimental" and as such have only been evaluated in animals. However, the common goal within the scientific community is to contribute to the development of a product that will be evaluated in humans and hopefully licensed for use. We have therefore opened the book with several chapters describing immunological, formulation, public health, safety, regulatory, and clinical considerations relevant to the design and development of subunit vaccines. These topics are critical concerns for those who manufacture vaccines as well as for those who receive them.

Most prominent in this book are chapters describing new adjuvants and vaccine delivery systems. Our concentration on this area not only represents our personal biases but also illustrates the breadth of interest in these products. New adjuvants have potential for use with numerous vaccines, including some that are currently approved for human use. Many of the vaccine delivery systems are adjuvant active and also have potential for altering the mode of vaccine administration. For example, the use of new technologies may allow vaccines to be administered orally, rather than by needle injection, and controlled release systems may allow "single-shot" delivery, thus avoiding booster immunizations. Many of the adjuvant products described in this book have been or will soon be evaluated in human clinical trials and we fully believe our excitement will be justified.

Although new adjuvants will have an impact on the vaccine industry, they are useless without the appropriate vaccine immunogen. Here again, we have selected topics based on novel technologies for designing immunogens with potential for widespread application. We have also included products for many new applications for which commercially viable vaccines do not exist. Examples include the development of synthetic polysaccharide–protein conjugates and recombinant lipid–protein conjugates for use in vaccines against bacteria as well as recombinant protein and synthetic-peptide immunogens for use against parasites, viruses, cancer, and even pregnancy!

This field is evolving rapidly and, by definition, the information provided will not long remain current. We urge the interested readers to contact the authors directly with their scientific questions and suggestions. Finally, we have made every attempt to be comprehensive but it is impossible to include all of the subunit vaccine technologies under development. To the inventors and advocates of technologies that we may have missed, we apologize.

MARK J. NEWMAN

Georgia

MICHAEL F. POWELL

San Diego

Contents

Chapter 5
Clinical Considerations in Vaccine Trials with Special Reference to Candidate HIV Vaccines
Patricia E. Fast, Leigh A. Sawyer, and Susan L. Wescott

Chapter 6
Laboratory Empiricism, Clinical Design, and Social Value: The Rough Road toward Vaccine Development
Donald P. Francis

Chapter 7
A Compendium of Vaccine Adjuvants and Excipients
Frederick R. Vogel and Michael F. Powell

Chapter 10

MF59: Design and Evaluation of a Safe and Potent Adjuvant for Human Vaccines

Gary Ott, Gail L. Barchfeld, David Chernoff, Ramachandran Radhakrishnan, Peter van Hoogevest, and Gary Van Nest

Chapter 11

Development of Vaccines Based on Formulations Containing Nonionic Block Copolymers

Robert N. Brey

Chapter 12

Development of an Emulsion-Based Muramyl Dipeptide Adjuvant Formulation for Vaccines

Deborah M. Lidgate and Noelene E. Byars

Chapter 20
Water-Soluble Phosphazene Polymers for Parenteral and Mucosal Vaccine Delivery
Lendon G. Payne, Sharon A. Jenkins, Alexander Andrianov, and Bryan E. Roberts

Chapter 21
Monophosphoryl Lipid A as an Adjuvant: Past Experiences and New Directions
J. Terry Ulrich and Kent R. Myers

Chapter 24
Vaccine Adjuvants Based on Gamma Inulin
Peter D. Cooper

Chapter 25
**A New Approach to Vaccine Adjuvants: Immunopotentiation by Intracellular
T-Helper-Like Signals Transmitted by Loxoribine**
Michael G. Goodman

Contents

xxxv

Chapter 38

**Design and Testing of Peptide-Based Cytotoxic T-Cell-Mediated
Immunotherapeutics to Treat Infectious Diseases and Cancer**

*Robert W. Chesnut, Alessandro Sette, Esteban Celis, Peggy Wentworth,
Ralph T. Kubo, Jeff Alexander, Glenn Ishioka, Antonella Vitiello, and Howard M. Grey*

List of Abbreviations

Ab   antibody
ACP   alternative complement pathway
AFV   antiferility vaccine
Ag   antigen
AIDS   acquired immunodeficiency syndrome
APCs   antigen-presenting cells
ASI   active specific immunity (immunotherapy)
ATL   adult T-cell leukemia/lymphoma

β_2M β_2-microglobulin
BCG   bacillus Calmette–Guérin
BHV   bovine herpesvirus
BSA   bovine serum albumin
BuA$_2$ 1,4-butanediamine

CBER   Center for Biologics Evaluation and Research
CDC   Centers for Disease Control
CDER   Center for Drugs Evaluation and Research
CDI   carbonyl diimidazole
CDV   canine distemper virus
CFA   complete Freund's adjuvant
CFR   Code of Federal Regulations
CG   chorionic gonadotropin
C.I.   confidence interval
CMI   cell-mediated immunity
CMV   cytomegalovirus
CRM$_{197}$ genetic mutant of diptheria toxin
CSF   colony-stimulating factor
CT   cholera toxin
CTB   B subunit of cholera toxin
CTLs   cytotoxic T lymphocytes
CTTH N-benzyloxycarbonyl-L-tyrosyl-L-tyrosine hexyl ester
CVID   common variable immunodeficiency disease
CWS   cell wall skeleton

D	diptheria toxoid
DEC	diethylcarbamazine
DMF	dimethylformamide
DNP	dinitrophenol
DNP-Pn	dinitrophenylated pneumococcus antigen
DP	degree of polarization
DPT	diphtheria–pertussis–tetanus
DT	diphtheria toxoid
	diphtheria–tetanus
DTH	delayed-type hypersensitivity
DTP	diphtheria–tetanus–pertussis
8BrGuo	8-bromoguanosine
8MGuo	8-mercaptoguanosine
EBV	Epstein–Barr virus
ED_{50}	50% effective dose
EDAC	1-ethyl-3-(3-dimethylaminopropyl) carbodiimide
EDTA	ethylenediaminetetraacetic acid
ELA	establishment license application
ELISA	enzyme-linked immunosorbent assay
ER	endoplasmic reticulum
E:T	effector-to-target ratio
EVAc	ethylene-vinyl acetate
EYPC	egg yolk phosphatidylcholine
F(ab)	antigen-binding fragment
FACS	fluorescence-activated cell sorter
FCS	fetal calf serum
FDA	Food and Drug Administration
FHA	filamentous hemagglutinin
FITC	fluorescein isothiocyanate
FIV	feline immunodeficiency virus
FMDV	foot-and-mouth disease virus
FSH	follicle-stimulating hormone
F-MuLV	Friend murine leukemic helper virus
γ-In	gamma-inulin
GALT	gut-associated lymphoid tissue
gB	glycoprotein B
G-CSF	granulocyte colony-stimulating factor
GM-CSF	granulocyte–macrophage colony-stimulating factor
GMP	Good Manufacturing Practices
GnRH	gonadotropin-releasing hormone
GPC	gel permeation chromatography
GXM	glucuronoxylomannan

HA	hemagglutinin
HAV	hepatitis A virus
HbOC	Lederle–Praxis Hib conjugate
HBsAg	hepatitis B surface antigen
HBV	hepatitis B virus
hCG	human chorionic gonadotropin
HCl	hydrochloric acid
HCV	hepatitis C virus
HEPES	N-2-hydroxyethylpiperazine-N'-2-ethanesulfonic acid
HGG	human gamma globulin
Hib	*Haemophilus influenzae* type b
HIV	human immunodeficiency virus
HLA	histocompatibility leukocyte antigen
HLB	hydrophile–lipophile balance
HMO	health maintenance organization
hPIV-1	human parainfluenza virus type 1
HPLC	high-pressure liquid chromatography
HPV	human papilloma virus
HRP	horseradish peroxidase
HSP	heat-shock protein
HSV	herpes simplex virus
HTLV	human T-cell leukemia/lymphotropic virus
ID_{50}	50% infective dose or 50% inhibiting dose
IEF	isoelectric focusing
IFA	incomplete Freund's adjuvant
IFN	interferon
Ig	immunoglobulin
IL	interleukin
i.m.	intramuscular
IND	investigational new drug
i.p.	intraperitoneal
IPV	inactivated polio vaccine
IRIVs	immunopotentiating reconstituted influenza virosomes
ISCOMs	immune-stimulating complexes
i.v.	intravenous
kD	kilodaltons
KLH	keyhole limpet hemocyanin
LAL	*Limulus* amoebocyte lysate
LCMV	lymphocyte choriomeningitis virus
LD_{50}	50% lethal dose
LH	luteinizing hormone
LHRH	luteinizing hormone-releasing hormone

LPS	lipopolysaccharide
LT	lymphotoxin
	heat-labile toxin of *E. coli*

MAb	monoclonal antibody
MAF	macrophage activation factor
MAP	multiple antigen peptide
M-CSF	macrophage colony-stimulating factor
MDP	muramyl dipeptide
MELs	microencapsulated liposomes
MHC	major histocompatibility complex
mIgA	membrane-bound IgA
MLA	4′-monophosphoryl lipid A
MMR	measles–mumps–rubella
MPL	monophosphoryl lipid A
MPL-A	monophosphoryl lipid A
MTP-PE	muramyl tripeptide phosphatidylethanolamine

NA	neuraminidase
NIAID	National Institute of Allergy and Infectious Diseases
NK	natural killer
NMR	nuclear magnetic resonance

OD	optical density
OMPC	outer membrane protein complex from *Neisseria meningitidis* B
OPV	oral poliovirus vaccine
Osp	outer surface protein
Ova	ovalbumin
OVA	ovalbumin

p	probability
PA	protective antigen
PAGE	polyacrylamide gel electrophoresis
PBLs	peripheral blood lymphocytes
PBMCs	peripheral blood mononuclear cells
PBS	phosphate-buffered saline
PCPP	poly[di(carboxylatophenoxy)phosphazene]
PE	phosphatidylethanolamine
PFCs	plaque-forming cells
PGA	polyglycolic acid
PK-C	protein kinase C
PLA	polylactic acid
	product license application
PLGA	polylactic coglycolic acid (poly-lactide-co-glycolide)
PLL	poly-L-lysine

PMMA	polymethyl methacrylate
p.o.	per oral or oral
POE	polyoxyethylene
POP	polyoxypropylene
Pr	protein
PRP	polyribosyl ribitol phosphate
PRP-D	Connaught Hib conjugate
PRP-OMPC	Merck Hib conjugate
PRP-T	Pasteur Merieux Hib conjugate
Ps	capsular polysaccharide
PVA	polyvinyl alcohol
PVP	polyvinylpyrrolidone
PZC	point of zero charge
r	recombinant (e.g., rIFN-γ)
R	receptor (e.g., IL-2R)
RBCs	red blood cells
RIA	radioimmunoassay
RP-HPLC	reverse phase HPLC
RSV	respiratory syncytial virus
RT	reverse transcriptase
7a8oGuo	7-allyl-8-oxoguanosine
7m8oGuo	7-methyl-8-oxoguanosine
SAF-1	Syntex Adjuvant Formulation-1
s.c.	subcutaneous
SCMHC	S-carboxymethylhomocysteine
SCMS	S-carboxymethylcysteamine
SD	standard deviation
SDS	sodium dodecyl sulfate
SE	standard error
SEB	staphylococcal enterotoxin B
SEC	size-exclusion chromatography
SEM	standard error of the mean
SFCs	spot-forming cells
sIgA	secretory IgA
SIV	simian immunodeficiency virus
SLA	soluble leishmania antigen
ST	stearyl tyrosine
STn	sialyl Tn
$t\frac{1}{2}$	half-life, half-time
Ta	T amplifier
TAA	tumor-associated antigen
TAP	transporter protein

TCA	trichloroacetic acid
TCR	T-cell receptor
TD	thymus-dependent
TDM	trehalose dimycolate
TF	Thomsen–Friedenreich
TGF	transforming growth factor
TGR	trans-Golgi reticulum
Th	T-helper cell (e.g., Th1)
TI	thymus-independent
TIL	tumor-infiltrating lymphocyte
TLC	thin-layer chromatography
TNF	tumor necrosis factor
TNP-OVA	trinitrophenyl ovalbumin
TPE	tropical pulmonary eosinophilia
TPI	triose phosphate isomerase
Ts	T suppressor
TSP/HAM	tropical spastic paraparesis/HTLV-associated myelopathy
TT	tetanus toxoid
UV	ultraviolet
VDPs	virus-derived particles
VLPs	viruslike particles
VSV	vesicular stomatitis virus
WHH	width at half height
WHO	World Health Organization

Vaccine Design

The Subunit and Adjuvant
Approach

Chapter 1

Immunological and Formulation Design Considerations for Subunit Vaccines

Mark J. Newman and Michael F. Powell

1. INTRODUCTION

Vaccination represents the most successful attempt yet to protect humans and domestic animals from infectious diseases. Most vaccines operate by limiting infections, not necessarily by preventing them; it is the host immune system that mediates control and ultimate clearance of the infectious agent. Many of the most widely used vaccines developed for use in humans are based on live replicating organisms that have been attenuated. Vaccination with these agents results in a limited infection, but measurable disease pathogenesis is usually avoided and recovery is complete. The resultant immune responses are protective against the fully virulent pathogens and long-term immunological memory is induced. Today, attenuated vaccines are still used and efforts to develop the next generation are active.

Inactivated vaccines differ considerably from standard attenuated vaccines since they use "killed" pathogenic organisms, such as viral particles or bacterial cells. Subunit vaccines represent further reduction or simplification of these inactivated products since only a limited number of components from the appropriate pathogen are formulated into the vaccine. Both inactivated and subunit vaccines are considered to be much safer than their attenuated counterparts because they contain absolutely no infectious agents. The safety profile is further enhanced for subunit vaccines because of their defined physical and chemical characteristics. This is the main reason for continued research into vaccines of this type.

Although inactivated and subunit vaccines have been used successfully against some diseases, historically, their utility has been limited. Their limitations include overall low levels of immunogenicity and failure to induce the types of immune responses that occur following natural infections or vaccination with attenuated vaccines. Modern biotechnol-

Mark J. Newman • Vaxcel, Inc., Norcross, Georgia 30071. *Michael F. Powell* • Genentech, Inc., South San Francisco, California 94080.

Vaccine Design: The Subunit and Adjuvant Approach, edited by Michael F. Powell and Mark J. Newman. Plenum Press, New York, 1995.

1

ogy techniques now provide alternate methods of producing subunit vaccine immunogens and adjuvant-active compounds that can be added to vaccine formulations to augment immune responses. With these advances, the promise of new subunit vaccines for use against a wide variety of pathogenic organisms, and possibly even cancer, is increasing dramatically.

The design of subunit vaccines is directed by numerous considerations that include immunogenicity, safety, and stability. However, it is the qualitative and quantitative characteristics of immune responses induced by vaccination that are the most crucial aspects of subunit vaccine design. There are five major factors affecting immune responses that are induced by subunit vaccines:

1. The nature and the dose of the immunogens
2. The adjuvant or carriers used in the formulation
3. The immunization schedule
4. The route of administration
5. The immune status of the host being immunized

This last factor, the immune status of the vaccine recipient, can be affected by age, genetic constraints, and preexisting deficits in the immune system. These variables are outside of the control of scientists who design vaccines for general prophylactic use and will not be considered further in this review; however, the interested reader is referred elsewhere (MacKenzie, 1977; Fulginiti, 1982; Bruguera *et al.*, 1992). The other factors represent the driving force behind much of the recent and current research on subunit vaccine design and formulation optimization.

In this introductory chapter, we attempt to review the most critical research and development issues associated with the design and production of new subunit vaccines. This includes basic descriptions of the compartments and/or properties of the immune system that are invoked through vaccination and that are critical to efficacy, such as antigen processing and presentation, cytokine production, and the establishment of immunological memory. We also briefly review the types of immune responses that are induced by infectious pathogens and that are relevant to current subunit vaccine research efforts. Manufacturing issues such as the choice and characterization of the optimal vaccine immunogens, the use of adjuvants and immunization schedule to alter immune responses, and product formulation and stability concerns are also reviewed. This chapter does not represent an inclusive review of the history or current status of vaccine development; for this the reader is referred to two excellent books (Plotkin and Mortimer, 1988; Brown *et al.*, 1993). Rather, it sets the stage for the more focused chapters in this book that contain descriptions of current biotechnology research into subunit vaccine development.

2. CHARACTERIZATIONS OF IMMUNE RESPONSES RELEVANT TO VACCINE DESIGN

Many of the earliest vaccines were developed using a trial-and-error approach, without detailed knowledge of the mammalian immune system. Today, vaccine researchers have an enormous data base on the immune system, both in general terms and for specific infectious pathogens. It is from this level of understanding that the research efforts into subunit vaccine immunogens and the associated delivery systems, carriers, and adjuvants are being directed.

2.1. Adaptive and Innate Immunity

The different types of immune responses that are induced following infection with pathogenic organisms are commonly categorized as either "adaptive" or "innate." The adaptive immune responses are antigen-specific and the effects are mediated directly by lymphocytes or their products, such as antibodies and cytokines. The specificity of adaptive immune responses is determined by the antigen-specific T-cell receptor (TCR) or B-lymphocyte cell-surface expressed antibodies. These types of responses are classified as adaptive because antigen stimulation induces cellular activation, replication, and differentiation of naive or precursor lymphocytes into functional effector cells and immunological memory is then established. Thus, the individual has "adapted" to fend off a particular pathogen. It is the adaptive segment of the immune system that is targeted through the use of vaccines.

Innate immune responses are mediated by cells that do not have antigen-specific receptors such as natural killer (NK) cells, macrophages, and neutrophils. These types of cells are also activated in response to many pathogenic challenges but the replication and differentiation steps that are common to the adaptive immune system are not induced and immunological memory is not established. The split between the innate and adaptive components of the immune system is not always definitive and interactions between antigen-specific and nonspecific cells are required for the induction of fully functional immune responses.

2.2. Antigen Processing and Presentation to the Immune System

The T-lymphocyte compartment of the immune system does not routinely encounter and react to intact native proteins when initially responding to infectious organisms. Instead, proteins are "processed" into antigenic peptides and then "presented" in a complex with either class I or class II major histocompatibility complex (MHC) molecular complexes. Peptides presented by class I MHC molecules are generally 8–10 amino acids in length and contain specific contact amino acids for use as anchor residues; these vary for different MHC allelic products (Falk *et al.*, 1990, 1991; van Bleek and Nathonson, 1990; Rotzschke *et al.*, 1990). Peptides expressed in association with class II MHC molecules are typically longer, 12–25 amino acids in length, but they also appear to contain specific motifs that are preferentially bound by different class II MHC allelic products (Sette *et al.*, 1988; Hunt *et al.*, 1992; Rudensky *et al.*, 1992). The peptides that are expressed in association with either the class I or II MHC molecules are generated through two intracellular processing pathways that are differentially utilized. The selective use of each pathway is dictated primarily by the route through which the immune system encounters the antigen, either exogenously or endogenously.

Proteins delivered to the immune system exogenously are endocytosed by antigen-presenting cells (APCs), such as macrophages, dendritic cells, or B lymphocytes. Proteins

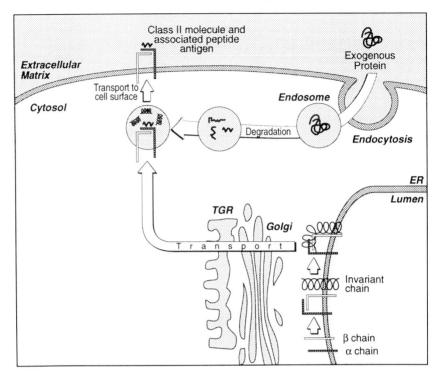

Figure 1. Simplified representation of the assembly and transport of MHC class II molecules with antigenic peptides. Proteins delivered exogenously are endocytosed into acidic endosomes where they are reduced and proteolytically cleaved into peptides. MHC class II α, β, and invariant chains are synthesized and assembled in the endoplasmic reticulum (ER) and then transported through the Golgi to the *trans*-Golgi reticulum (TGR). Here the endosomal processing and class II MHC molecule biosynthetic pathways intersect and the peptides bind to the α and β subunits of the class II molecular complex, displacing the invariant chain, which is subsequently degraded. Only the peptide-loaded class II MHC molecular complex is transported to the cell surface.

are delivered into acidic endosomes where they are first reduced (Collins *et al.*, 1991) and then proteolytically cleaved into peptides (van Noort *et al.*, 1991; Vidard *et al.*, 1991; Bennett *et al.*, 1992). The endosomal processing and class II MHC molecule biosynthetic pathways intersect (Peters *et al.*, 1991; Harding *et al.*, 1991) and the peptides bind to the α and β subunits of the class II molecular complex, displacing the invariant chain (Neefjes *et al.*, 1990; Anderson and Miller, 1992). It is this peptide-loaded class II MHC molecular complex that is expressed on the cell surface (Fig. 1).

Proteins delivered to the cytosol of cells are processed by the endogenous pathway. In this pathway proteins are proteolytically degraded into peptides, presumably by proteasome structures (Brown *et al.*, 1991; Martinez and Monaco, 1991; Goldberg and Rock, 1992), and then transported to the endoplasmic reticulum (Monaco *et al.*, 1990; Kelly *et al.*, 1992; Spies *et al.*, 1992; Suh *et al.*, 1994). In the endoplasmic reticulum, the peptides bind selectively to particular class I MHC heavy chains and are assembled into a stable

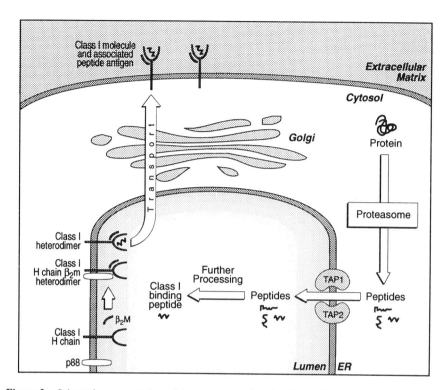

Figure 2. Schematic representation of the generation of antigenic peptides through the endogenous pathway and peptide-loading of MHC class I molecules. Cytosolic proteins are degraded by proteasomes and transported by transporter proteins (TAP1 and TAP2) to the lumen of the endoplasmic reticulum (ER) where they are degraded further. In the ER, newly synthesized MHC class I heavy (H) chains and β2-microglobulin (β2M) are assembled into heterodimeric MHC class I molecules through the activity of accessory proteins, such as p88. Each of these units can bind a peptide and the peptide-loaded MHC class I heterodimers are transported to the cell surface.

complex that includes β_2-microglobulin. This complex is then transported to the cell surface by intracellular chaperons (Schumacher *et al.*, 1991; Degen and Williams, 1991; Jackson *et al.*, 1994) (Fig. 2).

The class of MHC molecule that presents antigenic peptides to T lymphocytes dictates what type of immune effectors are induced. Peptides presented in association with class I MHC molecules will induce predominantly CD8[+] T-lymphocyte responses whereas peptides presented in association with class II MHC molecules will induce CD4[+] T-lymphocyte-mediated responses and antibody responses (Braciale *et al.*, 1987). It is this division of the immune system that represents one of the most significant obstacles for individuals attempting to design subunit vaccines since these products are typically administered parenterally and, as such, present the protein immunogen only to the endosomal processing pathway. Most simple subunit vaccines only induce antibodies and CD4[+] T-lymphocyte responses and these are not sufficient to protect against intracellular pathogens, such as viruses where CD8[+] T-lymphocyte responses are also needed.

Several observations indicate that the different pathways may not be totally separate. Endogenously processed viral antigens, such as influenza virus matrix protein, can be presented in association with class II MHC molecules (Nuchtern *et al.*, 1990), and hepatitis B virus proteins, presented to the immune system either as viral infection or vaccine, appear to be processed using both endosomal and nonendosomal processing pathways (Jin *et al.*, 1988). These findings demonstrate overlap between the two pathways, a property that may be of use to subunit vaccine designers.

2.3. Cytokines

The actual effectors of the immune system are mediated by a variety of cell types and interactions between cells are critical. Some of these interactions take the form of cell-to-cell contact, as occurs during antigen presentation. However, the immune system is also regulated through the action of numerous soluble factors or cytokines, referred to as interleukins (IL). The number of cytokines that have been identified and at least partially characterized is large and growing as is our understanding of their contributions to immune system protection against infectious pathogens (Paul and Seder, 1994).

Cytokines produced by murine T lymphocytes are probably the best characterized with respect to protective immune responses. It is known that different types of T-helper (Th) lymphocytes exist and that they can be categorized based on the specific cytokines that they produce. This was demonstrated initially using cloned murine CD4$^+$ helper T lymphocytes that were classified as either T-helper 1 (Th1) or T-helper 2 (Th2) cells (Mosmann *et al.*, 1986). Murine Th1 cells produce IL-2 and interferon-γ (IFN-γ) whereas Th2 cells produce IL-4, IL-5, IL-6, and IL-10. Cells of the Th0 phenotype produce a mixture of these cytokines (Mosmann and Coffman, 1989).

These different types of CD4$^+$ T lymphocytes can also be classified based on their functions. The Th1 cells preferentially mediate certain types of cellular immune responses, such as delayed-type hypersensitivity (DTH), and support other types of immune responses, such as CD8$^+$ CTL responses, whereas the Th2 cells provide support for antibody production (Cher and Mosmann, 1987; Boon *et al.*, 1988; Coffman *et al.*, 1988). Regulatory interactions between these two types of T lymphocytes are also known to exist. The Th1 cells provide helper activity to B lymphocytes that produce antibodies of the IgG2a isotype and increase the activity of Th2 cells (Stevens *et al.*, 1988). The reverse is true for Th2 cells since some of the cytokines they produce, such as IL-4 and IL-10, downregulate immune responses by suppressing antigen presentation activities of macrophages and the production of Th1 cytokines such as IFN-γ (Mosmann and Coffman, 1989).

Comparable types of CD4$^+$ helper T lymphocytes have been identified in humans, based on similar cytokine profiles (Del Prete *et al.*, 1991, 1994; Parronchi *et al.*, 1991; De Waal-Malefyt *et al.*, 1991). However, the separation into readily distinguishable Th1 and Th2 phenotypes is not as obvious since considerable cytokine production can be attributed to other types of mononuclear cells, such as CD8$^+$ T lymphocytes and macrophages (Salgame *et al.*, 1991; Tsutsui *et al.*, 1991). In this review we refer to these different types of responses simply as Type 1 and Type 2 responses or Type 1 and Type 2 cytokine profiles and do not use the Th1 and Th2 nomenclature developed for mice.

Protective immunity produced in response to pathogenic challenge in both mice and humans can be characterized by the cytokines that are produced. Infection with intracellular pathogens or tumors typically induces Type 1 responses and, as would be expected, the effector cells are CD8$^+$ T lymphocytes (Pamer, 1993; Kaufmann, 1993). The induction of Type 2 responses in these types of infections may actually exacerbate disease, probably by downregulating the Type 1 response (Graham *et al.*, 1993a; Modlin and Nutman, 1993). When antibody responses are critical to the control of pathogens, such as in certain parasitic infections, the Type 2 responses are likely to dominate (Urban *et al.*, 1992).

Probably the most important justification for studies of T-lymphocyte regulation and cytokines is their relevance to vaccine development since different types of vaccine immunogens and adjuvants induce production of different cytokines (Michalek *et al.*, 1989; Alwan *et al.*, 1993). Only certain types of lymphocytes and cytokines will contribute to the production of protective immune responses and vaccines that differ significantly from the actual infectious pathogen may fail. By design, subunit vaccines are quite different from the infectious pathogens against which they are supposed to induce protective immunity. Failure to induce the production of appropriate cytokines may be associated with nonresponsiveness, as was recently demonstrated for a hepatitis B vaccine (Vingerhoets *et al.*, 1994). Subunit vaccines may also fail because they induce irrelevant or even harmful immune responses, including inappropriate cytokines (Graham *et al.*, 1993a). Obviously, the challenge is to design subunit vaccines that will induce only the appropriate, protective, immune responses.

2.4. Immunological Memory

Immune responses are commonly described using the terms *primary* and *memory*. It is now widely accepted that memory immune responses are more vigorous and more rapidly induced than are primary immune responses (Gray and Sprent, 1990). The most direct measure of immunological memory is an increase in the numbers of antigen-committed B and T lymphocytes; it is this property that allows for both a more vigorous and immediate immune response on secondary challenge. Both B and T lymphocytes can be memory cells (Sprent, 1994).

Memory B lymphocytes are typically described as having the highest affinity antibodies for a particular antigen (Berek *et al.*, 1991; Rolink and Melchers, 1991; Rajewsky, 1992) and are thought to arise from a subpopulation different from those involved in the primary immune responses (Linton *et al.*, 1989; Yin and Vitetta, 1992). They can be phenotypically differentiated from naive B lymphocytes by their cell-surface expression of IgG instead of IgM, their high-level expression of certain differentiation and activation antigens, such as class II MHC antigens and CD44, and their low-level expression of the heat-stable antigen (Linton and Klinman, 1992; Gray, 1993; Mackay, 1993).

Unlike memory B lymphocytes, memory T lymphocytes are thought to arise or differentiate from naive T lymphocytes following antigen-specific stimulation and may exist as partially activated lymphocytes (Swain *et al.*, 1990; Bradley *et al.*, 1991). These two functional states can be distinguished by cell surface antigen phenotypes. Naive T lymphocytes express high levels of CD45R and L-selectin molecules and low levels of CD44. Memory T lymphocytes express the reciprocal phenotype, increased levels of CD44 and CD45RO, decreased levels of L-selectin, and increased levels of adhesion molecules, such as CD2 and LFA-3 (Akbar *et al.*, 1988; Butterfield *et al.*, 1989; Lee and Vitetta, 1991; Beverly, 1992; Swain *et al.*, 1992).

Memory B and memory T lymphocytes reside within the recirculating lymphocyte pool and are widely disseminated throughout the secondary lymphoid tissues of the body. However, they must recirculate differently than naive cells because they express low levels of the homing receptor for lymph node high endothelial venules, L-selectin or Mel-14. Data from recent studies suggest that memory lymphocytes migrate or recirculate through the afferent lymphatic system (Mackey, 1993; Mackay *et al.*, 1990).

The exact biological mechanisms required to establish and maintain immunological memory are not well defined, which is unfortunate for those involved in vaccine development since the induction of immunological memory is crucial to vaccine efficacy. One hypothesis is that persistent, low-level in vivo antigenic stimulation is required so that memory lymphocytes are maintained in an activated state (Gray and Skarvall, 1988; Gray and Matzinger, 1991; Oehen *et al.*, 1992). This hypothesis is based largely on the observation that transfer of memory B or T lymphocytes to a naive animal resulted in the establishment of a memory response only when antigen was transferred concomitantly. In an infectious disease model, one would predict that less than total clearance of the pathogen would maintain memory (Moskophidis *et al.*, 1993). The alternative hypothesis is that memory cells are long-lived and committed without the requirement for continued antigenic stimulation (Jamieson and Ahmed, 1989; Ahmed, 1992; Hou *et al.*, 1994; Lau *et al.*, 1994). The possible overlap between these two hypotheses is that continued exposure to antigen may occur in the form of cross-reacting environmental antigens (Beverly, 1990).

3. IMMUNE RESPONSES TO INFECTIOUS PATHOGENS, TUMORS, AND VACCINES

3.1. Immune Responses against Extracellular Bacteria

Different species of pathogenic bacteria infect and replicate in different sites of the body and this dictates the types of immune responses that are required to mediate control and clearance in vivo. Bacteria that replicate extracellularly can usually be controlled by antibodies through one or more mechanisms. First, antibodies bind to bacteria or their toxins and block attachment to receptors on host tissues. This directly interferes with the establishment of infection and cellular pathogenesis. Second, antibodies bind to bacteria and increase the efficiency with which they are phagocytosed and subsequently destroyed by macrophages and neutrophils, a process termed *opsonization*. Third, antibodies can kill bacteria directly or indirectly by activating complement. In all of these cases the bacterial antigens recognized by antibodies are usually surface expressed or, in the case of toxins, they may be soluble.

Subunit vaccines have proved effective in those instances where antibodies alone mediate protection, which is the case with some bacterial toxins and pathogenic extracellular bacteria. Examples include the toxoid vaccines that protect against the effects of *Clostridium tetani* (Wassilak and Orenstein, 1988) and *Corynebacterium diphtheriae* exotoxins (Mortimer, 1988a) and the inactivated *Bordetella pertussis* vaccine that is used to prevent whooping cough (Mortimer, 1988b). These vaccines not only represent some of the most successful and widely used vaccine products, but were also relatively simple to develop and manufacture.

Unfortunately, vaccines based on inactivated bacteria, such as the *B. pertussis* vaccine, can cause local, or rarely systemic, toxic reactions (Mortimer, 1988b) and the current research focus is on better subunit formulations. All of the adjuvants described in this book can be added to bacterial subunit vaccine formulations to increase their immunogenicity and these supplemented formulations are likely to function well. However, there is also a need to evaluate additional technologies. The example that we have included in this book is a subunit vaccine for the causative agent of lyme disease, *Borrelia burgdorferi*. This vaccine is based on recombinant proteins that were expressed so that a fatty acid molecule was attached to each protein molecule. The presence of this covalently attached fatty acid significantly increased the immunogenicity of the proteins and adjuvants could still be added (Chapter 32). This novel approach is likely to have widespread applicability for bacterial subunit vaccines, especially as the use of recombinant DNA technologies to produce protein immunogens gains acceptance.

Many types of bacteria evade the host immune system by presenting surface structures that are weakly immunogenic, most commonly polysaccharide capsules. Capsules can effectively protect bacteria by masking immunogenic outer membrane proteins that would otherwise be exposed and the polysaccharides themselves are usually only poorly immunogenic because they are not recognized by T lymphocytes. These are termed T-lymphocyte-independent antigens. One of the best characterized bacterial pathogens that is encapsulated with polysaccharides is *Haemophilus influenzae*. The polysaccharide capsule of this bacterium, polyribosyl ribitol phosphate (PRP), was used for a short time as a vaccine for *H. influenzae* but it did not induce the production of appropriate antibody isotypes or induce immunological memory in the critical target population, children under 2 years of age (Smith *et al.*, 1973; Makela *et al.*, 1977; Kayhty *et al.*, 1984; Deveikis *et al.*, 1988). This failure prompted the development of a second generation of vaccines based on the capsular polysaccharide conjugated to protein carriers (Anderson, 1983; Schneerson *et al.*, 1986; Tai *et al.*, 1987). Conjugation of the PRP to proteins converts it to a T-lymphocyte-dependent antigen and vaccines based on conjugates have proved superior to those containing unconjugated PRP (Anderson *et al.*, 1985; Insel and Anderson, 1986; Einhorn *et al.*, 1986).

The increased immunogenicity of polysaccharide–protein conjugates is related to the way that they are processed and presented to B and T lymphocytes. Initial antigen recognition by B lymphocytes occurs through cell-surface antibodies that are specific for the polysaccharide portion of the conjugate. The cell-surface-bound conjugate is then internalized by pinocytosis and the protein carrier is processed and presented to $CD4^+$ helper T lymphocytes in association with class II MHC molecules (Lanzavecchia, 1990). This process selects and activates Th lymphocytes that induce B lymphocytes to mature into antibody-secreting plasma cells and memory cells. Subsequent induction of antibodies by bacterial infections does not require the same carrier because of the existence of specific B-lymphocyte memory cells. There are several ways to produce polysaccharide conjugate vaccines and we have included two chapters describing both the history and the technical aspects relevant to the production of these types of vaccines (Chapters 30 and 31).

Many pathogenic bacterial infections are established through mucosal surfaces of the gastrointestinal tract. Examples of pathogens of this type that cause severe health problems worldwide include *Vibrio cholerae* and enterotoxigenic and enteropathogenic *Escherichia coli*; both are causative agents of severe and sometimes fatal diarrhea (Levine *et al.*, 1986). Immune system-mediated control and clearance of these types of pathogens typically requires the production of antigen-specific secretory IgA. The requirement for secretory IgA poses a unique problem because this antibody isotype is not normally induced by vaccines administered via parenteral injection, the standard route of delivery for subunit vaccines. Data to support the use of nonreplicating vaccines against enteric bacteria are sparse, but still encouraging. To date, the most successful vaccine of this type is for *V. cholerae*. The vaccine is based on a heat/formalin-inactivated whole bacteria formulation that is supplemented by the addition of the nontoxic B subunit of cholera toxin and is administered orally (Svennerholm *et al.*, 1984). Field trials indicate that the efficacy of this vaccine was reasonably good, as up to 85% of the test population was protected (Clemens *et al.*, 1986, 1990). Unfortunately, the need to develop vaccines against numerous other enteric bacteria still exists.

The development of carriers and adjuvants that will allow vaccines to be delivered directly to mucosal surfaces using the oral route of delivery is the main research focus of those working in this area. The use of polymer-based particulate delivery systems (Chapters 17 and 20) and liposomes (Chapters 14 and 15) has been evaluated experimentally with promising results. The potential of using these carrier or delivery systems and adjuvants with many different vaccine immunogens suggests that the development of vaccines for most enteric pathogens may soon be a reality.

3.2. Immune Responses against Intracellular Bacteria

While antibodies contribute to effective immune-mediated control of bacteria that replicate extracellularly, this type of response is not effective against intracellular bacteria. Immunologically mediated control of intracellular bacterial infections requires the production of cytokines that either downregulate bacterial replication or that activate phagocytic cells and enhance their ability to kill ingested bacteria. Also, the induction of CTLs that kill infected cells may be required. These are properties most commonly associated with Type 1 cytokines and the immune responses that they control. Another difference associated with immune responses produced against intracellular bacteria is their specificity. Antibodies that are effective against extracellular bacteria are typically specific for intact, surface-expressed proteins or polysaccharides, whereas the intracellular bacterial antigens recognized by the immune system are often internal, nonstructural components that are secreted from the bacterium (Kaufmann, 1993).

Some of the best characterized intracellular bacteria of concern for human health are the *Mycobacterium* species, such as *M. tuberculosis* and *M. leprae*. In the case of *M. leprae* infection, the clinical and immunological manifestations present as a spectrum from tuberculoid to lepromatous states, indicating control of disease and active disease, respectively (Ridley and Jopling, 1966). Antibody responses are correlated to disease with highest levels of antibodies observed coincident with the lepromatous state. Thus, antibodies appear to afford little protection against this pathogen but rather only reflect disease presence. Evaluation of cellular immune responses has documented the production of IL-2 and IFN-γ by CD4$^+$ T lymphocytes in tuberculoid lesions and only low levels of IL-4, IL-5, and IL-10, suggesting that a Type 1 cytokine profile is required for protection from progressive disease. The production of IL-4 by CD8$^+$ T lymphocytes and IL-10 by macrophages is common in the lepromatous state, suggesting that a Type 2 cytokine profile correlates with the progression of disease (Salgame *et al.*, 1991; Yamamura *et al.*, 1991, 1992; Sieling *et al.*, 1993).

Experimental infection of laboratory animals with *M. tuberculosis* induces potent, antigen-specific T-lymphocyte responses, including CD8$^+$ CTLs. The heat-shock protein (HSP65) and other internal or secreted bacterial proteins are the most commonly recognized targets (Anderson *et al.*, 1991, 1992; Anderson and Heron, 1993; Orem *et al.*, 1992). Humans infected with *M. tuberculosis* appear to respond similarly. This includes recognition of secreted bacterial antigens by T lymphocytes, induction of DTH responses, and the production of IFN-γ by antigen-specific lymphocytes (Daugelat *et al.*, 1992; Tsicopoulos *et al.*, 1992). The definitive contributions of different types of lymphocytes and their associated cytokines remain only poorly characterized in humans since many responses are of the mixed or Type 0 phenotype (Boom *et al.*, 1991; Barnes *et al.*, 1993; Del Prete *et al.*, 1993, 1994).

The most successful vaccines developed against intracellular bacteria have been based on the use of replication-competent, avirulent or attenuated bacteria. Again, the best example is *M. tuberculosis* where the bacillus Calmette–Guérin (BCG) strain of *M. bovis*, which is avirulent in most strains of mice and in humans, was used as a vaccine. Vaccination studies in mice demonstrated that cross-reactive protective immune responses could be induced (Orme and Collins, 1982; Gheorghiu *et al.*, 1985; Smith *et al.*, 1988). Although the reasons for the success are not well defined, the use of a live vaccine probably induced the required Type 1 cellular immune responses and CD8$^+$ CTLs (Flynn *et al.*, 1992). Similar types of immune responses have been observed in BCG-vaccinated humans (Pithie *et al.*, 1992; Mustafa *et al.*, 1993). Unfortunately, the results of large BCG vaccine clinical trials have been highly variable; protective immune responses were induced in up to 80% of some test populations whereas insignificant levels of protection were documented in other groups (Smith *et al.*, 1988; Colditz *et al.*, 1994). Recently, subunit vaccines based on secreted *M. tuberculosis* proteins have been tested in laboratory animals with some success (Hubbard *et al.*, 1992a,b; Pal and Horwitz, 1992). The need for new vaccines against intracellular bacteria is critical and these data suggest that their development may be feasible.

The critical limitation associated with subunit vaccines for intracellular bacteria is their failure to induce appropriate cell-mediated immune responses, particularly CD8$^+$ CTLs. New adjuvants and carriers that can induce effective cellular immune responses are now becoming available. These include adjuvants such as MF59 and QS-21 (Chapters 10 and 22) and carriers such as liposomes (Chapters 13–15). New subunit vaccines containing these adjuvants are likely to be safer, more efficacious, and easier to use than live BCG.

12 Mark J. Newman and Michael F. Powell

3.3. Immune Responses to Viruses

When described in structural or genetic terms, viruses are among the simplest of organisms. However, the number of different types of viruses is large; currently about 1400 viruses have been characterized well enough to be assigned to the appropriate "taxa" (Murphy and Kingsbury, 1990). The number of different diseases and disorders that pathogenic viruses cause is similarly expansive. Viral infections result in either acute disease pathogenesis, such as diarrhea and respiratory influenza, or chronic diseases, such as viral hepatitis. Disease pathogenesis may be mild or even without obvious symptoms, as with cytomegalovirus infections in healthy persons. Alternatively, viral infection may routinely result in fatal diseases, such as in human immunodeficiency virus type-1 (HIV-1) infections. Pathogenic viruses remain a major problem throughout the world, occurring with comparable prevalence in developed and developing nations.

Because viruses replicate intracellularly, it is generally assumed that CD8$^+$ CTLs are critical to effectively control and clear most viral pathogens in vivo. However, experiments in mice with targeted gene disruptions or using passive cellular transfer techniques have convincingly demonstrated the ability of the immune system to control many viral infections with either CD4$^+$ or CD8$^+$ T lymphocytes, although recovery was generally slower (Kast et al., 1986; Eichelberger et al., 1991; Muller et al., 1992; Hou et al., 1992; Scherle et al., 1992; Doherty et al., 1993; Epstein et al., 1993). It is now known that the processing and presentation of viral antigens occurs through both the class I and class II MHC-associated pathways in the infected host. The class I MHC-associated pathway is utilized by infected cells but professional APCs, such as macrophages and dendritic cells, can process and present secreted proteins and intact virus particles in association with the class II MHC molecules (Long and Jacobson, 1989; Murray and McMichael, 1992; Doherty et al., 1992). Based on these observations, it seems likely that both CD4$^+$ and CD8$^+$ T-lymphocyte responses and antibody responses are needed to optimally control most viral infections.

The balance between the Type 1 and Type 2 immune response profiles is also likely to be critical for the in vivo control and clearance of viral pathogens, as was recently demonstrated for respiratory syncytial virus (RSV) using a mouse model (Graham et al., 1993a). The induction of Type 1 responses is typically considered to be the most positive type of response because of the CD8$^+$ CTL component. However, CD8$^+$ CTLs may not be beneficial in all disease states since they may directly contribute to the pathogenesis of certain diseases, as has been demonstrated for lymphocytic choriomeningitis virus, again using mice (Buchmeier et al., 1980; Doherty et al., 1990). In humans, this type of association is still speculative. It has been suggested that Type 2 responses may be associated with progression of disease in HIV-1-infected persons whereas Type 1 responses may mediate some type of protection and slow the onset of AIDS (Shearer and Clerici, 1992; Clerici and Shearer, 1993), although this theory remains unproven (Graziosi et al., 1994; Maggi et al., 1994).

Many of the virus vaccines in use today are live attenuated and these are commonly considered to be superior to inactivated virus or subunit vaccines (Ada, 1990). The increased performance of attenuated vaccines is thought to be related to the fact that they actually infect the vaccinated individual and thus are likely to induce the Type 1 immune responses that are required to control subsequent natural infections, including $CD4^+$ Th lymphocytes and $CD8^+$ CTLs. However, inactivated whole virus vaccines have been used successfully against some human viral pathogens, including influenza virus (Kilbourne, 1988) and poliovirus (Salk and Drucker, 1988). The demonstrable efficacy of these vaccines indicates that antibodies and $CD4^+$ T-lymphocyte responses are sufficient in certain instances to mediate protection in vaccinated persons and this success has been used to justify continued research in this area, e.g., vaccines against hepatitis B virus. Subunit vaccines for this virus are not based on whole virus particles but rather on self-assembling Dane particles consisting of viral surface (S) protein, commonly referred to as HBsAg. These particles can be purified from the plasma of chronic carriers or produced by recombinant DNA technologies. Subunit vaccines based on both the natural and recombinant forms of these immunogens have proved efficacious (Hilleman *et al.*, 1975; Maupas *et al.*, 1976; McAleer *et al.*, 1984; Emini *et al.*, 1986).

Unfortunately, limitations are often associated with inactivated and subunit virus vaccines and attempts to develop products of this type against a number of viral pathogens have been unsuccessful. The most common limitation is lack of appropriate immunogenicity. Measles virus and mumps virus vaccines are classical examples of poor immunogenicity, the inactivated virus vaccines inducing only short-term immunity (Preblud and Katz, 1988; Weibel, 1988). Limitations with immunogenicity have also been associated with hepatitis B virus vaccines where up to 10% of the vaccinated populations fail to respond (Craven *et al.*, 1986; Eddleston, 1990). This lack of response can be characterized by a failure to produce Type 1 cytokines (Vingerhoets *et al.*, 1994) and is correlated with certain human MHC (HLA) types (Kruskall *et al.*, 1992).

Safety problems have also been associated with some inactivated virus vaccines. The best known cases of safety problems occurred during the development of inactivated virus vaccines for RSV and measles virus. These vaccines induced immune responses that enhanced pathogenesis of subsequent natural infection (Feldman, 1962; Fulginiti and Kempe, 1963; Kapikian *et al.*, 1969; Kim *et al.*, 1969). The mechanisms behind vaccine-induced enhancement have not been defined but inactivated virus preparations may be more likely to establish dominant Type 2 immune responses and, as was shown for intracellular bacteria, this type of immune response could contribute to disease pathogenesis. Support for this hypothesis has recently been obtained using a murine vaccine model (Graham *et al.*, 1993a). Also, technical problems associated with the manufacture of totally safe inactivated virus vaccines have remained complicated and expensive (Budowsky, 1991). When these limitations are considered together, the need for a new generation of safer and more efficacious subunit vaccines becomes obvious.

The next generation of virus subunit vaccines has yet to be defined and research efforts continue into both adjuvants and immunogens. Adjuvants that augment both antibody and cellular immune responses are most likely to prove useful. Some of the top candidate adjuvants are MF59 and QS-21 (Chapters 10 and 22) but any product that can induce cellular immunity is likely to be beneficial, such as liposomes and ISCOMs (Chapters 13–15 and 23). The design of novel immunogens using synthetic peptides or peptide complexes is also a major focus. The use of peptides to construct immunogens allows for the inclusion of individual antibody, helper T-lymphocyte, and CTL epitopes as well as the exclusion of unwanted epitopes. In this format only critical epitopes are presented to the immune system and in a concentrated form and this form of immunogen requires little or no processing prior to their presentation to the immune system. Examples of peptide-based virus vaccines are described in Chapters 36–38.

3.4. Immune Responses against Parasites

Parasitic protozoa and helminths continue to be a major cause of morbidity in both animals and humans. Parasitic infections of humans are most significant in the tropical and subtropical parts of the world, especially in developing nations, but parasites of domestic animals are common throughout the world. These types of organisms represent a very difficult target for the immune system because their complex life cycles often include multiple host species and developmental stages. Even their complex physical structure and large size contribute to the difficulty of immune system control.

Helminthic parasites include many different types of worms that generally infect the intestines, and associated organs, or the lymphatics. Immune responses to helminth infections are typically characterized by IgE production, increases in the numbers of circulating eosinophils, and an influx of mast cells into the infected tissues. Beyond this basic set of rules, the types of immune mechanisms that contribute to the control of parasitemia vary with each parasite.

The eosinophilia and IgE production are classified as Type 2 immune responses and have been thought to contribute to the in vivo control of parasites (Urban *et al.*, 1992). However, experiments with mice have not supported this dogma and now actual cause-and-effect relationships are questionable. For example, in vivo treatments of mice with monoclonal antibodies against cytokines, such as IL-4 and IL-5, significantly reduce the level of IgE and the numbers of eosinophils without negative impact on the parasite-infected animals (Madden *et al.*, 1991; Urban *et al.*, 1991, 1992). In the case of filarid and schistosomal infections, there appears to be a need for Type 1 immune responses for control of parasitemia whereas parasite-induced downregulation of immune responses is associated with Type 2 cytokine profiles (Mahanty *et al.*, 1992; King and Nutman, 1992; King *et al.*, 1993). These variable experimental results only make it more difficult to design prototype parasite subunit vaccines.

There are currently two opposing hypotheses regarding the roles of Type 1 and Type 2 cytokines in the control and clearance of helminthic parasites. The first hypothesis maintains that if Type 1 responses are required for immunologically mediated control of infection, then the predominance of a Type 2 response would reflect the incorrect response. Type 2 responses may actually be induced by the parasite as a defense mechanism, since this would downregulate the protective Type 1 response (Sher and Coffman, 1992). The alternative hypothesis is that a Type 2 response does in fact represent the host's protective response with IgE and mast cells representing the immune effectors (Urban *et al.*, 1992). When one considers the complex nature of helminthic parasites it is not surprising to find that the immune responses that they induce are similarly complex (Wilson, 1993).

Vaccine development for helminthic parasites is only in the experimental stage but optimism comes from two sources. First, resistance to reinfection by many parasites is correlated with past exposure and this suggests that adaptive immune responses may contribute to protection. For example, adults are typically much more resistant to reinfection with *S. mansoni* than are children and this protection correlates with increased serum IgE levels and antigen-specific cellular immunity (Hagan *et al.*, 1991; Dessein *et al.*, 1992; Dune *et al.*, 1992; Ribero *et al.*, 1993). Second, radiation-attenuated helminthic parasites have been used to vaccinate laboratory animals and the resultant immune responses protected these animals against secondary experimental challenge (Costant and Wilson, 1992; Mountford *et al.*, 1992; Smythies *et al.*, 1992a; Weil *et al.*, 1992). The physiological mechanisms that contributed to the control of parasitemia have only been partially described but it seems likely that cellular immune responses, particularly the action of IFN-γ, were involved (Smythies *et al.*, 1992b). These results, although preliminary in nature, support continued research directed at helminthic parasite vaccine development. The current status of experimental efforts against helminthic parasites is described in Chapter 33.

Because protozoan parasites exist primarily as intracellular pathogens, immune responses produced following infection are somewhat different than those raised against helminthic parasites. Most of the research effort has been directed into those systems where experimental animal models are available to complement human studies, such as *Leishmania* (Reed and Scott, 1993) and *Plasmodium* species, the latter being the example that we have chosen for this review.

The life cycles of *Plasmodium* species can be divided into discrete stages based on their host, mosquito or mammal, and the type of tissue that is infected, hepatocytes or erythrocytes. The parasites are transmitted from the mosquito to humans as sporozoites that rapidly infect the liver where they differentiate into merozoites; this is the stage that can productively infect erythrocytes. Some of the merozoites will develop into gametocytes, the sexual stage that can be taken up by mosquitos, and the cycle continues. Most vaccine efforts have focused on the preerythrocytic and blood stage organisms, since these are the stages that occur in infected humans (Nardin and Nussenzweig, 1993). The preerythrocytic stage is also a prime candidate for vaccine intervention because this represents that stage where parasite burden is lowest and therefore most readily controlled.

The feasibility of vaccinating against plasmodium species was established using irradiation-attenuated sporozoites to infect persons via the bite of infected mosquitos. The exposure-induced immune responses were capable of protecting "vaccinated" individuals from subsequent infectious challenge (Herrington *et al.*, 1991). Although this approach is not commercially feasible, it has proved useful for characterizing protective immune responses in both humans and experimental animals (Nardin *et al.*, 1989, 1991; Moreno *et al.*, 1991; Millet *et al.*, 1991; Malik *et al.*, 1991). These studies have demonstrated the need for cellular immune responses with the effector mechanisms including IFN-γ, produced by both CD4$^+$ and CD8$^+$ T lymphocytes, and CD8$^+$ CTL-mediated killing of infected hepatocytes. Antibodies also appear to be critical, with the circumsporozoite protein representing the immunodominant protein.

The in vivo functions of protective T lymphocytes are not yet characterized but they are likely to include CTL activity and cytokine production, similar to the types of responses used against viruses and intracellular bacteria. The contribution of antibodies remains uncharacterized but their activity may decrease the mobility of the parasite thus limiting its infectivity and increasing the likelihood of phagocytosis by macrophages (Stewart *et al.*, 1986). As was suggested for virus vaccines, the induction of both antibody and cellular based responses will likely be needed for optimum vaccine efficacy. A description of both the historical and current aspects of vaccine development for malarial parasites is presented in Chapter 35.

3.5. Nontraditional Uses of Vaccine Technologies

Vaccines are typically used in a prophylactic manner, to protect individuals from diseases caused by infectious pathogens such as bacteria and viruses. However, new technologies for producing vaccine immunogens and adjuvants have spurred efforts to develop vaccines for a variety of nontraditional uses. These include products designed to control ectoparasites such as ticks, fleas, and biting flies, as well as the allergies that they induce (Wikel, 1988; Dryden and Blakemore, 1989; Willadsen *et al.*, 1993), products to treat cancer (Bystryn *et al.*, 1993), and even a vaccine to be used as a form of fertility control (Jones *et al.*, 1988; Stevens and Jones, 1990). Most of the experimental vaccines that are being developed against ectoparasites are designed for domestic animals and will not be reviewed here. However, the use of vaccines to treat cancer and as a form of birth control have been evaluated for use in humans and we have included three chapters on these topics (Chapters 38, 39, and 41).

The use of vaccines in cancer patients differs from the more standard use of vaccines since the goal is to induce immune responses against existing tumors rather than to protect the healthy individual. As such, these vaccines are typically referred to as immunotherapeutic vaccines. One of the major difficulties associated with the development of vaccines for the treatment of cancer is the identification of a suitable immunogen. Some tumors have a viral etiology or are associated with viral infection, such as hepatitis B virus and hepatocarcinoma, human T-cell lymphotropic virus type I (HTLV-I) and certain T-lymphocyte leukemia or human papilloma virus (HPV) and cervical cancer. In these instances, the evaluation of vaccines containing selected virus components as immunogens is a logical approach (Hilleman, 1993; Chapter 38). Unfortunately, tumors without an established viral etiology are far more common in humans and this makes the design of suitable vaccines a more difficult task.

One of the most promising approaches is to use altered or mutated proteins that are expressed on tumors as the immunogens in subunit vaccine formulations (Hellstrom and Hellstrom, 1989). Experiments using synthetic peptides containing portions of mutated p53 and the *ras* oncogene to immunize mice have demonstrated that this approach can be used to generate both antibody and T-lymphocyte responses (Pullano *et al.*, 1989; Cheever *et al.*, 1990; Peace *et al.*, 1991; Fenton *et al.*, 1993; Yanuck *et al.*, 1993). Similar immune responses have been measured against p53, *ras* and other oncogene products in humans with certain types of tumors (Houbiers *et al.*, 1993; Nijman *et al.*, 1993; Pupa *et al.*, 1993; Schlichtolz *et al.*, 1993; Disis *et al.*, 1994). A slightly different approach is the use of mucin, which is expressed on tumors in altered forms that make it immunogenic (Chapter 39). Immune responses to tumor-expressed mucins have been detected in humans (Bard *et al.*, 1989; Jerome *et al.*, 1991, 1993; Domenech *et al.*, 1993; Ioannides *et al.*, 1993) and protective immune responses have been induced in mice by vaccination (Fung *et al.*, 1990; Acres *et al.*, 1993). These data clearly demonstrate the immunogenicity of altered proteins expressed by tumors and support further research in this area.

An alternative strategy is to target markers that are expressed at high levels on tumors but absent from most normal tissues. An example of this is human chorionic gonadotropin (hCG) which is expressed on many different types of tumors but not on normal tissues, with the exception of embryonic placental tissues. It is this limited tissue expression that has allowed hCG to be used as an immunogen in therapeutic cancer vaccines. Additional examples of tumor immunotherapy based on this approach are described by Bystryn *et al.*, (1993). Interestingly, the use of hCG for cancer immunotherapy is actually secondary; vaccines containing immunogenic forms of this hormone were originally developed as a form of birth control for use in developing nations (Chapter 41).

4. DESIGN CRITERIA FOR SUBUNIT VACCINES

4.1. Selection of Vaccine Immunogen

Pathogenic organisms typically contain numerous immunogenic components including proteins, glycoproteins, polysaccharides, and glycolipids. Only a finite number of these are likely to induce immune responses that will contribute to prophylactic immunity. Therefore, selection of the "correct" immunogen and delivery of this immunogen in an appropriate form are essential for the development of an effective subunit vaccine.

The definition of a correct immunogen is operational and likely to vary considerably for different vaccines, but a simple set of guidelines can be employed. First, the immunogen must be the appropriate target and induce immune responses that are effective against the pathogen. This can be highly variable since pathogens that replicate intracellularly will induce immune responses with different specificity than those that replicate extracellularly. Relevant examples were described previously for extracellular and intracellular bacteria. The second guideline has to do with structure or confirmation of the immunogen with respect to antibodies, which recognize native or discontinuous epitopes, and T lymphocytes, which only recognize small linear epitopes. The conformation of the immunogen may dictate the appropriateness of the responses, as was demonstrated for experimental HIV-1 vaccines where only native proteins induced high-titered neutralizing antibodies (Berman *et al.*, 1990; Haigwood *et al.*, 1992). Finally, the immunogen should be of the relevant antigenic type, also called serotype. Here the relevance is dictated by the prevalence of different serotypes in the population. A good example is the design of influenza virus vaccines, which require modifications every few years to match variation of the virus in infected populations (Kilbourne, 1988).

Other factors that may alter the utility of vaccines are the physical nature and the dose of the immunogen. For example, baboons immunized with recombinant hepatitis B vaccine produced long-lasting antibody responses, whereas animals immunized with an experimental HIV-1 vaccine containing recombinant gp120 produced antibody responses that waned rapidly (Anderson *et al.*, 1989). The critical difference in this example is likely the physical nature of the immunogen; the HBsAg was in particulate form and nonglycosylated whereas the HIV-1 gp120 was a soluble and heavily glycosylated protein. Obviously, the number of variables that need to be addressed for each new vaccine contribute significantly to both the cost and time required to develop these products.

4.2. The Use of Adjuvants to Alter Vaccine Immunogenicity

Adjuvants and certain carriers are compounds that when used in combination with specific vaccine immunogens, augment the resultant immune responses (Ramon, 1926). The use of adjuvants to augment immune responses is a well-established practice in experimental immunology and in our opinion, represents one of the best approaches for developing the next generation of subunit vaccines. Because of this, we have devoted significant attention to the topic in this book and Chapters 7–29 describe most of the newest adjuvants and carriers. We also refer interested persons to the recent review by Cox and Coulter (1992). However, we must stress that adjuvants only augment responses against the immunogen contained in the vaccine formulation, making the selection of immunogen and adjuvant a "hand-in-hand" process. To quote Edelman and Tacket (1990), "The best adjuvant will never correct the choice of the wrong epitope."

Adjuvants come in many different forms so their classification can be difficult. One method of classifying adjuvants is by their mechanism of action. Adjuvants such as alum, stearyl tyrosine, and biodegradable polymer microspheres provide sustained release of immunogen (Chapters 8, 9, and 16–20). Others, such as emulsions, liposomes, saponins, monophosphoryl lipid-A (MPL-A), and muramyl tripeptide phosphatidylethanolamine (MTP-PE), can be classified as surfactant-like (Chapters 10–15 and 21–23). Unfortunately, this simple approach to adjuvant classification is misleading because many adjuvants function through more than a single mechanism and many have overlapping mechanistic properties but unique physical properties (Fig. 3).

The augmentation of immune responses by adjuvants is commonly measured as an increase in antibody levels in the immunized animals. However, adjuvants may also induce other significant changes such as increasing the numbers of epitopes that are recognized, altering the antibody isotype profiles and the induction of cellular immune responses. Some adjuvants that change the numbers of epitopes recognized and alter antibody isotype are liposomes, saponins, and block polymers (Alving *et al.*, 1986; Gregoriadis *et al.*, 1987;

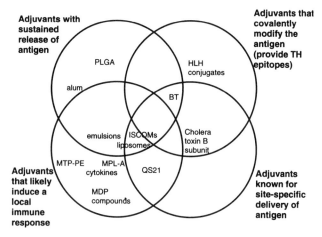

Figure 3.   Schematic representation showing the classification of adjuvants based on their mechanism of action. This approach can be misleading since many adjuvants operate through more than one mechanism.

Kenney *et al.*, 1989; Karagouni and Hadjipetrou-Kourounakis, 1990; Cohen *et al.*, 1991; Kalish *et al.*, 1991; Kensil *et al.*, 1991; Bennett *et al.*, 1992; Wu *et al.*, 1992). Antigen-specific cellular immune responses, including $CD8^+$ CTL responses, can be induced using formulations containing adjuvants, such as the saponins (Wu *et al.*, 1992; Newman *et al.*, 1992; Chapters 22 and 23) or using carriers, such as liposomes (Miller *et al.*, 1992; see also Chapters 13–15).

The use of microspheres to deliver vaccine immunogens represents a nontraditional adjuvant approach. Proteins or glycoproteins encapsulated into polymer microsphere formulations are delivered and released to the immune system more slowly than are soluble immunogens (Eldridge *et al.*, 1991). Slow-release microsphere formulations have the potential for reducing the number of immunizations required to achieve the desired responses, with the ultimate goal of developing formulations requiring only a single immunization (Preis and Langer, 1979; Gilley *et al.*, 1992; Cleland *et al.*, 1994; Chapters 16 and 18–20).

Cytokines represent another nontraditional type of adjuvant with totally different mechanisms of action (Chapters 27–29). Although there is little consensus concerning the optimal way of using cytokines as vaccine adjuvants, several researchers have demonstrated that the direct addition of certain cytokines to formulations is beneficial (Weinberg and Merigan, 1988; Stürchler *et al.*, 1989; Alfonso *et al.*, 1994). The development of cytokines as adjuvants is likely to be much more complicated than the development of small molecule adjuvants. This is because cytokines need to be delivered to the appropriate cell at the correct time during the maturation of immune responses. Many cytokines exert more than one effect, some having both down- and upregulatory effects, as well as undesirable side effects such as the induction of acute inflammatory responses (Ogle *et al.*, 1990; Heath and Playfair, 1991; Gillott *et al.*, 1993). A major technical problem is the species-specificity of many cytokines. This will limit the utility of experimental animal models that are commonly used to characterize and optimize formulations and to evaluate

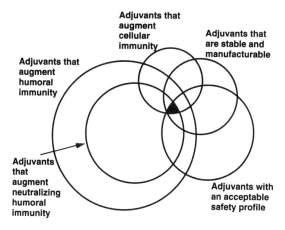

Figure 4. Venn diagram showing a few of the desirable traits for vaccine adjuvants. Many adjuvants have some of the desirable characteristics but few meet all criteria, shown here as the darkened intersection of all circles.

Table I
Design of an "Optimal" Subunit Vaccine for HIV-1 Prophylaxis

Desired characteristic	Possible solution
Several different isotypes of recombinant antigen (or polypeptides of known B-cell and T-cell epitope function)	Use of rgp120 from different clades (A–E), as well as different isotypes from the same clade (MN, SF2, IIIB). Use core proteins (p17, p24).
Antigen encapsulated in large microspheres for slow release of antigen	PLA microspheres, 20–40 μm, (autoboost release at 100–120 days) of 3–5% loading.
Antigen encapsulated in submicron microspheres to induce rapid macrophage uptake and processing	PLGA microspheres, < 1 μm, of 7–10% loading.
Stable emulsion of optimized composition to induce both cellular and humoral immunity	Squalane-based emulsion compatible with other components, including PLA, PLGA, and cytokine(s).
Components added to induce cellular immunity	Addition of QS-21 or MPL-A (either soluble or encapsulated).
Cytokines added to boost both the humoral and cellular responses	Addition of gamma interferon and IL-12.
Local anesthetic to reduce pain upon injection	Lidocaine, or other local anesthetics.

safety (Green and Terrell, 1992; Terrell and Green, 1993). An alternative to cytokine use may be the use of compounds that are nonspecific immune system stimulators (Chapters 21 and 24) or that directly induce cellular activation pathways and thereby replace cytokines (Chapter 25).

To date, many compounds with adjuvant activity have been identified but none are considered to be "the best." It is likely that a "best" adjuvant for all subunit vaccines does not exist since each immunogen and the targeted pathogen will have their own requirements. For example, an adjuvant that significantly increases antibody titers and induces isotype switching would be very useful in vaccines against extracellular bacteria but of no benefit for vaccines against intracellular organisms where cellular immune responses are critical. An adjuvant with some toxicity would not be acceptable as a replacement of an existing pediatric vaccine but may be considered acceptable for use in cancer immunotherapy. This interconnection of desirable and undesirable traits is shown in Fig. 4.

Adjuvants are most commonly evaluated and characterized in vaccine formulations individually. These types of studies are important even when a particular adjuvant proves inadequate because they provide the framework for the design of more complex formulations containing several adjuvant components. Because individual adjuvants alter different biological responses, the use of combinations of adjuvants may provide for even more potent immune responses than any single adjuvant. We feel that it is likely that the next generation of adjuvant formulations will consist of several different adjuvant components, where each component is added to augment a particular type of immune response with the final effect being an additive or synergistic one. An example of a theoretical subunit vaccine containing many adjuvants and carriers is described in Table I.

4.3. Immunization/Vaccination Schedule

The type, magnitude, and duration of the immune response are strongly affected by the immunization schedule, which can be defined as the spacing between the initial immunization and subsequent or booster immunizations. For many vaccines, the maximum antibody response is induced by delaying one or more of the booster immunizations for several months. The time between booster immunizations, called a rest period, appears to be necessary for the induction of antigen-specific memory lymphocytes, particularly memory B lymphocytes.

This effect has been demonstrated in several species, including humans, using both experimental and approved vaccines (Table II). For example, baboons immunized with recombinant HIV-1 gp120 using alum as the adjuvant and a 0, 4, 24 week schedule produced significantly higher antibody titers than animals that received the same vaccine using a 0, 4, 8 week immunization schedule (Anderson *et al.*, 1989). In clinical trials with the recombinant hepatitis vaccine, higher levels of antibodies were produced by persons receiving the vaccine on a 0, 4, 24 week schedule, compared to those vaccinated using a 0, 4, 8 week schedule (Hess *et al.*, 1992). Immune responses induced by the inactivated hepatitis A vaccine formulated with alum were also found to vary significantly with vaccination schedules (Jilg *et al.*, 1992; Westblom *et al.*, 1994). Most experiments designed to optimize immunization schedules have been done using antibody production as the end point, and it is possible that the optimization of a cellular immune response may require a different schedule (Gorse *et al.*, 1993).

The effect of the dosing schedule on antibody responses may be dependent on whether suboptimal or optimal amounts of vaccine are given. For example, very small doses given repeatedly will usually increase the affinity of the resultant antibody responses (Eisen and Siskind, 1964; Steiner and Eisen, 1967). Examples of this phenomenon were seen in clinical trials for inactivated poliovirus (Salk *et al.*, 1984) and disaggregated W138 rabies virus (Cabasso *et al.*, 1978) vaccines. Although high-affinity antibodies are likely to be advantageous, larger doses of vaccine may be required to establish immunological memory and repeated booster immunizations are not practical.

The duration of vaccine-induced antibody titers is typically measured as a function of circulating antibodies and this can be independent of the maximum antibody levels.

Table II
Effect of Species on the Duration of Antibody to an HIV-1 gp120 Vaccine

Species	Schedule (weeks)	Anti-gp120 Ab half-life (weeks)[a]	Reference
Human	0, 4, 24	~26	Berman *et al.* (1993)
Chimpanzee	0, 4, 32	~2 ± 0.5	Berman *et al.* (1990)
Baboon	0, 4, 24	~3 ± 1	Anderson *et al.* (1989)
Guinea pig	0, 4, 8	~20 ± 4	Powell *et al.* (1994)

[a]The decrease in gp120 specific antibody titers following the third immunization was fit to the first-order rate law, and the decay constant fit by nonlinear least squares analysis. Where antibody half lives were not reported directly in the references given, the decay constants and half lives were calculated from the raw data given in the reference.

Table III
Selected Immunization Schedules Used in Human Vaccines

Vaccine	Schedules (weeks)[a]	Reference
Longer schedule better		
Hepatitis B	0, 4, 24 > 0, 4, 8	Hess et al. (1992)
Rabies	0, 4, 8 > 0, 1, 3	Cabasso et al. (1978)
Acellular DPT	0, 8, 16 ≥ 0, 4, 8	Just et al. (1991)
SPf66 malaria	0, 3, 32 > 0, 3, 13	Rocha et al. (1992)
Polio	0, 3, 24 > 0, 3, 8[b]	Salk (1955)
Hepatitis A	0, 4 > 0, 2 > 0, 0	Jilg et al. (1992)
	0, 1, 12 > 0, 1, 2[b]	Westblom et al. (1994)
Shorter schedule better		
Rabies	0, 1, 3 > 0, 4, 8	Cabasso et al. (1978)

[a]The immunization schedules are shown, where the superior schedule giving the higher immune response is left of the ">." Where only a marginal schedule superiority was found, the "≥" sign is used.
[b]Several immunization schedules were tested and in all cases, longer total schedules induced higher titers of specific antibodies.

Experiments designed to measure this aspect of vaccine-induced responses have been done in both animals and humans. Unfortunately, the differences between species are significant and this has made it difficult to extrapolate data from experimental animals to human vaccines. For example, the levels of circulating antibodies produced following vaccination with recombinant HIV-1 gp120 have been determined for several species, all of which have remarkably different antibody persistence kinetics (Table III). The most relevant data therefore must be obtained in clinical trials.

The persistence of antibodies in vaccinated humans was found to be variable and different for each vaccine and dosing schedule. The levels of circulating antibodies produced in response to several experimental HIV-1 vaccines containing different immunogens and adjuvants were all maintained for comparable times; antibody "half lives" ranged from 11 to 17 ± 3–4 weeks (Belshe et al., 1993; Graham et al., 1993b; McElrath et al., 1994). In the case of hepatitis B vaccination, antibody persistence was dependent on the immunization schedule; antibodies produced using a 0, 4, 24 week immunization schedule decreased to their half-maximal level in 14 ± 2 weeks (Just et al., 1993) whereas antibodies produced using the 0, 4, 8 week schedule were maintained longer with the half-maximal level occurring approximately 24 weeks after the final booster immunization (Wiedermann et al., 1987). Antibodies produced following hepatitis A vaccination were maintained longer, with the half-maximal level observed 36 weeks after the third immunization and in this case, the responses were independent of vaccine dose (Wiedermann et al., 1990). Interestingly, the use of only two hepatitis A immunizations produced antibody responses that were maintained even longer (Müller et al., 1992). The antibody levels produced following vaccination with a Neisseria meningitidis polysaccharide vaccine, containing both A and C polysaccharides, were extremely stable and reached their half-maximal level a full 100 weeks after the final immunization (Zangwill et al., 1994).

Although it may be possible to design and formulate subunit vaccines that induce sustained antibody responses in most people, it will be difficult to induce optimal responses in everyone because of interindividual variation and genetic limitations. For example, a subset of persons that have been vaccinated with the hepatitis B virus vaccine have failed to respond and this appears to represent an MHC-linked defect in the immune system (Craven *et al.*, 1986; Eddleston, 1990; Kruskall *et al.*, 1992). Even in the responder population, the duration of functional antibody levels ranged from 40 to 280 days, independent of the magnitude of the initial immune responses (Nommensen *et al.*, 1989). These types of variations will likely continue to pose problems and limit the utility of some vaccines.

4.4. Vaccine Delivery Route

The immunization route used to deliver subunit vaccines can dramatically influence both the type and magnitude of the resulting immune responses (Webster, 1968; Pierce, 1984; Fadda *et al.*, 1987). Probably the most significant advance in nonparenteral delivery has been the development of vaccine formulations that can be targeted to the mucosa, typically through oral delivery. The advantage of the oral delivery route over parenteral administration is that it can lead to the induction of mucosal immunity, including secretory IgA (Holmgren *et al.*, 1992; Marx *et al.*, 1993; McGhee *et al.*, 1993). This type of immune response is critical for the control and clearance of enteric bacteria such as *V. cholerae* and pathogenic *E. coli*. Another advantage is the ease with which oral vaccine formulations can be delivered, for example, the oral polio vaccine (Salk *et al.*, 1984).

There are several compounds with adjuvant activity and vaccine carrier or delivery systems that have been used successfully to induce mucosal immunity. One of the most widely studied compounds is cholera toxin (CT) or its B subunit (CTB). This protein can significantly enhance mucosal immune responses and induce IgA production and secretion when administered in vaccine formulations (Elson and Ealding, 1984; McKenzie and Halsey, 1984; McGhee *et al.*, 1993). The mechanisms of CT and CTB adjuvant activity are poorly defined but both are known to bind to GM1 ganglioside receptors in the gut-associated lymphoid tissue, possibly targeting the immunogen for increased uptake. This phenomenon has been exploited for poorly immunogenic antigens by covalently binding the antigen to CT or CTB (Czerkinsky *et al.*, 1989; Liang *et al.*, 1988). The reader interested in mucosal versus parenteral immunization is referred to Chapters 15, 17, and 20.

4.5. Vaccine Formulation Stability

To properly design a successful subunit vaccine product, one must consider several critical formulation and regulatory issues. Most importantly, a vaccine must be both efficacious and safe but it must also be stable and relatively easy to use. An ideal subunit vaccine formulation designed for parenteral delivery should consist of a liquid formulation that does not require cold or frozen storage and can be used directly from a single vial. This ideal vaccine formulation should also be stable to agitation and exposure to light.

These ideal characteristics are not achieved by most vaccines available on the market and hence, the opportunity for marketing new vaccines is great, even if competitive products exist.

Vaccine stability can be defined in numerous ways and under many storage conditions. A reasonable standard of stability is a shelf life of 2 years or more, where the shelf life is defined as the time point for which the product remains at least 90% active or efficacious. The design of stable vaccine formulations requires that all of the components be stable in the final formulation. This is a challenging task indeed, because the stability requirements for the individual components are usually radically different.

Degradation of vaccine components results in a reduction in effectiveness. Two distinct types of degradation are of concern: chemical and physical. A common form of chemical degradation is proteolytic cleavage of the vaccine immunogen. An example of this is cleavage of the V3 loop of the HIV-1 gp120 protein that contains the dominant neutralizing epitope (LaRosa *et al.*, 1989). The gp120 molecule may undergo proteolytic cleavage within the V3 loop and when this occurs, the immunogenicity of the protein is altered so that neutralizing antibodies are not produced thus reducing the effectiveness of the vaccine. Physical degradation can also occur in the form of denaturation of protein immunogens resulting in the loss of conformationally dependent epitopes, such as was observed for another HIV-1 gp120-based vaccine (Haigwood *et al.*, 1992). To better understand the factors affecting the stability of subunit vaccines design, we recommend several excellent reviews on protein stability in parenteral formulations covering general stability concerns for pharmaceuticals (Mollica *et al.*, 1978; Manning *et al.*, 1989), effects of formulation stabilizers on peptide stability (Wang and Hanson, 1988), and protein degradation pathways (Chen, 1988). Here, we briefly summarize only the major degradation pathways for both the immunogens and several adjuvants.

Chemical degradation of protein immunogens can occur by several mechanisms that include hydrolysis, deamidation, oxidation and reduction, racemization, and photodegradation. Proteins are quite susceptible to chemical degradation because they have an enormous number of potential reaction sites. Reactivity of sites can be caused by their proximity to reaction groups or to formal catalysis by a neighboring group, such as general acid or base catalysis. For example, proteins containing the Asp residue are susceptible to acid-catalyzed hydrolysis (Piszkiewicz *et al.*, 1970), particularly if linked Asp-Pro are present (Schultz, 1967). This Asp-Pro linkage is sufficiently labile to degradation to limit the room temperature shelf life of subunit vaccine formulations, even at pH 5–7, the pH range that should provide maximum stability (Powell *et al.*, 1994). Proteins containing linked Asp-Gly are also susceptible to hydrolysis. In fact, this linkage group may be too reactive for use in aqueous vaccine formulations where a 2-year, room temperature shelf life is desired (Geiger and Clark, 1987).

Deamidation of proteins at the amino acid residues Asn and Gln is another example of degradation that can alter the immunogenicity of proteins used in subunit vaccines. The deamidation rate for Asn is usually greater than for Gln, and is greatest when Asn or Gln is adjacent to Gly (Robinson *et al.*, 1973). In general, polar amino acids in the position X-Asn or X-Gln accelerate the deamidation rate, whereas hydrophobic or bulky amino acids in the position Asn-X appear to slow the deamidation rate considerably. Adjacent amino acids X = Gly, Ser, Thr, Ala, or His show the greatest rates. Several reviews of protein deamidation have been published (Robinson and Rudd, 1974; Cleland *et al.*, 1993; Wright, 1991).

Oxidation and reduction represent still additional degradation pathways that may alter immunogenicity of proteins depending on the site of oxidation and the nature of the immune response being studied (Cleland *et al.*, 1993). Methionine and cysteine are the predominant amino acids subject to oxidation under conditions used to formulate subunit vaccines, such as pH 5–7 (Stadtman *et al.*, 1988). The reactivity of methionine residues in a protein can vary significantly because some are protected from oxidation by steric effects. This is particularly true if the residues are buried in the hydrophobic core of the intact protein molecule (Teh *et al.*, 1987). Cysteine is also easily oxidized to yield cystine disulfide and this reaction is usually accelerated at higher pH where the thiol is deprotonated (Philipson, 1962). Histidine, tryptophan, and tyrosine also oxidize under these conditions.

Initiation of oxidative and reductive degradation can usually be attributed to the presence of metal ions, exposure to light, or exposure to certain bases (Johnson and Gu, 1988). The rate of this type of degradation is often governed by trace amounts of peroxide, commonly present in the surfactants used to prepare emulsions. Because this reaction is fairly rapid, it is unlikely that proteins containing free cysteinyl groups can be formulated in aqueous solution and remain stable at room temperature for 2 years. In instances like this, a lyophilized formulation may be preferred but this assumes that the freeze/thaw process does not denature the protein and thereby alter immunogenicity.

Physical instability of proteins that are used as immunogens may compromise vaccine formulation stability. This can occur in several ways such as loss of protein via adsorption of the protein immunogen to the surface of the container or possibly by protein aggregation and subsequent denaturation. Surface adsorption usually occurs at low concentrations of protein and in the absence of carriers. The adsorption of protein has more profound implications than just the simple loss of a component in the formulation because adsorption increases protein susceptibility to denaturation (Steadman *et al.*, 1992). A well-characterized example is insulin which readily adsorbs to hydrophobic surfaces and subsequently denatures. Denatured insulin molecules then accumulate resulting in the formation of nonfunctional aggregates (Sluzky *et al.*, 1991; Sato *et al.*, 1984). Other effects associated with protein adsorption and aggregation have been extensively reviewed (Kiefhaber *et al.*, 1991; Norde and Lyklema, 1991; Andrade *et al.*, 1992; Sadana, 1992).

Protein adsorption can be prevented by increasing the protein concentration in the formulations or by the addition of appropriate carrier molecules, such as particulate alum or surfactants. Surfactants, such as those used in many emulsion-based adjuvant formulations, are useful because they bind to the hydrophobic areas of both the soluble protein and the container surfaces and inhibit protein adsorption. Examples of these types of compounds are the block copolymers and the polysorbate polymers, both of which have been used in vaccine formulations as adjuvants. The polysorbate polymers consist of a sorbitol–polyethylene oxide head group and a hydrocarbon tail, whereas the block copolymers consist of a polyethylene oxide–polypropylene oxide copolymer. Unfortunately, some surfactants also have the ability to denature proteins and this can alter immunogenicity (Ertürk *et al.*, 1989). This property is directly associated with the chemical nature of the surfactant. For example, ionic surfactants, such as sodium dodecyl sulfate, cause protein denaturation at relatively low concentrations (<0.1% w/v) whereas nonionic surfactants generally do not cause denaturation even at greater concentrations (1% w/v). Careful selection of the correct surfactant for individual formulations is essential.

4.6. Adjuvant Formulation Concerns

Adjuvant stability is also crucial in subunit vaccine design. Like vaccine immunogens, adjuvants may degrade through chemical and physical pathways. Chemical degradation can occur by several mechanisms based on the chemical and physical properties of the adjuvant. Cytokine adjuvants, such as IL-1, IL-2, and IFN-γ, are susceptible to the same types of degradation as protein immunogens, namely proteolytic cleavage, denaturation, and adsorption (Gu *et al.*, 1991; Hora *et al.*, 1992), and they must be stabilized when used in vaccine formulations (Brewster *et al.*, 1991; Hora *et al.*, 1992).

Hydrolysis can be a major problem for many adjuvant-containing formulations. The small molecule adjuvants such as muramyl dipeptide compounds, which include MDP, threonyl-MDP, murabutide, and MTP-PE, are susceptible to amide hydrolysis (Powell *et al.*, 1988). Saponin adjuvants, such as QS-21, have ester bonds that hydrolyze rapidly at room temperature at pH > 7.0 or pH < 4. This degradation can be controlled in the pH range 5–6 and by cold storage (Lim *et al.*, 1994). Stearyl tyrosine may be similarly susceptible to ester hydrolysis if stored in aqueous solution at high temperature and high or low pH (Penney *et al.*, 1986). Poly-lactide-co-glycolide (PLGA) polymers used in microsphere-based adjuvant formulations are also susceptible to hydrolysis if not stored absolutely dry. In this case, hydrolysis lowers the polymer mean molecular weight and this can result in release of the vaccine immunogen (Alonso *et al.*, 1993). In all of these examples, the hydrolyzed products retain only a fraction of the function of the parent compounds and the result is a rapid decrease in product shelf life.

Degradation through oxidation can also be a problem, especially for the current generation of emulsion-based formulations that are made using unsaturated squalene as the oil phase of the emulsion. Squalene can be highly susceptible to oxidation (Saint-Leger *et al.*, 1986) and this reaction can be catalyzed by peroxides found in the surfactants used in the formulations (Hamburger *et al.*, 1975; Donbrow *et al.*, 1978). This may result in physical degradation of the adjuvant, again resulting in a reduction of shelf life.

Adjuvants, such as alum, are prone to physical denaturation that results in a change of particle size or protein binding capacity (Chapters 8 and 9). This can occur when alum ages or is frozen (Nail *et al.*, 1976; Morefield *et al.*, 1986; Callahan *et al.*, 1991). Since the adjuvant effect of alum is the result of the depoting and sustained release of antigen over time (Aprile and Wardlaw, 1966), any degradation that alters the protein binding capacity can decrease adjuvant activity. The reverse situation, where protein cannot undergo normal desorption in vivo, can also be a problem in aged alum-containing formulations (Seeber *et al.*, 1991; Mordenti *et al.*, 1994).

Physical degradation can also be a problem in emulsion and liposome formulations where particle or droplet size is critical to immunogenicity (Van Nest *et al.*, 1992; Chapter 10) and physical stability (Lidgate *et al.*, 1989; Chapter 12). In these cases, smaller particle or droplet sizes are associated with higher levels of immunogenicity and better physical stability of the product (Van Nest *et al.*, 1992). Emulsion stability is determined largely by two factors, particle size and the amount and nature of the emulsifiers used. A description of emulsion stabilization conditions can be found in Chapter 10.

The most desirable formulation of a subunit vaccine should address many factors including stability, ease of administration, cost, and the types of immune responses that are required. Most vaccines are currently administered intramuscularly by needle injection and this is likely to continue as the standard route. The exception is for vaccines designed specifically to induce mucosal and gut-associated immune responses, which must be delivered to a mucosal surface and are therefore administered orally.

Aqueous, single vial vaccine formulations that are ready to use are highly desirable because of their biocompatibility and ease of administration. Unfortunately, their development is fraught with major stability hurdles. Often it is not possible to develop a stable liquid vaccine formulation because of chemical or physical instability, thus necessitating the development of a stable lyophilized formulation. However, lyophilization is a complex process involving freezing and drying and protein stability in lyophilized formulations is crucially dependent on several factors including: moisture content (Liu *et al.*, 1991; Pikal *et al.*, 1991a), excipients (Pikal, 1990; Carpenter *et al.*, 1990; Pikal *et al.*, 1991b), and method of freezing (Pikal, 1993).

Even when extreme caution is used, many vaccine formulations may not be stable to the lyophilization process. For example, alum-containing formulations cannot be lyophilized because freezing destroys the particulate structure of the alum (Shi. ¬dkar *et al.*, 1990). Most emulsion-based formulations cannot be lyophilized because the drying step changes the critical "water-to-oil" ratio thus destroying the balance required to maintain emulsion droplets (Lidgate *et al.*, 1989). Polymer microspheres may be sensitive to both the freezing and drying steps since these often cause cracks to form in the microsphere structure, thus altering the release profile. Lyophilization can also induce aggregation and denaturation, as occurs for certain cytokines (Pearlman and Nguyen, 1992; Prestrelski *et al.*, 1993). Because of the significant benefits associated with lyophilization of products, specifically storage and shipping, the development of new methods or stable formulations will remain a high developmental priority.

5. CONCLUSIONS

The design and development of new subunit vaccines is a complex issue. We have reviewed many of the preclinical concerns, those that can be addressed early in the design and development phases. However, many regulatory considerations must also be addressed before a new product can be tested in field trials and released for use in the public sector. Because most vaccines are designed to be used in healthy persons, the safety is paramount and must be evaluated in extremely conservative ways. This is particularly true for pediatric vaccines. Other regulatory issues include development and validation of manufacturing processes and licensing or registration. All of these issues have been addressed elsewhere in this book and will not be addressed here (Chapters 2–6).

The ability to manufacture a product in a way that is profitable is an issue that is seldom considered during the early phases of vaccine design and development. Unfortunately, there is little hope for any vaccine unless it can be manufactured in a cost-effective manner using current technology. This point may seem trivial to the uninitiated, but it often represents one of the greatest "real-life" barriers to vaccine design. Fortunately, solutions to many cost-related manufacturing problems may be found indirectly as scientists work to develop better subunit vaccines. For example, inexpensive adjuvant-active compounds may decrease the quantity of protein immunogen needed in a formulation or reduce the number of doses that will be required. Efforts of this type require collaboration between industry and academic institutions as well as collaborations between companies. Although not formally the focus of this text, we hope that this body of information, including the adjuvant component compendium (Chapter 7), will promote further collaborative advances in subunit vaccine design.

REFERENCES

Acres, R. B., Hareuveni, M., Balloul, J.-M., and Kieny, M.-P., 1993, Vaccinia virus MUC1 immunization of mice: Immune response and protection against the growth of murine tumors bearing the MUC1 antigen, *J. Immunother.* **14**:136–143.

Alfonso, L. C. C., Sharton, T. M., Vierira, L. Q., Wysocka, M., Thinchieri, G., and Scott, P., 1994, The adjuvant effect of interleukin-12 in a vaccine against *Leishmania major*, *Science* **263**:235–237.

Alving, C. R., Richards, R. L., and Moss, J., 1986, Effectiveness of liposomes as potential carriers of vaccines: Applications to cholera toxin and human malarial sporozoite antigen, *Vaccine* **4**:166–172.

Alwan, W. H., Record, F. M., and Openshaw, P. J. M., 1993, Phenotypic and functional characterization of T cell lines specific for individual respiratory syncytial virus proteins, *J. Immunol.* **150**:5211–5218.

Anderson, K. P., Lucas, C., Hanson, C. V., Londe, H. F., Izu, A., Gregory, T., Ammann, A., Berman, P. W., and Eichberg, J. W., 1989, Effect of dose and immunization schedule on immune response of baboons to recombinant glycoprotein 120 of HIV-1, *J. Infect. Dis.* **160**:960–969.

Anderson, M. S., and Miler, J., 1992, Invariant chain can function as a chaperon protein for class II major histocompatibility complex molecules, *Proc. Natl. Acad. Sci. USA* **89**:2282–2286.

Anderson, P., 1983, Antibody responses to *H. influenzae* type b and diphtheria toxin induced by conjugates of oligosaccharides of the type b capsule with the nontoxic protein CRM197, *Infect. Immun.* **39**:233–238.

Anderson, P., and Heron, I., 1993, Specificity of a protective immune response against *Mycobacterium tuberculosis*, *Infect. Immun.* **61**:844–851.

Anderson, P., Pichichero, M. E., and Insel, R. A., 1985, Immunization of 2-month-old infants with protein-coupled oligosaccharides derived from capsule of *H. influenzae* type b, *J. Pediatr.* **107**:346–351.

Anderson, P., Askgaard, D., Ljungqvist, L., Bentzon, M. W., and Heron, I., 1991, T-cell proliferative response to antigens secreted from *Mycobacterium tuberculosis*, *Infect. Immun.* **59**:1558–1563.

Anderson, P., Askgaard, D., Gottschau, A., Bennedsen, J., Nagai, S., and Heron, I., 1992, Identification of immunodominant antigens during infection with *Mycobacterium tuberculosis*, *Scand. J. Immunol.* **36**:823–831.

Andrade, J. D., Hlady, V., Wei, A.-P., Ho, C.-H., Lea, A. S., Jeon, S. I., Lin, Y. S., and Stroup, E., 1992, Proteins at interfaces: Principles, multivariate aspects, protein resistant surfaces, and direct imaging and manipulation of adsorbed proteins, *Clin. Mater.* **11**:67–70.

Aprile, M. A., and Wardlaw, A. C., 1966, Aluminum compounds as adjuvants for vaccines and toxoids in man: A review, *Can. J. Public Health* **57**:343–360.

Barnd, D. L., Lan, M. S., Metzgar, R. S., and Finn, O. J., 1989, Specific, major histocompatibility complex-unrestricted recognition of tumor-associated mucins by human cytotoxic T cells, *Proc. Natl. Acad. Sci. USA* **86**:7159–7164.

Barnes, P. F., Abrams, J. S., Lu, S. Z., Sieling, P. A., Rea, T. H., and Modlin, R. L., 1993, Patterns of cytokine production by mycobacterium-reactive human T-cell clones, *Infect. Immun.* **61**:197–203.

Belshe, R. B., Clements, M. L., Dolin, R., Graham, B. S., McElrath, J., Gorse, G. J., Schwartz, D., Keefer, M. C., Wright, P., Corey, L., Bolognesi, D. M., Matthews, T. J., Stablein, D. M., O'Brien, F. S., Eibl, M., Dorner, F., Koff, W., and the NIH NIAID AIDS VEG., 1993, Safety and immunogenicity of a fully glycosylated recombinant gp160 human immunodeficiency virus type 1 vaccine in subjects at low risk of infection, *J. Infect. Dis.* **168**:1387–1395.

Bennett, B., Check, I. J., Olsen, M. R., and Hunter, R. L., 1992, A comparison of commercially available adjuvants for use in research, *J. Immunol. Methods* **153**:31–40.

Bennett, K., Levine, T., Ellis, J. S., Peanasky, R. J., Samloff, I. M., Kay, J., and Chain, B. M., 1992, Antigen processing for presentation by class II major histocompatibility complex requires cleavage by cathepsin E, *Eur. J. Immunol.* **22**:1519–1524.

Berek, C., Berger, A., and Apel, M., 1991, Maturation of the immune response in germinal centers, *Cell* **67**:1121–1129.

Berman, P. W., Gregory, T. J., Riddle, L., Nakamura, G. R., Champe, M. A., Porter, J. P., Wurm, F. M., Hershberg, R. D., Cobb, E. K., and Eichberg, J. W., 1990, Protection of chimpanzees from infection by HIV-1 after vaccination with recombinant gp120 but not gp160, *Nature* **345**:622–625.

Berman, P. W., Matthews, T., Eastman, D., Nakamura, G., Murthy, K., and Schwartz, D., 1993, Comparison of the immune response to recombinant gp120 in man and chimpanzees, IX International Conference on AIDS, Berlin, Germany, Abstract PO-B27-2135.

Beverly, P. C. L., 1990, Is T cell memory maintained by cross-reactive stimulation? *Immunol. Today* **11**:203–205.

Beverly, P. C. L., 1992, Functional analysis of human T cell subsets defined by CD45 isoform expression, *Semin. Immunol.* **4**:35–41.

Boon, W. H., Liano, D., and Abbas, A. K., 1988, Heterogeneity of helper/inducer T lymphocytes. II. Effects of interleukin 4- and interleukin 2-producing T cell clones on resting B lymphocytes, *J. Exp. Med.* **167**:1352–1363.

Boon, W. H., Wallis, R. S., and Chervenak, K. A., 1991, Human mycobacterium tuberculosis-reactive CD4[+] T-cell clones: Heterogeneity in antigen recognition. Cytokine production and cytotoxicity for mononuclear phagocytes, *Infect. Immun.* **59**:2737–2743.

Braciale, T. J., Morrison, L. A., Sweetser, M. T., Sambrook, J., Gething, M.-J., and Braciale, V. L., 1987, Antigen presentation pathways to class I and class II MHC-restricted T lymphocytes, *Immunol. Rev.* **98**:95–114.

Bradley, L. M., Duncan, D. D., Tonkonogy, S., and Swain, S. L., 1991, Characterization of antigen-specific CD4[+] effector T cells *in vivo*: Immunization results in a transient population of Mel-14[−] CD45RB[−] helper cells that secrete interleukin-2 (IL-2), IL-3, IL-4 and interferon-γ, *J. Exp. Med.* **174**:547–559.

Brewster, M. E., Hora, M. S., Simpkins, J. W., and Bodor, N., 1991, Use of 2-hydroxypropyl-beta-cyclodextrin as a solubilizing and stabilizing excipient for protein drugs, *Pharm. Res.* **8**:792–795.

Brown, F., Dougan, G., Hoey, E. M., Martin, S. J., Rima, B. K., and Trudgett, A., 1993, *Vaccine Design*, Wiley, New York.

Brown, M. G., Driscoll, J., and Monaco, J. J., 1991, Structural and serological similarity of MHC-linked LMP and proteosome (multicatalytic proteinase) complexes, *Nature* **353**:335–357.

Bruguera, M., Cremades, M., Salinas, R., Costa, J., Grau, M., and Sans, J., 1992, Impaired response to recombinant hepatitis B vaccine in HIV-infected persons, *J. Clin. Gastroenterol.* **14**:27–30.

Bu, D., Domenech, N., Lewis, J., Taylor-Papadimitriou, J., and Finn, O. J., 1993, Recombinant vaccinia mucin vector: In vitro analysis of expression of tumor-associated epitopes for antibody and human cytotoxic T-cell recognition, *J. Immunother.* **14**:127–135.

Butterfield, K., Fathman, C. G., and Budd, R. C., 1989, A subset of memory CD4[+] helper T-lymphocytes identified by expression of Pgp-1, *J. Immunol.* **169**:1461–1466.

Bystryn, J.-C., Ferrone, S., and Livingston, P., (eds.), 1993, *Specific Immunotherapy of Cancer with Vaccines*, Vol. 690, New York Academy of Sciences, New York.

Cabasso, V. J., Louie, B. L., and Dobkin, M. B., 1978, Antibody levels following W138 rabies vaccine, *Dev. Biol. Stand.* **40**:231–235.

Callahan, P. M., Shorter, A. L., and Hem, S. L., 1991, The importance of surface charge in the optimization of antigen–adjuvant interactions, *Pharm. Res.* **8**:851–858.

Carpenter, J. F., Arakawa, T., and Crowe, J. H., 1990, Interactions of stabilizing additives with proteins during freeze-thawing and freeze-drying, *Dev. Biol. Stand.* **74**:225–238.

Cheever, M. A., Chen, W., Nelson, H., Greenberg, P. D., Lee, V. K., Crossland, K. D., and Peace, D. J., 1990, T cell immunity to the oncogenic form of *ras* protein can be induced by immunization with synthetic peptides, in: *Cellular Immunity and Immunotherapy of Cancer* (M. T. Lotze and O. J. Finn, eds.), Wiley–Liss, New York, pp. 295–302.

Chen, T., 1992, Formulation concerns of protein drugs, *Drug Dev. Ind. Pharm.* **18**:1311–1354.

Cher, D. J., and Mosmann, T. R., 1987, Two types of murine helper cell clones: 2. Delayed-type hypersensitivity is mediated by TH1 clones, *J. Immunol.* **138**:3688–3694.

Cleland, J. L., Powell, M. F., and Shire, S., 1993, The development of stable protein formulations: A close look at protein aggregation, deamidation and oxidation, *Crit. Rev. Ther. Drug Carrier Syst.* **10**:307–377.

Cleland, J. L., Powell, M. F., Lim, A., Barrón, L., Berman, P. W., Eastman, D. J., Nunberg, J. H., Wrin, T., and Vennari, J. C., 1994, Development of a single shot subunit vaccine for HIV-1, *AIDS Res. Hum. Retroviruses* **10**:521–526.

Clerici, M., and Shearer, G. M., 1993, A TH1–TH2 switch is a critical step in the etiology of HIV infection, *Immunol. Today* **14**:107–111.

Coffman, R. L., Seymour, B. W., Lebman, D. A., Hiraki, D. D., Christiansen, J. A., Shrader, B., Cherwinski, H. M., Savelkoul, H. F. J., Finkelman, F. D., Bond, M. W., and Mosmann, T. R., 1988, The role of helper T cell products in mouse B cell differentiation and isotype regulation, *Immunol. Rev.* **102**:5–28.

Cohen, S., Bernstein, H., Hewes, C., Chow, M., and Langer, R., 1991, The pharmacokinetics of, and humoral responses to, antigen delivered by microencapsulated liposomes, *Proc. Natl. Acad. Sci. USA* **88**:10440–10444.

Colditz, G. A., Brewer, T. F., Berkey, C. S., Wilson, M. E., Burdick, E., Fineberg, H. V., and Mosteller, F., 1994, Efficacy of BCG vaccine in the prevention of tuberculosis: Meta-analysis of the published literature, *J. Am. Med. Assoc.* **271**:698–702.

Collins, D. S., Unanue, E. R., and Harding, C. V., 1991, Reduction of disulfide bonds within lysosomes is a key step in antigen processing, *J. Immunol.* **147**:4054–4059.

Constant, S. L., and Wilson, R. A., 1992, *In vivo* responses in the draining lymph nodes of mice exposed to *Schistosoma mansoni*: Preferential proliferation of T cells is central to the induction of protective immunity, *Cell. Immunol.* **139**:145–161.

Cox, J., and Coulter, A., 1992, Advances in adjuvant technology and application, in: *Animal Parasite Control Utilizing Biotechnology* (W. K. Yong, ed.), CRC Press, Boca Raton, pp. 49–111.

Craven, D. E., Awdeh, R., Kunches, L. M., Yunis, E. J., Dienstag, J. L., Werner, B. G., Polk, B. F., Syndman, D. R., Platt, R., and Crumpacker, C. S., 1986, Nonresponsiveness to hepatitis B vaccine in health care workers. Results of revaccination and genetic typings, *Ann. Intern. Med.* **105**:356–360.

Czerkinsky, C., Russell, M. W., Lycke, N., Lindbad, M., and Holmgren, J., 1989, Oral administration of a streptococcal antigen coupled to cholera toxin B subunit evokes strong antibody responses in salivary glands and extramucosal tissues, *Infect. Immun.* **57**:1072–1077.

Daugelat, S., Gulle, H., Schoel, B., and Kaufmann, S. H. E., 1992, Secreted antigens of *Mycobacterium tuberculosis*—Characterization with T-lymphocytes from patients and contacts after two-dimensional separation, *J. Infect. Dis.* **166**:186–190.

Degen, E., and Williams, D. B., 1991, Participation of a novel 88 KD protein in the biogenesis of murine class I histocompatibility molecules, *J. Cell Biol.* **112**:1099–1115.

Del Prete, G. F., De Carli, M., Mastromauro, C., Biagiotti, R., Macchia, D., Falagiani, P., Ricci, M., and Romagnani, S., 1991, Purified protein derivative of *Mycobacterium tuberculosis* and excretory-secretory antigen(s) of *Toxocara canis* expand *in vitro* human T cells with stable and opposite (type 1 T helper or type 2 T helper) profile of cytokine production, *J. Clin. Invest.* **88**:346–350.

Del Prete, G. F., De Carli, M., Almerigogna, F., Grazia-Giudizi, M., Biagiotti, R., and Romagnani, S., 1993, Human IL-10 is produced by both type 1 helper (TH1) and type 2 helper (TH2) T cell clones and inhibits their antigen-specific proliferation and cytokine production, *J. Immunol.* **150**:353–360.

Del Prete, G. F., Maggi, E., and Romagnani, S., 1994, Biology of disease: Human Th1 and Th2 cells: Functional properties, mechanisms of regulation, and role in disease, *Lab. Invest.* **70**:299–306.

Dessein, A. J., Couissinier, P., Demeure, C., Rihet, P., Kohlstaedt, S., Carneiro-Carvalho, D., Ouattara, M., Goudot-Crozel, V., Dessein, H., Bourgois, A., Carvallo, E. M., and Prata, A., 1992, Environmental, genetic and immunological factors in human resistance to *Schistosoma mansoni*, *Immunol. Invest.* **21**:423–453.

Deveikis, A., Kim, K. S., and Ward, J. I., 1988, Prevention of *H. influenzae* type b in infant rats by human antibody induced by the capsular polysaccharides and polysaccharide-conjugate vaccines, *Vaccines* **6**:14–18.

De Waal-Malefyt, R., Haanen, J., Spits, H., Roncarolo, M. -G., Velde, A., Figdor, C., Johnson, K., Kastelein, R., Yssel, H., and De Vries, J., 1991, Interleukin 10 (IL-10) and viral IL-10 strongly reduce antigen-specific human T cell proliferation by diminishing the antigen-presenting capacity of monocytes via down regulation of class II major histocompatibility complex expression, *J. Exp. Med.* **174**:915–924.

Disis, M. L., Calenoff, E., McLaughlin, G., Murphy, A. E., Chen, W., Groner, B., Jeschke, M., Lydon, N., McGlynn, E., Livingston, R. B., Moe, R., and Cheever, M. A., 1994, Existent T-cell and antibody immunity to HER-2/neu protein in patients with breast cancer, *Cancer Res.* **54**:16–20.

Doherty, P. C., 1993, Virus infections in mice with targeted gene disruptions, *Curr. Opin. Immunol.* **5**:479–483.

Doherty, P. C., Allan, W., Eichelberger, M., and Carding, S. R., 1992, Roles of $\alpha\beta$ and $\gamma\delta$ T cell subsets in viral immunity, *Annu. Rev. Immunol.* **10**:123–151.

Donbrow, M., Azaz, E., and Pillersdorf, A., 1978, Autoxidation of polysorbates, *J. Pharm. Sci.* **67**:1676–1681.

Dryden, M. W., and Blakemore, J. C., 1989, A review of flea allergy dermatitis in the dog and cat, *Compan. Animal Pract.* **19**:10–17.

Dunne, D. W., Butterworth, A. E., Fulford, A. J. C., Kariuki, H. C., Langley, J. G., Ouma, J. H., Capron, A., Pierce, R. J., and Sturrock, R. F., 1992, Immunity after treatment of human schistosomiasis: Association between IgE antibodies to adult worm antigens and resistance to reinfection, *Eur. J. Immunol.* **22**:1483–1494.

Eddleston, A., 1990, Modern vaccines. Hepatitis, *Lancet* **1**:1142–1145.

Edelman, R., and Tacket, C. O., 1990, Adjuvants, *Int. Rev. Immunol.* **7**:51–66.

Eichelberger, M., Allan, W., Zijlstra, M., Jaenisch, R., and Doherty, P. C., 1991, Clearance of influenza virus respiratory infection in mice lacking class I major histocompatibility complex-restricted CD8[+] T cells, *J. Exp. Med.* **174**:875–880.

Einhorn, M. S., Weinberg, G. A., Anderson, E. L., Granoff, P. D., and Granoff, D. M., 1986, Immunogenicity in infants of *H. influenzae* type b polysaccharide in a conjugate vaccine with *Neisseria meningitidis* outer-membrane protein, *Lancet* **2**:299–302.

Eisen, H. N., and Siskind, G. W., 1964, Variations in affinities of antibodies during the immune response, *Biochemistry* **3**:996–400.

Eldridge, J. H., Staas, J. K., Meulbroek, J. A., McGhee, J. R., Rice, T. R., and Gilley, R. M., 1991, Biodegradable microspheres as a vaccine delivery system, *Mol. Immunol.* **28**:287–294.

Elson, C. O., and Ealding, W., 1984, Cholera toxin feeding did not induce oral tolerance in mice or abrogated oral tolerance to an unrelated oral antigen, *J. Immunol.* **133**:2892–2897.

Emini, E. A., Ellis, R. W., Miller, W. J., McAleer, W. J., Scolnick, E. M., and Gerety, R. J., 1986, Production and immunological analysis of recombinant hepatitis B virus vaccine, *J. Infect.* **13(A)**:31–38.

Epstein, S. L., Misplon, J. A., Lawson, C. M., Subbarao, E. K., Connors, M., and Murphy, B. R., 1993, β2-microglobulin-deficient mice can be protected against influenza A infection by vaccination with vaccinia–influenza recombinants expressing hemagglutinin and neuraminidase, *J. Immunol.* **150**:5484–5493.

Ertürk, M., Wellch, M. J., Phillpotts, R. J., and Jennings, R., 1989, Protection and serum antibody responses in guinea pigs and mice immunized with HSV-1 antigen preparations obtained with different detergents, *Vaccine* **7**:431–436.

Fadda, G., Maida, A., Masia, C., Obino, G., Romano, G., and Spano, E., 1987, Efficacy of hepatitis B immunization with reduced intradermal doses, *Eur. J. Epidemiol.* **3**:176–189.

Falk, K., Rotzschke, O., and Rammensee, H. -G., 1990, Cellular peptide composition governed by major histocompatibility complex class I molecules, *Nature* **348**:248–251.

Falk, K., Rotzschke, O., Stevanovic, S., Jung, G., and Rammensee, H. G., 1991, Allele-specific motifs revealed by sequencing of self-peptides eluted from MHC molecules, *Nature* **351**:290–295.

Feldman, H. A., 1962, Protective value of inactivated measle vaccine, *Am. J. Dis. Child.* **103**:423–424.

Fenton, R. G., Taub, D. D., Kwak, L. W., Smith, M. R., and Longo, D. L., 1993, Cytotoxic T-cell response and in vivo protection against tumor cells harboring activated ras proto-oncogenes, *J. Natl. Cancer Inst.* **85**:1294–1302.

Flynn, J. L., Goldstein, M. M., Triebold, K. J., Koller, B., and Bloom, B. R., 1992, Major histocompatibility complex class I-restricted T cells are required for resistance to *Mycobacterium tuberculosis* infection, *Proc. Natl. Acad. Sci. USA* **89**:12013–12017.

Fulginiti, V. A., 1982, Immunizations: Current controversies, *J. Pediatr.* **101**:487–494.

Fulginiti, V. A., and Kempe, C. H., 1963, Measles exposure among vaccine recipients, *Am. J. Dis. Child.* **106**:450–461.

Fung, P. Y. S., Madej, M., Koganty, R., and Longenecker, B. M., 1990, Active specific immunotherapy of a murine mammary adenocarcinoma using a synthetic tumor-associated glycoconjugate, *Cancer Res.* **50**:4308–4314.

Geiger, T., and Clarke, S., 1987, Deamidation, isomerization, and racemization of asparaginyl and aspartyl residues in peptides. Succinimide-linked reactions that contribute to protein degradation, *J. Biol. Chem.* **262**:785–794.

Gheorghiu, M., Mouton, D., Lecoeur, H., Lagranderie, M., Mevel, J. C., and Biozzi, G., 1985, Resistance of high and low antibody responder lines of mice to the growth of avirulent (BCG) and virulent (H37Rv) strains of mycobacteria, *Clin. Exp. Immunol.* **59**:177–184.

Gilley, R. M., Staas, J. K., Tice, T. R., Morgan, J. D., and Eldridge, J. H., 1992, *Proc. Int. Symp. Control. Rel. Bioact. Mater.* **19**:110–111.

Gillott, D. J., Nouri, A. M., Compton, S. J., and Oliver, R. T., 1993, Accurate and rapid assessment of MHC antigen upregulation following cytokine stimulation, *J. Immunol. Methods* **165**:231–239.

Goldberg, A. L., and Rock, K. L., 1992, Proteolysis, proteosomes and antigen presentation, *Nature* **357**:375–379.

Gorse, G. J., Patel, G., Mandava, M., Belshe, R., and the NIH NIAID AIDS Vaccine Clinical Trials Network, 1993, Cellular responses to T cell epitopes of HIV-1 envelope glycoprotein after vaccination with recombinant gp160 (rgp160), 33rd Interscience Conference on Antimicrobial Agents and Chemotherapy, New Orleans, Abstract 1135.

Graham, B. S., Henderson, G. S., Tang, Y.-W., Lu, X., Neuzil, K. M., and Colley, D. G., 1993a, Priming immunization determines T helper cytokine mRNA expression patterns in lungs of mice challenged with respiratory syncytial virus, *J. Immunol.* **151**:2032–2040.

Graham, B. S., Keefer, M. C., McElrath, J., Matthews, T. J., Schwartz, D., Gorse, G. J., Sposto, R., Chernoff, D., and the NIH NIAID AIDS Vaccine Clinical Trials Network, 1993b, Phase I trial of native HIV-1$_{SF2}$ rgp120 candidate vaccine, IX International Conference on AIDS, Berlin, Germany, Abstract PO-A29-0692.

Gray, D., 1993, Immunological memory, *Annu. Rev. Immunol.* **11**:49–77.

Gray, D., and Matzinger, P., 1991, T cell memory is short-lived in the absence of antigen, *J. Exp. Med.* **174**:969–974.

Gray, D., and Sharvall, H., 1988, B-cell memory is short-lived in the absence of antigen, *Nature* **336**:70–73.

Gray, D., and Sprent, J., 1990, Immunological memory, *Curr. Top. Microbiol. Immunol.* **159**:1–141.

Graziosi, C., Pantaleo, G., Gantt, K. R., Fortin, J. -P., Demarest, J. F., Cohen, O. J., Sekaly, R. P., and Fausi, A. S., 1994, Lack of evidence for the dichotomy of T_H1 and T_H2 predominance for HIV-infected individuals, *Science* **265**:248–252.

Green, J. D., and Terrell, T. G., 1992, Utilization of homologous proteins to evaluate the safety of recombinant human proteins—case study: Recombinant human interferon gamma (rhIFN-g), *Toxicol. Lett.* **64/65**:321–327.

Gregoriadis, G., Davis, D., and Davis, A., 1987, Liposomes as immunological adjuvants, *Vaccine* **5**:145–151.

Gu, L. C., Erdos, E. A., Chiang, H. S., Calderwood, T., Tsai, K., Visor, G. C., Duffy, J., Hsu, W. C., and Foster, L. C., 1991, Stability of interleukin 1 beta (IL-1 beta) in aqueous solution: Analytical methods, kinetics, products, and solution formulation implications, *Pharm. Res.* **8**:485–490.

Hagan, P., Blumenthal, U. J., Dunne, D. W., Simpson, A. J. G., and Wilkins, H. A., 1991, Human IgE, IgG4 and resistance to reinfection with *Schistosoma haematobium*, *Nature* **349**:243–245.

Haigwood, N. L., Nara, P. L., Brooks, E., Van Nest, G. A., Ott, G., Higgins, K. W., Dunlop, N., Scandella, C. J., Eichberg, J. W., and Steimer, K. S., 1992, Native but not denatured recombinant human immunodeficiency virus type I gp120 generates broad-spectrum neutralizing antibodies in baboons, *J. Virol.* **66**:172–182.

Hamburger, R., Azaz, E., and Donbrow, M., 1975, Autoxidation of polyoxyethylenic non-ionic surfactants and of polyethylene glycols, *Pharm. Acta Helv.* **50**:10–17.

Harding, C. V., Collins, D. S., Slot, J. W., Geuze, H. J., and Unanue, E. R., 1991, Liposome-encapsulated antigens are processed in lysomes, recycled and presented to T-cells, *Cell* **64**:393–401.

Heath, A. W., and Playfair, J. H. L., (eds.), 1991, *Vaccines 91*, Cold Spring Harbor Press, Cold Spring Harbor, NY, pp. 351–354.

Hellstrom, K. E., and Hellstrom, I., 1989, Oncogene-associated tumor antigens as targets for immunotherapy, *FASEB J.* **3**:1715–1722.

Herrington, D., Davis, J., Nardin, E. H., Beier, M., Cortese, J., Eddy, H., Losonsky, G., Hollingdale, M., Sztein, M., Levine, M., Nussenzweig, R. S., Clyde, D., and Edelman, R., 1991, Successful immunization of humans with irradiated malaria sporozoites: Humoral and cellular responses of the protected individuals, *Am. J. Med. Hyg.* **45**:539–547.

Hess, G., Hingst, V., Cseke, J., Bock, H. L., and Clemens, R., 1992, Influence of vaccination schedules and host factors on antibody response following hepatitis B vaccination, *Eur. J. Clin. Microbiol. Infect. Dis.* **11**:334–340.

Hilleman, M. R., 1993, The promise and the reality of viral vaccines against cancer, *Ann. NY. Acad. Sci.* **690**:6–18.

Hilleman, M. R., Buynak, E. B., Roehm, R. R., Tytell, A. A., Bertland, A. U., and Lampson, G. P., 1975, Purified and inactivated human hepatitis B vaccine: Progress report, *Am. J. Med. Sci.* **270**:401–404.

Holmgren, J., Dzerkinsky, C., Lycke, N., and Svennerholm, A.-M., 1992, Mucosal immunity: Implications for vaccine development, *Immunobiology* **184**:157–179.

Hora, M. S., Rana, R. K., Wilcox, C. L., Katre, N. V., Hirtzer, P., Wolfe, S. N., and Thomson, J. W., 1992, Development of a lyophilized formulation of interleukin-2, *Dev. Biol. Stand.* **74**:295–303.

Hou, S., Doherty, P. C., Zijlstra, M., Jaenisch, R., and Katz, J. M., 1992, Delayed clearance of Sendai virus in mice lacking class I MHC-restricted CD8+ T cells, *J. Immunol.* **149**:1319–1325.

Hou, S., Hyland, L., Ryan, K. W., Portner, A., and Doherty, P. C., 1994, Virus-specific CD8+ T-cell memory determined by clonal burst size, *Nature* **369**:652–654.

Houbiers, J. G. A., Nijman, H. W., van der Burg, S. H., Drijfhout, J. W., Kenemans, P., van de Velde, C. J. H., Brand, A., Momburg, F., Kast, W. M., and Melief, C. J. M., 1993, *In vitro* induction of human cytotoxic T lymphocyte responses against peptides of mutant and wild-type p53, *Eur. J. Immunol.* **23**:2072–2077.

Hubbard, R. D., Flory, C. M., and Collins, F. M., 1992a, Immunization of mice with mycobacterial culture filtrate proteins, *Clin. Exp. Immunol.* **87**:94–98.

Hubbard, R. D., Flory, C. M., Collins, F. M., and Cocito, C., 1992b, Immunization of mice with the antigen A60 of *Mycobacterium bovis* BCG, *Clin. Exp. Immunol.* **88**:129–131.

Hunt, D. F., Michel, H., Dickinson, T. A., Shabanowitz, J., Cox, A. L., Sakaguchi, K., Appella, E., Grey, H. M., and Sette, A., 1992, Peptides presented to the immune system by the murine class II major histocompatibility complex molecule I-A^d, *Science* **256**:660–662.

Inazu, K., and Shima, K., 1992, Freeze drying and quality evaluation of protein drugs, *Dev. Biol. Stand.* **74**:307–322.

Insel, R. A., and Anderson, P. W., 1986, Oligosaccharide–protein conjugate vaccines induce and prime for oligoclonal IgG antibody responses to the *H. influenzae* b capsular polysaccharide in human infants, *J. Exp. Med.* **163**:262–269.

Ioannides, C. G., Fisk, B., Jerome, K. R., Irimura, T., Wharton, T., and Finn, O. J., 1993, Cytotoxic T cells from ovarian malignant tumors can recognize polymorphic epithelial mucin core peptides, *J. Immunol.* **151**:3693–3703.

Jackson, M. R., Cohen-Doyle, M. F., Peterson, P. A., and Williams, D. B., 1994, Regulation of MHC class I transport by the molecular chaperon, calnexin (p88, IP90), *Science* **263**:384–387.

Jamieson, B. D., and Ahmed, R., 1989, T cell memory: Long-term persistence of virus-specific cytotoxic T cells, *J. Exp. Med.* **169**:1993–2005.

Jerome, K. R., Barnd, D. L., Bendt, K. M., Boyer, C. M., Taylor-Papadimitriou, J., McKenzie, I. F. C., Bast, R. C., and Finn, O. J., 1991, Cytotoxic T-lymphocytes derived from patients with breast adenocarcinoma recognize an epitope present on the protein core of a mucin molecule preferentially expressed by malignant cells, *Cancer Res.* **51**:2908–2916.

Jerome, K. R., Domenech, N., and Finn, O. J., 1993, Tumor-specific cytotoxic T cell clones from patients with breast and pancreatic adenocarcinoma recognize EBV-immortalized B cells transfected with polymorphic epithelial mucin complementary DNA, *J. Immunol.* **161**:1654–1662.

Jertborn, M., Svennerholm, A.-M., and Holmgren, J., 1993, Evaluation of different immunization schedules for oral cholera B subunit–whole cell vaccine in Swedish volunteers, *Vaccine* **11**:1007–1012.

Jilg, W., Bittner, R., Bock, H. L., Clemens, R., Schatzl, H., Schmidt, M., Andre, F. E., and Deinhardt, F., 1992, Vaccination against hepatitis A: Comparison of different short-term immunization schedules, *Vaccine* **10(Suppl.)**:126–128.

Jin, Y., Shih, J. W. K., and Berkower, I., 1988, Human T cell response to the surface antigen of hepatitis B virus (HBsAg). Endosomal and nonendosomal processing pathways are accessible to both endogenous and exogenous antigen, *J. Exp. Med.* **168**:293–296.

Johnson, D. M., and Gu, L. C., 1988, in: *Encyclopedia of Pharmaceutical Technology*, Vol. 1 (J. Swarbrick and J. C. Boylan, eds.), Dekker, New York, pp. 414–449.

Jones, A. J. S., 1993, Analysis of polypeptides and proteins, *Adv. Drug Deliv. Rev.* **10**:29–90.

Jones, W. R., Bradley, J., Judd, S. J., Denholm, E. H., Ing, R. M. Y., Mueller, U. W., Powell, J., Griffin, P. D., and Stevens, V. C., 1988, Phase I clinical trial of a World Health Organization birth control vaccine, *Lancet* **1**:1295–1298.

Just, M., Kanra, G., Bogaerts, H., Berger, R., Ceyhan, M., and Pêtre, J., 1991, Two trials of an acellular DTP vaccine in comparison with a whole-cell DTP vaccine in infants: Evaluation of two PT doses and two vaccination schedules, *Dev. Biol. Stand.* **73**:275–283.

Just, M., Berger, R., and Just, V., 1993, Reactogenicity and immunogenicity of a recombinant hepatitis B vaccine compared with a plasma-derived vaccine in young adults, *Postgrad. Med. J.* **63**:121–123.

Kalish, M. L., Check, I. J., and Hunter, R. L., 1991, Murine IgG isotype responses to the *Plasmodium cynomolgi* circumsporozoite peptide (NAGG)5. I. Effects on carrier, copolymer adjuvants, and lipopolysaccharide on isotype selection, *J. Immunol.* **146**:3583–3590.

Kapikian, A. Z., Mitchell, R. H., Chanock, R. M., Shvedoff, R. A., and Stewart, C. E., 1969, An epidemiological study of altered clinical reactivity to respiratory syncytial (RS) virus infection in children previously vaccinated with an inactivated RS vaccine, *Am. J. Epidemiol.* **89**:405–421.

Karagouni, E. E., and Hadjipetrou-Kourounakis, L., 1990, Regulation of isotype immunoglobulin production by adjuvants in vivo, *Scand. J. Immunol.* **31**:745–754.

Kast, W. M., Bronkhorst, A. M., de Waal, L. P., and Melief, C. J. M., 1986, Cooperation between cytotoxic and helper T lymphocytes in protection against lethal Sendai virus infection, *J. Exp. Med.* **164**:723–738.

Kaufmann, S. H. E., 1993, Immunity to intracellular bacteria, *Annu. Rev. Immunol.* **11**:129–164.

Kayhty, H., Karanko, V., Peltola, H., and Makela, P. H., 1984, Serum antibodies after vaccination with *H. influenzae* type b capsular polysaccharide and responses to reimmunization: No evidence of immunological tolerance or memory, *Pediatrics* **74**:857–865.

Kelly, A., Powis, S. H., Kerr, L.-A., Mockridge, I., Elliott, T., Bastin, J., Uchanska-Ziegler, B., Ziegler, A., and Townsend, A., 1992, Assembly and function of the two ABC transporter proteins encoded in the human major histocompatibility complex, *Nature* **355**:641–644.

Kenney, J. S., Huges, B. W., Masada, M. P., and Allison, A. C., 1989, Influence of adjuvants on the quantity, affinity, isotype and epitope specificity of murine antibodies, *J. Immunol. Methods* **121**:157–166.

Kensil, C. H., Patel, U., Lennick, M., and Marciani, D., 1991, Separation and characterization of saponins with adjuvant activity from *Quillaja saponaria* molina cortex, *J. Immunol.* **146**:431–437.

Kiefhaber, T., Rudolph, R., Kohler, H.-H., and Buchner, J., 1991, Protein aggregation *in vitro* and *in vivo*: A quantitative model of the kinetic competition between folding and aggregation, *Biotechnology* **9**:825–830.

Kilbourne, E. D., 1988, Inactivated influenza vaccines, in: *Vaccines* (S. A. Plotkin and E. A. Mortimer, eds.), Saunders, Philadelphia, pp. 420–434.

Kim, H. W., Canchola, J. G., Brandt, C. D., Pyles, G., Chanock, R. M., Jensen, K., and Parrott, R. H., 1969, Respiratory syncytial virus disease in infants despite prior administration of antigenic inactivated vaccine, *Am. J. Epidemiol.* **89**:422–434.

King, C. L., and Nutman, T. B., 1992, Biological role of helper T-cell subsets in helminth infections, *Chem. Immunol.* **54**:136–165.

King, C. L., Low, C. C., and Nutman, T. B., 1993, IgE production in human helminth infection. Reciprocal interrelationship between IL-4 and IFNγ, *J. Immunol.* **150**:1873–1880.

Kruskall, M. S., Alper, C. A., Awdeh, Z., Yunis, E. J., and Marcus-Bagley, D., 1992, The immune response to hepatitis B vaccine in humans: Inheritance patterns in families, *J. Exp. Med.* **175**:495–502.

Lanzavecchia, A., 1990, Receptor-mediated antigen uptake and its effect on antigen presentation to class II-restricted T lymphocytes, *Annu. Rev. Immunol.* **8**:773–793.

LaRosa, G. J., David, J. P., Weinhold, K., Waterbury, J. A., Profy, A. T., Lewis, J. A., Langlois, A. J., Dreesman, G. R., Boswell, R. N., Shedduck, P., Holley, L. H., Kamplus, M., Bolognesi, D. P., Mathews, T. J., Emini, E. A., and Putney, S. D., 1990, Conserved sequences and structural elements in the HIV-1 principal neutralizing determinant, *Science* **249**:932–935.

Lau, L. L., Jamieson, B. D., Somasundaram, T., and Ahmed, R., 1994, Cytotoxic T-cell memory without antigen, *Nature* **369**:648–652.

Lee, W. T., and Vitetta, E. S., 1991, The differential expression of homing and adhesion molecules on virgin and memory T cells in the mouse, *Cell. Immunol.* **132**:215–222.

Lehmann-Grube, F., Lohler, J., Utermohlen, O., and Gegin, C., 1993, Antiviral immune responses of lymphocytic choriomeningitis virus-infected mice lacking CD8[+] T lymphocytes because of disruption of the β2-microglobulin gene, *J. Virol.* **67**:332–339.

Levine, M. M., Losonsky, G., Herrington, D., Kaper, J. B., Tacket, C., Rennels, M. B., and Morris, J. G., 1986, Pediatric diarrhea: The challenge of prevention, *J. Pediatr. Infect. Dis.* **5(Suppl.)**:29–43.

Liang, X., Lamm, M. E., and Nedrud, J. G., 1988, Oral administration of cholera toxin–Sendai virus conjugate potentiates gut and respiratory immunity against Sendai virus, *J. Immunol.* **141**:1495–1501.

Lidgate, D. M., Fu, R. C., Byars, N. E., Foster, L. C., and Fleitman, J. S., 1989, Formulation of vaccine adjuvant muramyldipeptides. 3. Processing optimization, characterization, and bioactivity of an emulsion vehicle, *Pharm. Res.* **6**:748–752.

Lim, A., Cleland, J. L., Powell, M. F., Jacobsen, N., Basa, L., Spellman, M., Bedore, D., and Kensil, C. R., 1994, QS21 formulation stability and degradation products, Am. Assoc. Pharm. Sci. Meet., San Francisco.

Linton, P.-J., and Klinman, N. R., 1992, The generation of memory B cells, *Semin. Immunol.* **4**:3–9.

Linton, P.-J., Decker, D. J., and Klinman, N. R., 1989, Primary antibody forming cells and secondary B cells are generated from separate precursor cell subpopulations, *Cell* **59**:1049–1059.

Liu, W. R., Langer, R., and Klibanov, A. M., 1991, Moisture-induced aggregation of lyophilized proteins in the solid state, *Biotechnol. Bioeng.* **37**:177–180.

Long, E. O., and Jacobson, S., 1989, Pathways of viral antigen processing and presentation to CTL, *Immunol. Today* **10**:45–48.

Lubin, R., Schlichtholz, B., Bengoufa, D., Zalcman, G., Tredaniel, J., Hirsch, A., Caron de Fromentel, C., Preudhomme, C., Fenaux, P., Fournier, G., Mangin, P., Laurent-Puig, P., Pelletier, G., Schlumberger, M., Desgrandchamps, F., Le Duc, A., Peyrat, J. P., Janin, N., Bressac, B., and Soussi, T., 1993, Analysis of p53 antibodies in patients with various cancers define B cell epitopes of human p53: Distribution on primary structure and exposure on protein surface, *Cancer Res.* **53**:5872–5876.

McAleer, W. J., Buynak, E. B., Maigetter, R. Z., Wampler, D. E., Miller, W. J., and Hilleman, M. R., 1984, Human hepatitis B virus vaccine from recombinant yeast, *Nature* **307**:178–180.

McElrath, M. J., Corey, L., Berger, D., Hoffman, M. C., Klucking, S., Dragavon, J., Peterson, E., and Greenberg, P. D., 1994, Immune responses elicited by recombinant vaccinia–human immunodeficiency virus (HIV) envelope and HIV envelope protein: Analysis of the durability of responses and effect of repeated boosting, *J. Infect. Dis.* **169**:41–47.

McGhee, J. R., Fujihashi, K., Wu, A. -J., Elson, C. O., Beagley, K. W., and Kiyono, H., 1993, New perspectives in mucosal immunity with emphasis on vaccine development, *Semin. Hematol.* **30**(4):3–12.

Mackay, C. R., 1993, Immunological memory, *Adv. Immunol.* **53**:217–265.

MacKenzie, J. S., 1977, Influenza subunit vaccine: Antibody responses to one and two doses of vaccine and length of response, with reference to the elderly, *Br. Med. J.* **1**:200–202.

McKenzie, S. J., and Halsey, J. F., 1984, Cholera toxin B subunit as a carrier protein to stimulate a mucosal immune response, *J. Immunol.* **133**:1818–1824.

Madden, K. B., Urban, J. F., Ziltener, H. J., Schrader, J. W., Finkelman, F. D., and Katona, I. M., 1991, Antibodies to IL-3 and IL-4 suppress helminth-induced intestinal mastocytosis, *J. Immunol.* **147**:1387–1391.

Maggi, E., Mazzetti, M., Ravina, A., Annunziato, F., De Carli, M., Piccinni, M. P., Manetti, R., Carbonari, M., Pesce, A. M., Del Prete, G., and Romagnani, S., 1994, Ability of HIV to promote a T_H1 to T_H0 shift and to replicate preferentially in T_H1 to T_H0 cells, *Science* **265**:244–248.

Mahanty, S., Abrams, J. S., King, C. L., Limaye, A. P., and Nutman, T. B., 1992, Parallel regulation of IL-4 and IL-5 in human helminth infections, *J. Immunol.* **148**:3567–3571.

Makela, P. H., Peltola, H., Kayhty, H., Jousimies, H., Pettay, O., Ruoslahti, E., Sivonen, A., and Renkonen, 1977, Polysaccharide vaccines of group A *Neisseria meningitidis* and *Haemophilus influenzae* type b: A field trial in Finland, *J. Infect. Dis.* **136**(Suppl.):43–50.

Malik, A., Egan, J. E., Houghten, R. A., Sadoff, J. C., and Hoffman, S. L., 1991, Human cytotoxic T lymphocytes against the *Plasmodium falciparum* circumsporozoite protein, *Proc. Natl. Acad. Sci. USA* **88**:3300–3304.

Manning, M. C., Patel, K., and Borchardt, R. T., 1989, Stability of protein pharmaceuticals, *Pharm. Res.* **6**:903.

Martinez, C. K., and Monaco, J. J., 1991, Homology of proteasome subunits to a major histocompatibility complex-linked LMP gene, *Nature* **353**:664–667.

Marx, P. A., Compans, R. W., Gettie, A., Staas, J. K., Gilley, R. M., Mulligan, M. J., Yamshchikov, G. V., Chen, D., and Eldridge, J. H., 1993, Protection against SIV transmission with microencapsulated vaccine, *Science* **260**:1323–1327.

Maupas, P., Goudeau, A., Coursaget, P., Drucker, J., and Bagros, P., 1976, Immunization against hepatitis B in man, *Lancet* **1**:1367–1370.

Miller, M. D., Gould-Fogerite, S., Shen, L., Woods, R. M., Koenig, S., Mannino, R. J., and Letvin, N. L., 1992, Vaccination of rhesus monkeys with synthetic peptide in a fusogenic proteoliposome elicits simian immunodeficiency virus-specific $CD8^+$ cytotoxic T lymphocytes, *J. Exp. Med.* **176**:1739–1744.

Millet, P., Collins, W. E., Broderson, J. R., Bathurst, I., Nardin, E. H., and Nussenzweig, R. S., 1991, Inhibitory activity against *Plasmodium vivax* sporozoites induced by plasma from Saimiri monkeys immunized with circumsporozoite recombinant proteins or irradiated sporozoites, *Am. J. Trop. Med. Hyg.* **45**:44–48.

Modlin, R. L., and Nutman, T. B., 1993, Type 2 cytokines and negative immune regulation in human infections, *Curr. Opin. Immunol.* **5**:511–517.

Mollica, J. A., Ahuja, S., and Cohen, J., 1978, Stability of pharmaceuticals, *J. Pharm. Sci.* **67**:443–465.

Monaco, J. J., Cho, S., and Attaya, M., 1990, Transport proteins in the murine MHC: Possible implications for antigen processing, *Science* **250**:1723–1726.

Mordenti, J., Nguyen, T., Eastman, D., Osaka, G., Frie, S., Weissburg, R. P., Berman, P. W., Abramowitz, P., DiStefano, J., III, and Powell, M. F., 1994, Effects of alum on i.m. absorption and immunogenicity of MN rgp120 in rabbits, Am. Assoc. Pharm. Sci. Meet., San Francisco.

Morefield, E. M., Peck, G. E., Feldkamp, J. R., White, J. L., and Hem., S. L., 1986, Role of water in the aging of aluminum hydroxide suspensions, *J. Pharm. Sci.* **75**:403–406.

Moreno, A., Clavijo, P., Edelman, R., Davis, J., Sztein, M., Herrington, D., and Nardin, E., 1991, Cytotoxic CD4$^+$ T cells from a sporozoite-immunized volunteer recognize the *Plasmodium falciparum* CS protein, *Int. Immunol.* **3**:997–1003.

Mortimer, E. A., 1988a, Diphtheria toxoid, in: *Vaccines* (S. A. Plotkin and E. A. Mortimer, eds.), Saunders, Philadelphia, pp. 31–44.

Mortimer, E. A., 1988b, Pertussis vaccine, in: *Vaccines* (S. A. Plotkin and E. A. Mortimer, eds.), Saunders, Philadelphia, pp. 74–97.

Moskophidis, D., Lechner, F., Pircher, H., and Zinkernagel, R. M., 1993, Virus persistence in acutely infected immunocompetent mice by exhaustion of antiviral cytotoxic effector T cells, *Nature* **362**:758–761.

Mosmann, T. R., and Coffman, R. L., 1989, TH1 and TH2 cells: Different patterns of lymphokine secretion lead to different functional properties, *Annu. Rev. Immunol.* **7**:145–173.

Mosmann, T. R., Cherwinski, H., Bond, M. W., Gieldlin, M. A., and Coffman, R. L., 1986, Two types of murine helper T cell clones: 1. Definition according to profiles of lymphokine activities and secreted proteins, *J. Immunol.* **136**:2348–2357.

Mountford, A. P., Coulson, P. S., Pemberton, R. M., Smythies, L. E., and Wilson, R. A., 1992, The generation of interferon-γ-producing T lymphocytes in skin-draining lymph nodes, and their recruitment to the lungs, is associated with protective immunity to *Schistosoma mansoni*, *Immunology* **75**:250–256.

Muller, D., Koller, B. H., Whitton, J. L., LaPan, K. E., Brigman, K. K., and Frelinger, J. A., 1992, LCMV-specific, class II-restricted cytotoxic T cells in β2-microglobulin-deficient mice, *Science* **255**:1576–1578.

Müller, R., Chriske, H., Deinhardt, J. J., Jilg, J., Theilmann, L., Hess, G., Hofmann, F., Hopf, U., Stickl, H., and Mainwald, H., 1992, Hepatitis A vaccination: Schedule for accelerated immunization, *Vaccine* **10(Suppl.)**:124–145.

Murphy, F. A., and Kingsbury, D. W., 1990, Virus taxonomy, in: *Virology*, Vol. 1 (B. N. Fields and D. M. Knipe, eds.), Raven Press, New York, pp. 9–35.

Mustafa, A. S., Lundin, K. E. A., and Oftung, F., 1993, Human T cells recognize mycobacterial heat shock proteins in the context of multiple HLA-DR molecules: Studies with healthy subjects vaccinated with *Mycobacterium bovis* BCG and *Mycobacterium leprae*, *Infect. Immun.* **61**:5294–5301.

Nail, S. L., White, J. L., and Hem, S. L., 1976, Structure of aluminum hydroxide gel II. Aging mechanism, *J. Pharm. Sci.* **65**:1192–1195.

Nardin, E. H., and Nussenzweig, R. S., 1993, T cell responses to pre-erythrocytic stages of malaria: Role in protection and vaccine development against pre-erythrocytic stages, *Annu. Rev. Immunol.* **11**:687–727.

Nardin, E. H., Herringon, D. A., Davis, J., Levine, M., Stuber, D., Takacs, B., Caspers, P., Barr, P., Altszuler, R., Clavijo, P., and Nussenzweig, R. S., 1989, Conserved repetitive epitope recognized by CD4$^+$ clones from a malaria immunized volunteer, *Science* **246**:1603–1606.

Nardin, E. S., Clavijo, P., Mons, B., van Belkum, A., Ponnudurai, T., and Nussenzweig, R. S., 1991, T cell epitopes of the circumsporozoite protein of *Plasmodium vivax*. Recognition by lymphocytes of a sporozoite-immunized chimpanzee, *J. Immunol.* **146**:1674–1678.

Neefjes, J. J., Stollorz, V., Peters, P. J., Geuze, H. J., and Ploegh, H. L., 1990, The biosynthetic pathway of MHC class II but not class I molecules intersects the endocytic route, *Cell* **61**:171–183.

Newman, M. J., Wu, J.-Y., Gardner, B. H., Munroe, K. J., Leombruno, D., Recchia, J., Kensil, C. R., and Coughlin, R. T., 1992, Saponin adjuvant induction of ovalbumin-specific CD8$^+$ cytotoxic T lymphocyte responses, *J. Immunol.* **148**:2357–2362.

Nijman, H. W., Houbiers, J. G. A., van der Burg, S. H., Vierboom, M. P. M., Kenemans, P., Kast, W. M., and Melief, C. J. M., 1993, Characterization of cytotoxic T lymphocyte epitopes of a self-protein, p53, and a non-self-protein, influenza matrix: Relationship between major histocompatibility complex peptide binding affinity and immune responsiveness to peptides, *J. Immunother.* **14**:121–126.

Nommensen, F. E., Go, S. T., and MacLaren, D. M., 1989, Half-life of HBs antibody after hepatitis B vaccination: An aid to timing of booster vaccination, *Lancet* **2**:847–849.

Norde, W., and Lyklema, J., 1991, Why proteins prefer interfaces, *J. Biomater. Sci. Polym. Ed.* **2**:183–202.

Nuchtern, J. G., Biddison, W. E., and Klausner, R. D., 1990, Class II MHC molecules can use the endogenous pathway of antigen presentation, *Nature* **343**:74–77.

Oehen, S., Waldner, H., Kundig, T. M., Hengartner, H., and Zinkernagel, R. M., 1992, Antivirally protective cytotoxic T cell memory lymphocytic choriomeningitis virus is governed by persisting antigen, *J. Exp. Med.* **176**:1273–1281.

Ogle, J. D., Noel, J. G., Balasubramaniam, A., Sramoski, R. M., Ogle, C. K., and Alexander, J. W., 1990, Comparison of abilities of recombinant interleukin-1 alpha and -beta and noninflammatory IL-1 beta fragment 163–171 to upregulate C3b receptors (CR1) on human neutrophils and to enhance their phagocytic capacity, *Inflammation* **14**:185–194.

Orme, I. M., and Collins, F. M., 1983, Protection against Mycobacterium tuberculosis infection by adoptive immunotherapy. Requirement for T cell-deficient recipients, *J. Exp. Med.* **158**:74–83.

Pal, P. G., and Horwitz, M. A., 1992, Immunization with extracellular proteins of *Mycobacterium tuberculosis* induces cell-mediated immune responses and substantial protective immunity in a guinea pig model of pulmonary tuberculosis, *Infect. Immun.* **60**:4781–4792.

Pamer, E. G., 1993, Cellular immunity to intracellular bacteria, *Curr. Opin. Immunol.* **5**:492–496.

Parronchi, P., Macchia, D., Piccinni, M. P., Biswas, P., Simonelli, C., Maggi, E., Ricci, M., Ansari, A. A., and Romagnani, S., 1991, Allergen- and bacterial antigen-specific T cell clones established from atopic donors show a different profile of cytokine production, *Proc. Natl. Acad. Sci. USA* **88**:4538–4542.

Paul, W. E., and Seder, R. A., 1994, Lymphocyte responses and cytokines, *Cell* **76**:241–251.

Peace, D. J., Chen, W., Nelson, H., and Cheever, M. A., 1991, T-cell recognition of transforming proteins encoded by mutated *ras* proto-oncogenes, *J. Immunol.* **146**:2059–2065.

Pearlman, R., and Nguyen, T., 1992, Pharmaceutics of protein drugs, *J. Pharm. Pharmacol.* **44**:178–185.

Penney, C. L., Landi, S., Shah, P., Leung, K. H., and Archer, M. C., 1986, Analysis of the immunoadjuvant octadecyl tyrosine hydrochloride, *J. Biol. Stand.* **14**:345–349.

Peters, P. J., Neefjes, J. J., Oorschot, V., Ploegh, H. L., and Geuze, H. J., 1991, Segregation of MHC class II molecules from MHC class I molecules in the Golgi complex for transport to the lysosomal compartments, *Nature* **349**:669–676.

Philipson, L., 1962, Oxidation of 2,3-dimercaptopropranol, *Biochim. Biophys. Acta* **56**:375–381.

Pierce, N. F., 1984, Induction of optimal mucosal antibody responses: Effects of age, immunization route(s), and dosing schedule in rats, *Infect. Immun.* **43**:341–346.

Pikal, M. J., 1990, Freeze-drying of proteins—Part II: Formulation selection, *Biopharm.* **3**:26–30.

Pikal, M. J., 1993, Freeze drying of proteins: Process, formulation, and stability, Protein Formulations and Delivery Symposium, 205th American Chemical Society Meeting (abstract).

Pikal, M. J., Dellerman, K., and Roy, M. L., 1991a, Formulation and stability of freeze-dried proteins: Effects of moisture and oxygen on the stability of freeze-dried formulations of human growth hormone, *Dev. Biol. Stand.* **74**:21–27.

Pikal, M. J., Dellerman, K. M., Roy, M. L., and Riggin, R. M., 1991b, The effects of formulation variables on the stability of freeze-dried human growth hormone, *Pharm. Res.* **8**:427–436.

Piszkiewicz, D., Landon, M., and Smith, E. L., 1970, Anomalous cleavage of aspartyl-proline peptide bonds during amino acid sequence determinations, *Biochem. Biophys. Res. Commun.* **40**:1173–1178.

Pithie, A. D., Rahelu, M., Kumararatne, D. S., Drysdale, P., Gaston, J. S. H., Iles, P. B., Innes, J. A., and Ellis, C. J., 1992, Generation of cytolytic T cells in individuals infected by *Mycobacterium tuberculosis* and vaccinated with BCG, *Thorax* **47**:695–701.

Plotkin, S. A., and Mortimer, E. A., (eds.), 1988, *Vaccines*, Saunders, Philadelphia.

Powell, M. F., 1994, Peptide stability in aqueous parenteral formulations: Prediction of chemical stability based on primary sequence, in: *Protein Formulations and Delivery* (J. L. Cleland and R. S. Langer, eds.), American Chemical Society Symposium Series **567**:100–117.

Powell, M. F., Foster, L. C., Becker, A. R., and Lee, W., 1988, Formulation of vaccine adjuvant muramyldipeptides (MDP). 2. The thermal reactivity and pH of maximum stability of MDP compounds in aqueous solution, *Pharm. Res.* **5**:528–532.

Powell, M. F., Eastman, D. J., Lim, A., Lucas, C., Peterson, M., Vennari, J., Weissburg, R. P., Wrin, T., Kensil, C., Newman, M. J., Nunberg, J. H., Cleland, J. L., Gregory, T., and Berman, P. W., 1995, Effect of adjuvants on the immunogenicity of the MN rgp120 vaccine in guinea pigs, *AIDS Res. Hum. Retroviruses* (in press).

Preblud, R., and Katz, S. L., 1988, Measles vaccine, in: *Vaccines* (S. A. Plotkin and E. A. Mortimer, eds.), Saunders, Philadelphia, pp. 182–234.

Preis, I., and Langer, R. S., 1979, A single shot immunization by sustained antigen release, *J. Immunol. Methods* **28**:193–197.

Prestrelski, S. J., Tedeschi, N., Carpenter, J. F., and Arakawa, T., 1993, Dehydration-induced conformational transitions in proteins and their inhibitors, *Biophys. J.* **65**:661–671.

Pullano, T. G., Sinn, E., and Carney, W. P., 1989, Characterization of monoclonal antibody R256, specific for the activated *ras* p21 with arginine at 12, and analysis of breast carcinoma for v-Harvey-*ras* transgenic mouse, *Oncogene* **4**:1003–1008.

Pupa, S. M., Menard, S., Andreola, S., and Colnaghi, M. I., 1993, Antibody response against the c-*erb*B-2 oncoprotein in breast carcinoma patients, *Cancer Res.* **53**:5864–5866.

Rajewsky, K., 1992, Early and late B-cell development in the mouse, *Curr. Opin. Immunol.* **4**:171–176.

Ramon, G., 1926, Procedes pour accroitre la production des antioxines, *Ann. Inst. Pasteur* **40**:1–10.

Reed, S. G., and Scott, P., 1993, T cell and cytokine responses in leishmaniasis, *Curr. Opin. Immunol.* **5**:524–531.

Ribero, D. E., Jesus, A. M., Almeida, R. P., Bacelar, O., Araujo, M. I., Demeure, C., Bina, J. C., Dessein, A. J., and Carvalho, E. M., 1993, Correlation between cell-mediated immunity and degree of infection in subjects living in an endemic area of schistosomiasis, *Eur. J. Immunol.* **23**:152–158.

Ridley, D. S., and Jopling, W. H., 1966, Classification of leprosy according to immunity. A five-group system, *Int. J. Lepr.* **34**:255–273.

Robinson, A. B., and Rudd, C. J., 1974, in: *Current Topics in Cellular Regulations*, Vol. 8 (B. L. Horecker and E. R. Stadtman, eds.), Academic Press, New York, pp. 247–295.

Robinson, A. B., Scotchler, J. W., and McKerrow, J. H., 1973, Rates of nonenzymatic deamidation of glutaminyl and asparaginyl residues in pentapeptides, *J. Am. Chem. Soc.* **95**:8156–8159.

Rocha, C. L., Murillo, L. A., Mora, A. L., Rojas, M., Franco, L., Cote, J., Valero, M. V., Moreno, A., Amador, R., Nunez, F., Coronell, C., and Patarroyo, M. C., 1992, Determination of the immunization schedule for field trials with the synthetic malaria vaccine SPf 66, *Parasite Immunol.* **14**:95–109.

Rolink, A., and Melchers, F., 1991, Molecular and cellular origins of B lymphocyte diversity, *Cell* **66**:1081–1094.

Rotzschke, O., Falk, K., Deres, O., Schild, H., Norda, M., Metzger, J., Jung, G., and Rammensee, H.-G., 1990, Isolation and analysis of naturally processed viral peptides as recognized by cytotoxic T cells, *Nature* **348**:252–253.

Rudensky, A. Y., Preston-Hurlburt, P., Al-Ramadi, B. K., Rothbard, J., and Janeway, C. A., 1992, Truncation of variants of peptides isolated from MHC class II molecules suggest sequence motifs, *Nature* **359**:429–431.

Sadana, A., 1992, Protein adsorption and inactivation on surfaces. Influence of heterogeneities, *Chem. Rev.* **92**:1799–1807.

Saint-Leger, D., Bague, A., Cohen, E., and Chivot, M., 1986, A possible role for squalene in the pathogenesis of acne. I. In vitro study of squalene oxidation, *Br. J. Dermatol.* **114**:535–542.

Salgame, P., Abrams, J. S., Clayberger, C., Goldstein, H., Convit, J., Modlin, R. L., and Bloom, B. R., 1991, Differing lymphokine profiles of functional subsets of human CD4 and CD8 T cell clones, *Science* **254**:279–282.

Salk, D., van Wezel, A. L., and Salk, J., 1984, Induction of long term immunity to paralytic poliomyelitis by use of a non-infectious vaccine, *Lancet* **2**:1317–1321.

Salk, J. E., 1955, Considerations in the preparation and use of poliomyelitis virus vaccine, *J. Am. Med. Assoc.* **158**:1239–1248.

Salk, J., and Drucker, J., 1988, Noninfectious poliovirus vaccine, in: *Vaccines* (S. A. Plotkin and E. A. Mortimer, eds.), Saunders, Philadelphia, pp. 158–181.

Sato, S., Ebert, C. D., and Kim, S. W., 1984, Prevention of insulin self-association and surface adsorption, *J. Pharm. Sci.* **72**:228–232.

Scherle, P. A., Palladino, G., and Gerhard, W., 1992, Mice can recover from pulmonary influenza virus infection in the absence of class I-restricted cytotoxic T cells, *J. Immunol.* **148**:212–217.

Schneerson, R., Robbins, J. B., Parke, J. C., Parke, J. C., Bell, C., Schlesselman, J. J., Sutton, A., Wang, Z., Schiffman, G., Karpas, A., and Shiloach, J., 1986, Quantitative and qualitative analyses of serum antibodies elicited in adults by *H. influenzae* type b and pneumococcus type 6A capsular polysaccharide-tetanus toxoid conjugates, *Infect. Immun.* **52**:519–528.

Schultz, J., 1967, Cleavage at aspartic acid, *Methods Enzymol.* **11**:255–263.

Seeber, S. J., White, J. L., and Hem, S. L., 1991, Solubilization of aluminum-containing adjuvants by constituents of interstitial fluid, *J. Parenter. Sci. Technol.* **45**:156–159.

Sette, A., Buus, S., Colon, C., Miles, C., and Grey, H. M., 1988, I-A^d binding peptides derived from unrelated proteins share a common structural motif, *J. Immunol.* **141**:45–48.

Shearer, G. M., and Clerici, M., 1992, T helper cell immune dysfunction in asymptomatic, HIV-1-seropositive individuals: The role of TH1–TH2 cross-regulation, *Chem. Immunol.* **54**:21–43.

Sher, A., and Coffman, R. L., 1992, Regulation of immunity to parasites by T cells and T cell-derived cytokines, *Annu. Rev. Immunol.* **10**:385–409.

Shirodkar, S., Hutchinson, R. L., Perry, D. L., White, J. L., and Hem, S. L., 1990, Aluminum compounds used as adjuvants in vaccines, *Pharm. Res.* **7**:1282.

Sieling, P. A., Abrams, J. S., Yamamura, M., Salgame, P., Bloom, B. R., Rea, T. H., and Modlin, R. L., 1993, Immunosuppressive roles for interleukin-10 and interleukin-4 in human infection: In vitro modulation of T cell responses in leprosy, *J. Immunol.* **150**:5501–5510.

Sluzky, V., Tamada, J., Klibanov, A. M., and Langer, R., 1991, Kinetics of insulin aggregation in aqueous solutions upon agitation in the presence of hydrophobic surfaces, *Proc. Natl. Acad. Sci. USA* **88**:9377–9381.

Smith, D. H., Peter, G., and Ingram, D. L., 1973, Responses of children immunized with the capsular polysaccharide of H. influenza, type b, *Pediatrics* **52**:637–644.

Smith, D. W., Wiegeshaus, E. H., and Edwards, M. L., 1988, The protective effects of BCG vaccination against tuberculosis, in: *Mycobacterium tuberculosis Interactions with the Immune System* (M. Bendinelli and H. Friedman, eds.), Plenum Press, New York, pp. 341–370.

Smythies, L. E., Coulson, P. S., and Wilson, R. A., 1992a, T cell-derived cytokines associated with pulmonary immune mechanisms in mice vaccinated with irradiated cercariae of *Schistosoma mansoni*, *J. Immunol.* **148**:1512–1518.

Smythies, L. E., Coulson, P. S., and Wilson, R. A., 1992b, Monoclonal antibody to IFN-γ modifies pulmonary inflammatory responses and abrogates immunity to Schistosoma mansoni in mice vaccinated with attenuated cercariae, *J. Immunol.* **149**:3654–3658.

Spies, T., Cerundolo, V., Colonna, M., Cresswell, P., Townsend, A., and DeMars, R., 1992, Presentation of viral antigen by class I MHC molecules is dependent on a putative peptide transporter heterodimer, *Nature* **355**:644–646.

Sprent, J. T., 1994, T and B memory cells, *Cell* **76**:315–322.

Stadtman, E. R., 1990, Metal ion-catalyzed oxidation of proteins: Biochemical mechanism and biological consequences, *Free Radical Biol. Med.* **9**:315–325.

Steadman, B. L., Thompson, K. C., Middaugh, C. R., Matsuno, K., Vrona, S., Lawson, E. Q., and Lewis, R. V., 1992, The effects of surface adsorption on the thermal stability of proteins, *Biotechnol. Bioeng.* **40**:8–12.

Steiner, L. A., and Eisen, H. N., 1967, The relative affinity of antibodies synthesized in the secondary response, *J. Exp. Med.* **126**:1185–1205.

Stevens, T. L., Bossie, A., Sanders, V. M., Fernandez-Botran, R., Coffman, R. L., Mosmann, T. R., and Vitetta, E. S., 1988, Regulation of antibody isotype secretion by subsets of antigen-specific helper T cells, *Nature* **334**:255–258.

Stevens, V. C., and Jones, W. R., 1990, Vaccines to prevent pregnancy, in: *New Generation Vaccines* (G. C. Woodrow and M. M. Levine, eds.), Dekker, New York, pp. 879–990.

Stewart, M. J., Nawrot, R., Schulman, S., and Vanderberg, J. P., 1986, Plasmodium berghei sporozoite invasion is blocked in vitro by sporozoite-immobilizing antibodies, *Infect. Immun.* **51**:859–864.

Stürchler, D., Berger, R., Etlinger, H., Matile, H., Pink, R., Schlumbom, and Just, M., 1989, Effects of interferons on immune response to a synthetic peptide malaria sporozoite vaccine in non-immune adults, *Vaccine* **7**:457–461.

Suh, W.-K., Cohen-Doyle, M. F., Fruh, K., Wang, K., Peterson, P. A., and Williams, D. B., 1994, Interaction of MHC class I molecules with the transporter associated with antigen processing, *Science* **264**:1322–1326.

Swain, S. L., Weinberg, A. D., and English, M., 1990, CD4$^+$ T cell subsets: Lymphokine secretion of memory cells and of effector cells that develop from precursors *in vitro*, *J. Immunol.* **144**:1788–1799.

Swain, S. L., Bradley, L. M., Croft, M., Tonkonogy, S., Atkins, G., Weinberg, A. D., Duncan, D. D., Hedrick, S. M., Dutton, R. W., and Huston, G., 1991, Helper T-cell subsets: Phenotype, function and the role of lymphokines in regulating their development, *Immunol. Rev.* **123**:115–144.

Tai, J. Y., Vella, P., McLean, A. A., Woodhour, A. F., McAleer, W. J., Sha, A., Dennis-Sykes, C., and Hilleman, M. R., 1987, *H. influenzae* type b polysaccharide–protein conjugate vaccine, *Proc. Soc. Exp. Biol. Med.* **184**:154–161.

Teh, L. C., Murphy, L. J., Huq, N. L., Surus, A. S., Friesen, H. G., Lazarus, L., and Chapman, G. E., 1987, Methionine oxidation in human growth hormone and human chorionic somatomammotropin. Effects on receptor binding and biological activities, *J. Biol. Chem.* **262**:6472.

Terrell, T. G., and Green, J. D., 1993, Comparative pathology of recombinant murine interferon-g in mice and recombinant human interferon-g in cynomolgus monkeys, *Int. Rev. Exp. Pathol.* **34B**:73–101.

Tsicopoulos, A., Hamid, Q., Varney, V., Ying, S., Moqbel, R., Durham, S. R., and Kay, B., 1992, Preferential messenger RNA suppression of Th 1-type cells (IFN-γ^+, IL-2$^+$) in classical delayed-type (tuberculin) hypersensitivity reaction in human skin, *J. Immunol.* **148**:2058–2061.

Tsutsui, H., Mizoguchi, Y., and Morisawa, S., 1991, There is no correlation between function and lymphokine production of HBs-antigen-specific human CD4($^+$)-cloned T cells, *Scand. J. Immunol.* **34**:433–444.

Urban, J. F., Katona, I. M., Paul, W. E., and Finkelman, F. D., 1991, Interleukin 4 is important in protective immunity to a gastrointestinal nematode infection in mice, *Proc. Natl. Acad. Sci. USA* **88**:5513–5517.

Urban, J. F., Madden, K. B., Svetic, A., Cheever, A., Trotta, P. P., Gause, W. C., Katona, I. M., and Finkelman, F. D., 1992, The importance of TH2 cytokines in protective immunity to nematodes, *Immunol. Rev.* **127**:205–220.

van Bleek, G. M., and Nathenson, S. G., 1990, Isolation of an endogenously processed immunodominant viral peptide from the class I H-2K^b molecule, *Nature* **348**:213–216.

Van Nest, G. A., Steimer, K. S., Haigwood, N. L., Burke, R. L., and Ott, G., 1992, Advanced adjuvant formulations for use with recombinant subunit vaccines, in: *Vaccines 92*, Cold Spring Harbor Laboratory Press, Cold Spring Harbor, NY, pp. 57–62.

van Noort, J. M., Boon, J., Van der Drift, A. C. M., Wagenaar, J. P. A., Boot, A. M. H., and Goog, C. J. P., 1991, Antigen processing by endosomal proteases determines which sites on sperm-whale myoglobin are eventually recognized by T cells, *Eur. J. Immunol.* **21**:1989–1996.

Vidard, L., Rock, K. L., and Benacerraf, B., 1991, The generation of immunogenic peptides can be selectively increased or decreased by proteolytic enzyme inhibitors, *J. Immunol.* **147**:1786–1791.

Vingerhoets, J., Vanham, G., Kestens, L., Penne, G., Leroux-Roels, G., and Gigase, P., 1994, Deficient T-cell responses in non-responders to hepatitis B vaccination: Absence of TH1 cytokine production. *Immunol. Lett.* **39**:163–168.

Wang, Y.-C. J., and Hanson, M. A., 1988, Parenteral formulations of proteins and peptides. Stability and stabilizers, *J. Parenter. Sci. Technol.* **42(Suppl.)**:2–26.

Wassilak, S. G. F., and Orenstein, W. A., 1988, Tetanus, in: *Vaccines* (S. A. Plotkin and E. A. Mortimer, eds.), Saunders, Philadelphia, pp. 45–73.

Webster, R. G., 1968, The immune response to influenza virus: II. Effect of the route and schedule of vaccination on the quantity and avidity of antibodies, *Immunology* **14**:29–37.

Weibel, R. E., 1988, Mumps vaccine, in: *Vaccines* (S. A. Plotkin and E. A. Mortimer, eds.), Saunders, Philadelphia, pp. 223–234.

Weinberg, A., and Merigan, T. C., 1988, Recombinant interleukin-2 as an adjuvant for vaccine induced protection, *J. Immunol.* **140**:294–299.

Westblom, T. U., Gudipati, S., DeRousse, C., Midkiff, B. R., and Belshe, R. B., 1994, Safety and immunogenicity of an inactivated hepatitis A vaccine: Effect of dose and vaccination schedule, *J. Infect. Dis.* **169**:996–1001.

Wiedermann, G., Ambrosch, F., Kremsner, P., Kunz, C., Hauser, P., Simoen, E., André, F., and Safary, A., 1987a, Reactogenicity and immunogenicity of different lots of a yeast-derived hepatitis B vaccine, *Postgrad. Med. J.* **63**:109–112.

Wiedermann, G., Ambrosch, F., Kollaritsch, H., Hofmann, H., Kunz, C., Hondt, E. D., Delem, A., André, F. E., Safary, A., and Stephenne, J., 1987b, Safety and immunogenicity of an inactivated hepatitis A candidate vaccine in healthy adult volunteers, *Postgrad. Med. J.* **63**:109–112.

Wikel, S. K., 1988, Immunological control of hematophagous arthropod vectors: Utilization of novel antigens, *Vet. Parasitol.* **29**:235–264.

Willadsen, P., Eisemann, C. H., and Tellam, R. L., 1993, "Concealed" antigens: Expanding the range of immunological targets, *Parasitol. Today* **9**:132–135.

Wilson, R. A., 1993, Immunity and immunoregulation in helminth infections, *Curr. Opin. Immunol.* **5**:538–547.

Wright, H. T., 1991, Nonenzymatic deamidation of asparaginyl and glutaminyl residues in proteins, *CRC Crit. Rev. Biochem. Mol. Biol.* **26**:1–52.

Wu, J.-Y., Gardiner, B. H., Murphy, C. I., Seals, J. R., Kensil, C. H., Recchia, J., Beltz, G. A., Newman, G. W., and Newman, M. J., 1992, Saponin adjuvant enhancement of antigen-specific immune responses to an experimental HIV-1 vaccine, *J. Immunol.* **148**:1519–1525.

Yamamura, M., Uyemura, K., Deans, R. J., Weinberg, K., Rea, T. H., Bloom, B. R., and Modlin, R. L., 1991, Defining protective responses to pathogens: Cytokine profiles in leprosy lesions, *Science* **254**:277–279.

Yamamura, M., Wang, X.-H., Ahmen, J. D., Uyemura, K., Rea, T. H., Blom, B. R., and Modlin, R. L., 1992, Cytokine patterns of immunologically mediated tissue damage, *J. Immunol.* **149**:1470–1475.

Yanuck, M., Carbone, D. P., Pendleton, C. D., Tsukui, T., Winter, S. F., Minna, J. D., and Berzofsky, J. A., 1993, A mutant p53 tumor suppressor protein is a target for peptide-induced CD8[+] cytotoxic T cells, *Cancer Res.* **53**:3257–3261.

Yin, X.-M., and Vitetta, E. S., 1992, The lineage relationship between virgin and memory B cells, *Int. Immunol.* **6**:691–698.

Zangwill, K. M., Stout, R. W., Carlone, G. M., Pais, L., Harekeh, H., Mitchell, S., Wolfe, W. H., Blackwood, V., Plikaytis, B. D., and Wenger, J. D., 1994, Duration of antibody response after meningococcal polysaccharide vaccination in US Air Force personnel, *J. Infect. Dis.* **169**:847–852.

Chapter 2

Public Health Implications of Emerging Vaccine Technologies

*Dale N. Lawrence, Karen L. Goldenthal,
John W. Boslego, Donna K. F. Chandler, and
John R. La Montagne*

1. INTRODUCTION

This book provides insight into recent innovations or improved applications of existing technologies in the design of vaccines for the prevention of several specific diseases. It makes a broader contribution to the understanding of the vast array of technologies that support modern vaccinology. The objectives of this chapter are: (1) to provide an overview of how advances in vaccine-related technologies have fostered the development of vaccines with highly desirable characteristics for current and future public health vaccination programs; (2) to explore how the development and availability of such vaccines will shape public health concepts, policies, and practices; and (3) to explore how institutional and procedural changes may alter vaccine research and development, manufacture, and delivery to populations in need of immunization.

No official support or endorsement by the FDA or other agencies is intended or should be inferred regarding the views summarized in this report. The views of the authors do not purport to reflect the position of the Department of the Army or the Department of Defense. The use of registered trade names does not constitute endorsement.

Dale N. Lawrence • Division of AIDS, National Institute of Allergy and Infectious Diseases, National Institutes of Health, Bethesda, Maryland 20892. *Karen L. Goldenthal and Donna K. F. Chandler* • Division of Vaccines and Related Products Applications, Center for Biologics Evaluation and Research, Food and Drug Administration, Rockville, Maryland 20852. *John W. Boslego* • Walter Reed Army Institute of Research, Washington, D.C. 20307. *John R. La Montagne* • Division of Microbiology and Infectious Diseases, National Institute of Allergy and Infectious Diseases, National Institutes of Health, Bethesda, Maryland 20892.

Vaccine Design: The Subunit and Adjuvant Approach, edited by Michael F. Powell and Mark J. Newman. Plenum Press, New York, 1995.

1.1. The Children's Vaccine Initiative

The goals as outlined in the Children's Vaccine Initiative (CVI) have provided a remarkable stimulus for research and development of novel vaccine strategies and technological advances. In a "Declaration of New York" following the World Summit for Children, New York City, September, 1990, it was proposed that vaccines be developed that: (1) require one or two rather than multiple doses; (2) are able to be given early in life; (3) are able to be combined in novel ways so as to reduce the number of required injections or visits; (4) are stable, retaining potency during transport and storage; (5) are effective against a wide variety of diseases, including AIDS, acute respiratory infections, diarrheas, and parasites of public health importance that are not currently included in mass immunization campaigns; and (6) are affordable (V. S. Mitchell *et al.*, 1993; La Montagne and Rabinovich, 1994). Some or all of the new technologies discussed in this chapter can contribute to achieving the goals of the CVI.

1.2. Unconquered Pathogens and Other Clinical Indications

While currently available vaccines have proven to be extremely powerful tools for disease prevention, many infectious diseases remain poorly controlled by available public health measures because of an absence of effective, safe, and licensed vaccines. Effective vaccines that prevent the diseases caused by an "unconquered pathogen" can provide the core for implementing a comprehensive control program. After more than a century of international attempts to develop vaccines to prevent many of these diseases, including the use of increasingly sophisticated technologies, many serious pathogens of humans and animals remain uncontrolled (Plotkin and Plotkin, 1994). Such microbial adversaries include organisms causing afflictions described for hundreds or thousands of years, i.e., *Neisseria gonorrhoeae*, *Treponema pallidum* (syphilis), *Mycobacterium leprae*, *Trypanosoma* sp. (African sleeping sickness, Chagas disease), *Plasmodium* sp. (malaria), and the schistosomes. Pathogens such as rotavirus, streptococcus (Groups A and B, *S. pneumoniae*), respiratory syncytial virus (RSV), and parainfluenza continue to cause considerable pediatric morbidity and mortality worldwide. CMV infections in utero can cause devastating damage to the fetus. Shigella continues to be a major cause of diarrhea. Substantial efforts to develop improved vaccines against organisms such as *M. tuberculosis* and *Vibrio cholerae* are still incomplete (National Institute of Allergy and Infectious Diseases, 1993). Moreover, there is a need to develop strategies of control for a number of emerging diseases and syndromes such as Lyme disease, hemolytic uremic syndrome caused by *Escherichia coli* 0157:H7, drug-resistant pneumococcal disease, and the recently recognized hantavirus pulmonary syndrome (Centers for Disease Control and Prevention, 1993). Significant societal and economic benefit would be realized if the worldwide struggle to develop effective vaccines against the human immunodeficiency virus, type 1 (HIV-1), the cause of AIDS, is successful.

Special attributes of the "unconquered pathogens" or limitations in the repertoire of host immune responses probably account for their having eluded vaccine preventive efforts to date. Perhaps the new biotechnologies can overcome these obstacles through novel vaccine antigen presentation, formulation, or delivery. Identification of immunological response impediments, such as antigenic mimicry, immune tolerance, autoimmune reactogenicity, immunodominant and suppressor epitopes, and intracellular replication, may lead to potentially productive strategies in vaccine development.

While the focus of this book will be predominantly infectious disease vaccines, other indications for vaccines of public health importance that might utilize these technologies are noteworthy. Investigational vaccines for birth control have utilized both novel adjuvants and conjugation (Jones *et al.*, 1988; Aitken *et al.*, 1993). One tumor vaccine with an investigational adjuvant (M. S. Mitchell *et al.*, 1993) is being tested in efficacy trials.

1.3. Historical Model of Disease Eradication: Smallpox

The eradication of smallpox in October, 1977, has been justifiably acclaimed as one of mankind's greatest accomplishments. The history of that feat highlights the interdependence of medical research, epidemiology, technological development, public health administration, and community participation in achieving success (Henderson and Fenner, 1994). The essential requirement was that an effective smallpox vaccine be available. Thereafter, technical modifications dramatically increased vaccine yield, and the introduction of freeze-dried vaccinia in 1949 afforded greater stability than had been obtained with earlier drying methods and the use of glycerin preservatives (Hopkins, 1983). Repeated expression of public health commitments to a worldwide eradication campaign eventually generated public and political acceptance. A critical shortage of vaccine in West Africa in 1967 stimulated the discovery and rigorous implementation of a "surveillance and containment" strategy, which resulted in extensive savings in vaccine, time, and labor, resulting in a more efficient campaign. A simplified, reliable instrument for vaccination—the bifurcated needle—allowed field staff to easily and cheaply perform scarification following brief training (Hopkins, 1983). Were the worldwide campaign still under way, a molecularly attenuated vaccinia strain, able to avoid the rare but serious complications of generalized vaccinia or spread to close contacts, might be under evaluation as an improved vaccine.

1.4. Recent Model for Disease Control Approaching Eradication: *Haemophilus influenzae* Type b

The development and licensure of conjugate vaccines to prevent *Haemophilus influenzae* type b (Hib) invasive disease is one of the greatest recent public health achievements, and has been summarized by Ward *et al.* (1994). Invasive Hib disease was the most common cause of bacterial meningitis in U.S. children prior to the licensure of Hib conjugate vaccines (National Institute of Allergy and Infectious Diseases, 1993), and was also an important cause of pediatric pneumonia, bacteremia, epiglottitis, septic arthritis, and cellulitis. The initially available unconjugated polyribosylribitol phosphate (PRP) polysaccharide vaccines proved to be insufficiently immunogenic and efficacious in younger children and infants, the groups at highest risk for Hib invasive disease. This limitation was the impetus for the development of the glycoconjugate vaccine (see Chapter 30), based on the principle that coupling a polysaccharide to an immunogenic protein carrier can stimulate T-dependent immunity to the carbohydrate hapten. The resultant immune response has been shown to confer protection even to infants.

Interestingly, the December, 1987, introduction in the United States of the first Hib conjugate vaccine for children 18 months of age and older was followed by a decline in invasive disease not only in vaccinees, but also in unimmunized younger children and infants. This observation was presumably the result of vaccine-related reductions in asymptomatic Hib carriage in vaccinees and decreased transmission to the younger children and infants. The introduction in 1990 of Hib conjugate vaccine immunization for infants ≥ 2 months of age has been associated with further reductions, to the point of virtual elimination, of pediatric invasive Hib disease in the United States (Centers for Disease Control and Prevention, 1994a,b). The success with Hib conjugate vaccines has stimulated the investigation of this approach for the pneumococcus, *S. typhi*, and *C. neoformans* (V. S. Mitchell *et al.*, 1993; National Institute of Allergy and Infectious Diseases, 1993).

2. REEVALUATION OF THE PREMISES UNDERLYING PUBLIC HEALTH VACCINE PRACTICES

2.1. Premises Underlying Public Health Vaccine Programs and Practices

- The more inaccessible the population to be vaccinated, the greater the problem of maintaining vaccine potency, since potency for many vaccines is dependent on preservation of the "cold chain," i.e., consistent maintenance of the product within the manufacturer's recommended cold temperature range by freezing or refrigeration until the time of administration.
- Achieving the greatest level of protection from vaccine-preventable diseases in a population is impeded by many inconvenient requirements: adherence to vaccine-specific priming and boosting schedules; adherence to recommended sequencing of various vaccines/combinations; and alteration or elimination of certain vaccinations based on the vaccinee's characteristics, including age, maternal antibody, concurrent illnesses, hypersensitivities, or residence in a household with members at risk from spread of live-virus or live-vectored vaccines.
- Responses to vaccines may differ widely among populations depending on the genetic, nutritional, and disease state of the individual and the presence of other pathogens. For example, in some developing countries, trivalent oral polio vaccine (OPV) recipients had reduced antibody responses to vaccine-associated virus types 1 and 3; proposed explanations include, but are not limited to, interference from pre-existing intestinal tract enteric viruses or interference from polio vaccine type 2 virus (Patriarca *et al.*, 1991; Melnick, 1994).
- The biology of host immune responses is such that induction of a long-lasting, fully protective immune response is usually not attainable after a single administration.
- The more limited the transportation or public health infrastructure of a region, the less likely that full protection will be achieved by vaccines requiring "boosting"

since a diminishing proportion of the target population will receive the second, third, and subsequent doses.

- The logistics of immunization campaigns must accommodate the need to dispose safely of large quantities of used needles and syringes to prevent the spread of blood-borne pathogens (HIV-1, hepatitis B).
- The costs and logistics for campaigns using needle-injectable vaccines must incorporate either high per-unit price for use of prefilled syringes or the added labor and time to fill syringes in the field under conditions that maintain vaccine sterility.
- Inclusion of antigens representing newly identified, epidemiologically important variants into reformulated vaccines is a slow process. For influenza vaccines used in the United States, this process has been condensed to less than a year and depends on having a worldwide surveillance network for emerging strains, a manufacturing process adaptable to incorporation of new strains, and appropriate animals available for preclinical study.

2.2. New Technologies Altering the Public Health Vaccine Premises

2.2.1. IMMUNOGEN STABILITY

Maintaining the stability of vaccine immunogens requires attention to the manufacturer's recommended conditions of storage or shipment. For many vaccines, a cold chain must be maintained to assure potency. Vaccines that have been preserved by lyophilization require resolubilization for ease of administration, and immunogens suspended in liquid medium are thought to present the most biologically natural configuration of charge and conformational structure. Stabilizers such as lactose or other saccharides may be added to both lyophilized and liquid vaccines to improve stability during storage. Moreover, vaccines that are formulated in multidose containers must contain an antibacterial preservative agent (e.g., thimerosal, phenoxyethanol). Precautions must be taken that any added preservatives or stabilizers are compatible with all the components of the vaccine formulation, especially for combination vaccines.

Experience in the Americas has demonstrated that adequately maintained OPV can effectively interdict the transmission of polio (de Quadros *et al.*, 1994). However, a heat-stable (i.e., less than 0.5 $\log_{10}$ loss in titer when held at 45°C for 7 days) oral polio vaccine could offer decided advantages to a polio eradication campaign, particularly in countries where documented problems in maintenance of a cold chain have hampered vaccine campaigns. Modifications proposed for polio vaccine to achieve thermostability would, in theory, assure efficacy for this vaccine and would provide more flexibility in vaccine storage and handling prior to administration (de Quadros *et al.*, 1994; Lemon and Milstien, 1994). The World Health Organization (WHO) has supported, as the Secretariat, the Childhood Vaccine Initiative's Product Development Group as it has actively pursued ways to promote development of thermostable oral polio vaccines. The use of deuterium oxide is being evaluated for thermostabilization of OPV. Progress continues to be made on the development of other techniques, such as physicochemical procedures, that contribute to the thermostability of vaccines under field conditions.

If a vaccine product can be stored under ambient field conditions, the added costs for maintaining the cold chain might be reduced. Without the limitation imposed by cold chain maintenance, the decision whether to achieve high levels of population protection through consistent timely attention to regular immunization schedules, or through mounting a massive vaccination campaign, can be based on such other elements as cost of vaccine and transport, community motivational factors, and the status of the existing medical and public health infrastructure.

2.2.2. COMBINATION VACCINES: NEW APPLICATIONS

A combination vaccine consists of two or more vaccine immunogens in a physically mixed preparation for administration. Combination vaccines have been used for over 40 years. Examples of combination vaccines available for use in many countries include diphtheria–tetanus–pertussis (DTP), measles–mumps–rubella (MMR), trivalent oral poliovirus (OPV) and inactivated poliovirus (IPV), and 23-valent pneumococcal vaccines. In 1993, the first DTP–Hib conjugate combination vaccine for single injection was licensed in the United States.

Intense global interest continues in new combination vaccines. One of the goals of the CVI is "to combine vaccines in novel ways." Among the advantages are protection against more diseases in a single administration. Also, decreasing the number of needle-sticks and/or the number of times that vaccine needs to be administered may improve coverage in all populations, may offer special advantages for populations inaccessible because of geography or because of sociodemographic and behavioral factors, and may reduce costs (V. S. Mitchell *et al.*, 1993). The advantages of combination vaccines will become even more important as vaccines for new indications are licensed (Ellis and Douglas, 1994). However, it should be remembered that even combination vaccines have certain disadvantages; for example, determining which component(s) was associated with an adverse event can be problematic.

The stability of new combination vaccines must be determined for each product, even if the components consist of already-licensed vaccines. The characteristics of the immune responses that are induced, including the potential for interference among components, and the altered pattern of reactogenicity of the host to new combinations of vaccines, cannot be predicted. This is true even if the immune responses and safety profile of the individual components have been previously characterized. Therefore, direct evidence from adequate preclinical studies and subsequent clinical trials for safety and immunogenicity of each new combination is needed for licensure.

For combination vaccines with already licensed components (e.g., DTP–Hib), an efficacy trial with clinical end points is usually not necessary. In these cases, comparative immunological data between the already licensed product and the respective component in the new combination are used to support efficacy. However, determining the clinical meaning of statistically significant differences in immunogenicity between products can be difficult, particularly when there is no clear quantitative relationship between immu-nological responses and clinical protection (Clemens *et al.*, 1994). Often, adequate data to compare the immunogenicity of vaccines can be obtained with sample sizes of Phase 2 magnitude, i.e., several hundred per study group. Thus, the extensive clinical safety data base that one often derives from a large field efficacy trial with thousands of individuals will not "automatically" be available in such situations. Therefore, one of the most important questions that frequently arises in the development of combination vaccines is how much clinical safety data are required. The answer to this question should consider such factors as the safety questions being posed and the intended population for vaccination, i.e., usually healthy infants and children. The availability of large health maintenance organizations (HMOs) with organized data bases can be helpful in this regard, for both pre- and postmarketing assessments (Black and Shinefield, 1994; Wassilak *et al.*, 1994).

2.2.3. NOVEL ADJUVANTS AND SUSTAINED STIMULATION

The immunogenicity of a vaccine is influenced by the dose, route of administration, timing of priming and booster immunizations, the adjuvant, and other features of the vaccine preparation that may influence homing to lymphoid tissues, antigen processing, and persistence of antigen in tissues. A single dose of immunogen is generally not as effective for stimulating durable immune responses as repeated administration. The persistence of immunogen either through tissue depots or by repeated boosting of immunological memory may make a substantial contribution to the level of immunity attained. Also, the ability to stimulate cell-mediated immune responses may be important for some immunogens.

Currently, the only adjuvants included in U.S.-licensed vaccines are aluminum compounds. New adjuvants or other methods, to enhance the immunogenicity of "weak" antigens or to allow the administration of fewer doses of "adequate" immunogens, are needed. The formulation of vaccines with these adjuvants, as described throughout this book, may yield greatly increased vaccine immunogenicity and ideally be tolerable clinically. The compensatory reduction in the number of vaccination visits required for protection and the resulting potential public health benefits justify the extensive research in this area (Edelman and Tacket, 1990).

The development of biodegradable polymers and devices to slow the release of bioactive pharmaceuticals has led to intense efforts to apply this technology toward single dose vaccines or implants in humans. There has been particular interest in using this approach to immunize women to prevent neonatal tetanus. The principle of sustained release has been demonstrated for drugs such as the contraceptive Norplant® and luteinizing hormone-releasing hormone (Zoladex®) for prostate cancer. The goals are to eliminate the requirement for repeated visits, especially for inaccessible populations, and to attain desired levels of immune responses without incurring an unacceptable level of reactogenicity as can be associated with extremely potent adjuvants and/or high doses of immunogen (Aguado, 1993; Cohen *et al.*, 1994). Clinical use of these novel approaches to enhance immunogenicity will require appropriate preclinical studies and a careful risk-benefit assessment (Goldenthal *et al.*, 1993; Edelman and Tacket, 1990).

2.2.4. ENVIRONMENTAL HAZARDS AND CONVENIENT DELIVERY SYSTEMS

Vaccination campaigns or trials have included: scarification with bifurcated needles; injection (intramuscular, subcutaneous, intradermal) with hypodermic needles; intradermal injection using high-pressure jet injector guns; and oral or intranasal administration of vaccines in the form of droplets or capsules. Each technique has been developed to deal with specific considerations and has advantages and disadvantages. The scar following vaccinia (smallpox) or BCG (tuberculosis vaccine) intradermal scarification often provided a lifelong visual marker that vaccine had been administered—a useful feature when single vaccination conferred long-lasting immunity. However, the scar was slow to heal, could be superinfected with skin bacteria, and could serve as the source of intrahousehold spread, particularly for vaccinia virus.

The invention of the bifurcated needle for use in the worldwide smallpox eradication campaigns of the 1960s and 1970s allowed skin penetration and scarification with a simple object that reliably delivered the predicted quantity of vaccine, was reusable after boiling for sterilization, presented far less bulk for disposal, and was not likely to be used for unintended purposes.

In contrast, injection of vaccine by hypodermic needle in the field is one of the most labor-intensive procedures and generates a high volume of hazardous biomedical waste. Facilities for safe handling and secure disposal of hypodermic needles are rarely available outside medical or public health facilities and are costly. In some field settings, needles must be destroyed as well as disinfected to prevent their being salvaged later for reuse by those uninformed or unmindful of the hazards.

Jet injector guns are unnecessary in settings of infrequent or selective vaccine administration. However, when used in large field campaigns where the labor, cost, environmental hazards, and inconveniences associated with hypodermic needles are prohibitive, the jet injector gun's ability to vaccinate as many as 1000 persons per hour makes it worth the effort to perform usage standardization and perform the necessary field maintenance and associated vaccination hygiene. However, reports of spread of infectious disease through the use of jet injector guns are of concern (Centers for Disease Control, 1986).

The development of orally administered polio vaccine not only circumvented many of the above-mentioned inconveniences and costs but, by avoiding an injection, also enhanced the acceptability to individuals of all ages. However, the oral polio vaccine requires a cold chain, whereas the more recently developed oral typhoid vaccine is more tolerant of ambient temperatures. Failure of the cold chain is responsible for vaccine failures, although the potential exists for the immunogenicity of orally administered live vaccines to be diminished by common intestinal infections which may vary by geographic location. Oral administration of vaccines, whether live-attenuated or live-vectored, theoretically affords one of the most effective ways to direct relevant immunogens to the mucosal immune system for induction of intestinal- and mucosal system-specific immunological memory, although the regimens and routes for maximal stimulation of mucosal immunity are not well established. Adequate mucosal immunity induced by vaccination could play a critical role in the prevention of sexually transmitted diseases such as those caused by HIV-1 (Mestecky *et al.*, 1994; Miller *et al.*, 1994).

Intranasal administration of several vaccines, including experimental influenza vaccines, has demonstrated the feasibility of this route of administration. The intranasal route, along with oral administration, may offer a more popular approach to developing mucosal immunity than the less thoroughly studied rectal and intravaginal routes, which are far less likely to be acceptable or applicable to the general population.

2.2.5. RAPID ANTIGEN SUBSTITUTION: EXPRESSION SYSTEMS AND VACCINES

The annual worldwide collaborative reevaluation of influenza A and B virus strains as candidates for inclusion in the traditional trivalent influenza vaccine seems to be a model for rapid assessment of clinically and epidemiologically relevant pathogens, expeditious manufacture of new vaccine according to established methods, and animal testing. This 8- to 12-month process is generally considered to be maximally efficient.

The new technologies under exploration for application to vaccines hold the promise that a similar timetable, if needed, could be instituted for many other organisms if genetic variation warranted. The use of synthetic peptide vaccines might be a feasible mechanism for rapidly incorporating antigens from variants considered critical for disease prevention, as with HIV-1, and which have important differences in regional prevalence. Methods by which live-vector recombinants could be adapted to changing epidemiological circumstances would also be noteworthy. Of course, techniques that facilitate rapid insertion of genes encoding newly identified protective antigens into manufacturing expression systems to produce large amounts of the desired immunogens would greatly enhance vaccine production capability.

2.2.6. VECTORS AND OTHER APPROACHES

While not the focus of this book, there is also the potential of expressing immunogens by recombinant technologies in vectors such as vaccinia or other poxviruses, BCG, salmonella, and adenovirus, for example. It is believed that vector-administered immunogens, by virtue of presenting antigens for processing in the context of active infection, would be more likely to stimulate broader based responses (e.g., cell-mediated immunity, humoral immunity, and antibodies of wider specificity) than might be obtained using subunit or inactivated vaccine antigens alone. However, the advantages of using live-vectored vaccines, e.g., oral delivery and potential mucosal stimulation, may be offset by the need for maintaining a cold chain and in some instances, by safety concerns.

The induction of a broad and long-lasting immune response may be a consequence of natural exposures and clinically attenuated infections following immunization with infection-permissive immunogens (Johansson et al., 1993). Live-attenuated vaccines that modify the clinical disease or prevent infection have a similar goal. Results of preclinical animal studies of DNA immunogens using "naked DNA," propelled into intradermal, subdermal, subcutaneous, or intramuscular locations, suggest that this approach may offer promise (Fynan et al., 1993; Cheng et al., 1993).

3. PUBLIC HEALTH IMPACT OF NEW TECHNOLOGIES

3.1. Research and Development

It is apparent that the extraordinary productivity in the molecular biologic and basic sciences has heightened excitement for the future roles of vaccines in medicine and public health. If new vaccines based on the novel approaches described in this book are eventually licensed, the general public will have available an array of personal and societal benefits derived from innovative medical research. A hopeful consequence is that the fear and financial uncertainties that prevailed during the decade following the National Influenza Immunization Program (NIIP) and the association of Guillain–Barre syndrome with the 1976 inactivated, killed influenza vaccines (Safranek *et al.*, 1991) will be replaced by public supportiveness. Nonetheless, as vaccines and immunization programs become successful, and targeted diseases are brought under control, the risks associated with the vaccines are more readily appreciated. Thus, issues of liability and compensation for adverse events following vaccination will continue to need substantial administrative and legal review.

3.2. Government Agency Activities

Recognizing that the focus of this chapter is to encourage the vaccine research and development community to imagine ways by which new vaccine technologies will shape public health policies and practices or be influenced by agency procedural changes, the roles of several U.S. government agencies are highlighted here: the Food and Drug Administration (FDA), the National Institute of Allergy and Infectious Diseases, and the Army Medical Research and Development Command.

The chapter does not review the valuable role of the Centers for Disease Control and Prevention (CDC) because the CDC's most frequent contributions have been to epidemiology, identification of emerging pathogens, postlicensure evaluation of safety and effectiveness of vaccines, and in the formulation, revision, and promulgation of public health recommendations of the Advisory Committee on Immunization Practices (ACIP) for use of licensed vaccines. It is presumed here that the CDC's role in vaccines will remain relatively unchanged over the next several years.

3.2.1. REGULATORY AGENCIES

The Center for Biologics Evaluation and Research (CBER) of the FDA is responsible for regulating vaccines in the United States. FDA's legal authority derives from Section 351 of the Public Health Service Act in addition to parts of the Federal Food, Drug and Cosmetic Act. As part of the premarketing process, the U.S. FDA must review a challenging assortment of Investigational New Drug applications (INDs). Generally, proposed clinical studies are designated as Phase 1 (initial studies in humans), Phase 2 (larger studies to obtain more definitive dose-ranging and safety information, with hundreds of subjects), or Phase 3 studies (efficacy studies or expanded safety studies, with thousands of subjects). Product issues such as safety, purity, identity, and potency must be addressed prior to any studies in humans, although it is expected that many of the assays will undergo refinement or modification during the drug development process. It is desirable that the product potency assay be correlated to an effect, normally immunogenicity, in the human recipient. The FDA, as part of its vaccine-related laboratory activities, may assist the sponsor in developing and evaluating assays.

The sponsor has the responsibility to coordinate the manufacturing, animal testing, and clinical evaluation, allowing product development to advance in a timely manner, and to provide adequate data so that FDA can make a satisfactory risk/benefit assessment. The imposition by the FDA of a "clinical hold," preventing human study(s) from proceeding, tends to occur most commonly with the original IND submission where a Phase 1 study is proposed (common reasons: inadequate manufacturing or animal data to assess safety), and at the Phase 3 stage (common reasons: inadequate efficacy protocol). When the sponsor has responded satisfactorily to FDA's questions, the "clinical hold" is removed, and human studies may proceed. It is noted that FDA letters to the IND sponsor may identify items to be addressed that are not an immediate reason for clinical hold, but could ultimately impede product development and licensure if not addressed in a timely manner, e.g., lot-to-lot consistency, scaleup.

In the event that a successful clinical efficacy trial of a product is performed and a manufacturer wishes to obtain approval for marketing, a Product License Application (PLA) and a companion Establishment License Application (ELA) are concurrently submitted to the Agency. Approval will depend on the acceptability of (1) the data to support clinical safety and efficacy for the intended use, and the corresponding labeling, (2) the data to document the adequacy and consistency of the manufacturing process, including lot-to-lot consistency, and (3) the manufacturing facility(s).

One approach that FDA has taken to assist the manufacturer in the preparation of high-quality INDs and PLAs has been the development of "Points to Consider" documents. These documents allow the Agency some appropriate flexibility beyond the Title 21 Code of Federal Regulations and "Guidelines." However, even updated "Points to Consider" documents cannot keep pace with all of the novel products that FDA must regulate, especially if the Agency has no prior experience with a particular type of product. For example, the introduction of novel adjuvants or polynucleotide vaccines raises issues of toxicology that have not been typical for vaccines in the past. In these instances, the sponsors must work with the FDA to devise appropriate preclinical testing and manufacturing controls. An organized approach to this testing can minimize the burden on manufacturers while maximizing the amount of information and ensuring the public safety.

The FDA has also hosted workshops on topics of current interest, including the recent "Combined Vaccines and Simultaneous Administration: Current Issues and Perspectives" (Center for Biologics Evaluation and Research, 1993).

Prior to licensure of a new vaccine or the approval of a significant new clinical indication for a currently licensed vaccine, manufacturers will usually present their data before the Vaccines and Related Biological Products (VRBP) Advisory Committee. FDA staff formulate relevant questions for the committee and may also make presentations before the committee. This process is not limited to the immediate prelicensure stage, however, as issues may be referred to the VRBP Advisory Committee or other appropriate FDA advisory committees at any time during preclinical or clinical development.

Because of their worldwide public health importance, vaccines comprise one area that promises to benefit from recent efforts at international harmonization of regulatory requirements and approaches. Joint reviews of PLAs between the FDA and other regulatory authorities also promise to increase the global efficiency of approvals.

For a broader review of the FDA functions applicable to the regulation of vaccines and other biologics, addressing the approach to clinical development and pre- and post-marketing activities see Chapter 4 by Davenport in this book and the overviews by

Parkman and Hardegree (1994) and Goldenthal and McVittie (1993). It is noteworthy that organizations such as various CVI task forces, WHO, and other national regulatory agencies have also provided guidance to the private sector in bringing products to the marketplace. Some of these regulatory agencies are described by Brown and Douglas (1994).

3.2.2. MILITARY MEDICAL RESEARCH AND DEVELOPMENT

Personnel in the U.S. military forces, whether serving as part-time reservists or on full-time active duty, are drawn from the general U.S. population and return to civilian status after completion of service. Infectious disease and other health hazards associated with military service are threats to the national security and occasionally to the general public. Civilian spouses and other dependent family members of military personnel are known to have become infected, on occasion, with pathogens for which the military member of the household served as the index. These pathogens have included meningo-coccus, bacterial and viral diarrheal agents, and agents of sexually transmitted diseases, including HIV-1. Initiation of vaccination programs (e.g., measles) in military personnel has provided an indirect benefit to members of the household, community, and nation (Centers for Disease Control, 1982).

Most military medical research and development activities are, of course, focused on infectious diseases associated with military deployments to geographic regions in which there is a substantial risk of exposure of the forces to debilitating or fatal pathogens. The history of military conflict is replete with examples of the major impact on military operations of malaria (Coates *et al.*, 1963), bacterial diarrheas (Ognibene and Barrett, 1982), plague (Ognibene and Barrett, 1982), hepatitis (Bancroft and Lemon, 1984), and other diseases for which vaccines or adequate control measures did not exist. For these reasons, over the past 75 years the Walter Reed Army Institute of Research, the Medical Research Institute of Infectious Diseases, and other components of the U.S. Army Medical Research and Development Command have had a continuing commitment to identify, develop, and evaluate new or improved vaccines to prevent many well-known scourges (malaria, shigellosis, enterotoxigenic *E. coli*, hepatitis A, typhoid, dengue, plague, menin-gococcus) and other less well-known organisms relevant to specific regions of the world (Rift Valley fever, Japanese B encephalitis, Argentine hemorrhagic fever).

It would be immensely valuable if military personnel who are subject to sudden deployment throughout the world were able to receive combination vaccines affording prolonged efficacy against the widest possible array of potential hazardous organisms following single administration. Sympathetic to the goals of the CVI, the military would be keenly interested in adaptations of relevant technologies to vaccines for pathogens of concern to deployable troops.

There are several examples of military vaccine research that have advanced vaccine science at times when civilian vaccine research lagged because of higher civilian priority assigned to therapeutic drug development, or because of concerns about litigation and vaccine injury compensation (Safranek *et al.*, 1991). Recent examples include military vaccine research into malaria (Oaks *et al.*, 1991) and hepatitis A (Hoke *et al.*, 1992). Lastly, many regions of the world are poor, and their populations are clinically afflicted with the same endemic pathogens that would pose substantial hazards to deployed U.S. military forces. There are many examples in which military medical scientists and host country public health officials have joined in collaborative clinical evaluations of candidate vaccines. For example, cooperation between Thailand and the U.S Army resulted in the provision of efficacy data supporting the licensure in the United States of the Japanese B encephalitis virus vaccine and hepatitis A vaccine. Of great importance, such collaborations have resulted in technology transfer, acquisition of training and indigenous vaccine production capability, and the commencement of campaigns to rid the host country of specific pathogens.

3.2.3. NATIONAL INSTITUTES OF HEALTH

The National Institute of Allergy and Infectious Diseases (NIAID) of the NIH has a major commitment to the research and clinical development of preventive vaccines, in addition to performing certain postmarketing studies. The intramural and extramural activities have included basic microbiological research and the development of certain vaccines that are in Phase 1/2 trials or are being commercially developed by manufacturers (e.g., a tetravalent rhesus reassortant rotavirus vaccine currently in human efficacy trials).

The Division of AIDS, NIAID, has sponsored much of the clinical research on preventive HIV vaccines in the United States. This support for preclinical and clinical development has promoted clinical testing of new promising vaccine approaches. Included in these efforts is an ongoing Phase 2 study in high-risk adults and a Phase 2 study in neonates of indeterminate infection status born to HIV-infected mothers.

It is expected that when candidate HIV vaccine(s) are selected for efficacy trials, NIAID will sponsor both domestic and foreign trials. In preparation for this, and in consultation with the Global Programme on AIDS of the World Health Organization, the Division of AIDS has provided funding support for preefficacy "Preparations for Vaccine Efficacy Trials" at international sites. Similar research has begun at U.S. sites through collaborations with other U.S. government agencies (NIDA/NIH, CDC, Department of Veterans Affairs). Through the recent establishment of Domestic (DMC) and International (IMC) Master Contractors for the HIV Vaccine Efficacy Trials Network, the Division of AIDS plans to support vaccine and nonvaccine HIV prevention research both in the United States and abroad.

NIH plays a leading role in pertussis vaccine-related research and clinical development, responding to the public health need for a less reactogenic pertussis vaccine for infants. NIAID currently supports two large trials in Sweden, and one in Italy, designed to test the safety and efficacy of a total of five candidate acellular pertussis vaccines* for infant immunization. Swedish Trial Part 1 and the Italian trial, which will likely be terminated within the next 6 months, have an adequate statistical design to evaluate *absolute* efficacy (versus placebo) of the respective acellular pertussis vaccines included in each trial and a whole cell pertussis vaccine. Swedish Trial Part 2, which has no placebo group, is designed to evaluate *comparative* efficacy of three acellular pertussis vaccines and a whole cell pertussis vaccine. It is hoped that, in addition to finding one or more effective vaccines, an immunological correlate(s) of protection for acellular pertussis vaccines will be identified.

---

*Two of the vaccines from the same manufacturer have the same antigens, but some quantitative differences.

NIAID is providing support to investigate maternal immunization to prevent neonatal and infant infections with pathogens such as Hib and Group B streptococcus (National Institute of Allergy and Infectious Diseases, 1993).

3.3. Private and Other Manufacturers of Vaccines and Possible International Partnerships

The development and availability of new vaccines to benefit the world's population requires both the viability of vaccine sponsors engaged in research and development (R and D) and the manufacturers who supply specific markets. In general, vaccine manufacturers who sponsor R and D and seek product licensure are in the private sector and hope to obtain a financial return from their investments. Therefore, they must continuously evaluate critically the benefits, risks, costs, and possible financial return from vaccines that, if successful, would be given, for example, only once or on a few occasions throughout the lifetime of the annual world "birth cohort" of 150 million potential recipients (Brown and Douglas, 1994). Vaccine coverage broadened to nearly the full "birth cohort" would require increased production of more doses of the relevant vaccines. If affordable, the large sales volume might compensate for smaller per-unit pricing. Transferring the technology of research and vaccine production to developing nations, where labor and transportation costs are less, are among additional ways proposed or used to reduce costs, and thereby increase access for these countries. Technology transfer also builds the local economic infrastructure and population resources to benefit the developing nations collaborating in such ventures (Martinez-Palomo *et al.*, 1994; Robbins and Arita, 1994).

The low expected "rate of return" is a substantial impediment for vaccine manufacturers in industrialized countries and hinders their commitment to research, testing, and production of vaccines for the developing world. In fact, the typical rate of return for marketed vaccines is not comparable to that for important pharmaceuticals nor does it reflect vaccines' public health importance. Currently, vaccine R and D and marketing for the developing world depend heavily on the profits from marketing in industrialized countries.

3.4. Opportunities for Scientific and Economic Advancement

As vaccine technologies improve the quality of vaccine products in use throughout the world, new epidemiological approaches may be needed to assess the efficiency of various strategies of vaccine usage—reminiscent of the "surveillance and containment" strategy in the smallpox eradication program. Development of novel analytical methods to assess vaccine immunogenicity (Smith *et al.*, 1984) might also be required.

As we approach the objectives of the CVI, each potential beneficiary country may recognize the opportunity for achieving significant reduction in mortality and morbidity and respond by mobilizing national political and popular will to fulfill public health and economic promise afforded by such advanced vaccines (National Academy of Science, Institute of Medicine, 1986; The International Bank for Reconstruction and Development/World Bank, 1993; Parker and Hill, 1994). This tremendous global investment in vaccine research has led to a proliferation of prototype vaccines. These promising new vaccines will pose significant challenges for their optimal integration into public health usage: (1) How will the vaccines be evaluated and the best products selected? (2) Which ones will fit into existing vaccination schedules? (3) How will the new vaccines be integrated into general use? Future attempts to resolve technical and policy issues (V. S. Mitchell *et al.*, 1993) will continue to test the imaginations of people in industry, academia, and government.

4. SUMMARY

The field of public health and medicine stands to benefit immensely from the emerging vaccine technologies and improved application of existing technologies. Technological advances may promote: (1) greater flexibility and simplicity in the design and operation of immunization campaigns or ongoing prevention programs, including reduction in number of vaccine doses, cold chain elimination, slow-release/prolonged antigenic stimulation, reduced cost and hazard and increased ease of administration through noninvasive, oral delivery systems, greater population levels of immunization and health; (2) the development of documents by FDA, WHO, and other regulatory authorities and groups, to assist the manufacturer in the appropriate manufacturing, preclinical, and clinical development of these new vaccines; (3) a greater array of vaccines to protect the civilian and military populations; (4) increased vaccine potency; (5) vaccines eliciting mucosal immunity, cytotoxic T cells, and/or neutralizing antibody.

At the end of the 20th century there remain many unconquered pathogens and noninfectious indications for which medical science suggests that vaccines could be effective. New technologies may provide the best hope to address this wide array of public health needs.

ACKNOWLEDGMENTS

The authors wish to express appreciation for the valuable guidance received either during the preparation of this manuscript or on earlier occasions from the following persons: Dr. Regina Rabinovich, National Vaccine Program and Division of Microbiology and Infectious Diseases, NIAID; Drs. Walter Orenstein and Alan Hinman, National Center for Prevention Services, Centers for Disease Control and Prevention; Dr. Alexis Shelokov, Government Services Division, Salk Institute; Dr. Daniel Thor, Chief Medical Officer, California State Department of Corrections (during his professorship at the University of Texas Health Sciences Center, San Antonio); Dr. Lewellys Barker, Division of AIDS, NIAID; Dr. Edmund C. Tramont, Medical Biotechnology Center, University of Maryland; Dr. Philip Russell, Johns Hopkins University School of Hygiene and Public Health; Dr. William L. Moore, Jr., U.S. Army Medical Department Center and School; Dr. Pat Keegan, CBER/FDA; Dr. William Habig, CBER/FDA; Dr. Peter Patriarca, CBER/FDA; Dr. David Karzon, Vanderbilt University Medical School; and Ms. Polly Harrison, Director, Division of International Health, Institute of Medicine, National Academy of Sciences. Editorial and secretarial assistance was provided by Ms. Patti Phillips.

REFERENCES

Aguado, M. T., 1993, Future approaches to vaccine development: Single-dose vaccines using controlled-release delivery systems, *Vaccine* **10**:596–597.

Aitkin, R. J., Paterson, M., and Koothan, P. T., 1993, Contraceptive vaccines, *Br. Med. Bull.* **49**:88–99.

Bancroft, W. H., and Lemon, S. M., 1984, Hepatitis A from the military perspective, in: *Hepatitis A* (R.J. Garety, ed.), Academic Press, New York, pp. 81–100.

Black, S., and Shinefield, H., 1995, Comprehensive evaluation of vaccine safety: Assessment of local and systemic side effects as well as emergency and hospitalization utilization. Proceedings of the combined vaccines and simultaneous administration: Current issues and perspectives workshop, *Ann. N.Y. Acad. Sci.* (in press).

Brown, K. R., and Douglas, R. G., Jr., 1994, New challenges in quality control and licensure: Regulation, *Int. J. Tech. Assess. Health Care* **10**:55–64.

Center for Biologics Evaluation and Research/FDA, 1995, Combined vaccines and simultaneous administration: Current issues and perspectives (Workshop sponsored by CBER/FDA, NVPO, NIAID/NIH, CDC, WHO, and held in Bethesda, MD, July 28–30, 1993), Proceedings to be published in *Ann. N.Y. Acad. Sci.*

Centers for Disease Control, 1982, *Measles Surveillance Report No. 11*, 1977–1981; Issued September, 1982.

Centers for Disease Control, 1986, Hepatitis B associated with jet gun injection—California, *Morbid. Mortal. Weekly Rep.* **35**:373–376.

Centers for Disease Control and Prevention, 1993, Hantavirus infection—Southwestern United States: Interim recommendations for risk reduction, *Morbid. Mortal. Weekly Rep.* **42**(Suppl. RR-11):1–13.

Centers for Disease Control and Prevention, 1994a, General recommendations on immunization. Recommendations of the Advisory Committee on Immunization Practices (ACIP), *Morbid. Mortal. Weekly Rep.* **43**(Suppl. RR-1):1–38.

Centers for Disease Control and Prevention, 1994b, Progress toward elimination of *Haemophilus influenzae* type b disease among infants and children—United States, 1987–1993, *Morbid. Mortal. Weekly Rep.* **43**(No. 8):144–148.

Cheng, L., Ziegelhoffer, P. R., and Yang, N.-S., 1993, *In vivo* promoter activity and transgene expression in mammalian somatic tissues evaluated by using particle bombardment, *Proc. Natl. Acad. Sci. USA* **90**:4455–4459.

Clemens, J., Brenner, R., and Rao, M., 1995, Interactions between PRP-T vaccine against *Haemophilus influenzae* type b and conventional infant vaccines: Lessons for further studies of simultaneous immunization and combined vaccines. Proceedings of the combined vaccines and simultaneous administration: Current issues and perspectives workshop, *Ann. N.Y. Acad. Sci.* (in press).

Coates, J. B., Hoff, E. C., and Hoff, P. M., (eds.), 1963, *Preventive Medicine in World War II. Vol. VI. Communicable Diseases: Malaria*, Office of the Surgeon General, Department of the Army, Washington, DC.

Cohen, S., Alonso, J. J., and Langer, R., 1994, Novel approaches to controlled-release antigen delivery, *Int. J. Tech. Assess. Health Care* **10**:121–130.

de Quadros, C. A., Carrasco, P., and Olive, J.-M., 1994, The desired field-performance characteristics of new improved vaccines for the developing world, *Int. J. Tech. Assess. Health Care* **10**:65–70.

Edelman, R., and Tacket, C. O., 1990, Adjuvants, *Int. Rev. Immunol.* **7**:51–66.

Ellis, R. W., and Douglas, R. G., Jr., 1994, New vaccine technologies, *J. Am. Med. Assoc.* **271**:929–931.

Fynan, E. F., Webster, R. G., Fuller, D. H., Haynes J. R., Santoro, J. C., and Robinson, H. L., 1993, DNA vaccines: Protective immunizations by parenteral, mucosal, and gene-gun inoculations, *Proc. Natl. Acad. Sci. USA.* **90**:11478–11482.

Goldenthal, K. L., and McVittie, L. D., 1993, The clinical testing of preventive vaccines, in: *Biologics Development: A Regulatory Overview* (M. Mathieu, ed.), Parexel International Corp., Waltham, MA, pp. 119–130.

Goldenthal, K. L., Cavagnaro, J. A., Alving, C. R., and Vogel, F. R., 1993, Safety evaluation of vaccine adjuvants: National cooperative vaccine development meeting working group, *AIDS Res. Hum. Retroviruses* **9**:S47–S51.

Henderson, D.A., and Fenner, F., 1994, Smallpox and vaccinia, in: *Vaccines*, 2nd ed. (S.A. Plotkin and E.A. Mortimer, Jr., eds.), Saunders, Philadelphia, pp. 13–40.

Hoke, C. H., Jr., Binn, L. N., Egan, J. E., DeFraites, R. F., MacArthy, P. O., Innis, B. L., Eckels, K. H., Dubois, D., D'Hondt, E., Sjogren, M. H., Rice, R., Sadoff, J. C., and Bancroft, W. H., 1992, Hepatitis A in the US Army: Epidemiology and vaccine development, *Vaccine* **10**(Suppl. 1):S75–S79.

Homma, A., and Knouss, R. F., 1994, The transfer of vaccine technology to developing countries. The Latin American experience, *Int. J. Tech. Assess. Health Care* **10**:47–54.

Hopkins, D. R., 1983, *Princes and Peasants: Smallpox in History*, University of Chicago Press, Chicago.

The International Bank for Reconstruction and Development/World Bank, 1993, *World Development Report 1993. Investing in Health*, Oxford University Press, London.

Johansson, B. E., Grajower, B., and Kilbourne, E. D., 1993, Infection-permissive immunization with influenza virus neuraminidase prevents weight loss in infected mice, *Vaccine* **11**:1037–1039.

Jones, W. R., Bradley, J., Judd, S. J., Denholm, E. H., Ing, R. M. Y., Mueller, U. W., Powell, J., Griffin, P. D., and Stevens, V. C., 1988, Phase 1 clinical trial of a World Health Organization birth control vaccine, *Lancet* **1**:1295–1298.

La Montagne, J. R., and Rabinovich, N. R., 1994, The promise of new technologies, *Int. J. Tech. Assess. Health Care* **10**:7–13.

Lemon, S. M., and Milstien, J. B., 1994, The thermostability of vaccines: Technologies for improving the thermostability of the oral poliovirus vaccine, *Int. J. Tech. Assess. Health Care* **10**:177–184.

Martinez-Palomo, A. M., Lopez-Cervantes, M., and Freeman, P., 1994, The role of vaccine research and development in the scientific development of middle-income countries, *Int. J. Tech. Assess. Health Care* **10**:30–38.

Melnick, J. L., 1994, Live attenuated poliovirus vaccines, in: *Vaccines*, 2nd ed. (S A. Plotkin and E. A. Mortimer, Jr., eds.), Saunders, Philadelphia, pp. 155–204.

Mestecky, J., Kutteh, W. H., and Jackson, S., 1994, Mucosal immunity in the female genital tract: Relevance to vaccinations efforts against the human immunodeficiency virus, *AIDS Res. Hum. Retroviruses* **10**(Suppl. 1) (in press).

Miller, C. J., Alexander, N. J., and McChesney, M. B., 1994, Vaccines to prevent sexually transmitted diseases: The challenge of generating protective immunity at genital mucosal surfaces, in: *Strategies in Vaccine Design* (G.L. Ada, ed.), R.G. Landes Company, Austin, TX, pp. 193–212.

Mitchell, M. S., Harel, W., Kan-Mitchell, J., LeMay, L. G., Goedegebuure, P., Huang, X. Q., Hofman, F., and Groshen, S., 1993, Active specific immunotherapy of melanoma with allogeneic cell lysates. Rationale, results, and possible mechanisms of action, *Ann. N.Y. Acad. Sci.* **690**:153–166.

Mitchell, V. S., Philipose, N. M., and Sanford, J. P., (eds.), 1993, *The Children's Vaccine Initiative. Achieving the Vision*, Institute of Medicine, National Academy Press, Washington, DC.

National Academy of Science, Institute of Medicine, 1986, *New vaccine development: Establishing priorities. Diseases of importance in the developing countries*, National Academy Press, Washington, DC.

National Institute of Allergy and Infectious Diseases, 1993, The Jordan Report. Accelerated Development of Vaccines—1993, Bethesda, MD.

Oaks, S. C., Mitchell, V. S., Pearson, G. W., and Carpenter, C. C. J., (eds.), 1991, *Malaria: Obstacles and Opportunities*, National Academy Press, Washington, DC.

Ognibene, A. J., and Barrett, O., Jr., (eds.), 1982, *Internal Medicine in Vietnam. Vol. II. General Medicine and Infectious Diseases*, Office of the Surgeon General and Center of Military History, United States Army, Washington, DC.

Parker, D., and Hill, T., 1994, The contribution of immunization to economic development, *Int. J. Tech. Assess. Health Care* **10**:21–29.

Parkman, P. D., and Hardegree, M. C., 1994, Regulation and testing of vaccines, in: *Vaccines*, 2nd ed. (S. A. Plotkin and E. A. Mortimer, Jr., eds.), Saunders, Philadelphia, pp. 889–901.

Patriarca, P. A., Wright, P. F., and John, T. J., 1991, Factors affecting the immunogenicity of oral poliovirus vaccine in developing countries: A review, *Rev. Infect. Dis.* **13**:926–939.

Plotkin, S. L., and Plotkin, S. A., 1994, A short history of vaccination, in: *Vaccines*, 2nd ed. (S. A. Plotkin and E. A. Mortimer, Jr., eds.), Saunders, Philadelphia, pp. 1–11.

Robbins, A., and Arita, I., 1994, The global capacity for manufacturing vaccines. Prospects for competition and collaboration among producers in the next decade, *Int. J. Tech. Assess. Health Care* **10**:39–46.

Safranek, T. J., Lawrence, D. N., Kurland, L. T., Culver, D. H., Wiederholt, W. C., Hayner, N. S., Osterholm, M. T., O'Brien, P., Hughes, J. M., and the Expert Neurology Group, 1991, Reassessment of the association between Guillain–Barre syndrome and receipt of swine influenza vaccine in 1976–1977: Results of a two-state study, *Am. J. Epidemiol.* **133**:940–951.

Smith, S. J., Lawrence, D. N., and Noble, G. R., 1984, An immune response profile model for immunogenicity quantitation, *J. Theor. Biol.* **110**:1–10.

Ward, J., Lieberman, J. M., and Cochi, S. L., 1994, *Haemophilus influenzae* vaccines in: *Vaccines*, 2nd ed. (S.A. Plotkin and E.A. Mortimer, Jr., eds.), Saunders, Philadelphia, pp. 337–386.

Wassilak, S. G. F., Glasser, J. W., Chen, R. T., and Hadler, S. C., 1995, Utility of large-linked databases in vaccine safety, particularly in distinguishing independent and synergistic effects, in: Proceedings of the workshop on combined vaccines and simultaneous administration: Current issues and perspectives, *Ann. N.Y. Acad. Sci.* (in press).

Chapter 3

Preclinical Safety Assessment Considerations in Vaccine Development

Jeanine L. Bussiere, George C. McCormick, and James D. Green

1. INTRODUCTION

No vaccine is totally safe and totally effective, and adverse reactions have been reported with all. However, adverse reactions to vaccines are generally mild, and severe events resulting in death or permanent damage are rare. Historically, for every approved vaccine, the benefits to the public of preventing the target disease far outweigh the risks and costs of vaccination (Duclos and Bentsi-Enchill, 1993). As the target disease disappears, however, rare adverse reactions to vaccines alter the risk:benefit ratio. Individuals become more concerned with the risk of adverse reactions to the vaccine than the risk of contracting the disease. Concern regarding adverse events from vaccination can have serious detrimental impact, as illustrated by events in the United Kingdom in the mid-1970s. Fear of the whole-cell pertussis vaccine was linked with vaccine complications ranging from fever to seizures, and the vaccine was even blamed for causing brain damage and death. This fear led to a 50% decline in immunizations. Several years later, pertussis cases began to increase significantly, which then led to a subsequent return to vaccination (Stuart-Harris, 1979). This event was, and still is, the subject of worldwide controversy.

Preclinical safety assessment programs for vaccine candidates are significantly different from those designed for traditional drugs (i.e., small organic molecules). The study of small molecules focuses on identifying target organ changes, assessing the pharmacokinetic profile and initial tissue disposition, and establishing a projected therapeutic ratio. For vaccines, programs emphasize mimicking the dose and dose interval of the intended clinical regimen. In addition, general health status, local tolerance, and immunogenicity are assessed, and comprehensive postmortem evaluations may or may not be conducted.

Jeanine L. Bussiere, George C. McCormick, and James D. Green • Department of Pathobiology and Toxicology, Genentech, Inc., South San Francisco, California 94080.

Vaccine Design: The Subunit and Adjuvant Approach, edited by Michael F. Powell and Mark J. Newman. Plenum Press, New York, 1995.

61

This chapter will examine historical safety issues associated with various types of vaccines, and will review and recommend key elements of preclinical safety assessment programs that are designed to support the safe clinical use of new vaccine candidates. Recommended safety evaluation studies for new vaccine adjuvants have been reviewed previously (Goldenthal *et al.*, 1993).

2. POTENTIAL ADVERSE EFFECTS ASSOCIATED WITH VACCINES

Potential toxic effects associated with vaccines include general systemic toxicity, enhancement of disease, antigenic competition, adverse immunologic effects, and teratogenic or reproductive effects. These potential adverse effects are summarized in Table I, and addressed in detail below.

2.1. General Toxicity of Vaccines

Adverse systemic effects in response to vaccination may range from mild to severe, and typically include chills, fever, malaise, and nausea. Local reactions at the injection site may range from mild tenderness and induration, to severe pain, granuloma or abscess

Table I
Summary of Potential Toxic Effects Associated with Vaccines

Systemic toxicity
    Chills, fever, malaise, nausea, etc.
    Local injection site pain and induration/adjuvant-induced toxicity
    Encephalopathy/neurotoxicity
Enhancement of disease/infection
    Insufficient attenuation of virus or reversion to virulence
    Antibody-dependent enhancement
    Incomplete immunity
    Infection from live-carriers for vaccines
Interactions
    Drug–vaccine
    Vaccine–vaccine
Induction of inappropriate immune responses
Alteration of cytokine profiles
Hypersensitivity
Sensitivity of immunosuppressed populations
Cross-reactive antibodies
    Development of autoantibodies to endogenous ligands
        Immunosuppression
        Immune complex formation
        Immunopathogenesis
    Teratogenicity

formation, and limb use impairment (Goldenthal *et al.*, 1993; Zunich *et al.*, 1992). Much of the local reaction is likely related to the adjuvant used in the vaccine formulation (Allison and Byars, 1992; Gupta *et al.*, 1993). In addition, anterior chamber uveitis has been associated with some muramyl peptide analogues used as adjuvants (Allison and Byars, 1992).

The most serious neurologic event attributable to immunization is encephalopathy, which has been seen following pertussis vaccination (Fenichel *et al.*, 1989). In addition, AIDS vaccines that include the major surface glycoprotein of HIV-1, gp120, may potentially be neurotoxic. Studies on cultured neuronal cells suggest that gp120 induces neurotoxicity (Lipton *et al.*, 1991; Savio and Levi, 1993), and s.c. injection of gp120 in neonatal rats (Hill *et al.*, 1993) or intracerebroventricular injection in adult rats (Glowa *et al.*, 1992) leads to learning and behavioral defects. The gp120 protein expressed in astrocytes of transgenic mice induced a spectrum of neuronal and glial changes similar to those found in brains of HIV-1-infected humans (Toggas *et al.*, 1994). Thus, vaccination with HIV-1 envelope glycoproteins may cause neurotoxicity in situations where the blood–brain barrier is compromised (i.e., in neonates, in certain disease states, with certain concurrent drug therapies, etc.), resulting in entry of the gp120 into the central nervous system.

2.2. Enhancement of Disease/Infection

One of the major concerns with vaccine safety is the possibility of increased incidence of infection (i.e., higher rates of infection on exposure to the virus, increased rate of disease progression following infection). In one example, cats were vaccinated with three different vaccine preparations of feline immunodeficiency virus (FIV); purified FIV incorporated into immune-stimulating complexes (ISCOMs; Quil-A–cholesterol complex), recombinant FIV p24 ISCOMs, or fixed, inactivated cell vaccine in Quil-A (saponin extracted from *Quillaja saponaria*). None of the vaccinated cats were protected from infection after i.p. challenge with FIV, and there appeared to be enhancement of infection, as the vaccinated cats became viremic sooner than unvaccinated controls. Additionally, 100% of the vaccinated cats became infected compared with only 78% of the controls (Hosie *et al.*, 1992). These authors speculate that any procedure that activates the immune system increases the expression of FIV receptor on T cells, and may enhance infection after challenge. In addition, Jiang and Neurath (1992) reported that antisera directed against V3 peptides from 21 different HIV-1 isolates can enhance HIV-1 infection of U937 cells, a $CD4^+$ human monocytoid cell line.

Enhancement of disease following infection may lead to immunopathogenic responses following vaccination. Horses vaccinated with a subunit equine infectious anemia virus vaccine experienced severe clinical signs (i.e., febrile episodes, marked depression, loss of appetite, and weight loss) following a challenge with a heterologous strain of the virus (Issel *et al.*, 1992). Thus, this subunit vaccine had a high potential to enhance disease that was induced by a subsequent challenge with heterologous virus. In addition, experiments on a murine lymphocyte choriomeningitis model indicated that vaccination with whole virus protected the mice from infection following challenge, while vaccination with a recombinant vaccinia virus vaccine caused an increased susceptibility to T-cell-mediated immunopathology which was triggered by a subsequent challenge infection (Oehen *et al.*, 1991).

Antibody-dependent enhancement of disease may occur by inducing antibodies (Abs) to a nonneutralizing epitope on the antigen, which then combine with viral antigens during subsequent natural infection to produce severe and sometimes fatal immunopathological disease (Kimman, 1992). For example, Abs to gp41 of HIV-1 enhance HIV-1 infection of PBMCs (Cohen, 1994). In addition, enhancing Abs and neutralizing Abs may be induced by distinct epitopes on gp120, and the ratio of these Abs may determine the outcome of enhanced infection or protection (Takeda *et al.*, 1991). The enhanced infection of influenza-A virus is mediated by Abs induced at subneutralizing concentrations by vaccination, and is Fc receptor mediated (Tamura *et al.*, 1991). In addition, antigens that induced infection-enhancing Abs drifted less quickly during the evolution of the virus strain than neutralizing epitopes.

2.3. Antigenic Competition

A second possible mechanism of increased risk of infection is the phenomenon of original antigenic sin (Schwartz, 1994). This is described as the predominance of Abs directed against a specific strain of virus (or vaccine) from an initial exposure, which then are expressed on a subsequent exposure to a different strain, and may prevent development of Abs to the new strain, or may not be cross-protective. Although an increased risk of infection may theoretically be a serious safety concern, this has not been identified historically with the use of vaccines. There may be a significant risk, however, if immunosuppression is induced by the vaccine, or when the population to be vaccinated is immunosuppressed (e.g., HIV-positive patients).

Interactions between a particular vaccine and other vaccines or drugs may result in serious adverse effects as reviewed previously (Grabenstein, 1990). Studies of numerous combinations of live vaccines have failed to show interference in developing an appropriate immune response. The only significant reciprocal antagonism seen following coadministration of two or more vaccines occurred between cholera and yellow fever vaccines, and between measles vaccine and meningococcal A&C vaccine. A decreased seroconversion rate to both vaccines was seen following coadministration (Grabenstein, 1990). Live poliovirus vaccine contains three distinct strains of the poliovirus, which tend to interfere with each other during their multiplication in the intestine; thus, the same vaccine is given three times to ensure a satisfactory response to each of the virus strains (Mims, 1986). In addition, naturally occurring enterovirus infections in children in developing countries can interfere with the response to the live poliovirus vaccine. A review of the use and standardization of combined vaccines can be found in *Developments in Biological Standardization* (van Wezel and Hennessen, 1986).

Immunosuppressive drugs may or may not suppress the anticipated immune response to vaccines, depending on the drug and the vaccine used. One example of a vaccine–drug interaction is the impairment of the anamnestic response to tetanus toxoid booster by chloramphenicol (Grabenstein, 1990). In addition, influenza vaccine may be able to depress certain drug-metabolizing pathways (hepatic cytochrome P-450) by induction of endogenous interferon (IFN) production. This alteration in drug metabolism capabilities may significantly influence the patient's response to certain medications. Vaccine interactions with other medications are typically not assessed preclinically; however, such interactions may be important to consider especially if any drug treatment is expected during the course of vaccination, or for vaccines designed as therapeutics (Cohen, 1994).

2.4. Unwanted Immune Responses

Induction of cellular immune responses following vaccination for HIV-1 [e.g., antigen-specific cytotoxic T lymphocytes (CTLs)] may lead to immunopathogenic changes. A strong correlation exists between the presence of HIV-specific CTLs in the lungs and the appearance of clinical abnormalities, and in skin rashes associated with AIDS viruses (Letvin, 1993; Letvin *et al.*, 1993). Thus, vaccination with potential AIDS vaccines designed to induce HIV-1-specific CTLs may or may not be advantageous: there may exist a fine balance between the induction of HIV-specific CTLs needed to protect against cell-associated virus, and CTLs that may play a role in the immunopathogenesis of HIV-induced disease.

Inducing a specific immune response with a vaccine may also be counterproductive if the vaccine alters cytokine profiles. Altered cytokine production may antagonize other immune responses necessary to prevent infection, or cause a general immune suppression. For example, induction of Th2 cells, which are crucial for Ab production, produces cytokines that antagonize the induction of Th1 cells. Th1 cells are important in the induction of CTL-mediated immunity and may play a role in the prevention of infection (Schwartz, 1994). A significant alteration of cytokine release has been observed in HIV-positive patients (Sinicco *et al.*, 1993), and potential AIDS vaccines such as recombinant gp120 induced IFN-γ and IFN-α production in peripheral mononuclear cells from healthy donors (Capobianchi *et al.*, 1993). HIV-1-derived gp160 induced specific CTLs to release sufficient tumor necrosis factor to induce upregulation of HIV-1 gene expression in chronically infected cells (Bollinger *et al.*, 1993). Thus, changes in cytokine profile, through induction of the cytokines themselves, or autoantibodies to the cytokines, can alter host immunocompetence.

2.5. Cross-Reactive Antibodies

Inappropriate immune reactions may be caused by cross-reactive Abs as demonstrated with both vaccines and adjuvants. Molecular mimicry between vaccines and endogenous proteins may lead to altered immune responses by inducing cross-reactive Abs to endogenous antigens such as MHC class I heavy chains (Lopalco *et al.*, 1993). For example, autoantibodies specific to HLA class I antigens were detected in the sera of subjects vaccinated with HIV-1-derived recombinant vaccines (De Santis *et al.*, 1993). Antibodies to gp120 cross-react with vasoactive intestinal peptide (Velikovic *et al.*, 1993), which may lead to an altered immune response. In addition, cross-reactive Abs to an antifertility vaccine are likely to react with luteinizing hormone (Mauck and Thau, 1990). Unfortunately, little is known about the adverse clinical consequences of generating cross-reactive autoantibodies in response to vaccination. Other examples of antigenic mimicry involved in induction of an autoimmune response are shown in Table II.

Table II
Examples of Antigenic Mimicry Involved in Autoimmunization[a]

Exogenous antigen	Autoantigen	Disease
Streptococcal M	Cardiac myosin	Rheumatic carditis
Mycobacterium tuberculosis	Cartilage proteoglycan	Rheumatic arthritis
Klebsiella nitrogenase	HLA-B27	Reiter's syndrome
Yersenia 19-kDa protein	HLA-B27	Reiter's syndrome
Yersenia protein	TSH receptor	Graves' disease
Adenovirus 72-kDa protein	La (SS-B)	Sjögren's syndrome
Poliovirus VP2	Acetylcholine receptor	Myasthenia gravis
Measles virus P3	Myelin basic protein	Encephalitis
Papilloma virus E2	Insulin receptor	Type I diabetes mellitus
Visna polymerase	Myelin basic protein	Encephalitis
Hepatitis B polymerase	Myelin basic protein	Encephalitis
Retroviral p30 protein	U1RNA	Systemic lupus erythematosus
Bacterial phospholipid	DNA	Systemic lupus erythematosus
Microbial tRNA	Jo	Polymyositis
Trypanosoma cruzi	Cardiac muscle	Chagas' disease
Mycoplasma	I-antigen	Hemolytic anemia
Adenovirus E1B protein	A-gliadin	Celiac disease

[a]From Robey *et al.* (1992).

Cross-reactive Abs generated in response to vaccination may cause immune suppression. One possible mechanism of immune suppression induced by molecular mimicry is a block of the interaction between the CD4 molecule and MHC class II. An interaction between these molecules and similar peptides found in HIV-1 gp120 has been demonstrated (Zagury *et al.*, 1993). Additionally, immune suppression by HIV-1 gp120 may occur by induction of apoptosis in CD4 cells expressing membrane-associated HIV envelope glycoproteins (Laurent-Crawford *et al.*, 1993). Whether these cross-reactive Abs would develop following vaccination with an HIV-1 gp120 AIDS vaccine is unknown.

Cross-reactive Abs may play a role in the immunopathogenesis of AIDS-related neurological disease. Antibodies generated to gp120 cross-react with three prominent human brain proteins (Trujillo *et al.*, 1993), and Abs to gp41 cross-react with human astrocytes (Yamada *et al.*, 1991). In addition, the induction of cross-reactive Abs following vaccination may alter cytokine production. For example, autoantibodies to IFN-γ have been detected in the serum of HIV-infected patients and other virus-infected patients (Turano and Caruso, 1993). These autoantibodies interfered with the immunomodulating activity, but not the antiviral or antiproliferative activity of IFN-γ. The clinical significance of these potential immunosuppressive effects has not yet been defined, nor has evidence yet suggested that vaccination with an HIV-1 vaccine will induce these cross-reactive Abs.

2.6. Teratogenic and Reproductive Effects

Another safety concern associated with vaccination is potential teratogenicity that may occur via transplacental passage of vaccine components, metabolites, or elicited Abs. For example, antisperm Abs, which develop in response to an antifertility vaccine, have been associated with early pregnancy loss (Mauck and Thau, 1990). Potential AIDS vaccines, which induce Abs to the V3 loop of the primary neutralizing domain of HIV-1, may play a role in maternal–fetal transmission of HIV-1 as mothers who transmitted infection to the offspring had significantly higher IgG1 Abs to the V3 loop of gp160 than mothers who were nontransmitters (Markham *et al.*, 1994). Some live vaccines, although safe for use in nonpregnant women, may cause fetal infection resulting in malformations or abortions, such as those seen clinically with the rubella virus vaccine (Tizard, 1990). This may be related to an immature immune system in the fetus, which may be unable to control the resulting infection. For example, newborn monocyte/macrophages are functionally immature relative to adult cells (e.g., decreased phagocytosis, chemotaxis) and are more susceptible to HIV-1 infection (Sperduto *et al.*, 1993).

Endocrinological effects following vaccination are another safety concern. Reproductive toxicity testing has not typically been conducted with vaccines because of the infrequent dosing schedule, the critical nature of the targeted disease, or because the intended patient population does not include women of childbearing age. There is currently a focus on including women earlier in clinical trials, which may put more emphasis on reproductive toxicity testing. In addition, for vaccines where pregnant women are a target population (i.e., for an AIDS vaccine), potential reproductive and teratogenic effects should be assessed with modified reproductive toxicity tests.

3. RISKS EXPERIENCED WITH SPECIFIC TYPES OF VACCINES AND ADJUVANTS

Risks associated with live vaccines, killed vaccines, live carrier vaccines, or adjuvants are reviewed below. Although adverse events associated with genetically engineered vaccines lack the long history of clinical use, these vaccines benefit from the advances in technology and understanding of problems found with use of earlier vaccine strategies. A summary of reported adverse events associated with the various types of vaccines and specific adjuvants is presented in Table III.

3.1. Live Vaccines

The risk of live (attenuated) vaccines such as MMR (mumps/measles/rubella) and polio lies in attaining the balance between minimal virulence and maximal immunogenicity. This balance may be achievable in a normal population, but may not be the same in a population with even minor defects in immune competence. Even different strains of a particular vaccine may have a varied potential for reversion to virulence or other associated toxicities. For example, an increased risk of meningitis following immunization with the mumps vaccine has been reported with the Urabe strain, but not the Jeryl-Lynn strain

Table III
Summary of Reported Adverse Events Associated with Vaccines

Live vaccines	
Mumps	Increased risk of meningitis
Rabies	Postvaccinal rabies
Rubella	Fetal infections, fetal/newborn malformations/death
Killed vaccines	
Measles	Immunopathogenic responses following natural infection, delayed hypersensitivity
Pertussis	Increased risk of encephalopathies
Influenza	Autoimmune postvaccinal encephalitis or peripheral neuritis, Reye's syndrome, Guillain–Barré syndrome?
RSV	Autoimmune Arthus reaction following natural infection
Live carrier vaccines	
Vaccinia	Eczema vaccinatum, generalized and progressive vaccinia, ophthalmic vaccinia
	Encephalitis, meningoencephalitis, encephalomyelitis
Adjuvants	
Alum, ISCOMs	Contact hypersensitivity
Alum, IFA	Injection site abscesses, granulomatous inflammation
LPS, MDP	Pyrogenicity
MDP	Uveitis, arthritis, Reiter's syndrome

(Duclos and Bentsi-Enchill, 1993). Modified live vaccines, such as the pseudorabies vaccine, may not cause obvious disease, but may still cause changes in the host's immunity, resistance to other infections, and/or growth (Hahn, 1992). Postvaccinal rabies has been reported in individuals immunized with a modified-live rabies vaccine (Tizard, 1990). Insufficient attenuation can lead to serious consequences beyond the original disease.

Insufficient, or reversion of, attenuation and spread to unvaccinated individuals also represent a major safety concern. For example, where use of the oral poliovirus vaccine has resulted in elimination of wild poliovirus, the only remaining poliomyelitis cases appear to be vaccine-associated (Racaniello, 1992). Adverse events have also been associated with faulty production of vaccines (e.g., bacterial or viral contamination) or faulty administration (e.g., use of nonsterile equipment). Mycoplasmal contamination is another potential problem in tissue culture vaccines that use fetal bovine serum without preservative (Tizard, 1990). Thus, several major disease episodes have been associated with inadequate quality control. Recommendations for neurovirulence testing of poliovirus vaccines and other live vaccine preparations should be considered when testing new batches of a vaccine (Brown and Lewis, 1993; Medicines Committee, 1993; Racaniello, 1992).

3.2. Killed Vaccines

Killed vaccines, such as an inactivated measles vaccine and a respiratory syncytial virus (RSV) vaccine, have given rise to harmful immunopathological complications following natural infection with the pathogen. A formalin-inactivated RSV vaccine induced an unbalanced immune response in children (i.e., a large proportion of the Abs were directed against nonneutralizing epitopes). Further, the functional Abs that inhibit syncytium formation were found to be lacking (Granström, 1991). The RSV-induced Abs that failed to neutralize RSV infection combined with viral antigens during subsequent natural infection and produced severe and sometimes fatal immunopathological disease (Kim *et al.*, 1969). Instead of providing protection against infection, these Abs initiated an Arthus reaction on subsequent infection (Murphy *et al.*, 1987).

Immunopathological responses, such as an increase in relative risk of encephalopathies subsequent to vaccination, have also been seen with DPT (diphtheria, pertussis, tetanus vaccine), but not DT vaccines, so this effect is likely related to the pertussis component (Fine and Chen, 1992; Duclos and Bentsi-Enchill, 1993). Adverse reactions following vaccination with a killed measles virus were associated with natural measles virus reinfection, and local reactions at the injection site (Karzon, 1983). Thus, it appeared that immunization with the killed measles virus established an altered immune state in which reinfection with the wild virus resulted in an unusual pathological response, including severe systemic and local reactions (i.e., fever, rash, malaise, and erythema, induration, swelling, and vesicle formation, respectively).

In 1976, following the largest A/New Jersey (swine) influenza vaccination program in the United States, there was an increase in the number of reports of Guillain–Barré syndrome, which provided strong epidemiological evidence that there was an excess risk related to vaccination (Schonberger *et al.*, 1979). In contrast, the 1978–1979 influenza vaccine was not associated with a statistically significant risk (Hurwitz *et al.*, 1981). However, Guillain–Barré syndrome has also been reported following polio, measles, hepatitis B, *Haemophilus influenzae* type b, MMR, and rabies immunizations; thus, a direct causal effect of the influenza vaccine has not been proven (Gervaix *et al.*, 1993; Grose and Spigland, 1976; Knittel *et al.*, 1989; Morris and Rylance, 1994; Tuohy, 1989; Uhari *et al.*, 1989). Other serious adverse reactions following an influenza virus infection are rare, but include myositis, myocarditis, encephalopathy, febrile convulsions, and toxic shock syndrome (Clements, 1992). Reye's syndrome has also been associated with influenza A and B outbreaks (Corey *et al.*, 1978; LaMontagne, 1980).

Because killed vaccines are not as immunogenic as live vaccines, adjuvants are coadministered to increase antigenicity. Safety concerns regarding adjuvant effects are described in Section 3.5.

3.3. Live Carrier Vaccines

For live modified viral vectors, the main safety concern is whether the vector is virulent. Replication-competent retroviruses can cause malignancies, particularly under adverse conditions such as complete bone marrow immunosuppression or extended retroviremia in monkeys (Holt *et al.*, 1987). It is important to test for these retroviruses in any vaccine preparation. Since herpesviruses have been proposed as vaccine vectors, the potential for delayed persistence and oncogenesis must be examined (Shih *et al.*, 1984). Both herpes simplex (Galloway and McDougall, 1990) and cytomegalovirus (Boldogh *et al.*, 1991) have been shown to activate endogenous retroviral expression and induce cellular changes through interactions at cell surface receptors, that may perturb normal cellular functions (Preston, 1990). Other viruses have also been associated with human cancers, including retroviruses and T-cell leukemias, hepatitis B virus and hepatocellular carcinoma, Epstein–Barr virus and nasopharyngeal carcinoma, and HIV and AIDS-related Kaposi's sarcoma (Haverkos *et al.*, 1991). The possible association of herpes simplex virus-2 vaccine with cervical carcinoma has also been suggested (Granström, 1991; Whitley and Meignier, 1992). The proven safety of adenoviruses as oral vaccines for over 20 years provides evidence of the potential of human adenoviruses as vaccine vectors. However, concerns about potential oncogenicity and potential pathogenicity in infants and immunocompromised individuals must be addressed before adenoviruses can be considered as potential recombinant vaccine vectors (Graham and Prevec, 1992).

A vaccinia-vectored HIV-1 vaccine is currently being tested in human clinical trials. Adverse effects of the vaccinia vector seen previously have included eczema vaccinatum, generalized vaccinia, progressive vaccinia, and ophthalmic vaccinia (Marcus-Sekura and Quinnan, 1989). These were found mainly in individuals with immunodeficiencies, eczema, or following direct exposure of virus in the eye. Thus, special populations may be more at risk of these adverse effects. For example, relatively severe reactions often occur in adults since the interval between vaccinations in most adults is generally more than 10 years. A 12-year study in the USSR found significant neurological complications associated with smallpox vaccine including encephalitis, meningoencephalitis, and encephalomyelitis with a fatality rate of 24% (Gurvich, 1992). The postviral encephalomyelitis had more to do with the abnormal immune status of the host than with the strain or type of virus involved (Collier, 1991); however, the incidence of encephalitis varied greatly in different countries and with different strains of the vaccinia virus (Moss, 1992). An extensive review of these postvaccinal complications can be found elsewhere (Regamey and Cohen, 1973).

3.4. Genetically Engineered Vaccines

As genetically engineered vaccines are relatively new, a long history of their safe use in humans does not yet exist. However, there does not appear to be anything intrinsically more dangerous in the development of vaccines by recombinant methods than by any other method, and in general, the noninfectious nature of these synthetic biologics reduces the issue of safety to that of the product and not the process (rDNA technology) (Hahn, 1992). Emphasis is placed on controlling production and meeting defined specifications throughout the process. Pathogens attenuated by recombinant techniques, recombinant vectors used for antigen expression, reversion to virulence, potential for oncogenesis, and recombination concerns are similar to those with other vaccine strategies. Genetically engineered vaccines are also generally poor immunogens and require adjuvants to evoke the desired immune response (Gupta *et al.*, 1993).

The hazards associated with the hepatitis B virus (HBV) are one of several reasons why conventional techniques were not suitable to produce a vaccine; rDNA techniques have made it possible to produce a nonvirulent recombinant organism capable of synthesizing large amounts of HBV surface antigen, thus circumventing the direct dangers of HBV (Issaacson, 1992). The advantage of an rDNA vaccine for hepatitis B over the earlier plasma-derived vaccine is the reduction of risk that the preparation would contain infective agents (residual HBV, HIV, etc.) or normal human serum protein, and the reduction of cost (Dreesman *et al.*, 1984). Besides having limited availability because of the small number of appropriate patients to use as donors, extensive safety testing was required for the plasma-derived vaccine (Issaacson, 1992). Strict quality control guidelines have been recommended by the Biologics Division of the FDA for monitoring the safety, purity, and potency of rDNA products, including characterization of the expression system, the master cell bank, production procedure, purification procedure, and the final product (i.e., tests for pyrogen, viral, nucleic acid, antigen, or microbial contamination) (Liu *et al.*, 1985).

3.5. Adjuvants

As with all drug and biological products, the absolute safety of adjuvants can never be guaranteed. Inherent toxicities can be ascribed in part to the unintended stimulation of various aspects of the immune response. Consequently, safety and adjuvanticity must be balanced between obtaining maximum immune stimulation with minimum side effects. The first concern when using an adjuvant is acute or subacute tissue damage at the injection site, or a later granulomatous reaction. The second undesirable side effect is pyrogenicity. It should be noted, however, that systemic effects such as uveitis, an influenza-like syndrome, generalized joint discomfort (i.e., Reiter's symptoms), and arthritis have also been identified as safety concerns (Allison and Byars, 1992; Goldenthal *et al.*, 1993).

Alum is presently the only adjuvant in products approved by the FDA for use in humans, but it is not active with every antigen and stimulates mostly humoral immunity (Audibert and Lise, 1993). During the 1930s, the superiority of alum-adjuvanted diphtheria and tetanus toxoids was established in humans (Aprile and Wardlaw, 1966), and used in DTP in billions of doses in children and infants. Side effects from the use of alum adjuvants include erythema, subcutaneous nodules, contact hypersensitivity, and granulomatous inflammation (Ross *et al.*, 1991). Little or no systemic toxicity is typically seen and the safety of alum adjuvants has been demonstrated with extensive clinical use.

Incomplete Freund's adjuvant (IFA)-based bacterial vaccines (e.g., cholera, tetanus) have produced side effects of sterile abscesses, ulcers, and delayed-type local reactions. These severe reactions at the injection site were considered to be related to the presence of lipopolysaccharide (LPS), and to certain enzymes in the bacterial vaccine components which degraded the Arlacel A component of IFA to release toxic fatty acids (Gupta *et al.*, 1993). Also, the presence of short-chain hydrocarbons may have the capacity to cause severe tissue destruction because of their lipid solvent action and consequent disruption of cell membranes. IFA is not currently used in humans because of these previously reported side effects, including carcinogenicity in mice (Murray *et al.*, 1972; Potter and Boyce, 1962; Potter and MacCardle, 1964). However, long-term follow-up of thousands of individuals vaccinated with IFA showed no apparent increase in mortality, tumor occurrence, or autoimmune disease (Gupta *et al.*, 1993).

Other, more recent adjuvants [e.g., muramyl dipeptide (MDP)] have been extensively evaluated for adjuvanticity. However, significant side effects including pyrogenicity, leukocytosis, uveitis, and adjuvant arthritis prevent MDP's use in human vaccines. A formulation of threonyl MDP with squalane–Pluronic polymer emulsion known as Syntex

Adjuvant Formulation-1 (SAF-1), is nonpyrogenic and has greatly reduced toxicity compared with MDP, and is currently being evaluated as an adjuvant for an HIV-1 vaccine (Allison and Byars, 1992).

Adjuvants such as Quil-A and ISCOMs elicit IgE Abs and can cause an acute hypersensitivity reaction (Allison and Byars, 1992). Quil-A and ISCOMs are used in veterinary vaccines, but have the additional side effects of hemolytic activity, and minor local reactions related to the detergent activity of the Quil-A molecule. These side effects are reduced when the Quil-A is incorporated into ISCOMs (Gupta *et al.*, 1993). Monkeys immunized with SIV in ISCOMs were sensitized in that they showed an acute hypersensitivity response when challenged with virus. Animals immunized with SAF-1 showed protection, but were not sensitized. This hypersensitivity response caused by the ISCOMs may be related to the production of IgE Abs (Allison and Byars, 1992). A purified fraction of Quil-A, QS-21, is also currently being evaluated as an adjuvant for several vaccines (Clark *et al.*, 1991).

4. BALANCING RISKS AND BENEFITS

The question of vaccine safety is a dynamic one; as more sensitive measures of pathogen persistence (e.g., polymerase chain reaction), immunosuppression, or induced oncogenesis arise, existing vaccines must be reassessed for potential safety, and future vaccines evaluated with these technology considerations in mind. The risks and benefits of vaccination must be examined for each vaccine. The risk/benefit analysis will vary depending on the disease itself (life-threatening or not), the population at risk (adult, child, high-risk behavior groups), and risks from the antigen versus the adjuvant/carrier or process. Most people are prepared to take more risks with vaccination when the disease itself is very harmful. For example, the benefit of an effective vaccinia–HIV preparation would far outweigh the risk of neuroparalytic accidents. Even though a live attenuated vaccine of SIV has been shown to be protective in rhesus monkeys (Daniel *et al.*, 1992), the use of a live attenuated vaccine against HIV is probably not appropriate, because of the high risk of the attenuated strain reverting to virulence and the serious nature of the disease. Adverse events not readily acceptable in normal patients (i.e., chills, fever, malaise, and nausea) may be deemed acceptable to oncology or HIV-seropositive patients.

The risk of childhood vaccinations has focused on a correlation with certain severe adverse events (i.e., encephalopathies, sudden infant death syndrome); however, these may be coincidental because of a similar age of vaccination with the onset of these events, rather than because of an effect of the vaccine (Fine and Chen, 1992). Risks may be underestimated since factors that predispose children to severe adverse events may also lead to postponement of vaccination.

Immunizations have a dual purpose: a direct protective effect for the individual, and an indirect effect of herd immunity (i.e., possible spread of the antigen to induce immunity in others, decreased spread of a disease by preventing infection in an individual). Also, vaccine administration is for prevention of a disease in a healthy individual and therefore is an elective procedure. Both of these have major implications in terms of accepting adverse effects. Thus, there may be a conflict of interest between the risks to an individual (associated with the vaccination) and the risks to a population (related to low level of herd immunity). For example, the greater apparent safety of the Jeryl-Lynn strain mumps vaccine (fewer vaccine-induced complications) is offset by the greater apparent efficacy of the Urabe strain (fewer complications because of natural infection) (Nokes and Anderson, 1991). Individual perception of risk may influence public acceptance of a vaccine.

5. PRECLINICAL SAFETY TESTING CONSIDERATIONS

Considerations for preclinical safety testing of vaccines are different than for small molecules. Infrequent dosing schedules and an expected immune response to the antigen make it difficult to assess safety concerns preclinically. In addition, the lack of appropriate animal models of disease and/or correlates of protection from infection makes predicting potential toxicities in the clinic a tenuous task. Some adverse events can be examined based on historical toxicities associated with certain types of vaccines; however, many potential toxicities may have been overlooked or unrecognized with past vaccines.

A review of the information presented in a number of Summary for Basis of Approval documents for certain representative marketed vaccines (recombinant Hepatitis B Vaccine; Pneumococcal Vaccine, Polyvalent; Rabies Vaccine; Rabies Vaccine, Adsorbed; Haemophilus b Conjugate Vaccine; BCG Vaccine U.S.P.) has indicated a paucity of preclinical safety/toxicity investigations conducted in support of vaccine approval and registration. With the exception of occasional reports of antigenicity (efficacy) testing in nonhuman primates and/or the conduct of final container tests normally required for biological products (general safety tests in rodents; pyrogenicity testing), preclinical toxicity testing with vaccines was not reported in these documents. Likewise, information contained in the AHFS 94 Drug Information Formulary (McEvoy, 1994) provides no description of preclinical toxicity evaluations for vaccines indicating that animal safety investigations invariably were not utilized in the testing program for these products. Guidelines have been established in the European community that suggest measuring certain safety parameters in preclinical studies for vaccines (Committee for Proprietary Medicinal Products, 1989).

The preclinical and clinical safety of each vaccine should be evaluated on an individual product basis; preclinical testing requirements should reflect the unique risks and benefits of each potential vaccine candidate. The clinical status of the recipient is also important as stated previously, since immunocompromised individuals may be more at risk for adverse events associated with vaccination. However, depending on the seriousness of the disease, and the available alternatives, certain adverse events may be more acceptable, especially if these events are reversible. The prophylactic, therapeutic, or diagnostic indication of the antigen should determine the extent of preclinical safety testing (particularly for conducting multiple-dosing studies), especially with regard to the recent use of vaccines to treat disease rather than prevent it (Cohen, 1994). In this regard, valuable information can be obtained by expanding multiple-dose efficacy studies to include measurements normally conducted in preclinical toxicity studies (i.e., body weight, food consumption, clinical pathology, ophthalmology, gross necropsy and histopathology). The potential for long-term effects such as carcinogenesis and autoimmune disease are difficult to assess in preclinical animal safety studies for most vaccine preparations, because of limitations in animal models or dosing schedules. Other preclinical safety studies that may provide useful information include: assessment of immune function, local deposition at the injection site, developmental/reproductive toxicology and protection studies against a viral challenge. In addition, since many new adjuvants are being investigated, information regarding the toxicity profile of the new adjuvant must be developed independently.

Studies that evaluate immune function should involve the evaluation of expected immunogenicity (level of Ab production, class and subclass of Ab produced, cell-mediated immunity, and duration of immune response). In addition, the formation of neutralizing Abs, cross-reactive Abs, immune complex formation, interactions with immune cells to cause dysfunction, and release of other molecules that affect the immune system should also be investigated. In particular, the cross-reactivity of Abs with intrinsic human antigens should be assessed.

Local deposition studies would assess the retention of the product at the site of injection and its further distribution. It is not current practice in vaccine testing to conduct pharmacokinetic studies on antigens, which are administered in very small amounts and may have a very short half-life. However, in certain cases, pharmacokinetic studies may provide useful information, especially with new formulation strategies, such as controlled-release delivery systems (Ellis and Douglas, 1994). The mechanism of action, intended dosage, and route of administration (including effects of the adjuvant) should be taken into consideration. For novel adjuvants, the safety of the adjuvant alone should be determined. Multidose studies of 2–4 weeks' duration in two species and information regarding mutagenic potential would be considered appropriate. In addition, Segment II studies to assess potential effects of new adjuvants on reproduction and development are considered important. The safety of the adjuvant in combination with the intended antigen should be evaluated in dosing protocols that mimic the clinical dosing regimen in a pharmacologically responsive species. Local tolerance testing with the final product formulation should be conducted, including measures other than gross or microscopic tissue examination (e.g., serum creatine phosphokinase) to assess local tissue damage (Allison and Byars, 1992). Special evaluations for problems known to be associated with a specific type of product should be considered, for example, slit-lamp ophthalmological examinations to investigate the potential for the induction of uveitis (Goldenthal *et al.*, 1993).

Reproductive toxicity studies are not normally conducted unless the vaccine is intended for use in women of childbearing age or during pregnancy. For the latter case, modified Segment II studies should assure coverage of the sensitive periods of development. Mutagenicity and tumorigenicity have not been assessed or required primarily because of infrequent use, as well as historical clinical data showing no increase in carcinogenicity in vaccine recipients. For formulation changes in the final product, use of different adjuvants, changes in cell lines, etc., appropriate bridging safety studies should be conducted prior to the initiation of clinical testing.

Challenge studies to provide evidence of protection are usually conducted for determining efficacy rather than safety; however, increased risk of infection is a significant concern. The FDA has recently recommended the inclusion of animal protection studies, notably a nonhuman primate challenge study, to justify initiation of Phase III efficacy trials with potential AIDS vaccines in high-risk volunteers (F-D-C Reports, Nov. 8, 1993). As stated previously, appropriate animal models of the disease are often not available, but protection studies may still provide some evidence of efficacy and/or safety before the onset of clinical trials. As much information as possible should be gathered in these efficacy

Table IV
Summary of Recommended Preclinical Safety Studies
That Should Be Considered with New Vaccines

Local tolerance and assessment of hypersensitivity

Immune function, including both specific and nonspecific Ab production and
  cell-mediated immune responses

Local deposition of the antigen and its distribution from the injection site

Studies to evaluate adjuvant-associated toxicity, with and without the intended antigen

Multiple-dose toxicity studies

Reproductive/developmental toxicity testing (if vaccine is to be used during pregnancy)

Challenge study to predict protection from infection

Miscellaneous studies as appropriate:

  Drug interactions

  Sensitivity of special populations

  Pharmacokinetic studies

  Safety studies in an appropriate animal model of the disease

trials to reduce the need for additional safety studies and conserve the use of animals (i.e., nonhuman primates).

As the risks associated with vaccination become more recognized, appropriate animal models may be developed to better predict toxicities. Recommended safety studies that should be considered in the design of a safety assessment program are summarized in Table IV. A preclinical safety testing program of a vaccine candidate should be tailored to the unique considerations associated with the conditions of use. Considerations should be related to the individual properties of the vaccine, the anticipated clinical protocols, the target population, and associated adjuvants or carriers.

REFERENCES

Allison, A. C., and Byars, N. E., 1992, Immunological adjuvants and their mode of action, in: *Vaccines: New Approaches to Immunological Problems* (R. W. Ellis, ed.), Butterworths–Heinemann, London, pp. 431–449.

Aprile, M. A., and Wardlaw, A. C., 1966, Aluminium compounds as adjuvants for vaccines and toxoids in man: A review, *Can. J. Public Health* **57(8)**:343–360.

Audibert, F. M., and Lise, L. D., 1993, Adjuvants: Current status, clinical perspectives and future prospects, *Immunol. Today* **14(6)**:281–284.

Boldogh, I., Abubakar, S., Fons, M. P., Deng, C. Z., and Albrecht, T., 1991, Activation of cellular oncogenes by clinical isolates and laboratory strains of human cytomegalovirus, *J. Med. Virol.* **34**:241–247.

Bollinger, R. C., Quinn, T. C., Liu, A. Y., Stanhope, P. E., Hammond, S. A., Viveen, R., Clements, M. L., and Siliciano, R. F., 1993, Cytokines from vaccine-induced HIV-1 specific cytotoxic T lymphocytes: Effects on viral replication, *AIDS Res. Hum. Retroviruses* **9(11)**:1067–1077.

Brown, F., and Lewis, B. P., 1993, *Poliovirus Attenuation: Molecular Mechanisms and Practical Aspects*, Vol. 78, Karger, Basel.

Capobianchi, M. R., Ameglio, F., Fei, P. C., Castilletti, C., Mercuri, F., Fais, S., and Dianzani, F., 1993, Coordinate induction of interferon α and γ by recombinant HIV-1 glycoprotein 120, *AIDS Res. Hum. Retroviruses* **9(10)**:957–962.

Clark, N., Kushner, N. N., Barrett, C. B., Kensil, C. R., Salsbury, D., and Cotter, S., 1991, Efficacy and safety field trials of a recombinant DNA vaccine against feline leukemia virus infection, *J. Am. Vet. Med. Assoc.* **199(10)**:1433–1443.

Clements, M. L., 1992, Influenza vaccines, in: *Vaccines: New Approaches to Immunological Problems* (R.W. Ellis, ed.), Butterworths–Heinemann, London, pp. 129–150.

Cohen, J., 1994, Vaccines get a new twist, *Science* **264**:503–505.

Collier, L. H., 1991, Safety of recombinant vaccinia vaccines, *Lancet* **337**:1035–1036.

Committee for Proprietary Medicinal Products, 1989, Notes to applicants for marketing authorizations on the pre-clinical biological safety testing of medicinal products derived from biotechnology (and comparable products derived from chemical synthesis), *J. Biol. Stand.* **17**:203–212.

Corey, L., Rubin, R. J., Hattwick, M. A. W., Noble, G. R., and Cassidy, B. A., 1978, A nationwide outbreak of Reye's syndrome: Its epidemiological relationship to influenza B, *Am. J. Med.* **61**:615–625.

Daniel, M. D., Kirchoff, F., Czajak, S. C., Sehgal, P. K., and Desrosiers, R. C., 1992, Protective effects of a live attenuated SIV vaccine with a deletion in the *nef* gene, *Science* **258**:1938–1941.

De Santis, C., Robbioni, P., Longhi, R., Lopalco, L., Siccardi, A. G., Beretta, A., and Roberts, N. J. J., 1993, Cross-reactive response to human immunodeficiency virus type 1 (HIV-1) gp120 and HLA class I heavy chains induced by receipt of HIV-1-derived envelope vaccines, *J. Infect. Dis.* **168**:1396–1403.

Dreesman, G. R., Ionescu-Matiu, I., Sanchez, Y., Kennedy, R. C., Sparrow, J. T., and Melnick, J. L., 1984, Hepatitis B surface antigen polypeptide and synthetic peptide vaccines, in: *Hepatitis B: The Virus, the Disease, and the Vaccine* (I. Millman, T. K. Eisenstein, and B. S. Blumberg, eds.), Plenum Press, New York, pp. 215–224.

Duclos, P., and Bentsi-Enchill, A., 1993, Current thoughts on the risks and benefits of immunisation, *Drug Safety* **8(6)**:404–413.

Ellis, R. W., and Douglas, R. G. J., 1994, New vaccine technologies, *J. Am. Med. Assoc.* **271(12)**:929–931.

Fenichel, G. M., Lane, D. A., Livengood, J. R., Horwitz, S. J., Menkes, J. H., and Schwartz, J. F., 1989, Adverse events following immunization: Assessing probability of causation, *Pediatr. Neurol.* **5(5)**:287–290.

Fine, P. E. M., and Chen, R. T., 1992, Confounding in studies of adverse reactions to vaccines, *Am. J. Epidemiol.* **136(2)**:121–135.

Galloway, D. A., and McDougall, J. K., 1990, Alterations in the cellular phenotype induced by herpes simplex viruses, *J. Med. Virol.* **31**:36–42.

Gervaix, A., Caflisch, M., Suter, S., and Haenggeli, C. A., 1993, Guillain–Barré syndrome following immunisation with *Haemophilus influenza* type b conjugate vaccine, *Eur. J. Pediatr.* **152**:613–614.

Glowa, J. R., Panlilio, L. V., Brenneman, D. E., Gozes, I., Fridkin, M., and Hill, J. M., 1992, Learning impairment following intracerebral administration of the HIV envelope protein gp120 or a VIP antagonist, *Brain Res.* **570**:49–53.

Goldenthal, K. L., Cavagnaro, J. A., Alving, C. R., and Vogel, F. R., 1993, Safety evaluation of vaccine adjuvants: National Cooperative Vaccine Development Meeting Working Group, *AIDS Res. Hum. Retrovir.* **9(1)**:S47–S51.

Grabenstein, J. D., 1990, Drug interactions involving immunologic agents. Part I. Vaccine–vaccine, vaccine–immunoglobulin, and vaccine–drug interactions, *DICP, Ann. Pharmacother.* **24**:67–81.

Graham, F. L., and Prevec, L., 1992, Adenovirus-based expression vectors and recombinant vaccines, in: *Vaccines: New Approaches to Immunological Problems* (R. W. Ellis, ed.), Butterworths–Heinemann, London, pp. 363–390.

Granström, M., 1991, Viral vaccines, in: *Immunotherapy and Vaccines* (S. J. Cryz, ed.), VCH Publishers, New York, pp. 68–70.

Grose, C., and Spigland, I., 1976, Guillain–Barré syndrome following administration of live measles vaccine, *Am. J. Med.* **60**:441–443.

Gupta, R. K., Relyveld, E. H., Lindblad, E. B., Bizzini, B., Ben-Efraim, S., and Gupta, C. K., 1993, Adjuvants—a balance between toxicity and adjuvanticity, *Vaccine* **11**(3):293–306.

Gurvich, E. B., 1992, The age-dependent risk of postvaccination complications in vaccines with smallpox vaccine, *Vaccine* **10**(2):96–97.

Hahn, E. C., 1992, Safety of recombinant vaccines, in: *Recombinant DNA Vaccines* (R. E. Isaacson, ed.), Dekker, New York, pp. 387–400.

Haverkos, H. W., Amsel, Z., and Drotman, D. P., 1991, Adverse virus–drug interactions, *Rev. Infect. Dis.* **13**:697–704.

Hill, J. M., Mervis, R. F., Avidor, R., Moody, T. W., and Brenneman, D. E., 1993, HIV envelope protein-induced neuronal damage and retardation of behavioral development in rat neonates, *Brain Res.* **603**:222–233.

Holt, J. T., Morton, C. C., Nienhuis, A. W., and Leder, P., 1987, Molecular mechanisms of hematologic neoplasms, in: *The Molecular Basis of Blood Diseases* (G. Stamatoyannopulos, A. W. Nienhuis, P. Leder, and P. W. Majerus, eds.), Saunders, Philadelphia, pp. 347–376.

Hosie, M. J., Osborne, R., Reid, G., Neil, J. C., and Jarrett, O., 1992, Enhancement after feline immunodeficiency virus vaccination, *Vet. Immunol. Immunopathol.* **35**:191–197.

Hurwitz, E. S., Schonberger, L. B., Nelson, D. B., and Holman, R. C., 1981, Guillain–Barré syndrome and the 1978–1979 influenza vaccine, *N. Engl. J. Med.* **305**(26):1557–1561.

Issaacson, R. E., 1992, The rationale for rDNA vaccines, in: *Recombinant DNA Vaccines: Rationale and Strategy* (R. E. Issaacson, ed.), Dekker, New York, pp. 1–17.

Issel, C. J., Horohov, D. W., Lea, D. F., Adams, W. V. Jr., Hagius, S. D., McManus, J. M., Allison, A. C., and Montelaro, R. C., 1992, Efficacy of inactivated whole-virus and subunit vaccines in preventing infection and disease caused by equine infectious anemia virus, *J. Virol.* **66**:3398–3408.

Jiang, S., and Neurath, A. R., 1992, Potential risks of eliciting antibodies enhancing HIV-1 infection of monocytic cells by vaccination with V3 loops of unmatched HIV-1 isolates, *AIDS* **6**:331–332.

Karzon, D. T., 1983, The immune basis for hypersensitivity to viral vaccines, in: *Human Immunity to Viruses* (F. A. Ennis, ed.), Academic Press, New York, pp. 111–130.

Kim, H. W., Canchola, J. G., Bradt, C. D., Pyles, G., Chanock, R. M., Jensen, K., and Parrot, R. H., 1969, Respiratory syncytial virus disease in infants despite prior administration of antigenic vaccine, *Am. J. Epidemiol.* **89**:422–434.

Kimman, T. G., 1992, Risks connected with the use of conventional and genetically engineered vaccines, *Vet. Q.* **14**(3):110–118.

Knittel, T., Ramadori, G., Mayet, W. J., Löhr, H., and Meyer zum Büschenfelde, K.-H., 1989, Guillain–Barré syndrome and human diploid cell rabies vaccine, *Lancet* **1**:1334–1335.

LaMontagne, J. R., 1980, Summary of a workshop on influenza B viruses and Reye's syndrome, *J. Infect. Dis.* **142**(3):452–465.

Laurent-Crawford, A. G., Krust, B., Riviere, Y., Desgranges, C., Muller, S., Kieny, M. P., Dauguet, C., and Hovanessian, A. G., 1993, Membrane expression of HIV envelope glycoprotein triggers apoptosis in CD4 cells, *AIDS Res. Hum. Retroviruses* **9**(8):761–773.

Letvin, N. L., 1993, Vaccines against human immunodeficiency virus—Progress and prospects, *N. Engl. J. Med.* **329**(19):1400–1405.

Letvin, N. L., Yasutomi, Y., Yamamoto, H., Ringler, D. J., and Chen, Z. W., 1993, The role of cytotoxic T lymphocytes in the immunopathogenesis of SIV-induced disease, in: *Animal Models of HIV and Other Retroviral Infections* (P. Racz, N. L. Letvin, and J. C. Gluckman, eds.), Karger, Basel, pp. 24–38.

Lipton, S. A., Sucher, N. J., Kaiser, P. K., and Dreyer, E. B., 1991, Synergistic effects of HIV coat protein and NMDA receptor-mediated neurotoxicity, *Neuron* **7**:111–118.

Liu, D. T., Gates, F. T. I., and Goldman, N. D., 1985, Quality control of biologicals produced by rDNA technology, in: *Developments in Biological Standardization*, Vol. 59 (F. T. Perkins and W. Hennessen, eds.), Karger, Basel, pp. 161–166.

Lopalco, L., De Santis, C., Meneveri, R., Longhi, R., Ginelli, E., Grassi, F., Siccardi, A. G., and Beretta, A., 1993, Human immunodeficiency virus type 1 gp120 C5 region mimics the HLA class I α1 peptide-binding domain, *Eur. J. Immunol.* **23**:2016–2021.

Marcus-Sekura, C. J., and Quinnan, G. V. J., 1989, Risks and benefits of vaccinia-vectored vaccine use from the regulatory perspective, *Res. Virol.* **140(5)**:467–469.

Markham, R. B., Coberly, J., Ruff, A. J., Hoover, D., Gomez, J., Holt, E., Desormeaux, J., Boulos, R., Quinn, T. C., and Halsey, N. A., 1994, Maternal IgG1 and IgA antibody to V3 loop consensus sequence and maternal–infant HIV-1 transmission, *Lancet* **343**:390–391.

Mauck, C. P., and Thau, R. B., 1990, Safety of anti-fertility vaccines, *Curr. Opin. Immunol.* **2**:728–732.

McEvoy, G. K., 1994, *AHFS 94 Drug Information, Vol. 80,* Americas Society of Hospital Pharmacists, Inc., Bethesda, MD, pp. 2184–2247.

Medicines Committee, 1993, Vaccines, in: *British Pharmacopoeia,* Vol. II (Medicines Committee, ed.), HMSO, London, pp. 1185–1210.

Mims, C. A., 1986, Vaccines—an addendum, in: *The Pathogenesis of Infectious Disease* (C. A. Mims, ed.), Academic Press, New York, pp. 303–321.

Morris, K., and Rylance, G., 1994, Guillain–Barré syndrome after measles, mumps, and rubella vaccine, *Lancet* **343**:60.

Moss, B., 1992, Vaccinia virus vectors, in: *Vaccines: New Approaches to Immunological Problems* (R.W. Ellis, ed.), Butterworths–Heinemann, London, pp. 345–362.

Murphy, B. R., Prince, G., Chanock, R. M., Wagner, D. K., and Walsh, E. E., 1987, Immune response of humans and cotton rats to respiratory syncytial virus infection or formalin-inactivated vaccine, in: *Vaccines 87: Modern Approaches to New Vaccines* (R. M. Chanock, R. A. Lerner, F. Brown, and H. Ginsberg, eds.), Cold Spring Harbor Laboratory Press, Cold Spring Harbor, NY, pp. 290–295.

Murray, R., Cohen, P., and Hardegree, M. C., 1972, Mineral oil adjuvants: Biological and chemical studies, *Ann. Allergy* **30**:146–151.

Nokes, D. J., and Anderson, R. M., 1991, Vaccine safety versus vaccine efficacy in mass immunisation programmes, *Lancet* **338**:1309–1312.

Oehen, S., Hengartner, H., and Zinkernagel, R. M., 1991, Vaccination for disease, *Science* **251**:195–198.

Potter, M., and Boyce, C. R., 1962, Induction of plasma cell neoplasmas in strain BALB/c mice with mineral oil and mineral oil adjuvants, *Nature* **193**:1086–1087.

Potter, M., and MacCardle, R. C., 1964, Histology of developing plasma cell neoplasia induced by mineral oil in BALB/c mice, *J. Natl. Cancer Inst.* **33**:497–515.

Preston, V. G., 1990, Herpes simplex virus activates expression of a cellular gene by specific binding to the cell surface, *Virology* **176**:474–482.

Racaniello, V. R., 1992, Poliovirus vaccines, in: *Vaccines: New Approaches to Immunological Problems* (R.W. Ellis, ed.), Butterworths–Heinemann, London, pp. 205–222.

Regamey, R. H., and Cohen, H., 1973, *International Symposium on Smallpox Vaccine,* Vol. 19, Karger, Basel.

Robey, F. A., Harris, T. A., Nguyen, A. K., Heegaard, N. H. H., and Batinic, D., 1992, Peptomers as vaccine candidates, in: *Genetically Engineered Vaccines* (J. E. Ciardi, J. R. McGhee, and J. M. Keith, eds.), Plenum Press, New York, pp. 209–215.

Ross, J. R., Smith, N. P., and White, I. R., 1991, Role of aluminium sensitivity in delayed persistent immunisation reactions, *J. Clin. Pathol.* **44**:876–878.

Savio, T., and Levi, G., 1993, Neurotoxicity of HIV coat protein gp120, NMDA receptors and protein kinase C: A study with rat cerebellar granule cell cultures, *J. Neurosci. Res.* **34**:265–272.

Schonberger, L. B., Bregman, D. J., and Sullivan-Bolyai, J. Z., 1979, Guillain–Barré syndrome following vaccination in the National Influenza Program, United States, 1976–1977, *Am. J. Epidemiol.* **110**:105–123.

Schwartz, D. H., 1994, Potential pitfalls on the road to an effective HIV vaccine, *Immunol. Today* **15(2)**:54–57.

Shih, M. F., Arsenakis, M., Tiollas, P., and Roizman, B., 1984, Expression of hepatitis B virus S gene by herpes simplex virus type 1 vectors carrying α-β-regulated gene chimeras, *Proc. Natl. Acad. Sci. USA* **81**:5867–5870.

Sinicco, A., Biglino, A., Sciandra, M., Forno, B., Pollono, A. M., Raiteri, R., and Gioannini, P., 1993, Cytokine network and acute primary HIV-1 infection, *AIDS* **7**:1167–1172.

Sperduto, A. R., Bryson, Y. J., and Chen, I. S. Y., 1993, Increased susceptibility of neonatal monocyte/macrophages to HIV-1 infection, *AIDS Res. Hum. Retrovir.* **9(12)**:1277–1285.

Stuart-Harris, C., 1979, Benefits and risks of immunisation against pertussis, *Dev. Biol. Stand.* **43**:75–83.

Takeda, A., Ennis, F. A., Robinson, J. E., Ho, D. D., and Debouck, C., 1991, Characterization of enhancement of HIV-1 infection by human monoclonal antibodies to HIV-1, in: *Vaccines 91: Modern Approaches to New Vaccines Including Prevention of AIDS* (R. M. Chanock, H. S. Ginsberg, F. Brown, and R. A. Lerner, eds.), Cold Spring Harbor Laboratory Press, Cold Spring Harbor, NY, pp. 23–27.

Tamura, M., Ennis, F. A., and Webster, R. G., 1991, Analysis of neutralizing and infection-enhancing antibodies of influenza-A viruses, in: *Vaccines 91: Modern Approaches to New Vaccines Including Prevention of AIDS* (R. M. Chanock, H. S. Ginsberg, F. Brown, and R. A. Lerner, eds.), Cold Spring Harbor Laboratory Press, Cold Spring Harbor, NY, pp. 217–220.

Tizard, I., 1990, Risks associated with use of live vaccines, *J. Am. Vet. Med. Assoc.* **196(11)**:1851–1858.

Toggas, S. M., Masliah, E., Rockenstein, E. M., Rall, G. F., Abraham, C. R., and Mucke, L., 1994, Central nervous system damage produced by expression of the HIV-1 coat protein gp120 in transgenic mice, *Nature* **367**:188–193.

Trujillo, J. R., McLane, M. F., Lee, T., and Essex, M., 1993, Molecular mimicry between the human immunodeficiency virus type 1 gp120 V3 loop and human brain proteins, *J. Virol.* **67(12)**:7711–7715.

Tuohy, P. G., 1989, Guillain–Barré syndrome following immunisation with synthetic hepatitis B vaccine, *N. Z. Med. J.* **102**:114–115.

Turano, A., and Caruso, A., 1993, The role of human autoantibodies against γ-interferon, *J. Antimicrob. Chemother.* **32A**:99–105.

Uhari, M., Rantala, H., and Niemelä, M., 1989, Cluster of childhood Guillain–Barré cases after an oral poliovaccine campaign, *Lancet* **2**:440–441.

van Wezel, A. L., and Hennessen, W., 1986, *Use and Standardization of Combined Vaccines*, Vol. 65, Karger, Basel.

Velikovic, V., Metlas, R., Danilo, V., Cavor, L., Pejinovic, N., Dujuc, A., Zakhariev, S., Guarnaccia, C., and Pongor, S., 1993, Natural autoantibodies cross-react with a peptide derived from the second conserved region of HIV-1 envelope glycoprotein gp120, *Biochem. Biophys. Res. Commun.* **196(3)**:1019–1024.

Whitley, R. J., and Meignier, B., 1992, Herpes simplex vaccines, in: *Vaccines: New Approaches to Immunological Problems* (R. W. Ellis, ed.), Butterworths–Heinemann, London, pp. 223–254.

Yamada, M., Zurbriggen, A., Oldstone, M. B. A., and Fujinami, R. S., 1991, Common immunologic determinant between human immunodeficiency virus type 1 gp41 and astrocytes, *J. Virol.* **65**:1370–1376.

Zagury, J. F., Bernard, J., Achour, A., Astgen, A., Lachgar, A., Fall, L., Carelli, C., Issing, W., Mbika, J.P., Picard, O., Carlotti, M., Callebaut, I., Mornon, J. P., Burny, A., Feldman, M., Bizzini, B., and Zagury, D., 1993, Identification of CD4 and major histocompatibility complex functional peptide sites and their homology with oligopeptides from human immunodeficiency virus type 1 glycoprotein gp120: Role in AIDS pathogenesis, *Proc. Natl. Acad. Sci. USA* **90**:7573–7577.

Zunich, K. M., Lane, H. C., Davey, R. T., Falloon, J., Polis, M., Kovacs, J. A., and Masur, H., 1992, Phase I/II studies of the toxicity and immunogenicity of recombinant gp160 and p24 vaccines in HIV-infected individuals, *AIDS Res. Hum. Retroviruses* **8(8)**:1335.

Chapter 4

Regulatory Considerations in Vaccine Design

Lawrence W. Davenport

1. INTRODUCTION

Vaccines, both those now approved and those that are in development, represent a variety of technologies, as shown in Table I. Earlier vaccines were preparations of killed, or inactivated, bacterial cells or viruses. Other early vaccines were preparations of bacterial toxoids. Often, it was not known why a vaccine worked, it was only known that it did. As knowledge of disease, immunology, and protection increased, vaccines became more sophisticated. Advances in technology led to vaccines that consisted of purified bacterial or viral antigens, and to live, attenuated viral vaccines. Conjugate technology allows a poorly immunogenic antigen to be coupled to a highly immunogenic carrier molecule. Recombinant technology allows an isolated antigen to be produced without the involvement of the pathogenic organism. Examples of approved vaccines and vaccines in development that illustrate the various technologies used to produce today's vaccines are also shown in Table I.

A single set of basic regulatory approval criteria apply to vaccines, regardless of the technology used to produce a vaccine. Vaccines are regulated in the United States by the Center for Biologics Evaluation and Research (CBER) of the Food and Drug Administration (FDA). The FDA requires that safety, purity, and potency must be established, as defined by the U.S. Code of Federal Regulations (CFR Title 21, Part 601), in order for a vaccine to be approved. As further defined in CFR Title 21, Part 600, safety is "the relative freedom from harmful effect to persons affected, directly or indirectly, by a product when prudently administered, taking into consideration the character of the product in relation to the condition of the recipient at the time." Purity is "relative freedom from extraneous matter in the finished product, whether or not harmful to the recipient or deleterious to the

Lawrence W. Davenport • Genentech, Inc., South San Francisco, California 94080.

Vaccine Design: The Subunit and Adjuvant Approach, edited by Michael F. Powell and Mark J. Newman. Plenum Press, New York, 1995.

Table I

Types of Vaccines[a]

Type of vaccine	Examples of approved vaccines		Examples of vaccines in development	
	Bacterial	Viral	Bacterial	Viral
Killed bacteria or viruses	Pertussis[2,4]	Influenza[2]		
	Typhoid[8]	Polio[2]		
Live, attenuated viruses		Yellow fever[2]		
		Polio[4]		
		Measles–mumps–rubella[5]		
Bacterial toxoids	Tetanus[2,4]			
	Diphtheria[2,4]			
Purified subunit (bacterial or viral)	Meningococcal polysaccharide (Groups A, C, Y, W135)[2,5]	Influenza[2,4,6,8]	Meningococcal polysaccharide (Group B)[2,5]	
			Pertussis (infants)[2,4]	
	Pertussis (children)[2,4]			
Conjugate	Haemophilus influenzae type b[2,4,5]			
Recombinant		Hepatitis B[5,7]		HIV-1 (gp120)[1,3]
				HSV[1,7]

[a] 1, Chiron; 2, Connaught; 3, Genentech; 4, Lederle; 5, Merck; 6, Parke–Davis; 7, SmithKline; 8, Wyeth.

product." Potency is "the specific ability or capacity of the product, as indicated by appropriate laboratory tests or by adequately controlled clinical data obtained through the administration of the product in the manner intended, to effect a given result." Simply put, in order to be approved, a vaccine must be a preparation of known characterization and purity that has been demonstrated to be safe and effective. The exact standards required to meet these criteria for a particular vaccine are dependent on the specific vaccine and the technology used to produce it. Specific "Additional Standards" exist in the CFR for certain vaccines.

This chapter will discuss the regulation of vaccines. Its purpose is to provide a background on the regulatory process involved in bringing a new vaccine through the clinical development and licensing processes. It is primarily intended as an introduction for individuals who are unfamiliar with the regulatory issues, and will focus on the regulation of vaccines in the United States. The principles of regulation as applied in the United States, however, are similar for other countries. Some details differ from country to country since, historically, each country has its own set of standards. However, as the development and use of drugs and biologics has become more global, so has the regulation of drugs and biologics become more global. Major efforts are currently under way to develop guidelines for the worldwide harmonization of regulations. Such guidelines, and international agreements, will eventually provide a basis for one set of rules for the development, regulatory evaluation, and approval of new drugs and biologics.

2. VACCINE DEVELOPMENT AND REGULATORY ISSUES

A general overview of vaccine development, outlining the significant steps of the process, is shown in Fig. 1. When a decision has been made that a candidate vaccine is ready to move into development, two parallel activities then take place. The process for making the vaccine in research must be developed into a process that is appropriate for the manufacture of clinical material. For example, purification procedures used in the manufacture must be amenable to scaleup and to regulatory approval. Modification of facilities may be required, and facility and process validation must meet the needs of the clinical program and, ultimately, the guideline for licensing. Manufacturing, quality (assurance and control), and regulatory input should be incorporated early in the development process.

Regulatory issues should be considered as early in the development process as possible, since ultimately, regulatory compliance is the basis for approval. While this may seem like an obvious statement, it is too often overlooked. A product that does not or cannot meet regulatory requirements for manufacturing and purity cannot be approved, regardless of the quality of the safety and efficacy data. Safety and efficacy data from studies that do not or cannot meet regulatory requirements for adequate, well-controlled studies do not lead to approval. Early attention to regulatory issues, including early and often contact with the FDA, avoids many of the problems that can lead to delays in the approval process.

The first regulatory requirements that must be considered are purity and preclinical safety, the two prerequisites to move a vaccine from the laboratory to the clinic. Both must be demonstrated prior to beginning clinical trials. The candidate vaccine must be well characterized and its purity demonstrated. The Investigational New Drug (IND) submission, which is described below in more detail, contains descriptions of the vaccine, the manufacture of the vaccine, control tests for release, and stability tests. Also included are a discussion of the scientific rationale for the vaccine, preclinical animal safety data, and the proposed Phase I clinical protocol. Control tests for release of the product include assays required by the CFR (general safety, sterility, pyrogens or endotoxin as appropriate) and assays developed by the manufacturer for characterization, chemical purity, and potency. Specifications for these latter tests must be developed as a basis for release of the vaccine for clinical study. Some specifications, such as for potency, will of necessity be preliminary, pending later correlation to clinical data. Characterization and chemical purity tests are chosen for their relevancy to the product, and may include various chromatography and electrophoresis techniques, specific ELISA procedures, protein assays, and the like. Potency assays measure biological activity or correlate to biological activity. Many potency assays are animal tests, involving the immunization of an appropriate animal species and evaluating the immune response by direct challenge of the animal or titration of the antibody concentration in the serum. For some vaccines, the total amount of antigen, or size of the antigen, or some other chemical parameter may correlate to biological activity.

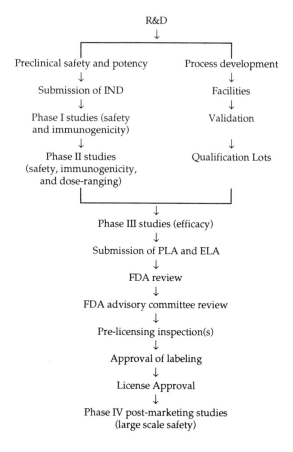

Figure 1. Vaccine development overview.

The general safety and sterility tests required by the FDA are required for all vaccines. Some vaccines, where appropriate, are also required to be tested for pyrogenic substances by intravenous injection into rabbits. The limulus amoebocyte lysate (LAL) assay for endotoxins may be substituted for the pyrogen test with the approval of the FDA when validation of the LAL assay in the presence of the product has been demonstrated. The general safety test, performed using guinea pigs and mice, is for the detection of extraneous toxic contaminants. The animals are injected with final product and observed over a 7-day period for survival, response, and weight gain. The test is satisfactory if all of the animals survive the test period, do not exhibit any response that is not specific for or expected from the product, and weigh no less at the end of the test period than at the time of injection. The sterility test is performed using a culture medium that provides favorable aerobic and anaerobic conditions for growth of microorganisms. The culture medium required in the test performed for the FDA is Fluid Thioglycolate Medium. Two types of test procedures can be used, direct inoculation and membrane filtration. In the direct inoculation test, product is inoculated into appropriate containers of growth media, which are then incubated for a period of no less than 14 days. In the membrane filtration test, product is filtered, the filtrate is discarded, and the filter (containing any retained microorganisms) is incubated in appropriate growth media for a period of no less than 7 days. The direct inoculation test requires that the ratio of media volume to test sample be large enough so that any preservative in the product will be diluted sufficiently so as not to interfere with the growth of any microorganisms that might be present. The membrane filtration test has the advantage of removing any preservative, and requires less incubation time. However, not all products are compatible with the membrane filtration procedure. For either procedure, a satisfactory test is where no growth is observed at any time during the test period.

Working with CBER during the time that control assays and preclinical safety protocols are being developed is critical since biologics in general, and vaccines specifically, tend to be unique products, with unique requirements. Guidelines exist for the general principles in developing and testing biologics, particularly biotechnology products. Specific standards of purity, potency, and preclinical safety, however, are often tailored to the specific product, and it is important that the manufacturer and the FDA are in agreement on the requirements that will be met. Additional controls are applied for characterizing purified antigen products and biotechnology products than are applied to killed bacteria vaccines, for instance. For example, the manufacturing process applied to recombinant vaccines must eliminate cell-associated impurities as technically feasible. Control assays must demonstrate the absence of these impurities, to the highest degree of sensitivity that is possible, and validation studies must demonstrate the safety of the final preparations. For less defined vaccines, such as killed whole bacteria preparations, demonstration of the absence of toxicity becomes the critical purity parameter. Obtaining prospective agreement with the FDA on these purity standards avoids many later problems.

Stability data for the IND must demonstrate that the vaccine is stable for the duration of the clinical study. Assays used to monitor stability may be the same or different than those used for product release. The key is that the stability-indicating assay(s) are relevant. An assay that assures high chemical purity of the vaccine antigen may be a critical product release test for freedom from extraneous matter, for instance, but may not be a relevant stability-indicating assay if degradation of the antigen over time does not correlate with potency of the vaccine. For example, an antigen that degrades over a 2-year shelf life to 50% of original chemical purity is stable, if the potency of the vaccine continues to meet specification. The vaccine must meet the minimum required potency specification, i.e., contain sufficient active antigen, that assures that the vaccine has satisfactory potency when administered at any time throughout the shelf life of the product. Another consideration when evaluating product stability is whether any of the degradation products are toxic. For instance, in the above example, if the breakdown products of the antigen cause toxicity, then chemical purity would be stability-indicating even though it does not correlate with potency. Stability-indicating assays must demonstrate that the vaccine remains both safe and effective throughout the dating period.

The clinical development of vaccines is carried out in four phases, as is the case for any drug or biologic. Vaccine development follows the same general scheme as drugs and other biologics, with some significant differences that will be discussed below. The general clinical development scheme for drugs and biologics is as follows. Initial studies, referred to as Phase I studies, are safety studies. Phase II studies are dose ranging studies that may provide early indications of efficacy. Phase I and II studies provide clinical research information that directs the development of the final formulation and dosing schedule; development may cycle between laboratory research and clinical research. Phase II studies are conducted in populations that provide an optimal opportunity to detect efficacy. Phase III studies are large-scale efficacy trials conducted in populations that represent the target population for the marketed product. Phase III studies provide the pivotal efficacy data that are required for licensing. For drugs and many biologics, the agency requires two adequate and well-controlled efficacy trials. The fourth phase, Phase IV, is generally a larger-scale postmarketing study conducted to obtain data on adverse events that may occur at very low frequency. Phase IV studies are not always required.

Vaccine clinical development, because of the nature of vaccines (which are designed to prevent infections, rather than to treat existing medical conditions), is unique compared to many other drugs and biologics, in that efficacy is not usually determined until Phase III. Phase I vaccine studies are safety and immunogenicity studies. The first studies are conducted in a small number of normal, healthy subjects who are at low risk for infection. Additional Phase I studies are conducted, as necessary, to provide safety data for evaluating the vaccine in additional populations. If the intended target population for the vaccine is infants, for instance, initial studies are usually conducted in adults, and additional studies are consecutively conducted in increasingly younger groups until the target population is reached. Such a scheme may include adults, followed by teens, followed by children, before testing in infants. In addition to safety data (local and systemic reactogenicity), Phase I studies provide initial human immunogenicity data. The objectives of Phase I and II studies tend to "blend together," with the distinction often being size of the study. For instance, evaluation of dose and schedule in the target population(s) may begin in Phase I and continue into Phase II. Phase II studies tend to include larger numbers of subjects as safety and immunogenicity are evaluated in subjects who are likely to be included in efficacy trials (Phase III). Phase II trials for vaccines are usually not sized large enough to obtain efficacy data.

The objective of Phase II vaccine trials is to determine the optimum dose and schedule to obtain maximum immunogenicity. If a laboratory correlate of protection for the target disease is known, either based on data derived from convalescent sera or derived from previous efficacy trials, estimates of efficacy can be made based on data for that correlate obtained during Phase I/II studies that provide support data for making the decision to proceed to Phase III. If no correlate information is available, such as in the case of HIV-1 where no convalescent sera are available to date (Haynes, 1993) or acellular pertussis where efficacy has been demonstrated but no correlate of protection has been found (Edwards, 1993), the decision to move to Phase III can be more difficult. The strength of the research data supporting the rationale for the vaccine, including animal models of protection, becomes critical.

Phase III efficacy trials for vaccines are conducted in large numbers of subjects. A small Phase III trial involves several hundred to several thousand participants; a large trial may involve tens of thousands of participants. The size and duration of the trial are determined by many factors, including the incidence of the infection (to allow detection of statistically significant efficacy), and a desire to understand the duration of protection afforded by a vaccine. In a double-blind, placebo-controlled trial, efficacy is calculated as the number of infections in the placebo group, minus the number of infections in the vaccinated group, divided by the number of infections in the placebo group. The number of infections needed to evaluate efficacy can be obtained by increasing the number of subjects or the duration of the trial. The higher the rate of infection in the high-risk study population, the smaller the study size and possibly the shorter the trial duration can be. The placebo group may be a true placebo, or may be another vaccine, as appropriate. Factors to be considered in the selection of a placebo include: (1) no approved vaccine currently exists that would preclude the use of a placebo, (2) no approved vaccine currently exists but another vaccine appropriate for the study population could be used as the placebo (subjects randomized to the placebo group will receive the benefit of the vaccine utilized as the placebo), or (3) an approved vaccine exists that must be used in comparison with the test vaccine.

A single large, multicenter vaccine efficacy trial that shows a high level of efficacy within reasonable 95% confidence limits is usually considered to be adequate efficacy data to support licensure in the United States. However, many vaccine efficacy trials must be conducted in foreign countries because of epidemiological considerations. In such cases, additional "bridging studies" must be conducted to provide a link between the vaccine-induced immune response elicited in the foreign efficacy study population and that elicited in the target population in the United States. Such comparisons of immunological data are easiest to interpret when an immunological correlate of protection was identified in the efficacy trial. The premise for the acceptability of the foreign efficacy data is the finding that the vaccine-induced immune response(s) in the U.S. target population is considered to be satisfactory in this comparison (Horne and Goldenthal, 1994).

Given the potential regulatory problems that can occur when vaccine efficacy trials are not conducted in the target population for which approval is sought, the question arises as to why such an efficacy trial would be conducted. The major reason is that situations exist where efficacy cannot be directly tested in the desired population, e.g., traveler's vaccines. Cohorts to study may not exist, incidences may be too low to design an adequate trial, or other approved vaccines may exist that preclude conducting a placebo-controlled trial, etc. In these cases, the efficacy trial may be conducted in another population, such as in another country, and bridging data are later developed for the primary target population.

A combination of an efficacy study and bridging study(studies) may provide the clearest route to approval. Approval of vaccines in the United States has been based on efficacy trials conducted in appropriate populations outside the United States. Bridging studies have provided safety and immunogenicity comparisons between the U.S. and outside the U.S. populations, as was the case with acellular pertussis vaccines (Marcinak *et al.*, 1993). Strategy considerations for clinical development of an AIDS vaccine also illustrate the point. Incidences of HIV-1 infection are higher outside the United States than inside. An efficacy trial conducted outside the United States may be smaller, and completed in a shorter period of time, than an efficacy trial conducted in the United States. Bridging data linking the outside the U.S. population to the U.S. population could provide the route to approval in the United States.

The final phase of clinical testing, Phase IV, is conducted after approval of the vaccine. Its primary purpose is to provide additional safety data for events that occur infrequently. Phase IV trials may also be used to evaluate breakthrough infections.

Evaluation of vaccine safety continues after the conclusion of formal clinical studies. Reports of adverse events for licensed vaccines are entered into the Vaccine Adverse Events Reporting System (VAERS), which is maintained by the FDA and the Centers for Disease Control and Prevention (CDC). These reports to VAERS can come from physicians,

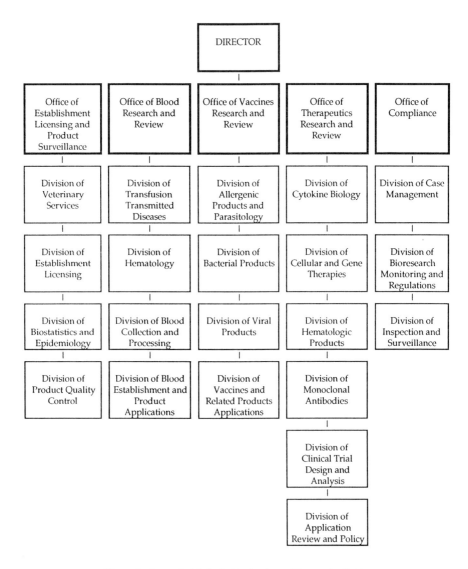

Figure 2. Center for Biologics Evaluation and Research (CBER)

manufacturers, and others. CBER and CDC staff monitor this data base for incidents of concern and patterns of events that appear to be vaccine-related. (Adverse reaction reports for investigational vaccines under IND are submitted to the IND.)

3. CENTER FOR BIOLOGICS EVALUATION AND RESEARCH

Vaccines in the United States are regulated as biologics by the Food and Drug Administration, Center for Biologics Evaluation and Research, Bethesda, Maryland. CBER, which was previously known as the Bureau of Biologics prior to the early 1980s, and as the Office of Biologics Research and Review during the 1980s, was created by the Public Health Service Act and was combined with the FDA in the 1970s. The pharmaceutical counterpart to CBER is the Center for Drugs Evaluation and Research (CDER). The FDA was created through the Federal Food, Drug, and Cosmetic Act (Parkman and Hardegree, 1994).

CBER is headed by a director who reports to the Commissioner of the FDA, and is organized into the following offices: the Office of Establishment Licensing and Product Surveillance, the Office of Blood Research and Review, the Office of Vaccines Research and Review, the Office of Therapeutics Research and Review, and the Office of Compliance (see Fig. 2). Each office is further organized into divisions. The Office of Vaccines Research and Review, which is responsible for the regulation of vaccines, consists of the Division of Allergenic Products and Parasitology, the Division of Bacterial Products, the Division of Viral Products, and the Division of Vaccines and Related Products Applications.

4. CODE OF FEDERAL REGULATIONS

Current authority for the regulation of vaccines resides in the Public Health Service Act and the Food, Drug, and Cosmetic Act (1980). The regulations used in implementing these acts are contained in Title 21 of the Code of Federal Regulations (1993). Title 21 of the Code of Federal Regulations (21CFR) consists of nine volumes (parts 1–99, 100–169, 170–199, 200–299, 300–499, 500–599, 600–799, 800–1299, and 1300–end). Table II lists parts of 21CFR that are applicable to the development, manufacture, licensure, and use of vaccines.

The CFR regulations cover the methods to be used in, and the facilities or controls to be used for, the manufacture, processing, packing, or holding of a drug to assure that such drug meets the requirements of the act as to safety, and has the identity and strength and meets the quality and purity characteristics that it purports or is represented to possess [21CFR210.1(a)]. These regulations detail the minimum requirements for the preparation of drug products for administration to humans or animals, and are referred to as the minimum Current Good Manufacturing Practices, or CGMPs (21CFR210 and 21CFR211). Minimum requirements for conducting nonclinical laboratory safety studies are termed Good Laboratory Practices, or GLPs (21CFR58). Minimum requirements for conducting clinical studies are referred to as Good Clinical Practices, or GCPs. There is no formal section in the CFR referred to as the GCPs; the requirements are taken from appropriate CFR sections covering protection of human subjects (21CFR50), institutional review

Table II
Code of Federal Regulations

21CFR parts 1–99, Subchapter A—General	
21CFR50	Protection of human subjects
21CFR56	Institutional review boards
21CFR58	Good laboratory practice for nonclinical laboratory studies
21CFR parts 200–299, Subchapter C—Drugs	
21CFR210	Current good manufacturing practice in manufacturing, processing, packing, or holding of drugs; general
21CFR211	Current good manufacturing practice for finished pharmaceuticals
21CFR parts 300–499, Subchapter D—Drugs For Human Use	
21CFR312	Investigational new drug application
21CFR parts 600–680, Subchapter F—Biologics	
21CFR600	Biological products: general
21CFR601	Licensing
21CFR610	General biological products standards
21CFR620	Additional standards for bacterial products
21CFR630	Additional standards for viral vaccines

boards (21CFR56), investigational new drug applications (21CFR312), and the Guideline for the Monitoring of Clinical Investigations issued by the FDA in 1988.

The minimum requirements (CGMPs, GLPs, and GCPs) emphasize practices to be followed, and documentation required to demonstrate that facilities, processes, studies, and products are in compliance with FDA regulations. Compliance with agency requirements for documentation is critical for establishing the validity of data submitted to the agency. The agency can establish the scientific merit of the data submitted in support of a vaccine only when the documentation demonstrates that the data are relevant to the facility, process, or study being reviewed.

5. INVESTIGATIONAL NEW DRUG APPLICATION

Ultimately, the goal of any vaccine development plan is to lead to an approved safe, efficacious vaccine. To this end, focusing on regulatory issues related to vaccines is important during the early research and development phases. Early and ongoing contact with CBER can therefore greatly facilitate making correct development decisions. The first formal contact with the agency requiring submission of documentation occurs when the vaccine under development is ready to move into clinical investigation. The documentation is referred to as the Investigational New Drug (IND) application, and the interaction with the FDA during the clinical investigation stage is often referred to as the IND process. The contents of the IND application are outlined in Table III.

The sponsor of an IND is the person or organization who is responsible for and initiates the clinical investigation. An organization sponsoring a clinical investigation may be a

Table III

IND Content and Format

Cover Sheet (Form FDA-1571)

Table of Contents

Introductory Statement and General Investigational Plan

Investigator's Brochure

Protocols

Chemistry, Manufacturing and Controls Information

Drug substance, including:

- Description, including its physical, chemical, or biological characteristics
- Name and address of the manufacturer
- General method of preparation
- Acceptable limits and analytical methods (identity, strength, quality, and purity)
- Data to support stability during the toxicological studies and the planned clinical studies

Drug product, including:

- List of all components used in the manufacture, and, where applicable, the quantitative composition of the investigational drug product
- Name and address of the manufacturer
- Brief general description of the manufacturing and packaging procedure
- Acceptable limits and analytical methods (identity, strength, quality, and purity)
- Data to assure the product's stability during the planned clinical studies
- Description of the composition, manufacture, and control of any placebo

Labeling

Environmental analysis requirements

Pharmacology and Toxicology Information

Previous Human Experience with the Investigational Drug

pharmaceutical company, governmental agency, academic institution, private organization, or other organization. The sponsor may or may not be the manufacturer of the vaccine. An investigator is an individual who actually conducts a clinical investigation. A sponsor-investigator is an individual who both initiates and conducts a clinical investigation.

As previously discussed, the vaccine must meet criteria for purity and safety prior to initiating a clinical investigation and the IND is the mechanism by which this information is submitted to CBER for review. Purity was discussed earlier in this chapter. Safety is determined in preclinical toxicity studies in one or more animal species. Traditionally, formal toxicity studies required for vaccines have been minimal, with a great deal of the preclinical safety data being derived from studies whose primary objective was immunogenicity. As vaccines from new technologies are being evaluated, traditional toxicity studies in one or more appropriate animal species, meeting GLP standards, have been required. The GLP regulations are contained in 21CFR58.

First contact with the agency should occur well in advance of the actual submission to allow time to resolve questions concerning the IND and its content. Submission of a complete document, containing all required studies and data, will eliminate avoidable delays in initiating clinical studies. A pre-IND meeting can be arranged with CBER to review available data and to discuss plans for completing the IND submission. This meeting should be used to determine that sufficient data have been developed, or are being developed, for the vaccine. This is also an opportunity to discuss the proposed clinical plan with the agency. Prospective agreement on the supporting data and clinical plan greatly facilitates the IND review process.

The agency has 30 days following receipt of the original IND application in which to complete the initial review. At the end of that time, a decision will be made either to approve the initiation of clinical studies, or to request that the sponsor supply additional information. In the event that additional information is required before approval to initiate the clinical investigation can be granted, the agency will place the initiation of clinical studies on hold until all outstanding issues are resolved. An IND can be placed on "clinical hold" at any time during the IND process. Furthermore, individual studies may be placed on hold, and others may be allowed to proceed, at the same time in the same IND. For example, Phase I and II studies may be ongoing while a Phase III study is not allowed to proceed until design issues are resolved.

The IND process is an interactive process, and the sponsor should take advantage of the opportunity to discuss issues with the agency. Many clinical investigations are placed on hold because a question was not asked of the agency early enough. The people at CBER are some of the best sources that companies can obtain input from for guiding their vaccine development programs.

6. PRODUCT LICENSE AND ESTABLISHMENT LICENSE APPLICATIONS

Although this chapter focuses primarily on regulatory considerations during the clinical investigation stage of vaccine development, some discussion of the license application is appropriate. The license application for biologics regulated by CBER actually consists of two submissions, the Product License Application (PLA) and the Establishment License Application (ELA). This contrasts with the New Drug Application (NDA) regulations required for drugs regulated by CDER.

Table IV
PLA Requirements

Data demonstrating that the manufactured product meets prescribed standards of safety, purity, and potency
    Nonclinical animal studies meet GLP requirements (Title 21, Part 58)
    Clinical studies meet requirements for institutional review (Title 21, Part 56) and informed consent (Title 21, Part 50)
Full description of manufacturing methods
Data establishing stability of the product through the dating period
Sample(s) representative of the product
Summaries of results of tests performed on the lot(s) represented by the submitted sample(s)
Specimens of the labels, enclosures, and containers proposed to be used for the product

Table V
ELA Requirements

Building and facilities
  Specific design and construction features of the various manufacturing areas
  Functions carried out in each room where storage, labeling, or manufacturing, including testing, occurs
  Construction of areas where sterile operations are performed (including functions, contamination control, and monitoring)
  Flow of personnel into and out of each area
  Water supply (including specifications and system validation)
  Air systems (including specifications and system validation)
Animal facilities
  What animals are used in the production or testing of products
  Animal quarantine procedures
  Disposal of animal waste
Work with microorganisms
  Microorganisms, including viruses, brought into or kept in the establishment
  Precautions taken with these microorganisms
Equipment
  Profile of major equipment used in manufacture and testing
  Materials and equipment sterilized by autoclave, dry heat, or other methods (including specifications and system validation)
  Methods of recording temperature of refrigerators, freezers, and incubators and frequency of calibration
  Methods used to clean and validate equipment used in processing and frequency of cleaning and calibration
Production and testing
  Products and methods used to prevent cross contamination in multiuse rooms
  Filling rooms and methods used to prevent contamination
  Storage and handling of unlabeled finished products
  Methods used to prevent errors during the labeling of products
  Selection and storage of retention samples
Records
  Manufacturing, sterilization, distribution records, and duration of retention
  Lot numbering system

The submission of the PLA and ELA, and subsequent steps in the review process, are shown in Fig. 1. The biological licensing regulations are contained in 21CFR601. The PLA contains data derived from nonclinical laboratory and clinical studies which demonstrate that the manufactured product meets prescribed standards of safety, purity, and potency. The PLA describes the manufacture of the vaccine and the results of the clinical trials conducted with the vaccine. Data from three or more qualification lots are provided in the application to demonstrate consistency of the manufacturing process. The ELA describes the facilities and controls for the facilities in which the product is manufactured. An overview of PLA requirements is shown in Table IV. ELA requirements are shown in Table V.

The license application review process includes (1) initial CBER review, (2) written dialog with CBER to respond to questions generated by the review, (3) meetings with

CBER as appropriate to discuss and resolve issues, (4) review by the CBER Vaccines Advisory Committee at one or more meetings, (5) prelicensing inspections of the manufacturing facilities and key clinical investigation sites, (6) review and approval of labeling, and (7) release of vaccine lots submitted with the license application. The Vaccines Advisory Committee reviews the data supporting the safety, purity, and potency of the vaccine, and provides nonbinding recommendations to the agency on the approvability of the product. While a vaccine that receives a recommendation for approval from the Vaccines Advisory Committee may not necessarily receive approval from CBER, pending the outcome of CGMP issues, a vaccine that does not receive a recommendation for approval will not gain regulatory approval.

7. GUIDELINE AND POINTS TO CONSIDER DOCUMENTS

In addition to the CFR the FDA has also issued guidelines that establish principles or practices of general applicability. Guidelines state procedures or standards of general applicability that are not legal requirements but are acceptable to the FDA. Guidelines have been issued that relate to performance characteristics, preclinical and clinical test procedures, manufacturing practices, product standards, scientific protocols, compliance criteria, and so forth. Guidelines relevant to the manufacture and testing of vaccines are listed below. In general the guidelines are issued by CDER. As such they are most relevant to the regulation of drugs, although many of the guidelines encompass issues relevant to both drugs and biologics. Points to Consider documents issued by CBER cover issues specific to biologics.

Following is a listing and brief outline of some of the Guidelines and Points to Consider that are relevant to vaccines:

- Guideline for the Format and Content of the Chemistry, Manufacturing, and Controls Section of an Application (1987). This guideline is intended to assist manufacturers in preparing the chemistry, manufacturing, and controls section of applications. While the guideline was written in support of New Drug Applications (NDA) for drugs, it is nevertheless useful in preparing similar information for biologics applications. The section covers composition, manufacture, and specifications of the product, including its physical and chemical characteristics and stability.
- Guideline for Submitting Documentation for the Stability of Human Drugs and Biologics (1987). This guideline provides guidance in submitting documentation for the stability of human drugs and biologics. The guideline provides a means of developing expiration dating from at least three different batches of the drug product. Estimated expiration dating periods must be confirmed by the manufacturer by continual assessment of stability properties.
- Guideline for Submitting Documentation for Packaging for Human Drugs and Biologics (1987). This guideline provides manufacturers with criteria for use in the preparation of information on the fabrication and quality of containers and container components.

- Guideline on the Preparation of Investigational New Drug Products (Human and Animal) (1991). This guideline provides information on certain practices and procedures for the preparation of sterile drug products by aseptic processing relevant to compliance with sections of the CGMP regulations for finished pharmaceuticals (21CFR210 and 211). Although specific for drugs, it does provide useful information that can be applied to biologics.
- Guideline on Sterile Drug Products Produced by Aseptic Processing (1987). This guideline provides information relevant to compliance with sections of the CGMP regulations for finished pharmaceuticals (21CFR210 and 211). Biological products comply with 21CFR parts 600 through 680 where they are different from 21CFR Parts 210 and 211.
- Guideline on General Principles of Process Validation (1987). This guideline discusses process validation elements and concepts that are considered by the FDA as acceptable parts of a validation program. Although specific for drugs, it does provide useful information that can be applied to biologics.
- Guideline on Validation of the Limulus Amebocyte Lysate Test as an End-Product Endotoxin Test for Human and Animal Parenteral Drugs, Biological Products, and Medical Devices (1987). This guideline sets forth acceptable conditions for use of the LAL test, providing for the use of the LAL test in lieu of the rabbit pyrogen test.
- Guideline for the Monitoring of Clinical Investigations (1988). This guideline presents acceptable approaches to monitoring clinical investigations. Proper monitoring is necessary to assure adequate protection of the rights and safety of human subjects involved in clinical investigations. Compliance ensures the quality and integrity of the resulting data submitted to the FDA.
- Points to Consider in the Characterization of Cell Lines Used to Produce Biologicals (1987). This guideline describes tests that are pertinent to demonstrating the acceptability of a cell line for use in production of a biological product. Because advances in biotechnology are occurring at a rapid pace, the information provided represents general expectations of manufacturers.
- Points to Consider in the Production and Testing of New Drugs and Biologicals Produced by Recombinant DNA Technology (1985). This guideline provides information for evaluating safety, purity, and potency of new drugs and biologics produced by recombinant DNA technology. Because advances in biotechnology are occurring at a rapid pace, the information provided represents general expectations of manufacturers.

8. SUMMARY

To summarize, vaccines are regulated in the United States as biologics by CBER and must meet requirements for safety, purity, and potency (efficacy). Although general requirements exist for safety, purity, and potency, specific standards for each vaccine are agreed to by the manufacturer and CBER. The final standards for any vaccine are relevant to the technology used to produce the vaccine. Vaccine efficacy is demonstrated through conducting one or more Phase III trials. A single, definitive, well-controlled, double-blind, placebo-controlled Phase III trial often provides sufficient efficacy data for licensing a vaccine. Pivotal efficacy data may be derived from U.S. or outside the U.S. studies. Bridging studies may be required to link the efficacy data to the intended marketing target population.

In the United States, approval for conducting clinical trials is obtained from the FDA through the mechanism of the IND application. Marketing approval is obtained through the mechanism of the PLA and ELA. Postmarketing Phase IV clinical trials are generally requested to develop large-scale field data for safety. Timely communication with the FDA throughout the development and approval process is the most efficient mechanism for meeting all regulatory requirements in the shortest possible time.

REFERENCES

Code of Federal Regulations, Title 21, 1993, Government Printing Office, Washington, DC.

Edwards, K. M., 1993, Acellular pertussis vaccines—A solution to the pertussis problem? *J. Infect. Dis.* **168**:15–20.

Federal Food Drug and Cosmetic Act: amended to include PHS, Biological Products Section 351 and 352, 1980, Government Printing Office, Washington, DC.

Haynes, B. F., 1993, Scientific and social issues of human immunodeficiency virus vaccine development, *Science* **260**:1279–1286.

Horne, A. D., and Goldenthal, K. L., 1994, Clinical and statistical considerations for evaluating preventive vaccines: Selected current topics, Presented at the 15th Annual Meeting of the Society for Clinical Trials, Houston, TX, May 10, 1994.

Marcinak, J. F., Ward, M., Frank, A. L., Boyer, K. M., Froeschle, J. E., and Hosbach, P. H., 4th, 1993, Comparison of the safety and immunogenicity of acellular (BIKEN) and whole-cell pertussis vaccines in 15- to 20-month-old children, *Am. J. Dis. Child.* **147**:290–294.

Parkman, P. D., and Hardegree, M. C., 1994, Regulation and testing of vaccines, in: *Vaccines*, 2nd ed. (S. A. Plotkin and E. A. Mortimer, Jr., eds.), Saunders, Philadelphia, pp. 889–901.

Chapter 5

Clinical Considerations in Vaccine Trials with Special Reference to Candidate HIV Vaccines

Patricia E. Fast, Leigh A. Sawyer, and Susan L. Wescott

1. INTRODUCTION

Clinical research on HIV-1 vaccine candidates, which began less than a decade ago, illustrates many facets of vaccine trials in general. At each step, however, from gaining public acceptance for the trial and recruiting volunteers to evaluation of data, unique problems have arisen. In this chapter, we will discuss clinical evaluation of HIV-1 vaccines as both a paradigm and a special case of vaccine clinical trials. We will emphasize prophylactic use of vaccines.

Discovery, development, and use of an HIV-1 vaccine will be a formidable task even though recent advances in immunology and molecular virology have given scientists powerful tools with which to explore HIV-1 pathogenesis and develop an AIDS vaccine. As do all retroviruses, HIV-1 has an RNA genome that is reverse transcribed by a viral enzyme to produce a DNA copy; this copy is then integrated into the host's genome, where it may remain quiescent or actively produce new viral RNA which then codes for viral proteins or is incorporated into new viral particles. Several unique features of HIV-1 will make vaccine development difficult: (1) there is, apparently, no recovery from the disease, so vaccines cannot be designed to mimic a state of naturally induced immunity to reinfection; (2) there are at least five to seven major groups (clades) of HIV-1, and novel viral variants continually arise within these clades by mutation; (3) the virus can travel directly between cells; and (4) the immune responses that would protect against HIV-1

Patricia E. Fast, Leigh A. Sawyer, and Susan L. Wescott • Vaccine and Prevention Research Program, Division of AIDS, National Institute of Allergy and Infectious Diseases, National Institutes of Health, Bethesda, Maryland 20892.

Vaccine Design: The Subunit and Adjuvant Approach, edited by Michael F. Powell and Mark J. Newman. Plenum Press, New York, 1995.

infection, especially by sexual transmission or by exposure to infected cells (rather than free virus), are unknown.

Successful vaccines usually prevent disease rather than infection. After successful vaccination, most pathogens can establish an initial infection, but their growth is arrested by the immune system before they cause significant pathology (Ada *et al.*, 1992). In some situations, passively administered preformed antibody can be protective, suggesting that antibodies may completely prevent the pathogen from establishing an infection and replicating, so-called "sterilizing immunity." Subclinical infection may, nevertheless, occur in individuals protected by passive immunization. For example, individuals suboptimally immunized against hepatitis B may develop antibody to core antigens, indicating that they have been infected, without clinical manifestations or chronic infection (Francis *et al.*, 1982; Szmuness *et al.*, 1981). Some scientists feel that sterilizing immunity, i.e., the prevention of infection of even one cell, is necessary for protection against HIV-1 disease (Sabin, 1993); recent evidence that simian immunodeficiency virus (SIV) infection can be transient (Pauza *et al.*, 1994; Miller *et al.*, 1994) and that immunologic responses to HIV-1 can be found in some exposed but "uninfected" individuals (Clerici, 1993) has called this view into question. See recent reviews (Ada, 1992a,b; Bolognesi, 1993; Letvin, 1993; Karzon *et al.*, 1992; Haynes, 1993; Oxford *et al.*, 1993; Hoth, 1993; Katzenstein *et al.*, 1988) for a more complete discussion. In this chapter, we will discuss how the complex issues of HIV-1 biology and epidemiology affect vaccine clinical trials. We will present background information on AIDS vaccines, then in subsequent sections we will discuss general issues related to clinical trials and their specific application to HIV-1 vaccines.

2. VACCINE CANDIDATES CURRENTLY IN CLINICAL TRIALS

2.1. Vaccine Candidates Other Than HIV-1

At present, more than 30 vaccines are licensed and distributed for use in the United States, and several others are used worldwide. Most are attenuated or killed whole organisms, bacterial capsular polysaccharides, or inactivated toxins. Table I describes currently licensed viral vaccines. Immunization with smallpox vaccine is no longer recommended because of successful eradication of smallpox by vaccination campaigns (Smallpox Vaccine, 1985). Many candidate vaccines (viral and bacterial) are now in clinical trials; some trials include licensed vaccines for comparison (Table II). Some candidate vaccines will be, if effective, the first vaccine against a particular disease; others are being developed as safer, less expensive, or more effective versions of existing vaccines or as combined vaccines (Ellis and Douglas, 1994; Douglas, 1993; Combined Vaccines and Simultaneous Administration, 1995).

The first human vaccine was a live bovine virus, relatively nonpathogenic in humans, used to protect against the closely related smallpox virus (Jenner, 1959). Similarly, bacillus Calmette–Guérin (BCG) is a bovine strain of *Mycobacterium* with some immunologic resemblance to agents of human tuberculosis and leprosy (Fine, 1988). Most vaccines, however, have been produced from human pathogens. Attenuated pathogens were traditionally produced by empiric means, without a detailed understanding of the molecular

Table I

Viral Vaccines Licensed and Currently Distributed in the United States

Vaccine	Description (virus, component, treatment)	Source	Manufacturer
Adenovirus (types 4 & 7)[a]	Live, oral trilayered tablet	W1-38 (human diploid fibroblasts)	Wyeth[b]
Hepatitis A	Whole virus, formalin	MRC-5 (human diploid fibroblasts)	SK[c]
Hepatitis B	Recombinant, HBsAg	Saccharomyces cerevisiae	Merck,[d] SK
Influenza A & B	Whole virus, formalin	Chick embryo allantoic fluid	CLI[e]
Influenza A & B	Split virus, formalin/Triton X-100	Chick embryo allantoic fluid	CLI
Influenza A & B	Split virus, formalin/ether	Chick embryo allantoic fluid	Parke-Davis[f]
	Split virus, formalin/tri-n-butylphosphate	Chick embryo allantoic fluid	Wyeth
Influenza A & B	Surface Ag, β-propiolactone/Triton N101	Chick embryo allantoic fluid	Evans[g], Lederle[h]
Japanese encephalitis	Nakayama NIH strain, formalin	Mouse brain	BIKEN[i]
Measles[j]	Live, Edmonston B	1° chick embryo fibroblasts	Merck
Mumps[j]	Live, Jeryl Lynn	1° chick embryo fibroblasts	Merck
Rubella[j]	Live, RA 27/3	W1-38 (human diploid fibroblasts)	Merck
Poliovirus trivalent	Live, oral Sabin types 1, 2, and 3	1° Cercopithecus kidney cells	Lederle
Poliovirus trivalent	Mahoney, MEF-1, Saukett, formalin	MRC-5 (human diploid fibroblasts)	CLL[k]
Poliovirus trivalent	Mahoney, MEF-1, Saukett, formalin	VERO (Cercopithecus kidney cells)	PM[l]
Rabies	Pitman-Moore strain, β-propiolactone	MRC-5 (human diploid fibroblasts)	PM
Rabies	SAD strain, β-propiolactone	MRC-5 (human diploid fibroblasts)	CLL
Rabies, adsorbed	CVS strain, β-propiolactone	Fetal rhesus lung cells	Michigan[m]
Smallpox (vaccinia)	Live, NYBH strain	Calf lymph	Wyeth[n]
Yellow fever	Live, 17D strain	Chick embryo	CLI

[a] Recommended for use in the United States Armed Forces.
[b] Wyeth-Ayerst Laboratories, Inc.
[c] SmithKline Beecham Biologicals.
[d] Merck Sharp & Dohme, Division of Merck & Co., Inc.
[e] Connaught Laboratories, Inc., A Pasteur Merieux Company.
[f] Parke–Davis, Division of Warner–Lambert Company.
[g] Evans Medical Limited.
[h] Lederle–Praxis Biologicals, A Cyanamid Business Unit.
[i] BIKEN, The Research Foundation for Microbial Diseases of Osaka University.
[j] Available as combined vaccines: measles/rubella, measles/mumps, measles/mumps/rubella, rubella/mumps.
[k] Connaught Laboratories Limited. A Pasteur Merieux Company.
[l] Pasteur Merieux Serums et Vaccins, S. A.
[m] Michigan Department of Public Health.
[n] Distribution is restricted by the National Centers for Disease Control.

Table II
Vaccines Other than HIV, in Clinical Trials[a]

Target agent	Vaccine approaches	Target agent	Vaccine approaches
		BACTERIAL	
Bordetella pertussis	Purified pertussis antigens, pertussis toxin (PT), filamentous hemagglutinin (FHA), pertactin, agglutinogens in various combinations[b]	*Mycobacterium leprae*	BCG plus heat-killed *Mycobacterium leprae* Heat-killed, purified *Mycobacterium leprae* Live, cross-reacting atypical mycobacteria
	Inactivated, nontoxic, PT vaccine and PT recombinant	*Mycobacterium tuberculosis*	*Mycobacterium vaccae*
	Purified PT and FHA[b]	*Neisseria meningitidis* A and C	Several glycoconjugates
	Purified PT, FHA, pertactin, agglutinogen 2 and 3	*Neisseria meningitidis* B	Glycoconjugate plus *Neisseria meningitidis* protein antigens
	Purified PT, FHA, pertactin and recombinant PT, FHA, pertactin	*Pseudomonas aeruginosa* and *P. cepacia*	Purified bacterial proteins, including flagellar antigen, LPS-O, porins, several inactivated bacterial toxins, and high-molecular-weight polysaccharide antigens and glycoconjugate
	Diphtheria–Tetanus–Pertussis (DTP) (whole cell)-Hib (conjugate)[b]		
	DTP (whole cell)-Hib (conjugate)-hepatitis B vaccine (HBV)	*Salmonella typhi*	Vi carbohydrate[c]
	DTP (whole cell)-inactivated poliovirus vaccine (IPV)		Vi carbohydrate–protein conjugate Live, attenuated Ty21a[c] Live, attenuated auxotrophic mutants
	DTP (whole cell)-Hib (conjugage)-HBV-IPV	*Shigella* (all species)	Polysaccharide–protein conjugate
Borrelia burgdorferi	Purified Osp A	*Shigella flexneri/sonnei*	*E. coli* hybrids
Enterotoxigenic *E. coli* (ETEC)	Nontoxigenic ETEC derivative, live, attenuated	*Streptococcus* Group A	M peptides linked to toxin subunit carrier M protein expressed in bacterial vector Multivalent M peptide hybrid constructs
	Killed cell and B subunit	*Streptococcus* Group B	Glycoconjugate vaccines of type 1a, 1b, II, III, and V to a carrier protein
Haemophilus influenzae type b (Hib)	Glycoconjugate of Hib capsular oligosaccharide linked to diphtheria CRM197 (HbOC)[c]		
	Glycoconjugate of Hib pure polysaccharide (PRP) and diphtheria toxoid (PRP-D)[c]	*Streptococcus pneumoniae*	Glycoconjugate vaccine (4,6B,9N,14,18C, 19F,23F) conjugated to meningococcal B OMP
	Glycoconjugate of Hib PRP and tetanus toxoid (PRP-TT)[c]		Glycoconjugate vaccine (6B,14,19,23F) conjugated to tetanus toxoid

	VIRAL

Organism / Disease	Vaccine
	Glycoconjugate of Hib capsular polysaccharide and *Neisseria meningitidis* outer membrane protein complex (Hib-OMPC)[c]
	Glycoconjugate vaccine (6B,14,18C,19F) conjugated to CRM197
Vibrio cholerae (01)	Killed bacteria (type 01) plus toxin B subunit
	Live (type 01), recombinant
Vibrio cholerae (0139)	Live (type 0139), recombinant
Cytomegalovirus	Live, attenuated
	Glycoprotein subunit vaccine
Dengue	Live, attenuated
Encephalitis virus	
Venezuelan equine	Inactivated, whole virus particles
	Infectious clones
Eastern equine	Inactivated, whole virus particles
Western equine	Inactivated, whole virus particles
Epstein–Barr	Glycoprotein subunit (gp350)
	Vaccinia recombinant virus expressing gp350
	Peptide induction of CTL
Hepatitis A	Inactivated HAV particles[c]
	Live, attenuated
Hepatitis B	HBV proteins expressed in yeast cells by rDNA[c]
	Salmonella
Herpes simplex types 1 and 2	Attenuated/recombinant
	Extract
	gD/recombinant
Influenza	Cold-adapted live, attenuated
	Purified viral hemagglutin (HA) subunit
	Purified "CTL" specific peptides
	Microencapsulated inactivated vaccine
	Liposome containing viral HA
	Purified, inactivated viral neuraminidase
	Baculovirus expressed recombinant HA subunit
Japanese B encephalitis	Whole, inactivated virus particles[c]
Measles	Live, attenuated[c]
	High titer, live (multiple strains)
	Poxvirus vector, live
Parainfluenza	Cold-adapted PIV3 attenuated virus
	Bovine attenuated
	Purified HN and F protein subunit vaccine
Poliovirus	Live, attenuated (oral)[c]
	Inactivated[c]
	Enhanced potency inactivated[c]
	Inactivated cell culture[c]
Rabies	Purified, F protein
Respiratory syncytial virus	Live, attenuated ts and/or ca strains
Rotavirus	Attenuated human/rhesus reassortant viruses
	Attenuated human rotavirus (cold-adapted)
	Attenuated bovine/human virus reassortants (WC3)
	Human nursery strains
Rubella	Live, attenuated[c]
Varicella zoster	Live, attenuated
Yellow fever	Live, attenuated[c]

(continued)

Table II
(Continued)

Target agent	Vaccine approaches		Target agent	Vaccine approaches
	FUNGAL			
Coccidioides immitis	Formalin-killed spherules			
	PARASITIC			
Leishmania sp.	Attenuated and killed whole parasites			Blood stage antigens
Plasmodium sp.	Circumsporozoite antigen expressed in several vectors			Circumsporozoite (CS) antigen
				Combination vaccines incorporating different stage specific antigens
	Gametocyte antigens			

[a]Adapted from the Jordan Report. Accelerated Development of Vaccines, 1994, Division of Microbiology and Infectious Diseases, NIAID, NIH, Bethesda, pp. 90–99.
[b]One form of this formulation exists as a licensed product.
[c]Vaccine licensed for use in the United States.

basis for the attenuation; an example is Sabin strain poliovirus (Sabin *et al.*, 1954). Now, scientists may be able to identify genes that are required for virulence, but not for growth, and remove or alter them selectively; examples include the transformation of vaccinia to NYVAC (Tartaglia *et al.*, 1992), the deletion of *nef* from SIV (Desrosiers, 1992), and development of attenuated *Salmonella typhi* (see Levine, 1991; Cardenas and Clements, 1992, for review).

Recently, newer methods for making viral vaccines have been developed: production of recombinant proteins (subunits) or viruslike particles (pseudovirions) by genetic engineering techniques, deliberate attenuation by deletion of known genetic sequences, introduction of genes from pathogens into live bacteria or replication-competent viruses (recombinant vectors), and synthesis of peptides that represent critical antigenic determinants (epitopes). A novel vaccine approach, direct introduction of DNA coding for one or more proteins into muscle or skin, is in preclinical development (Liu and Vogel, 1994; Wang *et al.*, 1993; Haynes *et al.*, 1993).

2.2. Types of HIV-1 Vaccine Trials: Preventive, Therapeutic, and Perinatal

HIV-1 vaccines are being evaluated for two different uses: prevention and therapy. The traditional, *preventive* approach will be to administer the HIV-1 vaccines to uninfected individuals in order to prevent subsequent infection and/or disease. In contrast, vaccination could be used to prevent infection of potentially exposed individuals, i.e., *postexposure* vaccination as for rabies and tetanus. These interventions might include the use of immune globulin to provide passive antibody protection until active immunity could develop. In *therapeutic* vaccination, individuals infected with HIV-1 may be vaccinated in an attempt to modulate the immune system and prevent disease progression after HIV-1 infection has been established. Another potential goal of vaccination is to *prevent* mother-to-infant HIV-1 transmission. This might be achieved either by vaccinating HIV-1-infected women, prior to or during pregnancy, to stimulate the immune response to their own virus or by vaccinating their newborn infants (Section 4.11). In this chapter, we will emphasize development of vaccines intended for uninfected individuals, because there is a strong historical precedent for success in disease prevention through prophylactic use of vaccines. Therapeutic vaccine trials will be discussed separately (Section 5.2).

2.3. HIV-1 Vaccine Candidates

The most extensively evaluated HIV-1 vaccines are recombinant envelope vaccines. Several recombinant envelope proteins have been evaluated in Phase I/II trials, including both gp160 and gp120, produced in baculovirus, yeast, and mammalian expression systems. These vaccines appear to be safe, all induce cell-mediated immunity as revealed by lymphocyte proliferation and immunologic memory, and all induce antibodies that bind the antigen (Dolin *et al.*, 1991; Kovacs *et al.*, 1993; Schwartz *et al.*, 1993b; Wintsch *et al.*, 1991; Belshe *et al.*, 1993, 1994c). The mammalian gp120 vaccines (Schwartz *et al.*, 1993b; Belshe *et al.*, 1994c; Kahn *et al.*, 1993; Graham *et al.*, 1993a) and at least one mammalian gp160 (Salmon *et al.*, 1993) consistently induce antibodies that neutralize HIV-1 in conventional assays using laboratory strains of HIV-1 grown in transformed T cells. Neutralization of fresh isolates of HIV-1 grown in PBMC has proved much more difficult (reviewed in Golding *et al.*, 1994).

The more than 20 HIV-1 vaccine candidates undergoing active evaluation in clinical trials are listed in Table III. Several recent reviews discuss these trials in detail (Walker and Fast, 1994; Birx *et al.*, 1994; Burke, 1993; Fast and Walker, 1993; Slade, 1993; Haynes, 1993; Letvin, 1993; Cease and Berzofsky, 1994; Hoth, 1993; Karzon, 1994). The vaccine candidates have been produced by a variety of methods, including inactivation and purification of whole HIV-1 (Race *et al.*, 1993; Salk, 1991; Trauger *et al.*, 1994). Cloning and expression of the recombinant envelope proteins gp160 (Barrett *et al.*, 1989; Kieny *et al.*, 1986; Cochran *et al.*, 1987) and gp120 (Lasky *et al.*, 1986; Haigwood *et al.*, 1992) or the core protein p24 either alone or as a self-assembling viruslike particle (Adams *et al.*, 1987), have employed yeast, bacterial, insect, and mammalian cells. In addition, poxviruses (vaccinia, attenuated vaccinia and canarypox) have been genetically engineered to express gp160 or multiple genes including envelope, core proteins, and some portions of the virus-encoded enzymes and regulatory genes (Adams and Paoletti, 1993; Hu *et al.*, 1986, 1991; Tartaglia *et al.*, 1993; Hesselton *et al.*, 1992; Earl *et al.*, 1991). New vaccine strategies that may soon enter trials include HIV-1 pseudovirions produced by mammalian cell lines transfected with portions of the HIV-1 genome (Rovinski *et al.*, 1992; Panicali *et al.*, 1992) and "T-B" peptides that incorporate T-cell and B-cell epitopes either from discontiguous portions of the envelope or from two different HIV-1 proteins (Palker *et al.*, 1988; Berzofsky *et al.*, 1988).

In addition, many recombinant live bacterial and viral vectors bearing one or more HIV-1 gene(s) are in preclinical development (see Walker and Fast, 1994, for review). Recently, natural or artificially produced attenuated mutants of SIV have protected monkeys against superinfection with virulent SIV (Marthas *et al.*, 1992; Daniel *et al.*, 1992). Work with the HIV-1 analogue has begun in chimpanzees (R. Desrosiers, personal communication). Another novel vaccine strategy, DNA (or genetic or polynucleotide) vaccination, is being developed for HIV-1. Polynucleotides coding for the vaccine antigen of interest are either injected intramuscularly (Robinson *et al.*, 1993; Wang *et al.*, 1993; Wolff *et al.*, 1990) or coated onto tiny gold spheres and propelled from a "gun" into the epidermis (Haynes *et al.*, 1994). DNA vaccines offer the potential ability to design a vaccine using any number of desired sequences and to deliver it with a small amount of heat-stable, relatively inexpensive material. The ease with which the nucleic acid sequence of DNA can be altered makes it ideally suited for vaccination against a pathogen as variable as HIV-1.

2.4. Sequential Use of Different Vaccines in One Regimen

One feature of the search for an HIV-1 vaccine has been highly unusual: the sequential use of different types of vaccines in one vaccination regimen. The goal is to enlist both antibodies and cell-mediated immunity to combat HIV-1. In theory, neutralizing antibodies would prevent the entry of most virus particles into cells. Addition of cytotoxic lymphocytes may be necessary to destroy infected cells expressing HIV-1 antigens, although cells harboring integrated HIV-1 DNA and expressing no viral antigens would not be destroyed. Primary immunization with recombinant vaccinia-gp160 (Graham *et al.*, 1992; Cooney *et*

Table III

AIDS Vaccine Candidates Undergoing Evaluation in Clinical Trials

Vaccine candidate	Expression system/production method	HIV strain	Adjuvant or delivery system	Vaccine developer
Envelope proteins/peptides:				
rgp160	Insect/baculovirus	LAI[a]	alum	MicroGeneSys
rgp160	Monkey kidney/vaccinia	LAI	alum + DOC[b]	Immuno AG
rgp160	Monkey kidney/vaccinia	MN	alum + DOC	Immuno AG
rgp160	Mammalian	MN/LAI[c]	alum or IFA[d]	Pasteur–Merieux–Connaught (Transgene)
rgp120 (Env 2-3)	Yeast	SF2	MF59 ± MTP-PE	Biocine
rgp120	Chinese hamster ovary	SF2	MF59 ± MTP-PE[e]	Biocine
rgp120	Chinese hamster ovary	LAI	alum	Genentech
rgp120	Chinese hamster ovary	MN	alum ± QS21	Genentech
V3–PPD	Synthetic peptide coupled to PPD[f]	MN	—	Swiss Serum & Vaccine Institute
		5 strains	—	Swiss Serum & Vaccine Institute
V3–toxin A	Synthetic peptide coupled to *Pseudomonas aeruginosa* toxin A	MN	—	Swiss Serum & Vaccine Institute
V3	Synthetic	MN	alum or IFA	Pasteur–Merieux–Connaught
V3–MAPS[g]	Synthetic	MN	alum	United Biomedical, Inc.
		15 strains	alum	United Biomedical, Inc.
V3 peptide	Synthetic[h] (RP400c)	MN	alum	Repligen
Core protein/peptides				
HGP-30	Synthetic p17 peptide	LAI	alum	Viral Technologies, Inc.
Ty.p24.VLP	Portion p17/p24 + yeast transposon product	LAI	alum/none	British Bio-tech. Ltd.
Lipopeptide	Synthetic peptide	LAI	DMSO/glycerol	United Biomedical, Inc.

(continued)

Table III
(continued)

Vaccine candidate	Expression system/production method	HIV strain	Adjuvant or delivery system	Vaccine developer
Recombinant poxvirus				
vac–gp160	Recombinant vaccinia	LAI	—	Bristol–Myers
CP–gp160	Recombinant canarypox	MN	—	Pasteur–Merieux–Connaught
CP–env, gag, protease	Recombinant canarypox	MN/LAI	—	Pasteur–Merieux–Connaught
Retroviral vectors				
MoMLV-HIV-1 env, rev	Recombinant murine retrovirus[h]	LAI	—	Viagene, Inc.
Whole inactivated HIV-1				
Whole inactivated HIV-1, envelope depleted	Inactivated with β-propiolactone and γ-irradiation[h]	Z321	IFA	Immune Response Corp.
CD4 as immunogen				
Recombinant CD4	*E. coli*[h]	—	IFA	Biogen, Inc.
Anti-idiotype approach				
Anti-gp120 (C39)	Murine monoclonal antibody[h]	—	SAF-M[i]	IDEC
Anti-CD4 idiotype (IOT4a)	Murine monoclonal antibody[h]	—	alum	Immunotech SA

[a]LAI, group of closely related HIV-1 isolates which includes LAV, IIIB, BRU, etc.
[b]Deoxycholate.
[c]Hybrid molecule.
[d]Incomplete Freund's adjuvant.
[e]Also with 5 other adjuvants.
[f]Purified protein derivative of *Mycobacterium*.
[g]Multiple Antigen Presentation System.
[h]Trials enrolling HIV-infected volunteers only.
[i]Syntex adjuvant formulation.

al., 1993) followed by boosting with recombinant gp160 protein antigen can induce, in humans (Cooney *et al.*, 1993; Graham *et al.*, 1993b) and nonhuman primates (Hu *et al.*, 1993), both neutralizing antibodies and CD8$^+$ cytotoxic lymphocytes (the lymphocyte class thought most likely to kill infected cells). In macaques, vaccinia-expressed envelope, core, and polymerase protein priming followed by a pseudovirion boost induced both neutralizing antibody and gag-specific CTL (Panicali *et al.*, 1992). Thus far, in clinical trials employing this strategy, only a fraction of immunized volunteers have produced CD8$^+$ CTL. This approach is now being extended to multiple components of HIV-1; a recombinant vaccinia containing *env, gag*, and a portion of *pol* and an analogous canarypox vaccine have just entered Phase I trials.

3. CLINICAL STUDIES OF VACCINE CANDIDATES

3.1. Approach to Vaccine Trials

The most desirable means of developing a vaccine is to understand which immune response protects against the infection or disease and to learn to produce that response, known as the *correlate of immunity* or *correlate of protection*, first in animals and then in humans. To employ this rational approach, vaccine developers must be able to measure an immune response that represents the true mechanism of immunity or a surrogate immune response that accompanies the development of protective immunity (even though it is not the actual mechanism). The approach may succeed, even if the response measured is not truly responsible for protection, provided the vaccine induces other, unmeasured, immune responses that can protect. An alternative approach is more empiric in nature. A vaccine resembling the pathogen may be produced, shown to be safe, and to induce some measurable immune response in animal and small-scale human trials, then it is field tested (Ada, 1992b). In retrospect, it seems that vaccine developers have usually attempted to develop vaccines rationally. From our modern vantage point, however, we can see that vaccine development has often been based on very limited knowledge of pathogenesis and immunity.

3.2. Phases of Clinical Development

The design of clinical trials is driven by the questions to be answered. The first step is to define the objectives of the trial, the outcome measures, and the number of participants required to answer the questions with an acceptable degree of precision. Vaccine evaluation begins with small trials designed to answer, in a limited way, the questions of safety and immunogenicity. Does the vaccine induce the anticipated immune response in most volunteers without unacceptable side effects? Intermediate trials expand the knowledge of safety and determine the optimal route of administration, dose, immunization schedule, and formulation. Some intermediate trials enroll volunteers from the populations that will be involved in the planned efficacy trials, to provide assurance that age, genetic and nutritional factors, prior exposure to vaccines or microbial infections, and other factors will not alter safety or immune responses significantly.

The following section will address several factors in trial design, including volunteer selection and informed consent, logistic considerations, and some special aspects of trials involving individuals who may need special protection, including children, pregnant women, and prisoners. Trials in developing countries will also be mentioned briefly. Careful planning for the statistical analysis of a trial, in advance, is a critical part of trial design, but is beyond the scope of this chapter. Several excellent texts discuss statistical analysis of trials in general (Smith and Morrow, 1991; Meinert, 1986); statistical considerations for planning of HIV-1 vaccine efficacy trials have been discussed elsewhere (Dixon *et al.*, 1993; Rida and Lawrence, 1994; Koff and Hoth, 1988; Rida *et al.*, 1993).

3.2.1. PHASE I AND II TRIALS

Clinical testing of vaccines is divided into three phases (Phases of an Investigation, 1993). Phase I trials are the first to begin with a small number of people, usually healthy adults. The primary focus of these studies is safety. Phase I studies may include dose escalation, based on the dose range found to be optimal in preclinical studies, but it is not necessary to define a maximum tolerated dose.

Phase II trials are considerably larger than Phase I, often involving hundreds of volunteers. These may involve dose and schedule variations and different routes of immunization. Ideally, the final formulation is used for at least some Phase II studies. Both safety and immune responses are measured in the Phase II trial(s). Individuals at higher risk for disease (like those to be enrolled in efficacy trials) may be included, but in the absence of a well-established correlate of immunity, no hint of efficacy can be obtained.

Phase I trials of candidate HIV-1 vaccines have often been dose-escalation studies that, after eventual expansion, have included dozens of volunteers. Most investigators have attempted to enroll healthy individuals at *low risk* for infection with HIV-1. There are several reasons for excluding high-risk individuals from Phase I trials:

1. Initially, investigators were uncertain whether inadvertent immunization of individuals who had just become infected with HIV-1 might cause rapid disease progression; the excellent safety record of vaccines in therapeutic trials, where HIV-1-infected individuals are enrolled (Redfield *et al.*, 1991), has minimized this concern for subunit or killed vaccines, but live recombinant vectors such as vaccinia may cause disseminated (Redfield *et al.*, 1987) or perhaps progressive infection in HIV-1-infected vaccinees (Zagury, 1991).
2. Prior exposure to HIV-1 (without productive infection) might alter the response to vaccine.
3. Subsequent infection in a vaccinated individual might falsely suggest that the vaccine either infected the volunteer or predisposed him/her to infection.
4. Vaccination might truly predispose to infection (immunologic enhancement). For a thorough discussion of this potential problem see Burke (1992) and Mascola *et al.* (1993).

In the first Phase II trial of HIV-1 vaccine candidates the AIDS Vaccine Evaluation Group (AVEG) enrolled individuals who reported low-risk or high-risk behavior. The volunteers were repeatedly counseled about avoidance of exposure to HIV-1 and told that they cannot expect to be protected by the vaccine. Subsequent risk-taking behavior was evaluated to determine the effects of participation in the trial and counseling. This trial included two gp120 candidate vaccines and their respective placebos (approximately 15% of recipients received placebo). The goal was to compare the immune responses of volunteers at low risk of HIV-1 exposure to responses of volunteers with a history of higher-risk behavior, including recent use of injection drugs and unprotected sexual exposure (homosexual or heterosexual). No significant differences in reactions or immune responses have been identified to date (McElrath *et al.*, 1994).

Infection with an infectious agent is not unexpected during Phase I and II vaccine trials, especially prior to the completion of a full immunization course. However, in HIV vaccine trials, intercurrent HIV infections have attracted considerable attention. A small number of volunteers have become infected while participating in Phase I and II HIV vaccine trials; these people have engaged in high risk behaviors despite repeated counseling (Belshe *et al.*, 1994a; Cohen, 1994). Not all of these individuals were initially classified as high-risk individuals, underscoring the fact that behavior may change over time. Some of the popular press coverage of these infections was unfortunate because it gave the impression that the vaccine caused the infections.

3.2.2. PHASE III TRIALS

The size and complexity of trials required to establish the efficacy of a vaccine can vary greatly. A critical factor is the frequency and severity of the disease. For mild or easily treatable diseases, initial trials may involve challenge of vaccinated volunteers with the infectious agent. For diseases that are, or may be, fatal or permanently disabling despite attempted treatment, challenge studies cannot be performed. Even if challenge studies give some indication that the vaccine is efficacious, field trials to prove the level of efficacy of the vaccine in actual practice are needed. A sufficient number of events (i.e., infections or disease) must occur to ensure that statistically significant results are obtained. The number of events needed for significance will depend on the vaccine efficacy; for the 60% efficacy envisioned for an early HIV-1 vaccine, the trial will have to be large enough to anticipate approximately 100 HIV-1 infections. If protection does not develop until after several immunizations or wanes rapidly, trial design must accommodate these temporal limitations. For a detailed discussion, see Dixon *et al.* (1993), Rida *et al.* (1993), and Rida and Lawrence (1994).

Participants in controlled trials are usually randomized on an individual basis into treatment groups that are designated at the outset of the trial, with one group for each treatment. Alternative designs for individual randomization include factorial designs and adaptive or "rolling" trials (see Rida and Lawrence, 1994). In cluster randomization, groups of individuals rather than single individuals would be randomized (Duffy *et al.*, 1992). Case-control studies may be used, particularly for post-marketing surveillance or comparison of vaccines (Comstock, 1994). For certain epidemic diseases, such as influenza or cholera, vaccine trials must coincide with epidemics. Those designing trials may need to consider heterogeneity either in the population's response to vaccines or in exposure to infection (e.g. if vaccinated individuals take greater risks or if only a subset of the population is at high risk) (Halloran *et al.*, 1994; Sheon, 1994).

The goal of Phase III trials is to prove that vaccination prevents or ameliorates disease. Prevention of transmission of the pathogen from vaccinated individuals to others, during disease or asymptomatic carriage, may be an equally important goal of vaccination, but it is difficult or impossible to incorporate as a trial end point. *Haemophilus influenzae* type b vaccine, for example, appears to reduce the incidence of invasive, symptomatic disease, as well as asymptomatic carriage of the pathogen; as a result, the reduction in disease incidence in the general population is greater than predicted based on the number of vaccinated infants and children. By definition, Phase III trials must enroll individuals at risk for infection and disease; however, if the disease is sufficiently common they need not enroll *particularly* high-risk populations. Trial population(s) should be representative, to the extent possible, of those who will be vaccinated in practice after the vaccine is licensed. Vaccine efficacy may be greatest when exposure to the pathogen is moderate or low.

Design of Phase III trials for HIV-1 candidates will be difficult; although trials may not be large by comparison with trials of polio, hepatitis A, or Japanese encephalitis virus vaccine, they will be complex (Lawrence *et al.*, 1993; Rida and Lawrence, 1994; Rida *et al.*, 1993; Vermund *et al.*, 1993, 1994). Trials in adults will involve recruiting individuals who engage in high-risk sex or injection drug use. Many of these individuals may have little trust in the trial's organizers or sponsors, and they may have many more immediate concerns than compliance with trial requirements. Some of them may deliberately attempt to determine whether they are in the experimental or placebo arm of the trial by antibody testing, and their behavior may change accordingly (Sheon, 1994). Extensive epidemiologic studies of HIV-1 are under way now, sponsored by several U.S. government agencies, the World Health Organization (WHO), and regional and national authorities. In addition to HIV-1 seroincidence data, information is being sought on the risk-taking behaviors of these populations and their willingness to participate in HIV-1 vaccine trials. Blood specimens are being collected from some volunteers from potential trial sites, and viruses isolated are being characterized with respect to genetic, biologic, and immunologic properties. The data generated will facilitate judgments regarding which populations should be involved in trials and which vaccines are appropriately matched to the local HIV-1 virus strains. The lack of appropriate vaccine candidates based on strains endemic in developing countries may impede the development and testing of HIV-1 vaccines.

4. FACTORS IN DESIGN OF CLINICAL TRIALS

4.1. Ethical Considerations in Testing HIV Vaccines

The history of vaccine trials includes many controversies, and HIV-1 vaccine trials, both prophylactic and therapeutic in intent, have raised many concerns. The ethical considerations include two issues: first, as with any trial, the conduct of the trial must be fair and explanations to participants honest, with proper consideration of the ethical principles of beneficence, autonomy, and respect for the individual. Second, initiation of any trial requires that the risk/benefit ratio be carefully evaluated and the trial justified. These issues have been discussed in detail elsewhere (Grady, 1994; Fast *et al.*, 1994; AIDS Action Foundation, "HIV Preventive Vaccines: Social, Ethical, and Political Considerations for Domestic Efficacy Trials," May 9–10, 1994, Washington, DC).

4.2. Volunteer Selection

The characteristics of volunteers sought for vaccine trials depend on the phase of testing. Volunteers for Phase I trials are usually healthy, with no history or evidence of disease. Subjects for Phase II trials are often recruited from populations similar or identical to those who will participate in the Phase III trial(s) and receive the vaccine after licensure. Phase III trials must enroll volunteers with a significant risk of infection or disease.

In selecting volunteers for initial trials, the investigator should consider both potential risks to the volunteer and factors that might lead to an inaccurate appraisal of the vaccine. Care should be taken, while devising the forms for data collection, taking the medical history, and examining the volunteer, to identify any immune compromise or immunosuppressive treatment. Subjects who have had severe reactions to immunization or anaphylaxis from any antigen are usually excluded. Women should be tested for pregnancy and cautioned to avoid pregnancy for the duration of the trial. In National Institutes of Health (NIH)-sponsored trials, blanket exclusions of women are not acceptable and inclusion of minority volunteers is encouraged (NIH, 1994). Refer to Section 4.7 for additional discussion of potential risk to volunteers as it affects the selection process.

Age, nutritional status, genetic predisposition, or prior exposure to related pathogens may alter the immune response to a vaccine. Infants respond poorly to polysaccharide antigens such as pneumococcal and *H. influenzae* capsular antigens; conjugation of the polysaccharide to protein carriers has significantly overcome this problem (Santosham *et al.*, 1991; Santosham, 1993). Measles vaccine is less effective in children less than 1 year of age owing, at least in part, to transplacentally acquired antibody (Sato *et al.*, 1979). Recently, an attempt to increase the effectiveness of measles vaccination in Africa by increasing the titer of the measles vaccine and vaccinating prior to the age of 9 months led to a surprising finding of increased mortality in the ensuing 3 years, particularly in female infants (Halsey, 1993). In some cases, responsiveness to vaccines may decline during and after middle age (Clements, 1994).

Variability of the immune response to a vaccine may correlate with ethnic group. Pneumococcal and *H. influenzae* polysaccharide antigens are less immunogenic in Native Americans than in other racial groups tested (Siber *et al.*, 1990). The response to hepatitis B vaccine appears to be genetically controlled, although not distributed along racial lines (Arif *et al.*, 1988), and it is likely that immune responses to other vaccines may be controlled genetically. This is particularly true for peptide vaccines, which may be immunogenic only in the presence of appropriate class I or class II major histocompatibility molecules (Cease and Berzofsky, 1994; Palker *et al.*, 1988).

Passive acquisition of maternal antibodies, recent transfusion, treatment with immune globulin, or previous immunization with a related product may mimic or alter immune responses. Pooled human immunoglobulin, given for therapeutic reasons, can impair induction of a protective antibody response to live attenuated vaccines (Siber *et al.*, 1993). BCG has been much more effective in certain studies than others; one possible confounding factor is the prevalence of infection with cross-reacting atypical mycobacteria (Eickhoff, 1988). Responses to the product of a recombinant gene carried by a live bacterial or viral vaccine vector may be affected by previous exposure to that same vector or by infection with a related pathogen. When vaccinia is used as a vector, prior immunization with smallpox vaccine may blunt the response to the product of the new gene (Cooney *et al.*, 1993; Graham *et al.*, 1992). Prior experience with the vector has been reported to be irrelevant for canarypox, a vector for which mammalian cells are nonpermissive (Tartaglia *et al.*, 1993). Preexisting immunity to BCG may enhance immunization to recombinant gene products delivered via this vector (Stover *et al.*, 1992) or coupled to purified protein derivative (S. J. Cryz, Jr. and A. Rubenstein, personal communication, 1993). In general, prior experience that suppresses replication of the vector seems to reduce expression of exogenous gene product.

4.3. Special Populations

Certain individuals require particularly stringent guidelines for study. When some or all of the subjects in a trial are likely to be vulnerable to coercion or undue influence, such as children, prisoners, pregnant women, mentally disabled persons, or economically or educationally disadvantaged persons, additional safeguards have been formulated to protect their rights and welfare (Protection of Human Subjects, 1993a). These classes of individuals have been called "vulnerable" and conditions for ethical use have been narrowly defined.

For research involving children, the Institutional Review Board (IRB) will determine whether the child is capable of consenting or if the parent(s) may provide permission, and if the risk/benefit ratio justifies the research. Generally, initial experience with immunogenicity and safety is gained in adults prior to trials in children. If the child is old enough, he or she may be asked to assent in addition to the permission of the parent or guardian. For HIV-1 therapeutic trials, children who are wards of a state or court may be eligible, with appropriate permission, but some jurisdictions will not allow participation (Twomey and Fletcher, 1994).

For research involving pregnant women and fetuses, there are several additional requirements: (1) safety must have been demonstrated in animals and nonpregnant human subjects, (2) except where the purpose of the research is to meet the health needs of the mother or fetus, the risk to the fetus must be minimal, (3) researchers may have no part in decisions concerning termination of the pregnancy or determining viability of the fetus, and (4) no inducements, monetary or otherwise, may be offered to terminate a pregnancy. If the research is for the benefit of the fetus rather than the mother, the father (if available) must also give permission (Protection of Human Subjects, 1993a).

For research involving prisoners, additional criteria must be met: (1) the research must have the intent and reasonable probability of improving the health and well-being of the subjects, and (2) for research including placebo groups, the study may proceed only after the FDA has consulted appropriate experts and published notice in the *Federal Register* of its intent to approve the research. Research on conditions particularly affecting prisoners as a class (for example, vaccine trials on hepatitis, a disease that is highly prevalent in prisons) may proceed if the above conditions are met even though prisoners may be assigned to control groups. The majority of members of the IRB that reviews the protocol shall have no association with the prison involved, and at least one member of the IRB must be a prisoner or prisoner representative. There can be no coercion or special favors to the prisoners who participate (Protection of Human Subjects, 1993a,b).

4.4. Informed Consent

Informed consent is an integral part of the recruitment process. Consent must be obtained from the volunteer or a legally authorized representative. The prospective volunteer must be given sufficient opportunity to consider whether or not to participate, without coercion or undue influence. For anyone to give truly informed consent, he or she must understand what is proposed. The document must include all pertinent information, but be concise. The reading level should be at the high school level or below, a goal that is difficult to achieve if all scientific information about the product is included. For volunteers who are illiterate, the trial must be explained verbally, and a witness should affirm that the volunteer understands and consents. For those who do not read well and for children, a video presentation may be helpful. Consent forms in languages other than English may be needed.

The subject may not waive any legal rights or release from liability for negligence of the investigator, the sponsor, the institution, or its agents. An informed consent includes: (1) a statement that the study involves research, an explanation of the purpose and the expected duration of the research, a description and identification of any procedures that are experimental; (2) a description of risks or discomforts; (3) a description of benefits to the volunteer or to others; (4) any alternate procedures or treatment, if appropriate; (5) a description of the extent of confidentiality under which records identifying the volunteer will be kept; (6) for research involving more than minimal risk, an explanation of compensation and medical treatments that may be available; (7) the name of someone who will answer questions regarding the rights of the volunteer and to whom research-related injury should be reported; (8) a statement that participation is voluntary, that refusal to participate will involve no penalty or loss of benefits, and that the volunteer may discontinue participation at any time without penalty or loss of benefits; and other elements as appropriate (Protection of Human Subjects, 1993a,b).

Volunteers must understand that the experimental vaccine may not be protective. In AIDS vaccine trials, subjects are counseled to avoid behavior that may put them at risk of acquiring the disease. The necessity for avoiding high-risk behavior, the experimental nature of the vaccine, the possibility that the vaccine could increase risk, and the presence of placebo in the trial (if any) are stated clearly in the informed consent. Recruiters assure that potential volunteers understand these points before enrollment, and that they understand HIV-1 transmission and how to protect themselves. Counseling is repeated frequently during the trial. Volunteers who truly understand the purpose of the research, the procedures, the time commitment, and the risks and discomforts they may experience are more likely to complete the study. Volunteers who like and trust the clinic staff are easier to retain.

Additional items may be added to the informed consent to reflect the conditions of a particular clinical trial. For example, informed consents for HIV-1 vaccine trials include discussions regarding the possibility of social discrimination that may result from appearing to be HIV-1 positive, and an explanation of how the volunteer can obtain assistance in resolving any problems caused by false-positive HIV-1 tests (see Section 4.7.2).

4.5. Age of Volunteers for HIV-1 Vaccine Trials

It is traditional to begin Phase I testing of any agent in adults (at least 18 years old), since the unknown risks are best understood and consented to by the volunteer, rather than by a guardian. Most vaccines in general use are targeted to infants and children. Vaccination of this young population is ideal since protection may be established early in life and there is a worldwide system for immunization of infants. Therefore, it is important to develop vaccines for use in infants in parallel to the development of vaccines for use in adults. The sequence of testing vaccines is normally (1) adults with antibody, (2) children with antibody, and (3) naive children, if all goes well. This last step is potentially the most hazardous. Often, testing is done first in young children and toddlers before introducing a new vaccine into infants.

In testing HIV-1 vaccine candidates, the approach has been different. The risk of infection with HIV-1, as with other sexually transmitted diseases, is almost nil in toddlers and young children and increases as sexual activity begins. Infants born to HIV-1-infected mothers constitute one of the highest-risk groups; rates of mother-to-infant transmission range from about 15 to 40%, and a significant portion of the transmission is thought to occur at or near the time of birth (see reviews by Mofenson, 1992; Report of a Consensus Workshop, 1992a,b,1995). If immunization of infants may reduce perinatal HIV-1 transmission or ameliorate HIV-1 disease, then the risk/benefit ratio seems relatively favorable. Therefore, testing of HIV-1 vaccines for preventive use will probably be done only in adults, adolescents, and newborns. A Phase I study of immunization in neonates born to HIV-1-infected mothers has been initiated by the Pediatric AIDS Clinical Trials Group, sponsored by the National Institute of Allergy and Infectious Diseases (NIAID), NIH (McNamara *et al.*, 1994). Diagnosis of HIV-1 infection in infants often relies on the waning of maternal antibody which usually occurs by 18 months of age. Active immunization of the neonate may delay the time at which the maternal antibody against HIV-1 wanes and an accurate HIV antibody test can be performed; until then, care must be exercised to avoid labeling immunized children as HIV-1-infected. This care is particularly important because such children may be candidates for foster placement or adoption and an incorrect diagnosis may jeopardize their opportunities for placement. Children and adolescents will be important to include in any population-based HIV-1 immunization strategy. Eventually, immunization at birth to initiate immunologic memory against HIV-1 and protect against perinatal transmission of the virus may be followed by boosting prior to initiation of sexual activity.

4.6. Choice of Dose or Dose Range for Clinical Trials

When evaluating vaccines that do not consist of living organisms, data from dose-ranging studies in subhuman primates are usually available. The choice of animal model may be limited for live antigens, depending on the host range of the organism. For example, *Salmonella typhi* has a host range restricted almost entirely to humans, so preclinical work has been done with *S. typhimurium* in mice. Similarly, preclinical work with live attenuated retroviruses has been done with the simian virus, SIV, since there is no nonhuman primate in which HIV-1 induces disease. Predictions based on studies using vectors or pathogens other than those in the vaccine must be viewed with caution.

4.7. Risks of Vaccination

4.7.1. ADVERSE REACTIONS

Vaccines for prevention are generally safe. They are administered to healthy individuals, and if they are effective the public sees few cases of disease; therefore, a very strict risk/benefit ratio is applied (La Montagne and Curlin, 1992). Risks of vaccination depend on the type of vaccine. In general, local reactions are the most common, usually including only pain, tenderness, swelling, and erythema at the site of injection. Local necrosis or sterile abscess formation at the site of vaccination has been reported after use of alum-adjuvanted vaccines (Miliauskas *et al.*, 1993). Rarely, extravasation may cause inflammatory sequelae or necrosis at distant sites.

Some adverse reactions associated with live virus vaccines are those resulting from infection with the virus. Although the live oral poliovirus vaccine (OPV) is manufactured using *attenuated* Sabin strains of poliovirus, one case per 520,000 first doses of OPV administered, results in paralytic disease in recipient or contact(s) (Nkowane *et al.*, 1987). The risk of vaccine-associated disease is considered greater in immunocompromised individuals. In general, live, attenuated virus vaccines and live bacterial vaccines are not recommended for use in immunocompromised individuals (General Recommendations on Immunization, 1994).

Allergic reactions are associated with vaccines. The responsible vaccine components include: vaccine antigen, animal protein, antibiotics, preservatives, and stabilizers (General Recommendations on Immunization, 1994). These reactions can be local or systemic, including delayed-type, Arthus, or immediate hypersensitivity reactions. Anaphylactic shock, which can be fatal, is a significant risk in vaccine preparations used for hyposensitization (e.g., bee-sting vaccine). Egg protein, found in vaccines prepared using embryonated chicken eggs or chicken embryo cell cultures (Table I), is the most common animal protein allergen (General Recommendations on Immunization, 1994). Vaccines containing trace amounts of antibiotic (e.g., neomycin) to which individuals may be allergic may cause anaphylaxis; although a rare event, this risk to hypersensitive individuals must be considered as a possible reaction in all vaccine clinical trials. Not uncommonly, unexpected adverse reactions occur that are identified only after extensive use of the vaccine. Booster doses of human diploid-cell rabies vaccine were associated with symptoms similar to delayed hypersensitivity because of alterations by beta-propiolactone of the stabilizing agent creating an allergen (Anderson *et al.*, 1987). Unusual reactions characterized by urticaria and angioedema were associated with administration of Japanese encephalitis virus vaccine (Andersen and Ronne, 1991; Ruff *et al.*, 1991); the immunologic mechanism has not been elucidated.

Autoimmune reactions are a hypothetical risk of vaccination. Neurological complications possibly related to the presence of myelin basic protein were common with the crude rabbit spinal-cord derived rabies vaccine. Modern vaccines are far purer. For example, the recently licensed Japanese encephalitis virus vaccine derived from infected mouse brain is purified and vaccination is rarely associated with a neurologic event (Inactivated Japanese Encephalitis Virus Vaccine, 1993). Many human pathogens bear antigens that cross-react with components of the human body, a phenomenon called molecular mimicry. Each cross-reaction is a hypothetical source of auto-reactive antibody or delayed hypersensitivity. For HIV-1, cross-reactions have been identified between gp160 and both class I and II histocompatibility antigens, and antibodies to these epitopes have been identified in infected and vaccinated individuals (Golding *et al.*, 1988; de Santis *et al.*, 1993). No clinical significance of the anti-HLA antibodies has been identified in uninfected, vaccinated individuals. In one study, no changes in antinuclear antibodies were found after vaccination with gp160 (Belshe *et al.*, 1993). In general, clinical examination, history, blood counts, and kidney and liver function tests are used to screen for potential autoimmune disease. There is no clear basis for more specific testing. An additional theoretical consideration for HIV-1 is that immune reactions directed against the envelope might harm $CD4^+$ lymphocytes via gp120 attached to this receptor (Fauci *et al.*, 1991). No loss of CD4 cells has been identified in vaccine trials to date (Keefer *et al.*, 1994).

4.7.2. FALSE-POSITIVE TESTS FOR HIV-1 CAUSED BY VACCINATION

While AIDS vaccines are carefully designed so that subjects cannot become infected from receiving them, some of the subjects may make antibodies that will cause them to test positive on standard HIV-1 tests for a number of months (Dolin *et al.*, 1991; Belshe *et al.*, 1993; Belshe *et al.*, 1994b; Parekh *et al.*, 1994). False-positive test results may have serious repercussions for the volunteers, who may encounter problems with employment, health or life insurance, military service, foreign travel, blood donation, or any other situation where an HIV-1 test is mandatory (Porter *et al.*, 1989; Westblom *et al.*, 1990; Belshe *et al.*, 1994b). It is imperative that each subject understands the implications of participating in an AIDS vaccine trial and the social discrimination that he or she may face before entering the trial. Some of the AIDS Vaccine Evaluation Units have asked potential volunteers to take written tests to assure comprehension of this possible outcome.

False-positive screening ELISA tests for HIV-1 infection may be clarified by further testing using Western blot or polymerase chain reaction. At present, the vaccine units provide these tests for volunteers. If an HIV-1 vaccine enters general use, a readily available mechanism for resolving such uncertainties will be needed (if the vaccine produces false-positive reactions).

The Division of AIDS, NIAID, NIH, has undertaken a dialogue with the insurance industry and other government agencies about vaccine-induced seroconversion. Each uninfected volunteer is given a tamper-proof picture identification card at the time of vaccination. Personnel at each clinical site are available to help volunteers with any problems that arise. There is also a toll-free telephone number that the volunteer may call. As the public becomes better informed about AIDS and about HIV-1 vaccine trials, volunteers should face fewer problems caused by false-positive HIV-1 tests. Participation in efficacy trials may, however, create additional problems of discrimination because volunteers will be identified as high risk solely by virtue of their participation.

4.7.3. EXCLUSION CRITERIA

In Phase I trials, individuals with significant systemic disease, history of autoimmune disease, immune deficiency, or hypersensitivity to other vaccines should be excluded. Receipt of related experimental vaccines or recent transfusion or treatment with immune globulin are other causes for exclusion. Vaccination during pregnancy, particularly early in pregnancy, is generally avoided, both to prevent potential harm to the developing fetus and because of concern about liability for fetal abnormalities unrelated to vaccination. In the absence of known teratogens, fetal abnormalities occur in as many as 5% of newborns, and about 1% of newborns have serious anomalies. Consequently, manufacturers and investigators fear that the association of use of a product with these events will give the appearance of fetal harm, even though the risk may be small and may not be attributable to the product. For example, rubella vaccine was considered potentially harmful to the fetus, because the wild-type virus causes congenital rubella syndrome. A surveillance program conducted by the Centers for Disease Control registered more than 300 infants whose mothers were vaccinated with rubella vaccine during pregnancy. No case of vaccine-associated congenital rubella syndrome was identified (Rubella Vaccination during Pregnancy, 1989).

In the AVEG HIV-1 vaccine trials, women are asked to avoid pregnancy for the duration of the trial and counseled regarding birth control at each visit. In addition, pregnancy tests are generally conducted prior to each vaccination and, if positive, the vaccination is canceled. The rate of pregnancy in these studies, overall, is about 0.8%. No significant fetal harm associated with HIV-1 vaccine administration has been identified (Keefer *et al.*, 1994). Exclusion of women from vaccine trials would be contrary to the policy of the NIH, and scientifically inappropriate, since the vaccines will be used in sexually active women.

4.8. Reimbursement

While Phase I/II clinical trials are essential to development of vaccines, few if any medical benefits accrue to participants in early safety and immunogenicity trials. A general medical examination and counseling regarding risk factors, e.g., in HIV-1 vaccine trials, may be of benefit to some individuals. In fact, participation has disadvantages. Prescreening examinations, vaccination, and follow-up may be time-consuming and inconvenient, phlebotomy and injections may cause discomfort, and expected or unanticipated adverse reactions may occur. For these reasons, volunteers are often reimbursed for their participation in initial vaccine clinical trials. In efficacy trials, reimbursement beyond out-of-pocket expenses is seldom given (Spilker and Cramer, 1992). Payment may be adequate to compensate the volunteer for his/her time and trouble, but not so large as to constitute coercion. Generally, payment should be given as the volunteer completes each segment of the clinical trial (prescreen, vaccination, follow-up) so there is no undue financial pressure to remain in the trial. Each IRB reviews the amount of payment and some may allow only reimbursement for expenses. The policy should be clearly explained in the informed consent.

4.9. Motivation of Volunteers in HIV-1 Vaccine Trials

Individuals enroll in vaccine trials for a variety of reasons, including monetary considerations, belief that they may benefit from the experimental vaccine, and desire to contribute to scientific and medical knowledge. Recruitment for AIDS vaccine trials involves special considerations. Many of the volunteers have known individuals with AIDS and want to join in the fight against this disease. Others routinely respond to the needs of their communities, for example by donating blood and participating in civic organizations. It is important to exclude or reeducate volunteers who mistakenly believe that they will be protected from HIV-1 by an experimental vaccine, and who may therefore increase risk behavior during the trial (Sheon, 1994).

There are many obstacles to recruitment into HIV-1 trials. The general public is not well informed about HIV-1 or about vaccination itself. Potential volunteers may fear that they can become infected with the virus and must be assured that current candidate vaccines contain no HIV-1 and that getting AIDS from vaccination is not possible. Some potential volunteers (or their associates) fear that volunteers will be deliberately infected with HIV-1 to determine whether the vaccine is efficacious. Of course, deliberate challenge with HIV-1 is never considered. Others simply wish to avoid any association with AIDS or AIDS research (N. Ketter and L. Bye, personal communication, 1994).

4.10. Randomization, Placebos, and Blinding

Randomization between treatment and placebo groups is a critical part of trial design. Volunteers for vaccine trials are a self-selected group with biologic and/or psychologic characteristics that cannot be completely defined if no placebo group is included for comparison. Inclusion of placebo control groups is advisable, even in Phase I trials. Some of the side effects attributed to vaccines, such as moderate pain and tenderness at the injection site, may be related simply to the injection process itself, while others, such as malaise and headache, are sufficiently common that the comparison with placebo can determine whether the symptoms are, in fact, associated with the vaccine.

The placebo is usually the adjuvant alone, such as alum. When the adjuvant is itself novel, an additional placebo may be required to determine the effect of the adjuvant alone. In some trials, a different vaccine may be used as placebo (if its effects are well known), thus offering something of at least potential benefit to all participants. Blinding may be difficult if the volume, turbidity, color, or storage conditions differ from the experimental vaccine. In early HIV-1 vaccine trials, telling volunteers that they may have received a "blank" rather than the vaccine, helps in underscoring to volunteers the importance of continued avoidance of high-risk behaviors.

Blinding of trials is important to avoid bias in judgments or reports by volunteers or clinicians, but blinding may be difficult. When neither clinicians nor volunteers know to which group, i.e., placebo or vaccine, the individual is assigned, the trials are called "double-blind." When different formulations are being compared, some preparation or mixing may be required just prior to administration. For multicenter trials, the randomization code is generated by the data center and, as a rule, only the pharmacists at the site are aware of the identity of the vaccines given to each volunteer. For efficacy trials, the vaccine and placebo are ideally manufactured in such a way that even the site pharmacists do not know which preparation is the active one. Blinding may also be difficult if the vaccine has different, or more severe, side effects than the placebo or adjuvant alone. If immunologic analysis is done at the study site(s), the presence of antibodies, in vitro T-cell responses, or delayed-type hypersensitivity may inadvertently unblind the investigators. These concerns may be addressed by analysis of sera at a separate central laboratory site or establishment of independent teams of clinicians—one to administer the vaccine and the other to evaluate the subjects.

HIV-1 candidate vaccines introduce another level of complexity, in that vaccinees may unblind themselves. Some HIV-1 vaccines may transiently convert the screening and/or confirmatory HIV-1 antibody tests to positive. If so, subjects may deliberately or inadvertently obtain information that would unblind them, for example by submitting the HIV-1 antibody tests required to obtain life insurance or as a result of tests performed for donating blood, or by attending an HIV-1 screening clinic. If a question of true infection should arise in the mind of the volunteer or his/her employer, medical caretaker, government agency, etc., then either clinic staff or a specific individual or team must address this issue. The possibility that volunteers' risk-taking behavior might be altered by knowledge that he or she is in the vaccine or placebo group thus confounding the trial, is a concern for efficacy trials; if vaccinated individuals take more risks than those receiving placebo, a vaccine effect may be masked. Refer to Rida and Lawrence (1994), for further discussion of these issues.

4.11. Special Considerations for Vaccine Trials in Pregnant Women

Ideally, all women should be protected against infectious diseases before childbearing age so that vaccination during pregnancy would be unnecessary. However, in some cases, it may be prudent to vaccinate pregnant women. Vaccination may be warranted if the disease to be prevented is life-threatening, e.g., rabies; if the risk to the mother is greater during pregnancy than at other times, as it may be in influenza (Deinard and Ogburn, 1994); or if the disease may cause abortion, e.g., polio (McCord et al., 1955; Siegel and Greenberg, 1956). In special cases, it may be desirable to vaccinate the mother to protect the developing fetus. Combined tetanus and diphtheria toxoids are the only immunobiologic agents routinely indicated for susceptible pregnant women (General Recommendations on Immunization, 1994). Hormonal changes that occur during pregnancy may alter the maternal immune response (Saballus et al., 1987). Therefore, the maternal immune response should be documented after vaccination, if possible.

Pregnant women have been excluded from many clinical trials of candidate vaccines, and few vaccine teratogenicity studies have been done in animals. However, limited safety data do exist for some vaccines. Data have been collected either prospectively in pregnant women who were accidentally vaccinated, e.g., with rubella (Rubella Vaccination during Pregnancy, 1989), or retrospectively after large numbers of women were vaccinated with polio vaccine (Harjulehto et al., 1989; Ornoy and Ishai, 1993), rabies vaccine (Chutivongse and Wilde, 1989; Chabala et al., 1991; Varner et al., 1982), and influenza virus vaccine (Deinard and Ogburn, 1994). Rare cases of fetal infection by vaccinia have been reported in association with smallpox vaccination (Levine et al., 1974; Goldstein et al., 1975).

Because of the limited experience in pregnant women, vaccines are not routinely recommended for use in this population.

A few attempts have been made to prevent disease in the newborn child by vaccinating the mother. Maternal antibodies pass through the placenta, especially after the fifth month of pregnancy, and could prevent disease in the neonate. The WHO is conducting a campaign to prevent neonatal tetanus by immunizing pregnant women (Kim-Farley *et al.*, 1992). Immunization of pregnant women with a polysaccharide vaccine is a promising strategy for prevention of perinatal infections caused by group B streptococci. Forty pregnant women were vaccinated with purified Type III capsular polysaccharide; women who responded to the vaccine produced antibodies that crossed the placenta and sera of their infants contained protective levels of antibody (Baker *et al.*, 1988). A similar strategy has been attempted to prevent vertical transmission of hepatitis B infection. In one trial conducted in Africa, transmission of anti-hepatitis B antibodies occurred in 60% of infants born to immunized mothers, as opposed to 32% of infants born to nonimmunized mothers. However, antibody titers were short-lived (Coursaget *et al.*, 1983).

The Division of AIDS, NIAID, NIH, through the AVEG and the AIDS Clinical Trials Group, is currently conducting a Phase I trial of candidate AIDS vaccine in HIV-1-infected but asymptomatic pregnant women. Each vaccine has previously been tested in uninfected and infected subjects, including women. The trial excludes women who already show symptoms of disease or who have significant obstetrical risk factors. Use of zidovudine, which has recently been shown to reduce mother-to-infant transmission of HIV-1 (Zidovudine, 1994), is encouraged. Eventually, international trials will be needed to perform efficacy trials for evaluation of the most promising active and/or passive immunization strategies to block perinatal transmission of HIV-1, alone or combined with obstetric or pharmacologic interventions (Report of a Consensus Workshop, 1995).

Nonvaccine placebo arms are included in HIV-1 vaccine trials because immunization of HIV-1-infected individuals with currently available envelope vaccines has not been proven to ameliorate disease, so standard-of-care therapy is not being withheld from placebo recipients. A placebo group was important because many of the end points in the trial depend on evaluation of laboratory parameters that have not been defined in pregnant HIV-1-infected individuals, and the placebo arm is important as a control for unexpected and undesirable outcomes in vaccine recipients. To date, the recombinant envelope vaccine appears to be safe in both mothers and infants. The study size, however, is far too small to prove or disprove efficacy.

4.12. Special Considerations for Trials in Developing Countries

Clinical trials done in developing countries under foreign sponsorship may require special protection of the subjects. Individuals from the host country involved in all aspects of the trial should ensure that the unique legal, ethical, behavioral, and social issues of the country will be considered. Appropriate informed consent in other cultures may differ from the Western principles, which are based on autonomy of individuals. In some societies, more emphasis is placed on the individual within the society and in relation to other society members. In such a culture, the consent process may involve family members or the community, and it may be necessary to secure the permission of the subject's family or social group in addition to the consent of the subject as an individual (Lurie *et al.*, 1994). While the crisis of the AIDS pandemic has prompted reconsideration of some aspects of the ethics of research involving human subjects in order to address the urgency of the problem in some developing countries, the life-threatening and infectious nature of the disease does not justify any suspension of the rights of research subjects (International Ethical Guidelines, 1993).

If clinical trials of candidate AIDS vaccine are conducted abroad, the following should be considered: (1) selecting vaccine candidates active against the HIV-1 strains present in the host country; (2) establishing and maintaining an adequate technological infrastructure; (3) assessing the feasibility of recruitment; (4) designing methods to obtain truly informed consent from each individual subject and agreement of the family and community; (5) creating appropriate methods to measure risk behavior; (6) providing culturally appropriate behavioral intervention for all participants; (7) providing laboratory methods to distinguish natural HIV-1 infection from vaccine-induced seropositivity, and (8) making an effective vaccine available free of charge to the placebo group and resolving issues of access to affordable vaccine for the community/nation where the trial has been conducted (Lurie *et al.*, 1994).

Research that takes place in economically disadvantaged communities in the United States is subject to similar considerations. In such communities, it is equally important to ensure that: (1) they are not singled out for research that could be carried out reasonably well in more affluent communities, (2) the research is responsive to the health needs and priorities of the community, and (3) there is appropriate review by members of the community (International Ethical Guidelines, 1993). Several countries have established ethical/scientific committees to review and monitor HIV vaccine trials with the assistance of WHO. Issues of compensation or medical care for vaccine-related injury may have to be addressed.

5. TRIAL OUTCOME MEASURES

5.1. Laboratory Assays in HIV-1 Prophylactic Trials: The Dilemma of Unknown Correlate(s) of Immunity/Protection

Correlates of immunity have been well established for some diseases for which there are successful vaccines. Most frequently, these are antibody levels. If disease or infection can be prevented by administration of pooled immunoglobulin (Ig) from normal donors (gamma globulin) or specifically immune donors (hepatitis B Ig, varicella zoster Ig), then antibody titers in recipients can be measured and used as a guide to protective antibody titers. This may underestimate the contributions of immune memory and/or T-cell responses; as an example, recipients of hepatitis B vaccine may be protected from disease after antibody titers wane (Hadler *et al.*, 1986). Alternatively, correlates of immunity may be determined from analysis of efficacy trials. Immune responses that are present in protected individuals but lacking in those who are not protected are candidate correlates of immunity. This analysis is strengthened by comparison of trials using different vaccine candidates. Ongoing NIAID-sponsored trials of several different acellular pertussis vaccines, containing different numbers of bacterial antigens, may for the first time define one or more correlates of immunity to pertussis (The Jordan Report, 1994). Information may also be derived from studies of mother-to-infant transmission. For example, infants born to infected mothers were protected from perinatal transmission of herpes simplex type 2 (HSV-2) only if they had transplacentally derived neutralizing antibody specific for HSV-2 (Ashley *et al.*, 1992).

For HIV-1, the correlates of immunity are unknown. This dilemma is not unique, since the correlates of immunity for other diseases have been unknown (and may still remain uncertain) during and after development of effective vaccines. Several approaches are being taken to learn, or guess at, the correlates of immunity. Animal models may be helpful, but with limitations. Few isolates of HIV-1 infect chimpanzees; no disease has yet been observed in infected chimpanzees. Antibody that neutralizes challenge virus, when given passively, can protect chimpanzees against infection under optimal conditions (Emini *et al.*, 1992; Prince *et al.*, 1990), and chimpanzees that had been actively immunized against HIV-1 envelope antigens have been protected from infection (Berman *et al.*, 1990; Bruck *et al.*, 1993). New viral stocks grown in blood mononuclear cells are not easily neutralized, and challenge of chimpanzees with these stocks (which more closely resemble "wild-type" HIV-1) may shed some light on the ability of in vitro neutralization assays to predict protection.

HIV-1 is uniquely variable, and the relationship of genetic sequence to antigenic structure is only now being elucidated. Therefore, some measure of breadth of neutralizing ability for antisera is needed, i.e. how many strains of HIV-1 can be neutralized, and how closely are they related? Antisera from some (but not all) infected individuals will neutralize some (but not all) freshly isolated HIV-1 strains within the same clade; some cross-clade neutralization is also observed (Golding *et al.*, 1994; Mascola *et al.*, 1994). Some workers have found that mothers whose antibodies neutralize their own virus are less likely to transmit HIV-1 to their infants, suggesting that neutralizing antibody may be protective against "wild-type" HIV-1 (Bryson *et al.*, 1993; Scarlatti *et al.*, 1993), but this finding is controversial. Analogous studies, involving transfer of the putative protective element, are difficult to achieve for cell-mediated immunity. One system in which cell transfer may be attempted is the hu-PBL-SCID mouse; transfer of PBMCs from an immunized human was protective when the cells were derived relatively soon after immunization (Mosier *et al.*, 1993). It should be noted, however, that the transferred cells included cells capable of producing antibodies and lymphokines as well as those that might develop into killers that would lyse infected cells. In an experiment with transfer of a cytolytic, *nef*-specific clone to the same system, viral infection was blocked, but the effect was not HLA-restricted and may not be entirely antigen-specific (van Kuyk *et al.*, 1993).

5.2. Outcome Measures in HIV-1 Therapeutic Trials: The Dilemma of Unknown Surrogate Marker(s)

Phase I and II trials of HIV-1 vaccine candidates in infected individuals are designed to test safety and immunogenicity of the vaccines, but therapeutic trials raise entirely different questions than prophylactic trials. The risk/benefit ratio may be perceived to be quite different; although HIV-1-infected volunteers could potentially gain from ameliora-tion or substantial delay of the disease, they also may be particularly vulnerable. Pertur-bation of the immune system might be harmful to HIV-infected persons, while leaving uninfected individuals unharmed, perhaps by increasing replication of HIV-1, as has been demonstrated with influenza immunization (O'Brien *et al.*, 1993).

Although HIV-1 disease is highly variable, following the number of CD4$^+$ lympho-cytes in the circulation gives a crude measure of disease progression. A possible confound-ing factor is alteration of the CD4 count, acutely, by some feature of the immune response *per se*. For example, IL-2, which is induced during immune responses, can (when given exogenously) temporarily elevate the number of circulating CD4$^+$ lymphocytes (Kovacs *et al.*, 1993a). A second safety measurement is the quantitation of virus; free virus in plasma or virus production in lymphocytes can be measured by reverse-transcribed polymerase chain reaction (RNA-PCR) or quantitative culture, and latent virus can be measured by DNA-PCR detection of integrated provirus in circulating PBMCs. The lymphoid organs such as spleen and lymph nodes are significant reservoirs and targets of HIV-1 (Fauci *et al.*, 1991; Rosenberg and Fauci, 1991), but routine detection of events in these tissues is not currently possible.

In therapeutic vaccine trials, vaccine-induced immune responses must be measured against a background of response to the HIV-1 infection itself. Antibody responses to the vaccines may differ in fine specificity from the responses to the infecting virus (Pincus *et al.*, 1993). Novel responses to immunogen, including antibodies, lymphoproliferative responses, cytotoxicity, and delayed-type hypersensitivity, have been demonstrated in several trials (Redfield *et al.*, 1991; Allan *et al.*, 1993; McElrath *et al.*, 1993; Schwartz *et al.*, 1993a; Katzenstein *et al.*, 1992; Levine *et al.*, 1993; Valentine *et al.*, 1992; Zunich *et al.*, 1992; Bratt *et al.*, 1993). It is critical to determine whether these responses are directed against native HIV-1 proteins, and whether they benefit the vaccinated patient.

Efficacy trials of HIV-1 vaccines in infected individuals are difficult to design, because there is no reliable intermediate marker for ultimate disease outcome in the presence of immune manipulation. In addition, the disease moves slowly and its course is highly variable. Therefore, thousands of individuals must be followed for many years, at least initially, to confirm any effects on disease end points. Possible surrogate markers include immune responses, CD4 count, and—probably most convincing if shown—a modification of the amount of measurable virus. In the absence of promising data showing favorable trends in clinical welfare, immune responses, or viral load, it will be difficult to commit large numbers of volunteers and resources to such trials. These issues have been reviewed elsewhere in detail (Birx and Redfield, 1991; Slade, 1993; Stein *et al.*, 1993; Burke, 1993; Birx *et al.*, 1995).

6. CONCLUSIONS

Vaccine clinical trials are designed to determine initial safety and immune response, expanded safety, optimal dose, schedule, formulation, and ultimately efficacy of vaccines. These are followed by postlicensure surveillance. Recent advances in molecular biology and in knowledge regarding disease pathogenesis have provided a variety of new methods for making vaccines and targeting specific immune outcomes, and clinical trials are under way. In addition, the WHO Expanded Program on Immunization and national programs have stimulated research designed to facilitate immunization of every human being against many pathogens. This research relies on a blend of empiricism and rational predictions.

The development of a vaccine to prevent HIV-1 infection and AIDS is one of the greatest challenges modern medical science has faced. Limited understanding of the basis of potential immunity to HIV-1, several features of the virus and its pathogenesis, and the public perception of AIDS are among the obstacles to HIV-1 vaccine development. Nevertheless, in the decade since the causative agent of AIDS was identified, extensive efforts have been undertaken in academic laboratories, the private sector, and government to produce and test many novel vaccine candidates. HIV-1 vaccine trials do involve some unique problems, but uncertainty and controversy have been features of the development of many other vaccines over the past 200 years (Plotkin and Plotkin, 1988). Despite these obstacles, great progress has been achieved, including the eradication of smallpox (Fenner *et al.*, 1988) and the virtual elimination of polio from the Western Hemisphere (Robbins, 1993; Wright *et al.*, 1991). This history of achievement should serve as an inspiration for those struggling with HIV-1, malaria, and other scourges.

ACKNOWLEDGMENTS

We thank Theresa Jones and Steve Hirsch for their tireless assistance with references, and our colleagues at the Division of AIDS and AIDS Vaccine Evaluation Group for enlightening discussions. We are especially grateful to Drs. George Curlin, David Karzon, Robert Yetter, and Joan Porter for their helpful suggestions on the manuscript, as well as Jessica Burdman for technical editing.

REFERENCES

Ada, G., 1992a, The design and testing of HIV prophylactic vaccines, *AIDS Res. Hum. Retroviruses* **8**:758–763.
Ada, G. L., 1992b, Vaccine efficacy and the immune response, *Vaccine Res.* **1**:17–23.
Ada, G., Koff, W., and Petricciani, J., 1992, The next steps in HIV vaccine development, *AIDS Res. Hum. Retroviruses* **8**:1317–1319.
Adams, S. E., and Paoletti, E., 1993, Use of new vectors for the development of vaccines, *AIDS* **7**(Suppl. 1):S141–S146.
Adams, S. E., Dawson, K. M., Gull, K., Kingsman, S. M., and Kingsman, A. J., 1987, The expression of hybrid HIV:Ty virus-like particles in yeast, *Nature* **329**:68–70.
Allan, J. D., Conant, M., Lavelle, J., Mitsuyasu, R., Twaddell, T., and Kahn, J., 1993, Safety and immunogenicity of MN and IIIB rgp 120/HIV-1 vaccines in HIV-1 infected subjects with CD4 counts >500 cells/mm^3, *IX International Conference on AIDS/IV STD World Congress*, Berlin, abstract PO-B27-2137, p. 491.
Andersen, M. M., and Ronne, T., 1991, Side-effects with Japanese encephalitis vaccine, *Lancet* **337**:1044.
Anderson, M. C., Baer, H., Frazier, D. J., and Quinnan, G. V., 1987, The role of specific IgE and beta-propiolactone in reactions resulting from booster doses of human diploid cell rabies vaccine, *J. Allergy Clin. Immunol.* **80**:861–868.
Arif, M., Mitchison, N. A., and Zuckerman, A. J., 1988, Genetics of nonresponders to hepatitis B surface antigen and possible ways of circumventing "nonresponse," in: *Viral Hepatitis and Liver Disease* (A. J. Zuckerman, ed.), Liss, New York, pp. 714–716.

Ashley, R. L., Dalessio, J., Burchett, S., Brown, Z., Berry, S., Mohan, K., and Corey, L., 1992, Herpes simplex virus-2 (HSV-2) type-specific antibody correlates of protection in infants exposed to HSV-2 at birth, *J. Clin. Invest.* **90**:511–514.

Baker, C. J., Rench, M. A., Edwards, M. S., Carpenter, R. J., Hays, B. M., and Kasper, D. L., 1988, Immunization of pregnant women with a polysaccharide vaccine of Group B streptococcus, *N. Engl. J. Med.* **319**:1180–1185.

Barrett, N., Mitterer, A., Mundt, W., Eibl, J., Eibl, M., Gallo, R. C., Moss, B., and Dorner, F., 1989, Large-scale production and purification of a vaccinia recombinant-derived HIV-1 gp160 and analysis of its immunogenicity, *AIDS Res. Hum. Retroviruses* **5**:159–171.

Belshe, R. B., Clements, M. L., Dolin, R., Graham, B. S., McElrath, J., Gorse, G. J., Schwartz, D., Keefer, M. C., Wright, P., Corey, L., Bolognesi, D. P., Matthews, T. J., Stablein, D. M., O'Brien, F. S., Eibl, M., Dorner, F., Koff, W., and the National Institute of Allergy and Infectious Diseases AIDS Vaccine Evaluation Group Network, 1993, Safety and immunogenicity of a fully glycosylated recombinant gp160 human immunodeficiency virus type 1 vaccine in subjects at low risk of infection, *J. Infect. Dis.* **168**:1387–1395.

Belshe, R. B., Bolognesi, D. P., Clements, M. L., Corey, L., Dolin, R., Mestecky, J., Stablein, D., and Wright, P., 1994a, HIV infection in vaccinated volunteers [letter], *J. Am. Med. Assoc.* **272**:431.

Belshe, R. B., Clements, M. L., Keefer, M. C., Graham, B. S., Corey, L., Sposto, R., Wescott, S., Lawrence, D., and the NIAID AIDS Vaccine Clinical Trials Group, 1994b, Interpretating HIV serodiagnostic test results in the 1990's: Social risks of HIV vaccine studies in uninfected volunteers, *Ann. Intern. Med.* **121**:584–589.

Belshe, R. B., Graham, B., Keefer, M., Gorse, G. J., Wright, P., Dolin, R., Matthews, T., Weinhold, K., Bolognesi, D. P., Sposto, R., Stablein, D. M., Twaddell, T., Berman, P. W., Gregory, T. J., Izu, A. E., Walker, M. C., and Fast, P. E., 1994c, Neutralizing antibodies to HIV-1 in seronegative volunteers immunized with recombinant gp120 from the MN strain of HIV-1, *J. Am. Med. Assoc.* **272**:475–480.

Berman, P. W., Gregory, T. J., Riddle, L., Nakamura, G. R., Champe, M. A., Porter, J. P., Wurm, F. M., Hershberg, R. D., Cobb, E. K., and Eichberg, J. W., 1990, Protection of chimpanzees from infection by HIV-1 after vaccination with recombinant glycoprotein gp120 but not gp160, *Nature* **345**:622–625.

Berzofsky, J. A., Bensussan, A., Cease, K. B., Bourge, J. F., Cheynier, R., Lurhuma, Z., Salaun, J.-J., Gallo, R. C., Shearer, G. M., and Zagury, D., 1988, Antigenic peptides recognized by T lymphocytes from AIDS viral envelope-immune humans, *Nature* **334**:706–708.

Birx, D. L., and Redfield, R. R., 1991, HIV vaccine therapy, *Int. J. Immunopharmacol.* **13**(Suppl. 1):129–132.

Birx, D., Ketter, N., and Fast, P. E., 1995, HIV vaccine development, treatment and prevention, in: *Clinical Immunology* (R. R. Rich, ed.), Mosby, St. Louis (in press).

Bolognesi, D. P., 1993, The immune response to HIV: Implications for vaccine development, *Semin. Immunol.* **5**:203–214.

Bratt, G., Eriksson, L., Gilljam, G., Hinkula, J., Wahren, B., and Sandstrom, E., 1993, The one year results of vaccination with gp160 vaccine (VaxSyn HIV-1; MicroGeneSys) in asymptomatic HIV-carriers, *IX International Conference on AIDS/IV STD World Congress*, Berlin, abstract PO-B27-2138, p. 491.

Bruck, C., Thiriart, C., Delers, A., Fabry, L., Francotte, M., Van Opstal, O., Culp, J., Rosenberg, M., De Wilde, M., Heidt, P., and Heeney, J., 1993, Comparison of vaccine protection in chimpanzees immunized with two different forms of recombinant HIV-1 envelope glycoprotein, *AIDS Res. Hum. Retroviruses* **9**(Suppl. 1):S110 (abstract).

Bryson, Y. J., Lehman, D., Garratty, E., Dickover, R., Plaeger-Marshall, S., and O'Rourke, S., 1993, The role of maternal autologous neutralizing antibody in prevention of maternal fetal HIV-1 transmission, *J. Cell. Biochem.* (Suppl. 17E) abstract QZ005, p.95.

Burke, D. S., 1992, Human HIV vaccine trials: Does antibody-dependent enhancement pose a genuine risk? *Perspect. Biol. Med.* **35**:511–530.

Burke, D. S., 1993, Vaccine therapy for HIV: A historical review of the treatment of infectious diseases by active specific immunization with microbe-derived antigens, *Vaccine* **11**:883–891.

Cardenas, L., and Clements, J. D., 1992, Oral immunization using live attenuated *Salmonella* spp. as carriers of foreign antigens, *Clin. Microbiol. Rev.* **5**:328–342.

Cease, K. B., and Berzofsky, J. A., 1994, Toward a vaccine for AIDS: The emergence of immunobiology-based vaccine development, *Annu. Rev. Immunol.* **12**:923–989.

Chabala, S., Williams, M. M., Amenta, R., and Ognjan, A. F., 1991, Confirmed rabies exposure during pregnancy: Treatment with human rabies immune globulin and human diploid cell vaccine, *Am. J. Med.* **91**:423–424.

Chutivongse, S., and Wilde, H. H., 1989, Postexposure rabies vaccination during pregnancy: Experience with 21 patients, *Vaccine* **7**:546–548.

Clements, M. L., 1994, Effect of age on immune responses to vaccine, *J. Infect. Dis.* **170**:510–516.

Clerici, M., 1993, Cell mediated immunity in HIV infection, *AIDS* **8**:S135–S140.

Cochran, M. A., Ericson, B. L., Knell, J. D., and Smith, G. E., 1987, Use of baculovirus recombinants as a general method for the production of subunit vaccines, in: *Vaccines 87: Modern Approaches to New Vaccines, Prevention of AIDS and Other Viral, Bacterial, and Parasitic Diseases* (R. M. Chanock, R. A. Lerner, F. Brown, and H. Ginsberg, eds.), Cold Spring Harbor Laboratory Press, Cold Spring Harbor, NY, pp. 384–388.

Cohen, J., 1994, AIDS vaccines. Will media reports KO upcoming real-life trials? *Science* **264**:1660.

Combined vaccines and simultaneous administration: Current issues and perspectives, 1995, *Ann. N.Y. Acad. Sci.* (in press).

Comstock, G. W., 1994, Evaluating vaccination effectiveness and vaccine efficacy by means of case-control studies, *Epidemiol. Rev.* **16**:77–89.

Cooney, E. L., Collier, A. C., Greenberg, P. D., Coombs, R. W., Zarling, J., Arditti, D. E., Hoffman, M. C., Hu, S. L., and Corey, L., 1991, Safety and immunological response to a recombinant vaccinia virus vaccine expressing HIV envelope glycoprotein, *Lancet* **337**:567–572.

Cooney, E. L., McElrath, M. J., Corey, L., Hu, S. L., Collier, A. C., Arditti, D., Hoffman, M., Coombs, R. W., Smith, G. E., and Greenberg, P. D., 1993, Enhanced immunity to human immunodeficiency virus (HIV) envelope elicited by a combined vaccine regimen consisting of priming with a vaccinia recombinant expressing HIV envelope and boosting with gp160 protein, *Proc. Natl. Acad. Sci. USA* **90**:1882–1886.

Coursaget, P., Chiron, J. P., Yvonnet, B., Barin, F., Goudeau, A., Denis, F., Perrin, J., N'Doye, R., and Diop-Mar, I., 1983, Hepatitis B immunisation in pregnancy: Maternal immune response and transmission of anti-HBs antibodies to infants, *Int. J. Microbiol.* **1**:27–34.

Daniel, M. D., Kirchhoff, F., Czajac, S. C., Sehgal, P. K., and Desrosiers, R. C., 1992, Protective effects of a live-attenuated SIV vaccine with a deletion in the nef gene, *Science* **258**:1938–1941.

Deinard, A. S., and Ogburn, P., Jr., 1994, A/NJ/8/76 Influenza vaccination program: Effects on maternal health and pregnancy outcome, *Am. J. Obstet. Gynecol.* **140**:240–245.

de Santis, C., Robbioni, P., Longhi, R., Lopalco, L., Siccardi, A. G., Beretta, A., and Roberts, N. J., Jr., 1993, Cross-reactive response to human immunodeficiency virus type 1 (HIV-1) gp120 and HLA class I heavy chains induced by receipt of HIV-1-derived envelope vaccines, *J. Infect. Dis.* **168**:1396–1403.

Desrosiers, R. C., 1992, HIV with multiple gene deletions as a live attenuated vaccine for AIDS, *AIDS Res. Hum. Retroviruses* **8**:411–421.

Dixon, D. O., Rida, W. N., Fast, P. E., and Hoth, D. F., 1993, HIV vaccine trials: Some design issues including sample size calculation, *J. Acquir. Immune Defic. Syndr.* **6**:485–496.

Dolin, R., Graham, B. S., Greenberg, S. B., Tacket, C. O., Belshe, R. B., Midthun, K., Clements, M. L., Gorse, G. J., Horgan, B. W., Atmar, R. L., Karzon, D. T., Bonnez, W., Fernie, B. F., Montefiori, D. C., Stablein, D. M., Smith, G. E., Koff, W. C., and the NIAID AIDS Vaccine Clinical Trials Network, 1991, The safety and immunogenicity of a human immunodeficiency virus type 1 (HIV-1) recombinant gp160 candidate vaccine in humans, *Ann. Intern. Med.* **114**:119–127.

Douglas, R. G., Jr., 1993, The Children's Vaccine Initiative—will it work? *J. Infect. Dis.* **168**:269–274.

Duffy, S. W., South, M. C., and Day, N. E., 1992, Cluster randomization in large public health trials: The importance of antecedent data, *Statistics Med.* **11**:307–316.

Earl, P. L., Koenig, S., and Moss, B., 1991, Biological and immunological properties of human immunodeficiency virus type 1 envelope glycoprotein: Analysis of proteins with truncations and deletions expressed by recombinant vaccinia viruses, *J. Virol.* **65**:31–41.

Eickhoff, T. C., 1988, Bacille Calmette-Guerin (BCG) vaccine, in: *Vaccines* (S. A. Plotkin and E. A. Mortimer, Jr., eds.), Saunders, Philadelphia, pp. 372–386.

Ellis, R. W., and Douglas, R. G., Jr., 1994, New vaccine technologies, *J. Am. Med. Assoc.* **271**:929–931.

Emini, E. A., Schleif, W. A., Nunberg, J. H., Conley, A. J., Eda, Y., Tokiyoshi, S., Putney, S. D., Matsushita, S., Cobb, K. E., Jett, C. M., Eichberg, J. W., and Murthy, K. K., 1992, Prevention of HIV-1 infection in chimpanzees by gp120 V3 domain-specific monoclonal antibody, *Nature* **355**:728–730.

Fast, P. E., and Walker, M. C., 1993, Human trials of experimental AIDS vaccines, *AIDS* **7**(Suppl. 1):S147–S159.

Fast, P. E., Mathieson, B. J., and Schultz, A. M., 1994, Efficacy trials of AIDS vaccines: How science can inform ethics, *Curr. Opin. Immunol.* **6**:691–697.

Fauci, A. S., Schnittman, S. M., Poli, G., Koenig, S., and Pantaleo, G., 1991, NIH Conference. Immunopathogenic mechanisms in human immunodeficiency virus (HIV) infection, *Ann. Intern. Med.* **114**:678–693.

Fenner, F., Henderson, D. A., Arita, I., Jezek, Z., and Ladnyi, I. D., 1988, *Smallpox and its Eradication*, History of International Public Health, No. 6, World Health Organization, Geneva.

Fine, P. E. M., 1988, BCG vaccination against tuberculosis and leprosy, *Br. Med. Bull.* **44**:691–703.

Francis, D. P., Hadler, S. C., Thompson, S. E., Maynard, J. E., Ostrow, D. G., Altman, N., Braff, E. H., O'Malley, P., Hawkins, D., Judson, F. N., Penley, K., Nylund, T., Christie, G., Meyers, F., Moore, J. N., Jr., Gardner, A., Doto, I. L., Miller, J. H., Reynolds, G. H., Murphy, B. L., Schable, C. A., Clark, B. T., Curran, J. W., and Redeker, A. G., 1982, The prevention of hepatitis B with vaccine. Report of the Centers for Disease Control multi-center efficacy trial among homosexual men, *Ann. Intern. Med.* **97**:362–366.

General Recommendations on Immunization. Recommendations of the Advisory Committee on Immunization Practices (ACIP), 1994, *MMWR* **43**(RR-1):18–19.

Golding, H., Robey, F. A., Gates, F. T., III, Linder, W., Beining, P. R., Hoffman, T., and Golding, B., 1988, Identification of homologous regions in human immunodeficiency virus 1 gp41 and human MHC class II *B* 1 domain. I. Monoclonal antibodies against the gp41-derived peptide and patients' sera react with native HLA class II antigens, suggesting a role for autoimmunity in the pathogenesis of acquired immune deficiency syndrome, *J. Exp. Med.* **167**:914–923.

Golding, H., D'Souza, M. P., Bradac, J., Mathieson, B., and Fast, P., 1994, Meeting report. Neutralization of HIV-1, *AIDS Res. Hum. Retroviruses* **10**:633–643.

Goldstein, J. A., Neff, J. M., Lane, J. M., and Koplan, J. P., 1975, Smallpox vaccination reactions, prophylaxis, and therapy of complications, *Pediatrics* **55**:342–347.

Grady, C., 1994, Ethical issues in the development and testing of a preventive HIV vaccine, Ph.D. thesis, Georgetown University, Washington, DC.

Graham, B. S., Belshe, R. B., Clements, M. L., Dolin, R., Corey, L., Wright, P. F., Gorse, G. J., Midthun, K., Keefer, M. C., Roberts, N. J., Jr., Schwartz, D. H., Agosti, J. M., Fernie, B. F., Stablein, D. M., Montefiori, D. C., Lambert, J. S., Hu, S.-L., Esterlitz, J. R., Lawrence, D. N., Koff, W. C., and the AIDS Vaccine Trials Network, 1992, Vaccination of vaccinia-naive adults with human immunodeficiency virus type 1 gp160 recombinant vaccinia virus in a blinded, controlled, randomized clinical trial, *J. Infect. Dis.* **166**:244–252.

Graham, B., Keefer, M., McElrath, J., Matthews, T., Schwartz, D., Gorse, G., Sposto, R., Chernoff, D., and the NIAID AIDS Vaccine Clinical Trials Network, 1993a, Phase I trial of native HIV-1 SF2 rgp120 candidate vaccine, *IX International Conference on AIDS/IV STD World Congress*, Berlin, abstract PO-A29-0692, p. 250.

Graham, B. S., Matthews, T. J., Belshe, R. B., Clements, M. L., Dolin, R., Wright, P. F., Gorse, G. J., Schwartz, D. H., Keefer, M. C., Bolognesi, D. P., Corey, L., Stablein, D. M., Esterlitz, J. R., Hu, S.-L., Smith, G. E., Fast, P. E., Koff, W. C., and the NIAID AIDS Vaccine Clinical Trials Network, 1993b,

Augmentation of human immunodeficiency virus type 1 neutralizing antibody by priming with gp160 recombinant vaccinia and boosting with rgp160 in vaccinia-naive adults, *J. Infect. Dis.* **167**:533–537.

Hadler, S. C., Francis, D. P., Maynard, J. E., Thompson, S. E., Judson, F. N., Echenberg, D. F., Ostrow, D. G., O'Malley, P. M., Penley, K. A., Altman, N. L., Braff, E., Shipman, G. F., Coleman, P. J., and Mandel, E. J., 1986, Long-term immunogenicity and efficacy of hepatitis B vaccine in homosexual men, *N. Engl. J. Med.*, **315**:209–214.

Haigwood, N. L., Nara, P. L., Brooks, E., Van Nest, G. A., Ott, G., Higgins, K. W., Dunlop, N., Scandella, C. J., Eichberg, J. W., and Steimer, K. S., 1992, Native but not denatured recombinant human immunodeficiency virus type 1 gp120 generates broad-spectrum neutralizing antibodies in baboons, *J. Virol.* **66**:172–182.

Halloran, M. E., Longini, I. M., Jr., Haber, M. J., Struchiner, C. J., and Brunet, R. C., 1994, Exposure efficacy and change in contact rates in evaluating prophylactic HIV vaccines in the field, *Stat. Med.* **13**:357–377.

Halsey, N.A., 1993, Increased mortality after high titer measles vaccines: Too much of a good thing, *Pediatr. Infect. Dis. J.* **12**:462–465.

Harjulehto, T., Aro, T., Hovi, T., and Saxen, L., 1989, Congenital malformations and oral poliovirus vaccination during pregnancy, *Lancet* **1**:771–772.

Haynes, B. F., 1993, Scientific and social issues of human immunodeficiency virus vaccine development, *Science* **260**:1279–1286.

Haynes, J. R., Fuller, D. H., Eisenbraun, M. D., Ford, M. J., and Pertmer, T. M., 1994, Accell® particle-mediated DNA immunization elicits humoral, cytotoxic, and protective immune responses, *AIDS Res. Hum. Retroviruses* **10**(Suppl. 2):S43–S45.

Haynes, J. R., Yao, F.-L., Ma, J., Cao, S. X., and Klein, M. H., 1991, Strategy for developing a genetically-engineered whole-virus vaccine against HIV, *Mol. Immunol.* **28**:231–234.

Hesselton, R. M., Mazzara, G. P., Panicali, D., and Sullivan, J. L., 1992, HIV-specific immune responses in rabbits immunized with HIV-like particles and recombinant vaccinia virus, *VIII International Conference on AIDS/III STD World Congress*, Amsterdam, abstract MoA0045, p. Mo13.

Hoth, D. F., 1993, Issues in the development of a prophylactic HIV vaccine, *Ann. N.Y. Acad. Sci.* **685**:777–783.

Hu, S.-L., Kosowski, S. G., and Dalrymple, J. M., 1986, Expression of AIDS virus envelope gene in recombinant vaccinia viruses, *Nature* **320**:537–540.

Hu, S.-L., Stallard, V., Abrams, K., Barber, G. N., Kuller, L., Langlois, A. J., Morton, W. R., and Benveniste, R. E., 1993, Protection of vaccinia-primed macaques against SIVmne infection by combination immunization with recombinant vaccinia virus and SIVmne gp160, *J. Med. Primatol.* **22**:92–99.

Inactivated Japanese encephalitis virus vaccine. Recommendations of the Advisory Committee on Immunization Practices (ACIP), 1993, *MMWR* **42**(RR-1):1–13.

International ethical guidelines for biomedical research involving human subjects, 1993, Prepared by the Council for International Organizations of Medical Sciences (CIOMS) in collaboration with the World Health Organization (WHO), Geneva.

Jenner, E., 1959, An inquiry into the causes and effects of the variolae vaccinae, a disease discovered in some of the western counties of England, particularly Gloucestershire and known by the name of the cow pox, reprinted in: *Classics of Medicine and Surgery* (C. N. B. Camac, ed.), Dover, New York.

Kahn, J., Chernoff, D., Sinangil, F., Baenziger, J., Murcar, N., and Steimer, K., 1993, Phase 1 study of an HIV-1 gp 120 vaccine combined with MF59 and with dose escalation of MTP-PE, in sero-negative adults, *IX International Conference on AIDS/IV STD World Congress*, Berlin, abstract WS-B27-2, p. 70.

Karzon, D. T., 1994, Preventive vaccines, in: *Textbook of AIDS Medicine* (S. Broder, T. C. Merigan, Jr., and D. Bolognesi, eds.), Williams & Wilkins, Baltimore, pp. 667–692.

Karzon, D. T., Bolognesi, D. P., and Koff, W. C., 1992, Development of a vaccine for the prevention of AIDS, a critical appraisal, *Vaccine* **10**:1039–1052.

Katzenstein, D. A., Sawyer, L. A., and Quinnan, G. V., Jr., 1988, Human immunodeficiency virus, in: *Vaccines* (S.A. Plotkin and E. A. Mortimer, Jr., eds.), Saunders, Philadelphia, pp. 558–567.

Katzenstein, D., Valentine, F., Kundu, S., Haslett, P., Smith, G., and Merigan, T., 1992, Delayed-type-hypersensitivity reactions to intradermal gp160 in HIV infected individuals immunized with gp160, *VIII International Conference on AIDS/III STD World Congress*, Amsterdam, abstract PoA2192, p. A35.

Keefer, M. C., Belshe, R., Graham, B., McElrath, J., Clements, M. L., Sposto, R., Fast, P., and the NIAID AIDS Vaccine Clinical Trials Network, 1994, Safety profile of HIV vaccination: First 1000 volunteers of AIDS Vaccine Evaluation Group, *AIDS Res. Hum. Retroviruses* **10**(Suppl. 2):S139–S140.

Kieny, M. P., Rautmann, G., Schmitt, D., Dott, K., Wain-Hobson, S., Alizon, M., Girard, M., Chamaret, S., Laurent, A., Montagnier, L., and Lecocq, J. P., 1986, AIDS virus env protein expressed from a recombinant vaccinia virus, *Bio/Technology*. **4**:790–795.

Kim-Farley, R. J., and the Expanded Programme on Immunization team, 1992, EPI for the 1990s, *Vaccine* **10**:940–948.

Koff, W. C., and Hoth, D. F., 1988, Development and testing of AIDS vaccines, *Science* **241**:426–432.

Kovacs, J. A., Baseler, M., Dewar, R., Vogel, S., Davey, R. T., Fallon, J., Polis, M. A., Walker, R. E., Stevens, R., Salzman, N. P., Metcalf, J. A., Masur, H., and Lane, H. C., 1993a, Sustained increases in CD4+ lymphocytes in HIV-infected patients treated with intermittent interleukin-2 therapy, *1st National Conference on Human Retroviruses and Related Infections*, Washington, DC, abstract 301, p. 108.

Kovacs, J. A., Vasudevachari, M. B., Easter, M., Davey, R. T., Fallon, J., Polis, M. A., Metcalf, J. A., Salzman, N., Baseler, M., Smith, G. E., Volvovitz, F., Masur, H., and Lane, H. C., 1993b, Induction of humoral and cell-mediated anti-human immunodeficiency virus (HIV) responses in HIV sero-negative volunteers by immunization with recombinant gp160, *J. Clin. Invest.* **92**:919–928.

La Montagne, J. R., and Curlin, G. T., 1992, Vaccine clinical trials, in: *Vaccine Research and Developments*, Vol. 1 (W. C. Koff and H. Six, eds.), Dekker, New York, pp. 197–222.

Lasky, L. A., Groopman, J. E., Fennie, C. W., Benz, P. M., Capon, D. J., Dowbenko, D. J., Nakamura, G. R., Nunes, W. M., Renz, M. E., and Berman, P. W., 1986, Neutralization of the AIDS retrovirus by antibodies to a recombinant envelope glycoprotein, *Science* **233**:209–212.

Lawrence, D. N., Rida, W. N., Sheon, A., Fischer, R. D., and Hoff, R., 1993, Symposium on preparedness for HIV vaccine efficacy trials, *AIDS Res. Hum. Retroviruses* **9**(Suppl. 1):S125–S126.

Letvin, N. L., 1993, Vaccines against human immunodeficiency virus—progress and prospects, *N. Engl. J. Med.* **329**:1400–1405.

Levine, A. M., Allen, J., Munson, K. M., Carlo, D. J., Jensen, F. C., and Salk, J., 1993, Initial studies of active immunotherapy in HIV infected patients using a gp-120 depleted HIV-1 immunogen: A five year followup, *IX International Conference on AIDS/IV STD World Congress*, Berlin, abstract WS-B28-2, p. 71.

Levine, M. M., 1991, Vaccines and milk immunoglobulin concentrates for prevention of infectious diarrhea, *J. Pediatr.* 118: S129–S136.

Levine, M. M., Edsall, G., and Bruce-Chwatt, L. J., 1974, Live-virus vaccines in pregnancy—risks and recommendations, *Lancet* **2**:34–38.

Liu, M. A., and Vogel, F. R., 1994, Use of novel DNA vectors and immunologic adjuvants in HIV vaccine development, *AIDS* **8**(Suppl. 1):S195–S201.

Lurie, P., Bishaw, M., Chesney, M. A., Cooke, M., Fernandes, M. E. L., Hearst, N., Katongole-Mbidde, E., Koetsawang, S., Lindan, C. P., Mandel, J., Mhloyi, M., and Coates, T. J., 1994, Ethical, behavioral, and social aspects of HIV vaccine trials in developing countries, *J. Am. Med. Assoc.* **271**:295–301.

McCord, W. J., Alcock, A. J. W., and Hildes, J. A., 1955, Poliomyelitis in pregnancy, *Am. J. Obstet. Gynecol.* **69**:265–276.

McElrath, J., Keefer, M., Greenberg, P., Sposto, R., Chernoff, D., Steimer, K., and the NIAID AIDS Vaccine Evaluation Group, 1993, Evaluation of a nonglycosylated yeast-derived envelope vaccine on HIV-1-specific immunity in a randomized, blinded, controlled HIV-1 seropositive trial, *IX International Conference on AIDS/IV STD World Congress*, Berlin, abstract PO-A28-0670, p. 246.

McElrath, M. J., Corey, L., Clements, M. L., Belshe, R., Keefer, M., Graham, B., Fast, P., Duliege, A. M., Francis, D., and the NIAID AIDS Vaccine Clinical Trials Network, 1994, A Phase II HIV vaccine trial in seronegative volunteers: Expanded safety and immunogenicity evaluation of two recombinant gp120 vaccines, *J. Cell. Biochem.* (Suppl. 18B), abstract J412, p. 158.

McNamara, J. G., Rogers, M., Goldenthal, K., Jackson, J. B., Rossi, P., Fenton, T., and Fast, P. E., 1994, Report of the perinatal intervention working group, *AIDS Res. Hum. Retroviruses* **10**(Suppl. 2):S161–S164.

Marthas, M. L., Sutjipto, S., Miller, C. J., Higgins, J., Torten, J., Unger, R. E., Marx, P. A., Pedersen, N. C., Kiyono, H., and McGhee, J. R., 1992, Efficacy of live-attenuated and whole-inactivated SIV vaccines against intravenous and vaginal challenge, in: *Vaccines 92* (F. Brown, R. M. Chanock, H. S. Ginsberg, and R. A. Lerner, eds.), Cold Spring Harbor Laboratory Press, Cold Spring Harbor, NY, pp. 117–122.

Mascola, J. R., Mathieson, B. J., Zack, P. M., Walker, M. C., Halstead, S. B., and Burke, D. S., 1993, Summary report: Workshop on the potential risks of antibody-dependent enhancement in human HIV vaccine trials, *AIDS Res. Hum. Retroviruses* **9**:1169–1178.

Mascola, J., Weislow, O., Snyder, S., Belay, S., Yeager, M., McCutchan, F., McNeil, J., Burke, D., and Walker, M. C., 1994, Neutralizing antibody activity in sera from human immunodeficiency virus type-1 vaccine recipients from the AIDS Vaccine Clinical Trials Network, *AIDS Res. Hum. Retroviruses* **10**(Suppl. 1) (asbtr.) S55.

Meinert, C. L., 1986, *Clinical Trials: Design, Conduct and Analysis, Monographs in Epidemiology and Biostatistics*, Vol. 8 (A.M. Lilienfeld, ed.), Oxford University Press, London.

Miliauskas, J. R., Mukherjee, T., and Dixon, B., 1993, Postimmunization (vaccination) injection-site reactions. A report of four cases and review of the literature, *Am. J. Surg. Pathol.* **17**:516–524.

Miller, C. J., Marthas, M., Lohman, B., McChesney, M., Alexander, N. J., and Hendrickx, A. G., 1994, Effect of seminal plasma on vaginal transmission of cell-free SIV and dissemination of SIV following vaginal inoculation, in: *Retroviruses of Human A.I.D.S. and Related Animal Diseases: "Colloque des Cent Gardes 1993"* (M. Girard and L. Valette, eds.), Fondation Marcel Merieux, Lyon, pp. 145–150.

Mofenson, L. M., 1992, Preventing mother to infant HIV transmission: What we know so far, *AIDS Reader* March/April:42–51.

Mosier, D. E., Gulizia, R. J., MacIsaac, P. D., Corey, L., and Greenberg, P. D., 1993, Resistance to human immunodeficiency virus 1 infection of SCID mice reconstituted with peripheral blood leukocytes from donors vaccinated with vaccinia gp160 and recombinant gp160, *Proc. Natl. Acad. Sci. USA* **90**:2443–2447.

NIH guidelines on the inclusion of women and minorities as subjects in clinical research, March 28, 1994, 59 *FR* No. 59, part VIII, Office of the Federal Register, National Archives and Records Administration, U.S. Government Printing Office, Washington, DC, pp. 14508–14513.

Nkowane, B. M., Wassilak, S. G. F., Orenstein, W. A., Bart, K. J., Schonberger, L. B., Hinman, A. R., and Kew, O. M., 1987, Vaccine-associated paralytic poliomyelitis United States: 1973 through 1984, *J. Am. Med. Assoc.* **257**:1335–1340.

O'Brien, W. A., Ovcak, S., Kalhor, H., Mao, S. H., and Zack, J. A., 1993, HIV-1 replication can be increased in blood from seropositive patients following influenza immunization, *IX International Conference on AIDS/IV STD World Congress*, Berlin, abstract PO-A12-0209, p. 169.

Ornoy, A., and Ishai, P. B., 1993, Congenital anomalies after oral poliovirus vaccination during pregnancy, *Lancet* **341**:1162.

Oxford, J. S., Frezza, P., and Race, E., 1993, Challenges and strategies for AIDS vaccine development, *Vaccine* **11**:612–614.

Palker, T. J., Clark, M. E., Langlois, A. J., Matthews, T. J., Weinhold, K. J., Randall, R. R., Bolognesi, D. P., and Haynes, B. F., 1988, Type-specific neutralization of the human immunodeficiency virus with antibodies to env-encoded synthetic peptides, *Proc. Natl. Acad. Sci. USA* **85**:1932–1936.

Panicali, D. L., Mazzara, G., Sullivan, J. L., Hesselton, R., Shen, L., Letvin, N., Daniel, M., Desrosiers, R., and Stott, E. J., 1992, Use of lentivirus-like particles alone and in combination with live vaccinia-virus-based vaccines, *AIDS Res. Hum. Retroviruses* **8**:1449.

Parekh, B. S., Phillips, S., Granade, T. C., Schochetman, G., George, J. R., and AIDS Vaccine Clinical Trials Network, 1994, Evaluation of commercial assays to discriminate vaccinees from HIV-1 infected individuals, *AIDS Res. Hum. Retroviruses* **10**(Suppl. 1):S34.

Pauza, D., Trivedi, P., Johnson, E., Meyer, K. K., Streblow, D. N., Malkovsky, M., Emau, P., Schultz, K. T., and Salvato, M. S., 1994, Acquired resistance to mucosal SIV infection after low dose intrarectal inoculation: The roles of virus selection and CD8-mediated T cell immunity, in: *Retroviruses of Human A.I.D.S. and Related Animal Diseases: "Colloque des Cent Gardes 1993"* (M. Girard and L. Valette, eds.), Fondation Marcel Merieux, Lyon, pp. 151–156.

Phases of an investigation, 1993, 21 *CFR* 321.21, Office of the Federal Register, National Archives and Records Administration, U.S. Government Printing Office, Washington, DC, p. 68.

Pincus, S. H., Messer, K. G., Schwartz, D. H., Lewis, G. K., Graham, B. S., Blattner, W. A., and Fisher, G., 1993, Differences in the antibody response to human immunodeficiency virus-1 envelope glycoprotein (gp160) in infected laboratory workers and vaccinees, *J. Clin. Invest.* **91**:1987–1996.

Plotkin, S. L., and Plotkin, S. A., 1988, A short history of vaccination, in: *Vaccines* (S. A. Plotkin and E. A. Mortimer, Jr., eds.), Saunders, Philadelphia, pp. 1–7.

Porter, J. P., Glass, M. J., and Koff, W. C., 1989, Ethical considerations in AIDS vaccine testing, *IRB* **11**:1-4. A publication of the Hastings Center, 255 Elm Road, Briarcliff Manor, NY 10510.

Prince, A. M., Horowitz, B., Shulman, R. W., Pascual, D., Hewlett, I., Epstein, J., and Eichberg, J. W., 1990, Apparent prevention of HIV infection by HIV immunoglobulin given prior to low-dose HIV challenge, in: *Vaccines 90: Modern Approaches to New Vaccines Including Prevention of AIDS* (F. Brown, R. M. Chanock, H. S. Ginsberg, and R. A. Lerner, eds.), Cold Spring Harbor Laboratory Press, Cold Spring Harbor, NY, pp. 347–351.

Protection of human subjects, 1993a, 21 *CFR* 50, Office of the Federal Register, National Archives and Records Administration, U.S. Government Printing Office, Washington, DC, pp. 229–236.

Protection of human subjects, 1993b, 45 *CFR* 46, Office of the Federal Register, National Archives and Records Administration, U.S. Government Printing Office, Washington, DC, pp. 116–135.

Race, E., Frezza, P., and Oxford, J., 1993, A chemically inactivated whole virus HIV-1 vaccine induces cross-neutralising antibodies, *IX International Conference on AIDS/IV STD World Congress*, Berlin, abstract PO-A29-0685, p. 249.

Redfield, R. R., Wright, D. C., James, W. D., Jones, T. S., Brown, C., and Burke, D. S., 1987, Disseminated vaccinia in a military recruit with human immunodeficiency virus (HIV) disease, *N. Engl. J. Med.* **316**:673–676.

Redfield, R. R., Birx, D. L., Ketter, N., Tramont, E., Polonis, V., Davis, C., Brundage, J. F., Smith, G., Johnson, S., Fowler, A., Wierzba, T., Shafferman, A., Volvovitz, F., Oster, C., Burke, D. S., and The Military Medical Consortium for Applied Retroviral Research, 1991, A Phase I evaluation of the safety and immunogenicity of vaccination with recombinant gp160 in patients with early human immunodeficiency virus infection, *N. Engl. J. Med.* **324**:1677–1684.

Report of a consensus workshop, Siena, Italy, January 17–18, 1992, Maternal factors involved in mother-to-child transmission of HIV-1, 1992a, *J. Acquir. Immune Defic. Syndr.* **5**:1019–1029.

Report of a consensus workshop, Siena, Italy, January 17–18, 1992, Early diagnosis of HIV infection in infants, 1992b, *J. Acquir. Immune Defic. Syndr.* **5**:1169–1178.

Report of a consensus workshop, Siena, Italy, June 3–6, 1993, Strategies for prevention of perinatal transmission of HIV infection, 1995, *J. Acquir. Immune Defic. Syndr.* **8**:161–175.

Rida, W. N., and Lawrence, D. N., 1994, Some statistical issues in HIV vaccine trials, *Stat. Med.* **13**:2155–2177.

Rida, W., Meier, P., and Stevens, C., 1993, Design and implementation of HIV vaccine efficacy trials: A working group summary, *AIDS Res. Hum. Retroviruses* **9**(Suppl. 1):S59–S63.

Robbins, F. C., 1993, Eradication of polio in the Americas, *J. Am. Med. Assoc.* **270**:1857–1859.

Robinson, H. L., Hunt, L. A., and Webster, R. G., 1993, Protection against a lethal influenza virus challenge by immunization with a haemagglutinin-expressing plasmid DNA, *Vaccine* **11**:957–960.

Rosenberg, Z. F., and Fauci, A. S., 1991, Immunopathogenesis of HIV infection, *FASEB J.* **5**:2382–2390.

Rovinski, B., Haynes, J. R., Cao, S. X., James, O., Sia, C., Zolla-Pazner, S., Matthews, T. J., and Klein, M. H., 1992, Expression and characterization of genetically engineered human immunodeficiency virus-like particles containing modified envelope glycoproteins: Implications for development of a cross-protective AIDS vaccine, *J. Virol.* **66**:4003–4012.

Rubella vaccination during pregnancy—United States, 1971–1988, 1989, *MMWR* **38**:289–293.

Ruff, T. A., Eisen, D., Fuller, A., and Kass, R., 1991, Adverse reactions to Japanese encephalitis vaccine, *Lancet* **338**:881–882.

Saballus, M. K., Lake, K. D., and Wager, G. P., 1987, Immunizing the pregnant woman—Risks versus benefits, *Postgrad. Med.* **81**(8):103–109.

Sabin, A. B., 1993, HIV vaccination dilemma [letter], *Nature* **362**:212.

Sabin, A. B., Hennessen, W. A., and Winnser, J., 1954, Studies on variants of poliomyelitis virus. I. Experimental segregation and properties of avirulent variants of three immunologic types, *J. Exp. Med.* **99**:551–576.

Salk, J., 1991, Prospects for AIDS vaccines: The need for clinical trials in human populations, *Vaccine* **9**:791.

Salmon, D., Sicard, D., Gluckman, J. C., Autran, B., Plotkin, S., and Excler, J. L., 1993, Safety and immunogenicity of MN/BRU-rgp160 followed with a MN-V3 synthetic peptide in HIV negative volunteers (ANRS VAC02), *IX International Conference on AIDS/IV STD World Congress*, Berlin, abstract WS-B27-3, p. 70.

Santosham, M., 1993, Prevention of Haemophilus influenzae type b disease, *Vaccine* **11**(Suppl. 1):S52–S57.

Santosham, M., Wolff, M., Reid, R., Hohenboken, M., Bateman, M., Goepp, J., Cortese, M., Sack, D., Hill, J., Newcomer, W., Capriotti, L., Smith, J., Owen, M., Gahagan, S., Hu, D., Kling, R., Lukacs, L., Ellis, R. W., Vella, P. P., Calandra, G., Matthews, H., and Ahonkhai, V., 1991, The efficacy in Navajo infants of a conjugate vaccine consisting of *Haemophilus influenzae* type b polysaccharide and *Neisseria meningitidis* outer-membrane protein complex, *N. Engl. J. Med.* **324**:1767–1772.

Sato, H., Albrecht, P., Reynolds, D. W., Stagno, S., and Ennis, F.A., 1979, Transfer of measles, mumps, and rubella antibodies from mother to infant, *Am. J. Dis. Child.* **133**:1240–1243.

Scarlatti, G., Albert, J., Rossi, P., Hodara, V., Biraghi, P., Muggiasca, L., and Fenyo, E. M., 1993, Mother-to-child transmission of human immunodeficiency virus type 1: Correlation with neutralizing antibodies against primary isolates, *J. Infect. Dis.* **168**:207–210.

Schwartz, D., Clements, M. L., Belshe, R., Gorse, G., Wright, P., and Graham, B., 1993a, Interim results of rgp160 vaccine trial in HIV+ volunteers, *IX International Conference on AIDS/IV STD World Congress*, Berlin, abstract PO-A28-0668, p. 246.

Schwartz, D. H., Gorse, G., Clements, M. L., Belshe, R., Izu, A., Duliege, A. M., Berman, P., Twaddell, T., Stablein, D., Sposto, R., Siciliano, R., and Matthews, T., 1993b, Induction of HIV-1-neutralizing and syncytium-inhibiting antibodies in uninfected recipients of HIV-1 IIIB rgp120 subunit vaccine, *Lancet* **342**:69–73.

Sheon, A. R., 1994, Overview: HIV vaccine feasibility studies, *AIDS Res. Hum. Retroviruses* **10**(Suppl. 2): S195–S196.

Siber, G. R., Santosham, M., Reid, G. R., Thompson, C., Almeido-Hill, J., Morell, A., DeLange, G., Ketcham, J. K., and Callahan, E. H., 1990, Impaired antibody response to *Haemophilus influenzae* type b polysaccharide and low IgG2 and IgG4 concentrations in Apache children, *N. Engl. J. Med.* **323**:1387–1392.

Siber, G. R., Werner, B. G., Halsey, N. A., Reid, R., Almeido-Hill, J., Garrett, S. C., Thompson, C., and Santosham, M., 1993, Interference of immune globulin with measles and rubella immunization, *J. Pediatr.* **122**:204–211.

Siegel, M., and Greenberg, M., 1956, Poliomyelitis in pregnancy: Effect on fetus and newborn infant, *J. Pediatr.* **49**:280–288.

Slade, H. B., 1993, HIV infection: Approaches to post-infection active immunotherapy, *Curr. Opin. Invest. Drugs* **2**:875–897.

Smallpox vaccine. Recommendations of the Immunization Practices Advisory Committee (ACIP), 1985, *MMWR* **34**:341–342.

Smith, P. G., and Morrow, R. H., (eds.), 1991, *Methods for Field Trials of Interventions Against Tropical Diseases: A Toolbox*, Oxford University Press, London.

Spilker, B., and Cramer, J. A., 1992, Ethical issues in patient recruitment, in: *Patient Recruitment in Clinical Trials*, Raven Press, New York, pp. 150–158.

Stein, D. S., Timpone, J. G., Gradon, J. D., Kagan, J. M., and Schnittman, S. M., 1993, Immune-based therapeutics: Scientific rationale and the promising approaches to the treatment of the human immunodeficiency virus-infected individual, *Clin. Infect. Dis.* **17**:749–771.

Stover, C. K., Cruz, V. F., Bansal, G. P., Hanson, M. S., Fuerst, T. R., Jacobs, W. R., Jr., and Bloom, B. R., 1992, Use of recombinant BCG as a vaccine delivery vehicle, in: *Genetically Engineered Vaccines* (J. E. Ciardi, J. R. McGhee, and J. M. Keith, eds.), Plenum Press, New York, pp. 175–182.

Szmuness, W., Stevens, C. E., Harley, E. J., Zang, E. A., Taylor, P. E., Alter, H. J., and the Dialysis Vaccine Trial Group, 1981, The immune response of healthy adults to a reduced dose of hepatitis B vaccine, *J. Med. Virol.* **8**:123–129.

Tartaglia, J., Perkus, M. E., Taylor, J., Norton, E.K., Audonnet, J.-C., Cox, W. I., Davis, S. W., van der Hoeven, J., Meignier, B., Riviere, M., Languet, B., and Paoletti, E., 1992, NYVAC: A highly attenuated strain of vaccinia virus, *Virology* **188**:217–232.

Tartaglia, J., Cox, W. I., and Paoletti, E., 1993, NYVAC and ALVAC vectors in retrovirus vaccine development, *AIDS Res. Hum. Retroviruses* **9**(Suppl. 1):S27 (abstract).

The Jordan report. Accelerated development of vaccines, 1994, Division of Microbiology and Infectious Diseases, NIAID, NIH, Bethesda.

Trauger, R. J., Ferre, F., Daigle, A. E., Jensen, F. C., Moss, R. B., Mueller, S. H., Richieri, S. P., Slade, H. B., and Carlo, D. J., 1994, Effect of immunization with inactivated gp120-depleted human immunodeficiency virus type 1 (HIV-1) immunogen on HIV-1 immunity, viral DNA, and percentage of CD4 cells, *J. Infect. Dis.* **169**:1256–1264.

Twomey, J. G., Jr., and Fletcher, J. C., 1994, Ethical issues surrounding care of HIV-infected children, in: *Pediatric AIDS*, 2nd ed. (P. A. Pizzo and C. M. Wilfert, eds.), Williams & Wilkins, Baltimore, pp. 713–724.

Valentine, F., Katzenstein, D., Haslett, P., Beckett, L., Borucki, M., Vasquez, M., Smriti, K., Smith, G., Korvick, J., Kagan, J., and Merigan, T., 1992, A randomized, controlled study of immunogenicity of rgp160 vaccine in HIV-infected subjects, *VIII International Conference on AIDS/III STD World Congress*, Amsterdam, abstract TuB 0561, p. Tu39.

van Kuyk, R., Torbett, B., Gulizia, R., MacIsaac, P., Leath, S., Mosier, D., and Koenig, S., 1993, Human CTL specific for the NEF protein of HIV protect Hu-PBL-SCID mice from HIV infection, *AIDS Res. Hum. Retroviruses* **9**(Suppl. 1):S77.

Varner, M. W., McGuinness, G. A., and Galask, R. P., 1982, Rabies vaccination in pregnancy, *Am. J. Obstet. Gynecol.* **143**:717–718.

Vermund, S. H., Fischer, R. D., Hoff, R., Rida, W. N., Sheon, A. R., Lawrence, D. N., Hoth, D. F., and Barker, L. F., 1993, Preparing for HIV vaccine efficacy trials: Partnerships and challenges, *AIDS Res. Hum. Retroviruses* **9**(Suppl. 1):S127–S132.

Vermund, S. H., Schultz, A. M., and Hoff, R., 1994, Prevention of HIV/AIDS with vaccines, *Curr. Opin. Infect. Dis.* **7**:82–94.

Walker, M. C., and Fast, P. E., 1994, Clinical trials of candidate AIDS vaccines, *AIDS* **8**(Suppl. 1):S213–S236.

Wang, B., Ugen, K. E., Srikantan, V., Agadjanyan, M. G., Dang, K., Refaeli, Y., Sato, A. I., Boyer, J., Williams, W. V., and Weiner, D. B., 1993, Gene inoculation generates immune responses against human immunodeficiency virus type 1, *Proc. Natl. Acad. Sci. USA* **90**:4156–4160.

Westblom, T. U., Belshe, R. B., Gorse, G. J., Anderson, E. L., Berry, C. F., and the NIAID AIDS Clinical Trials Network, 1990, Characteristics of a population volunteering for human immunodeficiency virus immunization, *Int. J. STD AIDS* **1**:126–128.

Wintsch, J., Chaignat, C. L., Braun, D.G., Jeannet, M., Stalder, H., Abrignani, S., Montagna, D., Clavijo, F., Moret, P., Dayer, J. M., Staehelin, T., Doe, B., Steimer, K. S., Dina, D., and Cruchaud, A., 1991, Safety and immunogenicity of a genetically engineered human immunodeficiency virus vaccine, *J. Infect. Dis.* **163**:219–225.

Wolff, J. A., Malone, R. W., Williams, P., Chong, W., Acsadi, G., Jani, A., and Felgner, P. L., 1990, Direct gene transfer into mouse muscle in vivo, *Science* **247**:1465–1468.

Wright, P. F., Kim-Farley, R. J., de Quadros, C. A., Robertson, S. E., Scott, R. M., Ward, N. A., and Henderson, R. H., 1991, Strategies for the global eradication of poliomyelitis by the year 2000, *N. Engl. J. Med.* **325**:1774–1779.

Zagury, D., 1991, Anti-HIV cellular immunotherapy in AIDS, *Lancet* **338**:694–695.

Zidovudine for the prevention of HIV transmission from mother to infant, 1994, *MMWR* **43**:285–287.

Zunich, K. M., Lane, H. C., Davey, R. T., Falloon, J., Polis, M., Kovacs, J. A., and Masur, H., 1992, Phase I/II studies of the toxicity and immunogenicity of recombinant gp160 and p24 vaccines in HIV-infected individuals, *AIDS Res. Hum. Retroviruses* **8**:1335.

Chapter 6

Laboratory Empiricism, Clinical Design, and Social Value

The Rough Road toward Vaccine Development

Donald P. Francis

1. INTRODUCTION

Vaccine development is inherently different from therapeutic drug development. Each step in vaccine development is influenced by the perceived value of the vaccine to be developed. That perception of value begins with the public who, ultimately, determine how important they consider the prevention of a given disease. Unfortunately, the public commonly undervalues the impact, and therefore value, of disease prevention in general. As a result, the full disease prevention potential of vaccines has yet to be realized. Smallpox has been eradicated by vaccine. Polio may soon be eradicated by vaccine. Measles, tetanus, diphtheria, and pertussis have been markedly reduced. But, considering the potential for the control or elimination of diseases with vaccine, we have only scratched the surface.

2. DISCUSSION

For the public to render value to a preventive vaccine, they must feel personally threatened by the disease in question. Here an important survival technique—denial—often conflicts directly with the process of translating what is important. Because few diseases are so visible or common that most people feel personally threatened, most individuals can deny that they or their family are at risk. It is not unlike the 30-year smokers who say they will never get lung cancer and many times their prediction of disease avoidance will be correct.

Donald P. Francis • Genentech, Inc., South San Francisco, California 94080.

Vaccine Design: The Subunit and Adjuvant Approach, edited by Michael F. Powell and Mark J. Newman. Plenum Press, New York, 1995.

From the sociopolitical standpoint, those who have the power to determine the social importance of vaccine development often have the lowest risk of infection for the common infectious diseases. Generally, such diseases have their highest incidence in the lower socioeconomic strata. Therefore, those who wield the political or financial power to make vaccine development a government or business priority, often fail to recognize the social as well as the medical importance of such action.

There are, however, some exceptions. The most recent example of a disease where a strong social movement was mounted to generate public and private interest in developing a preventive vaccine was polio. In the mid-1950s polio, although having a relatively low incidence of severe disease, had great social impact and led to a strong commitment to develop a vaccine to prevent it. This unusual response was generated because the circumstances surrounding polio were unique compared to most vaccine-preventable diseases. First, it affected the middle class, an important power base. Second, it was visible. The images of previously healthy children and adults, now in iron lungs or with crippled limbs, were powerful. Finally, the President of the United States, Franklin Roosevelt, was severely afflicted himself. The combination of these circumstances led our society to value a preventive vaccine for polio. National fund-raising campaigns were organized. Mothers, on door-to-door campaigns, collected dimes from neighbors. This valuation led to intense vaccine research and development, successful clinical evaluations, and, ultimately, successful delivery of the vaccine—all of this at a time when our understanding of virology and immunology was in its infancy (Carter, 1966).

Such is not the usual case. Without understanding the immediate threat, without the easily recognized images, and without the social power base of the middle class and the political power brokers, the interest in vaccines is usually minimal. With such minimal interest, society undervalues the potential of vaccines. The private sector, stimulated by potential profits, will move to fill a vacuum of social demand (or value). With low social value afforded vaccines, the private sector has little incentive to invest resources to develop them. In this low value setting, there is little motivation to invest in vaccine development. And since the private sector is the major source of new vaccines, the result is that few vaccines are developed.

The situation with AIDS is a perfect example. Despite the huge worldwide public health impact and the obvious need for a vaccine there has not emerged a social movement like that with polio. There is a huge, highly political, and very accomplished social movement that has arisen around AIDS. However, this movement has been centered around infected people—the need for a treatment, the need for care. With the interest in "a cure," the interest in a prophylactic vaccine has been minimal. In other words, the political movement of AIDS has not valued prophylactic vaccines. As a result, the pharmaceutical industry has not responded aggressively to make one. Without the society placing a clear value on an HIV-1 vaccine, there is little stimulus for industry to produce one.

In addition to the social undervaluation of vaccines, there is a scientific issue with vaccines that discourages industry from developing them. Compared to other drugs used to treat diseases, vaccine research is far less predictable in determining the potential for success during the development process. For standard therapeutic drugs, there are often early preclinical data that show that the new drug may be efficacious. Such data encourage the developer to make the next step—clinical trials. Moreover, once therapeutic drugs are tested in clinical experiments with ill people, there is usually a confirmation of preclinical results that the drug is efficacious and safe. That is, ill patients treated with the drug get better. Thus, by the time Phase III efficacy trials are started, there is a high probability, usually 80–90%, that the product will be marketed.

For vaccines, there are usually less data on which to base advancement to clinical trials, especially Phase III trials. Vaccines are given to healthy people and therefore there is no immediate indication they are functioning as designed. There are often indirect indicators to help guide development such as laboratory tests or animal models which, in a surrogate sense, reflect the potential for success. However, the ultimate issue remains— does the vaccine protect from infection or disease after natural exposure?

This question usually cannot be answered without carrying out a lengthy Phase III efficacy trial. Obviously, those making investment decisions will be far more likely to follow a path, like therapeutic drug development, having clearly marked guideposts rather than the less well marked path toward vaccine development.

And so, in clinical vaccine research there is the constant call to go ahead and "try it." But such calls always have potential or real risks and costs attached to them that must be balanced against the potential benefits. The first consideration for the developer is the cost of the trial. Vaccine efficacy trials usually require thousands of participants and take years to complete. Even with widely spaced follow-up visits or minimal laboratory tests, such studies are expensive. Somebody, ultimately society, must pay for them. To make the decision to pay such a price, somebody must value the end product. The potential value will be weighted together with other downside issues such as potential safety risks, costs, and opportunities lost to pursue other drug products.

As mentioned above in the comparison with therapeutic drugs, making a calculation of potential success of a prototype vaccine is often difficult. Milestones in vaccine development might include success in protecting an animal from similar exposure, success in inducing immunity that is known to confer protection, and the presumed or measured level of adverse events. Vaccine developers use these milestones to determine if the downside issues are offset by the probability of success.

Furthermore, in the decision whether or not to move ahead, the feasibility of the efficacy trial is weighted substantially. Such feasibility depends on the availability of a high-incidence population, the potential for such a population to cooperate to ensure adequate enrollment and follow-up, and the availability of measurable end points be they clinical or laboratory. There are examples over the years that highlight the difficulties of each of these feasibility issues. For the polio efficacy trials of the Salk vaccine, high-incidence groups could not be identified. As a result, entire communities of children were recruited to be given vaccine or placebo. In addition, no easily available laboratory end point was available and so clinical end points were used (Carter, 1966; Smith, 1990).

Similar difficulties were more recently encountered in studies of the pertussis vaccine. In this situation no simple laboratory test applicable under field conditions could readily differentiate whooping cough caused by *B. pertussis* from similar clinical disease caused by other microorganisms. The challenge of testing the vaccine was immense and required a huge sample size before the true efficacy could be estimated (Blackwelder *et al.*, 1991).

The availability of "guideposts" in vaccine development varies for different infections. For some infections there are clear immunologic targets that assist vaccine development. For example, with hepatitis B virus (HBV), there was a group of infected individuals who recovered and a group who developed chronic viremia. Comparisons of the two groups showed that a laboratory test, antibody to the surface protein, correlated with recovery. Early chimpanzee experiments and human clinical trials showed that those given plasma having high levels of this antibody were protected from infection (Purcell and Gerin, 1975; Redeker *et al.*, 1975). Moreover, our knowledge of HBV pathogenesis was limited at the time, making decisions easier; there were few laboratory tests at the time to confuse the issue. Thus, the logic was that if a vaccine induces antibodies to the surface protein, it should also protect. And it did (Maupas *et al.*, 1976; Szmuness *et al.*, 1980; Francis *et al.*, 1982).

Unfortunately, it is more difficult with other infections. There was almost a total absence of guideposts for pertussis. Another current example is HIV-1. In contrast to HBV, essentially everyone infected with HIV-1 has progressive disease. There is no group that develops some marker of immunity that differentiates those protected from disease from those not. Without such a marker, vaccine developers have been forced to follow more presumptive than factual paradigms. Most have followed the surface glycoprotein model with the presumption that the immune response induced to it will be protective (Ada, 1993). Prototype vaccines have been developed that induce immune responses to these proteins. The question now is whether these vaccines will be efficacious.

More and more emphasis is being placed on preventing diseases that follow acute infection by years or decades. For HBV and HIV-1 a unique challenge is offered because of the long period before the late manifestations (cancer of the liver in the case of HBV and AIDS in the case of HIV-1) become apparent. In both cases researchers rely on surrogate markers as more immediate indicators of protection from diseases that take years or decades to develop. For HBV it was the prevention of chronic viremia, a condition known to be associated with the development of the late manifestations of the virus.

For HIV-1, a similar measurement reflecting chronic viremia will probably be used when efficacy trials are initiated since, like HBV, the immunologic demise associated with HIV is related to a chronic viremic state, which, if prevented, will presumably prevent the late manifestations such as AIDS.

The issue of safety is weighted heavily in deciding the *value* of a prototype vaccine and whether efficacy trials should be initiated. Indeed, the issue of vaccine safety is weighted more heavily than for therapeutic agents because vaccines, in contrast to therapeutic agents, are given to healthy people. Side effects among people without disease are far less acceptable to society than side effects among ill persons treated for disease. Thus, where severe side effects with drugs of a few per 100 recipients are often acceptable, for vaccines they must be orders of magnitude less frequent.

Finally, in terms of research and development, be it in an academic research laboratory or in a pharmaceutical firm, the opportunity costs of doing vaccine development are carefully weighed before following someone's advice to "jump in" or "let's try it." In this case, opportunity costs are measured in terms of the other drugs that one cannot develop or pursue because one is instead testing vaccines. The "value," either of manuscript publication for the academic researcher, or of a licensed product for the pharmaceutical firm, must balance the potential for success pursuing a vaccine compared to pursuing other available choices. Often, vaccines take second place.

3. CONCLUSION

In sum, our current model is a poor one. Immense laboratory power now exists to make vaccines that could alleviate the large costs and intense suffering for the world's people. Yet, given the current dependence on profit motive, this power is not being tapped. New models need to be established where, through social valuation, profit stimulation, and long-range planning, governments, nongovernmental organizations, and the private sector work together to make and deliver these lifesaving products.

REFERENCES

Ada, G., 1993, HIV-towards Phase III trials for candidate vaccines, *Nature* **364**:489–490.

Blackwelder, W. C., Storsaeter, J., Olin, P., and Hallander, H. O., 1991, Acellular pertussis vaccines. Efficacy and evaluation of clinical case definitions, *Am. J. Dis. Child.* **145**:1285–1289.

Carter, R., 1966, *Breakthrough. The Saga of Jonas Salk*, Trident Press, New York.

Francis, D. P., Hadler, S. C., Thompson, S. E., Maynard, J. E., Ostrow, D. G., Altman, N., Braff, E. H., O'Malley, P., Hawkins, D., Judson, F. N., Penley, K., Nylund, T., Christie, G., Meyers, F., Moore, J. N., Jr., Gardner, A., Doto, I. L., Miller, J. H., Reynolds, G. H., Murphy, B. L., Schable, C. A., Clark, B. T., Curran, J. W., and Redeker, A. G., 1982, The prevention of hepatitis B with vaccine. Report of the CDC multi-center efficacy trial among homosexual men, *Ann. Intern. Med.* **97**:362–366.

Maupas, P., Goudeau, A., Coursaset, P., and Druker, J., 1976, Immunisation against hepatitis B in man, *Lancet* **1**:289–292.

Purcell, R. H., Gerin, J. L., 1975, Hepatitis B subunit virus vaccine: A preliminary report of safety and efficacy tests in chimpanzees, *Am. J. Med. Sci.* **270**:395–399.

Redeker, A. G., Mosley, J. W., Gocke, D. J., McKee, A. P., and Pollack, W., 1975, Hepatitis B immune globulin as a prophylactic measure for spouses exposed to acute type B hepatitis, *N. Engl. J. Med.* **293**:1055.

Smith, J., 1990, *Patenting the Sun. Polio and the Salk Vaccine*, Morrow, New York.

Szmuness, W., Stevens, C. E., Harley, E. J., Zang, E. A., Oleszko, W. R., William, D. C., Sadovsky, R., Morrison, J. M., and Kellner, A., 1980, Hepatitis B vaccine. Demonstration of efficacy in a controlled clinical trial in a high-risk population in the United States, *N. Engl. J. Med.* **303**:833–841.

Chapter 7

A Compendium of Vaccine Adjuvants and Excipients

Frederick R. Vogel and Michael F. Powell

In the early 20th century, researchers experimented with diverse compounds such as alum (aluminum salts), mineral oil, and killed mycobacteria to improve the immunogenicity of vaccines. These first empirical studies demonstrated the adjuvant activity of many substances, but several products also elicited significant local and systemic adverse reactions that precluded their use in human vaccine formulations. Alum adjuvant, first described in 1926, remains the only immunologic adjuvant used in human vaccines licensed in the United States.

Since the advent of modern immunology twenty years ago, hundreds of immuno-modulatory compounds have been evaluated as vaccine adjuvants. After extensive safety and toxicity testing, many of these modern adjuvants have proven to be acceptable for clinical evaluation. During the same time, investigations into the mechanisms of action of adjuvants have increased. Today, a major goal of adjuvant research is to apply the increased understanding of adjuvant activities so adjuvants can be selected based on the immune response desired for a particular vaccine.

The purpose of this compendium is to provide a reference for investigators interested in accessing information on the variety of adjuvants available for study, and to foster collaboration between basic and applied vaccine researchers, and adjuvant developers. This compendium is extensive but by no means complete. It is our hope that vaccinologists will find this a useful resource and that it may help to advance adjuvant development as an integral part of a rational vaccine design.

Frederick R. Vogel • Division of AIDS, National Institute of Allergy and Infectious Diseases, National Institutes of Health, Bethesda, Maryland 20892. *Michael F. Powell* • Pharmaceutical Research & Development, Genentech, Inc., South San Francisco, California 94080.

Vaccine Design: The Subunit and Adjuvant Approach, edited by Michael F. Powell and Mark J. Newman. Plenum Press, New York, 1995.

COMPONENT/ADJUVANT NAME: Adju-Phos

OTHER NAME(S): Aluminum phosphate gel

STRUCTURE: Amorphous aluminum hydroxyphosphate. A schematic of the unit layer of amorphous aluminum hydroxyphosphate showing the surface hydroxyl, water, and phosphate groups. Key: Al, •; OH, ◉; H₂O, ○; PO₄, ⊘

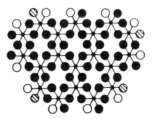

SOURCE: Obtained by precipitation. The degree of substitution of phosphate for hydroxyl depends on the concentration of reactants and precipitation conditions.

USES: Human applications: diphtheria, tetanus, and pertussis vaccines. Veterinary vaccine applications.

APPEARANCE: White gelatinous precipitate in aqueous suspension.

MOLECULAR WEIGHT: Not applicable.

RECOMMENDED STORAGE: 4–25°C. Never expose to freezing. Recommended 2 year shelf life.

CHEMICAL/PHYSICAL PROPERTIES: Primary particles have a platelike morphology and a diameter of 50–100 nm. The isoelectric point is acidic and is inversely related to the degree of substitution of phosphate for hydroxyl. Its high surface area gives it a high adsorptive capacity for antigens. Particle size range of final product 0.5–10 μm.

INCOMPATIBILITY: Dissolves in strong bases and acids.

SAFETY/TOXICITY: May cause mild local reactions at the site of injection (erythema and/or mild transient swellings).

- Yamanaka, M. *et al.*, 1992, Pathological studies on local tissue reactions in guinea pigs and rats caused by four different adjuvants, *J. Vet. Med. Sci.* **54**:685–692.
- Gupta, R. K., *et al.*, 1993, Adjuvants—A balance between toxicity and adjuvanticity, *Vaccine* **11**:293–306.

ADJUVANT PROPERTIES: The surface area, surface charge, and morphology of the amorphous aluminum hydroxyphosphate are major factors in its adjuvant characteristics. The use of aluminum adjuvants is accompanied by stimulation of IL-4 and stimulation of the T-helper-2 subsets in mice, with enhanced IgG1 and IgE production. Properties are described in:

- Seeber, S., *et al.*, 1991, Predicting the adsorption of proteins by aluminum-containing adjuvants, *Vaccine* **9**:201–203.
- Shirodkar, *et al.*, 1990, Aluminum compounds used as adjuvants in vaccines, *Pharm. Res.* **7**:1282–1288.
- Seeber, S. J., *et al.*, 1991, Solubilization of aluminum-containing adjuvants by constituents of interstitial fluid, *J. Parenteral Sci. Tech.* **45**:156–159.
- Gupta, R. K., *et al.*, Chapter 8, this volume.

CONTACT(S): E. B. Lindblad, Superfos Biosector a/s, DK-2950 Vedbaek, Denmark, Ph: 45 42 89 31 11; Fax: 45 42 89 15 95. Also: Al Reisch, Sergeant, Inc., Clifton, NJ 07012, Ph: 201-472-9111; Fax: 201-472-5686. Also: Stanley Hem, Purdue University, W. Lafayette, IN 47907-1336, Ph: 317-494-1451; Fax: 317-494-7880.

COMPONENT/ADJUVANT NAME: Algal Glucan

OTHER NAME(S): β-glucan; glucan

STRUCTURE: A linear β-D(1,3)-linked glucopyranose polymer having a triple-helical conformation.

SOURCE: Produced by an adapted strain of *Euglena gracilis* (SRI strain D86-G) grown heterotrophically in the dark. Obtained from the cytoplasm of the organism by methanol and chloroform extraction. Depyrogenized in hot 1 N HCl and washed sequentially in pyrogen-free water and pyrogen-free saline.

- Tusè, D., *et al.*, 1992, Production of β-1,3-glucan in *Euglena*, U.S. Patent No. 5,084,386.

USES: Administered with antigen for enhancement of both humoral and cell-mediated immunity. β-Glucans exert their immunostimulatory activities by binding to specific β-glucan receptors on macrophages. This ligand–receptor interaction results in macrophage activation and, in certain formulations, promotes antigen targeting.

- DiLuzio, N. R., *et al.*, 1979, Evaluation of the mechanism of glucan-induced stimulation of the reticuloendothelial system, *J. Reticuloendothel. Soc.* **7**:731–742.
- Czop, J. K., and Austen, K. F., 1985, A β-glucan inhibitable receptor on human monocytes: Its identity with the phagocytic receptor for particulate activators of the alternative complement pathway, *J. Immunol.* **134**:2588–2593.

APPEARANCE: White, odorless crystalline material. Forms a suspension in aqueous solutions.

MOLECULAR WEIGHT: Highest measured MW = 500,000.

RECOMMENDED STORAGE: Stable to light. Store solid Algal Glucan at room temperature and aqueous suspensions at 4°C. No apparent degradation after storage of aqueous suspension for 24 months at 4°C. Optimal storage conditions are to be determined.

CHEMICAL/PHYSICAL PROPERTIES: Native particulate material is water insoluble. Median particle size 3.7–4.6 μm, with specific gravity of 1.86–2.0 g/cm^3. Purified preparations contain 0.0001–0.35% phosphorus and 0.12–0.27% nitrogen.

INCOMPATIBILITY: Alkaline pH disrupts the triple-helical conformation.

SAFETY/TOXICITY: In preclinical studies, Algal Glucan has been intravenously administered at doses up to 25 mg/kg body weight and was well tolerated. Human clinical trials of β-glucans isolated from either plants or microorganisms indicate the feasibility of administering these compounds to humans without toxicity. Glucan particles bioerode over time in a physiological environment.

- Mansel, P. W. A., *et al.*, 1975, Macrophage-mediated destruction of human malignant cells in vivo, *J. Natl. Cancer Inst.* **54**:571–580.
- Okamura, K., *et al.*, 1986, Clinical evaluation of *Schizophyllan* combined with irradiation in patients with cervical cancer, *Cancer* **58**:865–872.
- Chihara, G., *et al.*, 1989, Lentinan as a host defense potentiator (HDP), *Int. J. Immunother.* **4**:145–154.
- Ostroff, G. R., 1994, Future therapeutic applications of Betafectin, a carbohydrate-based immunomodulator, The Second Annual Conference on Glycotechnology.

ADJUVANT PROPERTIES: Algal Glucan, a nonantigenic carbohydrate adjuvant, enhances both humoral and cell-mediated immunity to oligopeptides in experimental animal models. Mice immunized twice by coadministration of herpes virus glycoprotein D (gD2) and 100 μg Algal Glucan produced anti-gD2 antibodies that were significantly higher in titer and persisted longer ($p<0.01$) than those in animals injected with gD2 alone. Similarly, immunization of mice with either gD2- or HIV-1-gp120 with Algal Glucan added as an adjuvant heightened the antigen-specific response of splenic lymphocytes.

• Mohagheghpour, N., *et al.*, 1992, Adjuvant activity of an algal glycan, VIII International Conference on AIDS/III STD World Congress, Amsterdam.

CONTACT(S): Dr. Nahid Mohagheghpour, SRI International, Menlo Park, CA 94025, Ph: 415-859-3516; Fax: 415-859-3342. Also: Richard McIntosh, Genesis Technology Group, Inc., Cambridge, MA, Ph: 617-576-6610; Fax: 617-876-4002.

COMPONENT/ADJUVANT NAME: Algammulin

OTHER NAME(S): Gamma inulin/alum composite adjuvant

STRUCTURE: See entries under gamma inulin and Alhydrogel for primary materials. Inulin is crystallized in presence of Alhydrogel suspensions and transformed to gamma inulin at 37°C to form electron-dense ovoids that both adsorb antigen and activate complement.

- Cooper, P. D., and Steele, E. J., 1991, Algammulin: A new vaccine adjuvant comprising gamma inulin particles containing alum, *Vaccine* **9**:351–357.

USES: Included in adjuvant formulations as a primary adjuvant.

APPEARANCE: Milky white, nonviscous aqueous suspension, easily resuspended. Supplied at 50 mg/mL, sterile and pyrogen-free.

MOLECULAR WEIGHT: See entries under gamma inulin and Alhydrogel.

RECOMMENDED STORAGE: 2–8°C; maintain in aqueous medium. Do not freeze or heat over 45°C.

CHEMICAL/PHYSICAL PROPERTIES: See entries under gamma inulin and Alhydrogel for primary materials. Algammulin is stable for years under recommended storage. Unstable below pH 6 and above pH 10. Virtually insoluble at 37°C.

INCOMPATIBILITY: Degraded in strong acid. Adjuvants containing aluminum hydroxide gel may be incompatible with phosphate or anionic detergents.

SAFETY/TOXICITY: Nonpyrogenic, nonantigenic, and of very low toxicity in experimental animals and a Phase I clinical trial. Biodegradable to simple sugars and aluminum hydroxide gel. Large intravenous doses can cause acute complement-activation shock similar to that sometimes found in renal dialysis patients. Dissolved inulin is pharmacologically inert and is registered for human use; alum is also approved for human use.

ADJUVANT PROPERTIES: Expected to stimulate immune responses by causing ligation of leukocyte-surface complement receptors (CR) via known biochemical mechanisms, thus placing the antigen close to activated leukocytes. Addition of Algammulin is known to enhance both humoral and cell-mediated immunity from either Th1 or Th2 pathways, depending on the weight ratio of inulin to Alhydrogel.

- Cooper, P. D., *et al.*, 1991, The adjuvanticity of Algammulin, a new vaccine adjuvant, *Vaccine* **9**:408–415.
- Cooper, P. D., *et al.*, 1993, Gamma inulin and Algammulin: Two new vaccine adjuvants, in: *Vaccines 93, Modern Approaches to New Vaccines Including Prevention of AIDS* (H. S. Ginsburg, F. Brown, R. M. Chanock, and R. A. Lerner, eds.), Cold Spring Harbor Laboratory Press, Cold Spring Harbor, NY, pp. 25–30.
- Cooper, P. D., Chapter 24, this volume.

CONTACT(S): Dr. Peter D. Cooper, Division of Cell Biology, John Curtin School of Medical Research, Australian National University, Canberra, A. C. T., Australia 2601, Ph: 61-6-291-8670; Fax: 61-6-249-2595.

COMPONENT/ADJUVANT NAME: Alhydrogel

OTHER NAME(S): Aluminum hydroxide gel; alum

STRUCTURE: Crystalline aluminum oxyhydroxide AlOOH, known mineralogically as boehmite. The structure consists of corrugated sheets of aluminum octahedra.

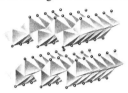

SOURCE: Obtained by precipitation of aluminum hydroxide under alkaline conditions.

USES: Human applications: diphtheria, tetanus, and pertussis vaccines. Veterinary vaccine applications.

APPEARANCE: White gelatinous precipitate in aqueous suspension.

MOLECULAR WEIGHT: Not applicable.

RECOMMENDED STORAGE: 4–25°C. Never expose to freezing. Recommended 2 year shelf life.

CHEMICAL/PHYSICAL PROPERTIES: Primary particles have a rodlike or fibril morphology and a high surface area. The isoelectric point is 11. Its high surface area gives it a high adsorptive capacity for antigen. Poorly soluble in solutions containing citrate ions. Normal particle size range 0.5–10 μm.

INCOMPATIBILITY: Dissolves in strong bases and acids.

SAFETY/TOXICITY: May cause mild local reactions at the site of injection (erythemas and/or mild transient swellings).

- Ganrot, P. O., 1986, Metabolism and possible health effects of aluminum, *Environ. Health Perspect.* **65**:363–441.
- Gupta, R. K., *et al.*, 1993, Adjuvants—A balance between toxicity and adjuvanticity, *Vaccine* **11**:293–306.

ADJUVANT PROPERTIES: Alhydrogel is the standard preparations for immunological research on aluminum hydroxide gels. The use of aluminum adjuvants is accompanied by stimulation of IL-4 and stimulation of the T-helper-2 subsets in mice, with enhanced IgG1 and IgE production. Further immunomodulation is accomplished by the aluminum content. Properties are described in:

- Shirodkar, S., *et al.*, 1990, Aluminum compounds used as adjuvant in vaccines, *Pharm. Res.* **7**:1282–1288.
- Stewart-Tull, D. E. S., 1989, Recommendations for the assessment of adjuvants (immunomodulators), in: *Immunological Adjuvants and Vaccines* (Gregoriadis, G., Allison, A. C., and Poste, G., eds.), Plenum Press, New York, pp. 213–226.
- Gupta, R., *et al.*, Chapter 8, this volume.
- Seeber, S., *et al.*, 1991, Predicting the adsorption of proteins by aluminum-containing adjuvants, *Vaccine* **9**:201–203.
- Seeber, S. J., *et al.*, 1991, Solubilization of aluminum-containing adjuvants by constituents of interstitial fluid, *J. Parenteral Sci. Tech.* **45**:156–159.
- Hem, S., and White, J. L., Chapter 9, this volume.

CONTACT(S): E. B. Lindblad, Superfos Biosector a/s, DK-2950 Vedbaek, Denmark, Ph: 45 42 89 31 11; Fax: 45 42 89 15 95. Also: Al Reisch, Sergeant, Inc., Clifton, NJ 07012, Ph: 201-472-9111; Fax: 201-472-5686. Also: Stanley Hem, Purdue University, West Lafayette, IN 47907-1336, Ph: 317-494-1451; Fax: 317-494-7880.

COMPONENT/ADJUVANT NAME: Antigen Formulation

OTHER NAME(S): SPT, AF

STRUCTURE: An emulsion of squalane (5%), Tween 80 (0.2%), Pluronic L121 (1.25%), phosphate-buffered saline pH 7.4, and antigen.

Polysorbate 80

Pluronic L121

Squalane

SOURCE: Oil-in-water microemulsion obtained by the microfluidization of the components at reduced temperature.

USES: A vaccine adjuvant vehicle that, when administered with antigen, induces both a cellular and humoral immune response.

APPEARANCE: Homogeneous, white milky liquid.

MOLECULAR WEIGHT: Not applicable.

RECOMMENDED STORAGE: 2–8 °C under inert gas. Avoid freezing.

CHEMICAL/PHYSICAL PROPERTIES: A microemulsion comprised of oil droplets of mean diameter around 150–175 nm. Vialed as a 3X formulation, AF is stable for up to 2 years when stored at 5°C, depending on the concentrations of the excipients used as well as the conditions of microfluidization. A uniform dispersion is achieved when diluting 1:3 with aqueous solution prior to administration.

INCOMPATIBILITY: None found.

SAFETY/TOXICITY: Pathology and toxicology studies completed in two species, including nonhuman primates. It is well tolerated at doses and schedules that exhibit immune stimulating activity. The safety and potency of the three-component microfluidized formulation has been demonstrated in Phase I/II clinical trials.

ADJUVANT PROPERTIES: Gives good humoral and CTL responses. A potent cytotoxic T cell response was induced when recombinant soluble antigens were injected with AF leading to the destruction of tumor cells or virally infected cells in vitro and in vivo.

- Raychaudhuri, *et al.*, 1992, Induction of antigen-specific class I-restricted cytotoxic T cells by soluble proteins in vivo, *Proc. Natl. Acad. Sci. USA* **89**:8308–8312.

CONTACT(S): Thomas Ryskamp, IDEC Pharmaceuticals Corporation, San Diego, CA 92121, Ph: 619-550-8500; Fax: 619-550-8750; Internet: tryskamp@idec.com.

COMPONENT/ADJUVANT NAME: Avridine®

OTHER NAME(S): N,N-dioctadecyl-N',N'-bis(2-hydroxyethyl) propanediamine; CP-20,961

STRUCTURE:

SOURCE: Chemical synthesis.

USES: Incorporation into a liposomal preparation, e.g., at a molar ratio of 1:2 Avridine:dimyristoyl phosphatidylcholine forms unilamellar liposomes; aqueous suspensions from alcoholic solution; in Intralipid, an aqueous soybean oil emulsion vehicle; other vegetable and mineral oil vehicles; Tween 80 dispersions in saline; saline suspension with alum-precipitated antigen.

APPEARANCE: White powder.

MOLECULAR WEIGHT: 667.17

RECOMMENDED STORAGE: Store as a powder at room temperature.

CHEMICAL/PHYSICAL PROPERTIES: Very insoluble in water, exhibits waxy properties at temperatures below 39°C; good solubility in absolute ethanol.

INCOMPATIBILITY: None known.

SAFETY/TOXICITY: Intranasal administration to humans induces interferon in nasal secretions and protection against rhinovirus challenge; injection site irritations; model for adjuvant arthritis in Lewis rats; antitumor properties in rodent tumor models.

- Niblack, J. F., 1977, Studies with low molecular weight inducers of interferon in man, *Toxicol. Rep. Biol. Med.* **35**:528–534.
- Waldman, R. H., and Ganguly, R., 1978, Effect of CP-20,961, an interferon inducer, on upper respiratory tract infections due to rhinovirus type 21 in volunteers, *J. Infect. Dis.* **138**:531–535.
- Chang, Y. H., *et al.*, 1980, Adjuvant polyarthritis. IV. Induction by a synthetic adjuvant: Immunologic, histopathologic, and other studies, *Arthritis Rheum.* **23**:62–71.

ADJUVANT PROPERTIES: Humoral and cellular immunity, proliferation of B and T lymphocytes, protective immunity, activation of macrophages, induction of interferon, enhancement of mucosal immunity when administered orally/enterically with antigen, adjuvanticity with a variety of antigens, induction of IgG2a and IgG2b isotypes.

- Niblack, J. F., *et al.*, 1979, CP-20,961: A structurally novel, synthetic adjuvant, *J. Reticuloendothel. Soc.* **26**(Suppl.):655–666.
- Kraaijeveld, C. A., *et al.*, 1982, Enhancement of delayed-type hypersensitivity and induction of interferon by the lipophilic agents DDA and CP-20,961, *Cell. Immunol.* **74**:277–283.
- Jensen, K. E., 1988, Synthetic adjuvants: Avridine and other interferon inducers, in: *Advances in Carriers and Adjuvants for Veterinary Biologics* (R. M. Nerwig, P. M. Gough, M. L. Kaeber, and C. A. Whetstone, eds.), Iowa State University Press, Ames, pp. 79–89.
- Anderson, A. O., *et al.*, 1987, Studies on anti-viral mucosal immunity with the lipoidal amine adjuvant Avridine, *Adv. Exp. Med. Biol.* **216B**:1781–1790.

CONTACT(S): Dr. Oksana K. Yarosh, VIDO, Saskatoon, Canada S7N 0W0, Ph: 306-966-7465; Fax: 306-966-7478; E mail: yarosh@sask.usask.ca. Also: Huw Hughes, M6 Pharmaceuticals, Inc., New York, NY 10701, Ph: 212-308-7200 ext. 14; E-mail: 74577.345@compuserve.com.

COMPONENT/ADJUVANT NAME: BAY R1005

OTHER NAME(S): *N*-(2-Deoxy-2-L-leucylamino-β-D-glucopyranosyl)-*N*-octadecyl-dodecanoylamide hydroacetate

STRUCTURE:

SOURCE: Chemical synthesis. Provided as the acetate salt.
- Lockhoff, O., 1991, Glycolipids as immunomodulators: Synthesis and properties, *Angew. Chem. Int. Ed. Engl.* **30**:1611–1620.

USES: Primary adjuvant.

APPEARANCE: White lyophilizate.

MOLECULAR WEIGHT: 726.1 + Acetate 60.1

RECOMMENDED STORAGE: Store at 2–8 °C in airtight containers.

CHEMICAL/PHYSICAL PROPERTIES: Slightly hygroscopic. No polymorphism detected. Chemically stable to air, light, at temperatures up to 50°C, and in aqueous solvents at pH 2–12 at ambient temperature. Amphiphilic molecule, forms micelles in aqueous solution. Formation of translucent liposomal dispersion by ultrasonic treatment.

INCOMPATIBILITY: None found.

SAFETY/TOXICITY: Exploratory studies in rats (doses 2.5, 25, or 100 mg/kg body weight) on acute i.p. toxicity according to "OECD Guidelines for Testing Chemicals, No. 401": no deaths, $LD_{50} > 100$ mg/kg b.w. subacute i.v. toxicity in rats (doses 2.5, 25, or 100 mg/kg body weight) for 14 days with subsequent 4-week follow-up period to test reversibility of possible effects: no-effect level at 2.5 mg/kg b.w.

ADJUVANT PROPERTIES: BAY R1005 in combination with purified virus vaccines or subunit vaccines led to increased protection of virus-challenged mice. Preclinical trials in other animal species (pig, sheep, horse) gave comparable results with respect to antibody production. The increase in antibody synthesis induced by BAY R1005 is specifically dependent on the antigen and is not the result of polyclonal stimulation. BAY R1005 acts on the proliferation of B lymphocytes as a second signal which has no effect until the antigen acts as a first signal. BAY R1005 is capable of activating B lymphocytes without the helper function of T lymphocytes.

- Stünkel, K. G., *et al.*, 1988, In vitro studies of synthetic glycolipids: A new class of compounds with immunomodulating activity, in: *Leucocyte Activation and Differentiation* (J. C. Mani and J. Dorn, eds.), de Gruyter, Berlin, pp. 421–425.
- Stünkel, K. G., *et al.*, 1988, Synthetic glycolipids: In vitro characterization of a new class of compounds with immunomodulating properties, *Adv. Biosci. (Oxford)* **68**:429–437.
- Stünkel, K. G., *et al.*, 1989, Synthetic glycolipids with immunopotentiating activity on humoral immunity: Evaluation in vivo, *Prog. Leukocyte Biol.* **9**:575–579.

CONTACT(S): Dr. O. Lockhoff, Bayer AG, D-51368 Leverkusen, Germany, Ph: 49-214-30-7958; Fax: 49-214-30-50070.

COMPONENT/ADJUVANT NAME: Calcitriol

OTHER NAME(S): $1\alpha,25$-dihydroxyvitamin D_3; 1,25-di(OH)$_2$D$_3$; 1,25-DHCC; $1\alpha,25$-dihydroxycholecalciferol; 9,10-seco(5Z,7E)-5,7,10(19)-cholestatriene-$1\alpha,3\beta,25$-triol

STRUCTURE:

SOURCE: Roche (Nutley, NJ) is the principal supplier to academic researchers. For citations involving the initial identification and methods of preparation see the *Merck Index* (Merck and Co., Inc., Rahway, NJ) under the entry for calcitriol.

USES: Promotes the induction of mucosal immunity when incorporated into vaccine formulations.

APPEARANCE: White, colorless powder or crystalline material.

MOLECULAR WEIGHT: 416.65

RECOMMENDED STORAGE: Air and light sensitive. Storage in a dry inert atmosphere at or below –20°C.

CHEMICAL/PHYSICAL PROPERTIES: Calcitriol is a hydrophobic molecule with limited solubility in water. It is soluble in organic solvents including alcohols. Solutions should be prepared in glass to avoid losses of the compound to plastic surfaces. Melting point: 111–115°C. Ultraviolet absorption maximum in ethanol is 264 nm (e = 19,000).

INCOMPATIBILITY: Avoid combining calcitriol with components capable of addition or oxidation reactions involving the conjugated *p* electron system. In particular, components capable of releasing free halogens should be avoided.

SAFETY/TOXICITY: Because calcitriol is the active form of vitamin D it should not be given to patients with hypercalcemia. Safety, toxicity, known metabolites, and dosage data are summarized under the entry for Rocaltrol in the *Physicians Desk Reference* (Medical Economics Data Production Co., Montvale, NJ).

ADJUVANT PROPERTIES: The incorporation of calcitriol (0.1–1.0 μg) directly into vaccine formulations containing protein or polysaccharide antigens promotes the induction of both systemic and common mucosal immune responses. Hormone modulation with immunization eliminates the need to apply immunizing antigens to mucosal surfaces for the induction of secretory antibodies.

- Daynes, R. A., *et al.*, 1994, Cytokine modulation in vivo with vitamin D3: Promotion of common mucosal immunity following a standard subcutaneous vaccination, *FASEB J.* **8**:A283.
- Daynes, R. A., and Araneo, B. A., 1994, The development of effective vaccine adjuvants employing natural regulators of T-cell lymphokine production in vivo, *Ann. N.Y. Acad. Sci.* **730**:144–161.
- Daynes, R. A., *et al.*, 1995, Steroids as regulators of the mammalian immune response, *J. Invest. Derm.* (in press).

CONTACT(S): Raymond A. Daynes, Department of Pathology, University of Utah Medical Center, Salt Lake City, UT 84132, Ph: 801-581-3013; Fax: 801-581-8946.

COMPONENT/ADJUVANT NAME: Calcium Phosphate Gel

OTHER NAME(S): Calcium phosphate

STRUCTURE: Hydrated calcium phosphate gel.

SOURCE: Precipitated by mixing soluble calcium and phosphate salts under carefully controlled conditions.

USES: Calcium phosphate has been used as adjuvant in vaccine formulations against diphtheria, tetanus, pertussis, and poliomyelitis. It has also been used for adsorption of allergenic extracts for hyposensitization of allergic patients.

APPEARANCE: White, gelatinous precipitate in aqueous suspension.

MOLECULAR WEIGHT: Not applicable.

RECOMMENDED STORAGE: 4–25°C. Never expose to freezing.

CHEMICAL/PHYSICAL PROPERTIES: Adsorbs soluble antigens and presents them in a particulate form to the immune system. Normal particle size range 0.5–15 μm.

INCOMPATIBILITY: Maintain neutral pH.

SAFETY/TOXICITY: Calcium phosphate adjuvant contains no components that are not natural constituents of the body and is very well tolerated.

- Gupta, R. K., *et al.*, 1993, Adjuvants—A balance between toxicity and adjuvanticity, *Vaccine* **11**:293–306.

ADJUVANT PROPERTIES: Properties are described in:

- Relyveld, E. H., 1986, Preparation and use of calcium phosphate-adsorbed vaccines, *Dev. Biol. Stand.* **65**:131–136.
- Relyveld, E. H., *et al.*, 1985, Calcium phosphate adjuvanted allergens, *Ann. Allergy* **54**:521–529.
- Gupta, R., *et al.*, Chapter 8, this volume.

CONTACT(S): E. B. Lindblad, Superfos Biosector a/s, DK-2950 Vedbaek, Denmark, Ph: 45 42 89 31 11; Fax: 45 42 89 15 95. Also: Al Reisch, Sergeant, Inc., Clifton, NJ 07012, Ph: 201-472-9111; Fax: 201-472-5686.

COMPONENT/ADJUVANT NAME: Cholera Holotoxin (CT)
Cholera Toxin B Subunit (CTB)

OTHER NAME(S): CT; CT B subunit; CT-B

STRUCTURE: The CT protein is composed of one enzymatically active, toxic A1 subunit which is linked to a pentamer of CTB subunits via the CTA2 fragment.

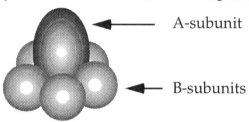

A-subunit

B-subunits

SOURCE: Bacterial protein is produced by *Vibrio cholerae*. CTB is the toxoid lacking the A subunit. Recombinant CTB is available. Suppliers include: List Biological Labs, Campbell, CA; Sigma Chemical Co, St. Louis, MO; Swedish National Vaccine Company, Stockholm, Sweden.

USES: CT is the prototype for an ADP-ribosylating bacterial toxin. It binds with high affinity via the CTB to its receptor ganglioside GM1 present on most mammalian cells. It is enzymatically active through its A1 subunit. The immunomodulating effect of CT is associated with the ADP-ribosylating ability, whereas effective delivery of antigen is achieved with the CTB as the carrier molecule. CT is the most effective adjuvant for mucosal immunity yet described for experimental use. CT in microgram doses may also be used experimentally to adjuvant systemic immune responses. Both humoral and cell-mediated immunity are known to be greatly augmented by CT-adjuvant. CT and CTB are used in soluble form simply by admixing with unrelated protein antigen or more effective as chemical conjugates with unrelated protein antigen. The CTB may be used as an efficient carrier molecule for other proteins or peptide fragments either chemically or genetically linked to CTB. CTB may be used in humans as an adjuvant/carrier molecule. Both CT and CTB are potent stimulators of immunological memory.

APPEARANCE: White lyophilized powder.

MOLECULAR WEIGHT: CT is 86,000, consisting of the A1 subunit (23,000), the CTA2 (5,000), and five subunits of CTB (11,000 each).

RECOMMENDED STORAGE: Store CT as a lyophilized powder under low humidity at 4°C. After reconstitution with water, store CT at –70°C, and CTB at 4°C.

CHEMICAL/PHYSICAL PROPERTIES: Good water solubility at neutral pH.

INCOMPATIBILITY: None found. Avoid proteases.

SAFETY/TOXICITY: CTB is nontoxic and has been used in humans without negative side effects. CT has not been used in humans because of its toxic effects, even at doses lower than 5 μg.

ADJUVANT PROPERTIES: CT exerts immunomodulating effects on T cells, B cells as well as antigen-presenting cells. Which of these effects is critical for adjuvant function is presently unknown. CTB lacks immunoenhancing effects after oral or intravenous administration, but may augment humoral response after intranasal administration. Although CTB is an effective carrier molecule, it appears that a small amount of ADP-ribosylation is required for an efficient adjuvant effect.

- Merrit, E., *et al.*, 1994, Crystal structure of cholera toxin B pentamer bound to receptor GM1-pentasaccharide, *Protein Sci.* **3**:166–175.
- Burnette, W. N., 1994, AB5 ADP-ribosylating toxins: Comparative anatomy and physiology, *Structure* **2**:151–158.
- Holmgren, J., *et al.*, 1994, Cholera toxin and cholera B-subunit as oral-mucosal adjuvant and antigen vector systems, *Vaccine* **11**:1179–1184.
- Hörnquist, E., *et al.*, 1994, Cholera toxin and cholera B-subunit as oral-mucosal adjuvant carrier systems, in: *Novel Delivery Systems for Oral Vaccines* (O'Hagan, ed.), CRC Press, Boca Raton, p. 153.
- Zhou, F., 1994, IgA-coated liposomes as a rectal vaccine delivery system for induction of secretory IgA in the rectal and colonic mucosa, Workshop on HIV/SIV Pathogenesis, NIH/DIADS March 14–17.

CONTACT(S): Nils Lycke, University of Göteborg, S-413 46 Göteborg, Sweden, Ph: 46-31-604936; Fax: 46-31-827-647. Also: Marian R. Neutra, Childrens Hospital/Enders 461, Boston, MA 02115, Ph: 617-735-6229; Fax: 617-730-0404.

COMPONENT/ADJUVANT NAME: CRL1005

OTHER NAME(S): Block Copolymer P1205

STRUCTURE: ABA block polymer with mean values of $x = 8$ and $y = 205$.

SOURCE: Linear chain polymers are synthesized by condensation of propylene oxide and ethylene glycol initiator in the presence of a cesium salt catalyst to form polyoxypropylene chain, followed by condensation of ethylene oxide on either end of the chain. Individual polymeric species of triblock nonionic block copolymers result from controlled synthesis of chains with predetermined length.

USES: A component of adjuvant formulations. The formulation is customized for particular uses. The water-in-oil emulsion typically contains 80% saline, and 20% oil phase consisting of squalene and Span 80. The copolymer is added to the aqueous phase in amounts sufficient for the required dose. It acts as both an adjuvant and stabilizer. The water-in-oil-in-water (w/o/w) multiple emulsion is prepared similarly with the addition of an outer aqueous phase.

APPEARANCE: Clear, colorless to slightly yellow, viscous liquid.

MOLECULAR WEIGHT: Approx. 12.5,000.

RECOMMENDED STORAGE: CRL1005 can be stored in tight amber glass containers with minimum headspace at 4°C for 2–3 years. Aqueous solutions (<10% w/v) stored at 4°C.

CHEMICAL/PHYSICAL PROPERTIES: CRL1005 is soluble in neutral or near neutral (pH 5.5–8) aqueous buffers at temperatures <4°C up to 10% (w/v). Above 4°C CRL1005 coalesces and forms large, stable micellelike structures 250–300 nm in diameter.

INCOMPATIBILITY: CRL1005 is compatible with aqueous buffering systems and can incorporate into the oil phase of oil-based emulsion vehicles. Compatible with a wide number of antigens, but more effective with intact proteins than peptides.

SAFETY/TOXICITY: Aqueous polymer suspensions of CRL1005 evaluated in rodent species in conjunction with influenza HA vaccines, with no adverse safety events noted. Microemulsions of CRL1005 with squalene evaluated in rodent species, with no adverse effects. Data not yet available for human safety.

ADJUVANT PROPERTIES: CRL1005 forms microparticulate structures that can bind a variety of antigens via a combination of hydrophobic interactions and surface charge. Available data suggest block copolymers influence epitope recognition and induce protective (e.g., IgG2a) antibody subclasses. Some formulations, particularly multiple emulsions, have potential as mucosal delivery vehicles. Data on cellular immunity not available.

- Hunter, R. L., *et al.*, 1981, Studies on the adjuvant activity of nonionic block polymer surfactants. I. The role of hydrophile–lipophile balance, *J. Immunol.* **127**:1244–1250.
- Hunter, R. L., *et al.*, 1991, Adjuvant activity of nonionic block copolymers, IV. Effect of molecular weight and formulation on titer and isotype of antibody, *Vaccine* **9**:250–256.
- Takayama, K., *et al.*, 1991, Adjuvant activity of nonionic block copolymers, V. Modulation of antibody isotype by lipopolysaccharides, lipid A and precursors, *Vaccine* **9**:257–265.

- Kalish, M. L., *et al.*, 1991, Murine IgG isotype responses to the *Plasmodium cynomolgi* circumsporozoite protein (NAGG)5. I. Effects of carrier, copolymer adjuvants, and nontoxic LPS on isotype distribution, *Infect. Immun.* **59**:2750–2757.
- van de Wijgert, J. H. H. M., *et al.*, 1991, Immunogenicity of *Streptococcus pneumoniae* type 14 capsular polysaccharide: Influence of carrier and adjuvants on isotype distribution, *Infect. Immun.* **59**:2750–2757.
- ten Hagen, T. L. M., *et al.*, 1993, The role of adjuvants in the modulation of antibody specificity and induction of protection by whole blood-stage *Plasmodium yoelii* vaccines, *J. Immunol.* **151**:7077–7085.
- Brey, R. N., Chapter 11, this volume.

CONTACT(S): Dr. Mark Newman, Vaxcel Corporation, GA 30092, Ph: 404-447-9330; Fax: 404-447-8875.

COMPONENT/ADJUVANT NAME: Cytokine-Containing Liposomes

OTHER NAME(S): Cytokine-containing Dehydration Rehydration Vesicles.

STRUCTURE: This is a dehydration–rehydration liposome composed of phosphatidyl-choline (PC) and cholesterol in a 1:1 molar ratio and recombinant cytokines. The following cytokines have been tested: IL-1α, IL-1β, IL-6, TNFα, and interferon-γ.

SOURCE: The lipids are purchased from Avanti Polar-Lipids, Inc., Alabaster, AL. Cytokines are purchased from commercial sources and should not be contaminated with endotoxin.

USES: Induces both cellular and humoral immunity.

APPEARANCE: Cloudy suspension when in solution or white powder when dried.

MOLECULAR WEIGHT: See below for physical properties.

RECOMMENDED STORAGE: Prepared immediately before use, but may be stored at 4°C.

CHEMICAL/PHYSICAL PROPERTIES: The size of the liposomes has been determined to be between 1 and 8 μm by electron microscopy.

INCOMPATIBILITY: None known.

SAFETY/TOXICITY: Multilamellar liposomes are in clinical trials in humans.

ADJUVANT PROPERTIES:

- Murray, J. L., *et al.*, 1989, Phase I trial of liposomal muramyl tripeptide phosphatidylethanolamine in cancer patients, *J. Clin. Oncol.* **7**:1915–1925.
- Fidler, I. J., 1988, Targeting of immunomodulators to mononuclear phagocytes for therapy of cancer, *Adv. Drug Deliv. Res.* **2**:69–83.
- Fogler, W. E., *et al.*, 1985, Distribution and fate of free and liposome-encapsulated [3H]nor-muramyl dipeptide and [3H]muramyl tripeptide phosphatidylethanolamine in mice, *J. Immunol.* **135**:1372–1377.
- Lopez Berestein, G., *et al.*, 1985, Liposomal amphotericin B for the treatment of systemic fungal infections in patients with cancer: A preliminary study, *J. Infect. Dis.* **151**:704–710.
- Gregoriadis, G., *et al.*, 1987, Liposomes as immunological adjuvants: Antigen incorporation studies, *Vaccine* **5**:145–151.
- Lachman, L., *et al.*, Chapter 29, this volume.

CONTACT(S): Lawrence B. Lachman, Ph.D., University of Texas M. D. Anderson Cancer Center, Department of Cell Biology, Houston, TX 77030, Ph: 713-792-8587; Fax: 713-797-9764; E-mail: AN10010@MDACC.MDA.UTH.TMC.EDU.

COMPONENT/ADJUVANT NAME: DDA

OTHER NAME(S): Dimethyldioctadecylammonium bromide; dimethyldistearylammonium bromide (CAS Registry Number 3700-67-2).

STRUCTURE:

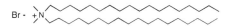

SOURCE: The chloride analogue of DDA is present in materials known as di(hydrogenate tallow)dimethylammonium salts available under various trade names (e.g., Quarternium-18, Adogen 442-110P, Cycloton D261 C/75). These salts comprise alkyl chains ranging from 12 to 18 carbon atoms with a typical distribution of C12:C14:C16:C18 = 1:4:31:64.

USES: For stimulation of immune responses against various antigens and especially delayed-type hypersensitivity. Oil-based emulsions in association with liposomes; also as a nonoil emulsion.

APPEARANCE: White, odorless powder.

MOLECULAR WEIGHT: 631

RECOMMENDED STORAGE: 4–20°C. Protect from light.

CHEMICAL/PHYSICAL PROPERTIES: Hydrophilic quaternary amine; positively charged surface-active substance with bromide (optionally chloride) as counterion. Gel–liquid transition temperature of 39.5°C. Poorly soluble in cold water but readily soluble/dispersible in warm water in which it forms liposomal structures. Soluble in organic solvents.

INCOMPATIBILITY: Complexes are formed with multivalent, negatively charged molecules (e.g., phosphate) in aqueous phase which might precipitate.

SAFETY/TOXICITY: Parenteral administration of DDA induces a mild inflammatory reaction at the site of injection (swelling and influx of polymorphonuclear neutrophils, macrophages, and lymphocytes). Effective dose range 1–10 mg/kg in small animals, and 0.01–1 mg/kg in large animals. Human trials include:

- Stanfield, J. P., et al., 1973, Single dose antenatal tetanus immunization, *Lancet* **301**:215–219.
- Chambers, J. D., et al., 1980, Induction of specific transplantation tolerance in man by autoblast immunization, *Blood* **41**:229–236.

ADJUVANT PROPERTIES: DDA stimulates both humoral and cell-mediated immune responses against a wide range of antigens and in various animal species. Especially delayed-type hypersensitivity reactions are augmented strongly by DDA after administration via subcutaneous for intracutaneous route. Functions as a carrier of antigen by direct binding of antigen, or modification at the oil/water interface.

- Hilgers, L. A. T., and Snippe, H., 1992, DDA as immunological adjuvant, *Res. Immunol.* **143**:494–503.
- Snippe, H., and Kraayeveld, C., 1989, The immunoadjuvant dimethyldioctadecylammonium bromide, in: *Immunological Adjuvants and Vaccines* (G. Gregoriadis, A. C. Allison, and G. Poste, eds.), Plenum Press, New York, pp. 47–59.

CONTACT(S): L. Hilgers, Solvay S.A., Research & Technology, Central Laboratory, Applied Immunology, Rue de Ransbeek 310, B-1120 Brussels, Belgium, or H. Snippe, University Utrecht, Eijkman-Winkler Laboratorium for Medical Microbiology, 3584 CX Utrecht, Netherlands. Also: Eastman Kodak Company, Rochester, NY 14650, Ph: 716-458-3702; Fax: 716-722-3172. Also: Huw Hughes, M6 Pharmaceuticals, Inc., New York, NY 10701, Ph: 212-308-7200 ext. 14; E-mail: 74577.345@compuserve.com.

COMPONENT/ADJUVANT NAME: DHEA

OTHER NAME(S): Dehydroepiandrosterone; 5-androsten-3β-ol-17-one; dehydroisoandrosterone; androstenolone; prasterone; transdehydroandrosterone; DHA

STRUCTURE:

SOURCE: Commercially available from numerous suppliers. For citations involving the initial identification and methods of preparation see the *Merck Index* (Merck and Co., Inc., Rahway, NJ) under the entry for prasterone.

USES: DHEA can be directly incorporated into vaccine formulations (2–10 μg/vaccination in mice, 100 μg/vaccination in dogs) and will enhance antibody formation.

APPEARANCE: White, colorless powder or crystals.

MOLECULAR WEIGHT: 288.4

RECOMMENDED STORAGE: DHEA is relatively stable; however, its double bond is susceptible to both addition and oxidation reactions. Long-term storage under dry inert gas at or below −20°C.

CHEMICAL/PHYSICAL PROPERTIES: DHEA is a hydrophobic molecule with limited solubility in water. It is soluble in organic solvents including alcohols and dimethylsulfoxide, and only slightly soluble in petroleum ether. Literature melting point varies: dimorphous needles 140–141°C, leaflets 152–153°C (*Merck Index*), crystals 149–151°C (Steraloids, Wilton, NH).

INCOMPATIBILITY: Do not combine DHEA with components capable of addition or oxidation reactions involving the *p* electron system, including components capable of releasing free halogens.

SAFETY/TOXICITY: Dosages up to 1600 mg per day have been given orally to humans with no adverse reaction.

ADJUVANT PROPERTIES: Administration of DHEA or its sulfate to animals that are immunologically compromised as a consequence of age rapidly restore normal immunologic competence. DHEA can be administered systemically (approximately 4 mg/kg/day) to animals at the time of vaccination, or can be directly incorporated into the vaccine formulation.

- Araneo, B. A., *et al.*, 1993, Reversal of the immunosenescent phenotype by dehydroepiandrosterone: Hormone treatment provides an adjuvant effect on the immunization of aged mice with recombinant hepatitis B surface antigen, *J. Infect. Dis.* **167**:830–840.
- Daynes, R. A., and Araneo, B. A., 1992, Prevention and reversal of some age-associated changes in immunologic responses by supplemental dehydroepiandrosterone sulfate therapy. Aging: *Immunol. Infect. Dis.* **3**:135–154.
- Araneo, B. A., *et al.*, 1993, Administration of DHEA to burned mice preserves normal immunologic competence, *Arch. Surg.* **128**:318–325.

CONTACT(S): Raymond A. Daynes, Department of Pathology, University of Utah Medical Center, Salt Lake City, UT 84132, Ph: 801-581-3013; Fax: 801-581-8946.

COMPONENT/ADJUVANT NAME: DMPC

OTHER NAME(S): Dimyristoyl phosphatidylcholine; sn-3-phosphatidylcholine-1, 2-dimyristoyl; 1, 2-dimyristoyl-sn-3-phosphatidylcholine (CAS Registry Number 18194-24-6).

STRUCTURE: $C_{36}H_{72}NO_8P$

SOURCE: Chemical synthesis.

• Walts, A. E., *et al.*, 1992, Applications of biocatalysts in the synthesis of phospholipids, in: *Chirality in Industry* (A. N. Collins, G. N. Sheldrake, and J. Crosby, eds.), Wiley, New York.

USES: Used in the manufacture of pharmaceutical-grade liposomes, typically in combination with DMPG and/or cholesterol. Also used in adjuvant systems for vaccine formulations. Applications in novel forms of drug delivery.

APPEARANCE: White powder.

MOLECULAR WEIGHT: 677.9

RECOMMENDED STORAGE: Keep airtight. Keep out of light. Store at 0–5°C.

CHEMICAL/PHYSICAL PROPERTIES: Amphiphilic solid. Poorly soluble in water. Solubility tends to increase as the pH is lowered within the range pH 3–8. Subject to hydrolysis below pH 3 and above pH 8.

INCOMPATIBILITY: Avoid strong bases.

SAFETY/TOXICITY: Has been used in numerous clinical trials without reported safety/toxicity issues.

ADJUVANT PROPERTIES:

• Alving, C. R., 1993, Immunologic presentation of liposomal antigens, *J. Liposome Res.* **3**:493–504.
• Just, M., *et al.*, 1992, A single vaccination with an inactivated hepatitis A liposome vaccine induces protective antibodies after only two weeks, *Vaccine* **10**:737–739.
• Glück, R., Chapter 13, this volume.
• Pietrobon, P. J. F., Chapter 14, this volume.

CONTACT(S): Tony Newton, Genzyme Pharmaceuticals and Fine Chemicals, Cambridge, MA 02139, Ph: 617-252-7783; Fax: 617-252-7772.

COMPONENT/ADJUVANT NAME: DMPG

OTHER NAME(S): Dimyristoyl phosphatidylglycerol; sn-3-phosphatidylglycerol-1, 2-dimyristoyl, sodium salt (CAS Registry Number 67232-80-8); 1, 2-dimyristoyl-sn-3-phosphatidylglycerol

STRUCTURE: $C_{34}H_{66}O_{10}PNa$

SOURCE: Chemical synthesis.

• Walts, A. E., *et al.*, 1992, Applications of biocatalysts in the synthesis of phospholipids, in: *Chirality in Industry* (A. N. Collins, G. N. Sheldrake, and J. Crosby, eds.), Wiley, New York.

USES: Used in the manufacture of pharmaceutical-grade liposomes, typically in combination with DMPC and/or cholesterol. Also used in adjuvant systems for vaccine formulations. Applications in novel forms of drug delivery.

APPEARANCE: White powder.

MOLECULAR WEIGHT: 688.9

RECOMMENDED STORAGE: Keep airtight. Keep out of light. Store at 0–5°C.

CHEMICAL/PHYSICAL PROPERTIES: Amphiphilic solid. Poorly soluble in water. Solubility tends to increase as the pH is lowered within the range pH 3–8. Subject to hydrolysis below pH 3 and above pH 8.

INCOMPATIBILITY: Avoid strong bases.

SAFETY/TOXICITY: Has been used in numerous clinical trials without reported safety/toxicity issues.

ADJUVANT PROPERTIES:

• Alving, C. R., 1993, Immunologic presentation of liposomal antigens, *J. Liposome Res.* **3**:493–504.
• Just, M., *et al.*, 1992, A single vaccination with an inactivated hepatitis A liposome vaccine induces protective antibodies after only two weeks, *Vaccine* **10**:737–739.
• Glück, R., Chapter 13, this volume.
• Pietrobon, P. J. F., Chapter 14, this volume.

CONTACT(S): Tony Newton, Genzyme Pharmaceuticals and Fine Chemicals, Cambridge, MA 02139, Ph: 617-252-7783; Fax: 617-252-7772.

COMPONENT/ADJUVANT NAME: DOC/Alum Complex

OTHER NAME(S): Deoxycholic Acid Sodium Salt; DOC/Al(OH)₃/mineral carrier complex

STRUCTURE:

DOC

SOURCE: DOC obtained from Sigma Chemicals.

USES: DOC has been used as a detergent. Complex used as adjuvant formulation.

APPEARANCE: White powder, or a clear, colorless solution.

MOLECULAR WEIGHT: 414.6

RECOMMENDED STORAGE: 4°C.

CHEMICAL/PHYSICAL PROPERTIES: Gives typical reactions common for all bile acids. Optical rotation $[\alpha]_D20 = +44 \pm 2°$ [c = 2% (w/v) in water].

INCOMPATIBILITY: Precipitates below pH 6 and in presence of divalent cations, forms gels at temperatures below 10°C (reversible).

SAFETY/TOXICITY: The DOC/Alum complex is non-toxic at adjuvant active doses, and has been used in humans without adverse side-effects.

- Nagy, L. K., 1972, The effect of deoxycholate on cholera vaccine, *Prog. Immunobiol. Stand.* **5**:341–347.
- Mussgay, M. and Weiland, E., 1973, Preparation of inactivated vaccines against alphaviruses using Semliki Forest virus–white mouse as a model. In Inactivation experiments and evaluation of double inactivated subunit vaccines, *Intervirology* **1**:259–268.

ADJUVANT PROPERTIES: Enhances immune response to membrane proteins.

- Barrett, N., *et al.*, 1989, Large-scale production and purification of a vaccinia recombinant-derived HIV-1 gp160 and analysis of its immunogenicity, *AIDS Res. Hum. Retroviruses* **5**:157–171.

CONTACT(S): Professor Friedrich Dorner, Immuno AG, Biomedical Research Center, A-2304 Ortha/Donau, Austria, Ph: 43-2212-2701/ext. 300; Fax: 43-2212-2716.

COMPONENT/ADJUVANT NAME: Freund's Complete Adjuvant

OTHER NAME(S): Complete Freund's adjuvant; CFA; FCA

STRUCTURE: Mixture of mineral oil (Marco 52) and emulsifier (Arlacel A [mannide monooleate]) as an emulsion of 85% mineral oil and 15% emulsifier with 500 μg heat-killed and dried *Mycobacterium tuberculosis* per mL of emulsifier mixture.

SOURCE: *M. tuberculosis* grown and adjuvant manufactured at the Statens Seruminstitut, Copenhagen, Denmark.

USES: The ethics of using Freund's complete adjuvant in animals is at present disputed, because of the profile of severe side effects.

APPEARANCE: Thick viscous liquid without color.

MOLECULAR WEIGHT: Not applicable.

RECOMMENDED STORAGE: Store at 2–8°C. Do not freeze the final emulsion, as it is disrupted by freezing.

CHEMICAL/PHYSICAL PROPERTIES: Mixing (usually syringe-to-syringe mixing) with an aqueous antigen phase in a 1:1 ratio makes a water-in-oil emulsion (w/o) ready for immunization.

INCOMPATIBILITY: Avoid freezing the final emulsion.

SAFETY/TOXICITY: May cause granulomas and abscesses at the site of injection. May cause arthritis, amyloidosis, and allergic reactions. Can cause ascites production in BALB/c mice when injected i.p. with or without antigen.

- Yamanaka, M., *et al.*, 1992, Pathological studies on local tissue reactions in guinea pigs and rats caused by four different adjuvants, *J. Vet. Med. Sci.* **54**:685–692.

ADJUVANT PROPERTIES:

- Freund, J., 1956, The mode of action of immunologic adjuvants, *Adv. Tuberc. Res.* **7**:130–148.
- Herbert, W. J., 1967, Methods for the preparation of water-in-oil, and multiple, emulsions for use as antigen adjuvants; and notes on their use in immunization procedures, in: *Handbook of Experimental Immunology* (D. M. Weir, ed.), Blackwell Scientific Publications, 1207–1214.
- Bomford, R., 1980, The comparative selectivity of adjuvants for humoral and cell-mediated immunity. II. Effect on delayed-type hypersensitivity in the mouse and guinea pig, and cell-mediated immunity to tumor antigens in the mouse of Freund's incomplete and complete adjuvants, Alhydrogel, *Corynebacterium parvum*, *Bordetella pertussis*, muramyl dipeptide and saponin, *Clin. Exp. Immunol.* **39**:435–441.

CONTACT(S): There are several contacts for CFA (see also Montanide ISA monographs). This product is by: Erik B. Lindblad, Superfos Biosector, DK-2950 Vedbaek, Denmark, Ph: 45 42 89 31 11; Fax: 45 42 89 15 95. Also: Al Reisch, Sergeant, Inc., Clifton, NJ 07012, Ph: 201-472-9111; Fax: 201-472-5686.

COMPONENT/ADJUVANT NAME: Freund's Incomplete Adjuvant
OTHER NAME(S): Incomplete Freund's Adjuvant; IFA; FIA
STRUCTURE: Mixture of mineral oil (Marcol 52) and emulsifier (Arlacel A [mannide monooleate]) as an 85% mineral oil and 15% emulsifier emulsion.
SOURCE: Manufactured by Statens Seruminstitut, Copenhagen, Denmark.
USES: Immunization of experimental animals.
APPEARANCE: Thick viscous liquid without color.
MOLECULAR WEIGHT: Not applicable.
RECOMMENDED STORAGE: Store at 2–8°C. Do not freeze the final emulsion, as it is disrupted by freezing.
CHEMICAL/PHYSICAL PROPERTIES: Mixing (usually syringe-to-syringe mixing) with an aqueous antigen phase in a 1:1 ratio makes a water-in-oil emulsion ready for immunization.
INCOMPATIBILITY: Avoid freezing the final emulsion.
SAFETY/TOXICITY: May cause granulomas and abscesses at the site of injection. Induces production of ascites in BALB/c mice when injected i.p. with or without antigen.

- Yamanaka, M., *et al.*, 1992, Pathological studies on local tissue reactions in guinea pigs and rats caused by four different adjuvants, *J. Vet. Med. Sci.* **54**:685–692.

ADJUVANT PROPERTIES:

- Herbert, W. J., 1967, Methods for the preparation of water-in-oil, and multiple, emulsions for use as antigen adjuvants; and notes on their use in immunization procedures, in: *Handbook of Experimental Immunology* (D. M. Weir, ed.), Blackwell Scientific Publications, 1207–1214.
- Bomford, R., 1980, The comparative selectivity of adjuvants for humoral and cell-mediated immunity. II. Effect on delayed-type hypersensitivity in the mouse and guinea pig, and cell-mediated immunity to tumor antigens in the mouse of Freund's incomplete and complete adjuvants, Alhydrogel, *Corynebacterium parvum*, *Bordetella pertussis*, muramyl dipeptide and saponin, *Clin. Exp. Immunol.* **39**:435–441.

CONTACT(S): There are several contacts for IFA (see also Montanide ISA monographs). This product is by: Erik B. Lindblad, Superfos Biosector, DK-2950 Vedbaek, Denmark, Ph: 45 42 89 31 11; Fax: 45 42 89 15 95. Also: Al Reisch, Sergeant, Inc., Clifton, NJ 07012, Ph: 201-472-9111; Fax: 201-472-5686.

COMPONENT/ADJUVANT NAME: Gamma Inulin

OTHER NAME(S): None

STRUCTURE: Linear (unbranched) β-D-(2→1) polyfructofuranosyl-α-D-glucose, as particles in the gamma polymorphic configuration. Typically $n = 50$–75.

SOURCE: Dahlia tubers. Obtained by aqueous extraction and crystallization of inulin, followed by adsorptive treatments, recrystallization, and conversion to the gamma form at 37°C.

- Cooper, P. D., and Carter, M., 1986, Anticomplementary action of polymorphic 'solubility forms' of particulate inulin, *Mol. Immunol.* **23**:895–901.

USES: Highly specific activator of the alternative pathway of complement in vitro and in vivo. Included in adjuvant formulations as a primary adjuvant and also as the immune stimulant when combined as composite particles with alum in the adjuvant Algammulin.

APPEARANCE: Milky white, nonviscous aqueous suspension, easily resuspended. Supplied at 50 mg/mL, sterile and pyrogen-free.

MOLECULAR WEIGHT: 8000–12,000. A typical preparation comprises a range of chain lengths corresponding to degrees of polymerization of 50–75 fructose residues.

RECOMMENDED STORAGE: 2–8°C in aqueous medium. Do not freeze or heat over 45°C.

CHEMICAL/PHYSICAL PROPERTIES: Neutral, edible polysaccharide of known primary structure, as ovoids about 1 μm diameter. Stable for years under recommended storage. Unstable below pH 6 and above pH 10. The gamma form is virtually insoluble at 37°C and is essential for biological activity.

INCOMPATIBILITY: Degraded in moderately strong acid.

SAFETY/TOXICITY: Nonpyrogenic, nonantigenic, and of very low toxicity in experimental animals. Biodegradable to simple sugars. Large intravenous doses can cause acute complement-activation shock similar to that sometimes found in human renal dialysis patients. Dissolved inulin is pharmacologically inert and is registered for human use.

ADJUVANT PROPERTIES: Expected to stimulate immune responses by causing ligation of leukocyte-surface complement receptors (CR) via known biochemical mechanisms. Addition of gamma inulin is known to enhance both humoral and cell-mediated immunity from mainly Th1 pathways. Gamma inulin also has an antitumor action and an effect on natural immunity.

- Cooper, P. D., and Steele, E. J., 1988, The adjuvanticity of gamma inulin, *Immunol. Cell Biol.* **66**:345–352.
- Cooper, P. D., *et al.*, 1993, Gamma inulin and Algammulin: Two new vaccine adjuvants, in: *Vaccines 93, Modern Approaches to New Vaccines Including Prevention of AIDS* (H. S. Ginsburg, F. Brown, R. M. Chanock, and R. A. Lerner, eds.), Cold Spring Harbor Laboratory Press, Cold Spring Harbor, NY, pp. 25–30.
- Cooper, P. D., Chapter 24, this volume.

CONTACT(S): Dr. Peter D. Cooper, Division of Cell Biology, John Curtin School of Medical Research, Australian National University, Canberra, A. C. T., Australia 2601, Ph: 61-6-291-8670; Fax: 61-6-249-2595.

COMPONENT/ADJUVANT NAME: Gerbu Adjuvant

OTHER NAME(S): None

STRUCTURE: Mixture of: (1) N-acetylglucosaminyl-(β1-4)-N-acetylmuramyl-L-alanyl-D-glutamine (GMDP), (2) dimethyl dioctadecylammonium chloride (DDA), (3) zinc L-proline salt complex (Zn-Pro$_{\sim 8}$) (shown below).

GMDP   DDA   Proline-Zinc (8:1)

SOURCE: (1) Semisynthetic, (2) synthetic, (3) semisynthetic.

USES: Proprietary adjuvant formulation intended for animal and human use.

APPEARANCE: White lyophilizate.

MOLECULAR WEIGHT: (1) GMDP = 695, (2) DDA = 631, (3) Pro$_{\sim 8}$:Zn complex = ~1000.

RECOMMENDED STORAGE: Store at 2–8°C.

CHEMICAL/PHYSICAL PROPERTIES: GMDP is a crystalline solid, easily dispersible in aqueous antigen solutions. DDA by itself is very sparsely soluble (2.5 mg/L) but in the zinc L-proline complex it is easily dispersible in water. At 37°C it remains in dispersion for at least 1 week. Frozen solutions can be thawed repeatedly and the dispersion of DDA remains stable. The material is soluble in 70% ethanol. The preparation is sterile and suitable for injection after reconstitution. It is kept in 5-mL glass vials with stoppers of butyl rubber. Once reconstituted, the storage must be in the frozen state to prevent microbial growth or "contamination."

INCOMPATIBILITY: None found.

SAFETY/TOXICITY: All components are extensively tested for oral and parenteral toxicity and found to be nontoxic in doses well above those recommended for immunization. Zinc and L-proline are widely used in infusions for a variety of human uses in doses larger as used in this adjuvant formula.

ADJUVANT PROPERTIES: Gerbu Adjuvant has already been tested in many applications, mainly with mice, hens, and rabbits.

• Gruhofer, N., 1994, An adjuvant based on GMDP with DDA and zinc–L-proline complex as synergists, *Immunology Lett.* (in press).

CONTACT(S): Dr. P. Cooper, CC Biotech Corporation, Poway, CA 92064, Ph: 619-451-9949; Fax: 619-487-8138; Dr. N. Grubhofer, Gerbu Biotecknik GmbH D69251 Gaiberg, Germany, Ph: 49 6223 47197; Fax 49 6223 47199.

COMPONENT/ADJUVANT NAME: GM-CSF

OTHER NAME(S): Granulocyte–macrophage colony stimulating factor; Sargramostim (yeast-derived rh-GM-CSF)

STRUCTURE: GM-CSF is a glycoprotein of 127 amino acids. Recombinant human GM-CSF is produced in yeast and it differs from the natural human GM-CSF by substitution of Leu for Arg at position 23.

- Walter, M. R., *et al.*, 1992, Three-dimensional structure of recombinant human granulocyte–macrophage colony stimulating factor, *J. Mol. Biol.* **224**:1075–1085.

Sequence of recombinant human GM-CSF (Sargramostin):

APARSPSPSTQPWEHVNAIQEALRLLNLSRDTAAEMNETVEVISEMFDLQEPTC
LQTRLELYKQGLRGSLTKLKGPLTMMASHYKQHCPPTPETSCATQIITFESFKE
NLKDFLLVIPFDCWEPVQE

SOURCE: Recombinant protein produced in yeast (*S. cerevisiae*).

USES: GM-CSF (Sargramostin) is an approved product indicated for acceleration of myeloid recovery in patients with non-Hodgkin's lymphoma, acute lymphoblastic leukemia, and Hodgkin's disease undergoing autologous bone marrow transplantation. Reports in the literature also suggest that GM-CSF is able to activate mature granulocytes and macrophages, and may have utility as co-adjuvant.

APPEARANCE: White, lyophilized powder (before reconstitution), or a clear colorless solution (after reconstitution).

MOLECULAR WEIGHT: 15,500, 16,800, and 19,500 (three bands on SDS-PAGE representing variation in glycosylation).

RECOMMENDED STORAGE: Both lyophilized GM-CSF (Sargramostin) and reconstituted product should be stored at 2–8°C. Lyophilized product may also be frozen at –20 or –70°C.

CHEMICAL/PHYSICAL PROPERTIES: GM-CSF (Sargramostin) exists as a major species (pI 5.2) and a minor species (pI 4.5–5.2). GM-CSF (Sargramostin) shows a specific activity of 5.6×10^6 IU/mg as measured in a TF-1 cell proliferation assay.

INCOMPATIBILITY: Avoid contact with proteases.

SAFETY/TOXICITY: Generally well tolerated when given for indications above. Safety data using GM-CSF as adjuvant have not been reported.

ADJUVANT PROPERTIES: This cytokine is a growth factor that stimulates normal myeloid precursors, and activates mature granulocytes and macrophages.

- Tao, M. H., and Levy, R., 1993, Idiotype/granulocyte–macrophage colony stimulating factor fusion protein as a vaccine for B-cell lymphoma, *Nature* **362**:755–758.
- Dranoff, G., *et al.*, 1993, Vaccination with irradiated tumor cells engineered to secrete murine granulocyte–macrophage colony stimulating factor stimulates potent, specific, and long-lasting anti-tumor immunity, *Proc. Natl. Acad. Sci. USA* **90**:3539–3543.

CONTACT(S): Dr. Michael Widmer, Immunex Corp., Seattle, WA 98101, Ph: 206-587-0430; Fax: 206-587-0606.

COMPONENT/ADJUVANT NAME: GMDP

OTHER NAME(S): N-Acetylglucosaminyl-(β1-4)-N-acetylmuramyl-L-alanyl-D-isoglutamine (CAS Registry Number 70280-03-4)

STRUCTURE:

CH$_2$OH / HO—O / HO / NHCOCH$_3$ / CH$_2$OH / O—O / OH / NHCOCH$_3$ / H O CONH$_2$ / N / N / OH / O H O

SOURCE: Semisynthetic. Disaccharide isolated from microbial source, dipeptide wholly synthetic. U.S. Patent No. 4,395,399.

USES: Primary adjuvant.

APPEARANCE: White, lyophilized powder.

MOLECULAR WEIGHT: 695. Contains defined low percentages of acetate and water.

RECOMMENDED STORAGE: Extremely stable at room temperature under dry conditions. For prolonged storage, desiccator at 4°C is recommended.

CHEMICAL/PHYSICAL PROPERTIES: Mp 166–170°C; pKa 5.48; optical rotation $[\alpha]_D20 = +2.8°$. Exists as an equilibrium mixture of two anomeric forms due to mutarotation of the -OH at C-1 of the muramic acid residue. Highly soluble in aqueous buffers, ethanol, methanol, DMF. Practically insoluble in chloroform, ether, and acetonitrile.

INCOMPATIBILITY: Avoid extremes of pH.

SAFETY: Extensive Phase I systemic safety data in humans (mostly after oral administration). Single oral doses of up to 50 mg given with no side effects. Intramuscular injections of 1 mg given with minimal local reaction. LD$_{50}$ in mouse = 7 g/kg. Less pyrogenic than prototype muramyl dipeptide. In Phase II clinicals for other applications.

ADJUVANT PROPERTIES: Highly effective primary adjuvant in a range of vehicles; aqueous buffers, mineral oil, pluronic/squalane/Tween emulsions. Also effective as oral adjuvant, enhancing mucosal IgA response.

- Andronova, T. M., and Ivanov, V. T., 1991, The structure and immunomodulating function of glucosaminylmuramyl peptides, *Sov. Med. Rev. D Immunol.* **4**:1–63.
- Bomford, R., *et al.*, 1992, The control of the antibody isotype response to recombinant human immunodeficiency antigen by adjuvants, *AIDS Res. Hum. Retroviruses* **8**:1765–1771.
- Campbell, M. J., *et al.*, 1990, Idiotype vaccination against murine B-cell lymphoma, *J. Immunol.* **145**:1029–1036.

CONTACT(S): Philip Ledger, Ph.D., Peptech(*UK*) Ltd., Cirencester, Glos GL7 2PF, United Kingdom, Ph: 44-285-643666; Fax: 44-285-644328.

COMPONENT/ADJUVANT NAME: Imiquimod

OTHER NAME(S): 1-(2-methypropyl)-1H-imidazo[4,5-c]quinolin-4-amine; R-837; S-26308

STRUCTURE:

SOURCE: Chemical synthesis.

• Gerster, J. F., 1987, U.S. Patent 4,680,338. Lagain, D., 1991, U.S. Patent 4,988,815.

USES: Included in adjuvant formulations as a primary adjuvant component.

APPEARANCE: White, fine crystalline solid.

MOLECULAR WEIGHT: 240.31 free base, 276.77 hydrochloride salt.

RECOMMENDED STORAGE: Solid is stable at room temperature. Shelf life is acceptable.

CHEMICAL/PHYSICAL PROPERTIES: Very limited solubility as the free base. The hydrochloride salt is soluble in water at concentrations up to 10 mg/mL. The optimal solubility for use is pH ~4.

INCOMPATIBILITY: None found.

SAFETY/TOXICITY: Imiquimod's safety package includes extensive evaluation with 4-month dermal and 6-month oral studies completed. In addition, no teratogenic or mutagenic effects were seen. Phase III trials as a topical antiviral agent using 5% cream, and Phase IIA trials as an oral antiviral agent using 50 and 200 mg doses of drug are ongoing.

ADJUVANT PROPERTIES: Addition of imiquimod known to induce both humoral and cell-mediated immunity via induction of cytokines from monocytes and macrophages.

• Bernstein, D. L., *et al.*, 1993, Adjuvant effects of imiquimod on a herpes simplex virus type 2 glycoprotein vaccine in guinea pigs, *J. Infect. Dis.* **167**:731–735.

• Sidky, Y. A., *et al.*, 1992, Inhibition of murine tumor growth by an interferon-inducing imidazoquinolinamine, *Cancer Res.* **52**:3528–3533.

• Reiter, M. J., *et al.*, 1994, Cytokine induction in mice by the immunomodulator imiquimod, *J. Leukocyte Biol.* **55**:234–240.

CONTACT(S): R. C. Hanson, Business Development, 3M Pharmaceuticals, St. Paul, MN 55144, Ph: 612-737-3137; Fax: 612-737-4556.

COMPONENT/ADJUVANT NAME: ImmTher™

OTHER NAME(S): *N*-Acetylglucosaminyl-*N*-acetylmuramyl-L-Ala-D-isoGlu-L-Ala-glycerol dipalmitate; DTP-GDP

STRUCTURE:

SOURCE: Synthetic (U.S. Patent 4,950,645).

USES: ImmTher™ is a potent macrophage activator, capable of inducing remission in human metastatic colorectal cancer. In vitro and in vivo it induces high levels of TNF, IL-1, and IL-6. The active drug compound is formulated as adjuvant in liposomes consisting of 175 mg of 1-palmitoyl-2-oleoyl phosphatidylcholine and 75 mg of 1,2-dioleoyl phosphatidylglycerol (per 2.5 mL).

APPEARANCE: White, odorless powder. The lyophilized product is reconstituted in 2.5 mL saline to produce an initial concentration of 400 μg/mL.

MOLECULAR WEIGHT: 1316.82

RECOMMENDED STORAGE: Stable as a lyophilized powder or in solution with saline or PBS at 3–8°C for 5 years.

CHEMICAL/PHYSICAL PROPERTIES: Amphoteric molecule soluble in chloroform:methanol (7:3), and tert-butanol. The ester bond between the peptide and the lipid is subject to hydrolysis.

INCOMPATIBILITY: Avoid strong acids and bases.

SAFETY/TOXICITY: Safe in humans up to single doses of 1.2 mg/m^2 and given weekly for up to 6 months at doses of 0.8 to 1.0 mg/m^2. Major toxicity is fever, chills, and hypotension at doses of 0.8 mg/m^2 or greater. There has been no observed hematological, hepatic, or neural toxicity.

ADJUVANT PROPERTIES: The formulation is a potent macrophage activator and enhances both cellular and humoral immunity.

- Vosika, G. J., *et al.*, 1991, Phase I trial of ImmTher™, a new liposome-incorporated lipophilic disaccharide tripeptide, *J. Immunother.* **10**:256–266.
- Vosika, G. J., *et al.*, 1990, Immunologic and toxicologic study of disaccharide tripeptide glycerol dipalmitoyl: A new lipophilic immunomodulator, *Mol. Biother.* **2**:50–56.

CONTACT(S): Gerald Vosika, M. D., ImmunoTherapeutics, Inc., Fargo, ND 58104, Ph: 701-232-9575; Fax: 701-237-9275.

COMPONENT/ADJUVANT NAME: Interferon-γ

OTHER NAME(S): Actimmune® (rhIFN-gamma, Genentech, Inc.); immune interferon; IFN-γ; gamma-interferon

STRUCTURE: Noncovalent dimer. Low-resolution crystal structure available. Monomer consists of 140 amino acids, no glycosylation or cysteines in human form. Murine form is a covalent dimer (one cysteine per monomer).

- Ealick, S. E., *et al.*, 1991, Three-dimensional structure of recombinant human interferon-γ, *Science* **252**:698–702.

Sequence of human interferon-gamma:

QDPYVKEAENLKKYFNAGHSDVADNGTLFLGILKNWKEESDRKIMQSQIVSF
YFKLFKNFKDDQSIQKSVETIKEDMNVKFFNSNKKKRDDFEKLTNYSVTDLN
VQRKAIHELIQVMAELSPAAKTGKRKRSQMLFRGRRASQ

SOURCE: Both human (rhIFN-gamma) and murine (rmuIFN-gamma) forms are expressed in *Escherichia coli* and distributed in a completely pure state.

USES: rhIFN-gamma (Actimmune®) is FDA-approved for use in chronic granulomatous disease (CGD). Currently, Actimmune® is in human clinical Phase III trials for renal cell carcinoma. rhIFN-gamma has been studied in humans as an adjuvant for hepatitis B subunit antigen (Quiroga *et al.*, 1990, *Hepatology* **12**:661–663).

APPEARANCE: Clear aqueous solution.

MOLECULAR WEIGHT: Monomer 16,440

RECOMMENDED STORAGE: 2–8°C (do not freeze).

CHEMICAL/PHYSICAL PROPERTIES: rhIFN-gamma: pI 9.9, absorptivity = 0.75 $(\text{mg/mL})^{-1}$ cm^{-1} at 280.4 nm, typical specific activity ~3–5 × 10^7 IU/mg. rmuIFN-gamma: absorptivity = 0.93 $(\text{mg/mL})^{-1}$ cm^{-1} at 280 nm, typical specific activity ~0.5–1 × 10^7 IU/mg.

INCOMPATIBILITY: Susceptible to shear-induced degradation (requires surfactants for stability), readily deamidates at high pH (> 6.5), and may be cleaved by proteases.

SAFETY/TOXICITY: rhIFN-gamma as Actimmune® is an FDA-approved commercial product for human use. Standard human dose is 100 μg. High doses can cause significant side effects such as nausea, fever, and other flulike symptoms. Effect of molecule is specific to species. Human form does not elicit toxicity in lower species at several mg/kg doses which are toxic to humans.

ADJUVANT PROPERTIES: Higher and earlier neutralizing antibody titers, increase in duration of neutralizing antibody titers, increase in MHC class II expression on antigen-presenting cells, increase in helper T cell levels, and an improved DTH response have all been observed when IFN-gamma was administered with an antigen. The IFN-gamma must be given at the same site and at the same time (within 6 h) as the antigen to have biological effect.

- Schijns, V. E. C. J., *et al.*, 1994, Modulation of antiviral immune responses by exogenous cytokines: Effects of tumour necrosis factor-α, interleukin-1α, interleukin-2 and interferon-γ on the immunogenicity of an inactivated rabies vaccine, *J. Gen. Virol.* **75**:55–63.
- Heath, A. W., and Playfair, J. H. L., 1992, Cytokines as immunological adjuvants, *Vaccine* **10**:427–434.
- Cao, M., *et al.*, 1992, Enhancement of the protective effect of inactivated influenza virus vaccine by cytokines, *Vaccine* **10**:238–242.
- Heath, A., Chapter 28, this volume.
- Dong, P., *et al.*, Chapter 27, this volume.

CONTACT(S): Dr. Jeffrey L. Cleland, Genentech, Inc., South San Francisco, CA 94080, Ph: 415-225-3921; Fax: 415-225-3979; E-mail: Cleland.Jeffrey@gene.com.

COMPONENT/ADJUVANT NAME: Interleukin-1β

OTHER NAME(S): IL-1β; IL-1; human interleukin-1β mature polypeptide 117-259

STRUCTURE: This protein is composed of 12 antiparallel β-strands folded into a six-stranded β barrel, with 3-fold symmetry about the axis of the barrel.

• Priestle, J. P., *et al.*, 1988, Crystal structure of the cytokine interleukin-1β, *EMBO J.* **7**:339–343.

Sequence of ILβ:

APVRSLNCTLRDSQQKSLVMSGPYELKALHLQGQDMEQQVVFSMSFVQGEES
NDKIPVALGLKEKNLYLSCVLKDDKPTLQLESVDPKNYPKKKMEKRFVFNKIE
INNKLEFESAQFPNWYISTSQAENMPVFLGGTKGGQDITDFTMQFVSS

SOURCE: Recombinant mature fragment 117–259 of human interleukin-1β, usually expressed in *E. coli* or other bacteria, derived from myeloid or placental libraries. Purified by sequential steps or ion-exchange chromatography and gel filtration.

USES: Primary adjuvant. Active by oral, intravenous, intraperitoneal, and subcutaneous routes. It can be administered admixed with antigen or separately.

APPEARANCE: White, odorless powder.

MOLECULAR WEIGHT: 17,377

RECOMMENDED STORAGE: Store lyophilized powder dry at –20 or 4°C. The concentrated solution must be aliquoted and stored at –80°C. Avoid freeze-thawing, which results in rapid loss of activity. If diluted in solution, it tends to adhere to the vessel walls: use siliconized glass, high protein concentrations, low temperature, stabilizing proteins.

CHEMICAL/PHYSICAL PROPERTIES: The recombinant protein is quite unstable: it does not stand storage in solution at 4°C nor does it stand freeze-thawing. The protein contains unreduced cysteines which form interchain disulfide bridges on prolonged storage (both in frozen and lyophilized conditions), with the appearance of multimeric molecules devoid of biological activity. pI 6.9.

INCOMPATIBILITY: Avoid proteases.

SAFETY/TOXICITY: IL-1 is a major inflammatory mediator; thus its use in vivo may have many unwanted effects. Phase I trials demonstrated severe hypotension as major side effect, as well as pain, respiratory and hematological alterations. However, the immunostimulatory effects of IL-1 are evident at doses much lower than those yielding toxicity.

ADJUVANT PROPERTIES: It increases both T-dependent and T-independent responses to different types of antigens. Active on both primary and secondary responses.

• Staruch, M. J., and Wood, D. D., 1983, The adjuvanticity of interleukin-1 in vivo, *J. Immunol.* **130**:2191–2194.

• Nencioni, L., *et al.*, 1987, In vivo immunostimulating activity of the 163–171 peptide of human IL-1β, *J. Immunol.* **139**:800–804.

• Frasca, D., *et al.*, 1988, In vivo restoration of T cell functions by human IL-1β or its 163–171 nonapeptide in immunodepressed mice, *J. Immunol.* **141**:2651–2655.

• McCune, C. S., and Marquis, D. M., 1990, Interleukin-1 as an adjuvant for active specific immunotherapy in a murine tumor model, *Cancer Res.* **50**:1212–1215.

• Heath, A., Chapter 28, this volume.

• Dong, P., *et al.*, Chapter 27, this volume.

CONTACT(S): Dr. Diana Boraschi, Dompè Research Center, Via Campo di Pile, 1-67100 L'Aquila, Italy, Ph: 39-862-338324; Fax: 39-862-338219.

COMPONENT/ ADJUVANT NAME: Interleukin-2

OTHER NAMES: IL-2; T-cell growth factor; aldesleukin (des-alanyl-1, serine-125 human interleukin-2); Proleukin®; Teceleukin®

STRUCTURE: Native human IL-2 contains 133 amino acids (see below); aldesleukin contains 132 amino acids. IL-2 exists as six alpha-helical domains, termed A to F. Glycosylation not essential for function.

- Rosenberg, S. A., *et al.*, 1983, Biological activity of recombinant human interleukin-2 produced in *Escherichia coli, Science* **223**:1412–1414.
- Brandhuber, B. J., *et al.*, 1987, Three dimensional structure of interleukin-2, *Science* **238**:1707–1709.
- Ju, G., *et al.*, 1987, Structure function analysis of human interleukin-2: Identification of amino acid residues required for biological activity, *J. Biol. Chem.* **262**:5723–5731.

Sequence of human IL-2:

APTSSSTKKTQLQLEHLLLDLQMILNGINNYKNPKLTRMLTFKFYMPKKATEL
KHLQCLEEELKPLEEVLNLAQSKNFHLRPRDLISNINVIVLELKGSETTFMCEY
ADETATIVEFLNRWITFCQSIISTLT

SOURCE: Recombinant protein expressed in *E. coli*.

USES: As a primary adjuvant, co-emulsified with antigens and lipids, with polyethylene glycol-modified long-acting form (PEG IL-2), or liposome-encapsulated sustained release dosage form. Aldesleukin (Proleukin®) is an FDA-licensed agent for treatment of metastatic renal cell carcinoma.

APPEARANCE: Lyophilized, white to off-white solid; reconstituted with water for injection to give a clear, colorless solution.

MOLECULAR WEIGHT: 15,300

RECOMMENDED STORAGE: Store lyophilized aldesleukin solid at 2–8°C. Store the reconstituted product at 2–8°C for no longer than 48 h. Reconstituted solution diluted with 5% dextrose to a 200 μg/mL IL-2 concentration stable in plastic syringes at 2–8°C for 14 days. Store lyophilized PEG IL-2 at –20°C and reconstituted PEG IL-2 at 2–8°C for up to 28 days. Storage stability of liposomal dosage form unknown.

CHEMICAL/ PHYSICAL PROPERTIES: Relatively hydrophobic protein with moderate aqueous solubility (~1 mg/mL). Major pI = 8.0. Adsorbs to glass and plastic surfaces below concentrations of 10 μg/mL or less, this can be prevented by having 0.1% human albumin present in the diluting solution prior to adding aldesleukin. Potential degradation pathways: methionine oxidation, aggregation, dimer and higher oligomer formation and deamidation.

INCOMPATIBILITY: Aldesleukin is not compatible with sodium chloride for injection, solutions with high ionic strength or containing preservatives. May degrade with proteases; avoid solutions of low or high pH extremes. Compatible with mineral oil and other lipoidal adjuvants (DDA, Avridine®).

SAFETY/TOXICITY: Frequency and severity of adverse reactions are generally dose-related. The most frequently reported serious adverse reactions include hypotension, renal dysfunction, dyspnea, and mental-state changes. Further descriptions are indicated in the Proleukin® (Aldesleukin for Injection) package insert (Chiron Corporation, Emeryville, CA).

- Rosenberg, S. A., *et al.*, 1985, Observations on the systemic administration of autologous lymphokine-activated killer cells and recombinant interleukin-2 to patients with metastatic cancer, *N. Engl. J. Med.* **313**:1485–1492.

- Kroemer, G., *et al.*, 1992, Interleukin-2, a pro-autoimmune lymphokine that interferes with post-deletional tolerance, *Semin. Immunol.* **4**:167–179.

ADJUVANT PROPERTIES: IL-2 supports the growth and proliferation of antigen-activated T lymphocytes and plays a central role in the cascade of cellular events involved in the immune response. Proliferating T cells also produce a variety of other lymphokines which may modulate other arms of the immune system. In view of these direct and indirect actions of IL-2 on the immune response, IL-2 may function as an adjuvant to vaccination by increasing the specific and durable response to vaccine immunogens. Low doses may give up to 25-fold increase in adjuvant effect, with inhibition of adjuvant effect at high doses. May induce cellular immunity when given systemically, and IgA when administered at a mucosal surface.

- Weinberg, A., and Merrigan, T. C., 1988, Recombinant interleukin-2 as an adjuvant for vaccine-induced protection, *J. Immunol.* **140**:294–299.
- Nunberg, J. H., *et al.*, 1989, Interleukin 2 acts as an adjuvant to increase the potency of inactivated rabies virus vaccine, *Proc. Natl. Acad. Sci. USA* **86**:4240–4243.
- Ho, R. J. Y., *et al.*, 1991, A potentially useful vaccine adjuvant, in: *Topics in Vaccine Adjuvant Research* (D. R. Spriggs and W. C. Koff, eds.), CRC Press, Boca Raton, pp. 69–76.
- Ho, R. J., *et al.*, 1992, Liposome-formulated interleukin-2 as an adjuvant for the treatment of recurrent genital HSV-2 in guinea pigs with recombinant HSV glycoprotein gD, *Vaccine* **10**:209–213.
- Hughes, H. P. A., *et al.*, 1991, Immunopotentiation of bovine herpes virus subunit vaccination by IL-2, *Immunology* **74**:461–466.
- Hughes, H. P. A., *et al.*, 1992, Multiple administration of with cytokines potentiates antigen specific responses to subunit vaccination with bovine herpes virus-1 glycoprotein IV, *Vaccine* **10**:226–230.
- Tan, L., and Gregoriadis, G., 1989, Effect of interleukin-2 on the immunoadjuvant action of liposomes, *Biochem. Soc. Trans.* **17**:693–694.
- Mbwuike, I. N., *et al.*, 1990, Enhancement of the protective efficacy of the inactivated influenza A virus vaccine in aged mice by IL-2 liposomes, *Vaccine* **8**:347–352.
- Heath, A., Chapter 28, this volume.
- Dong, P., *et al.*, Chapter 27, this volume.

CONTACT(S): Huw Hughes, M6 Pharmaceuticals, Inc., New York, NY 10701, Ph: 212-308-7200 ext. 14; E-mail 74577.345@compuserve.com. Also: Professional Services, Chiron Therapeutics, A Division of Chiron Corporation, Emeryville, CA.

COMPONENT/ADJUVANT NAME: Interleukin-7

OTHER NAME(S): IL-7

STRUCTURE:

- Goodwin, R. G., *et al.*, 1989, Molecular cloning and growth factor activity on human and murine B-lineage cells, *Proc. Natl. Acad. Sci. USA* **86**:302–306.

Sequence of IL-7:

MFHVSFRYIFGLPPLILVLLPVASSDCDIEGKDGKQYESVLMVSIDQLLDSMKEI
GSNCLNNEFNFFKRHICDANKEGMFLFRAARKLRQFLKMNSTGDFDLHLLKV
SEGTTILLNCTGQVKGRKPAALGEAQPTKSLEENKSLKEQKKLNDLCFLKRLL
QEIKTCWNKILMGTKEH

SOURCE: Recombinant protein expressed in *E. coli*. Immunex Corp., Sterling Winthrop Pharmaceuticals.

USES: Primary adjuvant, liposome-formulated sustained release form. Co-emulsified with antigen and lipids.

APPEARANCE: Clear aqueous solution.

MOLECULAR WEIGHT: 25,000

RECOMMENDED STORAGE: 4°C for both IL-7 and liposome-formulated IL-7.

CHEMICAL/PHYSICAL PROPERTIES: Reasonable solubility in water (~1 mg/mL).

INCOMPATIBILITY: Avoid proteases.

SAFETY/TOXICITY: Unknown.

ADJUVANT PROPERTIES:

- Bui, T., *et al.*, 1994, Biologic response of recombinant interleukin-7 on herpes simplex virus infection in guinea pigs, *Vaccine* **12**:646–652.
- Bui, T., *et al.*, 1994, Effect of MTP-PE liposomes and IL-7 on induction of antibody and cell-mediated immune responses to a recombinant HIV envelope protein, *J. AIDS* (in press).
- Heath, A., Chapter 28, this volume.
- Dong, P., *et al.*, Chapter 27, this volume.

CONTACT(S): Dr. Rodney Ho, University of Washington, Seattle, WA. Ph: 206-685-3914; Fax: 206-543-3204.

COMPONENT/ADJUVANT NAME: Interleukin-12

OTHER NAME(S): IL-12; natural killer cell stimulatory factor (NKSF); cytotoxic lymphocyte maturation factor (CLMF)

STRUCTURE: IL-12 is a heterodimeric protein composed of two disulfide-bonded glycoprotein subunits approximately 35 and 40 kDa in size. The two subunits represent two separate, unrelated gene products that have to be coexpressed to yield the secreted, bioactive, heterodimeric lymphokine.

- Gubler, U., *et al.*, 1991, Coexpression of two distinct genes is required to generate secreted, bioactive cytotoxic lymphocyte maturation factor, *Proc. Natl. Acad. Sci. USA* **88**:4143–4147.
- Wolf, S. F., *et al.*, 1991, Cloning of cDNA for natural killer cell stimulatory factor, a heterodimeric cytokine with multiple biologic effects on T and natural killer cells, *J. Immunol.* **146**:3074–3081.
- Schoenhaut, D. S., *et al.*, 1992, Cloning and expression of murine IL-12, *J. Immunol.* **148**:3433–3440.

Sequence of 40-kDa subunit of human IL-12:

IWELKKDVYVVELDWYPDAPGEMVVLTCDTPEEDGITWTLDQSSEVLGSGKT
LTIQVKEFGDAGQYTCHKGGEVLSHSLLLLHKKEDGIWSTDILKDQKEPKNKT
FLRCEAKNYSGRFTCWWLTTISTDLTFSVKSSRGSSDPQGVTCGAATLSAERVR
GDNKEYEYSVECQEDSACPAAEESLPIEVMVDAVHKLKYENYTSSFFIRDIIKP
DPPKNLQLKPLKNSRQVEVSWEYPDTWSTPHSYFSLTFCVQVQGKSKREKKD
RVFTDKTSATVICRKNASISVRAQDRYYSSSWSEWASVPCS

Sequence of 35-kDa subunit of human IL-12:

RNLPVATPDPGMFPCLHHSQNLLRAVSNMLQKARQTLEFYPCTSEEIDHEDITK
DKTSTVEACLPLELTKNESCLNSRETSFITNGSCLASRKTSFMMALCLSSIYEDL
KMYQVEFKTMNAKLLMDPKRQIFLDQNMLAVIDELMQALNFNSETVPQKSSL
EEPDFYKTKIKLCILLHAFRIRAVTIDRVTSYLNAS

SOURCE: Recombinant protein purified from the medium of cultures of CHO cells transfected with IL-12 cDNAs. Natural sources of the protein include activated monocyte/macrophages and B lymphocytes.

USES: Included as a primary adjuvant component to enhance Th1-dependent cell-mediated immunity.

MOLECULAR WEIGHT: Protein: 57,200; glycosylated protein: ~70,000.

RECOMMENDED STORAGE: Store IL-12 at –70°C in pH 7 buffer free of calcium, magnesium, and potassium salts (1 mg/mL). Maximum two freeze-thaws pending further investigation. Storage in opaque polypropylene containers is preferable.

CHEMICAL/PHYSICAL PROPERTIES: Three major bands in the pI range of 4.5 to 5.3. IL-12 is most stable at pH 7 at 10 μg/mL and greater. At lower and higher pH, significant loss occurs via either protein breakdown or protein adsorption to glass. Stress conditions such as heating and shaking promote aggregation and protein loss.

INCOMPATIBILITY: Avoid proteases.

SAFETY/TOXICITY: Clinical trials are in progress in AIDS and oncology (GI and Roche). In mice and primates repetitive daily dosing with ≥50 μg/kg may result in anemia, leukopenia, hepatotoxicity, skeletal muscle necrosis (seen only in mice), and vascular leak. It has also been shown in some species that repetitive daily dosing of >1 μg/kg results in the same side effects.

ADJUVANT PROPERTIES: Enhances Th1-dependent cell-mediated immune responses, including cytolytic T-lymphocyte responses. Suppresses Th2-dependent humoral immune responses such as IgE responses but may enhance production of Ig isotypes, such as IgG2a in mice, associated with Th1 responses.

- Afonso, L. C. C., *et al.*, 1994, The adjuvant effect of interleukin-12 in a vaccine against *Leishmania major*, *Science* **263**:235–237.
- Gately, M. K., *et al.*, 1994, Administration of recombinant IL-12 to normal mice enhances cytolytic lymphocyte activity and induces production of IFN-γ *in vivo*, *Int. Immunol.* **6**:157–167.
- McKnight, A. J., *et al.*, 1994, Effects of IL-12 on helper T cell-dependent immune responses in vivo, *J. Immunol.* **152**:2172–2179.
- Heath, A., Chapter 28, this volume.
- Dong, P., *et al.*, Chapter 27, this volume.

CONTACTS: Maury K. Gately or Alvin S. Stern, Hoffmann–LaRoche Inc., Nutley, NJ 07110-1199, Ph: 201-235-5720; Fax: 201-235-5279. Also: Stan Wolf, Genetics Institute, Cambridge, MA, Ph: 617-498-8134; Fax: 617-876-1504.

COMPONENT/ADJUVANT NAME: ISCOM(s)™

OTHER NAME(S): Immune stimulating complexes

STRUCTURE: ISCOMs are a complex composed of typically 0.5% Quillaja saponins, 0.1% cholesterol, 0.1% phospholipid, and antigen in PBS. Occasionally, surfactants are used to prepare ISCOMs (such as Mega 10) but are removed from the final formulation before use.

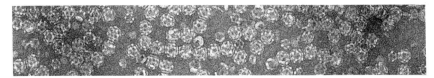

SOURCE: The adjuvant-active components of ISCOMs are derived by aqueous extraction of the bark of *Quillaja saponaria* and are further purified by chromatography. Quil A is a purified form of this. Further chromatographic purification provides components with high adjuvant activity and ISCOM-forming properties (see Iscoprep 7.0.3™).

USES: ISCOMs are powerful immunomodulators. Steric presentation of epitopes, and CTL responses are maximized by the incorporation of immunogens into ISCOMs. Iscotec holds patents covering the use of ISCOMs (ISCOM Basic, EPC 83850273; MATRIX, EPC 89911115.7).

APPEARANCE: ISCOMs form a clear product in solution.

MOLECULAR WEIGHT: A selection of components with various molecular weights: cholesterol, 386.7; Quil A, ~2000; DMPC, 677.9.

RECOMMENDED STORAGE: Store ISCOMs at conditions compatible with the incorporated antigen(s). In general, storage in physiological buffers 4–8°C or may be stored at –70°C.

CHEMICAL/PHYSICAL PROPERTIES: ISCOMs are stable complexes which show good suspendability (>100 mg/mL) in buffer.

INCOMPATIBILITY: Avoid exposure to alkaline pH > 8.0.

SAFETY/TOXICITY: Studies in progress have shown no adverse effects in several animal species. ISCOMs have not shown hemolytic activity at normally administered dose levels.

ADJUVANT PROPERTIES: The ISCOM is an antigen-presenting structure and has been studied for a number of antigens. ISCOMs generate long-lasting biologically functional antibody response, even in the presence of maternal antibodies. Protective immunity and a functional cell-mediated immune response, including class I-restricted CTLs, have been reported in several systems. ISCOMs have generally been administered subcutaneously or intramuscularly but nonparenteral administrations (intranasal and oral) have also proven to be effective.

- Morein, B., *et al.*, 1984, Iscom, a novel structure for antigenic presentation of membrane proteins from enveloped viruses, *Nature* **308**:457.
- Classen, I., and Osterhaus, A., 1992, The iscom structure as an immune enhancing moiety: Experiences in viral systems, *Res. Immunol.* **143**:531–541.
- Hoglund, S., *et al.*, 1989, Iscoms and immunostimulation with viral antigens, in: *Subcellular Biochemistry* (J. R. Harris, ed.), Plenum Press, New York, p. 39.
- Rimmelzwaan, G. F., and Osterhaus, A. D. M. E., Chapter 23, this volume.

CONTACT(S): ISCOTEC AB, Box 7418, S-10391 Stockholm, Sweden, Ph: 46-8-6797810; Fax: 46-18-674376. Also: Bror Morein, National Veterinary Institute, Uppsala, Sweden, Ph: 46-18-174571; Fax: 46-18-504-603.

COMPONENT/ADJUVANT NAME: Iscoprep 7.0.3™

OTHER NAME(S): None

STRUCTURE: Complex of saponin derivatives.

SOURCE: Purified by aqueous extraction of the bark of *Quillaja saponaria* and further purified by chromatography to produce Iscoprep 7.0.3™, a carefully selected mixture of saponin components with adjuvant activity and ISCOM-forming capacity.

USES: Iscoprep 7.0.3™ is used to produce ISCOMs.

APPEARANCE: Iscoprep 7.0.3™ is a light tan to white lyophilized powder.

MOLECULAR WEIGHT: Iscoprep 7.0.3™ is a selection of components with various molecular weights around 1800 to 2200.

RECOMMENDED STORAGE: Store powder at 4–8 °C in the dark, solutions at –20 °C.

CHEMICAL/PHYSICAL PROPERTIES: The mixture of saponin components in Iscoprep 7.0.3™ binds to cholesterol and phospholipid to form ISCOMs. ISCOMs are stable complexes made up of amphiphilic molecules.

INCOMPATIBILITY: Avoid exposure to alkaline pH >8.

SAFETY/TOXICITY: Studies are in progress. Iscoprep 7.0.3™ does not show hemolytic activity in ISCOMs at normally administered dose levels.

ADJUVANT PROPERTIES: Iscoprep 7.0.3™ is used to formulate ISCOMs. The IS-COM as an antigen-presenting structure and has been studied for a number of antigens. ISCOMs generate long-lasting biologically functional antibody response, even in the presence of maternal antibodies. Protective immunity and a functional cell-mediated immune response, including class I-restricted CTLs, have been reported in several systems. ISCOMs have generally been administered subcutaneously or intramuscularly but nonparenteral administrations (intranasal and oral) have also proven to be effective.

- Morein, B., *et al.*, 1984, Iscom, a novel structure for antigenic presentation of membrane proteins from enveloped viruses, *Nature* **308**:457.
- Classen, I., and Osterhaus, A., 1992, The iscom structure as an immune enhancing moiety: Experiences in viral systems, *Res. Immunol.* **143**:531–541.
- Hoglund, S., *et al.*, 1989, Iscoms and immunostimulation with viral antigens, in: *Subcellular Biochemistry* (J. R. Harris, ed.), Plenum Press, New York, p. 39.
- Rimmelzwaan, G. F., and Osterhaus, A. D. M. E., Chapter 23, this volume.

CONTACT(S): ISCOTEC AB, Box 7418, S-10391 Stockholm, Sweden, Ph: 46-8-6797810; Fax: 46-18-674376.

COMPONENT/ADJUVANT NAME: Liposomes

OTHER NAME(S): Liposomes (L) containing protein or Th-cell and/or B-cell peptides, or microbes with or without co-entrapped interleukin-2, BisHOP or DOTMA (see below). A, [L (Antigen)]; B, [L (IL-2 or DOTMA or BisHOP + Antigen)]; C, [L (Antigen)-mannose]; D, [L (Th-cell and B-cell epitopes)]; E, [L (microbes)].

STRUCTURE(S): A: Multilamellar liposomes prepared by the dehydration–rehydration method (average diameter 600–800 nm) composed of egg phosphatidylcholine (PC) or distearoyl phosphatidylcholine (DSPC) and equimolar cholesterol and containing antigens such as tetanus toxoid and synthetic Th-cell peptides. B: As in A with IL-2 (10^3–10^4 Cetus units) co-entrapped with the antigen in the aqueous phase or with 1,2-bis (hexadecylcycloxy)-3-trimethylaminopropane-HCL (BisHOP) or N-(2,3-dioleyloxy)-N,N,N-triethyl-ammonium (DOTMA) incorporated into the lipid phase of liposomes (0.8:1.0:0.2 molar ratio for PC or DSPC, cholesterol and DOTMA or BisHOP). C, as in A with mannosylated albumin covalently coupled to the surface of antigen-containing liposomes. D: As in A with Th-cell and B-cell peptides co-entrapped in the aqueous phase. E: Giant liposomes (average diameter 5–9 μm) prepared as in A or by a solvent-spherule evaporation method, composed of PC or DSPC, cholesterol, triolein (TO), and phosphatidylglycerol (PG) (4:4:1:2 molar ratio) and containing killed or live *Bacillus subtilis* or killed bacille Calmette-Guérin (BCG) with or without co-entrapped tetanus toxoid.

SOURCE: PC, DSPC, and PG in pure form from Lipid Products, Nuthill, Surrey, U.K.; TO in pure form from Sigma Chemical Co., Poole, Dorset, U.K.; recombinant interleukin-2 (des-Ala$_1$-Ser$_{125}$ mutein; 3×10^6 Cetus units/mg) obtained from Cetus Corporation, Emeryville, CA; BisHOP and DOTMA obtained from Syntex Research, Palo Alto, CA.

APPEARANCE: White, opalescent colloidal suspensions (A–E).

MOLECULAR WEIGHT: Equal to the sum of the molecular weights of the components used in each of the formulations. The molecular weight of antigen will vary according to its type.

RECOMMENDED STORAGE: Store formulations at 4 °C when in liquid form. Freeze-dried formulations stored at 4 or –20°C. Liquid formulations stable (in terms of entrapped antigen release) for at least 1 year when sterile. Precipitated liposomes made into suspended by light vortexing.

CHEMICAL/PHYSICAL PROPERTIES: Liposomes are stable at a pH range of 1–10; however, neutral pH is recommended when cytokines and certain antigens are present. Lipid components of liposomes are soluble in chloroform and are stable for at least 1 year at –20°C.

INCOMPATIBILITY: Formulations unstable in the presence of detergents (e.g., Triton X-100).

SAFETY/TOXICITY: Liposomes as such composed of PC and cholesterol have been administered to humans in numerous clinical trials with no adverse effects. None of the formulations (A–E) have been tested in humans.

IMMUNOLOGICAL ADJUVANT AND VACCINE CARRIER PROPERTIES: A, potentiation of immune responses (IgG1, IgG2a, IgG2b, or IgG3) to protein and peptide antigens; choice of phospholipid depends on antigen; a high mass ratio of phospholipid to antigen (e.g., 10^3) optimizes immune responses. B, IL-2, DOTMA, and BisHOP potentiate immune responses to antigens further, acting as co-adjuvants. C, targets liposomes to macrophages with immune responses being greater than with conventional liposomes. D, liposomes act as carrier of Th-cell peptide antigen which provides help for co-entrapped B-cell antigen to overcome genetic restriction and induce immunological memory. E, liposomes may act as carriers of attenuated or live microbial vaccines to deliver microbes and co-entrapped soluble antigens or cytokines simultaneously to antigen-presenting cells or to protect entrapped vaccines from interaction with maternal antibodies or antibodies to vaccine impurities in preimmunized subjects.

- Gregoriadis, G., 1990, Immunological adjuvants: A role for liposomes, *Immunol. Today* **11**:89–97.
- Davis, D., and Gregoriadis, G., 1987, Liposomes as adjuvants with immunopurified tetanus toxoid: Influence of liposomal characteristics, *Immunology* **61**:229–234.
- Gregoriadis, G., *et al.*, 1987, Liposomes as immunological adjuvants: Antigen incorporation studies, *Vaccine* **5**:143–149.
- Tan, L., and Gregoriadis, G., 1989, The effect of interleukin-2 on the immunoadjuvant action of liposomes, *Biochem. Soc. Trans.* **17**:693–694.
- Garcon, N., *et al.*, 1988, Targeted immunoadjuvant action of tetanus toxoid-containing liposomes coated with mannosylated albumin, *Immunology* **64**:743–745.
- Kahl, K. L., *et al.*, 1989, Vaccination against murine cutaneous leishmaniasis using L. Major antigen/liposomes: Optimization and assessment of the requirement for intravenous immunization, *J. Immunol.* **142**:4441–4449.
- Antimisiaris, S., *et al.*, 1993, Liposomes as vaccine carriers: Incorporation of soluble and particulate antigens in giant vesicles, *J. Immunol. Methods* **166**:271–280.
- Gregoriadis, G., *et al.*, 1993, Liposome-entrapped T-cell peptide provides help for co-entrapped B-cell peptide to overcome genetic restriction in mice and induce immunological memory, *Immunology* **80**:535–540.

CONTACT(S): Professor Gregory Gregoriadis, Centre for Drug Delivery Research, School of Pharmacy, University of London, 29-39 Brunswick Square, London WC1N 1AX, U.K., Ph:, +44-171-7535822; Phone/Fax +44-171-7535820.

COMPONENT/ADJUVANT NAME: Loxoribine
OTHER NAME(S): 7-Allyl-8-oxoguanosine
STRUCTURE:

SOURCE: Synthetic (U.S. Patent 5,011,828).

USES: Primary adjuvant for antibody responses to a wide variety of antigen types in a variety of species. Typical dose in mice: 1–3 mg/25 g mouse. In humans: 10 mg/kg has been used safely. Optimal dose unknown.

APPEARANCE: White, odorless crystalline powder.

MOLECULAR WEIGHT: 339

RECOMMENDED STORAGE: Store solid under low humidity at −20°C. Stable in solution for at least 4 weeks; found to be very stable at pH 8–11.

CHEMICAL/PHYSICAL PROPERTIES: Hydrophobic, lipophilic molecule. Soluble in DMSO, DMF, and aqueous media at alkaline pH. Mp = 234°C, pKa = 8.92.

INCOMPATIBILITY: Precipitates at low pH.

SAFETY/TOXICITY: Phase I clinical trial complete, without toxicity greater than grade I. No reported toxicity in a lower dose, Phase I/II clinical trial. Main side effects noted resemble those of interferon and are transient.

ADJUVANT PROPERTIES: Augmentation of CTL-mediated, NK cell-mediated, macrophage-mediated, and LAK cell-mediated cytotoxicity. Inducer of cytokines: IFN$\alpha/\beta/\gamma$, TNFα, TNFβ, IL-1α, IL-6. Upregulates humoral immune responses under conditions of normal immunity as well as in immunodeficiency. Acts as a surrogate Th signal.

- Goodman, M. G., and Weigle, W. O., 1985, Enhancement of the human antibody response by C8-substituted guanine ribonucleosides in synergy with interleukin 2, *J. Immunol.* **135**:3284–3288.
- Feldbush, T. L., and Ballas, Z. K., 1985, Lymphokine-like activity of 8-mercaptoguanosine: Induction of T and B cell differentiation, *J. Immunol.* **134**:3204–3211.
- Goodman, M. G., *et al.*, 1991, C-kinase independent restoration of specific immune responsiveness in common variable immunodeficiency, *Clin. Immunol. Immunopathol.* **59**:26–36.
- Goodman, M. G., and Weigle, W. O., 1983, T cell-replacing activity of C8-derivatized guanine ribonucleosides, *J. Immunol.* **130**:2042–2045.
- Pope, B. L., *et al.*, 1993, Loxoribine (7-allyl-8-oxoguanosine) activates natural killer cells and primes cytolytic precursor cells for activation by IL-2, *J. Immunol.* **151**:3007–3017.
- Goodman, M., Chapter 25, this volume.

CONTACT(S): Dr. Michael G. Goodman, Department of Immunology, The Scripps Research Institute, La Jolla, CA 92037, Ph: 619-554-8131; Fax: 619-554-6705.

COMPONENT/ADJUVANT NAME: LT-OA or LT Oral Adjuvant

OTHER NAME(S): *E. coli* labile enterotoxin protoxin

STRUCTURE: Polypeptide consisting of one 28-kDa A subunit (toxic component consisting of the A_1 chain of 21 kDa and the A_2 chain of 7 kDa) and five 11.6-kDa B subunits (binding component).

- Sixma, T. K., *et al.*, 1991, Crystal structure of a cholera toxin-related heat-labile enterotoxin from *E. coli*, *Nature* **351**:371–377.

Sequence of *E. coli* heat-labile enterotoxin subunit A:

NGDKLYRADSRPPDEIKRSGGLMPRGHNEYFDRGTQMNINLYDHARGTQTGF
VRYDDGYVSTSLSLRSAHLAGQSILSGYSTYYIYVIATAPNMFNVNDVLGVYS
PHPYEQEVSALGGIPYSQIYGWYRVNFGVIDERLHRNREYRDRYYRNLNIAPA
EDGYRLAGFPPDHQAWREEPWIHHAPQGCGDSSRTITGDTCNEETQNLSTIYL
RKYQSKVKRQIFSDYQSEVDIYNRIRNEL*
Sequence of *E. coli* heat-labile enterotoxin subunit B:
APQSITELCSEYRNTQIYTINDKILSYTESMAGKREMVIITFKSGATFQVEVPGS
QHIDSQKKAIERMKDTLRITYLTETKIDKLCVWNNKTPNSIAAISMEN*

SOURCE: Toxigenic *Escherichia coli*, either partially purified or recombinant, extracted under conditions that inhibit proteolysis and thus inhibit conversion to active toxin. Commercially available from Berna Products Corp., Coral Gables, FL.

USES: Sole active component of orally administered adjuvant.

APPEARANCE: White, odorless powder.

MOLECULAR WEIGHT: 84,000 to 94,000, depending on the assay method.

RECOMMENDED STORAGE: Store lyophilized solid at –20°C. Solutions of LT-OA at 1 mg/mL at pH 7.5 in nonphosphate buffers may be stored at 5°C for 1–2 years.

CHEMICAL/PHYSICAL PROPERTIES: Amphiphilic molecule with low solubility in water at neutral pH. pI 8.0. Not stable in phosphate buffers. Oxidizes on long-term storage to form intramolecular disulfide bonds.

INCOMPATIBILITY: Avoid proteases. Incompatible with phosphate buffer.

SAFETY/TOXICITY: Nontoxic at adjuvant-active doses in mouse, rabbit, and monkey. Human Phase I clinical trials began September, 1994.

- Majde, J. A., *et al.*, 1994, *Escherichia coli* heat-labile enterotoxin, an oral adjuvant for protection against mucosal pathogens, in: *Adjuvants—Theory and Practical Applications* (D. Stewart-Tull, ed.), Wiley, New York, pp. 337–351.

ADJUVANT PROPERTIES: For inducing mucosal and systemic immunity [both humoral (including IgA and IgG2a isotypes) and cell-mediated] to killed microorganism or peptide antigens mixed with it in neutral non-phosphate-buffered saline, with/without sodium bicarbonate.

- Clements, J. D., *et al.*, 1988, Adjuvant activity of *Escherichia coli* heat-labile enterotoxin and effect on the induction of oral tolerance in mice to unrelated protein antigens, *Vaccine* **6**:269–277.
- Walker, R. I., and Clements, J. D., 1993, Use of the heat labile toxin of enterotoxigenic *Escherichia coli* to facilitate mucosal immunization, *Vaccine Res.* **2**:1–10.
- Rollwagen, F. M., *et al.*, 1993, Killed *Campylobacter* elicits immune response and protection when administered with an oral adjuvant, *Vaccine* **11**:1316–1319.
- Baqar, S., *et al.*, 1995, Safety and immunogenicity of a prototype oral whole cell killed *Campylobacter* vaccine administered with a mucosal adjuvant in non-human primates, *Vaccine* (in press).

CONTACT(S): Dr. Jeannine A. Majde, Program Manager, Biomedical Science and Technology, Office of Naval Research, Arlington, VA 22217-5660, Ph: 703-696-4055; Fax: 703-696-1212; E-mail: majdej@onrhq.onr.navy.mil.

COMPONENT/ADJUVANT NAME: MF59

OTHER NAME(S): None

STRUCTURE: Squalene/water emulsion. Composition: 43 mg/mL squalene, 2.5 mg/mL polyoxyethylene sorbitan monooleate (Polysorbate 80), 2.4 mg/mL sorbitan trioleate (Span 85).

$HO(C_2H_4O)_w$ $(OC_2H_4)_xOH$

$CH(OC_2H_4)_yOH$
$CH_2(OC_2H_4)_zCOOC_{17}H_{33}$

Polysorbate 80

Span 85

HO

Squalene

SOURCE: The Biocine Company, Emeryville, CA.

USES: Intramuscular adjuvant.

APPEARANCE: White liquid.

MOLECULAR WEIGHT: Not applicable.

RECOMMENDED STORAGE: 2–8°C, inert gas overlay.

CHEMICAL/PHYSICAL PROPERTIES: Low-viscosity aqueous emulsion, biodegradable. Particle size 200–300 nm.

INCOMPATIBILITY: Unstable on freezing. Exposure to pH extremes results in hydrolysis of detergent components. Components are susceptible to oxidation in presence of O_2, peroxide, metals.

SAFETY/TOXICITY: Minor reactogenicity on intramuscular injection of humans in combination with HSV or HIV antigens.

ADJUVANT PROPERTIES: Intramuscular injection in combination with a variety of subunit antigens results in elevated humoral response, increased T cell proliferation, and presence of cytotoxic lymphocytes.

- Sanchez-Pestador, L., *et al.*, 1988, The effect of adjuvants on the efficacy of a recombinant herpes simplex glycoprotein vaccine, *J. Immunol.* **141**:1720–1727.
- Van Nest, G. A., *et al.*, 1992, Advanced adjuvant formulations for use with recombinant subunit vaccines, in: *Vaccines 92* (F. Brown, R. M. Chanock, H. S. Ginsberg, and R. A. Lerner, eds.), Cold Spring Harbor Press, Cold Spring Harbor, NY, p. 57.
- Ott, G., *et al.*, Chapter 10, this volume.

CONTACT(S): Dr. Gary Van Nest, Chiron Corporation, Emeryville, CA, Ph: 510-601-2965; Dr. Gary Ott, Chiron Corporation, Ph: 510-601-2964; Fax: 510-601-2586.

COMPONENT/ADJUVANT NAME: MONTANIDE ® ISA 51

OTHER NAME(S): Purified IFA; incomplete Freund's adjuvant

STRUCTURE: Mannide oleate (mostly mannide monooleate, esters of mannitol and oleic acids—an example is shown below) (MONTANIDE 80) in mineral oil solution (DRAKEOL 6VR).

SOURCE: Manufactured by SEPPIC.

USES: "Ready to use" oil for water-in-oil emulsion adjuvants. For human use. Final injection product usually 50% MONTANIDE ISA 51 (0.5–1 mL injection volume).

APPEARANCE: Limpid clear yellow liquid.

RECOMMENDED STORAGE: Store at 4°C or room temperature under nitrogen. Stable at room temperature for at least 1 year. Store at physiological pH.

CHEMICAL/PHYSICAL PROPERTIES: Acid value: 0.5 maximum; saponification value: between 16 and 20; hydroxyl value: between 9 and 13; peroxide value: 2 maximum; iodine value: between 5 and 9; water content: 0.5 maximum; refractive index at 25°C: between 1.455 and 1.465; density (at 20°C): about 0.85; viscosity (at 20°C): about 50 mPas. Water insoluble. DRAKEOL 6VR is a special pharmaceutical-grade mineral oil that contains paraffin oil with linear and ramified hydrocarbons in the range C_{14}–C_{26} (mean C_{24}).

INCOMPATIBILITY: Avoid strong bases.

SAFETY/TOXICITY: LD_{50} (mice) by i.p. route, > 22 g/kg. LD_{50} (rats) by oral route, > 2 g/kg. Nonirritating (skin) in rabbits, slight irritancy (ocular) in rabbits. No abnormal toxicity in mice or guinea pigs. Acute toxicity by i.m. injection (rats), > 5 g/kg. Pyrogen-free. Ames and mouse micronucleus test (Montanide 80)—no effect.

ADJUVANT PROPERTIES: Addition of MONTANIDE ISA 51 induces humoral and cell-mediated immunity with various antigens.

- Audibert, F. M., and Lise, L. D., 1993, Adjuvant: Current status, clinical perspectives and future prospects, *Immunol. Today* **14**:281–284.
- Ganne, V., *et al.*, 1994, Enhancement of the efficacy of a replication-defective adenovirus vectored pseudorabies vaccine by the addition of oil adjuvants, *Vaccine* (in press).

CONTACT(S): SEPPIC, 75321 Paris Cedex 07, France, Ph: 331 40 62 57 30; Fax: 331 40 62 52 53. See also monograph on Freund's incomplete adjuvant.

COMPONENT/ADJUVANT NAME: MONTANIDE ® ISA 720

OTHER NAME(S): Metabolizable oil adjuvant

STRUCTURE: A highly refined emulsifier from the mannide monooleate family (an example of mannide monooleate is shown below) in a natural metabolizable oil solution. The exact nature of the emulsifier and the metabolizable in MONTANIDE ISA 720 is proprietary, but can be disclosed under specific agreement with SEPPIC.

SOURCE: Manufactured by SEPPIC.

USES: "Ready to use" oil for water-in-oil emulsion adjuvants. Final injection product usually 70% Montanide ISA 720 (0.5–1 mL injection volume).

APPEARANCE: Yellow, odorless liquid.

RECOMMENDED STORAGE: Store at 4°C or room temperature under nitrogen. Stable at room temperature for at least 1 year. Store at physiological pH.

CHEMICAL/PHYSICAL PROPERTIES: Acid value 0.5 maximum; saponification value: between 17 and 21; hydroxyl value: between 9 and 12; peroxide value: 5 maximum; iodine value: between 320 and 350; water content: 0.5 maximum; refractive index (at 25°C) about 1.492; density (at 20°C): about 0.86; viscosity (at 20°C): about 15 mPas. Water insoluble. DRAKEOL 6VR is a special pharmaceutical-grade mineral oil that contains paraffin oil with linear and ramified hydrocarbons in the range C_{14}–C_{26} (mean C_{24}).

INCOMPATIBILITY: None found.

SAFETY/TOXICITY: LD_{50} (mice) by i.p. route, > 22 g/kg. LD_{50} (rats) by oral route, > 2 g/kg. Nonirritating (skin) in rabbits, slight irritancy (ocular) in rabbits. No abnormal toxicity in mice or guinea pigs. Acute toxicity by i.m. injection (rats), > 5 g/kg. Pyrogen-free. Ames and mouse micronucleus test (Montanide 80)—no effect.

ADJUVANT PROPERTIES: Addition of MONTANIDE ISA 720 induces humoral and cell-mediated immunity with various antigens.

- Jones, W. R., et al., 1988, Phase I clinical trial of World Health Organization birth control vaccine, *Lancet* 1:1295–1298.
- Jones, G. L., et al., 1990, Peptide vaccines derived from a malarial surface antigen: Effects of dose and adjuvants on immunogenicity, *Immunol. Lett.* **24**:253–260.
- Elliot, S., et al., 1994, Human compatible adjuvant induces protective cytotoxic T lymphocytes with peptide vaccine, Proceedings in CHI Vaccines—New Technologies and Applications, Alexandria, VA, March 21–23.

CONTACT(S): SEPPIC, 75321 Paris Cedex 07, France, Ph: 331 40 62 57 30; Fax: 331 40 62 52 53.

COMPONENT/ADJUVANT NAME: MPL®

OTHER NAME(S): 3-*O*-desacyl-4'-monophosphoryl lipid A; 3D-MLA

STRUCTURE: MPL® is composed of a series of 4'-monophosphoryl lipid A species that vary in the extent and position of fatty acid substitution. The hexaacyl structure shown below is the most highly acylated and most abundant component in MPL®. Species with five and four fatty acids are also present. All structures contribute to the adjuvant activity of MPL®.

SOURCE: Derived from the lipopolysaccharide (LPS) of *Salmonella minnesota* R595. Obtained by treatment of LPS with mild acid and base hydrolytic conditions, and chromatographic purification of the resulting 3D-MLA.

USES: As a primary adjuvant in adjuvant formulations. Adjuvant activity is manifested either alone in aqueous solution with antigen, or in combination with particulate vehicles (e.g., oil-in-water emulsions). Activity may be enhanced by use of vehicle that enforces close association with antigen.

APPEARANCE: Colorless, odorless white powder.

MOLECULAR WEIGHT: 1540–1670 (average).

RECOMMENDED STORAGE: Indefinite stability as lyophilized powder (in excess of 5 years if stored at 5°C). Available data indicate stability in aqueous solution is maximum between pH 5 and 6. An aqueous formulation was stable (<10% loss of most highly acylated component) for the equivalent of 2–3 years in an accelerated stability study.

CHEMICAL/PHYSICAL PROPERTIES: Composed of closely related 4'-monophosphoryl lipid A species that vary only in terms of fatty acid content (see above). All species in MPL® are highly amphiphilic. MPL® is probably aggregated in aqueous solution at concentrations above ~1 nM. Micelles or liposomes are formed depending on excipients and conditions of formulation. Solubility in water is greatest above pH 7, and is diminished below pH 5. Surfactants enhance solubility in water. Soluble in oils (e.g., squalene).

INCOMPATIBILITY: Solubility is diminished significantly in the presence of divalent metal cations.

SAFETY/TOXICITY: Has been studied in human Phase I/II clinical trials. Results to date indicate that MPL® is well tolerated at doses that exhibit beneficial immunostimulating activities. MPL® is pyrogenic at high doses.

- Rudbach, J. A., *et al.*, 1994, Prophylactic use of monophosphoryl lipid A in patients at risk for sepsis, in: *Bacterial Endotoxins: Basic Science to Anti-Sepsis Strategies-Proceedings of the International Conference on Endotoxins IV* (J. Levin, A. Sturk, T. Van Der Poll, and S. J. H. Van Deventer, eds.), Wiley, New York (in press).
- Thoelen, S., *et al.*, 1993, Immunogenicity of a recombinant hepatitis B vaccine with monophosphoryl lipid A administered following various two-dose schedules, Abstr. 340, 33rd Intersci. Conf. Antimicrob. Agents Chemother., p. 182.
- Van Damme, P., *et al.*, 1993, Safety, humoral and cellular immunity of a recombinant hepatitis B vaccine with monophosphoryl lipid A in healthy volunteers, Abstr. 667, 33rd Intersci. Conf. Antimicrob. Agents Chemother., p. 241.

ADJUVANT PROPERTIES: Numerous references have documented the adjuvant activity of MPL®.

- Ulrich, J. T., *et al.*, 1991, The adjuvant activity of monophosphoryl lipid A, in: *Topics in Vaccine Adjuvant Research* (D. R. Spriggs, and W. C. Koff, eds.), CRC Press, Boca Raton, pp. 133–143.
- Ivins, B. E., *et al.*, 1992, Immunization against anthrax with *Bacillus anthracis* protective antigen combined with adjuvants, *Infect. Immun.* **60**:662–668.
- Gustafson, G. L., and Rhodes, M. J., 1992, Bacterial cell wall products as adjuvants: Early interferon gamma as a marker for adjuvants that enhance protective immunity, *Res. Immunol.* **143**:483–488.
- Baker, P. J., 1990, Regulation of magnitude of antibody response to bacterial polysaccharide antigens by thymus-derived lymphocytes, *Infect. Immun.* **58**:3465–3468.
- Ulrich, J. T., and Myers, K. R., Chapter 21, this volume.

CONTACT(S): J. T. Ulrich/K. R. Myers, Ribi ImmunoChem Research, Inc., Hamilton, MT 59840, Ph: 406-363-6214; Fax: 406-363-6129; E-mail: 74043.1020@compuserve.com.

COMPONENT/ADJUVANT NAME: MTP-PE

OTHER NAME(S): N-acetyl-L-alanyl-D-isoglutaminyl-L-alanine-2-(1,2-dipalmitoyl-sn-glycero-3-(hydroxy-phosphoryloxy)) ethylamide, mono sodium salt.

STRUCTURE: $C_{59}H_{108}N_6O_{19}PNa \cdot 3\ H_2O$

SOURCE: Chemical synthesis by Ciba Geigy Ltd., Basel, Switzerland.

USES: Immunomodulator. Optionally a part of MF59.

APPEARANCE: White powder.

MOLECULAR WEIGHT: 1313.55

RECOMMENDED STORAGE: 2–8°C.

CHEMICAL/PHYSICAL PROPERTIES: Amphiphilic properties. Solubility in water 1%. Biodegradable.

INCOMPATIBILITY: Hydrolysis at high or low pH values.

SAFETY/TOXICITY: MTP-PE has been injected intravenously in a liposomal formulation in cancer patients and was safe up to 6 mg/m^2. Addition of MTP-PE to the MF59 adjuvant results in increased rates of local and systemic reactions over those seen in the absence of the muramyl peptide. No evidence of uveitis was seen in any patients receiving MF59 with MTP-PE.

- Wintsh, J., *et al.*, 1991, Safety and immunogenicity of a genetically engineered human immunodeficiency virus vaccine, *J. Infect. Dis.* **163**:219.

ADJUVANT PROPERTIES: In seronegative populations, humoral and cellular responses to HSV and HIV vaccine were not enhanced when MTP-PE was included in MF59. The addition of MTP-PE to the MF59-based HIV vaccine in HIV-seropositive individuals resulted in a marked increase in HIV antigen lymphocyte proliferation.

- Sanchez-Pestador, L., *et al.*, 1988, The effect of adjuvants on the efficacy of a recombinant herpes simplex glycoprotein vaccine, *J. Immunol.* **141**:1720–1727.
- Van Nest, G. A., *et al.*, 1992, Advanced adjuvant formulations for use with recombinant subunit vaccines, in: *Vaccines 92* (F. Brown, R. M. Chanock, H. S. Ginsberg, and R. A. Lerner, eds.), Cold Spring Harbor Press, Cold Spring Harbor, NY, p. 57.
- Ott, G., *et al.*, Chapter 10, this volume.

CONTACT(S): Dr. Peter van Hoogevest, Ciba Geigy Ltd., CH-4002 Basel, Switzerland, Ph: 41-61-6965651; Fax: 41-61-696-6981. Also: Gary Van Nest, Chiron Corp., Emeryville, CA, Ph: 510-601-2965; Fax: 510-601-2586.

COMPONENT/ADJUVANT NAME: MTP-PE Liposomes

OTHER NAME(S): MTP-PE antigen-presenting liposomes

STRUCTURE: $C_{59}H_{108}N_6O_{19}PNa \cdot 3H_2O$ (MTP)

SOURCE: Chemical synthesis.

- Phillip, N. C., *et al.*, 1985, Activation of alveolar macrophage tumoricidial activity and eradication of experimental metastases by freeze-dried liposomes containing a new lipophilic muramyl dipeptide derivative, *Cancer Res.* **45**:128–134.

USES: Primary adjuvant, liposome-formulated sustained release form, co-emulsified with antigen and lipids.

APPEARANCE: Lyophilized white powder.

MOLECULAR WEIGHT: MTP-PE, 1313.55

RECOMMENDED STORAGE: Store at 4°C for both the parent lyophilized compound and the liposome-formulated MTP-PE.

CHEMICAL/PHYSICAL PROPERTIES: Amphipathic molecule with good water solubility (1–2 mg/mL). It may form as mixed micelle suspension at high concentration. MTP-PE liposomes are multilamellar in nature, ranging from 1 to 5 μm in diameter.

INCOMPATIBILITY: Unknown.

SAFETY/TOXICITY: Liposome-formulated MTP-PE is currently under Phase II/III trials. Some systemic toxicity with MTP-PE given with gp120-based HIV-1 vaccines.

ADJUVANT PROPERTIES:

- Ho, R. J. Y., *et al.*, 1989, Antigen presenting liposomes are effective in treatment of recurrent herpes simplex genitalis in guinea pigs, *J. Virol.* **63**:2951–2958.
- Ho, R. J. Y., *et al.*, 1994, Disposition of antigen-presenting liposomes in vivo: Effect on presentation of HSV antigen rgD, *Vaccine* **12**:235–242.
- Bui, T., *et al.*, 1994, Effect of MTP-PE liposomes and IL-7 on induction of antibody and cell-mediated immune responses to a recombinant HIV envelope protein, *J. AIDS* **7**:799–806.

CONTACT(S): Rodney J. Y. Ho, Department of Pharmaceutics, University of Washington, Seattle, WA 98195, Ph: 206-543-9434; Fax: 206-543-3204. Also: Dr. Peter van Hoogevest, Ciba Geigy Ltd., CH-4002 Basel, Switzerland, Ph: 41-61-6965651; Fax: 41-61-696-6981.

COMPONENT/ADJUVANT NAME: Murametide

OTHER NAME(S): NAc-Mur-L-Ala-D-Gln-OCH3

STRUCTURE:

SOURCE: Synthesis.

USES: Administered in water-in-oil emulsion as adjuvant of humoral and cell-mediated immunity.

APPEARANCE: White powder.

MOLECULAR WEIGHT: 506.5

RECOMMENDED STORAGE: Stored as a powder at 4°C. Protect from light and humidity. Stable for more than 5 years.

CHEMICAL/PHYSICAL PROPERTIES: Hydrophilic molecule. Freely soluble in water. The solution is clear, colorless, and odorless, store at pH 5 to 7.5.

INCOMPATIBILITY: Avoid strong bases.

SAFETY/TOXICITY: Acute, subacute, and chronic toxicity studies in rats and monkeys allow administration in clinical studies of 1 to 4 s.c. injections at 2–4 week intervals at doses of 35–100 μg/kg. Pharmacokinetics was studied in rats and dogs. A Phase I clinical trial was completed that showed no toxicity at dosages up to 150 μg/kg.

ADJUVANT PROPERTIES: When administered in saline, Murametide is nonpyrogenic, induces granulocytosis, and enhances the humoral response. Murametide displays the same profile of adjuvant activity as MDP and has been chosen for development because of its favorable therapeutic ratio. When administered in 50% water-in-oil emulsion, it mimics the activity of Freund's complete adjuvant without its side effects. U.S. Patent #4,693,998.

- Audibert, F., *et al.*, 1985, Muramyl peptides as immunopharmacological response modifiers, in: *Biological Response Modifiers* (P. F. Torrence, ed.), Academic Press, New York, pp. 307–337.

CONTACT(S): Professor Louis Chedid, Dr. Françoise Audibert, VACSYN S.A., 75015 Paris, France, Ph: 331-40-60-75-92; Fax: 331-40-60-75-73.

COMPONENT/ADJUVANT NAME: Murapalmitine

OTHER NAME(S): NAc-Mur-L-Thr-D-isoGln-sn-glycerol dipalmitoyl

STRUCTURE:

SOURCE: Synthesis.

USES: Administered in water-in-oil emulsion as adjuvant of humoral and cell-mediated responses.

APPEARANCE: White powder.

MOLECULAR WEIGHT: 1072

RECOMMENDED STORAGE: Stored as a powder at 4°C. Protect from light and humidity.

CHEMICAL/PHYSICAL PROPERTIES: Lipophilic molecules giving homogeneous suspensions in mineral oil.

INCOMPATIBILITY: Avoid strong bases.

SAFETY/TOXICITY: Acute toxicity in mice, rats, rabbits, and guinea pigs satisfactorily completed. Preliminary subacute toxicity in dogs satisfactorily completed. Further toxicology studies in progress.

ADJUVANT PROPERTIES: Lipophilic MDPs are more active than hydrophilic MDPs. In saline, they are strong immunoadjuvants of humoral immunity and weaker adjuvants of cell-mediated immunity. In 50% w/o emulsions, they are strong immunoadjuvants and mimic Freund's complete activity. In contrast with other molecules of this subgroup, Murapalmitine is devoid of side effects and thus has been chosen for further development. U.S. Patents #4,939,122 and 5,210,072.

- Audibert, F., *et al.*, 1985, Muramyl peptides as immunopharmacological response modifiers, in: *Biological Response Modifiers* (P. F. Torrence, ed.), Academic Press, New York, pp. 307–337.

CONTACT(S): Professor Louis Chedid, Dr. Françoise Audibert, VACSYN S.A., 75015 Paris, France, Ph: 331-40-60-75-92; Fax: 331-40-60-75-73.

COMPONENT/ADJUVANT NAME: D-Murapalmitine

OTHER NAME(S): NAc-Mur-D-Ala-D-isoGln-sn-glycerol dipalmitoyl

STRUCTURE:

SOURCE: Synthesis.

USES: Administered in water-in-oil emulsion as adjuvant of humoral and cell-mediated immunity. To be developed as an adjuvant for vaccines likely to contain autoantigens.

APPEARANCE: White powder.

MOLECULAR WEIGHT: 1056

RECOMMENDED STORAGE: Stored as a powder at 4°C. Protect from light and humidity.

CHEMICAL/PHYSICAL PROPERTIES: Lipophilic molecules giving homogeneous suspensions in mineral oil.

INCOMPATIBILITY: Avoid strong bases.

SAFETY/TOXICITY: This MDP analogue is nonpyrogenic in rabbits and displays no acute toxicity when tested in mice, rats, guinea pigs, and rabbits. Further toxicology studies will be performed.

ADJUVANT PROPERTIES: D-Murapalmitine is a strong adjuvant of humoral and cell-mediated immunity when administered in a 50% mineral oil emulsion. However, in contrast with other MDPs, it does not induce experimental allergic encephalomyelitis (EAE) when administered with myelin basic protein. When given with an antigenic preparation containing hetero and autologous epitopes, it favors the response to the heterologous determinants. U.S. patent #4,939,122, French patent #9,207,126.

• Audibert, F., et al., 1985, Muramyl peptides as immunopharmacological response modifiers, in: *Biological Response Modifiers* (P. F. Torrence, ed.), Academic Press, New York, pp. 307–337.

CONTACT(S): Professor Louis Chedid, Dr. Françoise Audibert, VACSYN S. A., 75015 Paris, France, Ph: 331-40-60-75-92; Fax: 331-40-60-75-73.

COMPONENT/ADJUVANT NAME: NAGO

OTHER NAME(S): Neuraminidase–galactose oxidase

STRUCTURE: NAGO is a mixture of the enzymes neuraminidase and galactose oxidase at a 1:5 ratio in units of activity. The primary amino acid sequences of the two enzymes are appended.

- McPherson, M. J., *et al.*, 1992, Galactose oxidase of *Dactylium dendroides*: Gene cloning and sequence analysis, *J. Biol. Chem.* **267**:8146–8152.
- Galen, J. E., *et al.*, 1992, Role of *Vibrio cholerae* neuraminidase in the function of cholera toxin, *Infect. Immun.* **60**:406–415.

Sequence of neuraminidase (E.C. 3.2.18):

MRFKNVKKTALMLAMFGMATSSNAALFDYNATGDTEFDSPAKQGWMQDNT
NNGSGVLTNADGMPAWLVQGIGGRAQWTYSLSTNQHAQASSFGWRMTTEM
KVLSGGMITNYYANGTQRVLPIISLDSSGNLVVEFEGQTGRTVLATGTAATEYH
KFELVFLPGSNPSASFYFDGKLIRDNIQPTASKQNMIVWGNGSSNTDGVAAYRD
IKFEIQGDVIFRGPDRIPSIVASSVTPGVVTAFAEKRVGGGDPGALSNTNDIITRTS
RDGGITWDTELNLTEQINVSDEFDFSDPRPIYDPSSNTVLVSYARWPTDAAQNG
DRIKPWMPNGIFYSVYDVASGNWQAPIDVTDQVKERSFQIAGWGGSELYRRN
TSLNSQQDWQSNAKIRIVDGAANQIQVADGSRKYVVTLSIDESGGLVANLNGV
SAPIILQSEHAKVHSFHDYELQYSALNHTTTLFVDGQQITTWAGEVSQENNIQF
GNADAQIDGRLHVQKIVLTQQGHNLVEFDAFYLAQQTPEVEKDLEKLGWTKI
KTGNTMSLYGNASVNPGPGHGITLTRQQNISGSQNGRLIYPAIVLDRFFLNVMS
IYSDDGGSNWQTGSTLPIPFRWKSSSILETLEPSEADMVELQNGDLLLTARLDF
NQIVNGVNYSPRQQFLSKDGGITWSLLEANNANVFSNISTGTVDASITRFEQSD
GSHFLLFTNPQGNPAGTNGRQNLGLWFSFDEGVTWKGPIQLVNGASAYSDIYQ
LDSENAIVIVETDNSNMRILRMPITLLKQKLTLSQN

Sequence of galactose oxidase (E.C. 1.1.3.9):

MKHLLTLALCFSSINAVAVTVPHKAVGTGIPEGSLQFLSLRASAPIGSAISRNNW
AVTCDSAQSGNECNKAIDGNKDTFWHTFYGANGDPKPPHTYTIDMKTTQNV
NGLSMLPRQDGNQNGWIGRHEVYLSSDGTNWGSPVASGSWFADSTTKYSNFE
TRPARYVRLVAITEANGQPWTSIAEINVFQASSYTAPQPGLGRWGPTIDLPIVPA
AAAIEPTSGRVLMWSSYRNDAFGGSPGGITLTSSWDPSTGIVSDRTVTVTKHD
MFCPGISMDGNGQIVVTGGNDAKKTSLYDSSSDSWIPGPDMQVARGYQSSAT
MSDGRVFTIGGSWSGGVFEKNGEVYSPSSKTWTSLPNAKVNPMLTADKQGLY
RSDNHAWLFGWKKGSVFQAGPSTAMNWYYTSGSGDVKSAGKRQSNRGVAP
DAMCGNAVMYDAVKGKILTFGGSPDYQDSDATTNAHIITLGEPGTSPNTVFAS
NGLYFARTFHTSVVLPDGSTFITGGQRRGIPFEDSTPVFTPEIYVPEQDTFYKQN
PNSIVRVYHSISLLLPDGRVFNGGGGLCGDCTTNHFDAQIFTPNYLYNSNGNLA
TRPKITRTSTQSVKVGGRITISTDSSISKASLIRYGTATHTVNTDQRRIPLTLTNNG
GNSYSFQVPSDSGVALPGYWMLFVMNSAGVPSVASTIRVTQ

SOURCE: GO is biochemically purified from *Dactylium dendroides*. It has an activity of approximately 800 units per mg of protein and is commercially available from Sigma Chemical Co. (Cat. No. G3385) as a partially purified lyophilized powder containing 25% protein to be reconstituted in buffered saline. NA is biochemically purified from *Vibrio cholerae*. It has an activity of 25 units per μg of protein and is commercially available from Merck Ltd. (BDH Laboratory Supplies), Merck House, Poole, Dorset BH12 1BR, U.K.

USES: Primary adjuvant. A mixture of the two enzymes containing 10 units NA and 50 units GO per mL of aqueous solution and antigen is administered subcutaneously or intramuscularly. It is comparable in effectiveness to Freund's complete adjuvant, but is nonreactogenic. It is especially effective in the induction of CD8 cytotoxic T-cell responses.

APPEARANCE: GO: lyophilized off-white solid. NA: clear, colorless aqueous solution.

MOLECULAR WEIGHT: GO: 68,500. NA: 83,000.

RECOMMENDED STORAGE: Long-term storage: GO at $-20°C$, NA at $4°C$.

CHEMICAL/PHYSICAL PROPERTIES: Biologically active proteins in aqueous media.

INCOMPATIBILITY: Avoid denaturing conditions. Not compatible with alum. Activity reduced in oil emulsions.

SAFETY/TOXICITY: Histopathology studies in mice showed that NAGO is less inflammatory than alum and produced no adverse local or systemic reactions.

ADJUVANT PROPERTIES: NAGO generates cell surface Schiff base-forming aldehydes on antigen-presenting cells and Th cells, thereby amplifying physiologic Schiff base formation that occurs between cell-surface ligands as an essential element in APC:T-cell inductive interaction. It is a potent noninflammatory adjuvant with viral, bacterial, and protozoal subunit vaccines, and is especially effective in the generation of cytotoxic T cells.

- Zheng, B., et al., 1992, Galactose oxidation in the design of immunogenic vaccines, Science **256**:1560–1563.
- Zhong, G., et al., 1993, Immunogenicity evaluation of a lipidic amino acid based synthetic peptide vaccine for Chlamydia trachomatis, J. Immunol. **151**:3728–3736.

CONTACT(S): Dr. John Rhodes, Wellcome Foundation Ltd., Beckenham, Kent BR3 3BS, U.K., Ph: 44-81-639-5336; Fax: 44-81-663-6176.

COMPONENT/ADJUVANT NAME: Nonionic Surfactant Vesicles

OTHER NAME(S): NISV

STRUCTURE: Multilamellar vesicles comprising a mixture of nonionic surfactant (e.g., 1-monopalmitoyl-rac-glycerol), cholesterol, and dicetyl phosphate.

Dicetyl phosphate

Cholesterol   Monopalmitoyl-rac-glyceral

SOURCE: Synthetic/semisynthetic.
- Alexander, J., and Brewer, J. M., 1992, Vaccines containing non-ionic surfactant vesicles, PCT/GB93/00716, priority date 7 April 92.

USES: Used as a primary vaccine adjuvant for entrapped antigen. NISV adjuvant biodegrades in vivo with release of the entrapped antigen. NISV adjuvant induces humoral and cell-mediated immunity and probably functions by targeting the antigen to the macrophage population.

APPEARANCE: Milky, colloidal suspension.

MOLECULAR WEIGHT: 1-Monopalmitoyl glycerol: 329; cholesterol: 386; dicetyl phosphate: 547.

RECOMMENDED STORAGE: Component raw materials should be stored at low humidity. Refrigeration of NISV at 4°C is preferred for antigen-containing preparations. Optimal storage conditions are under evaluation.

CHEMICAL/PHYSICAL PROPERTIES: Stable at neutral and alkaline pH. Components are amphiphilic, insoluble in water, and soluble in chloroform. The T_c of NISV is approximately 55°C. NISV are formulated as a suspension in saline.

INCOMPATIBILITY: Most organic solvents and some detergents; osmotically sensitive.

SAFETY/TOXICITY: Extremely low toxicity of NISV has been demonstrated in rat studies after administration by either the subcutaneous or intramuscular route. At doses up to 575 mg/kg body weight there was no persistence of NISV at the site of injection (s.c.).
- Brewer, J. M., et al., 1994, Non-ionic surfactant vesicles as vaccine delivery systems, in: *Proceedings of the Second Conference on Industrial Immunology,* Chameleon Press, London, pp. 34–36.

ADJUVANT PROPERTIES: Induces both a humoral and cell-mediated immune response. Preferentially stimulates the Th1 subpopulation of T-helper cells. Effective with antigens within a broad size range, from short peptides to particulates. Adjuvant function is unrestricted by genetic background.
- Brewer, J. M., and Alexander, J., 1992, The adjuvant activity of non-ionic surfactant vesicles (niosomes) on the BALB/c humoral response to bovine serum albumin, *Immunology* **75**:570–575.
- Brewer, J. M., and Alexander, J., 1994, Studies on the adjuvant activity of non-ionic surfactant vesicles: Adjuvant-driven IgG2a production independent of MHC control, *Vaccine* **12**:613–619.
- Brewer, J. M., et al., 1994, The demonstration of an essential role for macrophages in the in vivo generation of IgG2a antibodies, *Clin. Exp. Immunol.* **97**:164–171.

CONTACT(S): Jurek S. Sikorski, Proteus Molecular Design Limited, Macclesfield, Cheshire SK11 0JL, U.K., Ph: 44-625-500555; Fax: 44-625-500666.

COMPONENT/ADJUVANT NAME: Pleuran

OTHER NAME(S): β-glucan; glucan

STRUCTURE: A β-1,3-linked glucose polymer having β-D-glucosyl side chains attached by alternate $\beta(1,6)$ or $\beta(1,4)$ bonds at the -0-6 position of every fourth anhydroglucose unit.

SOURCE: Isolated from the fruit-body of the oyster fungus *Pleurotus ostreatus* by alkali extraction at 95–100°C, followed by bleaching with sodium chlorite (pH 3.5–4.5) at 50–60°C. The bleached products were washed in water, dehydrated in organic solvent, and finally dried by vacuum at 60°C.

- Kuniake, L., *et al.*, 1993, A new fungal glucan and its preparation, W. I. P. O. Patent No. WO93/12243.
- Karacsonyi, S., and Kuniak, L., 1994, Polysaccharides of *Pleurotus ostreatus*: Isolation and structure of Pleuran, an alkali-insoluble β-D-glucan, *J. Biopolym.* (in press).

USES: Administered with antigen for enhancement of both humoral and cell-mediated immunity. β-glucans exert their immunostimulatory activities by binding to specific β-glucan receptors on macrophages. This ligand–receptor interaction results in macrophage activation and, in certain formulations, promotes antigen targeting.

- DiLuzio, N. R., *et al.*, 1979, Evaluation of the mechanism of glucan-induced stimulation of the reticuloendothelial system, *J. Reticuloendothel. Soc.* **7**:731–742.
- Czop, J. K., and Austen, K. F., 1985, A β-glucan inhibitable receptor on human monocytes: Its identity with the phagocytic receptor for particulate activators of the alternative complement pathway, *J. Immunol.* **134**:2588–2593.

APPEARANCE: White, odorless powder. Viscous in aqueous solution.

MOLECULAR WEIGHT: 762,000

RECOMMENDED STORAGE: Stable to light. Store solid Pleuran at room temperature and aqueous suspensions at 4°C. Optimal storage conditions are to be determined.

CHEMICAL/PHYSICAL PROPERTIES: Water insoluble. Median particle size of homopolymer is 150 μm. Purified preparations contain <0.57% chitin and <0.03% protein.

INCOMPATIBILITY: Alkaline pH disrupts the triple-helical conformation.

SAFETY/TOXICITY: In preclinical studies, Pleuran has been intravenously administered at doses up to 25 mg/kg body weight and was well tolerated. Human clinical trials of β-glucans isolated from either plants or microorganisms indicate the feasibility of administering these compounds to humans without toxicity. Glucan particles bioerode over time in a physiological environment.

- Mansel, P. W. A., *et al.*, 1975, Macrophage-mediated destruction of human malignant cells in vivo, *J. Natl. Cancer Inst.* **54**:571–580.
- Okamura, K., *et al.*, 1986, Clinical evaluation of Schizophyllan combined with irradiation in patients with cervical cancer, *Cancer* **58**:865–872.
- Chihara, G., *et al.*, 1989, Lentinan as a host defense potentiator (HDP), *Int. J. Immunother.* **4**:145–154.

- Ostroff, G. R., 1994, Future therapeutic applications of Betafectin, a carbohydrate-based immunomodulator, The Second Annual Conference on Glycotechnology.

ADJUVANT PROPERTIES: Rabbits as well as mice immunized once by coadministration of viral antigens and 60 μg of Pleuran produced at least 20-fold higher antibody titers than control animals injected with the immunogen alone.

CONTACT(S): Richard McIntosh, Genesis Technology Group, Inc., Cambridge, MA 02139, Ph: 617-576-6610; Fax: 617-876-4002. Also: Dr. Nahid Mohagheghpour, SRI International, Menlo Park, CA 94025, Ph: 415-859-3516; Fax: 415-859-3342.

COMPONENT/ADJUVANT NAME: PLGA, PGA, and PLA

OTHER NAME(S): Homo- and copolymers of lactic and glycolic acid; lactide/glycolide polymers; poly-lactic-co-glycolide

STRUCTURE: Structures shown below (left to right): PGA, homo-PLGA, and PLA.

SOURCE: Synthesized by the ring-opening polymerization of the cyclic dimers, lactide and glycolide.

- Deasy, P. B., *et al.*, 1989, Preparation and characterization of lactic/glycolic acid polymers and copolymers, *J. Microencapsul.* **6**:369–378.

USES: Antigens incorporated in PLGA microspheres have exhibited enhanced and prolonged immune responses compared to equivalent doses of free antigen.

APPEARANCE: Odorless, white to tan pellets.

MOLECULAR WEIGHT: Standard grades available from 10,000 to 500,000.

RECOMMENDED STORAGE: Store at 0°C or below and minimize exposure to moisture to maintain quality.

CHEMICAL/PHYSICAL PROPERTIES: Stable except in presence of moisture. Polymers react with water and degrade to glycolic and/or lactic acid.

INCOMPATIBILITY: Reacts with water and aqueous acids and bases. Hydrolyzes to form hydroxyacetic acid (glycolic acid) and lactic acid.

SAFETY/TOXICITY: Materials are used commercially as surgical suture, staples and clips, and sustained release delivery systems. FDA has approved specific applications using this family of polymers. Drug Master File (DMF) established with FDA.

ADJUVANT PROPERTIES: The adjuvant properties of polylactides have been ascribed to the size of the microspheres and small microspheres (<10 μm) may be phagocytosed to enhance antigen presentation. However, the major use of polylactides for vaccine delivery is based on their ability to control the release of antigen after administration, thereby eliminating or reducing the need for boost immunizations.

- Cleland, J. L., *et al.*, 1994, Development of a single shot subunit vaccine for HIV-1, *AIDS Res. Hum. Retroviruses* **10**:S21–S26.
- Eldridge, J. H., *et al.*, 1991, Biodegradable and biocompatible poly(DL-lactide-co-glycolide) microspheres as an adjuvant for staphylococcal enterotoxin B toxoid which enhances the level of toxin-neutralizing antibodies, *Infect. Immun.* **59**:2978–2986.
- Eldridge, J. H., *et al.*, 1991, Biodegradable microspheres as a vaccine delivery, *Mol. Immunol.* **28**:287–294.
- Singh, M., *et al.*, 1992, Immunogenicity studies on diphtheria toxoid loaded biodegradable microspheres, *Int. J. Pharm.* **85**:R5–R8.
- Hazrati, A. M., *et al.*, 1993, Studies of controlled delivery tetanus vaccine in mice, *Proc. Int. Symp. Control. Rel. Bioact. Mater.* **20**:67–68.
- Hazrati, A. M., *et al.*, 1993, *Salmonella enteritidis* vaccine utilizing biodegradable microspheres, *Proc. Int. Symp. Control. Rel. Bioact. Mater.* **20**:101–102.
- Aguado, M. T., and Lambert, P. -H., 1992, Controlled-release vaccines—biodegradable polylactide/polyglycolide (PL/PG) microspheres as antigen vehicles, *Immunobiology* **184**:113–125.
- Esparza, I., and Kissel, T., 1992, Parameters affecting the immunogenicity of microencapsulated tetanus toxoid, *Vaccine* **10**:176–180.

- Nellore, R. V., *et al.*, 1992, Evaluation of biodegradable microspheres as vaccine adjuvant for hepatitis B surface antigen, *J. Parenteral Sci. Tech.* **46**:176–180.
- Hanes, J., *et al.*, Chapter 16, this volume.
- Cleland, J. L., Chapter 18, this volume.

CONTACT(S): There are several suppliers of PLGA polymers. The monograph prepared by: Medisorb Technologies Intl. L. P., Cincinnati, OH 45242, Ph: 800-772-5091; Fax: 513-489-7244. Also: Jeffrey L. Cleland, Genentech, Inc., South San Francisco, CA 94080, Ph: 415-225-3921; Fax: 415-225-2866; E-mail: cleland.jeffrey@gene.com.

COMPONENT/ADJUVANT NAME: Pluronic L121
OTHER NAME(S): Poloxamer 401
STRUCTURE:

SOURCE: Synthetic block copolymer of ethylene oxide and propylene oxide.

USES: Component of IDEC Antigen Formulation (AF) present in final concentration of 0.05–1.25% (w/v) with antigen, and as a component of the Syntex Adjuvant Formulation (SAF) present in a final concentration of 2.5% (w/v) with antigen.

APPEARANCE: Off-white viscous liquid at room temperature.

MOLECULAR WEIGHT: Approximately 4400

RECOMMENDED STORAGE: Airtight container at room temperature.

CHEMICAL/PHYSICAL PROPERTIES: Water-insoluble surfactant with hydrophilic/lipophilic balance (HLB) of approximately 1.0 which classifies the compound as a spreading agent.

INCOMPATIBILITY: None found.

SAFETY: Currently under study.

ADJUVANT PROPERTIES: The amphipathic structure is hypothesized to enhance the presentation of antigen to cells of the immune system. Also see references for SAF-1 and Antigen Formulation.

- Allison, A. C., and Byars, N. E., 1992, Syntex Adjuvant Formulation, *Res. Immunol.* **143**:519–525.
- Hunter, R. L., *et al.*, 1981, The adjuvant activity of nonionic block polymer surfactants I. The role of hydrophile–lipophile balance, *J. Immunol.* **127**:1244–1250.
- Hunter, R. L., *et al.*, 1984, The adjuvant activity of nonionic block polymer surfactants II. Antibody formation and inflammation related to the structure of triblock and octablock copolymers, *J. Immunol.* **133**:3167–3175.
- Hunter, R. L., *et al.*, 1986, The adjuvant activity of nonionic block polymer surfactants III. Characterization of selected biologically active surfaces, *Scand. J. Immunol.* **23**:287–300.
- Lidgate, D. M., and Byars, N., Chapter 12, this volume.

CONTACT(S): Thomas Ryskamp, IDEC Pharmaceuticals Corporation, San Diego, CA 92121, Ph: 619-550-8500; Fax: 619-550-8750; Internet: tryskamp@idec.com. Also: Deborah M. Lidgate, Syntex Corp., Palo Alto, CA 94304, Ph: 415-852-1887; Fax: 415-852-1784.

COMPONENT/ADJUVANT NAME: PMMA
OTHER NAME(S): Polymethyl methacrylate
STRUCTURE:

SOURCE: Emulsion polymerization of methyl methacrylate.

USES: Primary adjuvant for all types of antigens. Added to the aqueous antigens in concentrations of 0.05% to 1.0% (w/w). Optimal adjuvant concentration in most cases 0.5%.

APPEARANCE: White odorless powder; forms a white milky suspension in water.

MOLECULAR WEIGHT: 30,000–400,000, depending on polymerization conditions.

RECOMMENDED STORAGE: Room temperature in solid powder form; between 2 and 8°C in aqueous suspension (pH range 2–11).

CHEMICAL/PHYSICAL PROPERTIES: Insoluble polymer, suspendable in aqueous solution. Forms a milky suspension on dispersion in water, easy to resuspend once hydrated. Polymer particle size 100–500 nm.

INCOMPATIBILITY: None found.

SAFETY/TOXICITY: PMMA has been used as an artificial bone material and bone cement in humans for over 50 years. Breakdown of these artificial bone materials leads to fragments with similar particle size to that of the adjuvant; no adverse reactions have been observed.

ADJUVANT PROPERTIES: Good adsorbate for a large number of antigens, particularly hydrophobic antigens. Antigen may be absorbed to previously polymerized particles, or may be incorporated into the polymer particles by polymerization in the presence of the antigen. PMMA is slowly biodegradable (40%/year in rats). PMMA enhances the temperature stability of a number of antigens.

- Kreuter, J., 1992, Physicochemical characterization of nanoparticles and their potential for vaccine preparation, *Vaccine Res.* **1**:93–98.
- Kreuter, J., *et al.*, 1981, Long-term studies of microcapsulated and adsorbed influenza vaccine nanoparticles, *J. Pharm. Sci.* **70**:367–371.
- Kreuter, J., Chapter 19, this volume.

CONTACT(S): Dr. Jorg Kreuter, Institut für Pharmazeutische Technologie, J. W. Goethe-Universität, D-60439 Frankfurt, Germany, Ph: 49-69-5800-9682; Fax: 49-69-5800-9694.

COMPONENT/ADJUVANT NAME: PODDS™

OTHER NAME(S): Proteinoid microspheres

STRUCTURE: Acylated amino acids (early experiments done with thermally condensed α-amino acids).

SOURCE: Chemical synthesis, purified by reprecipitation in acid. Microspheres are made in citric or acetic acid; compounds such as gum arabic, gelatin, or lactose may be added to formulate the material.

USES: Microspheres are being used as vehicles for oral immunization for the development of both mucosal and humoral responses. They are thought to protect antigens, target them to Peyer's patches, and/or facilitate transport of the protein antigens across mucosal epithelium.

APPEARANCE: Exists as liquid suspension or free flowing powder (after lyophilization).

MOLECULAR WEIGHT: 250–300

RECOMMENDED STORAGE: If lyophilized, store at room temperature under low humidity. Stability studies of suspension have not been conducted.

CHEMICAL/PHYSICAL PROPERTIES: Proteinoids have good water solubility at neutral pH, and precipitate out as microspheres at pH 2–3 at concentrations from 20 to 100 mg/mL. Particle size distribution of microspheres ranges from 0.1 to 10 μm, depending on the composition and formulation. Microspheres remain stable at acid pHs, soluble at neutral pHs. Proteinoids interact noncovalently with proteins, and have high encapsulation affinities.

INCOMPATIBILITY: None found.

SAFETY/TOXICITY: Toxicology data available on thermal condensate products in rats and dogs, following acute and subacute i.v. and p.o. dosing; dosing of human volunteers with the thermal condensate carrier resulted in good safety profile. Formal toxicology not completed with acylated amino acid microspheres; these carriers have been administered orally and intraduodenally to rodents and primates at doses up to 1000 mg/kg.

ADJUVANT PROPERTIES: Serves as a vehicle for oral immunization, protecting the antigen and allowing for co-encapsulation of adjuvants with antigens in microspheres.

- Santiago, N., *et al.*, 1993, Oral immunization of rats with proteinoid microspheres encapsulating influenza virus antigens, *Pharm. Res.* **10**:1243–1247.
- Santiago, N., *et al.*, Chapter 17, this volume.

CONTACT(S): Noemi Santiago or Robert Baughman, Emisphere Technologies, Inc., Hawthorne, NY 10532, Ph: 914-347-2220; Fax: 914-347-2498.

COMPONENT/ADJUVANT NAME: Poly rA: Poly rU

OTHER NAME(S): Polyadenylic acid-polyuridylic acid complex

STRUCTURE: Poly rA:poly rU is a double helix comprised of polyadenylic acid (left structure, two repeat units shown) and polyuridylic acid (right structure, two repeat units shown).

SOURCE: Synthetic. Polyribonucleotide complexes are formed following the action of the enzyme polynucleotide phosphorylase on the synthetic mononucleotide diphosphate. A hydrogen-bonded double helix forms following mixing of the opposite base pairs.

USES: Immunomodulation.

APPEARANCE: White, odorless powder.

MOLECULAR WEIGHT: Variable, ranging from 200,000 to 2,000,000. Sw_{20} values range from 4 to 11 units.

RECOMMENDED STORAGE: Stable for several years in sterile physiological saline at 4°C.

CHEMICAL/PHYSICAL PROPERTIES: Polyadenylate as potassium salt; polyuridylate as ammonium salt; readily water soluble at neutral pH (pH 7.2–7.6).

INCOMPATIBILITY: Destroyed by RNase.

SAFETY/TOXICITY: No toxicity in human trials at 600 mg/m^2/wk for 6 wks.

ADJUVANT PROPERTIES: Adjuvant to humoral and cell-mediated immunity when given with antigen; increases nonspecific immunity to microorganisms; antibody suppressant when given before antigen.

- Johnson, A. G., *et al.*, 1979, Modulation of the immune system by synthetic polynucleotides, *Springer Semin. Immunopathol.* **2**:149–168.
- Tursz, T. A., *et al.*, 1990, Poly A-poly U: An updated review, in: *Immunotherapeutic Prospects of Infectious Diseases* (K. N. Mashihi and W. Lange, eds.), Springer-Verlag, Berlin, pp. 263–272.
- Lacour, J., *et al.*, 1984, Adjuvant treatment with polyadenylic-polyuridylic acid in operable breast cancer: update results of a randomized trial, *Br. Med. J.* **288**:589–592.

CONTACT(S): Cynthia Ewel, Institute Henri Beaufour-USA, Washington, DC 20037, Ph: 202-973-2400; Fax: 202-887-5032. Also: A. G. Johnson, University of Minnesota, Duluth, MN 55812, Ph: 218-726-7561; Fax: 218-726-6235.

COMPONENT/ADJUVANT NAME: Polyphosphazene

OTHER NAME(S): PCPP; poly[di(carboxylatophenoxy)]phosphazene

STRUCTURE:

$$\left[\begin{array}{c} O\text{—}\bigcirc\text{—COOH} \\ | \\ P=N \\ | \\ O\text{—}\bigcirc\text{—COOH} \end{array} \right]_n$$

SOURCE: Synthetic.

USES: As an adjuvant for parenteral formulations. As a microsphere hydrogel for mucosal formulations.

APPEARANCE: White, odorless substance.

MOLECULAR WEIGHT: 3000–10,000,000

RECOMMENDED STORAGE: Store at a temperature not exceeding 30°C.

CHEMICAL/PHYSICAL PROPERTIES: Soluble in aqueous alkali solutions; ionically cross-linkable in aqueous media when treated with salts of di- or trivalent cations; T_g = –4.7°C.

INCOMPATIBILITY: None found.

SAFETY/TOXICITY: Subcutaneous injection of polyphosphazine in mice showed an intense inflammatory response without formation of a granuloma.

ADJUVANT PROPERTIES: Induces a sustained antibody response in mice after a single parenteral dose. High functional antibody titers are induced. The response is largely IgG1. Sustained IgG and IgA responses are also induced in mice after mucosal immunization.

• Payne, L. G., *et al*., Chapter 20, this volume.

CONTACT(S): Lendon G. Payne, Virus Research Institute, Cambridge, MA 02134, Ph: 617-864-6232; Fax: 617-864-6334.

COMPONENT/ADJUVANT NAME: Polysorbate 80

OTHER NAME(S): Tween 80; Sorbitan mono-9-octadecenoate poly(oxy-1,2-ethanediyl) derivatives

STRUCTURE:

$$HO(C_2H_4O)_w \quad (OC_2H_4)_xOH$$
$$CH(OC_2H_4)_yOH$$
$$CH_2(OC_2H_4)_zCOOC_{17}H_{33}$$

SOURCE: Polysorbate 80 is produced via copolymerization of ethylene oxide with an oleate ester of sorbitan and its anhydrides.

USES: A stabilizer in the MF59 and IDEC SPT formulations, present in final concentration of approximately 0.2% (w/v) with antigen. Commonly used surfactant in foods, cosmetics, and pharmaceuticals.

APPEARANCE: Amber, viscous liquid.

MOLECULAR WEIGHT: 1309.68

RECOMMENDED STORAGE: Airtight container at room temperature.

CHEMICAL/PHYSICAL PROPERTIES: HLB of 12–16 and therefore highly soluble in aqueous solution. The oleic acid esters are susceptible to oxidation.

INCOMPATIBILITY: Avoid strong oxidizing agents, bases, and heavy metal salts.

SAFETY/TOXICITY: Mild ocular irritant (rabbit eye test 150 mg). LD_{50} (rat) via i.v., 1.8 g/kg; LD_{50} (mouse) via oral, 25 g/kg. Generally considered safe (GRAS).

ADJUVANT PROPERTIES: Polysorbate 80 has no adjuvant properties on its own. Used in emulsion vaccine formulations including MF59, SAF-1, and Antigen Formulation. See those headings for additional references.

- Sanchez-Pestador, L., *et al.*, 1988, The effect of adjuvants on the efficacy of a recombinant herpes simplex glycoprotein vaccine, *J. Immunol.* **141**:1720–1727.
- Van Nest, G. A., *et al.*, 1992, Advanced adjuvant formulations for use with recombinant subunit vaccines, in: *Vaccines 92* (F. Brown, R. M. Chanock, H. S. Ginsberg, and R. A. Lerner, eds.), Cold Spring Harbor Press, Cold Spring Harbor, NY, p. 57.
- Ott, G., *et al.*, Chapter 10, this volume.
- Lidgate, D. M., and Byars, N., Chapter 12, this volume.

CONTACT(S): There are several suppliers of Polysorbate 80. For use in adjuvant formulations: Thomas Ryskamp, IDEC Pharmaceuticals Corporation, San Diego, CA 92121, Ph: 619-550-8500; Fax: 619-550-8750; Internet: tryskamp@idec.com. Also: Gary Van Nest, Chiron Corp., Emeryville, CA, Ph: 510-601-2965; Fax: 510-601-2586. Also: Deborah M. Lidgate, Syntex Research, Palo Alto, CA 94304, Ph: 415-852-1887; Fax: 415-852-1784.

COMPONENT/ADJUVANT NAME: Protein Cochleates

OTHER NAME(S): None

STRUCTURE: Protein cochleates are stable protein phospholipid–calcium precipitates, which are distinct from liposomes. They have a unique structure consisting of a large, continuous, solid, lipid bilayer sheet rolled up in a spiral, with no internal aqueous space. The calcium maintains the cochleate in its rolled-up form, bridging between successive layers. One of its positive charges interacts with a single negative charge on a phospholipid head group in one bilayer, and the other with a phospholipid in the opposing bilayer. Membrane proteins, or lipid-anchored peptides or proteins are tightly associated with the lipid bilayer.

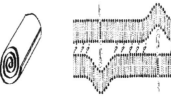

SOURCE: Cholesterol, phosphatidylethanolamine (egg or synthetic), and phosphatidylserine (bovine brain or synthetic) are obtained from Avanti Polar Lipids, Inc. Antigens which have been utilized include glycoproteins isolated directly from enveloped viruses, or expressed as recombinants in tissue culture, as well as synthetic peptides covalently linked to phosphatidylethanolamine. A mixture of phospholipids from the envelope will also be included when glycoproteins are isolated from viruses by our method of detergent extraction.

USES: Protein cochleates act as both carriers and adjuvants, providing multivalent presentation of antigens to the immune system, with maintenance of native conformation and biological activity. Protection of antigens from degradation following oral delivery. Probable controlled or slow release properties.

APPEARANCE: White, fine-grained suspension or precipitate. May be lyophilized to a white powder.

MOLECULAR WEIGHT: Macromolecular structure of varying size depending on antigen and lipid content.

RECOMMENDED STORAGE: Protein cochleates are stable for at least 6 months at 4°C. Alternatively, they may be lyophilized and stored at room temperature for 6 months as a powder, and reconstituted with liquid prior to administration. Storage for longer time periods and higher temperatures has not been assessed.

CHEMICAL/PHYSICAL PROPERTIES: Protein cochleates are formed at or near neutral pH. Their stability to extremes of pH has not been characterized, but they are capable of protecting associated antigens when given orally. This is probably related to their unique rolled-up solid precipitate structure which prevents the exposure of antigens within the interior of the spiral to the external milieu.

INCOMPATIBILITY: None found.

SAFETY/TOXICITY: The phospholipids used in the preparation of protein cochleates have been used in humans for vaccines and drug delivery with no significant negative side effects. Protein cochleates have been given to hundreds of mice by various routes including oral, intramuscular, and intranasal, with no negative local or systemic effects noted.

ADJUVANT PROPERTIES: Protein cochleates stimulate strong mucosal and systemic antibody, proliferative, and cytotoxic responses to associated antigens. They also afford protection from degradation following oral delivery and probable slow release properties.

- Gould-Fogerite, S., and Mannino, R. J., 1992, Targeted fusogenic liposomes: Functional reconstitution of membrane proteins into large unilamellar vesicles via protein-cochleate intermediates, in: *Liposome Technology* 2nd ed. (G. Gregoriadis, ed.), CRC Press, Boca Raton, Vol. III, pp. 262–275.
- Gould-Fogerite, S., *et al.*, 1994, Orally delivered protein cochleate vaccines stimulate mucosal and circulating immunity and protection from mucosal challenge with live influenza virus, (submitted).
- Mannino, R. J., and Gould-Fogerite, S., Chapter 15, this volume.

CONTACT(S): Dr. Susan Gould-Fogerite and Dr. Raphael J. Mannino, MuDNJ, New Jersey Medical School, Dept. of Laboratory Medicine and Pathology, Newark, NJ 07103-2714, Ph: 201-982-7836; Fax: 201-982-7293.

COMPONENT/ADJUVANT NAME: QS-21
OTHER NAME(S): Stimulon™ QS-21 Adjuvant
STRUCTURE:

SOURCE: Natural product of the bark of the *Quillaja saponaria* Molina tree (species native to Chile and Argentina). Extracted from the bark by aqueous extraction. Purified by normal phase and reverse phase chromatography.

- Kensil, C. R., *et al.*, 1991, Separation and characterization of saponins with adjuvant activity from *Quillaja saponaria* Molina cortex, *J. Immunol.* **146**:431–437.

USES: Used in vaccine formulations as a primary adjuvant component for enhancement of both humoral and cell-mediated immunity. Water soluble. No emulsification required. Can be used alone or combined with aluminum hydroxide adjuvant.

APPEARANCE: Solid: white, odorless powder. Aqueous solution: clear, colorless solution.

MOLECULAR WEIGHT: Parent: 1990, sodium salt: 2012.

RECOMMENDED STORAGE: Store solid QS-21 under low-humidity conditions at −20°C. Protect from light. Optimum storage conditions are under evaluation. No apparent degradation under low-humidity conditions after storage at 25°C for 8 weeks. Aqueous solutions are optimally stable between pH 5 and 6 and in micellar form. Solutions of QS-21 in 0.5 mg/mL solution may be stored in this pH range at 5°C for 2 or 3 years. Protect from light. In aqueous solution, the fatty acid ester bond migrates between the 3 and 4 position on fucose, with the ester at the 4 position being favored. Both forms are active as adjuvants. Primary degradation reaction is alkaline hydrolysis of the fatty acid ester bond at the 3 or 4 position on fucose. Due to alkaline-catalyzed degradation reaction, sterilization should be carried out by membrane filtration instead of autoclaving.

CHEMICAL/PHYSICAL PROPERTIES: Amphiphilic molecule with good water solubility above pKa of carboxyl group (solubility approximately 2 mg/mL to pH 4, 15 mg/mL at pH 5, 28 mg/mL at pH 6, and 32 mg/mL at pH 7 in buffered saline solutions). Forms micelles in aqueous solution (cmc approximately $50\,\mu g/mL$ in phosphate-buffered saline, pH 7.0).

INCOMPATIBILITY: Avoid strong bases.

SAFETY/TOXICITY: Studies in human Phase I clinical trial of therapeutic melanoma vaccine at doses up to 200 μg by subcutaneous route. Currently under study in human Phase I clinical trial of prophylactic HIV-1 subunit vaccine at doses up to 100 μg by intramuscular route.

- Livingston, P. O., *et al.*, 1994, Phase I trial of immunological adjuvant QS-21 with a GM2 ganglioside-KLH conjugate vaccine in patients with malignant melanoma, *Vaccine* **12(14)**:1275–1280.

ADJUVANT PROPERTIES: Shown to stimulate humoral immune responses in mice, including antigen-specific IgG1, IgG2b, and IgG2a titers. Augments production of IgG responses to ganglioside antigen in melanoma vaccine in human Phase I clinical trials. Shown also to stimulate CTL responses in mice.

- Kensil, C. R., *et al.*, 1993, The use of Stimulon adjuvant to boost vaccine response, *Vaccine Res.* **2(4)**:273–281.
- Newman, M. J., *et al.*, 1992, Saponin adjuvant induction of ovalbumin specific CD8+ cytotoxic T-lymphocyte responses, *J. Immunol.* **138**:2357–2362.
- Augments production of IgG responses to ganglioside antigen in melanoma vaccine in human Phase I clinical trial (Livingston, P. O., 1993, Approaches to augmenting the IgG antibody response to melanoma ganglioside vaccines, *Ann. N.Y. Acad. Sci.* **690**:204–213.
- Kensil, C., *et al.*, Chapter 22, this volume.
- Coughlin, R. T., *et al.*, Chapter 32, this volume.

CONTACT(S): Dr. Edward Balkovic, Cambridge Biotech Corporation, Worcester, MA 01605, Ph: 508-797-5777; Fax: 508-797-4014.

COMPONENT/ADJUVANT NAME: Quil A

OTHER NAME(S): Quil A saponin, *Quillaja* saponin

STRUCTURE: A complex but purified mixture of *Quillaja* saponins which are glycosides of quillaic acid and carbohydrates. The aglycone of Quil A is shown below.

COOR'
OH
RO
CHO

SOURCE: Purified extract from the bark of the South American tree *Quillaja saponaria* Molina.

USES: Quil A is used in veterinary vaccines and for production of ISCOMs.

APPEARANCE: Lyophilized powder. Color is light brownish, almost white.

MOLECULAR WEIGHT: Ranges from approximately 1400 to 2400

RECOMMENDED STORAGE: Dry storage in the lyophilized state. Can be stored frozen, refrigerated, or at room temperature.

CHEMICAL/PHYSICAL PROPERTIES: The mixture contains fractions that bind to cholesterol, are adjuvant active, are hemolytic, and are able to form ISCOMs.

INCOMPATIBILITY: Should not be exposed to alkaline conditions (pH > 8.0).

SAFETY/TOXICITY: Avoid inhalation and eye contact when handling Quil A. It is highly irritating to mucosa and contains hemolyzing saponins. Quil A is not used in human trials because of overt toxicity. It is, however, used extensively in veterinary vaccines.

- Speijers, G. J. A., *et al.*, 1988, Local reactions of the saponin Quil A and a Quil A containing iscom measles vaccine after intramuscular injection of rats: A comparison with the effects of DTP-polio vaccine, *Fundam. Appl. Toxicol.* **10**:425–430.

ADJUVANT PROPERTIES: Quil A is used as a part of a novel antigen presentation system called ISCOMs, as well as with antigen alone. It induces both humoral and cell-mediated responses.

- Morein, B., 1984, Iscom, a novel structure for antigenic presentation of membrane proteins from enveloped viruses, *Nature* **308**:457–460.
- Dalsgaard, K., *et al.*, 1977, Evaluation of the adjuvant "Quil-A" in the vaccination of cattle against foot-and-mouth disease, *Acta Vet. Scand.* **18**:349–360.
- Dalsgaard, K., 1984, Assessment of the dose of the immunological adjuvant Quil-A in mice and guinea pigs, using sheep red blood cells as model antigen, *Zbl. Vet. Med. B* **31**:718–720.
- Dalsgaard, K., and Jensen, M. H., 1977, The adjuvant activity of "Quil-A" in trivalent vaccination of cattle and guinea pigs against foot-and-mouth disease, *Acta Vet. Scand.* **18**:367–373.
- Rimmelzwaan, G. F., and Osterhaus, A. D. M. E., Chapter 23, this volume.

CONTACT(S): There are several suppliers of Quil A. The monograph prepared by: E. B. Lindblad, Superfos Biosector, DK-2950 Vedbaek, Denmark, Ph: 45 42 89 31 11; Fax: 45 42 89 15 95. Also: Al Reisch, Sergeant, Inc., Clifton, NJ 07012, Ph: 201-472-9111; Fax: 201-472-5686. Also: Accurate Chemical & Scientific Corp., Westbury, NY 11590, Ph: 800-645-6264; Fax: 516-997-4948.

COMPONENT/ADJUVANT NAME: Rehydragel HPA

OTHER NAME(S): High protein adsorbency aluminum hydroxide gel; alum

STRUCTURE: Crystalline aluminum oxyhydroxide AlOOH, known mineralogically as boehmite. The structure consists of corrugated sheets of aluminum octahedra.

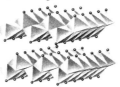

SOURCE: Synthetic oxyhydroxide of aluminum (aluminum hydroxide) prepared by acid–base precipitation.

USES: Primary adjuvant in parenteral vaccine formulations. Does not generally induce cell-mediated immunity.

APPEARANCE: Translucent, thixotropic, colloidal aqueous gel supplied sterile.

MOLECULAR WEIGHT: 60 (empirical formula)

RECOMMENDED STORAGE: Stable at room temperature for indefinite period. Freezing should be avoided.

CHEMICAL/PHYSICAL PROPERTIES: Contains 2% equivalent Al_2O_3 or 3% equivalent $Al(OH)_3$. Primary particles have a rodlike morphology and a high surface area. The isoelectric point is 11. Its high surface area gives it a high adsorptive capacity for antigens. Typical pH: 5.8 to 6.8. Insoluble in water between pH 4 and 8, and poorly soluble in solutions containing citrate ion. Average particle size: 0.3 μm. Pumpable suspension.

INCOMPATIBILITY: Do not freeze, otherwise chemically inert and stable.

SAFETY/TOXICITY: Aluminum compounds (aluminum hydroxide, aluminum phosphate, alum) are currently the only vaccine adjuvants used in U.S.-licensed vaccines. They can induce granulomas at the inoculation site. Supplied pyrogen free.

- Ganrot, P. O., 1986, Metabolism and possible health effects of aluminum, *Environ. Health Perspect.* **65**:363–441.
- Gupta, R. K., *et al.*, 1993, Adjuvants—A balance between toxicity and adjuvanticity, *Vaccine* **11**:293–306.

ADJUVANT PROPERTIES: Protein binding capacity: 2.5 mg BSA/mg Al_2O_3 minimum. The surface area, surface charge, and morphology of the aluminum hydroxide are major factors in its adjuvant characteristics. The use of aluminum adjuvants is accompanied by stimulation of IL-4 and stimulation of the T-helper-2 subsets in mice, with enhanced IgG1 and IgE production.

- Shirodkar, S., *et al.*, 1990, Aluminum compounds used as adjuvant in vaccines, *Pharm. Res.* **7**:1282–1288.
- Aprile, M. A., and Wardlaw, A. C., 1966, Aluminum compounds as adjuvants for vaccines and toxoids in man, *Can. J. Public Health* **57**:343–354.
- Gupta, R. K., *et al.*, Chapter 8, this volume.
- Seeber, S., *et al.*, 1991, Predicting the adsorption of proteins by aluminum-containing adjuvants, *Vaccine* **9**:201–203.
- Seeber, S. J., *et al.*, 1991, Solubilization of aluminum-containing adjuvants by constituents of interstitial fluid, *J. Parenteral Sci. Tech.* **45**:156–159.
- Hem, S., and White, J. L., Chapter 9, this volume.

CONTACT(S): Philip B. Klepak, Reheis Inc., Berkeley Heights, NJ 07922, Ph: 908-464-1500; Fax: 908-464-7726. Also: Stanley Hem, Purdue University, West Lafayette, IN 47907-1336, Ph: 317-494-1451; Fax: 317-494-7880.

COMPONENT/ADJUVANT NAME: Rehydragel LV

OTHER NAME(S): Low-viscosity aluminum hydroxide gel; alum

STRUCTURE: Crystalline aluminum oxyhydroxide AlOOH, known mineralogically as boehmite. The structure consists of corrugated sheets of aluminum octahedra.

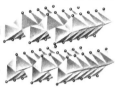

SOURCE: Synthetic oxyhydroxide of aluminum (aluminum hydroxide) prepared by acid–base precipitation.

USES: Primary adjuvant in parenteral vaccine formulations. Does not generally induce cell-mediated immunity.

APPEARANCE: White, fluid aqueous suspension supplied sterile.

MOLECULAR WEIGHT: 60 (empirical formula)

RECOMMENDED STORAGE: Stable at room temperature for indefinite period. Freezing should be avoided.

CHEMICAL/PHYSICAL PROPERTIES: Contains 2% equivalent Al_2O_3 or 3% equivalent $Al(OH)_3$. Primary particles have a rodlike or fibril morphology, but are larger than Rehydragel HPA. Surface area and antigen absorptive capacity diminished compared with Rehydragel HPA. Typical pH is 5.8 to 6.8. Insoluble in water between pH 4 and 8, and poorly soluble in solutions containing citrate ion. Average particle size: 1 μm. Has a low viscosity and is pumpable.

INCOMPATIBILITY: Do not freeze, otherwise chemically inert and stable.

SAFETY/TOXICITY: Aluminum compounds (aluminum hydroxide, aluminum phosphate, alum) are currently the only vaccine adjuvants used in U.S.-licensed vaccines. They can induce granulomas at the inoculation site. Supplied pyrogen free.

- Ganrot, P. O., 1986, Metabolism and possible health effects of aluminum, *Environ. Health Perspect.* **65**:363–441.
- Gupta, R. K., *et al.*, 1993, Adjuvants—A balance between toxicity and adjuvanticity, *Vaccine* **11**:293–306.

ADJUVANT PROPERTIES: Protein binding capacity: 1.5 mg BSA/mg equivalent Al_2O_3 minimum. The surface area, surface charge, and morphology are major factors in its adjuvant characteristics. The use of aluminum adjuvants is accompanied by stimulation of IL-4 and stimulation of the T-helper-2 subsets in mice, with enhanced IgG1 and IgE production.

- Aprile, M. A., and Wardlaw, A. C., 1966, Aluminum compounds as adjuvants for vaccines and toxoids in man, *Can. J. Public Health* **57**:343–354.
- Gupta, R. K., *et al.*, Chapter 8, this volume.
- Seeber, S., *et al.*, 1991, Predicting the adsorption of proteins by aluminum-containing adjuvants, *Vaccine* **9**:201–203.
- Seeber, S. J., *et al.*, 1991, Solubilization of aluminum-containing adjuvants by constituents of interstitial fluid, *J. Parenteral Sci. Tech.* **45**:156–159.
- Hem, S., and White, J. L., Chapter 9, this volume.

CONTACT(S): Philip B. Klepak, Reheis Inc., Berkeley Heights, NJ 07922, Ph: 908-464-1500; Fax: 908-464-7726. Also: Stanley Hem, Purdue University, West Lafayette, IN 47907-1336, Ph: 317-494-1451; Fax: 317-494-7880.

COMPONENT/ADJUVANT NAME: S-28463

OTHER NAME(S): 4-Amino-α,α-dimethyl-2-ethoxymethyl-1H-imidazo[4,5-c]quino-line-1-ethanol

STRUCTURE:

SOURCE: Chemical synthesis. International Publication 92/15582.

USES: Included in adjuvant formulations as a primary adjuvant component.

APPEARANCE: White, fine crystalline solid.

MOLECULAR WEIGHT: 314.39 free base, 350.85 hydrochloride salt.

RECOMMENDED STORAGE: Solid is stable at room temperature. Shelf life is acceptable.

CHEMICAL/PHYSICAL PROPERTIES: Somewhat limited solubility as the free base. The hydrochloride salt is soluble in water at concentrations at least to 10 mg/mL.

INCOMPATIBILITY: None found.

SAFETY/TOXICITY: In preclinical animal safety evaluation studies.

ADJUVANT PROPERTIES: Addition of S-28463 induces both humoral and cell-mediated immunity via induction of cytokines from monocytes and macrophages. Unpublished results indicate S-28463 is about 100-fold more potent than imiquimod in antiviral models and in cytokine induction from monocytes and macrophages.

CONTACT(S): R. C. Hanson, Business Development, 3M Pharmaceuticals, St. Paul, MN 55144, Ph: 612-737-3137; Fax: 612-737-4556.

COMPONENT/ADJUVANT NAME: SAF-1

OTHER NAME(S): SAF, SAF-m; Syntex Adjuvant Formulation

STRUCTURE: Composed of threonyl-MDP (0.05–~1%) in an emulsion vehicle [5% squalane, 2.5% Pluronic® L121, 0.2% Polysorbate 80, and phosphate-buffered saline (pH 7.4)].

Threonyl-MDP

Polysorbate 80

Pluronic L121

Squalane

SOURCE: See individual components.

USES: Adjuvant formulation.

APPEARANCE: White, fluid, oil-in-water emulsion.

MOLECULAR WEIGHT: Not applicable (see individual components).

RECOMMENDED STORAGE: ≤30°C.

CHEMICAL/PHYSICAL PROPERTIES: Particle size depends on the manufacturing method used. If the emulsion is manufactured using a Microfluidizer, then the mean particle size is ~160 nm.

INCOMPATIBILITY: None found.

SAFETY/TOXICITY: At therapeutic doses, no safety concern is anticipated. Dose is indication dependent, but a typical volume of injection is 1 mL.

ADJUVANT PROPERTIES: Antigens become arranged on the surface of the emulsion droplets partly because of their amphipathic nature, and partly because of hydrogen bonding with poloxamer 401. The emulsion droplets also activate complement, as demonstrated by consumption of C3 and production of C3b; the latter, on the surface of droplets, targets them to antigen-presenting cells (follicular dendritic cells and interdigitating cells) in lymph nodes of the drainage chain and possibly in more distant lymphoid tissues. In this way the emulsion facilitates the presentation of antigens to responding lymphocytes. See threonyl-MDP monograph.

- Allison, A. C., and Byars, N. E., 1992, Syntex Adjuvant Formulation, *Res. Immunol.* **143**:519–525.
- Byars, N. E., and Allison, A. C., 1987, Adjuvant formulation for use in vaccine to elicit both cell mediated and humoral immunity, *Vaccine* **5**:223–228.
- Allison, A. C., *et al.*, 1986, An adjuvant formulation that selectively elicits the formation of antibodies of protective isotypes and of cell-mediated immunity, *J. Immunol. Methods* **95**:157–168.
- Lidgate, D. M., and Byars, N., Chapter 12, this volume.

CONTACT(S): Deborah M. Lidgate, Syntex Research, Palo Alto, CA 94304, Ph: 415-852-1887; Fax: 415-852-1784.

COMPONENT/ADJUVANT NAME: Sclavo Peptide

OTHER NAME(S): IL-1β 163–171 peptide

STRUCTURE: VQGEESNDK •HCl

SOURCE: From human IL-1β amino acid sequence. Obtained by solid phase synthesis, purified by HPLC and ion-exchanged to the HCl salt.

USES: Primary adjuvant. Active either when administered separately from antigen, or admixed with antigen, or physically linked to antigen. Routes of administration: i.v., i.p., s.c., p.o.

APPEARANCE: White, odorless powder.

MOLECULAR WEIGHT: 1000

RECOMMENDED STORAGE: Stored lyophilized peptide dry at –20°C. Stable also at room temperature. The concentrated solution can be stored in siliconized glass at 4°C for at least 2–3 months. Do not freeze.

CHEMICAL/PHYSICAL PROPERTIES: Good solubility in water. Very acidic. Adjust pH to neutrality before use.

INCOMPATIBILITY: Avoid peptidases.

SAFETY/TOXICITY: No toxicity in mice when given i.v. as a bolus up to 100 mg/kg.

ADJUVANT PROPERTIES: It enhances immune response to T-dependent and T-independent antigens. Active also in increasing secondary responses. Active as adjuvant for a tumor vaccine. Antitumor activity through recruitment of host immune response.

- Nencioni, L., *et al.*, 1987, In vivo immunostimulating activity of the 163–171 peptide of human IL-1β, *J. Immunol.* **139**:800–804.
- Boraschi, D., *et al.*, 1988, In vivo stimulation and restoration of the immune response by the noninflammatory fragment 163–171 of human IL-1β, *J. Exp. Med.* **168**:675–686.
- McCune, C. S., and Marquis, D. M., 1990, Interleukin-1 as an adjuvant for active specific immunotherapy in a murine tumor model, *Cancer Res.* **50**:1212–1215.
- Rao, K. V. S., and Nayak, A. R., 1990, Enhanced immunogenicity of a sequence derived from hepatitis B virus surface antigen in a composite peptide which includes the immunostimulatory region from human interleukin-1, *Proc. Natl. Acad. Sci. USA* **87**:5519–5522.
- Beckers, W., *et al.*, 1993, Increasing the immunogenicity of protein antigens through the genetic insertion of VQGEESNDK sequence of human IL-1β into their sequence, *J. Immunol.* **151**:1757–1764.

CONTACT(S): Dr. P. Ghiara, IRIS-Biocine, Siena, Italy, Ph: 39-577-293111; Fax: 39-577-293564. Also: Drs. A. Tagliabue and D. Boraschi, Dompè Research Center, L'Aquila, Italy, Ph: 39-862-338324; Fax: 39-862-338219.

COMPONENT/ADJUVANT NAME: Sendai Proteoliposomes
Sendai-Containing Lipid Matrices

OTHER NAME(S): Sendai glycoprotein-containing vesicles; fusogenic proteo-liposomes; FPLs; Sendai lipid matrix-based vaccines

STRUCTURE: Sendai proteoliposome: The glycoproteins of Sendai virus (parainfluenza type 1) are integrated in the lipid bilayers of large, mainly unilamellar, liposomes. Native conformation and biological activities of receptor binding and membrane fusion are maintained. Other proteins containing hydrophobic regions or lipid-anchored proteins or peptides may be encapsulated in the lipid bilayer. Water-soluble proteins or other materials may be encapsulated in the aqueous interior of the vesicles.

Sendai-containing lipid matrices: Some peptides which are amphipathic (i.e., possess both hydrophilic and hydrophobic regions) have the ability to collapse lipid bilayers. When these peptides are encapsulated by adding EDTA to Sendai protein cochleates, lipid aggregates, rather than liposomes (with a continuous lipid bilayer encapsulating an internal aqueous space), are produced. Polymorphic lipid aggregates also form when plain lipid cochleates are converted by EDTA in the presence of high concentrations of these amphipathic peptides.

Sendai
proteoliposome 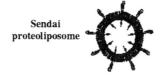   Sendai
containing
lipid matrix

SOURCE: Prepared from Sendai protein cochleates by chelation of Ca^{2+} with EDTA. See Protein cochleates for lipids and antigens used and sources. Material encapsulated includes chemically synthesized peptides, isolated and recombinant proteins, whole fixed viruses, small-molecule drugs, and DNA.

USES: Sendai proteoliposomes produced by these methods are highly effective immunogens in mice, rabbits, and monkeys. This includes the ability to stimulate strong T-helper and $CD8^+$ cytotoxic T-cell responses (CTL) to lipid bilayer-integrated glycoproteins as well as encapsulated peptides, proteins, and whole formalin-fixed viruses. These vesicles also act as effective delivery vehicles for drugs and proteins. They were used to achieve the first stable gene transfer in animals using a liposome-based system. These abilities probably arise from their membrane attachment and fusion activity which facilitates introduction into the cytoplasm and access to an MHC class I presentation pathway.

APPEARANCE: Opalescent suspension in aqueous isotonic buffer.

MOLECULAR WEIGHT: Macromolecular structure of varying size depending on antigen and lipid content.

RECOMMENDED STORAGE: Phospholipids used as raw materials are stored in chloroform at 20°C under nitrogen. Proteoliposomes should be stored at 4°C in isotonic buffer. They are generally used within a few days of preparation. Long-term stability has not been assessed.

CHEMICAL/PHYSICAL PROPERTIES: Proteoliposomes are stable in aqueous isotonic buffers. They are solubilized by detergents or organic solvents in sufficient quantities.

INCOMPATIBILITY: None found.

SAFETY/TOXICITY: The phospholipids used in the preparation of proteoliposomes have been used in humans for vaccines and drug delivery with no significant negative side effects. Proteoliposomes have been given to hundreds of mice, by intraperitoneal and intramuscular immunization, and many rabbits and 16 monkeys by intramuscular immunization with no negative local or systemic effects noted.

ADJUVANT PROPERTIES: Proteoliposomes stimulate strong antibody and proliferative responses to associated antigens. They are particularly powerful inducers of cytotoxic T lymphocytes. Antigens can be associated with the lipid bilayer or encapsulated within the aqueous interior.

- Gould-Fogerite, S., *et al.*, 1989, Chimerasome-mediated gene transfer in vitro and in vivo, *Gene* **84**:429–438.
- Gould-Fogerite, S., and Mannino, R. J., 1992, Targeted fusogenic liposomes: Functional reconstitution of membrane proteins into large unilamellar vesicles via protein-cochleate intermediates, in: *Liposome Technology*, 2nd ed. (G. Gregoriadis, ed.), CRC Press, Boca Raton, Vol. III, pp. 262–275.
- Miller, M. D., *et al.*, 1992, Vaccination of rhesus monkeys with synthetic peptide in a fusogenic proteoliposome elicits simian immunodeficiency virus-specific CD8[+] cytotoxic T lymphocytes, *J. Exp. Med.* **176**:1739–1744.
- Mannino, R. J., and Gould-Fogerite, S., Chapter 15, this volume.

CONTACT(S): Dr. Susan Gould-Fogerite and Dr. Raphael J. Mannino, UMDNJ, New Jersey Medical School, Dept. of Laboratory Medicine and Pathology, Newark, NJ 07103-2714, Ph: 201-982-7836; Fax: 201-982-7293.

COMPONENT/ADJUVANT NAME: Span 85

OTHER NAME(S): Arlacel 85, sorbitan trioleate

STRUCTURE: Spans are partial esters of common fatty acids (lauric, palmitic, stearic, and oleic) and hexitol anhydrides (hexitans and hexides), derived from sorbitol. An example structure is shown below.

SOURCE: Synthetic.

USES: Used as an emulsification agent in MF59 adjuvant formulation.

APPEARANCE: Viscous yellow liquid.

MOLECULAR WEIGHT: Most spans are actually mixtures with one particular span predominating.

RECOMMENDED STORAGE: Store in a cool dry place.

CHEMICAL/PHYSICAL PROPERTIES: Span products tend to be oil-soluble. Span 85 is insoluble in water but can be dispersed with a hydrophilic surfactant. Density 0.956.

INCOMPATIBILITY: Strong oxidizing agents.

SAFETY/TOXICITY: Vapor or mist is irritating to mucous membranes. Causes skin irritation.

ADJUVANT PROPERTIES: None described for the compound itself. See MF59.

• Ott, G., *et al.*, Chapter 10, this volume.

CONTACT(S): Several suppliers offer Span 85. Sigma Chemical Company, Ph: 800-325-3010. For vaccine formulation use: Gary Van Nest, Chiron Corp., Emeryville, CA, Ph: 510-601-2965; Fax: 510-601-2586.

COMPONENT/ADJUVANT NAME: Specol

STRUCTURE(S): Marcol 52 (mineral oil, paraffins, and cycloparaffins, chain length 13-22 C atoms)

Span 85 (emulsifier, sorbitan trioleate)

Tween 85 (emulsifier, polyoxyethylene-20-trioleate)

SOURCE: Ingredients are commercially available and all are individually FDA approved for veterinary use. Mineral oil and emulsifiers (Span and Tween) are thoroughly mixed 9:1 (v/v) and can be stored at 4°C for prolonged periods of time (several years).

USES: Specol can be obtained from ID-DLO in Lelystad and is a primary adjuvant (only antigen needed). The adjuvant mixture of mineral oil and emulsifiers is mixed with the water phase (physiological saline) containing the immunogen (water: oil = 0.44) and emulsified. A stable emulsion is obtained when the second of two drops, deposited on the surface of a water-containing tube, continues to float intact. When a stable (sterile) emulsion is obtained this can be stored for up to 1 year at 4–16°C or 3 months at 37°C (dependent on antigen). It functions as a depot (slow release of antigen) and a polyclonal activator (independent of presence of antigen) for cells of the immune system (cytokine release).

APPEARANCE: Specol is a clear oily fluid. The water-in-oil (w/o) emulsion resulting from mixing Specol with immunogen/water is white and gel-like.

MOLECULAR WEIGHT: Not applicable.

RECOMMENDED STORAGE: 4°C in low-oxygen conditions (e.g., in completely filled bottles or under N_2). As stated below, both Specol and the emulsion are relatively insensitive to temperature changes.

CHEMICAL/PHYSICAL PROPERTIES: The water-in-oil emulsion (Specol emulsified with immunogen in water) is resistant to temperature shifts (4–37°C). It has a low conductivity (indicative of proper separation of oil and water) of <0.6 siemens and a low viscosity (enabling easy application by injection) of 70–100 mPa/s (both measured at 20°C).

INCOMPATIBILITY: The Specol–water/immunogen emulsion is not compatible with natural rubber and is probably incompatible with most organic solvents as is common for w/o emulsions.

SAFETY: No known use in humans, registered for veterinary use by itself (nonspecific stimulation of immune system, e.g., in weanlings) or in combination with vaccines.

ADJUVANT PROPERTIES: The adjuvant properties of Specol, which are comparable to CFA, in rodents are reviewed in:

• Boersma, W. J. A., *et al.*, 1992, Adjuvant properties of stable water-in-oil emulsions, evaluation of the experience with Specol. 44th Forum in Immunology, *Res. Immunol.* **143**:503–512.

• Bokout, B. A., *et al.*, 1981, A selected water in oil emulsion: Composition and usefulness as an immunological adjuvant, *Vet. Immunol. Immunopathol*: **2**:491–500.

CONTACT(S): Source: Dr. B. Bokout, Institute of Animal Science and Health, POB 65, 8200 AB, The Netherlands, Ph: + 31 3200 73432; Fax: + 31 3200 73473; email: B.A.Bokhout@CDI.AGRO.NL. Rodent studies: Prof. Dr. E. Claassen, TNO-Prevention and Health, Fax + 31 71 181 276.

COMPONENT/ADJUVANT NAME: Squalane

OTHER NAME(S): Spinacane; Robane®; 2,6,10,15,19,23-hexamethyltetracosane

STRUCTURE:

SOURCE: Obtained by the total hydrogenation of the triterpene squalene, a component of shark liver oil and some vegetable oils.

USES: Component of Antigen Formulation (AF) and Syntex Adjuvant Formulation (SAF), present in final concentration of 5% w/v with antigen. Constitutes the oil component of the emulsion. A metabolizable oil, used in cosmetics, topicals, and as a vehicle for lipophilic drugs.

APPEARANCE: Clear oil.

MOLECULAR WEIGHT: 422.83

RECOMMENDED STORAGE: Airtight container at room temperature.

CHEMICAL/PHYSICAL PROPERTIES: Stable to air and oxygen. Readily soluble in organic solvents, slightly soluble in alcohol. Specific gravity 0.807–0.810 at 20°C.

INCOMPATIBILITY: None found.

SAFETY:

- Christian, M. S., 1982, Final report on the safety assessment of squalane and squalene, *J. Am. Coll. Toxicol.* **1**:37–56.

ADJUVANT PROPERTIES: Squalane itself is not an adjuvant. See monographs on SAF-1 and AF.

- Lidgate, D. M., and Byars, N., Chapter 12, this volume.

CONTACT(S): Supplied by several companies. For adjuvant use contact: Thomas Ryskamp, IDEC Pharmaceuticals Corporation, San Diego, CA 92121, Ph: 619-550-8500; Fax: 619-550-8750; Internet: tryskamp@idec.com. Also: Deborah M. Lidgate, Syntex Research, Palo Alto, CA 94304, Ph: 415-852-1887; Fax: 415-852-1784.

COMPONENT/ADJUVANT NAME: Squalene

OTHER NAME(S): Spinacene; Supraene; 2,6,10,15,19,23-hexamethyl-2,6,10,14,18,22-tetracosahexaene

STRUCTURE:

SOURCE: Found in shark liver oil and some vegetable oils. Intermediate in the biosynthesis of cholesterol.

USES: Bactericide, intermediate in the manufacturing of pharmaceuticals, component of MF59 emulsion formulation, constitutes the oil component of the emulsion.

APPEARANCE: Clear oil, colorless. Faint, agreeable odor.

MOLECULAR WEIGHT: 410.7

RECOMMENDED STORAGE: Store in a cool place.

CHEMICAL/PHYSICAL PROPERTIES: A metabolizable oil. Practically insoluble in water, highly soluble in organic solvents, may become viscous on absorbing oxygen. Specific gravity 0.858. Bp 285°C/25mm.

INCOMPATIBILITY: Avoid oxidizers.

SAFETY: May be harmful by inhalation, ingestion, or percutaneous adsorption. Oral LD$_{50}$ 5 g/kg, i.v. LD$_{50}$ 1.8 g/kg.

- Christian, M. S., 1982, Final report on the safety assessment of squalane and squalene, *J. Am. Coll. Toxicol.* **1**:37–56.

ADJUVANT PROPERTIES: Squalene itself is not an adjuvant. See monograph on MF59.

- Sanchez-Pestador, L., *et al.*, 1988, The effect of adjuvants on the efficacy of a recombinant herpes simplex glycoprotein vaccine, *J. Immunol.* **141**:1720–1727.
- Van Nest, G. A., *et al.*, 1992, Advanced adjuvant formulations for use with recombinant subunit vaccines, in: *Vaccines 92* (F. Brown, R. M. Chanock, H. S. Ginsberg, and R. A. Lerner, eds.), Cold Spring Harbor Laboratory Press, Cold Spring Harbor, NY, p. 57.
- Ott, G., *et al.*, Chapter 10, this volume.

CONTACT(S): Supplied by several companies. For example, Sigma Chemical Company, Ph: 800-325-3010. For vaccine formulation use: Gary Van Nest, Chiron Corp., Emeryville, CA, Ph: 510-601-2965; Fax: 510-601-2586.

COMPONENT/ADJUVANT NAME: Stearyl Tyrosine

OTHER NAME(S): Octadecyl tyrosine hydrochloride

STRUCTURE:

SOURCE: Chemical synthesis from tyrosine and stearyl alcohol (octadecanol).

• Penney, C. L., *et al.*, 1985, A simple method for the synthesis of long-chain alkyl esters of amino acids, *J. Org. Chem.* **50**:1457–1459.

USES: Primary vaccine adjuvant with minimal immunostimulatory properties. Some use in allergy desensitization therapy. Biocide.

APPEARANCE: White, amorphous free-flowing, odorless powder.

MOLECULAR WEIGHT: 470.14 (hydrochloride salt)

RECOMMENDED STORAGE: Store solid at room temperature. Aqueous suspensions may be stored at pH 4.0–7.5 at 4°C for several years.

CHEMICAL/PHYSICAL PROPERTIES: Sharp melting point (171–3°C). Insoluble (<0.01%) at neutral and alkaline pH; soluble at low pH in hot mineral acid.

INCOMPATIBILITY: Incompatible with strong base.

SAFETY/TOXICITY: Nontoxic up to 2500 mg/kg in many animals, including primates. Nonpyrogenic. No adjuvant arthritis (rats). No damage at site of injection (cats). Biodegradable.

ADJUVANT PROPERTIES: "Organic equivalent" of aluminum hydroxide, with likely carrier depot effect; adjuvancy similar to aluminum hydroxide with bacterial vaccines; superior to aluminum hydroxide with viral vaccines. Favorable isotype distribution. Biocompatible.

• Penney, C. L., *et al.*, 1993, Further studies on the adjuvanticity of stearyl tyrosine and ester analogues, *Vaccine* **11**:1129–1134.

• Penney, C. L., *et al.*, 1994, Further studies on the adjuvanticity of stearyl tyrosine and amide analogues, *Vaccine* **12**:629–632.

• Penney, C., Chapter 26, this volume.

CONTACT(S): Dr. Christopher L. Penney, BioChem Therapeutic, Inc., Laval, Quebec, Canada H7V 4A7, Ph: 514-978-7811; Fax: 514-978-7777.

COMPONENT/ADJUVANT NAME: Theramide™

OTHER NAME(S): *N*-acetylglucosaminyl-*N*-acetylmuramyl-L-Ala-D-isoGlu-L-Ala-dipalmitoxy propylamide (DTP-DPP)

STRUCTURE:

SOURCE: Synthetic.

USES: The drug compound is a potent macrophage activator and adjuvant. It induces IL-6, IL-12, TNF, IFN-γ, and relatively lesser quantities of IL-10. The compound preferentially induces cellular immunity. When reconstituted, it spontaneously forms liposomes in which lipopeptides may be incorporated.

APPEARANCE: White, odorless powder.

MOLECULAR WEIGHT: 1315.84

RECOMMENDED STORAGE: Stable as a lyophilized powder or in solution at room temperature for 5 years in saline or PBS at pH 7.4.

CHEMICAL/PHYSICAL PROPERTIES: Amphoteric molecule soluble in chloroform:methanol (7:3), and tert-butanol.

INCOMPATIBILITY: Avoid strong acids or bases.

SAFETY/TOXICITY: Human Phase I clinical trials at 200 μg/m^2 to 1000 μg/m^2 i.v. weekly have been initiated.

ADJUVANT PROPERTIES: The compound augments both cellular and humoral immunity and is active in murine models of CMV.

CONTACT: Gerald J. Vosika, M. D., ImmunoTherapeutics, Inc., Fargo, ND 58104, Ph: 701-232-9575; Fax: 701-237-9275.

COMPONENT/ADJUVANT NAME: Threonyl-MDP

OTHER NAME(S): Termurtide™ ; [thr[1]]-MDP; *N*-acetyl muramyl-L-threonyl-D-isoglutamine

STRUCTURE:

SOURCE: Synthetic.

• Jones, G. J., *et al.*, Novel immunological adjuvant compounds and methods of preparation thereof, Syntex, U.S.A., U.S. Patent #4,082,735.

USES: Threonyl-MDP is included in adjuvant formulations as a primary adjuvant component.

APPEARANCE: White to off-white, odorless powder.

MOLECULAR WEIGHT: 522.5

RECOMMENDED STORAGE: The powdered drug substance should be stored dessicated at or below 25°C. For optimal stability, solutions (0.5–10 mg/mL) of threonyl-MDP should be formulated between pH 3.5 and 5.5; under this condition, a 2-year shelf life at 25°C can be expected. Solutions of threonyl-MDP formulated in a broader pH range of 1.5 to 7.5 show a 2-year shelf life if stored at 5°C.

• Powell, M. F., *et al.*, 1988, Formulation of vaccine adjuvant muramyldipeptides. 2. Thermal reactivity and pH of maximum stability of MDP compounds in aqueous solution, *Pharm. Res.* **5**:528.

CHEMICAL/PHYSICAL PROPERTIES: Threonyl-MDP has an aqueous solubility of >600 mg/mL. The pKa of the isoglutamine carboxylic acid is 4.3. The compound is very hygroscopic and found to deliquesce at ≥ 68% relative humidity.

INCOMPATIBILITY: Avoid strong bases.

SAFETY/TOXICITY: At therapeutic doses, no safety concern is anticipated. The dose is indication dependent, but a guideline is 0.05–1% (w/w), with an injection volume of ~1 mL.

ADJUVANT PROPERTIES: Threonyl-MDP induces the production of a cascade of cytokines, including IL-1α, IL-1β and IL-6. Responding lymphocytes release IL-2 and IFN-γ. The latter increases the production of antibodies of certain isotypes, including IgG2a in the mouse. This isotype, and the homologous IgG1 in primates, interacts with high affinity Fcγ receptors, so that the antibodies can function efficiently in opsonizing viruses and other infectious agents for uptake by phagocytic cells.

• Allison, A. C., and Byars, N. E., 1992, Syntex Adjuvant Formulation, *Res. Immunol.* **143**:519–525.
• Allison, A. C., and Byars, N. E., 1986, An adjuvant formulation that selectively elicits the formation of antibodies of protective isotypes and of cell-mediated immunity, *J. Immunol. Methods* **95**:157–168.
• Lidgate, D. M., and Byars, N., Chapter 12, this volume.

CONTACT(S): Deborah M. Lidgate, Syntex, Palo Alto, CA 94304, Ph: 415-852-1887; Fax: 415-852-1784.

COMPONENT/ADJUVANT NAME: Ty Particles

OTHER NAME(S): Ty-VLPs (Virus Like Particles)

STRUCTURE: Amino acids 1–381 of the p1 protein encoded by the yeast retrotransposon Ty, followed by a unique restriction site for the insertion of foreign sequences and a translational stop codon.

Sequence of the p1 Ty protein:

MESQQLSQHSPISHGSACASVTSKEVHTNQDPLDVSASKTEECEKASTKANSQ
QTTTPASSAVPENPHHASPQTAQSHSPQNGPYPQQCMMTQNQANPSGWSFYG
HPSMIPYTPYQMSPMYFPPGPQSQFPQYPSSVGTPLRTPSPESGNTFTDSSSADS
DMTSTKKYVRPPPMLTSPNDFPNWVKTYIKFLQNSNLGGIIPTVNGKPVRQITD
DELTFLYNTFQIFAPSQFLPTWVKDILSVDYTDIMKILSKSIEKMQSDTQEANDI
VTLANLQYNGSTPADAFETKVTNIIDRLNNNGIHINNKVACQLIMRGLSGEYKF
LRYTRHRHLNMTVAELFLDIHAIYEEQQGSRNSKPNYRRNPSDEKNDSRSYTN
TTKPKAGS K*

SOURCE: Recombinant protein produced from *Saccharomyces cerevisiae*. Purified by filtration and chromatography techniques.

USES: As a carrier protein for expressing foreign antigens. Hybrid Ty particles induce cell-mediated immunity (without additional adjuvant) and humoral immunity (with aluminum hydroxide).

APPEARANCE: Clear aqueous solution.

MOLECULAR WEIGHT: Monomer 42,000

RECOMMENDED STORAGE: Store purified Ty particles at –20°C. Particles formulated with aluminum hydroxide should not be frozen, and can be stored at 4°C for 1–2 years.

CHEMICAL/PHYSICAL PROPERTIES: Approximately 300 monomers assemble to form a Ty particle.

INCOMPATIBILITY: Avoid contact with proteases.

SAFETY/TOXICITY: No systemic toxicity observed in human Phase I clinical trials (maximum dose 0.5 mg/subject, administered 4 times).

ADJUVANT PROPERTIES: Ty particles present antigen in a polyvalent, particulate form. Cytotoxic T lymphocytes are induced in the absence of any other adjuvant formulations.

- Adams, S. E., *et al.*, 1987, The expression of hybrid Ty virus-like particles in yeast, *Nature* **329**:68–70.
- Layton, G. T., *et al.*, 1993, Induction of HIV-1 specific cytotoxic T-lymphocytes in vivo by immunization with hybrid HIV-1: Ty virus-like particles, *J. Immunol.* **151**:1097–1107.
- Adams, S., and Kingsman, A., Chapter 34, this volume.

CONTACT(S): Dr. Sally E. Adams, British Biotech., Oxford, OX4 5LY, UK, Ph: 44-1235-551151; Fax: 44-1235-551155.

COMPONENT/ADJUVANT NAME: Walter Reed Liposomes

OTHER NAME(S): Liposomes containing lipid A adsorbed to aluminum hydroxide, [L(Lipid A + Antigen) + Alum]

STRUCTURE: Phospholipids: dimyristoyl phosphatidylcholine and dimyristoyl phosphatidylglycerol; cholesterol, Lipid A: from *Salmonella minnesota* R595, heterogeneous mixture of structures, molecular weight ranging from 1400 to 1800 depending on number of fatty acids and phosphate groups present, aluminum hydroxide gel.

SOURCE: Phospholipids and cholesterol are obtained in pure form, GMP grade, from Avanti Polar Lipids, Inc. Native lipid A, prepared by acid hydrolysis of the lipopolysaccharide of *S. minnesota* R595, is obtained from List Biological Laboratories. Monophosphoryl lipid A is obtained from Ribi ImmunoChem. Aluminum hydroxide gel is Alhydrogel or Rehydragel LV.

USES: Liposomes provide a vehicle for delivery of antigen to the immune system and also a mild adjuvant activity, but liposomes containing lipid A provide a very potent adjuvant activity. Adsorption of liposomes containing lipid A to aluminum hydroxide gel contributes additional strong adjuvant activity with many antigens. Liposomes containing lipid A have been shown to induce both humoral and cell-mediated immunity.

APPEARANCE: White, opalescent particulate suspension.

MOLECULAR WEIGHT: Equal to the sum of the molecular weights of the components used in the formulation, e.g., antigen molecular weight will vary with the vaccine formulation.

RECOMMENDED STORAGE: Store liquid liposome formulations at 4–6°C. Lyophilized liposomes prior to reconstitution with antigen may be stored at either 4–6°C or –20°C. Liposomes in the liquid form reconstituted with antigen are stable for at least 1–2 years.

CHEMICAL/PHYSICAL PROPERTIES: Liposomes are stable at pH from 1 to 10. Solubility and stability will depend on the antigen encapsulated. Phospholipids, cholesterol, and native lipid A are soluble in chloroform. Monophosphoryl lipid A is soluble in chloroform–methanol 9:1. All liposomal components are stable in organic solvents for at least 1 year when stored at –20°C.

INCOMPATIBILITY: None found.

SAFETY/TOXICITY: Liposomal vaccine formulations have been administered to humans in four Phase I or Phase I/IIa clinical trials (three containing recombinant antigens derived from the *Plasmodium falciparum* sporozoite and one containing gp120 derived from the envelope of HIV). The vaccine formulations used in all four trials passed all preclinical safety and toxicity tests and no adverse side reactions have been observed.

- Fries, L. F., *et al.*, 1992, Liposomal malaria vaccine in humans: A safe and potent adjuvant strategy, *Proc. Natl. Acad. Sci. USA* **89**:358–362.

ADJUVANT PROPERTIES:

- Alving, C. R., and Richards, R. L., 1990, Liposomes containing lipid A: A potent nontoxic adjuvant for a human malaria sporozoite vaccine, *Immunol. Lett.* **25**:275–280.
- Verma, J. N., *et al.*, 1992, Adjuvant effects of liposomes containing lipid A: Enhancement of liposomal antigen presentation and recruitment of macrophages, *Infect. Immun.* **60**:2438–2444.
- Alving, C. R., *et al.*, 1992, Liposomes containing lipid A as a potent non-toxic adjuvant, *Res. Immunol.* **143**:249–251.
- Alving, C. R., *et al.*, 1993, Novel adjuvant strategies for experimental malaria and AIDS vaccines, *Ann. N.Y. Acad. Sci.* **690**:265–275.

CONTACT(S): Dr. Carl Alving, Dr. Nabila Wassef and Dr. Roberta Richards, Department of Membrane Biochemistry, Walter Reed Army Institute of Research, Washington, DC 20307-5100, Ph: 202-782-3248; Fax: 202-782-0721.

3. ACKNOWLEDGMENTS AND UPDATE SUMMARY

This compendium would not have been possible without the enormous support we received from vaccinologists, formulators, immunologists, and others worldwide. We are indebted to the following contributors for both general guidance and, in many cases, sending us up-to-date information on specific vaccine adjuvants and components: Sally Adams (British BioTechnology, Oxford, UK); Carl Alving (Walter Reed Army Institute of Research, Washington, DC); Françoise Audibert (Vacsyn SA, Paris, France); Gail Barchfeld (Chiron Corp., Emeryville, CA); Bob Baughman (Emisphere Technologies, Hawthorne, NY); Joan Bell (Genetics Institute, Cambridge, MA); Diana Boraschi (Dompè S.p.A., L'Aquila, Italy); Eugene Bortnek, (Seppic, Fairfield, NJ); James N. Brewer (University of Strathclyde, Glasgow, UK); Robert Brey (Vaxcel, Inc., Norcross, GA); Louis Chedid (Vacsyn SA, Paris, France); Robert Chesnut (Cytel Corp., San Diego, CA); Linda C. Clarke (Washington Research Foundation, Seattle, WA); Jeffrey Cleland (Genentech, Inc., S. San Francisco, CA); John Clements (Tulane University, New Orleans, LA); Peter D. Cooper (John Curtin School of Medical Research, Canberra, Australia); Peter Cooper (CC Biotech, Poway, CA); Raymond Daynes (University of Utah, Salt Lake City, UT); Phillipe DeLafaire (Seppic SA, Paris, France); David Dodds (Schering Corp., Bloomfield, NJ); Friedrich Dorner (Immuno AG, Ortha Donau, Austria); Johann Eibl (Immuno AG, Vienna, Austria); Vincent Ganne (Seppic SA, Paris, France); Maury Gately (Hoffmann–LaRoche, Nutley, NJ); Karen Goldenthal (FDA, Washington, DC); Michael Goodman (Scripps Research Institute, La Jolla, CA); Geoffrey Gorse (Saint Louis University, St. Louis, MO); Susan Gould-Fogerite (UMDNJ, NJ Medical School, Newark, NJ); Rajesh Gupta (Mass. Institute of Public Health, Jamaica Plain, MA); Nabil Hanna (IDEC Pharmaceuticals, San Diego, CA); Robert Hanson (3M Pharmaceuticals, St. Paul, MN); Andy Heath (University of Sheffield Medical School, Sheffield, UK); Stanley Hem (Purdue University, West Lafayette, IN); Cliff Hendrick (Genzyme Corp., Cambridge, MA); Luuk Hilgers (Solvay SA, Brussels, Belgium); Rodney Ho (University of Washington, Seattle, WA); Maninder Hora (Chiron Corp., Emeryville, CA); Huw Hughes (M6 Pharmaceuticals, Yonkers, NY); Robert Hunter (Emory University, Atlanta, GA); Arthur Johnson (University of Minnesota, Duluth, MN); Stephen Kaminsky (United Biomedical Inc., Hauppauge, NY); Charlotte Kensil (Cambridge Biotech, Worcester, MA); Philip B. Klepak (Reheis Inc., Berkeley Heights, NJ); Jorg Kreuter (Johann Wolfgang Goethe-Universität, Frankfurt, Germany); Lawrence Lachman (M. D. Anderson Cancer Center, Houston, TX); Robert Leather (Reheis, Inc., Berkeley Heights, NJ); Philip Ledger (Peptech (UK) Ltd., Cirencester, Glos, UK); Deborah Lidgate (Syntex Research, Palo Alto, CA); Amy Lim (Genentech, Inc., South San Francisco, CA); Erik B. Lindblad (Superfos Biosector a/s, Vedbaek, Denmark); Oswald Lockhoff (Bayer AG, Leverkusen, Germany); Nils Lycke (University of Göteborg, Göteborg, Sweden); Jeannine Majde (Office of Naval Research, Arlington, VA); Raphael Mannino (UMDNJ, NJ Medical School, Newark, NJ); Richard McIntosh (Genesis Tech. Group, Cambridge, MA); Richard Miller (3M Pharmaceuticals,

St. Paul, MN); Nahid Mohagheghpour (SRI International, Menlo Park, CA); Bror Morein (National Veterinary Institute, Uppsala, Sweden); Kent R. Myers (Ribi ImmunoChem, Hamilton, MT); Tattanahalli Nagabhushan (Schering Corp., Bloomfield, NJ); Marian Neutra (Harvard Medical School, Boston, MA); Tony Newton (Genzyme Corp., Cambridge, MA); Jack Nunberg (Genentech, Inc., S. San Francisco, CA); Keiko Oishi (Genentech, Inc., Japan); Albert Osterhaus (Erasmus University, Rotterdam, Sweden); Gary Ott (Chiron Corp., Emeryville, CA); Lendon Payne (VRI, Cambridge, MA); Christopher Penney (BioChem Therapeutic Inc., Quebec, Canada); Ramachandran Radhakrishnan (Chiron Corp., Emeryville, CA); Mike Ramstack (Medisorb Tech. Intl., Cincinnati, OH); Al Reisch (Sargeant, Inc., Clifton, NJ); John Rhodes (The Wellcome Research Labs, Kent, UK); Roberta L. Richards (Walter Reed Army Institute of Research, Washington, DC); Bryan Roberts (VRI, Cambridge, MA); Thomas Ryskamp (IDEC Pharmaceuticals Corp., San Diego, CA); Noemi Santiago (Emisphere Technologies, Hawthorne, NY); Paul Sleath (Immunex Corp., Seattle, WA); Christine Smart (Proteus International, PLC, Macclesfield, UK); H. Snippe (University Utrecht, Utrecht, Netherlands); Alvin S. Stern (Hoffmann–LaRoche, Nutley, NJ); Bo G. Sundqvist (Iscotec, Uppsala, Sweden); Aldo Tagliabue (Dompè S.p.A., L'Aquila, Italy); J. Terry Ulrich (Ribi ImmunoChem, Hamilton, MT); Peter van Hoogevest (Ciba Geigy, Basel, Switzerland); Gary Van Nest (Chiron Corp., Emeryville, CA); Gerald Vosika (ImmunoTherapeutics, Inc., Fargo, ND); Nabila M. Wassef (Walter Reed Army Institute of Research, Washington, DC); Robert Weissburg (Genentech, Inc., South San Francisco, CA); Stan Wolf (Genetics Institute, Cambridge, MA).

We also thank Jessica Burdman for technical editing and organizational aspects, and Mili Chin for secretarial assistance. Tom Patapoff played a key role in translating several summaries from "unusual" format to Mac or PC format. A special thanks to Rodney Pearlman for supporting this work, and to Igor Gonda for his help. A great deal of adjuvant support and advice was also provided by Phil Berman, Tim Gregory, and Jack Obijeski, all of Genentech.

Finally, it is our goal to update this compendium in 1996–1997. Our goal is to present an accurate listing of vaccine adjuvants available for use in basic research, and preclinical and clinical evaluation. In some cases, we have shown only a few of the possible contacts or suppliers available for a particular adjuvant, of consideration in keeping this compendium as short as possible. Many suppliers often exist for a particular adjuvant and its components. If you would like to update a monograph in the next edition of this compendium, or contribute a new one, please send your information to:

Dr. Michael F. Powell
Genentech, Inc. MS#82
460 Pt. San Bruno Blvd.
South San Francisco, CA 94080
Ph: 415-225-1389
Fax: 415-225-2866
E-mail: powell.mike@gene.com

Chapter 8

Adjuvant Properties of Aluminum and Calcium Compounds

Rajesh K. Gupta, Bradford E. Rost,
Edgar Relyveld, and George R. Siber

1. INTRODUCTION

Aluminum compounds, including aluminum phosphate ($AlPO_4$), aluminum hydroxide [$Al(OH)_3$], and alum-precipitated vaccines (historically referred to as protein aluminate), are currently widely used with human vaccines. These adjuvants have often been referred to as "alum" in the literature. Alum, which chemically is potassium aluminum sulfate [$KAl(SO_4)_2 \cdot 12H_2O$], has not been used as an adjuvant as such. Rather, it was used to partially purify protein antigens, mainly tetanus toxoid (TT) and diphtheria toxoid (DT) by precipitating them in the presence of anions including phosphate and bicarbonate ions resulting in a mixture of compounds, mainly aluminum phosphate and aluminum hydroxide (Holt, 1950; Aprile and Wardlaw, 1966). The amounts of aluminum phosphate and aluminum hydroxide in the mixture depended on the amount and nature of anions present in the reaction mixture and adjustment of pH of the final product with sodium hydroxide (Relyveld, 1986; Nicklas, 1992). Although alum-precipitated TT and DT had been used for human immunization for many years, their use has declined considerably because of variations in production of alum-precipitated toxoids (van Ramshorst, 1949; Holt, 1950; Aprile and Wardlaw, 1966; Gupta *et al.,* 1993). Referring to all aluminum adjuvants as "alum" is misleading because aluminum hydroxide and aluminum phosphate have different physical characteristics (see Chapter 9) and differ in their adjuvant properties.

Aluminum adjuvants have a long history of use with routine childhood vaccines since it was discovered that a suspension of alum-precipitated DT had much higher immunogenicity than the soluble toxoid (Glenny *et al.,* 1926). During the 1930s the superiority of

Rajesh K. Gupta, Bradford E. Rost, and George R. Siber • Massachusetts Public Health Biologic Laboratories, State Laboratory Institute, Boston, Massachusetts 02130.   *Edgar Relyveld* • Office d'Etudes en Vaccinologie, Paris, France.

Vaccine Design: The Subunit and Adjuvant Approach, edited by Michael F. Powell and Mark J. Newman. Plenum Press, New York, 1995.

alum-precipitated DT and TT in humans was well established (White and Schlageter, 1934; Jones and Moss, 1936; Volk and Bunney, 1939, 1942; Aprile and Wardlaw, 1966) and use of aluminum adjuvants with diphtheria–tetanus–pertussis (DTP) vaccines became common.

Calcium phosphate is the other mineral salt adjuvant used with routine childhood vaccines. DTP and inactivated polio vaccines, and allergens adsorbed onto calcium phosphate have been used for many years mainly in France (Relyveld, 1980, 1986; Gupta *et al.,* 1993; Relyveld and Chermann, 1994). The use of calcium phosphate as an adjuvant was described during the 1960s by Relyveld and colleagues (Relyveld *et al.,* 1964, 1969; Relyveld and Raynaud, 1967).

2. ALUMINUM COMPOUNDS

Since aluminum compounds are the only adjuvants used for human vaccines, these have become the benchmark or reference preparations for evaluating new adjuvant formulations for human vaccines. Aluminum adjuvants have been described as difficult to manufacture in a physicochemically reproducible way, thus resulting in batch-to-batch variations (Edelman, 1980; Alving *et al.,* 1993). Adsorption of antigens on aluminum adjuvants depends on the physical and chemical characteristics of the antigen, type of aluminum adjuvant, and conditions of adsorption (van Ramshorst, 1949; Edelman, 1980; Lindblad and Sparck, 1987; Bomford, 1989; Nicklas, 1992). These conditions are often overlooked and a poorly formulated aluminum adjuvant preparation does not give optimal adjuvanticity. To minimize the variations and to avoid the nonreproducibility resulting from use of different preparations of aluminum compounds, a specific preparation (Alhydrogel®, aluminum hydroxide, from Superfos Biosector, Vedbaek, Denmark) was recommended as a scientific standard for evaluation of new adjuvant formulations (Stewart-Tull, 1989). However, complete adsorption of each antigen under study on aluminum adjuvants should be verified and the conditions of adsorption optimized, if necessary.

2.1. Method of Preparation

Two methods have commonly been used to prepare vaccines and toxoids with aluminum compounds: in situ precipitation of aluminum compounds in the presence of antigen, and adsorption of antigen onto preformed aluminum gel (Aprile and Wardlaw, 1966; Edelman, 1980). In situ precipitation of TT and DT in culture medium used for growing the organisms containing anions including phosphate and bicarbonate ions with potassium or sodium alum is the original method developed primarily for purifying toxoids (Seal and Johnson, 1941; Bomford, 1989). Vaccines prepared by this method were referred to as alum-precipitated toxoids and showed higher immunogenicity than the soluble preparations. Alum-precipitated vaccines were a mixture of aluminum compounds, mainly aluminum phosphate and aluminum hydroxide. This product was difficult to manufacture in a consistent and reproducible manner (van Ramshorst, 1949; Holt, 1950; Aprile and Wardlaw, 1966; Gupta *et al.,* 1993). In 1976, a World Health Organization report described this method as a laboratory procedure that did not define the nature of the material obtained either quantitatively or qualitatively. For these reasons this product is not very common now.

In situ adsorption of antigens on aluminum phosphate has also been carried out by suspending purified vaccine antigens in dibasic or tribasic sodium phosphate or phosphate buffer and precipitating it with aluminum chloride. This type of reaction is carried out under controlled conditions and results in a consistent product.

Currently the most commonly used method for preparation of aluminum-adsorbed vaccines is adsorption of antigens on preformed aluminum phosphate or aluminum hydroxide gels under controlled conditions (Bomford, 1989). These preparations are usually referred to as aluminum phosphate- or aluminum hydroxide-adsorbed or -adjuvanted vaccines. Gels of aluminum phosphate and aluminum hydroxide for human use (of clinical grade) are commercially available with a good uniformity. Adsorption of antigens is also carried out on freshly prepared aluminum phosphate gel (Gupta and Siber, 1994).

2.2. Factors Affecting the Adsorption

Adsorption of antigens on aluminum salts depends heavily on electrostatic forces between adjuvant and antigen. Other interactions including hydrophobic, van der Waals, and hydrogen bonding contribute to the adsorption of antigens on aluminum adjuvants. However, these forces may not suffice to cause adsorption of antigen if the same charge (electrostatic repulsive force) is present on antigen and adjuvant. The two most commonly used aluminum adjuvants, aluminum hydroxide and aluminum phosphate, have different points of zero charge (Al-Shakhshir et al., 1994). At neutral pH these gels have opposite charges, i.e., aluminum phosphate is negatively charged and aluminum hydroxide is positively charged. It is important to select the aluminum adjuvant carefully on the basis of the charge of the antigen at neutral pH. Physical conditions affecting adsorption of antigens on aluminum adjuvants include pH, temperature, and ionic strength of the reaction mixture (van Ramshorst, 1949; Lindblad and Sparck, 1987; Bomford, 1989).

Acidic pH of less than 6 has been found optimal for adsorption of antigens on aluminum adjuvants (van Ramshorst, 1949). The optimal pH for adsorption of TT and DT onto aluminum phosphate was 6.0–6.3 (Table I). The adsorption of DT was influenced by the presence of excess phosphate ions in the reaction mixture (Tables I and II). Lindblad and Sparck (1987) recommended avoiding phosphate-buffered saline in the reaction mixture for adsorption of antigen onto aluminum adjuvants. Freshly prepared aluminum phosphate gel appeared to give the highest absorption (Table I), but it is not clear whether this is related to the higher gel concentration or to higher adsorption capacity of fresh gels. In situ adsorption of DT resulted in higher adsorption than the commercial aluminum phosphate preparation. Adsorption of TT and DT onto aluminum hydroxide gel (Alhydrogel®) was not sensitive to the conditions of pH and excess phosphate ions. In contrast, a low ionic strength and absence of excess phosphate ions and impurities are recommended for optimal adsorption of antigens on aluminum phosphate gel (Bomford, 1989). Excess anions, particularly phosphate ions, and impurities (amino acids, peptides, and polysaccharides) reduce protein adsorption, probably by competing with antigen for adsorption sites (Lindblad and Sparck, 1987). The temperature of adsorption is important for complete adsorption of antigen onto aluminum phosphate although most of the adsorption (up to 80–90% of DT) occurred within a few minutes at temperatures ranging from 4 to 45°C (van Ramshorst, 1949).

Table I
Effect of pH and Excess Phosphate Ions on the Adsorption of
TT and DT onto Aluminum Adjuvants

Adjuvant type and concentration	Conditions of adsorption		% adsorption[a]	
	Medium	pH	Tetanus toxoid	Diphtheria toxoid
Aluminum phosphate in situ[b], 1.36 mg/mL	PBS[c]	7.2	71	0
		6.0–6.3	94	57
	Saline	7.2	75	13
		6.0–6.3	100	100
Aluminum phosphate freshly made[d], 4 mg/mL	PBS[c]	7.2	85	0
		6.0–6.3	99	93
	Saline	7.2	85	52
		6.0–6.3	99	93
Aluminum phosphate Adju-Phos[®e], 2 mg/mL	PBS[c]	7.2	60	0
		6.0–6.3	97	46
	Saline	7.2	83	0
		6.0–6.3	100	55
Aluminum hydroxide Alhydrogel[®e], 2 mg/mL	PBS[c]	7.2	100	99
		6.0–6.3	100	100
	Saline	7.2	100	100
		6.0–6.3	100	100

[a]Tetanus toxoid at 10 Lf/mL and diphtheria toxoid at 20 Lf/mL were adsorbed onto various gels at room temperature overnight and supernatants after centrifugation were assayed for unadsorbed antigen by a sandwich-type capture ELISA (Gupta and Siber, 1994).
[b]In situ adsorption on aluminum phosphate was carried out by suspending the antigens in phosphate buffer (1.0× concn., see Table II), precipitating with aluminum chloride, and adjusting pH with sodium hydroxide.
[c]PBS = phosphate-buffered saline with 0.01 M phosphate buffer.
[d]Prepared by precipitation of trisodium phosphate and aluminum chloride, adjusting pH with sodium hydroxide, followed by addition of antigens (Gupta and Siber, 1994).
[e]From Superfos Biosector, Vedbaek, Denmark.

There has been some discussion on the desorption of antigen from adjuvant after injection into the body where a physiologically neutral pH and presence of body fluids containing proteins and anions might desorb the antigen from the gel. Earlier studies showed that freshly made preparations of aluminum phosphate-adsorbed DT showed more antigen desorption than aged preparations when exposed to neutral pH or serum (van Ramshorst, 1949). Aging of aluminum-adsorbed vaccines improved their immunogenicity also (Holt, 1950).

Aluminum hydroxide (Alhydrogel[®]) showed higher adsorption of TT (273.4 Lf or ~820 μg/mg gel) and DT (126.6 Lf or ~380 μg/mg gel) than aluminum phosphate (Adju-phos[®]) (53.5 Lf or ~161 μg TT/mg gel) at room temperature overnight at a pH of 6.0 (R. K. Gupta, P. Griffin, and G. R. Siber, unpublished data). Nicklas (1992) described adsorption of 50–200 μg protein/mg aluminum hydroxide gel. Lindblad and Sparck (1987) found 10–20 times more adsorption of human serum albumin on aluminum hydroxide than on aluminum phosphate.

Table II
In Situ Adsorption of DT at 20 Lf/mL onto Aluminum Phosphate Gel (0.3 mg Aluminum/mL) with Varying Concentration of Excess Phosphate Ions Present during Precipitation

Excess phosphate buffer concn.[a]	pH	% adsorption
1.0×	6.00[b]	100
1.0×	6.40[b]	78
3.8×	6.00	60
5.0×	6.25	25
10.0×	6.75	0
10.0×	6.00[c]	34

[a]0.792 mL of 1.12 M phosphate buffer (a mixture of Na_2HPO_4, 12.5 g, and $NaH_2PO_4 \cdot H_2O$, 3.3 g, in 100 mL) for 100 mL of gel is 1.0× concn. For the preparation of in situ aluminum phosphate gel, antigens in a total volume of 100 mL with 0.792 mL of 1.12 M phosphate buffer are precipitated with 2.7 mL of 10% $AlCl_3 \cdot 6H_2O$ and pH adjusted immediately to 6 with sodium hydroxide.

[b]pH adjusted with sodium hydroxide immediately after forming the gel.

[c]pH adjusted with hydrochloric acid immediately after forming the gel.

2.3. Adjuvant Properties

The adjuvanticity of aluminum adjuvants for human vaccines, particularly TT and DT, was clearly established during the 1930s (White and Schlageter, 1934; Jones and Moss, 1936; Volk and Bunney, 1939, 1942). Thereafter, the use of aluminum adjuvants became common, although a few reports stated that alum-adjuvanted vaccines were not better than soluble vaccines (Aprile and Wardlaw, 1966). The major advantage of using aluminum adjuvants was the development of earlier, higher, and longer-lasting immunity after primary immunization compared to soluble vaccines (Volk and Bunney, 1939, 1942). There are numerous reports in humans and animals showing the superiority of aluminum-adsorbed TT and DT over soluble toxoids, particularly after the first dose or for primary immunization (Levine *et al.,* 1961, 1966; Aprile and Wardlaw, 1966; Levine, 1972; MacLennan *et al.,* 1973; Menon *et al.,* 1976; Ahuja *et al.,* 1986; Jensen and Koch, 1988; Bomford, 1989; Gupta and Siber, 1994). However, aluminum-adsorbed vaccines did not show any advantage over soluble preparations for the booster or secondary response (Ipsen, 1954; Haas and Thomssen, 1961; Collier *et al.,* 1979; Jensen and Koch, 1988; Gupta and Siber, 1994; Mark and Granstrom, 1994). The adsorbed TT was more reliable than soluble toxoid when given simultaneously with an injection of tetanus antitoxin (Suri and Rubbo, 1961; Fulthorpe, 1965; Levine *et al.,* 1966). Aluminum adjuvants are universally used with the DTP vaccine. However, the adjuvant effect of aluminum adjuvants on whole cell pertussis vaccine is not clear. Although serum agglutinins to *Bordetella pertussis* after immunization with aluminum-adjuvanted pertussis vaccine were higher than those obtained after inoculation with unadsorbed pertussis vaccine (Preston *et al.,* 1974; Preston, 1976, 1979; Cameron, 1985; Gupta *et al.,* 1990), there was no difference between unadsorbed and adjuvanted pertussis vaccine with regard to protection against disease (Butler *et al.,* 1962a). The adjuvant effect of aluminum phosphate or aluminum hydroxide on the mouse intracerebral potency of whole cell pertussis vaccine is controversial. In a few studies, the potency of adjuvanted vaccine was higher than the nonadjuvanted pertussis vaccine (Pittman, 1954; Cameron, 1976, 1979; Gupta *et al.,* 1987) and in other studies the adjuvant did not have any effect on potency (Aprile and Wardlaw, 1966; Cameron and Knight, 1972; Novotny and Brookes, 1975; Gupta *et al.,* 1992). Nevertheless, aluminum compounds are routinely used with the acellular pertussis vaccine (Sato *et al.,* 1984; Ad Hoc Group for the Study of Pertussis Vaccines, 1988; Krantz *et al.,* 1990; Siber *et al.,* 1991; Podda *et al.,* 1991). Aluminum compounds have also been used with inactivated polio vaccine (Butler *et al.,* 1962b), human diploid cell strain rabies vaccine (Kuwert *et al.,* 1978), hepatitis B vaccine (Murray *et al.,* 1984) and with the newly developed vaccine against hepatitis A (Andre *et al.,* 1990; Peetermans, 1992). Aluminum hydroxide-adsorbed cholera vaccine provided higher protection than the unadsorbed cholera vaccine (Saroso *et al.,* 1978).

The immunogenicity of antigens adsorbed onto aluminum adjuvants depends on a number of factors, most importantly on the degree of adsorption of antigen on the adjuvant and the dose of adjuvant. Table III shows that the immunogenicity in mice of DT adsorbed onto aluminum adjuvants depends on the degree of adsorption. The formulation which did not show any adsorption of DT onto aluminum phosphate because of the presence of a tenfold excess of phosphate did not elicit antibodies to DT after the first injection and showed a poor response after the second dose. Adsorption of 80% or more of TT and DT onto aluminum adjuvants is recommended by the World Health Organization (1977). The United States Minimum Requirements (1956) for adult tetanus and diphtheria toxoid specify at least 75% adsorption of DT component on the aluminum adjuvants.

The dose of aluminum adjuvant also affects the overall immunogenicity (Bomford, 1989). Although a small amount of aluminum adjuvant is required for complete adsorption of the antigen, such low doses, even though they completely adsorb the antigens, may not show an optimal adjuvant effect. There appears to be a need for excess free adjuvant to obtain an optimal adjuvant effect (Jensen and Koch, 1988; Cooper *et al.,* 1991). As the amount of aluminum adjuvant is increased, the adjuvant effect increased up to a certain concentration after which the adjuvant effect declined with further increases in aluminum adjuvant concentration (Prigge, 1942, 1949; Holt, 1955; Hennessen, 1965; Schmidt, 1967; Bomford, 1989). The reasons for this optimum concentration of adjuvant are unknown. We speculate that a certain minimum amount of aluminum compound is necessary to form a depot at the site of injection or to optimally stimulate macrophages. Excessive amounts of aluminum compounds may suppress immunity by covering the antigen completely with mineral compounds (Haas *et al.,* 1955; Haas and Thomssen, 1961) or by being toxic to macrophages as aluminum compounds are somewhat cytotoxic to macrophages (Munder *et al.,* 1969). Several studies showed lower immunogenicity/potency of aluminum-adsorbed vaccines diluted in saline in mice and guinea pigs than those diluted in the aluminum adjuvant (Hennessen, 1965, 1967; Relyveld, 1985). It has been stressed that dilution of adjuvanted vaccines may disturb the composition of the vaccine (Hennessen, 1965, 1967; J. Lyng, personal communication). We, therefore, recommend that for immunogenicity studies of aluminum compound-adsorbed antigens in animals, the formulation intended for human use should be injected with a minimum dilution, preferably undiluted. The usual dose of aluminum used for human vaccines is around 0.5 mg. The upper allowable limit of aluminum adjuvants for injection in humans is 1.25 mg aluminum as per World Health Organization regulations (1990) and 0.85 to 1.25 mg aluminum as per United States Food and Drug Administration guidelines (May *et al.,* 1984).

Aluminum hydroxide has been found to be a more potent adjuvant than aluminum phosphate (Levine *et al.,* 1955; Berman *et al.,* 1985). This may be related to higher adsorption capacity and better adsorption of certain antigens at neutral pH by aluminum hydroxide than aluminum phosphate (Table I). Aluminum hydroxide-adjuvanted antigens showed similar or superior antibody responses than the antigens given with complete Freund's adjuvant (CFA) (Bomford, 1980a; Woodard, 1989). We have observed that DT adsorbed onto aluminum phosphate under optimal conditions showed antibody levels in rabbits similar to those elicited by DT given with CFA (C. Varanelli, R. K. Gupta, D. Wallach, and G. R. Siber, unpublished data). Aluminum hydroxide is a good adjuvant for weak antigens in mice but saponin and CFA are more potent adjuvants than aluminum hydroxide for strong antigens (Bomford, 1984, 1989). We have observed that aluminum phosphate is a very strong adjuvant for TT and DT in outbred CD-1 mice (Table III and Fig. 1). The antibody response in mice obtained after a single dose of TT adsorbed onto aluminum phosphate was higher and longer lasting than after soluble toxoid (Fig. 1). Guinea pigs also showed similar high and long-lasting antibody responses after a single injection (Fig. 2).

Table III

Effect of Degree of Adsorption of DT onto Aluminum Adjuvants on Immunogenicity in Mice[a]

	Dose per mouse			GM[b] anti-DT IgG (μg/mL) after	
Adjuvant	Adjuvant (mg)	DT (μg)	Adsorption (%)	First dose	Second dose
Aluminum phosphate (in situ)	0.068	1.5	0	0.04 (0.01–0.22)	8.1 (1.4–46.8)
	0.068	1.5	90	11.0 (4.6–26.3)	380.9 (211.7–685.4)
	0.068	1.5	100	9.4 (3.9–22.4)	361.3 (169.8–769.1)
	0.068	3.0	78	2.9 (0.9–9.0)	157.8 (54.4–457.6)
Aluminum phosphate (freshly made)	0.200	3.0	100	62.6 (44.9–87.4)	919.3 (643.1–1314.1)
Aluminum hydroxide (Alhydrogel®)	0.033	1.5	100	49.1 (19.3–125.1)	424.6 (162.6–1108.6)
	0.033	3.0	100	29.2 (12.9–65.7)	791.8 (345.0–1817.3)
	0.100	1.5	100	45.0 (17.3–116.9)	1021.2 (573.2–1819.4)
None	—	1.5	—	0.03	0.3

[a]Four-week-old female outbred (CD-1 strain) mice were injected with diphtheria toxoid subcutaneously twice at an interval of 30 days. Mice were bled 4 weeks after the first and 2 weeks after the second dose. IgG antibodies to diphtheria toxoid were determined in the sera of individual mice by ELISA.

[b]GM = geometric mean with 95% confidence intervals in parentheses.

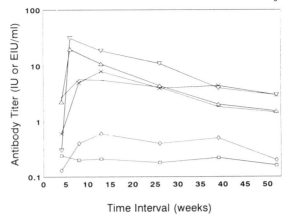

Figure 1. IgG and neutralizing antibodies to tetanus toxin in sera of mice (4-week-old female, CD-1) injected with a single dose (5 Lf or ~12.5 μg) of soluble TT (□, IgG to tetanus toxin by ELISA; ◇, tetanus antitoxin); of aluminum phosphate-adsorbed TT (+, IgG to tetanus toxin by ELISA; X, tetanus antitoxin); and two doses (0.5 Lf or ~1.25 μg each at an interval of 4 weeks) of aluminum phosphate-adsorbed TT (△, IgG to tetanus toxin by ELISA; ▽, tetanus antitoxin). The mice were bled at different intervals and IgG antibodies in the individual sera and neutralizing antibodies (tetanus antitoxin) on the pooled sera were determined by ELISA in ELISA International Units (EIU)/mL and toxin neutralization test in mice in IU/mL, respectively (Gupta and Siber, 1994).

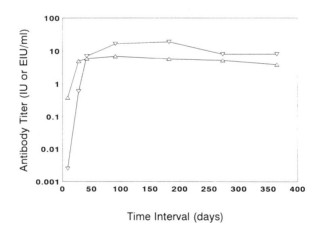

Figure 2. IgG and neutralizing antibodies to tetanus toxin in sera of guinea pigs (female, Hartley, 450–550 g) injected with a single dose (7.5 Lf or ~18.75 μg) of aluminum phosphate-adsorbed TT (△, IgG to tetanus toxin by ELISA; ▽, tetanus antitoxin). The guinea pigs were bled at different intervals and IgG antibodies in the individual sera and neutralizing antibodies (tetanus antitoxin) on the pooled sera were determined by ELISA in EIU/mL and toxin neutralization test in mice in IU/mL, respectively (Gupta and Siber, 1994).

2.4. Mechanism of Action

Glenny *et al.* (1931) proposed that aluminum adjuvants act by depot formation at the site of injection, allowing the slow release of antigen, and thus prolonging the time for interaction between antigen and antigen-presenting cells and lymphocytes. The local depot mechanism was challenged when Holt (1950) described that antibody formation continued even after removal of adjuvant–antigen depot from the site of injection. White *et al.* (1955) showed that antibody-producing cells in the regional (popliteal) lymph nodes of rabbits injected with 150 Lf of soluble DT completely disappeared in 3 weeks, whereas rabbits injected with 10 Lf of aluminum phosphate-precipitated toxoid showed antibody-producing cells in the node at 3–4 weeks. Aluminum adjuvants cause inflammation at the site of injection, attracting immunocompetent cells and thereby forming granulomas that contain antibody-producing plasma cells (White *et al.*, 1955).

The particle size of commercially available aluminum adjuvant gels is less than 10 μm [the average size for aluminum hydroxide (Alhydrogel[®]) was 3.07 μm and for aluminum phosphate (Adju-phos[®]) 4.26 μm; A. Chang and R. K. Gupta, unpublished data]. It has been shown that poly lactide glycolide (PLGA) microspheres less than 10 μm are taken up by antigen-presenting cells and show strong adjuvant effects (Eldridge *et al.*, 1991). Mannhalter *et al.* (1985) reported that antigen adsorbed onto aluminum hydroxide is more readily taken up by human monocytes than free antigen, and the human monocytes exposed to aluminum hydroxide secrete IL-1. Flebbe and Braley-Mullen (1986) showed an increased antibody response to a soluble antigen when aluminum adjuvant was injected at a different site, suggesting a systemic stimulatory effect on immunocompetent cells, possibly by release of cytokines. However, we could not reproduce these results in experiments comparing the immune responses of mice to DT and aluminum hydroxide injected at different sites versus soluble DT alone. Both elicited very low and similar antibody levels even after two doses (R. K. Gupta and P. Griffin, unpublished data).

The most direct evidence for a local depot effect comes from experiments in which local granulomas after injection of aluminum-adsorbed vaccines were excised from the site of injection 7 weeks later, macerated, and injected into other animals (Harrison, 1935). An immune response was observed in the recipients. Remarkably, the antigen in the granuloma was apparently not available to the animals for a secondary response, because minute doses of antigen injected adjacent to the granuloma produced a secondary antibody response (White, 1967). White (1967) postulated that antigen at this time is unable to penetrate the fibrous tissue surrounding the granuloma and antibody may react with antigen to form an antigen–antibody precipitate within the fibers of the peripheral zone of the granuloma thus preventing the diffusion of antigen from granuloma and sequestering it from antigen-presenting cells.

Aluminum compounds also induce eosinophilia (Walls, 1977) and activate complement (Ramanathan *et al.*, 1979) which may lead to a local inflammatory response, thus enhancing the antibody response. The aluminum adjuvants augment mainly humoral immunity, particularly IgG1 and IgE antibody responses, through IL-4 (Grun and Maurer, 1989) by activating Th2-type cells (Cooper, 1994). Aluminum adjuvants are generally not considered efficient in raising cell-mediated immune responses (Alving *et al.*, 1992, 1993). Cooper (1994) described aluminum adjuvants as good stimulants for Th2-type cell-mediated immune response, especially eosinophils. The induction of delayed-type hypersensitivity by aluminum adjuvants in mice and guinea pigs has not been clearly demonstrated (Bomford, 1980b, 1989). However, humans immunized with aluminum-adsorbed TT develop delayed-type hypersensitivity.

2.5. Limitations

Aluminum adjuvants have an extensive record of safety. Billions of doses of aluminum-adsorbed vaccines, particularly DTP with and without inactivated polio vaccine, have been inoculated into children and infants. Occasionally, however, these vaccines have been associated with severe local reactions such as erythema (Aprile and Wardlaw, 1966; Collier *et al.*, 1979), subcutaneous nodules (Frost *et al.*, 1985), contact hypersensitivity (Clemmenson and Knudsen, 1980), and granulomatous inflammation (White *et al.*, 1955; Erodohazi and Newman, 1971; Durand *et al.*, 1992). A few studies showed less reactions with aluminum-adsorbed DTP vaccine than unadsorbed vaccine (Hilton and Burland, 1970; Cameron, 1980) because of adsorption and subsequently slow release of reactogenic materials onto adjuvant. In animals, as well as in humans, aluminum adjuvants increase the levels of antigen-specific and total IgE antibodies (Nagel *et al.*, 1977; Vassilev, 1978; Matsuhasi and Ikegami, 1982; Cogne *et al.*, 1985; Relyveld, 1986; Gupta and Siber, 1994; Odelram *et al.*, 1994; Mark *et al.*, 1995) and may promote IgE-mediated allergic reactions. Nevertheless, aluminum adjuvants have been used for many years for hyposensitization of allergic patients with satisfactory results (Gupta *et al.*, 1993).

Studies on booster injections up to 10 years later with aluminum-adsorbed vaccines showed more local reactions such as redness, swelling, and itching in children who received aluminum-adsorbed vaccines for primary immunization than those who received unadsorbed vaccines for primary immunization (Hedenskog *et al.*, 1989; Blennow *et al.*, 1990, 1994). Antigen-specific IgE antibody levels after booster injections were higher in the group that received aluminum-adsorbed vaccines for primary immunization than in the group that received unadsorbed vaccine for primary immunization (Hedenskog *et al.*, 1989). On the other hand, there was no difference in the frequency of local reactions and IgG antibody response to a booster dose of soluble or aluminum phosphate-adsorbed diphtheria–tetanus toxoid in children who had primary immunization 10 years earlier with aluminum-adsorbed vaccines (Mark and Granstrom, 1994). However, the children boosted with aluminum phosphate-adsorbed vaccine developed higher levels of tetanus-specific IgE than those boosted with unadsorbed vaccine (Mark *et al.*, 1995). Higher levels of antigen-specific IgE correlated with local reactions (Blennow *et al.*, 1990; Mark *et al.*, 1995). Taken together these studies suggest that children who had primary immunization with aluminum-adsorbed vaccines develop more antigen-specific IgE and show a higher frequency of local reactions on booster injection with soluble or aluminum-adsorbed vaccines than children who had primary immunization with unadsorbed vaccines. There have been concerns, particularly in patients with impaired renal function, about systemic accumulation of aluminum, which has been associated with nervous system disorders and bone diseases (Food and Drug Administration, 1987; Gupta and Relyveld, 1991). However, the aluminum intake from vaccines is minor compared to that of diet and medications such as antacids.

Other limitations of aluminum adjuvants include their ineffectiveness for certain antigens (Alving *et al.*, 1992) and induction of mainly humoral immunity by eliciting primarily Th2-type responses in mice (Audibert and Lise, 1993). Aluminum compounds did not exhibit an adjuvant effect when used with typhoid vaccine (Cvjetanovic and Umera, 1965), influenza hemagglutinin antigen (Davenport *et al.*, 1968), and *Haemophilus influenzae* type b capsular polysaccharide–TT conjugate (Claesson *et al.*, 1988). However, aluminum hydroxide was used with a conjugate vaccine composed of capsular polysaccharide from *H. influenzae* type b linked to outer membrane proteins of *Neisseria meningitidis* as the adsorbed preparations produced fewer local and systemic reactions than the soluble preparation because of slow release of vaccine (Einhorn *et al.*, 1986). The inability of aluminum adjuvants to elicit cell-mediated immune responses, particularly cytotoxic T-cell responses, may be a major limitation, particularly for vaccines against intracellular parasites and viral infections such as human immunodeficiency virus. Further, aluminum is not "biodegradable" (Nixon *et al.*, 1992). We have detected aluminum adjuvants at the site of s.c. injection for up to 1 year in mice and guinea pigs (R. K. Gupta, P. Griffin, and R. Rivera, unpublished observations).

Aluminum adjuvants cannot be frozen or lyophilized (Warren *et al.*, 1986; Alving *et al.*, 1993). Freezing and lyophilization of aluminum adjuvants cause the collapse of the gel, resulting in gross aggregation and precipitation. Although TT with collapsed gel precipitates was immunogenic (Menon *et al.*, 1976), such a vaccine is not clinically acceptable. Successful lyophilization of aluminum adjuvants has been reported (Rethy *et al.*, 1985), but lyophilized vaccines containing aluminum adjuvants are not commercially used. We have found that the selection of stabilizers and cryopreservatives for lyophilization is very important because stabilizers desorb antigens from aluminum adjuvants on reconstitution of lyophilized vaccines (A. Chang, R. K. Gupta, and G. R. Siber, unpublished data).

3. CALCIUM PHOSPHATE

An alternative to aluminum adjuvants is calcium phosphate, which has been successfully used in France with routine childhood and adult vaccines for many years and has been found to be safe and efficacious in various field trials (Relyveld, 1980, 1986; Gupta *et al.*, 1993; Relyveld and Chermann, 1994). Calcium phosphate is a normal constituent of the body and is well tolerated and readily resorbed. Unlike aluminum adjuvants, calcium phosphate does not enhance IgE production in humans and animals (Relyveld *et al.*, 1974; Vassilev, 1978; Relyveld, 1980; Ickovic *et al.*, 1983).

3.1. Method of Preparation

Like aluminum adjuvants, two methods are used for adsorbing antigen onto calcium phosphate: in situ precipitation of gel in the presence of antigens (Relyveld *et al.*, 1985, 1991) and adsorption onto a preformed gel. Preformed calcium phosphate gel of clinical grade is commercially available from Superfos Biosector, Vedbaek, Denmark.

Table IV
Effect of Reactant Mixing Time (Equal Volumes of 0.07 M Disodium Hydrogen Phosphate and 0.07 M Calcium Chloride) on the Chemical Composition of Calcium Phosphate Gel

| Reaction time[a] | Concentration (mg/mL) in | | | | | |
| | Reactants | | Gel | | Decanted liquid | |
	Ca	P	Ca	P	Ca	P
10 s	1.41	1.07	1.38	0.76	0.03	0.32
10 min	1.47	1.15	1.40	1.03	0.07	0.12
20 min	1.43	1.12	1.39	0.92	0.04	0.20
30 min	1.44	1.07	1.39	0.90	0.05	0.17

[a]Time taken to pour calcium chloride into disodium hydrogen phosphate.

The quality of calcium phosphate gel depends on the concentration of the reactants, disodium hydrogen phosphate and calcium chloride, and the rate at which the reactants are mixed. Slow mixing of the reactants (longer than 3 min) results in a gel with a calcium-to-phosphorus ratio of 1.35 to 1.55 whereas quick mixing of the reactants (10 s) gives a calcium-to-phosphorus ratio of 1.83 (Table IV). There is more phosphorus in the supernatant of the gel prepared by fast mixing than in that prepared by slow mixing (Table IV). Calcium phosphate gel used as an adjuvant is prepared by quick mixing (within 3 min) of equimolar solutions (0.05 to 0.1 M), preferably 0.07 M of disodium hydrogen phosphate ($Na_2HPO_4 \cdot 12H_2O$) and calcium chloride ($CaCl_2 \cdot 2H_2O$) and adjusting the pH to 6.8–7.0 with sodium hydroxide. The gel is then washed with 0.9% sodium chloride to remove excess phosphate.

The rate of mixing of disodium hydrogen phosphate and calcium chloride also affects the physical characteristics and adsorption of antigens onto the gel. Table V shows that a gel prepared by rapid pouring of calcium chloride into disodium hydrogen phosphate and mixing within 10 s results in a gel that has a lower pH and sediments more slowly than the

Table V
Effect of Reactant Mixing Time (Equal Volumes of 0.07 M Disodium Hydrogen Phosphate and 0.07 M Calcium Chloride) on the Physical Characteristics of Calcium Phosphate Gel

| Reaction time[a] | pH of gel | Height[b] (mm) of clear solution in | | | | |
		5 min	10 min	20 min	75 min	17 h
10 s	5.7	2.5	3.8	6.3	21.2	85.0
10 min	6.5	48.0	82.0	92.0	100.0	105.0
20 min	6.0	48.0	83.0	91.0	95.0	105.0
30 min	6.1	57.0	89.0	95.0	105.0	109.0

[a]Time taken to pour calcium chloride into disodium hydrogen phosphate.
[b]Height of clear liquid at top of gel in 125-mm-long tube containing 50 mL of gel, held at 20°C.

gel made by slow mixing of reactants (≥ 10 min). These gels also have different adsorption capacities of DT. The gel prepared by fast mixing (10 s) adsorbed 100% of the DT from a solution containing 120 Lf/mL whereas the gel prepared by slow mixing (in 10 min) adsorbed only 58% of the toxoid.

In situ precipitation of antigens on calcium phosphate gel is carried out by dialyzing the antigens in 0.07 M disodium hydrogen phosphate and the equal volume of 0.07 M calcium chloride is poured as quickly as possible with fast stirring. The pH of the gel is adjusted immediately to 6.8–7.0 with sodium hydroxide. The gel with adsorbed antigen is washed with 0.9% sodium chloride and finally suspended in 0.9% sodium chloride containing 0.01% thimerosal. As with aluminum adjuvant gels, excess phosphate ions present in calcium phosphate gel inhibit adsorption of antigens and should be removed by washing the gel.

3.2. Adjuvant Properties

Calcium phosphate has been used with DTP, inactivated polio vaccines, and allergens for many years, particularly in France for the immunization of children and adults or hyposensitization of allergic patients (Relyveld et al., 1964; Relyveld and Raynaud, 1967; Ickovic et al., 1983; Relyveld, 1986). In humans as well as animals, calcium phosphate elicited similar or slightly lower neutralizing antibodies than aluminum adjuvants after a single injection of TT or DT (Relyveld et al., 1991; Gupta and Siber, 1994). After booster injection with TT, however, calcium phosphate elicited higher neutralizing antibodies than aluminum phosphate in pregnant women (Relyveld et al., 1991). Calcium phosphate was used successfully as an adjuvant for simultaneous immunizations with diphtheria, tetanus, polio, BCG, yellow fever, measles, and hepatitis B vaccines (Gateff et al., 1973; Relyveld et al., 1973; Coursaget et al., 1985, 1986). Adverse local and generalized reactions were rare and mild with calcium phosphate-adsorbed vaccines. Calcium phosphate has also been used with HIV-1 gp160 antigen in rabbits (Relyveld and Chermann, 1994).

Like aluminum adjuvants, calcium phosphate is believed to act mainly by depot formation at the site of injection, thus releasing the antigen slowly, and by targeting the antigen efficiently to antigen presenting cells as particulate antigens. Therefore, adsorption of the antigen is important for immunogenicity. As calcium phosphate does not elicit IgE production, it may stimulate less IL-4-mediated T-cell help than aluminum adjuvants.

4. COMBINATION OF ALUMINUM COMPOUNDS WITH OTHER ADJUVANTS

Aluminum compounds have also been used in combination with other adjuvants. However, these combinations are not described in detail in this chapter.

Historically, aluminum adjuvants have been used with DTP vaccine which has two other adjuvant-active components from pertussis organisms, lipopolysaccharide and pertussis toxin (Gupta et al., 1993). The adjuvant effect of pertussis vaccine is clearly evident on TT by increase in its potency in mice in the presence of pertussis vaccine (WHO, 1990). In recent years, aluminum compounds have been used along with liposomes and monophosphoryl lipid A (Alving *et al.*, 1993), γ-inulin (Cooper, 1994; see chapter 24), and QS-21 (Kensil *et al.*, 1991; see Chapter 22).

5. SUMMARY

It is likely that aluminum compounds will continue to be used with human vaccines for many years as a result of their excellent track record of safety and adjuvanticity with a variety of antigens. For infections that can be prevented by induction of serum antibodies, aluminum adjuvants formulated under optimal conditions are the adjuvants of choice. It is important to select carefully the type of aluminum adjuvant and optimize the conditions of adsorption for every antigen since the degree of adsorption of antigens onto aluminum adjuvants markedly affects immunogenicity. The mechanism of adjuvanticity of aluminum compounds includes formation of a depot at the site of injection from which antigen is released slowly; stimulation of immune-competent cells of the body through activation of complement, induction of eosinophilia, and activation of macrophages; and efficient uptake of aluminum-adsorbed antigen particles by antigen-presenting cells because of their particulate nature and optimal size ($< 10\,\mu$m). Limitations of aluminum adjuvants include local reactions, production of IgE antibodies, ineffectiveness for some antigens, and inability to elicit cell-mediated immune responses especially cytotoxic T-cell responses. Calcium phosphate, which has adjuvant properties similar to aluminum adjuvants, has the potential advantages of being a natural component of the body and of not increasing IgE production. There is a need for alternative adjuvants, particularly for diseases in which cell-mediated immune responses are important for prevention or cure.

ACKNOWLEDGMENTS

We thank Dr. Erik Lindblad, Superfos Biosector, Vedbaek, Denmark, for providing Alhydrogel® and Adju-phos® adjuvants, Paul Griffin for technical assistance in experiments described in this chapter, and Ann Day for assistance in completing the bibliography.

REFERENCES

Ad Hoc Group for the Study of Pertussis Vaccines, 1988, Placebo-controlled trial of two acellular pertussis vaccines in Sweden: Protective efficacy and adverse events, *Lancet* **1**:955–960.

Ahuja, S., Sharma, S. B., Gupta, R. K., Maheshwari, S. C., Bhandari, S. K., and Saxena, S. N., 1986, Antibody response of guinea pigs to fluid and adsorbed tetanus toxoids, *Indian J. Pathol. Microbiol.* **29**:285–292.

Al-Shakhshir, R., Regnier, F., White, J. L., and Hem, S. L., 1994, Effect of protein adsorption on the surface charge characteristics of aluminium-containing adjuvants, *Vaccine* **12**:472–474.

Alving, C. R., Glass, M., and Detrick, B., 1992, Summary: Adjuvants/Clinical Trials Working Group, *AIDS Res. Hum. Retroviruses* **8**:1427–1430.

Alving, C. R., Detrick, B., Richards, R. L., Lewis, M. G., Shafferman, A., and Eddy, G. A., 1993, Novel adjuvant strategies for experimental malaria and AIDS vaccines, *Ann. N.Y. Acad. Sci.* **690**:265–275.

Andre, F. E., Hepburn, A., and D'Hondt, E., 1990, Inactivated candidate vaccines for hepatitis A, *Prog. Med. Virol.* **37**:72–95.

Aprile, M. A., and Wardlaw, A. C., 1966, Aluminum compounds as adjuvants for vaccine and toxoids in man: A review, *Can. J. Public. Health* **57**:343–354.

Audibert, F. M., and Lise, L. D., 1993, Adjuvants: Current status, clinical perspectives and future prospects, *Immunol. Today* **14**:281–284.

Berman, P. W., Gregory, T., Crase, D., and Laski, L. A., 1985, Protection from genital herpes simplex virus type 2 infection by vaccination with cloned type 1 glycoprotein D, *Science* **227**:1490–1492.

Blennow, M., Granstrom, M., and Bjorksten, B., 1990, Immunoglobulin E response to pertussis toxin after vaccination with acellular pertussis vaccine, in: *Proceedings of the Sixth International Symposium on Pertussis* (C. R. Manclark, ed.), Department of Health and Human Services, Bethesda, DHHS Publication No. (FDA) 90-1164, pp. 184–188.

Blennow, M., Granstrom, M., and Strandell, A., 1994, Adverse reactions after diphtheria–tetanus booster in 10-year-old school children in relation to the type of vaccine given for the primary vaccination, *Vaccine* **12**:427–430.

Bomford, R., 1980a, The comparative selectivity of adjuvants for humoral and cell-mediated immunity. I. Effect on the antibody response to bovine serum albumin and sheep red blood cells of Freund's incomplete and complete adjuvants, Alhydrogel, *Corynebacterium parvum, Bordetella pertussis*, muramyl dipeptide and saponin, *Clin. Exp. Immunol.* **39**:426–434.

Bomford, R., 1980b, The comparative selectivity of adjuvants for humoral and cell-mediated immunity. II. Effect on delayed-type hypersensitivity in the mouse and guinea pig, and cell-mediated immunity to tumour antigens in the mouse of Freund's incomplete and complete adjuvants, Alhydrogel, *Corynebacterium parvum, Bordetella pertussis*, muramyl dipeptide and saponin, *Clin. Exp. Immunol.* **39**:435–443.

Bomford, R., 1984, Relative adjuvant efficacy of Al(OH)$_3$ and saponin is related to the immunogenicity of the antigen, *Int. Arch. Allergy Appl. Immunol.* **75**:280–281.

Bomford, R., 1989, Aluminium salts: Perspectives in their use as adjuvants, in: *Immunological Adjuvants and Vaccines* (G. Gregoriadis, A. C. Allison, and G. Poste, eds.), Plenum Press, New York, pp. 35–41.

Butler, N. R., Wilson, B. D. R., Benson, P. F., Dudgeon, J. A., Ungar, J., and Beale, A. J., 1962a, Response of infants to pertussis vaccine at one week and to poliomyelitis, diphtheria and tetanus vaccine at six months, *Lancet* **2**:112–114.

Butler, N. R., Wilson, B. D. R., Benson, P. F., Dudgeon, J. A., Ungar, J., and Beale, A. J., 1962b, Effect of aluminum phosphate on antibody response to killed poliomyelitis vaccine, *Lancet* **2**:114–115.

Cameron, J., 1976, Problems associated with control testing of pertussis vaccine, *Adv. Appl. Microbiol.* **20**:57–80.

Cameron, J., 1979, Pertussis vaccine: Control testing problems, in: *International Symposium on Pertussis* held at the National Institutes of Health, Bethesda, November 1–3, 1978 (C. R. Manclark and J. C. Hill, eds.), U.S. Government Printing Office, Washington, DC, pp. 200–207.

Cameron, J., 1980, The potency of whooping cough (pertussis) vaccines in Canada, *J. Biol. Stand.* **8**:297–302.

Cameron, J., 1985, in: Discussion, *Dev. Biol. Stand.* **61**:315.

Cameron, J., and Knight, P. A., 1972, Interaction of components of triple antigen (diphtheria, tetanus, pertussis, DTP), in: *Proceedings of the Symposium on Combined Vaccines*, Yugoslavian Academy of Science and Arts, Zagreb, pp. 55–67.

Claesson, B. A., Trollfors, B., Lagergard, T., Taranger, J., Bryla, D., Otterman, G., Crampton, T., Yang, Y., Reimer, C. B., Robbins, J. B., and Schneerson, R., 1988, Clinical and immunologic responses to the capsular polysaccharide of *Haemophilus influenzae* type b alone or conjugated to tetanus toxoid in 18- to 23-month-old children, *J. Pediatr.* **112**:695–702.

Clemmenson, O., and Knudsen, H. E., 1980, Contact sensitivity to aluminium in a patient hyposensitized with aluminium precipitated grass pollen, *Contact Dermatitis* **6**:305–308.

Cogne, M., Ballet, J. J., Schmitt, C., and Bizzini, B., 1985, Total and IgE antibody levels following booster immunization with aluminium adsorbed and non adsorbed tetanus toxoid in humans, *Ann. Allergy* **54**:148–151.

Collier, L. H., Polakoff, S., and Mortimer, J., 1979, Reactions and antibody responses to reinforcing doses of adsorbed and plain tetanus vaccines, *Lancet* **1**:1364–1368.

Cooper, P. D., 1994, The selective induction of different immune responses by vaccine adjuvants, in: *Strategies in Vaccine Design* (G. L. Ada, ed.), R. G. Landes Company, Austin, pp. 125–158.

Cooper, P. D., McComb, C., and Steele, E. J., 1991, The adjuvanticity of algammulin, a new vaccine adjuvant, *Vaccine* **9**:408–415.

Coursaget, P., Yvonnet, B., Relyveld, E. H., Barres, J. L., Dubourg, J. C., Diouf, C., Diopo-Mar, I., and Chiron, J. P., 1985, Simultaneous administration of hepatitis B vaccine with diphtheria/tetanus/pertussis/polio vaccine, in: *Proceedings of the Seventh International Conference on Tetanus* (G. Nistico, P. Maestroni, and M. Pitzurra, eds.), Gangemi, Rome, pp. 401–406.

Coursaget, P., Yvonnet, B., Relyveld, E. H., Barres, J. L., Diop-Mar, I., and Chiron, J. P., 1986, Simultaneous administration of diphtheria–tetanus–pertussis–polio and hepatitis B vaccines in a simplified immunization program: Immune response to diphtheria toxoid, tetanus toxoid, pertussis and hepatitis B surface antigen, *Infect. Immun.* **51**:784–787.

Cvjetanovic, B., and Umera, K., 1965, The present status of field and laboratory studies of typhoid and paratyphoid vaccines with special reference to studies sponsored by the World Health Organization, *Bull. W.H.O.* **32**:29–36.

Davenport, F. M., Hennessy, A. V., and Askin, F. B., 1968, Lack of adjuvant effect of $AlPO_4$ on purified influenza virus haemagglutinins in man, *J. Immunol.* **100**:1139–1140.

Durand, C., Pineau, A., Bureau, B., and Stalder, J. F., 1992, Complications cutanees des vaccinations diphterie, tetanos, coqueluche, poliomyelite (tetracoq) role de l'hydroxyde d'alumine, *Nouv. Dermatol.* **11**:523–526.

Edelman, R., 1980, Vaccine adjuvants, *Rev. Infect. Dis.* **2**:370–383.

Einhorn, M. S., Weinberg, G. A., Anderson, E. L., Granoff, P. L., and Granoff, D. M., 1986, Immunogenicity in infants of Haemophilus influenzae type b polysaccharide in a conjugate vaccine with Neisseria meningitidis outer-membrane protein, *Lancet* **2**:299–302.

Eldridge, J. H., Staas, J. K., Meulbroek, J. A., Tice, T. R., and Gilley, R. M., 1991, Biodegradable and biocompatible poly(DL-lactide-co-glycolide) microspheres as an adjuvant for staphylococcal enterotoxin B toxoid which enhances the level of toxin-neutralizing antibodies, *Infect. Immun.* **59**:2978–2986.

Erodohazi, M., and Newman, R. L., 1971, Aluminium hydroxide granuloma, *Br. Med. J.* **3**:621–623.

Flebbe, L. M., and Braley-Mullen, H., 1986, Immunopotentiating effects of the adjuvants SGP and Quil A. I. Antibody responses to T-dependent and T-independent antigens, *Cell. Immunol.* **99**:119–127.

Food and Drug Administration, 1987, Summary Minutes—Allergenic Products Advisory Committee and Report on Safety Considerations for the Aluminum Component of Alum-precipitated Allergenic Extracts, Office of Biologics Research and Review, Biologics Information Staff (NFN-20) FDA, Bethesda.

Frost, L., Johansen, P., Pedersen, S., Veien, N., Ostergaard, P. A., and Nielsen, M. H., 1985, Persistent subcutaneous nodules in children hyposensitized with aluminium-containing allergen extracts, *Allergy* **40**:368–372.

Fulthorpe, A. J., 1965, The influence of mineral carriers on the simultaneous active and passive immunization of guinea pigs against tetanus, *J. Hyg.* **63**:243–262.

Gateff, C., Relyveld, E. H., Le Gonidec, G., Vincent, J., Labusquiere, R., McBean, M., Monchicourt, D., and Chambon, L., 1973, Etude d'une nouvelle association vaccinale quintuple, *Ann. Microbiol. (Inst. Pasteur)* **124B**:387–409.

Glenny, A .T., Pope, C. G., Waddington, H., and Wallace, U., 1926, The antigenic value of toxoid precipitated by potassium alum, *J. Pathol. Bacteriol.* **29**:38–45.

Glenny, A. T., Buttle, G. A. H., and Stevens, M. F., 1931, Rate of disappearance of diphtheria toxoid injected into rabbits and guinea pigs: Toxoid precipitated with alum, *J. Pathol. Bacteriol.* **34**:267–275.

Grun, J. L., and Maurer, P. H., 1989, Different T helper cell subsets elicited in mice utilizing two different adjuvant vehicles: The role of endogenous interleukin-1 in proliferative responses, *Cell. Immunol.* **121**:134–145.

Gupta, R. K., and Relyveld, E. H., 1991, Adverse reactions after injection of adsorbed diphtheria–pertussis–tetanus (DPT) vaccine are not due only to pertussis organisms or pertussis components in the vaccine, *Vaccine* **9**:699–702.

Gupta, R. K., and Siber, G. R., 1994, Comparison of adjuvant activities of aluminum phosphate, calcium phosphate and stearyl tyrosine for tetanus toxoid, *Biologicals* 22:53–63.

Gupta, R. K., Sharma, S. B., Ahuja, S., and Saxena, S. N., 1987, The effect of aluminum phosphate adjuvant on the potency of pertussis vaccine, *J. Biol. Stand.* 15:99–101.

Gupta, R. K., Saxena, S. N., Sharma, S. B., and Ahuja, S., 1990, Immunogenicity of glutaraldehyde inactivated pertussis vaccine, *Vaccine* 8:563–568.

Gupta, R. K., Saxena, S. N., Sharma, S. B., and Ahuja, S., 1992, Comparative stabilities of glutaraldehyde & heat inactivated pertussis vaccine components of adsorbed DPT vaccine with different preservatives, *Indian J. Med. Res.* 95:8–11.

Gupta, R. K., Relyveld, E. H., Lindblad, E. B., Bizzini, B., Ben-Efraim, S., and Gupta, C. K., 1993, Adjuvants—A balance between toxicity and adjuvanticity, *Vaccine* 11:293–306.

Haas, R., and Thomssen, R., 1961, Uber den entwicklungsstand der in der immunbiologie gebrauch-lichen adjuvantien, *Ergeb. Mikrobiol.* 34:27–119.

Haas, R., Keller, W., and Kikuth, W., 1955, Grundsatzliches zur aktiven schutzimpfung gegen poliomyelitis, *Dtsch. Med. Wochenschr.* 80:273.

Harrison, W. T., 1935, Some observations on the use of alum-precipitated diphtheria toxoid, *Am. J. Public Health* 25:298–300.

Hedenskog, S., Bjorksten, B., Blennow, M., Granstrom, G., and Granstrom, M., 1989, Immunoglobulin E response to pertussis toxin in whooping cough and after immunization with a whole-cell and an acellular pertussis vaccine, *Int. Arch. Allergy Appl. Immunol.* 89:156–161.

Hennessen, W., 1965, The mode of action of mineral adjuvants, *Prog. Immunobiol. Stand.* 2:71–79.

Hennessen, W., 1967, Mode of action and consequences for standardization of adjuvanted vaccines, *Symp. Ser. Immunobiol. Stand.* 6:319–326.

Hilton, M. L., and Wurland, W. L., 1970, Pertussis containing vaccines: The relationship between laboratory toxicity tests and reactions in children, *Symp. Ser. Immunobiol. Stand.* 13:150–156.

Holt, L. B., 1950, *Developments in Diphtheria Prophylaxis,* Heinemann Medical Books, London, pp. 1–181.

Holt, L. B., 1955, Quantitative studies in diphtheria prophylaxis: An attempt to derive a mathematical characterization of the antigenicity of diphtheria prophylactic, *Biometric* 11:83–94.

Ickovic, M. R., Relyveld, E. H., Henocq, E., David, B., and Marie, F. N., 1983, Calcium phosphate adjuvanted allergens: Total and specific IgE levels before and after immunotherapy with house dust and *Dermatophagoides pteronyssinus* extracts, *Ann. Immunol. (Institut Pasteur)* 134D:385–398.

Ipsen, J., Jr., 1954, Immunization of adults against diphtheria and tetanus, *N. Engl. J. Med.* 251:459–466.

Jensen, O. M., and Koch, C., 1988, On the effect of Al(OH)3 as an immunological adjuvant, *Acta Pathol. Microbiol. Immunol. Scand.* 96:257–264.

Jones, F. G., and Moss, J. M., 1936, Studies on tetanus toxoid. I. The antitoxic titer of human subjects following immunization with tetanus toxoid and tetanus alum precipitated toxoid, *J. Immunol.* 30:115–125.

Kensil, C. R., Barrett, C., Kushner, N., Beltz, G., Storey, J., Patel, U., Recchia, J., Aubert, A., and Marciani, D., 1991, Development of a genetically engineered vaccine against feline leukemia virus infection, *J. Am. Vet. Med. Assoc.* 199:1423–1427.

Krantz, I., Sekura, R., Trollfors, B., Taranger, J., Zackrisson, G., Lagergard, T., Schneerson, R., and Robbins, J., 1990, Immunogenicity and safety of a pertussis vaccine composed of pertussis toxin inactivated by hydrogen peroxide, in 18- to 23-month-old children, *J. Pediatr.* 116:539–543.

Kuwert, E. K., Menzel, H., Marcus, I., and Majer, M., 1978, Antigenicity of low concentrated HDCS vaccine with and without adjuvant as compared to the standard fluid formulation, *Dev. Biol. Stand.* 40:29–34.

Levine, L., 1972, A predictive equation for the primary immune response of mice to adsorbed tetanus toxoid as a function of dose of antigen and dose of adjuvant, *J. Immunol.* 109:1138–1142.

Levine, L., Stone, J. L., and Wyman, L., 1955, Factors affecting the efficiency of the aluminum adjuvant in diphtheria and tetanus toxoids, *J. Immunol.* 75:301–307.

Levine, L., Ipsen, J., and McComb, J. A., 1961, Adult immunization: Preparation and evaluation of combined fluid tetanus and diphtheria toxoids for adult use, *Am. J. Hyg.* 73:20–35.

Levine, L., McComb, J. A., Dwyer, R. C., and Latham, W. C., 1966, Active–passive tetanus immunization, *N. Engl. J. Med.* **274**:186–190.

Lindblad, E. B., and Sparck, J. V., 1987, Basic concepts in the application of immunological adjuvants, *Scand. J. Lab. Anim. Sci.* **14**:1–13.

MacLennan, R., Levine, L., Newell, K. W., and Edsall, G., 1973, The early primary immune response to adsorbed tetanus toxoid in man, *Bull. W.H.O.* **49**:615–626.

Mannhalter, J. W., Neychev, H. O., Zlabinger, G. J., Ahmad, R., and Eibl, M. M., 1985, Modulation of the human immune response by the non-toxic and non-pyrogenic adjuvant aluminium hydroxide: Effect of antigen uptake and antigen presentation, *Clin. Exp. Immunol.* **61**:143–151.

Mark, A., and Granstrom, M., 1994, The role of aluminium for adverse reactions and immunogenicity of diphtheria–tetanus booster vaccine, *Acta Paediatr.* **83**:159–163.

Mark, A., Bjorksten, B., and Granstrom, M., 1995, Immunoglobulin E responses to diphtheria and tetanus toxoids after booster with aluminium-adsorbed and fluid DT-vaccines, *Vaccine* (in press).

Matsuhasi, T., and Ikegami, H., 1982, Elevation of levels of IgE antibody to tetanus toxin in individuals vaccinated with diphtheria–pertussis–tetanus vaccine, *J. Infect. Dis.* **146**:290.

May, J. C., Progar, J. J., and Chin, R., 1984, The aluminum content of biological products containing aluminum adjuvants: Determination by atomic absorption spectrometry, *J. Biol. Stand.* **12**:175–183.

Menon, P. S., Sahai, G., Joshi, V. B., Murthy, R. G. S., Boprai, M. S., and Thomas, A. K., 1976, Field trial on frozen and thawed tetanus toxoid, *Indian J. Med. Res.* **64**:25–32.

Munder, P. G., Ferber, E., Modolell, M., and Fischer, H., 1969, The influence of various adjuvants on the metabolism of phospholipids in macrophages, *Int. Arch. Allergy* **36**:117–128.

Murray, K., Bruce, S. A., Hinnen, A., Wingfield, P., van Erd, P. M. C. A., de reus, A., and Schellekens, H., 1984, Hepatitis B virus antigens made in microbial cells immunize against viral infection, *EMBO J.* **3**:645–650.

Nagel, J., Svec, D., Water, T., and Fireman, P., 1977, IgE synthesis in man. I. Development of specific IgE antibodies after immunization with tetanus–diphtheria (TD) toxoids, *J. Immunol.* **118**:334–341.

Nicklas, W., 1992, Aluminum salts, *Res. Immunol.* **143**:489–494.

Nixon, A., Zaghouani, H., Penney, C. L., Lacroix, M., Dionne, G., Anderson, S. A., Kennedy, R. C., and Bona, C. A., 1992, Adjuvanticity of stearyl tyrosine on the antibody response to peptide 503-535 from HIV gp160, *Viral Immunol.* **5**:141–150.

Novotny, P., and Brookes, J. E., 1975, The use of *Bordetella pertussis* preserved in liquid nitrogen as a challenge suspension in the Kendrick mouse protection test, *J. Biol. Stand.* **3**:11–29.

Odelram, H., Granstrom, M., Hedenskog, S., Duchen, K., and Bjorksten, B., 1994, Immunoglobulin E and G responses to pertussis toxin after booster immunization in atopy, local reactions and aluminium content of the vaccines, *Pediatr. Allergy Immunol.* **5**:118–123.

Peetermans, J., 1992, Production, quality control and characterization of an inactivated hepatitis A vaccine, *Vaccine* **10**(Suppl. 1):S99–S101.

Pittman, M., 1954, Variability of the potency of pertussis vaccine in relation to the number of bacteria, *J. Pediatr.* **45**:57–69.

Podda, A., Nencioni, L., Marsili, I., Peppoloni, S., Volpini, G., Donati, D., Di Tommaso, A., De Magistris, M. T., and Rappuoli, R., 1991, Phase I clinical trial of an acellular pertussis vaccine composed of genetically detoxified pertussis toxin combined with FHA and 69 KDa, *Vaccine* **9**:741–745.

Preston, N. W., 1976, Protection by pertussis vaccine: Little cause for concern, *Lancet* **1**:1065–1067.

Preston, N. W., 1979, Some unsolved problems with vaccines, *Prog. Drug Res.* **23**:9–26.

Preston, N. W., Mackay, R. I., Bomford, F. N., Crofts, J. E., and Burland, W. L., 1974, Pertussis agglutinins in vaccinated children: Better response with adjuvant, *J. Hyg.* **73**:119–125.

Prigge, R., 1942, Wirksamkeit und schutzkraft der diphtherie-impfstoffe, *Behringwerk Mitt.* **21**:75–99.

Prigge, R., 1949, Die beziehung zwischen dem antigengehalt der diphtherie-impfstoffe und ihrer wirksamkeit, *Klin. Wochenschr.* **27**:685–690.

Ramanathan, V. D., Badenoch-Jones, P., and Turk, J. L., 1979, Complement activation by aluminium and zirconium compounds, *Immunology* **37**:881–888.

Relyveld, E. H., 1980, Current developments in production and testing of tetanus and diphtheria vaccines, in: *New Developments with Human and Veterinary Vaccines* (A. Mizrahi, I. Hertman, M. Klingberg, and A. Kohn, eds.), Liss, New York, pp. 51–76.

Relyveld, E. H., 1985, Immunological, prophylactic and standardization aspects in tetanus, in: *Proceedings of the Seventh International Conference on Tetanus* (G. Nistico, P. Maestroni, and M. Pitzurra, eds.), Gangemi, Rome, pp. 215–227.

Relyveld, E. H., 1986, Preparation and use of calcium phosphate adsorbed vaccines, *Dev. Biol. Stand.* **65**:131–136.

Relyveld, E., and Chermann, J. C., 1994, Humoral response in rabbits immunized with calcium phosphate adjuvanted HIV-1 gp160 antigen, *Biomed. Pharmacother.* **48**:79–83.

Relyveld, E. H., and Raynaud, M., 1967, Etudes sur le phosphate de calcium comme adjuvant de l'immunite, *Symp. Ser. Immunobiol. Stand.* **6**:77–88.

Relyveld, E. H., Hencoq, E., and Raynaud, M., 1964, Etude de la vaccination antidiphterique de sujets alergiques avec une anatoxine pure adsorbee sur phosphate de calcium, *Bull W.H.O.* **30**:321–325.

Relyveld, E. H., Martin, R., Raynaud, M., Damas, J.-P., Therond, C., Henocq, E., Romain, F., Turpin, A., Ceolin, G., Cheve, J., Digeon, M., and Cheyroux, M., 1969, Le phosphate de calcium comme adjuvant dans les vaccinations chez l'homme, *Ann. Institut Pasteur* **116**:300–326.

Relyveld, E. H., Gateff, C., Chambon, L., Guerin, N., and, Charpin, M., 1973, Etudes sur le vaccinations en Afrique, *Symp. Series Immunobiol. Stand.* **22**:215–222.

Relyveld, E. H., Lavergne, M., and De Rudder, J., 1974, Taux d'immunogoblulines (IgG; IgA; IgM et IgE) apres stimulation antigenique ches des sujets europeens et africains, *Dev. Biol. Stand.* **27**:79–90.

Relyveld, E. H., Ickovic, M. R., Henocq, E., and Garcelon, M., 1985, Calcium phosphate adjuvanted allergens, *Ann. Allergy* **54**:521–529.

Relyveld, E., Bengounia, A., Huet, M., and Kreeftenberg, J. G., 1991, Antibody response of pregnant women to two different adsorbed tetanus toxoids, *Vaccine* **9**:369–372.

Rethy, L., Solyom, F., Bacskai, L., Geresi, M., Gerhardt, Z., Koves, B., Kriston, K., Magyar, T., Masek, I., Nagy, B., and Nemesi, M., 1985, Design and control of new type vaccines. Efficacy testing of adsorbed and freeze-dried toxoid–virus–bacterium combined vaccines, *Ann. Immunol. Hung.* **25**:49–57.

Saroso, J. S., Bahrawi, W., Witjaksono, H., Budiarso, R. L. P., Brotowasisto, B. Z., Dewitt, W. E., and Gomez, C. Z., 1978, A controlled field trial of plain and aluminum hydroxide-adsorbed cholera vaccines in Surabaya, Indonesia, during 1973–75, *Bull. W.H.O.* **56**:619–627.

Sato, Y., Kimura, M., and Fukumi, H., 1984, Development of a pertussis component vaccine in Japan, *Lancet* **1**:122–126.

Schmidt, G., 1967, The adjuvant effect of aluminum hydroxide in influenza vaccine, *Symp. Ser. Immunobiol. Stand.* **6**:275–282.

Seal, S. C., and Johnson, S. J., 1941, Studies on the purification of alum-precipitated diphtheria toxoid, *J. Infect. Dis.* **69**:102–107.

Siber, G. R., Thakrar, N., Yancey, B. A., Herzog, L., Todd, C., Cohen, N., Sekura, R. D., and Lowe, C. U., 1991, Safety and immunogenicity of hydrogen peroxide-inactivated pertussis toxoid in 18-month-old children, *Vaccine* **9**:735–740.

Stewart-Tull, D. E. S., 1989, Recommendations for the assessment of adjuvants (immunopotentiators), in: *Immunological Adjuvants and Vaccines* (G. Greogoriadis, A. C. Allison, and G. Poste, eds.), Plenum Press, New York, pp. 213–226.

Suri, J. C., and Rubbo, S. D., 1961, Immunization against tetanus, *J. Hyg.* **59**:29–48.

United States Minimum Requirements, 1956, Tetanus and Diphtheria Toxoids Combined Precipitated, Adsorbed (For Adult Use), Amendment No. 1, U.S. Department of Health, Education & Welfare, National Institutes of Health, Bethesda.

van Ramshorst, J. D., 1949, The adsorption of diphtheria toxoid on aluminum phosphate, *Recl. Trav. Chim. Pays-Bas* **68**:169–180.

Vassilev, T. L., 1978, Aluminium phosphate but not calcium phosphate stimulates the specific IgE response in guinea-pigs to tetanus toxoid, *Allergy* **33**:155–159.

Volk, V. K., and Bunney, W. E., 1939, Diphtheria immunization with fluid toxoid and alum precipitated toxoid. Preliminary report, *Am. J. Public Health* **29**:197–204.

Volk, V. K., and Bunney, W. E., 1942, Diphtheria immunization with fluid toxoid and alum precipitated toxoid, *Am. J. Public Health* **32**:690–699.

Walls, R. S., 1977, Eosinophil response to alum adjuvants: Involvement of T cells in non-antigen-dependent mechanisms, *Proc. Soc. Exp. Biol. Med.* **156**:431–435.

Warren, H. S., Vogel, F. R., and Chedid, L. A., 1986, Current status of immunological adjuvants, *Annu. Rev. Immunol.* **4**:369–388.

White, J. L., and Schlageter, E. A., 1934, Diphtheria toxoid. Comparative immunizing value with and without alum, as indicated by Schick test, *J. Am. Med. Assoc.* **102**:915.

White, R. G., 1967, Concepts relating to the mode of action of adjuvants, *Symp. Ser. Immunobiol. Stand.* **6**:3–12.

White, R. G., Coons, A.H., and Connolly, J. M., 1955, Studies on antibody production. III. The alum granuloma, *J. Exp. Med.* **102**:73–82.

Woodard, L. F., 1989, Adjuvant activity of water-insoluble surfactants, *Lab. Anim. Sci.* **39**:222–225.

World Health Organization, 1976, Immunological adjuvants, in: *Tech. Rep. Series 595*, World Health Organization, Geneva, pp. 3–40.

World Health Organization, 1977, *Manual for the Production and Control of Vaccines—Tetanus Toxoid*, BLG/UNDP/77.2 Rev. 1.

World Health Organization, 1990, Requirements for diphtheria, tetanus, pertussis and combined vaccines, in: *Technical Report Series 800*, World Health Organization, Geneva, pp. 87–179.

Chapter 9

Structure and Properties of Aluminum-Containing Adjuvants

Stanley L. Hem and Joe L. White

1. INTRODUCTION

The use of aluminum-containing adjuvants originated in 1926 with the observations of Glenny *et al.* (1926) that an alum-precipitated diphtheria vaccine had greater antigenic properties than the standard diphtheria vaccine. Other aluminum hydroxide gels used in the preparation of vaccines were shown by the early X-ray diffraction and electron microscopy studies of Souza Santos *et al.* (1958) to consist of crystalline phases ranging from poorly ordered boehmite (aluminum oxyhydroxide, AlOOH) to well-crystallized gibbsite and bayerite [aluminum hydroxide polymorphs, $Al(OH)_3$]. Aluminum hydroxide gels containing phosphate were also developed as adjuvants. Although aluminum compounds have a long history of use as adjuvants, inconsistent antibody production has been a recurrent problem (Warren and Chedid, 1988). The adjuvant action of aluminum hydroxide has been reviewed by Aprile and Wardlaw (1966), Edelman (1980), Warren *et al.* (1986), and Nicklas (1992). Although the mechanism of adjuvant action of aluminum hydroxide and related phases is not fully understood, it is likely that surface area, surface charge, and morphology of the aluminum hydroxide are important factors (Hem and White, 1984).

Aluminum hydroxide adjuvants and their derivatives have been widely used because of their reputation for safety in humans and, currently, are the only ones included in vaccines licensed by the Food and Drug Administration (Edelman, 1980).

2. CHARACTERIZATION

Vaccines containing aluminum compounds as adjuvants are prepared by two principal methods: (1) mixing of a commercially prepared adjuvant, usually labeled aluminum

Stanley L. Hem • Department of Industrial and Physical Pharmacy, Purdue University, West Lafayette, Indiana 47907.   *Joe L. White* • Department of Agronomy, Purdue University, West Lafayette, Indiana 47907.

Vaccine Design: The Subunit and Adjuvant Approach, edited by Michael F. Powell and Mark J. Newman. Plenum Press, New York, 1995.

hydroxide or aluminum phosphate, with the antigen, or (2) in situ precipitation in a solution of alum, $KAl(SO_4)_2 \cdot 12H_2O$, mixed with the antigen solution. The resulting precipitate has been described historically as protein aluminate and the vaccines prepared in this manner are termed "alum-precipitated" vaccines. In situ precipitations may also be performed using aluminum chloride in place of alum.

Among the attributes of a satisfactory aluminum-containing adjuvant are stability and high surface area. Precipitation of aluminum hydroxide at 25 °C from solutions containing anions that have a weak to moderate affinity for aluminum (e.g., chloride and sulfate, respectively) initially produces an amorphous aluminum hydroxychloride or hydroxysulfate with a very high surface area (Nail et al., 1976a; Hem and White, 1984). However, the precipitate ages quickly as the adsorbed chloride and sulfate anions are displaced by hydroxyl ions to form crystalline $Al(OH)_3$ (gibbsite) with a much lower surface area and reactivity (Nail et al., 1976b). These changes in surface area and associated properties would be unacceptable in a material used as an adjuvant as they would lead to instability and diminished efficacy of the vaccine on storage.

The following procedures have been used in efforts to achieve the required high surface area and stability of the adjuvant: (1) preparation of an amorphous aluminum hydroxide gel having a high surface area and use of an anion having moderate to high affinity for aluminum to inhibit crystallization (White and Hem, 1975; Hsu, 1979); (2) preparation of an amorphous aluminum hydroxide gel and use of hydrothermal treatment to transform the gel into a poorly crystalline phase which retains a high surface area. The crystalline phase does not change significantly during aging (Tettenhorst and Hofmann, 1980).

An important factor in the formulation and production of aluminum-containing adjuvants is the surface charge. The hydroxylated surfaces of aluminum hydroxide may become charged, either through amphoteric dissociation of the surface OH groups, or by adsorption of H^+ or OH^- or other potential-determining ions. Concentrations of the potential-determining ions and the net surface charge are pH-dependent and there will be a pH value at which the net surface charge is zero, i.e., the densities of positive and negative charge are equal. This pH is referred to as the isoelectric point (pI) or point of zero charge (PZC). The surface charge is described by the following equation:

$$\text{surface charge} = 59 \text{ mV (PZC} - \text{pH)}$$

Even though the pH of most vaccines is 7.4, the pI of aluminum-containing adjuvants may range from 5 to 11. Therefore, the surface charge may vary from strongly positive to strongly negative depending on the pI.

An important step in producing a consistent adjuvant effect is the thorough characterization of the aluminum compounds currently used as adjuvants (Hem and White, 1984). By use of X-ray diffraction, IR spectroscopy, transmission electron micrography, energy-dispersive spectrometry, Doppler electrophoretic light scattering analysis, rate of solubilization in constituents of interstitial fluid, and protein adsorptive capacity measurements, Shirodkar et al. (1990), Seeber et al. (1991a, b), and Al-Shakhshir et al. (1994) have established the amorphous or crystalline nature of these compounds, their morphology, solubilization rate in simulated interstitial fluid, protein adsorptive capacity, and surface charge. Commercial aluminum-containing adjuvants have been historically classified into aluminum hydroxide, aluminum phosphate, and alum-precipitated groups. As shown by Shirodkar *et al.* (1990), alum-precipitated adjuvants precipitated in the presence of a phosphate buffer contain significant amounts of phosphate. Because of the great similarities in composition, morphology, surface charge, and other physicochemical properties between aluminum phosphate and alum-precipitated adjuvants, it is possible to consider them both under the designation of aluminum hydroxyphosphate. Thus, the results of characterization studies and their implications will be discussed for categories of aluminum-containing adjuvants designated as either aluminum hydroxide or aluminum hydroxyphosphate.

2.1. Aluminum Hydroxide Adjuvants

Commercial adjuvants labeled as "aluminum hydroxide" show varying degrees of crystallinity when examined by X-ray diffraction and have diffraction bands at 6.46, 3.18, 2.35, 1.86, 1.44, and 1.31 Å (Fig. 1A) (Shirodkar *et al.*, 1990). These spacings correspond to those of boehmite (Tettenhorst and Hofmann, 1980), an aluminum oxyhydroxide, AlOOH. The degree of crystallinity is reflected in the width of the diffraction band at half height (WHH); poorly crystalline boehmite particles show greater line broadening as a result of smaller crystallite size (Tettenhorst and Hofmann, 1980). As would be predicted, the surface area and chemical reactivity of boehmite increase as the WHH increases. In a comparison of two commercial aluminum hydroxide adjuvants, Seeber *et al.* (1991b) observed enhanced albumin adsorption (1.77 versus 2.59 mg/mg Al) and a faster rate of solubilization (Seeber *et al.*, 1991a) in simulated interstitial fluid by the sample having the greater line broadening as measured by the WHH. In an examination of the adsorption of two malaria antigens by two aluminum hydroxide adjuvants, Callahan *et al.* (1991) observed greater adsorption for the boehmite sample having the greater WHH.

Using thermal treatment to control the primary crystallite size of aluminum hydroxide adjuvants, Masood *et al.* (1994) demonstrated that adsorption of BSA by boehmite is directly related to the WHH of the (020) reflection in the X-ray diffraction pattern (Table I). Thus, X-ray diffractograms of aluminum hydroxide adjuvants should be useful in predicting and controlling their properties.

The IR spectra of aluminum hydroxide adjuvants provide further evidence for their identification as boehmite. The IR spectrum of a typical aluminum hydroxide adjuvant is shown in Fig. 2A. The adsorption band at 1070 cm^{-1}, in the O–H deformation region, is indicative of boehmite (Fripiat *et al.*, 1967; Van der Marel and Beutelspacher, 1976). The strong shoulder at 3090–3100 cm^{-1} is also unique for boehmite and indicates the existence of structural hydroxyl environments which are characteristic of boehmite. Additional bands attributed to boehmite include those at 750, 640, and 485 cm^{-1} (Tettenhorst and Hofmann, 1980).

The fibrous morphology of aluminum hydroxide adjuvants is illustrated in the transmission electron micrograph in Fig. 3A and is characteristic of boehmite. Energy-dispersive spectrometry showed only the presence of aluminum, which is consistent with the composition of boehmite.

In a study of the solubilization of three commercially available aluminum-containing adjuvants by citrate anion, Seeber *et al.* (1991a) found that aluminum phosphate adjuvant

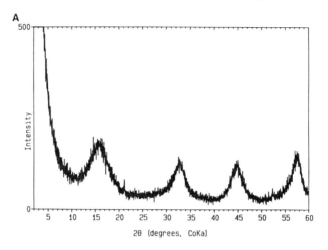

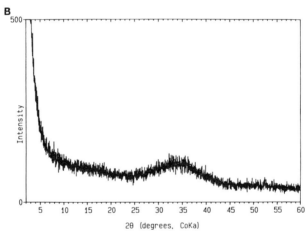

Figure 1. Typical X-ray diffraction pattern of aluminum hydroxide adjuvant (A) and aluminum phosphate adjuvant (B).

Table I
Relationship between Protein Adsorptive Capacity and Line Broadening
of the X-ray Diffraction Pattern of Aluminum Hydroxide Adjuvants[a]

Width at half height (° 2θ)	Albumin adsorptive capacity at pH 7.4 (mg/mg Al)
3.56	3.50
3.28	3.07
2.94	2.59
2.43	2.32
1.97	1.78

[a]From Masood *et al.* (1994).

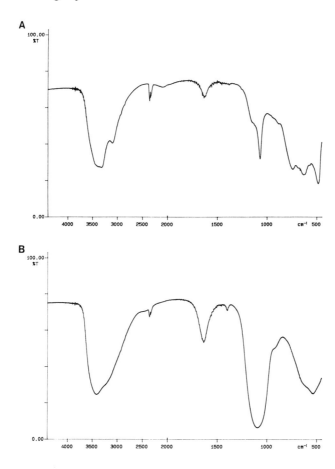

Figure 2. Typical IR spectrum of aluminum hydroxide adjuvant (A) and aluminum phosphate adjuvant (B).

and aluminum hydroxide adjuvant were both solubilized, but the aluminum phosphate adjuvant dissolved significantly faster than the aluminum hydroxide adjuvant. Thus, the slower rate of dissolution of aluminum hydroxide adjuvants may create more of a depot effect than is achieved with aluminum phosphate adjuvants.

The isoelectric point (pI) of aluminum hydroxide adjuvant is about 11. Thus, in a physiological pH range around 7.4, the adjuvant surface is positively charged and will adsorb negatively charged antigens by electrostatic attraction.

2.2. Aluminum Hydroxyphosphate Adjuvants

Since commercial alum-precipitated adjuvants and aluminum phosphate adjuvants both contain phosphate and have very similar properties, they can be considered as members of a continuous series of aluminum hydroxyphosphate compositions in which the molar PO_4/Al ratio ranges from 0.3 to 0.9.

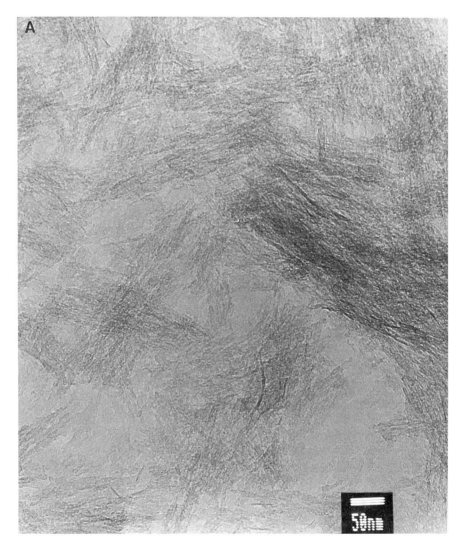

Figure 3. Typical transmission electron micrograph of aluminum hydroxide adjuvant (A) and aluminum phosphate adjuvant (B). (continued)

A critical factor in the differences between aluminum phosphate adjuvants and alum-precipitated adjuvants that are precipitated in the presence of a phosphate buffer is the relative affinity of anions other than phosphate for aluminum. Hsu (1989) proposed the following categories of anions based on their affinity for aluminum: weak affinity: nitrate, chlorate, and chloride; moderate affinity: sulfate; strong affinity: phosphate; and very strong affinity: fluoride. Thus, precipitates from solutions containing phosphate plus

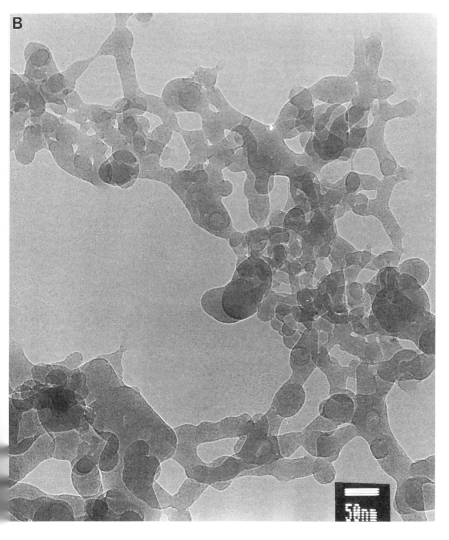

Figure 3. (continued)

anions having a weak affinity for aluminum would be expected to have a higher phosphate content than those from a solution having a comparable phosphate concentration but that contained anions having moderate affinity for aluminum. Aluminum phosphate adjuvants made using aluminum salts in which the anion has weak affinity for aluminum, such as aluminum chloride, have a higher phosphate content than alum-precipitated adjuvants prepared using a phosphate buffer, since in the latter the sulfate anion competes more effectively with phosphate for adsorption sites. Based on the relationship between molar PO_4/Al ratio and the isoelectric point of aluminum hydroxyphosphate adjuvants, aluminum phosphate adjuvants have a PO_4/Al ratio in the range of 0.8–0.9 whereas in alum-precipitated adjuvants the ratio is usually in the 0.3–0.6 range.

Cheung *et al.* (1986) employed X-ray diffraction and high-resolution solid-state NMR spectroscopy using both ^{27}Al and ^{31}P nuclei to study the structure of aluminum phosphates coprecipitated from solutions in which the PO_4/Al ratio was less than one. They concluded that the precipitates were amorphous structures in which the phosphate is randomly dispersed, and the aluminum exists in one octahedral and several different tetrahedral environments. Bleam *et al.* (1991) used ^{31}P solid-state NMR to study phosphate adsorption at the surface of aluminum oxyhydroxide and concluded that inner-sphere surface complexes form between phosphate and the surface aluminum atoms, and the phosphates in these complexes hydrolyze with varying pH. Liu *et al.* (1984) found that phosphate was specifically adsorbed by aluminum hydroxycarbonate through anion ligand exchange; IR analysis indicated that phosphate exchanged with specifically adsorbed carbonate. IR observations by Shirodkar *et al.* (1990) on alum-precipitated adjuvants precipitated at molar PO_4/Al ratios of 0.25, 0.50, and 1.0 showed that phosphate also exchanged with specifically adsorbed sulfate. Thus, changes in the solution environment can result in desorption or adsorption of phosphate by aluminum-containing adjuvant surfaces with concomitant changes in surface charge and antigen/adjuvant interactions.

2.2.1. ALUMINUM PHOSPHATE ADJUVANTS

Commercial adjuvants designated as "aluminum phosphate" show no X-ray diffraction bands characteristic of crystalline phases, indicating they are amorphous (Fig. 1B). Transmission electron micrographs of aluminum phosphate adjuvants show a network of platy particles as illustrated in Fig. 3B. Energy-dispersive spectra of samples of these adjuvants indicate the presence of both aluminum and phosphorus. The IR spectrum of an aluminum phosphate adjuvant is shown in Fig. 2B. The absorption band in the 1080–1090 cm^{-1} region is attributed to P–O stretching (Ross, 1974) and is characteristic for phosphate. Other bands in synthetic aluminum hydroxyphosphate occur in the 650, 700–730, and 510–550 cm^{-1} regions (Shirodkar *et al.*, 1990). In addition, the broad OH-stretching band in the 3420–3430 cm^{-1} region has a major component in the 3150 cm^{-1} region. A sample heated to 200°C showed a prominent OH-stretching frequency at 3164 cm^{-1} as well as a band at 3450 cm^{-1} (Shirodkar *et al.*, 1990). The band at 3164 cm^{-1} is evidence for the presence of structural hydroxyls. Thus, the aluminum phosphate adjuvants are more properly designated amorphous aluminum hydroxyphosphate.

Seeber *et al.* (1991a) found that an aluminum phosphate adjuvant was solubilized in simulated interstitial fluid significantly faster than an aluminum hydroxide adjuvant. It appears that dissolution patterns of aluminum-containing adjuvants in interstitial fluid vary widely and may influence the release pattern of the antigen.

Commercial aluminum phosphate adjuvants, such as Adju-phos, have isoelectric points around 5. However, in general the isoelectric point is inversely related to the phosphate content (Liu *et al.*, 1984). Thus, in solutions at the physiological pH of 7.4, these adjuvants have a negative charge. Electrostatic attraction occurs with antigens that are positively charged at pH 7.4.

2.2.2. ALUM-PRECIPITATED ADJUVANTS

Preparation of adjuvants by the alum-precipitation method normally requires the antigen to be in a buffered solution when it is mixed with the alum solution [$KAl(SO_4)_2 \cdot 12H_2O$]. Shirodkar et al. (1990) found that the aluminum hydroxide resulting from the precipitation process contained not only sulfate anion from the alum but also the anion from the buffer that was used to stabilize the antigen solution (acetate, carbonate, citrate, phosphate, etc.). The X-ray diffraction pattern of the alum-precipitated adjuvant prepared in the presence of phosphate or other buffers showed the solid phase to be amorphous as in aluminum phosphate adjuvant. IR spectra of these adjuvants contained bands associated with sulfate as well as the buffer anion. Thus, the adjuvant produced by the alum-precipitation process is an amorphous aluminum hydroxy (buffer anion) sulfate. The composition and properties of this type of adjuvant, such as the isoelectric point, depend on the precipitation conditions. Since phosphate buffers are widely used in vaccine production, alum-precipitated adjuvants prepared in a phosphate buffer are best described as amorphous aluminum hydroxyphosphatesulfate. Because of the much higher affinity of aluminum for phosphate, very little sulfate appears in the adjuvant. The degree of substitution of phosphate for hydroxyl depends on the concentration of the phosphate buffer and the precipitation conditions.

Alum-precipitated adjuvants that are precipitated in the presence of a phosphate buffer are essentially the same as aluminum phosphate adjuvants except that they contain a small amount of sulfate from the alum. The isoelectric point is inversely related to the phosphate content as was observed for aluminum phosphate adjuvants. Because of their amorphous nature, it is expected that alum-precipitated adjuvants will show the rapid rate of dissolution in simulated interstitial fluid that was observed for aluminum phosphate adjuvants. For the remainder of the chapter it will be assumed that alum-precipitated adjuvants that are precipitated in the presence of phosphate buffer exhibit the properties associated with aluminum phosphate adjuvants having a similar phosphate content.

2.3. Commercial Vaccines

The aluminum-containing adjuvants in three commercial diphtheria and tetanus toxoids, U.S.P., were examined by Shirodkar et al. (1990). These were identified as follows: vaccine A (Connaught, labeled as an alum-precipitated toxoid in an isotonic sodium chloride solution containing sodium phosphate to control the pH); vaccine B (Sclavo, labeled as a sterile suspension of toxoids adsorbed by aluminum hydroxide); and vaccine C (Wyeth, labeled as aluminum phosphate adsorbed). Characterization of the adjuvant in these commercial vaccines by X-ray diffraction, IR spectroscopy, transmission electron microscopy, and energy-dispersive spectrometry showed the adjuvant in vaccine A to be similar to amorphous aluminum hydroxyphosphatesulfate from the alum-precipitation process. The vaccine B adjuvant exhibited properties similar to those of aluminum hydroxide adjuvants. The vaccine C adjuvant was found to be amorphous aluminum hydroxyphosphate similar to the previously described aluminum phosphate adjuvants.

Aluminum-containing adjuvants can be categorized chemically as either crystalline aluminum oxyhydroxide (boehmite) or amorphous aluminum hydroxyphosphate. These

Table II

Some Physical and Chemical Properties of Aluminum-Containing Adjuvants

Commercial designation	Chemical formula	Structure	Morphology	pI	Protein adsorptive capacity, mg/mg Al, pH 7.4	Solubility in citrate[a]
Aluminum hydroxide	AlOOH	Crystalline boehmite	Thin fibrils	11	1.8–2.6^b	~0%
Aluminum phosphate	$Al(OH)_x(PO_4)_y^c$	Amorphous	Plate-like	5–7	0.7–1.5^d	55%
Alum-precipitated	$Al(OH)_x(PO_4)_y(SO_4)_z^c$	Amorphous	Plate-like	6–7	1.0–1.3^d	nd[e]

[a]Seeber et al. (1991a).
[b]BSA.
[c]The sum of the valence of each anion times its mole fraction is −3.
[d]Lysozyme.
[e]Not determined.

adjuvants are known as aluminum hydroxide or aluminum phosphate, respectively. Selected chemical and physical properties are summarized in Table II.

The surface charge and the rate of dissolution in simulated interstitial fluid are very different for aluminum hydroxide adjuvants and aluminum phosphate adjuvants. Thus, selection of an adjuvant for a vaccine formulation should be based on the net charge of the antigen and the desired dissolution rate of the adjuvant in interstitial fluid. Aluminum hydroxide adjuvants will adsorb negatively charged antigens by electrostatic forces and will dissolve relatively slowly in interstitial fluid. Aluminum phosphate adjuvants will adsorb positively charged antigens by electrostatic forces and will dissolve relatively rapidly in interstitial fluid.

3. OPTIMIZING ANTIGEN–ADJUVANT ADSORPTION

One objective in the formulation of vaccines using aluminum-containing adjuvants is to adsorb the antigen onto the adjuvant (Edelman, 1980). Although the adsorption of proteins by polymers has been extensively studied, the adsorption of proteins by aluminum-containing adjuvants has been neglected even though aluminum-containing adjuvants have been used in vaccines for decades (Glenny et al., 1926). Polymers and aluminum-containing adjuvants differ so significantly in properties that generalizations that apply to the adsorption of proteins by polymers cannot be applied to the adsorption of antigens by aluminum-containing adjuvants. For example, polymer surfaces are usually hydrophobic while the surface of aluminum-containing adjuvants is composed of hydrophilic groups such as hydroxyl, oxygen, or phosphate. A second major difference is that aluminum-containing adjuvants are amphoteric and thus may exhibit a net positive, neutral, or negative surface charge, depending on the pH. In contrast, the polymers used to study protein adsorption are usually uncharged.

3.1. Model Proteins

It is likely that electrostatic forces are important in the adsorption of antigens by aluminum-containing adjuvants, as both antigens and adjuvants have a pH-dependent surface charge (Seeber *et al.*, 1991b). This hypothesis was tested by determining the effect of ionic strength on the adsorptive capacity of several model systems (Al-Shakhshir *et al.*, 1995b). Aluminum hydroxide or aluminum phosphate adjuvants having isoelectric points of 11.1 and 5.0, respectively, were combined with either lysozyme (pI = 9.6) or BSA (pI = 5.0) at pH 7.4. The adsorption of negatively charged BSA by positively charged aluminum hydroxide adjuvant follows the Langmuir equation (Fig. 4). The adsorptive capacity was taken from the plateau value of the isotherm. As seen in Table III, the adsorptive capacity decreased from 1.7 to 1.4 mg BSA/mg Al as the ionic strength increased from 0.06 to 0.75 M. Since increasing the ionic strength shields the surface charge, this behavior indicates that electrostatic forces are contributing to adsorption.

The adsorption of positively charged lysozyme by negatively charged aluminum phosphate adjuvant is even more strongly dependent on ionic strength. At low ionic strength, 0.06 M, adsorption followed the Langmuir equation (Fig. 5). However, adsorption was drastically reduced at higher ionic strength and did not follow the Langmuir equation. Thus, electrostatic adsorptive forces are also important in the adsorption of lysozyme by aluminum phosphate adjuvant.

The adsorption of positively charged lysozyme by positively charged aluminum hydroxide adjuvant at 0.06 M ionic strength was much less than was observed for BSA. Only approximately 0.1 mg of lysozyme was adsorbed per milligram of aluminum even when the concentration of lysozyme in solution was 4–6 mg/mL (compare to Fig. 4). Likewise, virtually no adsorption of negatively charged BSA by negatively charged aluminum phosphate adjuvant was observed at ionic strength 0.06 M. It is clear that

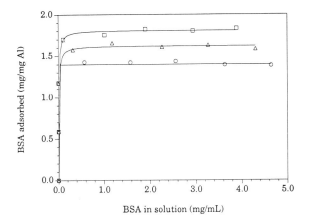

Figure 4. Effect of electrolyte concentration on the Langmuir adsorption isotherm for BSA by aluminum hydroxide adjuvant at pH 7.4 and 25°C. ○, 0.06 M NaCl; △, 0.25 M NaCl; □, 0.75 M NaCl. From Al-Shakhshir *et al.* (1995b).

Table III

Effect of Ionic Strength and Ethylene Glycol Concentration on the Adsorptive Capacity of
Bovine Serum Albumin (BSA) and Lysozyme by Aluminum-Containing Adjuvants[a]

Adjuvant	Protein	Adsorption solution	Adsorptive capacity, mg/mg Al	Langmuir equation R^2
Aluminum hydroxide	BSA	0.06 M NaCl	1.7	0.99
		0.25 M NaCl	1.6	0.99
		0.75 M NaCl	1.4	0.99
Aluminum phosphate	Lysozyme	0.06 M NaCl	0.7	6.99
		0.15 M NaCl	—[b]	0.74
		0.25 M NaCl	—[b]	0.69
Aluminum hydroxide	Lysozyme	0.06 M NaCl	—[b]	0.35
Aluminum phosphate	BSA	0.06 M NaCl	—[b]	—[c]
Aluminum hydroxide	BSA	0% ethylene glycol in 0.06 M NaCl	1.7	0.99
		20% ethylene glycol in 0.06 M NaCl	1.7	0.99
		40% ethylene glycol in 0.06 M NaCl	1.7	0.99
Aluminum phosphate	Lysozyme	0% ethylene glycol in 0.06 M NaCl	0.7	0.99
		20% ethylene glycol in 0.06 M NaCl	0.6	0.99
		40% ethylene glycol in 0.06 M NaCl	0.5	0.98

[a]From Al-Shakhshir et al. (1995b).
[b]Adsorption did not follow the Langmuir equation.
[c]Adsorption too low to calculate.

electrostatic repulsive forces in these systems are strong enough to prevent substantial adsorption by other attractive forces.

Hydrophobic attractive forces are a major force in determining the conformation of proteins. It is possible that hydrophobic interactions may contribute to the adsorption of antigens by aluminum-containing adjuvants. Ethylene glycol is frequently added to mobile phases in hydrophobic interaction chromatography to reduce the hydrophobic interaction between protein and sorbent (Srinivasan and Ruckenstein, 1980). It functions by stabilizing the hydration layer of the protein, rendering hydrophobic interactions thermodynamically unfavorable. As seen in Fig. 6 and Table III, the adsorption of BSA by aluminum hydroxide adjuvant at 0.06 M ionic strength was not affected by the presence of 20 or 40% ethylene glycol. In contrast, the adsorptive capacity of lysozyme by aluminum phosphate adjuvant was inversely related to the ethylene glycol concentration (Fig. 7 and Table III). The data in Figs. 6 and 7 indicate that hydrophobic forces contribute to the adsorption of lysozyme but not to BSA. This observation is consistent with the report (Gooding et al., 1984) that lysozyme has a longer retention time than BSA during hydrophobic interaction chromatography.

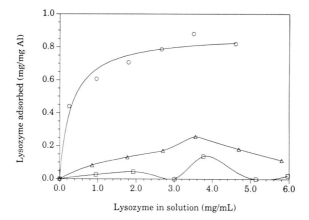

Figure 5. Effect of electrolyte concentration on the Langmuir adsorption isotherm for lysozyme by aluminum phosphate adjuvant at pH 7.4 and 25°C. ○, 0.06 M NaCl; △, 0.15 M NaCl; □, 0.25 M NaCl. From Al-Shakhshir *et al*. (1995b).

It can be concluded that electrostatic attractive forces and hydrophobic forces contribute to the adsorption of antigens by aluminum-containing adjuvants. It is likely that van der Waals forces and hydrogen bonding also contribute to adsorption in these systems. However, the attractive adsorption forces may not be sufficient to produce adsorption of an antigen if electrostatic repulsive forces are present.

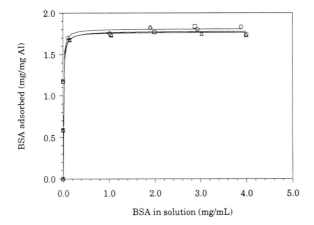

Figure 6. Effect of ethylene glycol on the Langmuir adsorption isotherm for BSA by aluminum hydroxide adjuvant at ionic strength 0.06 M, pH 7.4, and 25°C. ○, 0% ethylene; △, 20% ethylene glycol; □, 40% ethylene glycol. From Al-Shakhshir *et al*. (1995b).

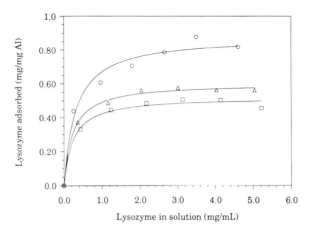

Figure 7. Effect of ethylene glycol on the Langmuir adsorption isotherm for lysozyme by aluminum phosphate adjuvant at ionic strength 0.06 M, pH 7.4, and 25°C. ○, 0% ethylene glycol; △, 20% ethylene glycol; □, 40% ethylene glycol. From Al-Shakhshir *et al.* (1995b).

3.2. Malaria Antigens

The importance of surface charge in the adsorption of antigens by aluminum-containing adjuvants was tested using recombinant malarial antigens (Callahan *et al.*, 1991). The antigens were based on the repeat regions of the sporozoite coat protein of the malarial parasites *Plasmodium falciparum* and *Plasmodium vivax*. Although the repeat region sequence is fairly similar, the tail regions result in distinctive isoelectric points. The R32NS181 and NS181V20 antigens have isoelectric points of 5.9 and 5.5, respectively, whereas the R32tet32 antigen is basic, with a pI of 12.8. The pH dependence of the extent of adsorption by aluminum hydroxide adjuvant is presented in Fig. 8. The data include experimental points obtained for both forward and reverse pH steps as indicated by the numerical sequence. The antigens with low pI values were adsorbed to a considerable extent. Adsorption was inversely related to pH for both NS181V20 and R32NS181 antigens. Electrostatic attractive forces are important because adsorption decreased as the pH approached the isoelectric point of the aluminum hydroxide adjuvant (pI = 9.8). The higher degree of adsorption observed for NS181V20 may be related to the contribution of other adsorption mechanisms such as hydrophobic bonding and hydrogen bonding.

The basic antigen, R32tet32, was not adsorbed to any significant degree by the aluminum hydroxide adjuvant (Fig. 8). In this case both the antigen and adjuvant are positively charged in the pH range of 5 to 9 and electrostatic repulsive forces apparently prevent adsorption by other mechanisms.

The aluminum phosphate adjuvant, whose isoelectric point was 4.5, had a negative surface charge over the pH range of 5–9. As seen in Fig. 9, antigen R32NS181 was not adsorbed by the aluminum phosphate adjuvant. In comparison, this antigen was 70% adsorbed at pH 5 by the aluminum hydroxide adjuvant. The electrostatic repulsive force

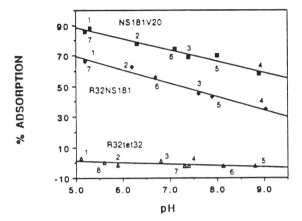

Figure 8. Effect of pH on the adsorption of three malarial antigens by aluminum hydroxide adjuvant. The numbers indicate the sequence in which the experiments were performed. From Callahan *et al.* (1991).

between the negatively charged antigen and the negatively charged adjuvant was apparently blocking adsorption.

Antigen NS181V20 displayed a higher degree of adsorption to aluminum phosphate adjuvant but its adsorption was decreased by approximately 50% relative to aluminum hydroxide adjuvant (compare Figs. 9 and 8). This is probably related to the contribution of hydrophobic adsorption forces as noted in Fig. 8.

The basic antigen, R32tet32, displayed pH-dependent adsorption to aluminum phosphate adjuvant (Fig. 10). Adsorption increased as the surface charge of the aluminum phosphate adjuvant became more negative. Antigen R32tet32 exhibited a positive surface charge in this pH region. In this system, adsorption was irreversible, as no desorption was observed when the pH was brought to pH 9 and then decreased.

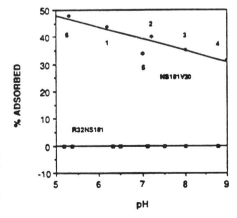

Figure 9. Effect of pH on the adsorption of two acidic malarial antigens by aluminum phosphate adjuvant. The numbers indicate the sequence in which the experiments were performed. From Callahan *et al.* (1991).

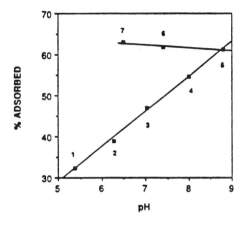

Figure 10. Effect of pH on the adsorption of a basic malarial antigen by aluminum phosphate adjuvant. The numbers indicate the sequence in which the experiments were performed. From Callahan *et al.* (1991).

It is possible to modify the surface charge characteristics of aluminum hydroxide adjuvant by substituting phosphate for hydroxyl at the surface. The substitution of the higher valence anion reduces the point of zero charge as seen in Fig. 11. The increased negative surface charge resulting from treatment with phosphate anion increased the adsorption of positively charged R32tet32 (Fig. 12) by aluminum hydroxide adjuvant. The adsorption of the negatively charged antigens, R32NS181 and NS181V20, was reduced by treatment of the aluminum hydroxide adjuvant with phosphate anion.

The adsorption of antigens by aluminum-containing adjuvants is significantly influenced by the electrostatic forces operating in the system. Electrostatic attractive forces result in adsorption of the antigen. Therefore, the choice of using either an aluminum hydroxide adjuvant or an aluminum phosphate adjuvant should be based on the pI of the antigen (assuming antigen binding and immunogenicity correlate). Antigens having a pI

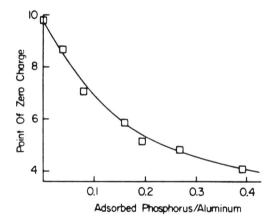

Figure 11. Effect of phosphate substitution for hydroxyl on the point of zero charge of aluminum hydroxide. From Liu *et al.* (1984).

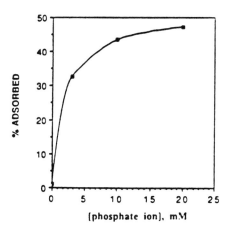

Figure 12. Effect of phosphate anion on the adsorption of the basic malarial antigen, R32tet32, by aluminum hydroxide adjuvant at pH 7 and constant ionic strength. From Callahan *et al.* (1991).

below 7.4 will be most strongly adsorbed by aluminum hydroxide adjuvant, while antigens whose pI is above 7.4 will be best adsorbed by aluminum phosphate adjuvant. It is also possible to modify the surface charge characteristics of aluminum hydroxide adjuvant by pretreating the adjuvant with phosphate anion. This will result in the substitution of phosphate for hydroxyl at the surface of the adjuvant and will lower the isoelectric point. Such pretreatment may permit aluminum hydroxide adjuvants to adsorb antigens having pI's above 7.4.

4. EFFECT OF PROTEIN ADSORPTION ON SURFACE PROPERTIES

The importance of electrostatic forces on the adsorption of antigens by aluminum-containing adjuvants was illustrated in the previous section. Knowledge of the pI of the antigen and adjuvant as well as the pH allows prediction of the degree of adsorption that will occur when the vaccine is prepared. However, examination of the pI values and pH may not be useful in predicting the physical properties of the completed vaccine because the physical properties will likely depend on the surface charge characteristics of the antigen–adjuvant complex (Al-Shakhshir *et al.*, 1994).

The surface charge characteristics of aluminum phosphate adjuvant and lysozyme are presented on the upper axis of Fig. 13. The isoelectric point of the aluminum phosphate adjuvant was 5.0 and the pI of lysozyme was 9.6. The aluminum phosphate adjuvant exhibits a smooth curve as the ionization state of surface hydroxyl groups changed from $-OH_2^+$ to $-O^-$. In contrast, the surface charge of lysozyme is relatively independent of pH between 5 and 9. This behavior occurs because histidine (pKa = 6.5) and cysteine (pKa = 8.5) are the only amino acids that ionize in this pH region. Lysozyme contains one histidine and eight cysteine amino acids out of 129 amino acids. The actual number of ionizable groups is even less, as all eight cysteines in lysozyme are part of disulfide bonds (Imoto *et al.*, 1972).

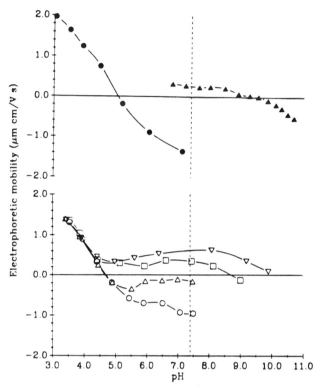

Figure 13. Effect of lysozyme adsorption on the surface charge characteristics of aluminum phosphate adjuvant at ionic strength 0.07 M and 25°C. The adsorptive capacity is 0.73 mg lysozyme/mg Al. ●, aluminum phosphate adjuvant; ▲, lysozyme; ○, 0.27 mg lysozyme adsorbed/mg Al; △, 0.39 mg lysozyme/mg Al; □, 0.54 mg lysozyme adsorbed/mg Al; ▽, 0.71 mg lysozyme adsorbed/mg Al. From Al-Shakhshir *et al.* (1994).

The adsorptive capacity of the aluminum phosphate adjuvant for lysozyme was 0.73 mg lysozyme/mg Al. The effect of lysozyme adsorption on the surface charge characteristics of the aluminum phosphate adjuvant is seen on the lower axis of Fig. 13. The adsorption of the positively charged lysozyme reduced and, at higher concentrations, reversed the negative electrophoretic mobility that the adjuvant exhibits at pH 7.4. It is also apparent from Fig. 13 that the electrophoretic mobility of the lysozyme–aluminum phosphate adjuvant complex became independent of pH between pH 5 and 9 when the amount of adsorbed lysozyme reached approximately 50% of the adsorptive capacity. At a surface coverage of approximately 75% of the adsorptive capacity, the surface charge characteristics of the complex were those of lysozyme. Similar behavior was observed when negatively charged BSA was adsorbed by positively charged aluminum hydroxide adjuvant. Thus, the surface charge characteristics of the aluminum-containing adjuvant dominate at low protein coverage. However, the surface charge characteristics of the adsorbed protein dominate at high protein coverage.

5. INTERACTIONS IN MULTIVALENT VACCINES USING MIXTURES OF ALUMINUM-CONTAINING ADJUVANTS

Optimum formulation of vaccines containing multivalent antigens may require that more than a single type of aluminum-containing adjuvant be used (Al-Shakhshir *et al.*, 1995a). In some cases, in order to maximize the binding of negatively charged antigen(s), a positively charged adjuvant such as aluminum hydroxide could be used. In other cases, if the antigen(s) were positively charged, a negatively charged adjuvant such as aluminum phosphate might be preferred. The multivalent vaccine would therefore be prepared by combining the individual monovalent bulks resulting in a suspension consisting of mixed aluminum-containing adjuvants. Questions arise regarding the potential for redistribution of antigens and adsorbed phosphate anions as well as the colloidal stability of multivalent vaccines that use different aluminum-containing adjuvants.

5.1. Redistribution of Antigens

The preparation of multivalent vaccines may require the mixing of monovalent suspensions. In order to study whether the antigen remained adsorbed on such dilution, model protein-adsorbed adjuvant suspensions were diluted 1:2, 1:10, and 1:100 in 0.07 M NaCl rather than with the other adjuvant suspension. The amount of protein in the supernatant was determined before and after dilution.

The dilution of the BSA–aluminum hydroxide adjuvant complex resulted in little or no desorption of the BSA after a 1:2 or 1:10 dilution and only 7% desorption after a 1:100 dilution (Table IV). On the other hand, a 1:2 dilution of the lysozyme–aluminum phosphate adjuvant complex resulted in the desorption of 26% of the adsorbed lysozyme. A 1:100 dilution caused 88% of the lysozyme to desorb. The higher degree of lysozyme desorption can be related to weaker binding to the adjuvant because of lysozyme's structural stability compared to BSA, which has a greater tendency to adapt conformationally and thus accommodate multiple binding sites (Norde and Anusiem, 1992).

Since the surface charge characteristics of the protein–adjuvant complex are dependent on the amount of adsorbed protein (Al-Shakhshir *et al.*, 1994), the desorption of positively charged lysozyme increased the net negative surface charge of the lysozyme–aluminum phosphate adjuvant complex at pH 7.4.

Table IV
Effect of Dilution on the Desorption of the Protein in Protein–Aluminum-Containing Adjuvant Suspensions at 0.07 M Ionic Strength, pH 7.4, and 25°C[a]

		% protein desorbed on dilution (dilution ratio)		
Adjuvant	Protein	1:2	1:10	1:100
Aluminum hydroxide	Bovine serum albumin	0	0	7
Aluminum phosphate	Lysozyme	26	58	88

[a]From Al-Shakhshir *et al.* (1995a).

Table V

Effect of Dilution on the Desorption of Phosphate Anion from an Aluminum Phosphate
Adjuvant at 0.07 M Ionic Strength, pH 7.4, and 25°C[a]

Concentration mg Al/mL	PO_4 in supernatant mg/mg Al	PO_4 desorbed by dilution, μg/ml Al
4.4	109	—
1.7	128	19
0.85	142	33
0.17	178	69
0.017	191	82

[a]From Al-Shakhshir et al. (1995a).

5.2. Redistribution of Phosphate Anions

The effect of dilution on the phosphate concentration of the supernatant of the aluminum phosphate adjuvant is shown in Table V. Dilution of the commercial adjuvant (4.4 mg Al/mL) to the maximum concentration allowed in a vaccine (0.85 mg Al/0.5 mL) resulted in the desorption of 19 μg PO_4/mg Al. The surface charge characteristics will be affected by the partial desorption of phosphate, i.e., the isoelectric point of the aluminum phosphate adjuvant will increase (Liu et al., 1984).

In order to simulate the dilution that occurs during the preparation of a multivalent vaccine, the dilution experiment was repeated using the same concentration of aluminum phosphate adjuvant but also including an equal concentration of aluminum hydroxide adjuvant in the mixture. As seen in Table VI, the level of phosphate in solution increased as the degree of dilution increased. However, the amount of phosphate in the supernatant was much less than observed when only the aluminum phosphate adjuvant was diluted (compare to Table V). It is believed that a fraction of the phosphate anion that desorbed from the aluminum phosphate adjuvant on dilution was adsorbed by the aluminum hydroxide adjuvant. This will lower the isoelectric point of the aluminum hydroxide adjuvant. Thus, the distribution of phosphate anion during the preparation of a multivalent vaccine is altered, as a result of desorption of phosphate anions from the aluminum phosphate adjuvant and their adsorption by the aluminum hydroxide adjuvant.

Table VI

Effect of Dilution on the Distribution of Phosphate Anion in a Mixed Suspension
Containing Equal Parts of Aluminum Phosphate Adjuvant and Aluminum Hydroxide
Adjuvant at 0.07 M Ionic Strength, pH 7.4, and 25°C[a]

Concentration, mg Al/mL	PO_4 remaining in supernatant μg/mg Al	PO_4 adsorbed by aluminum hydroxide adjuvant μg/mg Al
3.4	26	103
1.7	32	110
0.34	64	114
0.034	72	119

[a]From Al-Shakhshir et al. (1995a).

5.3. Colloidal Interactions

Colloidal interactions in mixtures can be determined by monitoring the electro-phoretic mobility of the populations in dilute mixed suspensions as a function of time. An aluminum hydroxide adjuvant and an aluminum phosphate adjuvant were oppositely charged at pH 7.4, having electrophoretic mobilities of 2.0 and –2.1 μm-cm/V-s, respec-tively (Fig. 14). Immediately after mixing the suspensions, the positive electrophoretic mobility of the aluminum hydroxide adjuvant decreased to 0.7 μm-cm/V-s, while the negative electrophoretic mobility of the aluminum phosphate adjuvant decreased to –0.3 μm-cm/V-s. The decreases in electrophoretic mobilities are likely related to the desorption of phosphate anions from the aluminum phosphate adjuvant and their adsorption by the aluminum hydroxide adjuvant. Both populations were observed in the mixture for approxi-mately 40 min after which a single population having an intermediate electrophoretic mobility was present.

The effect of adsorbed protein on the colloidal interactions was studied by preparing a BSA–aluminum hydroxide adjuvant complex in which 0.80 mg BSA was adsorbed/mg Al and a lysozyme–aluminum phosphate adjuvant complex containing 0.51 mg lysozyme/mg Al. Both of these model vaccines were prepared to be below the adsorptive capacity of each adjuvant. As seen in Fig. 15, the adsorption of BSA by the aluminum hydroxide adjuvant reduced the electrophoretic mobility of the aluminum hydroxide adjuvant from 2.0 to 1.0 μm-cm/V-s. The adsorption of lysozyme by the aluminum phosphate adjuvant reduced the electrophoretic mobility from –2.1 to –0.3 μm-cm/V-s. Following mixing of the two protein–adjuvant complex suspensions, two populations appeared, which had electrophoretic mobilities of approximately 0.5 and –0.4 μm-cm/V-s. It is believed that these populations arise as a result of the redistribution of lysozyme and phosphate anions following mixing. The desorption of lysozyme is expected to increase the negative electrophoretic mobility of the lysozyme–aluminum phosphate adjuvant complex, while desorption of phosphate anions will reduce the negative electrophoretic

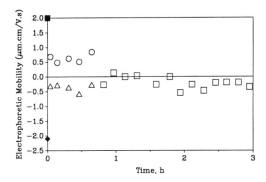

Figure 14. Electrophoretic mobility of populations present during the aging of a 1:1 elemental aluminum mixture of aluminum hydroxide adjuvant and aluminum phosphate adjuvant containing 0.017 mg Al/mL at pH 7.4, 0.01 M ionic strength, and 25°C. ■, aluminum hydroxide adjuvant alone; ♦, aluminum phosphate adjuvant alone; ○, △, □, populations observed during aging of the mixture. From Al-Shakhshir *et al.* (1995a).

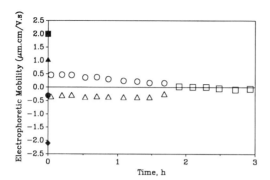

Figure 15. Electrophoretic mobility of populations present during the aging of a 1:1 elemental aluminum mixture containing 0.017 mg Al/mL of BSA–aluminum hydroxide adjuvant complex (0.80 mg BSA adsorbed/mg Al) and lysozyme–aluminum phosphate adjuvant complex (0.51 mg lysozyme/mg Al) at pH 7.4, 0.01 M ionic strength, and 25°C. The adsorptive capacities were 1.6 and 0.7 mg/mg Al, respectively. ■, aluminum hydroxide adjuvant alone; ♦, aluminum phosphate adjuvant alone; ▲, BSA–aluminum hydroxide adjuvant complex alone; ●, lysozyme–aluminum phosphate adjuvant complex alone; ○, △, □, populations observed during aging of the mixture. From Al-Shakhshir *et al.* (1995a).

mobility. No significant desorption of BSA from the BSA–aluminum hydroxide adjuvant complex is expected based on the data in Table IV. Furthermore, lysozyme desorbed from the lysozyme–aluminum phosphate adjuvant complex has been shown to be very poorly adsorbed by aluminum hydroxide adjuvant (Seeber *et al.*, 1991b). However, the phosphate anion desorbed from the aluminum phosphate adjuvant may be adsorbed by the BSA–aluminum hydroxide complex (Table VI) and increase its negative electrophoretic mobility.

The two populations of particles that are present in the mixture for approximately 100 min cannot be unequivocally identified, although it is believed that the population with an electrophoretic mobility of –0.4 μm-cm/V-s is the lysozyme–aluminum phosphate adjuvant complex following the desorption of some phosphate and lysozyme. The population with an electrophoretic mobility of 0.5 μm-cm/V-s may be the BSA–aluminum hydroxide adjuvant complex following adsorption of phosphate anions.

It is likely that the single population that ultimately formed in Figs. 14 and 15 is a result of aggregation. Adsorption of protein by the adjuvants appears to delay aggregation. The adsorbed protein may be providing a steric repulsive force.

6. EFFECT OF ANIONS

Some anions such as borate, sulfate, carbonate, and phosphate are specifically adsorbed by aluminum hydroxide. IR studies (Serna *et al.*, 1977) have illustrated the relative strength of these adsorption forces. Such specific adsorption lowers the isoelectric point of aluminum hydroxide (Parks, 1965). Other anions such as nitrate and chloride are not specifically adsorbed but are loosely held in the diffuse layer region of the double layer (Serna *et al.*, 1977). These anions do not affect the isoelectric point.

Vaccines come in contact with anions during their manufacture and use. Phosphate buffers are frequently included in vaccines to control the pH. Following intramuscular injection, vaccines come in contact with interstitial fluid which contains 114 mM chloride anion and 5 mM of phosphate and sulfate anions combined (McSweeney, 1988). Thus, an understanding of the effect of anions on antigen–aluminum-containing adjuvant complexes is important.

6.1. Aluminum Hydroxide Adjuvant

The effect of added nitrate, sulfate, or phosphate anion on a model vaccine composed of negatively charged ovalbumin adsorbed by positively charged aluminum hydroxide adjuvant at pH 7.4 was studied (Rinella *et al.*, 1995). As seen in Fig. 16, phosphate and sulfate anions caused desorption of ovalbumin while nitrate anion had no effect. In this example, the amount of ovalbumin in the system, 2.9 mg/mg Al, exceeded the adsorptive capacity of the aluminum hydroxide adjuvant, which was 2.6 mg/mg Al. Approximately 45% of the ovalbumin desorbed when 4 mM phosphate anion was added to the protein–adjuvant complex. The addition of 4 mM sulfate anion desorbed approximately 10% of the ovalbumin. The relative effect of phosphate, sulfate, and nitrate anions on the desorption of ovalbumin from the aluminum hydroxide adjuvant corresponds to the relative strength of their coordination to aluminum (Serna *et al.*, 1977; Hsu, 1989).

The amount of ovalbumin desorbed by the addition of phosphate or sulfate anion decreased as the protein–adjuvant complex aged. Figure 17 shows the effect of adding phosphate anion 0, 1, 3, 11, or 17 days after the ovalbumin–aluminum hydroxide adjuvant was prepared. The desorption of ovalbumin resulting from the addition of 4 mM phosphate anion decreased from 45 to 23% after the complex aged for 17 days. A similar phenomenon was observed for sulfate anion. It has been suggested that a protein may undergo conformational changes on adsorption to optimize its interaction with the surface (Norde *et al.*, 1986). This effect is believed to account for the decreasing ability of phosphate and sulfate anions to desorb ovalbumin as the complex ages.

The effect of phosphate, sulfate, and nitrate anions on the desorption of ovalbumin from the aluminum hydroxide adjuvant was also studied when the concentration of ovalbumin was approximately 50% of the adsorptive capacity. The behavior was similar except that much less ovalbumin was desorbed. For example, the addition of 4 mM phosphate anion or sulfate anion to a model vaccine at approximately 50% of adsorptive

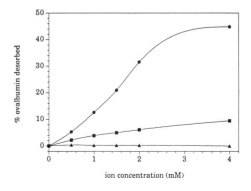

Figure 16. Effect of phosphate (●), sulfate (■), and nitrate (▲) on the desorption of ovalbumin from an aluminum hydroxide adjuvant. Desorption was performed on the day of adsorption. The amount of ovalbumin, 2.9 mg/mg Al, exceeded the adsorptive capacity of the adjuvant (2.6 mg ovalbumin/mg Al). The ionic strength was 15 mM and the pH was 7.4. From Rinella *et al.*, 1995.

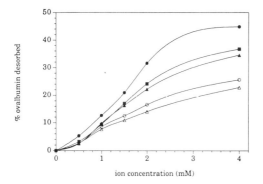

Figure 17. Effect of aging of the ovalbumin–aluminum hydroxide adjuvant complex on the desorption by phosphate anion. The amount of ovalbumin, 2.9 mg/mg Al, exceeded the adsorptive capacity of the adjuvant (2.6 mg ovalbumin/mg Al). The ionic strength was 15 mM and the pH was 7.4. Desorption when phosphate anion was added: 0 (●); 1 (■); 3 (▲); 11 (○); or 17 (△) days after the model vaccine was prepared. From Rinella *et al.*, 1995.

capacity resulted in 23 or 2% desorption, respectively. In addition, a much smaller aging effect was noted when the ovalbumin concentration was at approximately 50% of the adsorptive capacity.

The adsorption of proteins by aluminum hydroxide adjuvants is complex and probably involves contributions of electrostatic, hydrophobic, and other attractive forces. One mechanism that may contribute to the desorption of ovalbumin from aluminum hydroxide adjuvant is the adsorption of phosphate or sulfate anions by the adjuvant. Figure 18 illustrates this mechanism. The aluminum hydroxide adjuvant has a large positive zeta potential at pH 7.4, while ovalbumin has a negative zeta potential. This situation leads to electrostatic attractive forces that contribute to adsorption. However, the surface charge of the aluminum hydroxide adjuvant becomes less positive as phosphate or sulfate anions are adsorbed. In fact, when 4 mM phosphate anion was added to the aluminum hydroxide adjuvant, the surface charge of the adjuvant became negative at pH 7.4. An electrostatic repulsive force now exists between the negatively charged ovalbumin and the negatively charged adjuvant and desorption occurs.

6.2. Aluminum Phosphate Adjuvant

Aluminum phosphate adjuvants usually have an isoelectric point below 7.4 and are therefore negatively charged at physiological pH. The effect of adding phosphate, sulfate, or nitrate anions to a model vaccine composed of lysozyme adsorbed by aluminum phosphate adjuvant was also studied (Rinella *et al.*, 1995). As seen in Fig. 19, the addition of phosphate anion and to a lesser degree sulfate anion caused additional adsorption of positively charged lysozyme by the negatively charged aluminum phosphate adjuvant. Nitrate anion had no effect. The adsorption of additional phosphate anion by aluminum phosphate adjuvants lowered the isoelectric point of the adjuvant (Fig. 20). Thus, the adjuvant becomes more negative at pH 7.4. This change increases the electrostatic attraction for positively charged lysozyme.

The effect of phosphate anions on antigen–adjuvant complexes illustrated in Figs. 16 and 19 has practical implications. Following intramuscular injection, the antigen–adjuvant complex is immersed in interstitial fluid that contains up to 5 mM phosphate anion. An

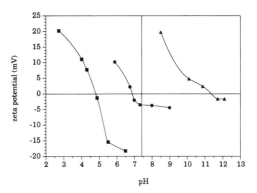

Figure 18. Effect of the adsorption of 4 mM phosphate anion on the surface charge characteristics of aluminum hydroxide adjuvant. ▲, aluminum hydroxide adjuvant; ●, aluminum hydroxide adjuvant following adsorption of 4 mM phosphate anions. The effect of pH on the surface charge of ovalbumin (■) is given for reference. From Rinella *et al.*, 1995.

antigen having a pI below 7.4, which is adsorbed by an aluminum hydroxide adjuvant, will likely be desorbed. In contrast, a vaccine composed of a basic antigen adsorbed by aluminum phosphate adjuvant binds the antigen more strongly, following adsorption of additional phosphate anion. Thus, the release profile of antigens from vaccines following intramuscular administration is influenced by the presence of phosphate anion in the interstitial fluid.

It is sometimes desirable to desorb the antigen for analysis during the quality control procedures required to release the vaccine for use. The addition of phosphate anion may be useful if the vaccine is composed of a negatively charged antigen and aluminum hydroxide adjuvant. On the other hand, the addition of phosphate to a vaccine composed of a positively charged antigen and aluminum phosphate adjuvant will result in stronger adsorption rather than desorption.

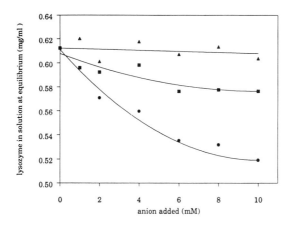

Figure 19. Effect of phosphate (●), sulfate (■), or nitrate (▲) anion on the concentration of lysozyme in solution for a lysozyme–aluminum phosphate adjuvant complex containing 0.50 mg lysozyme/mg Al at pH 7.4 and ionic strength of 105 mM. The adsorptive capacity under these conditions is 0.34 mg lysozyme/mg Al. From Rinella *et al.*, 1995.

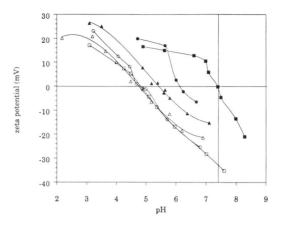

Figure 20. Effect of the addition of 10 mM phosphate anion (open symbols) on the surface charge characteristics of three aluminum phosphate adjuvants. The solid symbols are the controls. From Rinella *et al.*, 1995.

The effect of specifically adsorbed anions may also influence the formulation of a vaccine. The use of a phosphate buffer in the formula may alter the surface charge of the adjuvant. Aluminum hydroxide adjuvants will become less positive and aluminum phosphate adjuvants will become more negative as a result of adsorbing phosphate anion. Thus, one must consider the surface charge of the adjuvant after exposure to the buffer. In fact, as was seen in the studies with the malarial antigens, it is possible to adjust the surface charge of an adjuvant to the desired value by treatment with phosphate anion.

7. SUMMARY

This chapter is concerned with the identification, characterization, and behavior of aluminum-containing adjuvants with proteins and anions similar to those occurring in vaccines and interstitial fluid. Aluminum-containing adjuvants referred to commercially as aluminum hydroxide have been identified as poorly crystalline aluminum oxyhydroxide with the structure of the mineral boehmite. Relevant properties of this material include its high surface area and its high pI, which provide the adjuvant with a high adsorptive capacity for positively charged proteins. Aluminum phosphate and alum-precipitated adjuvants may be classified as amorphous aluminum hydroxyphosphate with little or no specifically adsorbed sulfate. Variations in the molar PO_4/Al ratio of amorphous aluminum hydroxyphosphates result in pI values that range from 5 up to 7; the materials are negatively charged at a physiological pH of 7.4. The amorphous nature of these compounds gives them high surface area and high protein adsorptive capacity for positively charged proteins.

Observations on the interactions of anions and charged proteins with charged adjuvant surfaces have provided a framework for predicting behavior of complex systems of vaccines and for designing specific combinations of adjuvants and antigens to optimize the stability and efficacy of vaccines.

ACKNOWLEDGMENTS

   The authors thank Dr. Ann L. Lee, Merck Research Laboratories, for helpful discussions especially relating to multivalent vaccines. We also thank Mr. Joseph V. Rinella, Jr., Purdue University, for his contributions to the section on the effect of anions.

REFERENCES

Al-Shakhshir, R. H., Lee, A. L., White, J. L., and Hem, S. L., 1995a, Interactions in model vaccines composed of mixtures of aluminum-containing adjuvants, *J. Colloid Interface Sci.* **169:**197–203.

Al-Shakhshir, R. H., Regnier, F. E., White, J. L., and Hem, S. L., 1995b, Contribution of electrostatic and hydrophobic interactions to the adsorption of proteins by aluminum-containing adjuvants, *Vaccine* **13:**41–44.

Al-Shakhshir, R., Regnier, F., White, J. L., and Hem, S. L., 1994, Effect of protein adsorption on the surface charge characteristics of aluminum-containing adjuvants, *Vaccine* **12:**472–474.

Aprile, M. A., and Wardlaw, A. C., 1966, Aluminum compounds as adjuvants for vaccines and toxoids in man: A review, *Can. J. Public Health* **57:**343–354.

Bleam, W. F., Pfeffer, P. E., Goldberg, S., Taylor, R. W., and Dudley, R., 1991, A ^{31}P solid-state nuclear magnetic resonance study of phosphate adsorption at the boehmite/aqueous solution interface, *Langmuir* **7:**1703–1712.

Callahan, P. M., Shorter, A. L., and Hem, S. L., 1991, The importance of surface charge in the optimization of antigen–adjuvant interactions, *Pharm. Res.* **8:**851–858.

Cheung, T. T. P., Willcox, K. W., McDaniel, M. P., and Johnson, M. M., 1986, The structure of coprecipitated alumino-phosphate catalyst supports, *J. Catal.* **10:**10–20.

Edelman, R., 1980, Vaccine adjuvants, *Rev. Infect. Dis.* **2:**370–383.

Fripiat, J. J., Bosmans, H., and Rouxhet, P. G., 1967, Proton mobility in solids. I. Hydrogenic vibration modes and proton delocalization in boehmite, *J. Phys. Chem.* **71:**1097–1112.

Glenny, A. T., Pope, C. G., Waddington, H., and Wallace, U., 1926, The antigenic value of toxoid precipitated by potassium alum, *J. Pathol. Bacteriol.* **29:**31–40.

Gooding, D. L., Schmuck, M. N., and Gooding, K. M., 1984, Analysis of proteins with new, mildly hydrophobic high performance liquid chromatography packing materials, *J. Chromatogr.* **296:**107–114.

Hem, S. L., and White, J. L., 1984, Characterization of aluminum hydroxide for use as an adjuvant in parenteral vaccines, *J. Parenteral Sci. Tech.* **38:**2–10.

Hsu, P. H., 1979, Effect of phosphate and silicate on the crystallization of gibbsite from OH-Al solutions, *Soil Sci.* **127:**219–226.

Hsu, P. H., 1989, Aluminum hydroxides and oxyhydroxides in: *Minerals in Soil Environments*, 2nd ed. (J. B. Dixon and S. B. Weed, eds.), Soil Science Society of America, Madison, WI, pp. 331–378.

Imoto, T., Johnson, L. N., North, A. C., Phillips, D. C., and Rupley, J. A., 1972, Vertebrate lysozymes, in: *The Enzymes*, Vol. 7 (P. D. Boyer, ed.), Academic Press, New York, pp. 665–868.

Liu, J. C., Feldkamp, J. R., White, J. L., and Hem, S. L., 1984, Adsorption of phosphate by aluminum hydroxycarbonate, *J. Pharm. Sci.* **73:**1355–1358.

McSweeney, G. W., 1988, Fluid and electrolyte therapy and acid–base balance, in: *Clinical Pharmacy and Therapeutics* (E. T. Herfindal, D. R. Gourley, and L. L. Hart, eds.), Williams & Wilkins, Baltimore, p. 2.

Masood, H., White, J. L., and Hem, S. L., 1994, Relationship between protein adsorptive capacity and the X-ray diffraction pattern of aluminum hydroxide adjuvants, *Vaccine* **12:**187–189.

Nail, S. L., White, J. L., and Hem, S. L., 1976a, Structure of aluminum hydroxide gel I: Initial precipitate, *J. Pharm. Sci.* **65:**1188–1191.

Nail, S. L., White, J. L., and Hem, S. L., 1976b, Structure of aluminum hydroxide gel II: Aging mechanism, *J. Pharm. Sci.* **65:**1192–1195.

Nicklas, W., 1992, Aluminum salts, *Res. Immunol.* **143:**489–494.

Norde, W., and Anusiem, A., 1992, Adsorption, desorption and re-adsorption of proteins on solid surfaces, *Colloids Surf.* **66:**73–80.

Norde, W., MacRitchie, F., Nowicka, G., and Lyklema, J., 1986, Protein adsorption at solid–liquid interfaces: Reversibility and conformation aspects, *J. Colloid Interface Sci.* **112:**447–456.

Parks, G. A., 1965, The isoelectric points of solid oxides, solid hydroxides, and aqueous hydroxo complex systems, *Chem. Rev.* **65:**177–198.

Rinella, J. V. Jr., White, J. L., and Hem, S. L., 1995, Effect of anions on model aluminum adjuvant containing vaccines, *J. Colloid Interface Sci.* (in press).

Ross, S. D., 1974, Phosphates and other oxy-anions of group V, in: *The Infrared Spectra of Minerals* (V. C. Farmer, ed.), Mineralogical Society, London, p. 400.

Seeber, S. J., White, J. L., and Hem, S. L., 1991a, Solubilization of aluminum-containing adjuvants by constituents of interstitial fluid, *J. Parenteral Sci. Tech.* **45:**156–159.

Seeber, S. J., White, J. L., and Hem, S. L., 1991b, Predicting the adsorption of proteins by aluminum-containing adjuvants, *Vaccine* **9:**201–203.

Serna, C. J., White, J. L., and Hem, S. L., 1977, Anion–aluminum hydroxide gel interactions, *Soil Sci. Soc. Am. J.* **41:**1009–1013.

Shirodkar, S., Hutchinson, R. L., Perry, D. L., White, J. L., and Hem, S. L., 1990, Aluminum compounds used as adjuvants in vaccines, *Pharm. Res.* **2:**1282–1288.

Souza Santos, P., Vallejo-Friere, A., Parsons, J., and Watson, J. H. L., 1958, The structure of Schmidt's aluminum hydroxide gel, *Experientia* **14:**318–320.

Srinivasan, R., and Ruckenstein, E., 1980, Role of physical forces in hydrophobic interaction chromatography, *Sep. Purif. Methods* **9:**267–370.

Tettenhorst, R., and Hofmann, D. A., 1980, Crystal chemistry of boehmite, *Clays Clay Miner.* **28:**373–380.

Van der Marel, H. W., and Beutelspacher, H., 1976, *Atlas of Infrared Spectroscopy of Clay Minerals and Their Admixtures*, Elsevier, Amsterdam, pp. 194, 228.

Warren, H. S., and Chedid, L. A., 1988, Future prospects for vaccine adjuvants, *CRC Crit. Rev. Immunol.* **8:**83–101.

Warren, H. S., Vogel, F. R., and Chedid, L. A., 1986, Current status of immunological adjuvants, *Annu. Rev. Immunol.* **4:**369–388.

White, J. L., and Hem, S. L., 1975, Role of carbonate in aluminum hydroxide gel established by Raman and infrared analysis, *J. Pharm. Sci.* **64:**468–469.

Chapter 10

MF59

Design and Evaluation of a Safe and Potent Adjuvant for Human Vaccines

Gary Ott, Gail L. Barchfeld, David Chernoff,
Ramachandran Radhakrishnan,
Peter van Hoogevest, and Gary Van Nest

1. RATIONALE FOR AND DESIGN OF MICROFLUIDIZED OIL/WATER EMULSIONS

Advances in recombinant DNA technology have made possible the advent of a new generation of safer, better-defined subunit vaccines. Because vaccines based on these weakly immunogenic antigens require an adjuvant for efficacy, we undertook the development of a safe and efficacious adjuvant suitable for widespread human administration. Vaccines formulated with aluminum salts (alum), the only adjuvant thus far utilized with vaccines approved in the United States for human administration, were necessarily adopted as a benchmark for the minimum acceptable activity of a new adjuvant. Our goal was to develop an adjuvant that significantly exceeded aluminum hydroxide in potency, while retaining equally low toxicity. By the early 1990s a wide variety of approaches to adjuvant development had been described (Allison and Byars, 1990; Edelman, 1980; Gregoriadis and Panagiotidi, 1989; Warren *et al.*, 1986). Two major mechanisms of adjuvant activity have been repeatedly cited in this literature: the depot effect, whereby long-term release of antigen results in increased immune response; and coadministration of immunostimulators, which specifically activate portions of the immune system in, as yet, incompletely defined fashions. The prototypic strong adjuvant, complete Freund's adjuvant (CFA),

Gary Ott, Gail L. Barchfeld, David Chernoff, Ramachandran Radhakrishnan, and Gary Van Nest • Chiron Corporation, Emeryville, California 94608. *Peter van Hoogevest* • Ciba Geigy, Ltd., Basel, Switzerland.

Vaccine Design: The Subunit and Adjuvant Approach, edited by Michael F. Powell and Mark J. Newman. Plenum Press, New York, 1995.

combined these functions by releasing a mixture of immunostimulatory mycobacterial cell wall components along with antigen from a water/mineral oil/Arlacel A emulsion depot over an extended period of time (Freund, 1956). CFA remains the reference standard for potent adjuvant activity; however, it is now considered too toxic in many cases for use even in laboratory animals. In addition to the aluminum salts, several adjuvants based on the depot effect alone have been studied. These include incomplete Freund's adjuvant (IFA), which lacks the potent, but toxic, cell wall components, and Adjuvant 65 (water/peanut oil/mannide monooleate), a yet further detoxified water/oil formulation (Hilleman *et al.*, 1972a,b). Despite extensive study, neither formulation was approved for human administration. We chose to avoid water/oil emulsions. A more recent version of the depot approach, controlled release of antigen from synthetic polymer microspheres, remains a promising area of study (Cohen *et al.*, 1991; O'Hagan *et al.*, 1991) but appears to have an unacceptably long development time for our purposes.

A major part of the long ongoing effort to develop immunostimulators as adjuvants has been devoted to characterization and synthesis of mycobacterial cell wall components and their analogues (White *et al.*, 1964). The most studied component of the cell wall, the muramyl peptide *N*-acetylmuramyl-L-alanyl-D-isoglutamine (MDP), was synthesized by 1975 (Kotani *et al.*, 1975; Merser *et al.*, 1975) and the activity of a number of analogues has since been described (Ott *et al.*, 1992). We initially set out to develop an adjuvant that used the amphiphilic muramyl tripeptide, MTP-PE [sodium *N*-acetyl-muramyl-L-alanyl-D-isoglutaminyl-L-alanyl-2-(1′,2′-dipalmitoyl-*sn*-glycero-3′-phospho)ethylamide] (Gisler *et al.*, 1986). MTP-PE was selected because of an established clinical record of high potency and low toxicity (Fidler, 1988; Fidler *et al.*, 1981) as well as the availability of sufficient quantities of injectable-grade material.

Because muramyl peptides alone have been reported to be no more effective an adjuvant than alum (Audibert *et al.*, 1980) they have been formulated with a variety of vehicles. The use of liposomes containing muramyl peptides has been described for several systems (Brynestad *et al.*, 1990; Gregoriadis and Manesis, 1980; Ullrich and Fidler, 1992). It has been our experience that more robust antibody responses are obtained with oil/water emulsions (Sanchez-Pescador *et al.*, 1988). Complex squalene/water emulsions containing a muramyl peptide component, trehalose dimycolates, and monophosphoryl lipid A have been shown to be effective adjuvants (Masihi *et al.*, 1986; Ribi *et al.*, 1976). A body of work has been devoted to generation of less complex and better defined variations of these formulations. Similar emulsions have been used to formulate a variety of hydrophobic spreading agents (Woodward, 1989). A family of potent synthetic hydrophobic agents, the pluronic block polymers, have been used with both squalene emulsions (Hunter and Bennett, 1984; Hunter *et al.*, 1981) and squalane emulsions in combination with the synthetic muramyl peptide, threonyl MDP (Byars and Allison, 1987; Byars, *et al.*, 1990). Finally, the hydrophobic muramyl peptide B30-MDP has also been formulated with a Ribi-like emulsion (Tsujimoto *et al.*, 1986).

Our initial formulations were designed with the intention of binding MTP-PE to the surface of a squalene/water emulsion. The formulation MTP-LO, a prototype formulation generated by multiple intersyringe passages, had excellent adjuvant activity in guinea pigs (Sanchez-Pescador *et al.*, 1988). Poor physical stability and the modest adjuvant activity observed in preclinical studies with large animals and clinical trials with the HIV coat protein antigen env2-3 (Wintsch *et al.*, 1991) led to a series of efforts to improve the emulsion by emulsification under higher shear forces and to modification of surfactant composition with the intent of generating a stable, sterile-filterable formulation that would be compatible with a variety of antigens and buffer systems. Higher shear forces were first applied to the MTP-LO formulation by passage through a Kirkland "knife-edge valve" homogenizer (Kirkland Instruments, El Cajon, CA). The emulsion, K-LO, had a mean droplet diameter of ~700 nm, but suffered from flocculation (creaming) after storage for 2 h. Homogenization of the same formulation with a Microfluidizer® (Microfluidics, Newton, MA) resulted in an emulsion, MF-LO, with a droplet diameter of ~ 400 nm. However, this emulsion coalesced on exposure to PBS (0.15 M NaCl, 0.01 M sodium phosphate). While higher energy homogenization produced improved emulsions, the original concentrations of Tween 80 and MTP-PE were not sufficient to obtain an oil/water emulsion with the desired characteristics.

In order to investigate the emulsifying potential of MTP-PE alone, a series of MTP-PE/squalene emulsions were prepared using the Microfluidizer®. Emulsion diameters were determined in water and in PBS after a 2-h incubation (Fig. 1). While stable MTP-PE/squalene emulsions of nearly constant diameter could be generated in water, the diameter in the presence of PBS was strongly dependent on the MTP-PE concentration. The interdependence of potentially critical parameters (squalene dose, MTP-PE dose, and droplet diameter) was a potential source of difficulty with these formulations. A single example, MF1, was employed for preclinical testing.

Stabilization with Tween 80, which had been used as a minor component in the squalene formulations previously described (Byars and Allison, 1987; Hunter *et al.*, 1981; Ribi *et al.*, 1976), was an attractive alternative to using MTP-PE as the emulsifier. In addition, emulsions stabilized with mixtures of Tween 80 and the homologous low HLB spreading agent Span 85 were studied. These emulsions offered the possibility of both greater long-term stability (Boyd *et al.*, 1972) and the potential for an adjuvant contribution from the spreading agent (Woodward, 1989). Figure 2 shows the mean droplet diameter

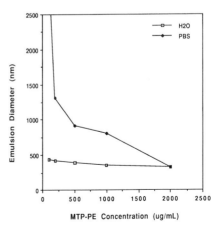

Figure 1. Dependence of emulsion diameter on MTP-PE concentration. 4.3% (w/v) squalene was emulsified with MTP-PE at 12,000 psi (Microfluidizer®) in water and emulsion diameters were determined by photocorrelation spectroscopy on samples in water or phosphate-buffered saline.

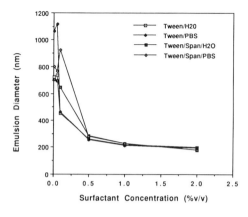

Figure 2. Dependence of emulsion diameter on total surfactant concentration. 4.3% (w/v) squalene was emulsified with either Tween 80 or a 50:50 mixture of Tween 80 and Span 85 at 12,000 psi (Microfluidizer®) in water and emulsion diameters were determined in water or phosphate-buffered saline.

obtained by microfluidization of a series of 4.3% (w/v) squalene emulsions stabilized with varying inputs of either Tween 80 or a 50:50 mixture of Tween 80 and Span 85. At total detergent concentrations greater than 0.5% (w/v), emulsions of <300 nm diameter were produced with either surfactant composition. The droplet diameter of these emulsions was not sensitive to incubation in the presence of physiological saline, and they showed no sign of either creaming or coalescence over a period of months. In addition, we were able to sterilize these emulsions by passage through a 0.22-μm filter. These properties led us to focus development on two of these formulations: MF59 (4.3% w/v squalene, 0.5% w/v Tween 80, 0.5% w/v Span 85) and MF69 (4.3% w/v squalene, 0.25% w/v Tween 80, 0.75% w/v Span 85). Homogenization of a modified MF59 formulation containing 100 μg/dose MTP-PE (MF59-100) resulted in an emulsion that was indistinguishable in size from the MF59-0 vehicle. A series of MTP-PE-containing formulations have been used and the MTP-PE dose is designated in hyphenated style. The MF59 emulsion system thus fulfilled our requirement for a vehicle where size and stability were independent of the presence of MTP-PE. Determination of the degree of interaction between the emulsion and MTP-PE was carried out by separating the emulsion droplets from the aqueous phase by flotation in a discontinuous sucrose gradient. MTP-PE concentration was determined both for the upper fraction where the emulsion had been concentrated and for the lower fractions where free MTP-PE remained. Figure 3 shows the distribution of MTP-PE in the gradient for microfluidized MF59-100 (Fig. 3A) and for a control containing 100 μg of MTP-PE alone (Fig. 3B). Approximately 50% of the MTP-PE is found in the uppermost fraction with the emulsified squalene droplets. This result was compared with the distribution achieved after incubation of 100 μg MTP-PE with MF59-0 (data not shown). After 48 h incubation, ~50% binding was observed. Incubation of the MTP-PE/MF59 complex isolated from the uppermost gradient fraction with PBS for 72 h resulted in dissociation of less than 10% of the bound MTP-PE. These in vitro experiments indicated that MF59 could function as an MTP-PE carrier and would be suitable for preclinical testing.

In summary, preliminary formulation work on squalene/H2O emulsions provided three candidates for second-generation preclinical testing in a variety of species: (1)

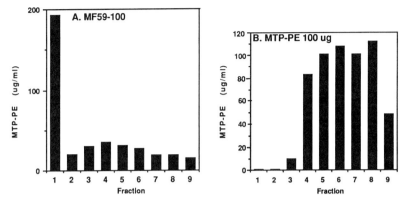

Figure 3. Sucrose gradient distribution of emulsion-bound and free MTP-PE. Either MF59-100 or 100 μg MTP-PE in 55% (w/v) sucrose was overlaid with phosphate-buffered saline and centrifuged for 60 min at 20,000 rpm in an SW55 Ti. Nine 0.5-mL fractions were collected from the top of the centrifuge tube and MTP-PE was determined by RP-HPLC.

well-homogenized versions of the parent MTP-LO formulation, (2) the rather closely related MTP-PE-stabilized MF-1 formulation, and (3) the nonionically stabilized MF59/69 emulsions, which can serve as carriers for MTP-PE but do not require it for stability.

2. PRECLINICAL EXPERIENCE WITH MF59

While testing the early low-oil-emulsion formulations, it became apparent that significant differences exist among animal species with respect to the ability of the animals to respond to particular adjuvant formulations. This is illustrated in Fig. 4, which shows the anti-gD2 responses of guinea pigs and baboons that received different adjuvant formulations. In guinea pigs, gD2 adsorbed to aluminum hydroxide produced low antibody titers (mean titer 140) compared to MTP-PE/LO (mean titer 5200), the insufficiently stable prototype emulsion formulation. The stable formulation MF59 produced titers equivalent to MTP-PE/LO (mean titer 4800). In baboons, however, both MTP-PE/LO and the MTP-PE-stabilized emulsion MF1 generated antibody titers (mean titers respectively 7385 and 7800) similar to aluminum hydroxide (4900). In contrast, immunization with MF59 resulted in fivefold higher titers (mean titer 26000) than the other three adjuvants (Van Nest *et al.*, 1992). We have consistently observed this species-dependent difference in response to low-oil-emulsion adjuvants. Mice, guinea pigs, and rabbits respond well to most of the low-oil formulations, regardless of the emulsion droplet size or stability. Goats, baboons, and chimpanzees require a stable, small-droplet-diameter emulsion for optimal responses. This requirement has also proven to be the case in human clinical trials. The particular antigen used does not alter this effect. It is not clear whether there is a simple physiological basis for this difference between small and large animals, or if perhaps there

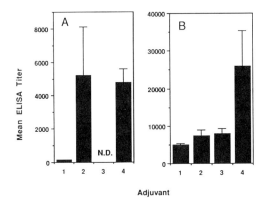

Figure 4. Performance of different adjuvant formulations with HSV gD2 in guinea pigs and baboons. Animals were immunized three times at 3-week intervals with recombinant gD2 produced in Chinese hamster ovary (CHO) cells combined with different adjuvant formulations. Adjuvants: (1) aluminum hydroxide (Alhydrogel); (2) MTP-PE-LO; (3) MF1; (4) MF59. gD2 doses used were 12.5 μg for guinea pigs and 25 μg for baboons. Aluminum hydroxide doses were 42 μg for guinea pigs and 85 μg for baboons. With MTP-PE-LO, MF1, and MF59 formulations, 50-μg doses of MTP-PE were used for guinea pigs and 100 μg for baboons. Two weeks after the third immunization, animals were bled, and anti-gD2 antibody titers were determined by ELISA. ELISA values represent the geometric mean and standard error of groups of five animals. (A) Guinea pig titers; (B) baboon titers. MF1 was not tested in guinea pigs. Reproduced by permission of Cold Spring Harbor Laboratory Press.

is an immunological basis for the differences. The pragmatic conclusion is that large animal models are more relevant for predicting adjuvant performance in humans.

MF59 has been extensively tested in a number of animal species with both recombinant and natural antigens. The animal models used include mice, guinea pigs, rabbits, goats, and several nonhuman primates including chimpanzees. The vaccine antigens tested include recombinant proteins and glycoproteins from HSV, HIV, HCV, CMV, HBV, HPV, and malaria as well as natural glycoproteins from the influenza virus. The specific animal and antigen combinations that have been studied are summarized in Table I. In all instances, the antigen/MF59 combinations generated high antigen-specific antibody titers and, where tested, high virus neutralizing titers. In cases where MF59 vaccines were compared with aluminum hydroxide-adsorbed antigen at equal antigen doses the MF59 titers were generally 3- to 50-fold higher than the alum titers. Several examples of the MF59 to alum comparisons are shown in Table II. In these examples, MF59 generated antibody titers 4- to 34-fold higher than alum, depending on both the antigen and the animal species studied. The potent CFA/IFA adjuvants have served as standards for effective adjuvants. When MF59 or other microfluidized low-oil emulsions that we have prepared were compared to CFA/IFA, different relative effects were seen with different animals and antigens. For instance, in rabbits immunized with HSV gD2 and CFA/IFA, titers at 2 weeks after the third immunization were 31,900 ± 1700, but for animals immunized with emulsion and MTP-PE titers were slightly higher at 50,500 ± 14,700. Conversely, *Aotus* monkeys

Table I
Experience with MF59 in Animal Models

Species	HSV	HIV	Influenza	HCV	CMV	HBV	HPV	Malaria
Mouse	+	+	+		+		+	+
Guinea pig	+	+	+		+			
Rabbit	+	+	+			+	+	
Goat	+	+	+			+		+
Aotus monkey								+
Rhesus macaque		+						
Baboon	+	+						
Chimp		+		+				

immunized with malaria SERA 1 antigen and either CFA/IFA or MF59 had titers of 692,000 ± 140,700 and 25,500 ± 11,200, respectively, 4 weeks after the third immunization (Inselberg *et al.*, 1993). MF59 gave higher antibody titers than IFA against gp120 when compared in baboons (Van Nest *et al.*, 1992). Overall, MF59 and related microfluidized low-oil emulsions generate antibody titers consistently higher than those obtained with aluminum hydroxide, equal to or higher than IFA, and equal to or lower than CFA/IFA.

The low-oil emulsions could function as MTP-PE carriers and MTP-PE was originally included as an immunostimulant in many MF59 formulations. In rabbits and guinea pigs with HSV and HIV antigens, MTP-PE has a demonstrable effect on specific antibody levels. A typical experiment is shown in Fig. 5 in which rabbits were immunized with HSV gD2 and MF59 containing from 0 to 1000 μg MTP-PE. At 2 weeks after the second immunization there is little difference in titers for animals immunized with 0 to 25 μg MTP-PE, but a marked increase is observed with 100 and 1000 μg of MTP-PE. After the third immunization, all MTP-PE doses show antibody titers higher than MF59-0, with the

Table II
Comparison of Alum and MF59 with Different Antigens in Several Animal Species[a]

Species	Antigen	ELISA titer with alum	ELISA titer with MF59	Ratio MF59:alum
Guinea pig[b]	HSV gD2	140 ± 30	4800 ± 400	34
Goat[b]	HSV gD2	170 ± 30	1600 ± 490	9
Goat[b]	HBVsAg	1500 ± 800	5300 ± 1900	4
Baboon[b]	HSV gD2	4900 ± 360	26,000 ± 9000	5
Baboon[c]	HIV gp120	1070 ± 590	28,300 ± 10,800	26

[a]Groups of five animals (except the HSV gD2–baboon experiment where groups of three were used) were immunized three times with the stated antigen and either alum or MF59 as adjuvant. Two weeks after the third immunization, the animals were bled and the antibody titers against the specific antigens were determined by ELISA.
[b]Experiments used MF59/MTP-PE (50 μg MTP-PE for guinea pigs, 100 for goats and baboons).
[c]Experiment used MF59-0.

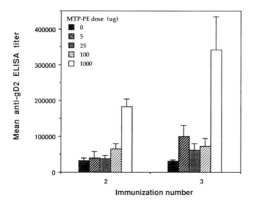

Figure 5. Effect of MTP-PE in the MF59 formulation on anti-gD2 antibody responses in rabbits. Groups of five animals were immunized three times at 3-week intervals with 25 μg gD2 and MF59 containing 0, 5, 25, 100, or 1000 μg MTP-PE. Two weeks after the second and third immunizations, animals were bled and anti-gD2 antibody titers were determined as in Fig. 4.

1000-μg dose clearly higher than the others. The MTP-PE dose effect was not found in experiments with larger animals. Table III shows the antibody responses of goats immunized three times at 4-week intervals with HSV gD2 and MF59, containing 10 to 1000 μg MTP-PE. Variability within the groups, indicated by standard errors, is greater than differences between the groups. MTP-PE provides no obvious benefit in this model. There is a similar absence of MTP-PE effect in baboons with both HSV and HIV antigens. Clinical studies (see Section 5) have confirmed the goat and baboon results and show no enhancement of antibody responses in humans with the inclusion of MTP-PE in the formulation. The immune-stimulating activities of MF59 are a property of the microfluidized emulsion and do not necessarily require the addition of other immunostimulatory factors.

The discovery that the emulsion was the primary adjuvant made squalene dose ranging studies advantageous. Preliminary preclinical studies utilized the prototypic emulsion (43 mg/mL squalene) in a 1:1 dilution with the antigen/PBS at the maximum volume appropriate for each species. Initial dose ranging consisted of varying squalene concentration around the prototypic value. Data from Fig. 6 show antibody titers obtained from guinea pigs vaccinated twice at a 3-week interval with 0.2 mL of MF59/influenza vaccine at doses

Table III

Effect of MTP-PE on the Antibody Response Induced
with MF59 and gD2 in Goats[a]

MTP-PE dose (μg)	Anti-gD2 ELISA titer after 2 immunizations	Anti-gD2 antibody titer after 3 immunizations
10	1318 ± 702	899 ± 253
100	717 ± 416	435 ± 286
500	960 ± 526	471 ± 204
1000	1194 ± 992	965 ± 700

[a]Groups of five animals were immunized three times at 4-week intervals with 25 μg gD2 and MF59 containing 10, 100, 500, or 1000 μg MTP-PE. Two weeks after the second and third immunizations, animals were bled and anti-gD2 antibody titers were determined by ELISA.

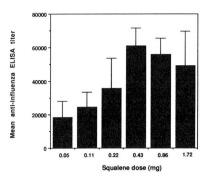

Figure 6. Effect of emulsion dose on antibody response to influenza vaccine in guinea pigs. Groups of five animals were immunized two times with a 3-week interval with 9 μg of trivalent influenza vaccine and MF59 containing 0.05, 0.11, 0.22, 0.43, 0.86, or 1.72 mg squalene. Two weeks after the second immunization the animals were bled and anti-influenza ELISA titers were determined as in Fig. 4.

ranging from 0.05 to 1.72 mg squalene. Antibody response increased with increasing doses up to 0.43 mg (mean titer 61,100) while larger doses of MF59 did not produce significantly higher titers (1.72 mg squalene produced a mean titer of 49,200). A similar plateau in the dose response was observed in goats immunized with 0.5 mL influenza/MF59-100 vaccine with doses ranging from 10.8 to 43 mg squalene. In this case, the prototypic dose of 10.8 mg squalene performed as well as the higher doses and was adopted for further studies.

A variety of toxicology tests have been done with both MF59 alone and in combination with HSV and HIV antigens. These studies have included both short-term protocols (2–3 immunizations at weekly or biweekly intervals or 14 daily immunizations) and long-term protocols (12 immunizations over 8 months). All studies were done using anticipated human doses and injection volumes in rabbits or dogs. The results of the studies indicate that while some changes in clinical laboratory parameters and histopathology were detected, all of the changes were minor and transient. Teratology studies in rats and rabbits indicated no embryotoxic or teratogenic effects of MF59 combined with HIV gp120. The overall conclusion from these studies is that the MF59 adjuvant formulation presents no safety problems either alone or combined with the antigens tested. The favorable toxicology profile of MF59 has allowed extensive clinical testing of the adjuvant in the general adult population and also in infants and children.

3. MECHANISM OF ADJUVANT ACTIVITY

To have rational adjuvant design, it is important to define the mechanism(s) of action for adjuvant systems that have significant efficacy. We have attempted to determine which features of MF59 contribute to its adjuvant activity. While a significant part of the activity of water/oil emulsions has been attributed to the long-term residence of antigen and adjuvant at the injection site (Freund, 1956), the depot effect does not appear to be significant for oil/water emulsions such as MF59. In a preliminary experiment to determine the rate of clearance of both MF59 emulsion and the HSV gD2 antigen from the injection site, either radiolabeled MF59 (^{125}I-iodinated squalene) or ^{125}I-HSV gD2 was administered to rabbits as a standard intramuscular injection. The muscle at the injection site was excised at times ranging from 6 to 120 h and radioactivity remaining in the tissue was determined. At 6 h, iodinated squalene at the injection site was only 10% of the input and decreased to

5% of the input over the 120-h period. For the antigen, 25% of the injected dose was found at the injection site after 6 h and this decreased to <0.05% at 120 h.

Despite our initial thought that MF59 could function as a carrier to transport MTP-PE to local lymph nodes, the data derived from large animal immunogenicity studies indicate a rather weak dependence of antibody titer on the dose of MTP-PE administered. While we have no data on actual delivery of MTP-PE to any critical site, substantial adjuvant effect is observed in the absence of any muramyl peptide; therefore, the emulsion vehicle is itself the source of adjuvant activity.

A potential basis for the adjuvant activity of MF59 was binding of antigen to the emulsion. The emulsion could be envisioned as a core for the formation of a pseudovirion particle. Such a particle might, like inactivated viruses, have increased immunogenicity derived from either facilitated transport to lymphoid tissues, or the effects of polyvalent arrayed antigen presentation. Adjuvant activity of synthetic particles has previously been discussed in terms of antigen binding (Kossovsky *et al.*, 1991; Kreuter *et al.*, 1986, 1988), and the SAF oil/water emulsion has been reported to bind antigen to the droplet surface (Allison and Byars, 1987). The interaction of the HSV antigens gD2 and gB2 with the MF59 emulsion was investigated by utilizing the sucrose gradient centrifugation method previously described for MTP-PE binding. After separation of the emulsion droplets from the original aqueous phase, no gD2 was found to be associated with the oil droplets. Since MF59 is effective at generating high-titer antibody to gD2, detectable binding of antigen to MF59 is not necessary for adjuvant activity. Incubation of HSV gB2 with MF59 for 48 h at 37°C resulted in ~10% binding and the MF59/gB2 complex was stable enough to be isolated by sucrose gradient centrifugation. Antibody titers generated by either free or bound gB2 (Fig. 7) indicate that at our typical antigen/emulsion ratio the effect of binding gB2 to MF59 is not significant. However, when the MF59 dose was reduced to 1% of the normal dose and gB2 was held constant, the titer obtained with bound protein was ~fourfold greater than that obtained with free gB2. Thus, at very low emulsion doses in which surface density of antigen is much greater, the effect of bound antigen becomes significant compared to the effect of emulsion alone, which dominates at higher MF59 doses. In order to further demonstrate the independent activities of antigen and adjuvant in vivo, the antigen and adjuvant portions of the vaccine were injected into proximate sites at different

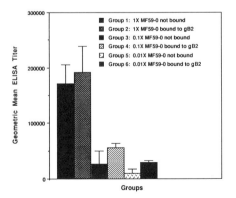

Figure 7. Effect on immunogenicity of binding HSV gB2 to MF59-0. Groups of eight animals were immunized three times at 3-week intervals with 4 μg gB2 and 4.3, 0.43, or 0.043 mg MF59-0. Protein was either bound to the emulsion by 48 h incubation or mixed with emulsion immediately prior to injection. Animals were bled 2 weeks after the third immunization and anti-gB2 titers determined by ELISA.

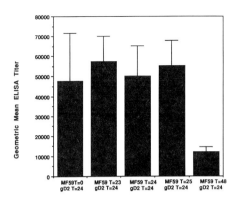

Figure 8. Effect on immunogenicity of temporally separated delivery of antigen and adjuvant. Five groups of eight rabbits were vaccinated with 25 μg HSV gD2 and 4.3 mg MF59-0 three times at 3-week intervals. Antigen and adjuvant were injected at proximal sites at times indicated. Animals were bled 2 weeks after the third immunization and anti-gD2 titers determined by ELISA.

times (Fig. 8). Administration of MF59 at times ranging from 24 h before antigen injection to 1 h after antigen injection resulted in indistinguishable antibody titers. Administration of MF59 24 h postinjection of gD2 resulted in a much reduced antibody titer. These results are consistent with the interpretation that MF59 droplets activate the immune system in the absence of antigen and that the activation persists for at least 24 h. Perhaps macrophage uptake of the emulsion droplets results in cytokine production, which leads to enhanced activity in the presence of antigen.

One clear feature in the action of MF59 vaccines is the ability of combined emulsion and antigen to stimulate production of a variety of cytokines. In one example of the cytokine responses to MF59, mice were immunized three times at weekly intervals with influenza vaccine alone or influenza vaccine combined with MF59-0. Three hours after the last immunization, animals were sacrificed. Draining lymph nodes were dissected and lymph node cell preparations were plated in culture medium without further stimulation. Twenty-four hours later, the culture media were collected and assayed for IL-2, IL-4, IL-5, and IL-6 levels by ELISA. As shown in Table IV, the vaccine alone did not induce production of detectable levels of IL-2 or IL-4 and induced only low levels of IL-5 and IL-6 (140 and 120 pg/ml, respectively). In contrast, vaccine plus MF59 induced much higher levels of

Table IV
Cytokine Response[a] at the Local Lymph Node after Injection of Mice with Influenza Vaccine Alone or Combined with MF59-0[b]

Immunogen	IL-2	IL-4	IL-5	IL-6
Influenza vaccine	<5	<5	140	120
Influenza vaccine + MF59	580	122	4050	825

[a]Cytokine responses are expressed as pg/mL in lymph node cell culture media.
[b]BALB/c mice were immunized subcutaneously three times at weekly intervals either with 9 μg of trivalent influenza vaccine alone or with the vaccine combined with MF59-0. Three hours after the third immunization, mice were sacrificed, draining lymph nodes were dissected, and lymph node cell suspensions were prepared. The lymph node cells were cultured 24 h without further restimulation and the media were assayed for IL-2, IL-4, IL-5, and IL-6 by ELISA.

all four cytokines. This stimulation was caused by the antigen and emulsion in the absence of any of the immunostimulatory molecules thus far associated with cytokine induction. The observation that an MF59-adjuvanted vaccine induces an elevated cytokine response is consistent with T-cell proliferation data obtained in clinical trials (R.L. Burke, personal communication). In this study, peripheral blood mononuclear cells were isolated at various times from individuals who were either naive with respect to HSV gD2, or had been vaccinated with gD2/alum or gD2/MF59. The frequency of gD2-responsive T cells was determined by a modified limiting dilution assay. Vaccination with MF59/gD2 resulted in 4- to 8-fold greater T-cell frequencies after two immunizations than those achieved with four vaccinations using gD2 adsorbed to aluminum hydroxide. In contrast to results obtained with alum, the MF59-induced gD2-dependent T-cell frequencies remained high during the 5-month interval between the second and third immunizations and were elevated to 6- to 15-fold over alum after that immunization.

While some data have been obtained concerning the mechanism of action of MF59 and related adjuvants, much more information is clearly needed. Up to this point, the primary efforts have been devoted to demonstration of clinical efficacy, which we hope will justify additional probes into the immunological mechanism of action.

4. MANUFACTURING AND SCALEUP OF MF59

The development of reliable high-pressure homogenization conditions was necessary to reproducibly manufacture large-scale submicron adjuvant emulsions for commercial use. Because no commercial instrument is suitable for the introduction of separate oil and aqueous phases, preemulsions were generated by mixing an oil phase, consisting of squalene and Span 85, with an aqueous solution of Tween 80 and homogenizing with a high-speed blade homogenizer. These preemulsions, which had droplet diameters in the range of 1 to 10 μm, were homogenized with a Microfluidizer® 110Y (Microfluidics, Newton, MA) to give the final submicron emulsions. Initially, 100- to 300-mL batches of emulsion were generated using five passes through the Microfluidizer® in a recycling mode. Droplet size distributions were determined by photocorrelation spectroscopy using a Coulter N4MD laser particle sizer. Droplet diameter data (pre and post sterile filtration)

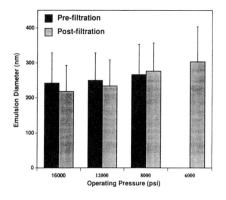

Figure 9. Effect of operating pressure on adjuvant emulsion droplet diameter. Emulsions were prepared by homogenization in a Microfluidizer® Model 110Y and were assayed for droplet diameter by photocorrelation spectroscopy using a Coulter N4MD submicron particle analyzer. Error bars indicate average standard deviation around the unimodal mean diameter.

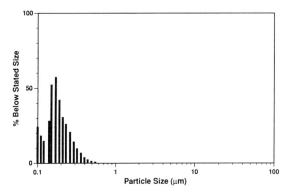

Figure 10. Droplet diameter distribution of MF59-100. MF59-100 was homogenized at 12,000 psi in the Microfluidizer® Model 110Y and size distribution was determined by laser light scattering with a Malvern Mastersizer X. Number average distribution is presented.

obtained by homogenization at pressures ranging from 6000 to 16,000 psi is shown in Fig. 9. The droplet diameters and moderate dependence of mean droplet diameter on operating pressure are consistent with data reported for the second generation microfluidized SAF emulsion (Lidgate *et al.*, 1992). Homogenization at 12,000 psi was adopted for continued development and emulsions were further characterized by light scattering with a Mastersizer X (Malvern Instruments, Southborough, MA) in order to determine contaminating levels of 1- to 10-μm droplets. Number-averaged data showed no detectable droplets in this range (Fig. 10).

In order to determine optimal process conditions for the preparation of adjuvant, 5-mL lots of MF59-0 were prepared by the previously described homogenization method using a number of process variations: (1) cooling to maintain product temperature at 25°C; (2) cooling to maintain product temperature at 40°C; (3) substitution of two serial passes for the recycle mode. The products were sterile filtered at the end of the runs through a 0.22-μm filter at a positive pressure of < 20 psi. The acceptability of the process was based on filterability of the product and yield of squalene as assessed by reverse-phase high-pressure chromatography (RP-HPLC) for the final squalene content. Results obtained from the series of runs are summarized in Table V. Adjuvants prepared at 25°C using the end-to-end process with two passes were somewhat difficult to filter, though no losses in squalene were observed. In contrast, emulsions made at 40°C using the recycling mode could be filtered at constant flow rates, and consistent lots of adjuvant emulsions were prepared and filtered with no change in composition. Therefore, a process employing 40°C runs at 12,000 psi using the recycling mode was adopted for the manufacture of 5-L lots of adjuvant.

Initial test vaccines were based on two vial formulations. Antigen was stored at –80°C and adjuvant at 2 to 8°C. Vials were mixed immediately before use. Therefore, a preliminary stability study was conducted with MF59-0 emulsion alone in either water for injection or 10 mM sodium citrate, pH 6.0, stored with or without nitrogen overlay for a period of 3 months at 4, 25, and 37°C. Adjuvant formulations stored at 2 to 8°C maintained pH and squalene content. Based on visual and microscopic appearance, morphology was unchanged during the study. On the other hand, emulsions prepared and stored in water at

Table V

Effects of Manufacturing Conditions on the Filterability and
Composition of Adjuvant Emulsions

Sample	Volume	Run type	Unfiltered/ filtered	Bath/product temp.	Percent squalene	Percent of starting	Filterability
1	5 L	Recycle	Unfiltered	4/28°C	3.891 ± 0.010	91.7%	Difficult
			Filter 1		3.495 ± 0.048	81.4%	
			Filter 2		3.310 ± 0.027	77.1%	
2	5 L	Recycle	Unfiltered	4/28°C	4.454 ± 0.003	104%	Difficult
			Filtered		4.284 ± 0.051	99.8%	
3	5 L	Recycle	Unfiltered	25/38°C	4.530 ± 0.033	105%	Constant flow
			Filtered		4.350 ± 0.015	101%	
4	5 L	Recycle	Unfiltered	25/38°C	4.404 ± 0.015	103%	Constant flow
			Filtered		4.228 ± 0.045	98.5%	
5	5 L	Recycle	Unfiltered	25/38°C	4.259 ± 0.070	99.2%	Constant flow
			Filtered		4.228 ± 0.045	90.5%	
6	5 L	Recycle	Unfiltered	25/38°C	4.382 ± 0.051	102%	Constant flow
			Filtered		4.094 ± 0.005	95.4%	
7	5 L	End-to-end	Unfiltered	25/38°C	4.220 ± 0.039	98.3%	Constant flow
			Filtered		3.940 ± 0.021	91.8%	

25 or 37°C showed a drop in pH during storage and a significant squalene loss. When the adjuvant was buffered in citrate, however, there was no drop in pH or loss in squalene at the higher temperatures in the presence or absence of nitrogen. It is of interest to note that stabilization with the citrate buffer was superior to nitrogen overlay of the vial. The mechanism of the pH drop observed with the emulsions in water is currently under investigation.

Two formats were tested for use with vaccine formulations for advanced clinical trials: a single-vial liquid format containing MF59 and antigen in buffer and a dual-vial liquid with antigen and adjuvant stored separately. In either case an acceptable formulation was required to be stable at 2 to 8°C for at least 1 year. Two stability problems with these formulations needed to be addressed. Antigens had been stored at –80°C for Phase I trials and required development of buffers suitable for 4°C storage. In addition, no data existed on long-term compatibility of antigen(s) with MF59. A 90-day stability study was conducted with the MF59/HSV gB2, gD2 vaccine at 4, 25, and 37°C in order to evaluate the stability of the single-vial formulation in comparison with the corresponding two-vial formulation. The formulations tested are described in Table VI. Citrate buffering was previously shown to provide both pH stability and protection against loss of squalene. The addition of glycine inhibits formation of nonreducible gB2 oligomers presumably by competition with lysine and additional sodium chloride is required to avoid protein adsorption at low antigen inputs. A minimum set of stability-indicating assays was used. Emulsion stability was assessed by determination of visual appearance, pH, squalene content (RP-HPLC), and droplet diameter (photocorrelation spectroscopy). Antigen stability was assessed by determination of protein content (BCA), molecular weight (SDS

Table VI

Vaccine Compositions

Component	Concentration (mg/mL)
HSV single-vial vaccine composition	
Squalene	21.5
Tween 80	2.5
Span 85	2.4
Sodium chloride	4.7
Trisodium citrate dihydrate	2.68
Citric acid monohydrate	0.19
Glycine	10.0
gB2	0.060
gD2	0.060
WFI q.s. to	1.0 mL
HSV double-vial vaccine compositions—antigen	
gB2	0.120
gD2	0.120
Sodium chloride	9.4
Trisodium citrate dihydrate	2.68
Citric acid monohydrate	0.19
Glycine	20.0
WFI q.s. to	1.0 mL
HSV double-vial vaccine compositions—MF59	
Squalene	43.0
Tween 80	2.5
Span 85	2.4
Trisodium citrate dihydrate	2.68
Citric acid monohydrate	0.19
WFI q.s. to	1.0 mL

PAGE), and conformation (ELISA). Critical data from the comparative study are presented in Table VII. These data indicate that both formulations were unchanged over the 90-day period at either 4 or 25°C. Antigens showed only minimal signs of degradation by SDS PAGE after 3 months at 37°C. No loss of sterility was observed for any sample.

Immunogenicity studies conducted in guinea pigs showed that the 90-day formulations gave equivalent anti-gD2 and anti-gB2 ELISA titers as the day 0 samples, as well as indistinguishable virus neutralization responses (Fig. 11). Thus, the potencies of the vaccines were retained in both formulations. An additional stability study conducted to simulate transport conditions confirmed that these formulations would survive conditions of shipping. Based on these experimental data and outcome of an analysis of the key product criteria such as convenience in shipping, storage, and ease of clinical administration, the single-vial liquid formulation was chosen as the prototype formulation for future clinical trials.

Adjuvant emulsion formulations, with or without MTP-PE, have been generated in 5- to 10-L quantities for clinical trials. Also, a useful single-vial liquid formulation

Table VII

Summary Results from the 3-Month Stability Study with MF59/HSV gB2–gD2 Vaccine Formulations

Stability criteria	Single-vial liquid	Two-vial format (antigen & buffered MF59-0)
Droplet diameter	Remained the same for formulations at 4, 25, and 37°C.	Remained the same at all temperatures.
Visual/microscopic appearance	Remained homogeneous. Few large particles were seen under microscope at 3 months and at 37°C.	MF59-0 in citrate was homogeneous by visual appearance. Few large particles under microscopic exam at 37°C and 3 months.
Squalene content	No compositional change at 4 and 25°C.	No change in squalene at 4 and 25°C.
Protein (SDS-PAGE)	No evidence of proteolysis at 4 and 25°C.	No evidence of proteolysis at 4 and 25°C.
ELISA	ELISA showed no drop for gD2 and gB2 with respect to time zero measurements.	ELISA showed no detectable changes in either antigen with respect to time zero activity.
pH	Stable.	No changes in the buffered adjuvant or antigens.

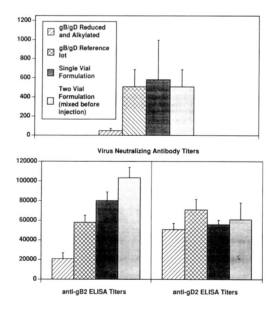

Figure 11. Virus neutralizing and ELISA antibody titers obtained in stability studies. Four groups of eight guinea pigs were immunized twice at a 2-week interval with MF59/gB,gD formulations which had been held 90 days at the time of the first injection. Reduced and alkylated gB2/gD2 were used with MF59 as a negative control for the virus neutralization assay.

containing the adjuvant and antigen(s) has been designed, and it provides physicochemical stability sufficient for performance of preclinical and clinical investigations. Further scaleup of the manufacturing process to produce 50- to 100-L quantities of the adjuvant and optimization of the different vaccine formulations are in progress.

5. CLINICAL RESULTS WITH THE MF59 ADJUVANT FORMULATION

The MF59 adjuvant formulation has been tested in over 3000 human volunteers in combination with recombinant HSV glycoproteins (gB and gD), recombinant HIV envelope proteins, and with commercially available influenza vaccines. These studies have been performed in both seronegative and seropositive volunteers with the HSV and HIV vaccines. Study populations have included normal adults (HSV, HIV, influenza) as well as elderly populations (influenza) and children and infants (HIV). The safety and immunogenicity of the MF59 adjuvant formulation have been clearly demonstrated in these clinical trials.

In HSV and HIV seronegative studies, recombinant antigens combined with the MF59 formulation generated high antibody responses as measured by ELISA or by virus neutralizing assays. In many cases the antibody titers achieved by vaccination with viral antigens combined with MF59 approached or even surpassed titers seen in seropositive, naturally infected individuals. In HSV trials, the antibody titers generated using MF59 were significantly higher than titers generated using alum. Very strong helper T-cell responses (lymphocyte proliferation) were also induced in HSV and HIV seronegative subjects with the MF59 formulation. In the seronegative populations, humoral and cellular responses to the vaccine were not enhanced when MTP-PE was included in the MF59 formulation. The MF59 formulation was also effective in stimulating immune responses with HSV, HIV, and influenza vaccines in seropositive subjects. Of interest, the addition of MTP-PE to the vaccine in HIV-seropositive individuals resulted in marked increases in HIV antigen-specific lymphocyte proliferation compared to results obtained in the absence of the muramyl peptide. This is the only circumstance where MTP-PE has been shown to have an immunological advantage over the emulsion-based formulation alone.

The clinical trials with MF59-0 have demonstrated that the adjuvant formulation is safe and well tolerated. The local reactions associated with the MF59 vaccine formulations include pain and tenderness at the injection site, and at a much lower frequency, erythema and induration which generally resolve within 24 to 48 h of immunization. Systemic reactions include a flu-like syndrome characterized by arthralgias, myalgias, headache, fever, and malaise. These symptoms also tend to resolve within 24 to 48 h of immunization. There does not appear to be a clear-cut relationship between local and systemic reactions associated with one immunization in terms of predicting the same side effect profile on subsequent immunizations. Other side effects that were noted very infrequently include transient elevation in liver function tests and rash. Safety has been clearly established with regard to hematologic parameters as well as renal function. The reaction profiles noted in HIV-1 seronegative subjects in a Phase II trial of gp120 MN with aluminum hydroxide versus gp120 SF2 with MF59 show identical low rates of reactions (mild local and systemic), further documenting the safety of the MF59 adjuvant. Ongoing Phase II prophylactic and Phase I/II therapeutic trials with HIV vaccine, Phase II trials with influenza vaccine, and Phase III prophylactic and therapeutic trials with HSV vaccines will continue to document the safety of the MF59-0 adjuvant formulation.

Early trials with influenza vaccine, HIV vaccine, and HSV vaccine have shown that the addition of MTP-PE to the MF59 adjuvant formulation results in increased rates of local and systemic reactions over those seen in the absence of the muramyl peptide. In particular, a majority of individuals immunized with influenza vaccine or HIV env 2-3 developed moderate to severe local and systemic reactions which generally resolved within 24 to 48 h. There did not appear to be a dose–response relationship in terms of reactogenicity when graded amounts of MTP-PE were used in vaccine trials using the env 2-3 antigen. Of interest, subjects who had local and systemic reactions associated with the MF59/MTP-PE vaccine formulation had better tolerance to the vaccine in subsequent immunizations when the MTP-PE was removed from the formulation. No evidence of uveitis (by slit lamp examination) was seen in any subjects receiving vaccines containing MF59-0 or MF59/MTP-PE.

In summary, the MF59 formulation is a safe and highly immunogenic adjuvant when used in combination with a variety of recombinant and natural subunit antigens derived from HSV, HIV, and influenza viruses. Both humoral and cellular responses have been elicited with the MF59 formulations. The addition of the muramyl peptide, MTP-PE, provides no obvious immunological advantage in seronegative subjects but does increase the antigen-specific T-cell responses in HIV-seropositive individuals and does increase reactogenicity of the vaccine.

6. SUMMARY

MF59 is a safe, practical, and potent adjuvant for use with human vaccines. The formulation is easily manufactured, may be sterilized by filtration, and is both compatible and efficacious with all antigens tested to date. MF59 has been shown to be a potent stimulator of cellular and humoral responses to subunit antigens in both animal models and clinical studies. Toxicology studies in animal models and Phase I–III studies in humans have demonstrated the safety of MF59 with HSV, HIV, and influenza vaccines.

REFERENCES

Allison, A., and Byars, N., 1987, Vaccine technology: Adjuvants for increased efficacy, *Biotechnology* **5**:1043–1045.

Allison, A. C., and Byars, N. E., 1990, Adjuvant formulations and their mode of action, *Semin. Immunol.* **2**:369–374.

Audibert, F. M., Parant, C., Damais, C., Lefrancier, P., Denien, M., Choay, J., and Chedid, L., 1980, Disassociation of immunostimulating activities of muramyldipeptide (MDP) by linking of amino acids or peptides to the glutaminyl residue, *Biochem. Biophys. Res. Commun.* **96**:915–923.

Boyd, J., Parkinson, C., and Sherman, P., 1972, Factors affecting emulsion stability and the HLB concept, *J. Colloid Interfac. Sci.* **41**:359–370.

Brynestad, K., Babbit, B., Huang, L., and Rouse, B. T., 1990, Influence of peptide acylation, liposome incorporation, and synthetic immunomodulators on the immunogenicity of a 1-23 peptide of glycoprotein D of herpes simplex virus: Implications for subunit vaccines, *J. Virol.* **64**:680–685.

Byars, N. E., and Allison, A. C., 1987, Adjuvant formulation for use in vaccines to elicit both cell-mediated and humoral immunity, *Vaccine* **5**:223–228.

Byars, N. E., Allison, A. C., Harmon, M. W., and Kendal, A. P., 1990, Enhancement of antibody responses to influenza B virus haemagglutinin by use of a new adjuvant formulation, *Vaccine* **8**:49–56.

Cohen, S., Yoshioka, T., Lucarelli, M., Hwang, L., and Langer, R., 1991, Controlled delivery systems for proteins based on poly (lactic/glycolic acid) microspheres, *Pharm. Res.* **8**:713–720.

Edelman, R., 1980, Vaccine adjuvants, *Rev. Infect. Dis.* **2**:370–383.

Fidler, I., 1988, Targetting of immunomodulators to mononuclear phagocytes for therapy in cancer, *Adv. Drug Deliv. Res.* **1**:69–76.

Fidler, I. J., Sone, S., Fogler, W. F., and Barnes, Z. L., 1981, Eradication of spontaneous metastases and activation of alveolar macrophages by intravenous injection of liposomes containing muramyl tripeptide, *Proc. Natl. Acad. Sci. USA* **78**:1680–1684.

Freund, J., 1956, The mode of action of immunologic adjuvants, *Adv. Tuberc. Res.* **7**:130–148.

Gisler, R. H., Shumann, G., Sackman, W., Pericin, C., Tarcsay, L., and Dietrich, F. M., 1986, A novel muramyl peptide, MTP-PE: Profile of biological activities, in: *Immunomodulation by Microbial Products and Related Synthetic Compounds* (Y. K. S. Yamamura, ed.), Excerpta Medica, Amsterdam, pp.167–170.

Gregoriadis, G., and Manesis, E. K., 1980, Liposomes as immunological adjuvants for hepatitis B surface antigens, in: *Liposomes and Immunology* (H. Six, ed.), Elsevier/North Holland, Amsterdam, pp. 271–283.

Gregoriadis, G., and Panagiotidi, C., 1989, Immunoadjuvant action of liposomes: Comparison with other adjuvants, *Immunol. Lett.* **20**:237–240.

Hilleman, M. R., Woodhour, A., Friedman, A., Weibel, R. E., and Stokes, J., Jr., 1972a, The clinical application of adjuvant 65, *Ann. Allergy* **30**:152–158.

Hilleman, M. R., Woodhour, A. F., Friedman, A., and Phelps, A. H., 1972b, Studies for safety of adjuvant 65, *Ann. Allergy* **30**:477–483.

Hunter, R., and Bennett, B., 1984, The adjuvant activity of nonionic block polymer surfactants. II. Antibody formation and inflammation related to the structure of triblock and octablock copolymers, *J. Immunol.* **133**:3167–3175.

Hunter, R., Strickland, F., and Kezdy, F., 1981, The adjuvant activity of nonionic block polymer surfactants. I. The role of hydrophile lipophile balance, *J. Immunol.* **127**:1244–1250.

Inselberg, J., Bathurst, I., Konsopon, J., Barchfeld, G., Barr, P., and Rosau, R., 1993, Protective immunity induced in *Aotus* monkeys by a recombinant SERA protein of *Plasmodium falciparum*: Adjuvant effects on induction of protective immunity, *Infect. Immun.* **61**:2041–2047.

Kossovsky, N., Gelman, A., Sponsler, E., and Millett, D., 1991, Nanocrystalline Epstein–Barr virus decoys, *J. Appl. Biomater.* **2**:251–259.

Kotani, S., Watanabe, Y., Kinoshita, F., Shimono, T., Morisaki, I., Shiba, T., Kusumoto, S., Tarumi, Y., and Ikenaka, K., 1975, Immunoadjuvant activities of synthetic N-acetylmuramyl peptides or amino acids, *Biken J.* **18**:105–111.

Kreuter, J., Berg, U., Liehl, E., Soliva, M., and Speiser, P. P., 1986, Influence of the particle size on the adjuvant effect of particulate polymeric adjuvants, *Vaccine* **4**:125–129.

Kreuter, J., Liehl, E., Berg, U., Soliva, M., and Speiser, P. P., 1988, Influence of hydrophobicity on the adjuvant effect of particulate polymeric adjuvants, *Vaccine* **6**:253–256.

Lidgate, D., Trattner, T., Schultz, R., and Maskiewicz, R., 1992, Sterile filtration of a parenteral emulsion, *Pharm. Res.* **9**:860–863.

Masihi, K. N., Lange, W., Brehmer, W., and Ribi, E., 1986, Immunobiological activities of nontoxic lipid A: Enhancement of nonspecific resistance in combination with trehalose dimycolate against viral infection and adjuvant effects, *Int. J. Immunopharmacol.* **8**:339–345.

Merser, C., Sinay, P., and Adam, A., 1975, Total synthesis and adjuvant activity of bacterial peptidoglycan derivatives, *Biochem. Biophys. Res. Commun.* **66**:1316–1322.

O'Hagan, D. T., Jeffery, H., Roberts, M. J., McGee, J. P., and Davis, S. S., 1991, Controlled release microparticles for vaccine development, *Vaccine* **9**:768–771.

Ott, G., Van Nest, G., and Burke, R. L., 1992, The use of muramyl peptides as vaccine adjuvants, in: *Vaccine Research and Developments* (W. Koff and H. Six, eds.), Dekker, New York, pp. 89–114.

Ribi, E., Takayama, K., Milner, K., Gray, G. R., Goren, M., Parker, R., McLaughlin, C., and Kelly, M., 1976, Regression of tumors by an endotoxin combined with trehalose mycolates of differing structure, *Cancer Immunol. Immunother.* **1**:265–270.

Sanchez-Pescador, L., Burke, R. L., Ott, G., and Van Nest, G., 1988, The effect of adjuvants on the efficacy of a recombinant herpes simplex virus glycoprotein vaccine, *J. Immunol.* **141**:1720–1727.

Tsujimoto, M., Kotani, S., Kinoshita, F., Karoh, S., Shiba, T., and Kusumoto, S., 1986, Adjuvant activity of 6-O-acyl-muramyldipeptides to enhance primary cellular and humoral immune responses in guinea pigs: Adaptability to various vehicles and pyrogenicity, *Infect. Immun.* **53**:511–516.

Ullrich, S., and Fidler, I., 1992, Liposomes containing muramyl tripeptide phosphatidylethanolamine (MTP-PE) are excellent adjuvants for induction of an immune response to protein and tumor antigens, *J. Leukocyte Biol.* **52**:489–494.

Van Nest, G., Steimer, K., Haigwood, N., Burke, R., and Ott, G., 1992, Advanced adjuvant formulations for use with recombinant subunit vaccines, in: *Vaccines 92*, Cold Spring Harbor Laboratory Press, Cold Spring Harbor, NY, pp. 57–62.

Warren, H. S., Vogel, F. R., and Chedid, L. A., 1986, Current status of immunological adjuvants, *Annu. Rev. Immunol.* **4**:369–388.

White, R. G., Jolles, P., Samour, D., and Lederer, E., 1964, Correlation of adjuvant activity and chemical structure of wax D fractions of mycobacteria, *Immunology* **7**:158–163.

Wintsch, J., Chaignat, C. L., Braun, D. G., Jeannet, M., Stalder, H., and Abrignani, S., 1991, Safety and immunogenicity of a genetically engineered human immunodeficiency vaccine, *J. Infect. Dis.* **163**:219–225.

Woodward, L., 1989, Adjuvant activity of water-insoluble surfactants, *Lab. Anim. Sci.* **39**:222–225.

Chapter 11

Development of Vaccines Based on Formulations Containing Nonionic Block Copolymers

Robert N. Brey

1. INTRODUCTION

This chapter focuses on the capacity of vaccine formulations containing synthetic nonionic block polymers to modify or augment immune responses to current vaccines and some vaccines under development. These polymers are surface-active agents that can be formulated alone with antigens or as part of hydrophobic delivery vehicles. In current licensed human vaccines, improvements can be made to increase vaccine immunogenicity so that they can be administered in fewer injections, or so that seroconversion rates can be increased in target populations. Subunit antigen vaccines under development can lack potency, which can be significantly enhanced if formulated with an adjuvant or given in the appropriate delivery system. The capacity to induce a protective immune response can be induced by incorporating immunogens into delivery systems. These delivery systems include molecules and preparations classified as adjuvants, antigen encapsulation strategies, antigen targeting techniques, pulsatile release vehicles, live vectors, and other systems.

New and improved vaccines are needed for a host of infectious diseases that affect populations in industrialized countries and in underdeveloped areas of the world (Institute of Medicine Committee on the Children's Vaccine Initiative, 1993) (see Chapter 2). Although numerous vaccines are under development to prevent disease in both pediatric and adult populations, many may have limited utility because of the complex immunization schedules and limited efficacy of some subunit antigens. For pediatric vaccines, strategies to combine antigens in single dosage formats, such as the MMR vaccine and the newly introduced DTP + *Haemophilus influenzae* combinations, have the potential to minimize the number of immunizations with increased compliance. However, even current combi-

Robert N. Brey • Vaxcel, Inc., Norcross, Georgia 30071.

Vaccine Design: The Subunit and Adjuvant Approach, edited by Michael F. Powell and Mark J. Newman. Plenum Press, New York, 1995.

nation vaccines with few exceptions require at least two immunizations to achieve protective immunity. Beyond combination strategies, improvement of current adult and pediatric vaccines centers around efforts to reduce the number of injections required to achieve protective immunity, or to raise seroconversion rates. On the other hand, the development of subunit protein, peptide, peptide/carrier, or saccharide-based vaccine candidates can be hampered by poor efficacy. The structure and epitope composition of the subunit obviously influences immunogenicity, but other factors related to antigen delivery also ultimately affect vaccine efficacy. These include targeting to lymphoid follicles, sub-cellular antigen presentation and processing pathways, the regulatory cytokine environment in the early stages of antigen processing and recognition, and the nature of T cells stimulated by antigen. The current interest in a variety of vaccine delivery systems is based on the notion that vaccines can be engineered to induce protective immunity by incorporating the protective immunogens in an effective delivery system.

An effective vaccine resulting in protective immunity must include in its design ways to induce the correct type of immune response. Protective immunity may require either a humoral antibody response, cellular immune response, the presence of secretory immunoglobulin at mucosal surfaces, or a combination of these responses. For T-dependent antigens, development of vaccine-induced humoral or cellular immunity is dependent on the nature of the T cells that are stimulated and how they differentiate after immunization. The current dogma suggests that induction of effector T cell mechanisms results from the stimulation of $CD8^+$ cytolytic T cells (CTLs) by peptides derived from the degradation of internally synthesized cytosolic proteins that are transported to the surface of an antigen-presenting cell (APC) in conjunction with nascent MHC class I molecules (Germain and Margulies, 1993; Townsend and Bodmer, 1989). On the other hand, $CD4^+$ T cells, which provide T cell help, selectively recognize endosomally processed antigen in association with MHC class II molecules, favoring development of humoral immunity (Lanzavecchia, 1993). Further, functional specialization of T cells has been implicated in control of several parasitic diseases in animals and humans, and may be involved in resistance to the AIDS virus (Clerici et al., 1993; Mosmann and Coffman, 1989). Activated T cells may differentiate into two specific types in response to regulatory cytokines and are classified according to the types of cytokines that they secrete. Protection against infection with *Leishmania* parasites in mice and humans is thought to result from polarization of T cell responses toward Th1, characterized by IFN-γ, and IL-2 synthesis, and susceptibility results from primarily host Th2 response, characterized by IL-4 and IL-10 synthesis (Ghalib et al., 1993; Scott, 1991; Scott et al., 1989). Th1 responses are characterized by cellular responses and the production of opsonizing antibodies such as IgG2a (in mice), whereas Th2 responses are characterized by production of IgE, IgA, and IgG1 (in mice). Cytokines such as IL-2, IFN-γ, lymphotoxin, and IL-12 tend to promote cell-mediated immunity whereas cytokines such as IL-4, IL-5, IL-6, and IL-10 promote the immune deviation from cellular to humoral, including the development of IgE-dependent allergic responses. Thus, both the subcellular pathway that an antigen enters and the cytokine milieu in the microenvironment of the APCs are important to the outcome of vaccination. Depending on the pathogenic mechanism of the infecting organism, the role of cellular immunity versus humoral immunity and the potential role of T cell subsets should be thoroughly considered in development of effective vaccines.

2. VACCINE DELIVERY SYSTEMS AND ADJUVANTS

Many subunit antigens may contain the appropriate primary or secondary structure necessary to induce protective immunity, but may ultimately fail because the antigen is incorrectly processed or stimulates inappropriate immunity. Subunit antigen vaccines may fail because antigens are presented to the immune system outside the context of the intact pathogen, or may be rapidly cleared. Further, subunit antigens may lack critical B-cell or T-cell epitopes or the epitope targets within the antigen structure may be subject to variation and immune selection, such as neutralizing domains of HIV-1 gp120 V3 loop region or T cell domains of the human malaria parasite *P. falciparum* circumsporozoite protein (Good *et al.*, 1988b). Many of these failures can be potentially overcome by delivering subunit antigens with adjuvants. The practical application of delivery and adjuvant technology to human vaccines is based on experimental observations that interactions between antigens and lymphoid tissue cells can be influenced by other factors than the primary and secondary structure of antigens. Still, the use of these agents and systems is largely empirical.

The conventional approach to enhance human vaccine candidates—and the only universally acceptable approach—is to formulate vaccines by adsorbing antigens to alum (salts of aluminum). Although widely used in pediatric and adult human vaccines, alum may not effectively augment immune responses necessary for a number of new subunit protein or peptide vaccines. Alum is an example of an agent that strongly interacts with most proteins and saccharides, adsorbing them to the surface or capturing them within the matrix of microcrystals. Adsorption of antigens to alum augments the immune response by allowing the formation of an antigen depot at the injection site in which antigen gradually desorbs from the microcrystalline structure, slowing clearance of the antigen and allowing extended interaction between the antigen and APCs. In current commercial parenterally administered human vaccines, alum is included in DTP, the DTP *Haemophilus influenzae* type b (Hib) combinations, one of the Hib conjugates (PRP–OMPC), the tetanus and diphtheria combinations, and hepatitis B vaccines. However, the MMR combination live attenuated vaccine, the multivalent pneumococcal saccharide vaccine, several Hib conjugates (HBOC and PRP-D), the *N. meningitidis* A/C/Y/W-135 vaccine, and the influenza vaccine are administered to humans without alum adsorption. For influenza vaccines, the vaccine components do not adsorb well to alum or only marginally affect immunogenicity (Potter *et al.*, 1977; Skea and Barber, 1993). Moreover, the capacity of alum salts to modulate effective immunity to several subunits such as HIV-1 gp120 and HSV gD is limited (Haigwood *et al.*, 1992; Sanchez-Pescador *et al.*, 1988). Alum as adjuvant may not be sufficient to aid in stimulating cellular immunity, and may selectively block development of CD8$^+$ CTLs by immunization with some antigens (Schirmbeck *et al.*, 1994).

To date, a number of promising adjuvants and delivery systems have been developed and tested with a number of vaccines. Some have been tested in human clinical trials and are candidates for inclusion in commercial vaccines. Adjuvants can include vehicles that may target or depot antigens, and can also include other components designed to interact with lymphoid cells. For example, nontoxic derivatives of saponins (such as QS-21) or lipopolysaccharide (LPS) can be potent adjuvants in aqueous solution or combined with vehicles (Kensil *et al.*, 1991). Some of them may function directly on macrophages and other cells by influencing the production of cytokines such as IL-1, TNF, and IL-6. These molecules include deacylated forms of LPS and monophosphoryl lipid A (Takayama *et al.*, 1991) and other components derived from bacterial cell walls, including the cell wall adjuvant of mycobacteria, muramyl dipeptide (MDP), and its derivatives (Allison and Byars, 1990; Audibert and Lise, 1993). Other strategies to modify immune responses have been based on modification of specific ligand–receptor interactions, sometimes in conjunction with adjuvant vehicles. For example, it has been demonstrated that a CTL epitope presented by injection as a soluble peptide with β_2-microglobulin can target a peptide CTL epitope to empty surface-localized class I MHC molecules and elicit a specific CTL response (Rock *et al.*, 1993). Further, intact protein antigens can be targeted to macrophages by capturing antigen with α_2-macroglobulin (Chu and Pizzo, 1993). Recent studies have demonstrated that purified cytokines can be used to modulate vaccine immunogenicity. IL-12 combined with *Leishmania* antigen extract, specifically directed immunity toward protective Th1 responses and replaced requirement for a whole-cell bacterial adjuvant *Corynebacterium parvum* (Afonso *et al.*, 1994). Formulation of IL-2 with a malaria sporozoite vaccine overcame genetic restriction in nonresponding mice (Good *et al.*, 1988a). Similarly, vaccination with HBsAg followed by treatment with IL-2 induced protective levels of anti-HB antibodies in previously nonresponsive hemodialysis patients (Meuer, 1989). These results suggest that other adjuvants and delivery vehicles may also permit preferential stimulation of protective Th1 subsets in other vaccines, modulate epitope recognition by MHC molecules, or otherwise modify regulatory cytokine profiles in APCs.

3. NONIONIC BLOCK POLYMERS IN VACCINE FORMULATIONS

Historically, the use of adjuvants in human vaccines has dated back many decades. Polyvalent influenza vaccines were formulated with incomplete Freund's adjuvant and administered intramuscularly as water-in-oil emulsions to over 18,000 military personnel in the early 1950s (Hilleman, 1967). A substitute incomplete Freund's adjuvant was developed in the 1960s containing vegetable oil and mannide monooleate as an emulsifier (Hilleman *et al.*, 1972). Long-term follow-up of people receiving these vaccines has revealed no significant increases in risks of acquiring neoplasms or risk of increased mortality (Page *et al.*, 1993). Side effects of the vaccine may have included an increased incidence of hospitalizations related to cysts at the site of injection and increased frequency of allergic responses.

More recently, a number of vaccine formulations based on emulsion vehicles have been developed and some have been evaluated or are currently undergoing evaluation in clinical trials. In addition to the immunomodulating capacity of cell wall derivatives and similar preparations, it is becoming increasing clear that vaccine formulation vehicles often have inherent adjuvant activity. Vehicles include a wide array of materials and formulations ranging from oil-based emulsions to liposomes to microparticulate pulsatile release systems (Eldridge *et al.*, 1991). Emulsion vehicles have been used in experimental vaccines for years, and variations on the formulations containing mineral oils and emulsifying agents have centered around replacements containing vegetable oils or other metabolizable oils. Current efforts to develop safe and effective emulsion vehicles have been based on low-oil formulations engineered as microdroplets for efficient uptake by APCs. These formulations include Syntex SAFm (Byars *et al.*, 1991), Chiron MF59 (Inselburg *et al.*, 1993; Keitel *et al.*, 1993), and IDEC AF (Raychaudhuri *et al.*, 1992). The common element of these formulations is that they consist of metabolizable oil vehicles, usually oils such as squalene or squalane, which are stabilized with emulsifying agents such as Span 85 or Tween 80. Formulations containing these compounds can be stabilized for long-term storage under refrigeration conditions by reducing the oil droplet size to less than 1 μm in diameter by expelling the compounded emulsion through small orifices under high pressure. Under usual conditions, an antigen can be mixed directly with the adjuvant formulation and injected. Several emulsion formulations have been evaluated clinically. The Chiron formulation MF59, optionally containing MTP-PE, has been evaluated in conjunction with several influenza vaccines. This vaccine combination induced significant toxicity in people, an effect that was attributable to MTP-PE (Keitel *et al.*, 1993; Wintsch *et al.*, 1991). The Syntex formulation SAFm, optionally containing threonyl MDP, has been evaluated in humans, surgically treated for advanced melanoma, in conjunction with an anti-idiotype MAb for an antigen expressed on melanoma cells (Livingston *et al.*, 1994). In that study, significant systemic side effects, such as profound fatigue and myalgia lasting up to 4 days, were associated with injection of the highest doses of threonyl MDP. Some local reactogenicity was associated with the vehicle component. High rates of seroconversion to the melanoma antigen were elicited by the SAFm vaccine, although antibody induction did not appear to be dependent on the inclusion of threonyl MDP in the vaccine (Livingston *et al.*, 1994). The side effects noted at intermediate levels of threonyl MDP in patients treated for melanoma may be acceptable for therapeutic vaccination of patients surgically treated for advanced melanoma. It is likely, however, that the same side effects would not be acceptable in people receiving routine influenza immunizations.

In addition to the common oil and emulsifier ingredients, the Syntex SAF and the IDEC AF emulsions contain a nonionic block copolymer, L121, as a vehicle component. This copolymer has been included in a number of other experimental adjuvant formulations that have been evaluated favorably in preclinical models (Byars *et al.*, 1990, 1991; Hunter *et al.*, 1991; Millet *et al.*, 1992; Takayama *et al.*, 1991). L121 and other nonionic block polymers are constructed synthetically with relatively simple chemistry from hydrophilic blocks of polyoxyethylene (POE) and hydrophobic blocks of polyoxypropylene (POP). Nonionic block polymers are currently used commercially in a wide number of over-the-counter products, including shampoos, mouthwashes, cosmetics, topical ointments, and contact lens solutions. These compounds are generally regarded as safe and are also used as wetting agents, dispersion agents, and thickening agents. These compounds are generally classified as "excipients" and are thought to have little or no inherent pharmacological action. A variety of nonionic block copolymer structures have been synthesized (Fig. 1). These structures include triblock (Fig. 1A), reverse triblock (Fig. 1B), octablock (Fig. 1C), and reverse octablock (Fig. 1D) molecules. The octablock class of molecules is constructed around an ethylene diamine core. These molecules essentially differ from each other in the number and orientation of oxyethylene and oxypropylene subunits.

The rationale for including nonionic block copolymers in vaccine formulations stems from the observation that L121 and similar molecules are amphipathic, are surface-active agents, and are apparently capable of binding proteins or other antigens. It has been

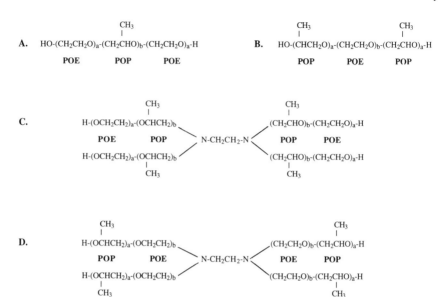

Figure 1. The structure and orientation of polyoxyethylene (POE) and polyoxypropylene (POP) of synthetic nonionic block copolymers: (A) triblock polymers; (B) reverse triblock polymers; (C) octablock polymers; and (D) reverse octablock polymers.

suggested that L121 binds antigen to the surface of the vehicle oil drops (in emulsions) or presumably to the surface of other hydrophobic vehicles, and hence promotes the interaction of antigen with cell surfaces (Hunter and Bennett, 1984; Hunter *et al.*, 1981). Scanning electron microscopy of oil-in-water emulsions containing L121 and BSA has indicated localization of BSA on the surface of oil droplets. Further, the interactions between hydrophobic milieu and oil droplets are thought to be mild, since presumably conformational aspects of protein structure can be retained by binding to surfaces artificially created by binding L121 to a plastic medium (Hunter and Bennett, 1986).

    L121 and other classes of nonionic block copolymers have been evaluated over the years for their capacity to enhance immunogenicity of a number of different antigens in animal models. It is apparent that a number of these molecules are not simply vehicles and probably have intrinsic activity on cells of the immune system as an outcome of their surface-active properties. L121 and other similar nonionic block polymers often enhance the immunogenicity of a variety of vaccines when formulated with other vehicles or in combination with other adjuvant materials, as the threonyl MDP in SAFm (see Chapter 12). The mechanism whereby copolymer adjuvants can influence immunogenicity is thought to result from enhancement of antigen presentation to macrophages or dendritic cells, where proteins could be presented as a condensed two-dimensional matrix with conformational B-cell epitopes intact. Similar to fusogenic liposomes, which may assist antigens in entering endogenous processing pathways (Alving, 1993; Alving *et al.*, 1992), vaccines containing nonionic block copolymers may influence subcellular antigen processing. The ability of copolymer to influence antigen processing via the class I pathway, inferred by induction of specific CTL, has not been explored. The mechanism of their action may also include a depot effect in some formulations containing oil. This may especially be true in formulations containing polydisperse oil droplet matrices, which could result in longer-term antigen retention. In addition, copolymers may have a more direct role in influencing the production of cytokines and other factors in APCs. It has been demonstrated that one of the triblock compounds, L81, in the context of oil-in-water emulsions with squalane, can enhance the expression of MHC class II molecules on the surface of macrophages and may increase complement activation (Howerton *et al.*, 1990).

Two early studies conducted with a spectrum of copolymers indicated that these compounds could enhance the antibody titers obtained by injection of formulations with either soluble proteins in oil-in-water emulsion vehicles or haptenated liposomes (Hunter and Bennett, 1984; Zigterman *et al.*, 1987). In studies conducted with BSA formulated in oil-in-water emulsions, results suggested that the ability of these compounds to enhance anti-BSA antibody responses depended both on the ratio of hydrophobic component to hydrophilic component and on the length of the hydrophobic central chain (Hunter and Bennett, 1984). The most effective compounds were ones in which the content of hydrophilic POE side chains was less than 10% of the total molecular weight of the polymer species. On the other hand, early antibody responses to haptenated liposomes demonstrated little correlation to the content of hydrophilic side chains and were more associated with higher total molecular weights and the structural class of the copolymer (Zigterman *et al.*, 1987). Octablock and triblock polymers having less than 10% POE side chains were effective with BSA, whereas reverse block molecules were ineffective. Reverse triblock molecules were more effective with haptenated liposomes. Haptenated liposomes were evaluated with insoluble copolymers mixed into the vaccine formulations immediately prior to injection. Vaccination of young mice with a BSA–*S. pneumoniae* type 3 hexasaccharide conjugate formulated in an oil-in-water emulsion with either an octablock molecule (T1501) or a triblock (L121) polymer resulted in significant protection against virulent challenge, which was not achieved by vaccination with the conjugate alone (Zigterman *et al.*, 1988). In ensuing studies, it was suggested that protection could be correlated to elevated levels of more avid IgG2a antibody against the type 3 capsule (Van Dam *et al.*, 1989). The level of IgG2a was influenced primarily by the block polymer; this could be demonstrated whether the vaccines were formulated in oil-in-water emulsions or with polymers in aqueous suspension. The tendency to induce IgG2a has also been demonstrated with *S. pneumoniae* type 14 polysaccharide–BSA conjugate when L121 was included in oil-in-water vaccines, independent of the presence of co-adjuvant molecules such as MDP or MPL (Van de Wijgert *et al.*, 1991). More recently, trinitrophenyl ovalbumin (TNP-OVA) was formulated with a series of high-molecular-weight triblock copolymers in oil-in-water emulsion vaccines (Hunter *et al.*, 1991). The results indicated that antibody titers observed 28 days following a single injection of the vaccines were proportional to increasing molecular weights of the central hydrophobic core. Further, the vaccines formulated with the highest-molecular-weight polymers induced higher proportions of IgG2b subclass antibodies to the hapten. The combined results of all of these basic studies have suggested that the most effective polymers were triblock molecules, containing less than 10% hydrophilic side chains, and having molecular weight above 8000.

Despite considerable barriers in synthetic methodology, several high-molecular-weight (> 10,000) triblock copolymers have been synthesized. Several of these have been tested recently in malaria vaccine models. Equivalent results indicating induction of IgG2 subclass antibodies have been obtained in mice with a *Plasmodium cynomolgi* (NAGG)$_5$–BSA conjugate vaccine candidate formulated with triblock polymers L121 or L141 in oil-in-water emulsions (Kalish *et al.*, 1991). Induction of functional IgG2a antibodies was independent of the inclusion of co-adjuvant molecules such as MDP and MPL. In other studies, this peptide vaccine was formulated with a high-molecular-weight triblock co-polymer, p1004, and used to immunize rhesus monkeys (Millet *et al.*, 1992). Monkeys were immunized three times with 200 μg of the CS peptide (NAGG)$_5$–diphtheria toxoid in squalene-in-water with either detoxified RaLPS or MTP-PE. All p1004 vaccines with RaLPS were well-tolerated, but mild local reactions were seen. Animals injected with the squalene/water vaccines with either MTP-PE or detoxified LPS produced higher antibody titers by immunofluorescence than those immunized similarly with the oil–copolymer vaccines. The animals were challenged with infected mosquito bites and the only group that showed significant protection was the one immunized with the conjugate in the p1004–RaLPS squalene/water vaccine. These animals had a significant delay in the onset of parasitemia, suggesting a 95 to 99% reduction in the inoculum.

Recently, these studies have been extended to an experimental blood stage malaria vaccine (using the *P. yoelii* murine malaria model). In this malaria model, protection against blood stage parasite challenge following immunization of mice with whole killed *P. yoelii* blood stage parasites has been shown to be adjuvant dependent (ten Hagen *et al.*, 1993). A whole blood stage parasite vaccine was formulated with p1004 in combination with a variety of emulsions, including water-in-oil, oil-in-water, and aqueous copolymer formu-lations. Protection against lethal or severe parasitemia appeared to depend on format of the vaccine vehicle. Vaccine formulations of p1004 in squalene-in-water or those with no oil induced protective responses, while all of the water-in-squalene formulations failed. Antibody titers to total parasite proteins were measured by ELISA and immunofluores-cence. Because of the staining techniques, immunofluorescence primarily detects surface-associated epitopes, whereas ELISA detects total parasite antigens. Protection was correlated with the induction of antibody of the IgG2a isotype detected by immunofluo-rescence. This antibody was effectively induced by squalene-in-water preparations or vaccines with no oil, but not by water-in-oil vaccines (including complete Freund's adjuvant). Water-in-squalene vaccines induced high titers of antibody detected by ELISA but not by immunofluorescence. Formulations without oil or squalene-in-water emulsions induced antibody against epitopes on the surface of the parasite, while water-in-oil vaccines preferentially induced antibody against epitopes on the interior of the parasite as detected by ELISA. Addition of deacylated RaLPS enhanced the production of immunofluores-cence-positive IgG2a antibody and the level of protection when used with the p1004 in saline formulation, but suppressed IgG2a (by immunofluorescence) in oil-containing vaccines. Vaccines composed of low doses of antigen (<12 μg of protein) induced persistent protection not accountable by antibody levels prior to challenge. However, these animals developed a strong anamnestic antibody response on challenge with virulent parasites. The anamnestic response was predominantly IgG2a as measured by immunofluorescence (Hunter *et al.*, 1994). Other formulations that had similar antibody profiles prior to

Figure 2. Anti-SPf66 antibodies in sera of immunized Balb/c mice obtained 2 weeks after second injection. Groups of five Balb/c mice were immunized with vaccines formulated with 400 μg of peptide SPf66 from human clinical lot 91002 (Walter Reed Army Institute of Research). Animals were immunized on day 0 and day 42. The vaccines administered on day 42 contained 100 μg peptide per dose. The water-in-oil (W/O) vaccine was prepared by admixing equal volumes of peptide with 10% p1205 (v/v) and adding that mixture at a ratio of 1:5 to squalene containing 10% Span 80. The oil-in-water (O/W) vaccine contained 2% squalane, 5% p1205, and 0.2% Tween 80 and was made by mixing lyophilized peptide with copolymer and squalane, followed by mixing into

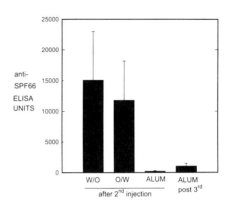

aqueous PBS. The alum SPf66 vaccine was made by coprecipitating the peptide in the presence of aluminum phosphate so that the final content of alum was approximately 1.7 mg/mL and the peptide was 2 mg/mL. Animals were injected with 0.1 mL of the indicated vaccines. Anti-SPf66 ELISA were performed by binding 1 mg SPf66/well in microtiter plates. Results are expressed as the arithmetic mean ± SEM.

challenge primed animals for increase of IgG1 and IgG2b on challenge and produced less protection. Protection was transferred by immune sera of protected animals to naive animals. These results suggested that the vaccine format can influence antigen presentation so that antibodies can be directed against surface-exposed or interior epitopes and can strongly influence the presentation of conformational epitopes.

Several potential human vaccines have been developed using formulations containing a 12-kDa triblock copolymer, termed p1205. In the past several years, the SPf66 peptide malaria vaccine has been undergoing field evaluation and has some potential for preventing malaria in endemic areas (Sempertegui *et al.*, 1994; Teusher *et al.*, 1994). This antigen is a chemically synthesized peptide composed of several *P. falciparum* merozoite epitopes. Unfortunately, this vaccine is prepared with 2 mg of peptide per dose and at least three doses are required to seroconvert naive humans. The vaccine is administered with approximately 0.7 mg of alum per dose, which adsorbs no more than 50% of the peptide (W. R. Ballou, personal communication). Hence, this vaccine is a good candidate for improvement with an adjuvant formulation which lowers the peptide dose and aids in the efficacy of the vaccine. To evaluate this possibility, SPf66 was formulated in several oil-based formulations with p1205. As shown in Fig. 2, either oil-in-water vaccine or water-in-oil vaccine was capable of inducing antipeptide antibodies after two injections, whereas a vaccine made by coprecipitation with aluminum phosphate induced poor serological response after three injections in Balb/c mice.

Another example has been obtained with a plasma-derived hepatitis B surface antigen (HBsAg) vaccine. The current recombinant or plasma-derived HBsAg vaccines are administered to people in a series of three injections over a 6-month period (Butterly *et al.*, 1989). Although HBsAg is a very effective vaccine, a significant number of immunized individuals fail to respond to the vaccine (10–15%), even after three immunizations (Weissman *et al.*, 1988). In a variety of clinical evaluations of recombinant and plasma-derived antigens, single injections of HBsAg induce seroconversion in 10-30% of vaccinees, whereas two

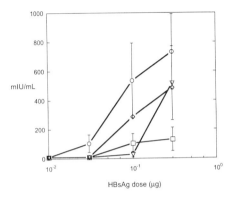

Figure 3. Anti-HBsAg in Balb/c mice. Balb/c mice were immunized with plasma-derived HBsAg at the indicated dosage in oil-in-water ◇, water-in-oil ○, alum ▽, or buffer □. Specific anti-HBsAg antibodies were measured by AUSAB (Abbott) in individual serum samples obtained 28 days following a single immunization. The vaccines were prepared according to Fig. 2. Calculations of milliinternational units (mIU) were made against a standard panel. Since mouse sera were diluted 1:10 for the assay, measurements < 100 mIU were assigned a value of 10 for purpose of calculating geometric mean titers. Results are expressed as the arithmetic mean ± SEM.

injections increase this rate to 50-80%. As shown in Fig. 3, HBsAg was formulated with p1205 in oil-in-water or water-in-oil formulations. In this case, water-in-oil formulations were more effective in inducing antibodies to the HBsAg in comparison to alum-adsorbed or antigen-alone vaccines. These responses occurred at lower antigen doses, which were at the threshold of responsiveness in Balb/c mice. Moreover, the increase in geometric mean titer as a function of the adjuvant formulation with HBsAg correlated to increased seroconversion rates within groups ($p < 0.01$), as shown in Table 1.

Table I

Seroconversion to Plasma-Derived HBsAg in Balb/c Mice Immunized with Formulations Containing Decreasing Doses of HBsAg

mIU per mL[a]	HBsAg dose	Proportion of animals seroconverting (%)			
		Week 4: W/O	Week 4: O/W	Week 4: alum adsorbed	Week 4: no adjuvant
<100	0.3 μg	1/5 (20)	0/5 (0)	0/5 (0)	3/5 (60)
100–999		2/5 (40)	5/5 (100)	4/5 (80)	2/5 (40)
>1000		2/5 (40)	0/5 (0)	1/5 (20)	0/5 (0)
<100	0.1	0/5 (0)	1/5 (20)	4/5 (80)	2/5 (40)
100–999		4/5 (80)	4/5 (80)	1/5 (20)	2/5 (40)
>1000		1/5 (20)	0/5 (0)	0/5 (0)	1/5 (20)
<100	0.03	3/5 (60)	5/5 (100)	5/5 (100)	5/5 (100)
100–999		2/5 (40)	0/5 (0)	0/5 (0)	0/5 (0)
>1000		0/5 (0)	0/5 (0)	0/5 (0)	0/5 (0)
<100	0.01	5/5 (100)	5/5 (100)	5/5 (100)	5/5 (100)
100–999		0/5 (0)	0/5 (0)	0/5 (0)	0/5 (0)
>1000		0/5 (0)	0/5 (0)	0/5 (0)	0/5 (0)

[a]AUSAB assays were performed with sera initially diluted at least 1:10. AUSAB values <10 mIU by assay were calculated to be <100 mIU/mL; AUSAB values >10 mIU in assay were multiplied by the serum dilution factor to calculate mIU per mL of mouse serum. All individual prebleed sera were below 100 mIU/mL.

4. PROPERTIES OF VACCINE FORMULATIONS CONTAINING NONIONIC BLOCK COPOLYMERS

The results discussed above have been primarily obtained with vaccines formulated with antigen and polymer, and squalene or squalane as oil-in-water emulsions. These emulsions can be obtained experimentally by combining antigen, copolymer, and oil vehicle in a single step, followed by mild emulsification in buffer. Usually, these vaccines have been made with lyophilized antigen. Although vaccines made like this could conceivably be made for commercial use by a reconstitution method, vaccines prepared as such in a single vial may not have the required stability characteristics. To overcome this potential problem, copolymer-containing oil-in-water vaccines have been stabilized by microfluidization. In a number of potential human vaccines, vaccines microfluidized with high-molecular-weight copolymers have provided much of the efficacy of the "lab format" oil-in-water vaccines and have the desired stability characteristics. Microfluidization is a physical method to disperse oil droplets through a small orifice under pressure to reduce them to a uniform small size (< 500 nm). Small-droplet vaccines may be the optimal composition and size for efficient uptake in APCs, and may allow CTL priming. Specific CTL induction to ovalbumin or HIV-1 gp120 has been demonstrated with microfluidized vaccines containing L121 (Raychaudhuri *et al.*, 1992). In other formats, antigens can be formulated directly with high-molecular-weight copolymers (oil-free) to yield vaccines in which proteins or antigens interact directly with copolymer microdroplets. In the *P. yoelii* blood stage malaria vaccine model, copolymer interactions with parasite antigens in the absence of an oil vehicle promoted IgG2a induction. Vaccines formulated with copolymers as water-in-oil emulsions have some properties similar to incomplete Freund's adjuvant in that they are high in oil, but differ since the copolymers seem to stabilize water-in-oil emulsions containing as little as 20% squalene. In these vaccines, the antigen is contained within the water phase, which is composed of droplets surrounded by oil. The view is that such formulations may be effective for enhancing certain antigens, possibly as single-shot vaccines.

Nonionic block copolymers have unusual properties that influence not only the immunological outcome of vaccination, but also the physical properties of vaccine formulations. Triblock and octablock copolymer molecules with a high content of hydrophilic POE are more soluble in water, as expected, whereas those with a decreasing proportion of POE are less soluble in water. Rather, they display limited solubility in water, dissolving in cold water up to 10 g/100 mL. The unusual property of these molecules is that they coalesce in water at "cloud point" temperatures, which are characteristic for each polymer. Typically, cloud points for polymers are above 0°C but less than 10°C. Depending on the particular molecule, the aggregates can be spherical droplets, or can assume other forms, such as L121, which is fibrous in aqueous media (Hunter and Bennett, 1986). For high-molecular-weight (> 8000) triblock copolymers, polymers form stable droplets. However, the polymer droplets are not traditional micelles, since they form in water independent of polymer concentration. Polymer droplets consist of aggregates of polymers with flexible hydrophobic parts of the chains directed inward and the hydrophilic ethylene oxide side chains interacting with water at the droplet surface. The copolymers having more hydrophobic character are freely soluble in many organic solvents and partition effectively into hydrophobic solvents such as oil.

5. SUMMARY

In summary, data indicate that nonionic block copolymers in several different delivery formats can effectively enhance antibody responses to a variety of viral, parasite, or bacterial antigens. Polymers have historically been evaluated as polymers alone in aqueous buffer, in oil-in-water and water-in-oil emulsions. Several of those formulations can induce protective antibodies in preerythrocytic or erythrocytic malaria vaccine models or in pneumococcal vaccine models. In those models, protective immunity is associated with the development of IgG2a subclass antibodies. These results tend to indicate that copolymer adjuvant can influence isotype development, possibly by stimulating the appropriate T-cell subsets. Although there are some data suggesting that microfluidized vaccines containing the L121 nonionic block copolymer can induce CTL, equivalent experimental results with larger block polymers, which are effective in induction of greater proportions of IgG2a, have not yet been obtained. Several of the basic formulations with an appropriate copolymer may be suitable for clinical evaluation in conjunction with either current or future subunit antigens. Other formulations containing copolymers may also be suitable for mucosal administration.

ACKNOWLEDGMENTS

I would like to thank Deborah Goodwyn and Margaret Olsen for developing the serological assays and for formulating the vaccines used in these studies.

REFERENCES

Afonso, L. C. C., Scharton, T. M., Vieira, L. Q., Wysocka, M., Trinchieri, G., and Scott, P., 1994, The adjuvant effect of interleukin-12 in a vaccine against *Leishmania major, Science* 263:235–237.
Allison, A. C., and Byars, N. E., 1990, Adjuvant formulations and their mode of action, *Semin. Immunol.* 2:369–374.
Alving, C. R., 1993, Lipopolysaccharide, lipid A, and liposomes containing lipid A as immunologic adjuvants, *Immunobiology* 187:430–446.
Alving, C. R., Verma, J. N., Rao, M., Krzych, U., Amselem, S., Green, S. M., and Wassef, N. M., 1992, Liposomes containing lipid A as a potent non-toxic adjuvant, *Res. Immunol.* 143:197–198.
Audibert, F. M., and Lise, L. D., 1993, Adjuvants: Current status, clinical perspectives and future prospects, *Immunol. Today* 14:281–284.
Butterly, L., Watkins, E., and Dienstag, J. L., 1989, Recombinant-yeast derived hepatitis B vaccine in healthy adults: Safety and two-year immunogenicity of early investigative lots of vaccine, *J. Med. Virol.* 27:155–159.
Byars, N. E., Allison, A. C., Harmon, M. W., and Kendal, A. P., 1990, Enhancement of antibody responses to influenza B virus haemagglutinin by use of a new adjuvant formulation, *Vaccine* 8:49–56.
Byars, N. E., Nakano, G., Welch, M., Lehman, D., and Allison, A. C., 1991, Improvement of hepatitis B vaccine by the use of a new adjuvant, *Vaccine* 9:309–318.
Chu, C. T., and Pizzo, S. V., 1993, Receptor-mediated antigen delivery into macrophages, *J. Immunol.* 150:48–58.

Clerici, M., Lucey, D. R., Berzovsky, J.A., Pinto, L. A., Wynn, T. A., Blatt, S. A., Dolan, M. J., Hendrix, C. W., Wolf, S. W., and Shearer, G. M., 1993, Restoration of HIV-specific cell-mediated immune responses by interleukin-12 in vitro, *Science* **262**:1721–1724.

Eldridge, J. H., Staas, J. K., Meulbroek, J. A., Tice, T. R., and Gilley, R. M., 1991, Biodegradable and biocompatible poly(DL-lactide-co-glycolide) microspheres as an adjuvant for staphylococcal enterotoxin B toxoid which enhances the level of toxin neutralizing antibodies, *Infect. Immun.* **59**:2978–2986.

Germain, R. N., and Margulies, D. H., 1993, The biochemistry and cell biology of antigen processing and presentation, *Annu. Rev. Immunol.* **11**:403–540.

Ghalib, H. W., Piuvezam, M. R., Skeiky, Y. A., Siddig, M., Hashim, F. A., el Hassan, A., Russo, D. M., and Reed, S. G., 1993, Interleukin 10 production correlates with pathology in human *Leishmania donovani* infections, *J. Clin. Invest.* **92**:324–329.

Good, M. F., Pombo, D., Lunde, M. N., Maloy, W. L., Halenbeck, R., Koths, K., Miller, L. H., and Berzofsky, J. A., 1988a, Recombinant human IL-2 overcomes genetic nonresponsiveness to malaria sporozoite peptides. Correlation of effect with biologic activity of IL-2, *J. Immunol.* **141**:972–977.

Good, M. F., Pombo, D., Quakyi, I. A., Riley, E. M., Houghten, R. A., Menon, A., Alling, D. W., Berzofsky, J. A., and Miller, L. H., 1988b, Human T-cell recognition of the circumsporozoite protein of *Plasmodium falciparum*: Immunodominant T-cell domains map to the polymorphic regions of the molecule, *Proc. Natl. Acad. Sci. USA* **85**:1199–1203.

Haigwood, N. L., Nara, P. L., Brooks, E., Van Nest, G., Ott, G., Higgins, K. W., Dunlop, N., Scandella, C. J., Eichberg, J. W., and Steimer, K. S., 1992, Native but not denatured recombinant human immunodeficiency virus type 1 gp120 generates broad-spectrum neutralizing antibodies in baboons, *J. Virol.* **66**:172–182.

Hilleman, M. R., 1967, Considerations for safety and application of emulsified oil adjuvants to viral vaccines, in: *International Symposium on Adjuvants of Immunity*, Utrecht, 1966, Karger, Basel, pp. 13–26.

Hilleman, M. R., Woodhur, A., and Friedman, A., 1972, The clinical application of adjuvant 65, *Ann. Allergy* **30**:152–158.

Howerton, D. A., Hunter, R. L., Ziegler, H. K., and Check, I. J., 1990, Induction of macrophage Ia expression in vivo by a synthetic block polymer, L81, *J. Immunol.* **144**:1578–1584.

Hunter, R. L., and Bennett, B., 1984, The adjuvant activity of nonionic block polymer surfactants. II. Antibody formation and inflammation related to the structure of triblock and octablock copolymers, *J. Immunol.* **133**:3167–3175.

Hunter, R. L., and Bennett, B., 1986, The adjuvant activity of nonionic block polymer surfactants. III. Characterization of selected biologically active surfaces, *Scand. J. Immunol.* **23**:287–300.

Hunter, R. L., Strickland, F., and Kezdy, F., 1981, The adjuvant activity of nonionic block polymer surfactants. I. The role of hydrophile–lipophile balance, *J. Immunol.* **127**:1244–1250.

Hunter, R., Olsen, M., and Buynitzky, 1991, Adjuvant activity of non-ionic block copolymers. IV. Effect of molecular weight and formulation on titre and isotype of antibody, *Vaccine* **9**:250–256.

Hunter, R. L., Kidd, M. R., Olsen, M. R., Patterson, P. S., and Lal, A. A., 1994, Induction of long-lasting immunity to *P. yoelii* malaria using whole blood-stage antigen and copolymer adjuvants, (submitted).

Inselburg, J., Bathurst, I. C., Kansopon, J., Barr, P. J., and Rossan, R., 1993, Protective immunity induced in *Aotus* monkeys by a recombinant SERA protein of *Plasmodium falciparum*: Further studies using SERA1 and MF75.2 adjuvant, *Infect. Immun.* **61**:2048–2052.

Institute of Medicine Committee on the Children's Vaccine Initiative, 1993, *The Children's Vaccine Initiative* (V. S. Mitchell, N. M. Philipose, and J. P. Sanford, eds.), National Academy Press, Washington, DC.

Kalish, M. L., Check, I. J., and Hunter, R. L., 1991, Murine IgG isotype responses to the *Plasmodium cynomolgi* circumsporozoite peptide (NAGG)5, *J. Immunol.* **146**:3583–3590.

Keitel, W., Couch, R., Bond, N., Adair, S., Van Nest, G., and Dekker, C., 1993, Pilot evaluation of influenza virus vaccine (IVV) combined with adjuvant, *Vaccine* **11**:909–913.

Kensil, C. R., Patel, U., Lennick, M., and Marciani, D., 1991, Separation and characterization of saponins with adjuvant activity from Quillaja saponaria Molina cortex, *J. Immunol.* **146**:431–437.

Lanzavecchia, A., 1993, Identifying strategies for immune intervention, *Science* **260**:937–944.

Livingston, P. O., Adluri, S., Raychaudhuri, S., Hughes, M. H., Calves, M. J., and Merritt, J. A., 1994, A phase I trial of the immunological adjuvant SAFm in melanoma patients vaccinated with the anti-idiotype antibody MELIMMUNE™, *Vaccine Res.* **3**:71–81.

Meuer, S. C., 1989, Low dose interleukin-2 induces systemic immune response against HBsAg in immunodeficient non-responders to hepatitis B vaccination in dialysis patients, *Lancet* **1**:15–18.

Millet, P., Kalish, M. L., Collins, W. E., and Hunter, R. L., 1992, Effect of adjuvant formulations on the selection of B-cell epitopes expressed by a malaria peptide vaccine, *Vaccine* **10**:547–550.

Mosmann, T. R., and Coffman, R. L., 1989, TH1 and TH2 cells: Different pattern of lymphokine secretion lead to different functional properties, *Annu. Rev. Immunol.* **7**:145–173.

Page, W. F., Norman, J. E., and Benenson, A. S., 1993, Long-term follow-up of army recruits immunized with Freund's incomplete adjuvanted vaccine, *Vaccine Res.* **2**:141–149.

Potter, C. W., Jennings, R., Phair, J. P., Clarke, A., and Stuart-Harris, C. H., 1977, Dose–response relationship after immunization of volunteers with a new, surface antigen-adsorbed influenza virus vaccine, *J. Infect. Dis.* **135**:423–431.

Raychaudhuri, S., Tonks, M., Carbone, F., Ryskamp, T., and Morrow, J.W., 1992, Induction of antigen-specific class I-restricted cytotoxic T cells by soluble protein *in vivo, Proc. Natl. Acad. Sci. USA* **89**:8308–8312.

Rock, K. L., Fleischacker, C., and Gamble, S., 1993, Peptide-priming of cytolytic T cell immunity in vivo using β_2-microglobulin as an adjuvant, *J. Immunol.* **150**:1244–1252.

Sanchez-Pescador, L., Burke, R. L., Ott, G., and Van Nest, G., 1988, The effect of adjuvants on the efficacy of a recombinant herpes simplex virus glycoprotein vaccine, *J. Immunol.* **141**:1720–1727.

Schirmbeck, R., Melber, K., Kuhrober, A., Janowicz, Z. A., and Reimann, J., 1994, Immunization with soluble hepatitis B virus specific surface protein elicits murine H-2 class-I restricted cytotoxic T lymphocyte responses in vivo, *J. Immunol.* **152**:1110–1119.

Scott, P., 1991, IFN-gamma modulates the early development of Th1 and Th2 responses in a murine model of cutaneous leishmaniasis, *J. Immunol.* **147**:3149–3155.

Scott, P., Pearce, E., Cheever, A. W., Coffman, R. L., and Sher, A., 1989, Role of cytokines and CD4⁺ T-cell subsets in the regulation of parasite immunity and disease, *Immunol. Rev.* **112**:161–182.

Sempertegui, F., Estrella, B., Moscoso, J., Piedrahita, L., Hernandez, D., Gaybor, J., Naranjo, P., Mancero, O., Arias, S., Bernal, R., Cordova, M. E., Suarez, J., and Zicker, F., 1994, Safety, immunogenicity and protective effect of SPf66 malaria synthetic vaccine against *Plasmodium falciparum* infection in a randomized double-blind placebo-controlled field trial in an endemic area of Ecuador, *Vaccine* **12**:337–342.

Skea, D. L., and Barber, B. H., 1993, Adhesion-mediated enhancement of the adjuvant activity of alum, *Vaccine* **11**:1018–1026.

Takayama, K., Olsen, M., Datta, P., and Hunter, R. L., 1991, Adjuvant activity of non-ionic block copolymers. V. Modulation of antibody isotype by lipopolysaccharides, lipid A and precursors, *Vaccine* **9**:257–265.

ten Hagen, T. L. M., Sulzer, A. J., Kidd, M. R., Lal, A. A., and Hunter, R. L., 1993, Role of adjuvants in the modulation of antibody isotype, specificity, and induction of protection by whole blood-stage *Plasmodium yoelii* vaccines, *J. Immunol.* **151**:7077–7085.

Teusher, T., Armstrong-Schellenberg, J. R. M., Bastos de Azvedo, I., Hurt, N., Smith, T., Hayes, R., Masanja, H., Silva, Y., Lopez, M. C., Kitua, A., Kilama, W., Tanner, M., and Alonzo, P. L., 1994, SPf66, a chemically synthesized subunit malaria vaccine, is safe and immunogenic in Tanzanians exposed to intense malaria transmission, *Vaccine* **12**:328–336.

Townsend, A., and Bodmer, H., 1989, Antigen recognition by class I-restricted T lymphocytes, *Annu. Rev. Immunol.* **7**:601–624.

Van Dam, G J., Verheul, A. F. M., Zigterman, G. J. W. J., De Reuver, M. J., and Snippe, H., 1989, Nonionic block polymer surfactants enhance the avidity of antibodies in polyclonal antisera against *Streptococcus pneumoniae* type 2 in normal and Xid mice, *J. Immunol.* **143**:3049–3053.

Van de Wijgert, J. H. H. M., Verheul, A. F. M., Snippe, H., Check, I. J., and Hunter, R. L., 1991, Immunogenicity of Streptococcus pneumoniae type 14 capsular polysaccharide: Influence of carriers and adjuvants on isotype distribution, *Infect. Immun.* **59**:2750–2757.

Weissman, J. Y., Tsuchiyose, M. M., Tong, M. J., Co, R., Chin, K., and Ettenger, R. B., 1988, Lack of response to recombinant hepatitis B vaccine in nonresponders to the plasma vaccine, *J. Am. Med. Assoc.* **260**:1734–1738.

Wintsch, J., Chaignat, C.-L., Braun, D.G., Jeannet, M., Stadler, H., and Abrignanai, S., 1991, Safety and immunogenicity of a genetically engineered human immunodeficiency virus vaccine, *J. Infect. Dis.* **163**:219–225.

Zigterman, G. J. W. J., Snippe, H., Jansze, M., and Willers, J. M. N., 1987, Adjuvant effects of nonionic block polymer surfactants on liposome-induced humoral immune response, *J. Immunol.* **138**:220–225.

Zigterman, G. J. W. J., Snippe, H., Jansze, M., Ernste, E. B. H. W., De Reuver, M. J., and Willers, J. M. N., 1988, Nonionic block polymer surfactants enhance immunogenicity of pneumococcal hexasaccharide-conjugate vaccines, *Infect. Immun.* **56**:1391–1393.

Chapter 12

Development of an Emulsion-Based Muramyl Dipeptide Adjuvant Formulation for Vaccines

Deborah M. Lidgate and Noelene E. Byars

1. INTRODUCTION

This chapter contains a summary of the development of a very effective adjuvant that contains a muramyl dipeptide (MDP) analogue (threonyl-MDP, temurtide) in an oil-in-water emulsion vehicle. The oil-in-water emulsion system contains squalane, Pluronic® L121, and polysorbate 80 in an isotonic, pH 7.4, phosphate-buffered saline solution. This adjuvant elicits both cell-mediated and humoral immune responses. While threonyl-MDP serves to increase antibody production and cell-mediated responses, the emulsion vehicle enhances immunogenicity by facilitating presentation of antigens to responding lymphocytes. Because threonyl-MDP does not exhibit toxicity usually associated with alanyl-MDP (pyrogenicity, uveitis, adjuvant-induced arthritis), no safety concerns are anticipated at therapeutic doses. In several animal species, this vehicle proved safe and efficacious, having been used successfully with a variety of antigens.

2. COMPOUND SELECTION

After the original muramyl dipeptide (*N*-acetyl muramyl-L-alanyl-D-isoglutamine; alanyl-MDP) was described (Ellouz *et al.*, 1974), chemists at Syntex synthesized over 120 MDP analogues. These compounds were screened for enhancement of antibody synthesis and cell-mediated immunity using an emulsion of incomplete Freund's adjuvant (IFA) as a vehicle for the MDP derivative. Guinea pigs were typically immunized with arsanilic tyrosine, bovine serum albumin, and a MDP analogue at 0 and 4 weeks, bled at 4 and 6

Deborah M. Lidgate and Noelene E. Byars • Syntex Research, Palo Alto, California 94304.

Vaccine Design: The Subunit and Adjuvant Approach, edited by Michael F. Powell and Mark J. Newman. Plenum Press, New York, 1995.

weeks for antibody determination, and skin tested at 2 weeks (arsanilic tyrosine) and 6 weeks (bovine serum albumin) for delayed hypersensitivity. Compounds that showed activity greater than alanyl-MDP were then further assayed in dose–response experiments, and for nonspecific immunity, and toxicity (e.g., pyrogenicity, induction of adjuvant arthritis, or uveitis) (Waters *et al.*, 1986). We selected *N*-acetyl muramyl-L-threonyl-D-iso-glutamine (threonyl-MDP, temurtide) from a group of approximately 20 active compounds because of its superior adjuvant activity compared to alanyl-MDP, and its lack of side effects. Threonyl-MDP is not pyrogenic at doses needed for adjuvant activity, is not uveogenic (Waters *et al.*, 1986), does not induce adjuvant arthritis (unpublished data), and is selective in the type of macrophage activation it induces (Fraser-Smith *et al.*, 1982). Threonyl-MDP is readily soluble in aqueous solutions, unlike some of the other analogues with good adjuvant activity, e.g., *N*-acetyl-4, 6-di-*O*-octanoyl-D-muramyl-L-alanyl-D-isoglutamine.

While our initial screening was done using IFA, it was obvious that an alternate vehicle would need to be developed for use in either human or veterinary vaccines. Both mineral oil and Arlacel® A (mannide monooleate, a nonionic surfactant with an HLB of 4.3) used in IFA had been shown to be carcinogenic in mice (Potter and Boyce, 1962; Murray *et al.*, 1972) and produce granulomas at injection sites (Allison and Byars, 1986). A number of metabolizable oils (e.g., coconut, olive, and peanut oil, lanolin) were screened as replace-ments for mineral oil; likewise, various surfactants were screened as alternatives to Arlacel® A. We developed an emulsion containing squalane and a pluronic polyol (Allison and Byars, 1992). Certain pluronic polyols possess adjuvant activity through their ability to bind protein antigen to oil droplets of emulsion vehicle (Hunter *et al.*, 1981, 1991; Hunter and Bennett, 1984, 1986). Emulsions prepared with either squalene or squalane were equally efficacious; squalane was chosen since it is more chemically stable because of the absence of the double bonds. The final emulsion (see Table I) contained Pluronic® L121, squalane, and polysorbate 80 in phosphate-buffered saline [Syntex adjuvant formulation (SAF)]. This vehicle proved to be a stable, nontoxic formulation, suitable for both human and veterinary vaccines. When serum CPK levels were assayed following intramuscular

Table I
The Syntex Adjuvant Formulation[a]

Excipient	% w/v
Emulsifiers	
Pluronic® L121	2.5
Polysorbate 80, USP	0.2
Oil Phase	
Squalane, NF	5.0
Aqueous Phase	
Sodium chloride, USP	0.736
Potassium chloride, USP	0.0184
Potassium phosphate monobasic, NF	0.0184
Sodium phosphate dibasic, anhydrous, USP	0.11
Water for injection, USP q.s.	100.0

[a]The above concentrations represent the final concentrations of each excipient after dilution with antigen and threonyl-MDP solution(s).

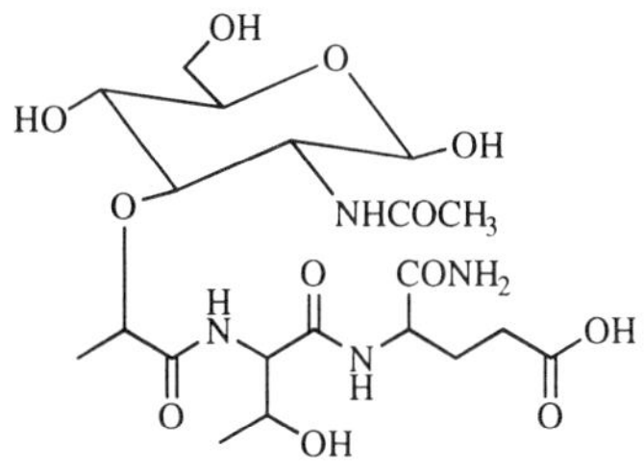

Figure 1. Threonyl-MDP.

injection of SAF with threonyl-MDP, only low levels were found, indicating that the formulation causes very little muscle irritation at the injection site (Lidgate *et al.*, 1989a).

3. CHEMISTRY OF THREONYL-MDP

Threonyl-MDP is comprised of a muramyl sugar derivative and two nonaromatic amino acids linked by amide bonds. It has a molecular weight of 522.52, and the structure is provided in Fig. 1. Threonyl-MDP is a white amorphous powder (Chan and Becker, 1988), containing approximately 3% surface moisture; the compound is highly hygroscopic, adsorbing 71% moisture at 93% relative humidity. Threonyl-MDP is extremely stable in light and requires no light protection.

The solubility of threonyl-MDP is greater than 600 mg/mL in aqueous solution over a wide pH range, and approximately 500 mg/mL in methanol, dimethylacetamide, and dimethylsulfoxide. The solubility in nonpolar solvents, such as chloroform, methylene chloride, and hexane, is less than 3 μg/mL. The apparent partition coefficient for threonyl-MDP in octanol/water was found to be 0.0044; and the methylene chloride/water partition coefficient was 0.00017.

The degradation rate of threonyl-MDP in aqueous solution was determined as a function of pH and temperature. The pH-logarithmic rate plot showed a symmetrical U-shaped profile with a minimum at pH 4.5 (the pH of maximum stability). Calculated activation energies predict a 2-year shelf life of threonyl-MDP when stored in a pH 4.5 aqueous solution at 25°C (Powell *et al.*, 1988). At physiological pH, the predicted shelf life of threonyl-MDP in aqueous solution at room temperature is less than 40 days; at 5°C, a shelf life of 2 years may be possible.

4. EMULSION FORMULATION CONSIDERATIONS

Designing an MDP vaccine adjuvant involves optimizing and understanding the chemistry of the MDP analogues and the physical aspects of the emulsion vehicle. The dilution vehicle for threonyl-MDP is composed of a finely dispersed metabolizable oil in an aqueous continuous phase. When combining two immiscible liquids, strong intermolecular forces promote minimized interfacial contact and area. To form an emulsion, the interfacial tension (or the force required to break the surface between these two phases) needs to be reduced. Emulsions form spontaneously when the interfacial tension is zero, producing a microemulsion (Prince, 1967, 1969). As interfacial tension decreases, interfacial contact, or area, between the two phases increases. Increased interfacial area leads to increased free energy of the system and results in thermodynamic instability. This instability can be attenuated by the choice and amount of emulsifier, the dispersed droplet particle size, the density difference between the internal and external phases, the viscosity of the external phase, and the manufacturing technique.

Typically, emulsion physical instability is evident by either creaming (or sedimenting, depending on density differences) and/or coalescence. Creaming occurs when the two phases of the emulsion have differing specific gravities and/or when the dispersed particles are initially large (and are not responsive to Brownian movement). If coalescence does not occur simultaneously, the emulsion can be redispersed with gentle mixing. Creaming can be minimized by adjusting the specific gravity of one or both phases, reducing the particle size, changing the particle charge, and/or increasing the viscosity of the continuous phase.

Coalescence occurs when the interfacial film ruptures between two particles of the internal phase. Larger particles have a greater tendency to coalesce. Often, coalescence is irreversible (unless an emulsifier is chosen to facilitate reemulsification on shaking). Coalescence can be minimized by reducing the tendency of emulsion creaming, increasing the charge on the particles, and increasing the viscosity of the continuous phase.

Through their action at the oil–water interface, emulsifiers promote stabilization of dispersed droplets by reducing interfacial free energy and creating physical or electrostatic barriers to droplet coalescence (Boyd et al., 1972). Nonionic emulsifiers orient at the interface and produce relatively bulky structures, which lead to steric avoidance of the dispersed droplets. Anionic/cationic emulsifiers induce formation of an electrical double layer by attracting counterions; the double layer repulsive forces cause droplets to repel one another when they approach.

Emulsifiers are typically categorized with an HLB number, or the hydrophile–lipophile balance (HLB) value. This value expresses the relative simultaneous attraction for water and oil. The HLB is determined by chemical composition and extent of ionization. The emulsifier HLB determines the type of emulsion formed: a low HLB promotes water-in-oil (w/o) emulsions, a high HLB promotes oil-in-water (o/w) emulsions.

5. SAF FORMULATION

Squalane (Robane®, 2,6,10,15,19,23-hexamethyltetracosane) is a free-flowing oil with a molecular weight of 422.80 and a density of approximately 0.811. Squalane is chemically saturated and is obtained by complete hydrogenation of squalene, found in shark liver oil. Squalane is a metabolizable oil and has been used in pharmaceuticals and cosmetics as a skin lubricant, as an ingredient in suppositories, and as a vehicle for lipophilic drugs. The squalane used in the SAF formulation conforms with National Formulary (NF) guidelines.

Pluronic® L121 is a block copolymer of ethylene oxide and propylene oxide. This particular nonionic surfactant (also referred to as poloxamer 401) contains 10% by weight of the hydrophilic ethylene oxide group. The average molecular weight for Pluronic® L121 is 4400; it is a liquid at room temperature and has an HLB close to 1.0. This low HLB value puts it in a class of water-insoluble surfactants known as spreading agents. Spreading agents do not stabilize emulsions and have no cleansing or detergent activity. Spreading agents adhere preferentially to hydrophobic surfaces in contact with aqueous media, and because of their distinct hydrophilic and hydrophobic portions, they promote interaction with (antigen) macromolecules at the oil–water interface of the emulsion. Researchers suggest that this characteristic of Pluronic® L121 contributes to the adjuvant activity by increasing the concentration of antigen presented to cells of the immune system (Hunter *et al.*, 1981; Woodard and Jasman, 1985).

Polysorbate 80 (Tween® 80) is an extensively used surfactant in foods, cosmetics, and pharmaceuticals (including parenteral formulations). The polysorbate 80 used in the SAF formulation conforms with United States Pharmacopeia (USP) guidelines. Polysorbate 80 has an HLB in the range of 12–16; it therefore is very soluble in aqueous media. Polysorbate 80 serves as an emulsifier in the formulation and helps stabilize the emulsion over longer-term storage.

The aqueous continuous phase is composed of isotonic phosphate-buffered saline (PBS) with a final formulation pH of 7.4. Based on the partition properties of threonyl-MDP, virtually all of the MDP remains in this aqueous phase of the emulsion.

6. SAF MANUFACTURING

Initial biological testing was performed with emulsions that were prepared by blending all excipients using a laboratory vortex. Although producing a biologically efficacious emulsion, the product was physically unstable, and the manufacturing method was clearly not suitable for large-scale manufacture. In order to reproducibly manufacture an acceptable product, the manufacturing equipment must be considered a critical counterpart to the formulation. Therefore, selection of specific manufacturing equipment should complement the formulation to enhance product quality. Emulsion manufacturing equipment must supply appropriate shear force in order to properly disperse the emulsion's internal phase to a sufficiently small particle size, in order to avoid coalescence and potential deterioration of the physical nature of the emulsion. Manufacturing equipment will facilitate better orientation of the emulsifier at the oil–water interface, thus providing a barrier to coalescence. The equipment will also provide a more uniform droplet size.

Factors affecting the formation of emulsions and dispersions are derived from the formulation (surface/interfacial tension; electrostatic attraction/repulsion; internal/external phase density differences) and from mechanical forces provided by the type(s) of mixing equipment available (shear, impact, cavitation). Typical mixing equipment includes a propeller mixer, a turbine rotor and stator, a colloid mill, a homogenizer, a sonicator. All of these mixers provide one or more of the mechanical forces mentioned above. Two mixers evaluated during formulation development provided all three forces; these mixers were (1) a high-pressure homogenizer (such as a Gaulin homogenizer) and (2) a Microfluidizer. After extensive evaluation of the various equipment options available for emulsion manufacture, the Microfluidizer was selected for its ability to reproducibly provide an elegant, physically stable emulsion with consistent particle size (Lidgate *et al.*, 1989a, b).

Emulsion formation using a Microfluidizer occurs as two fluidized streams interact at very high velocities within an interaction chamber. The Microfluidizer is air or nitrogen

Table II
Droplet Size of SAF-m[a]

No. of cycles through microfluidizer[b]	Mean droplet size (nm)[c]	Droplet size range (nm)
1	187	115–1000
2	157	81–405
4	164	118–315
5	164	90–308
7	165	81–270

[a]SAF-m is processed without antigen. For this study, 2 L of emulsion was manufactured.

[b]For this study, SAF-m was manufactured with a Microfluidizer M110Y having an internal operating pressure of 16,000–17,000 psi.

[c]Aliquots of SAF-m were diluted (as needed) with the emulsion's aqueous phase; particle size was then determined by laser photon correlation spectroscopy (using a Nicomp model 200 laser particle sizer and a Nicomp model TC-100 computing autocorrelator).

driven and can operate at internal pressures in excess of 20,000 psi with a throughput of 300–500 mL/min. The emulsion can be continuously recycled through a closed loop system.

With the appropriate mixing conditions, the SAF vehicle is a homogeneous, elegant emulsion, exhibiting little or no creaming. These characteristics coincide with the observation that SAF emulsion (designated SAF-m after being processed by the Microfluidizer) consists entirely of submicron droplets (see Table II).

Sterile manufacture of SAF emulsion can be achieved through either aseptic processing (Avallone, 1985) of the components and equipment or sterile filtration of the final emulsion (Lidgate *et al.*, 1992). Either technique produces a sterile emulsion, free of endotoxin. Sterile filtration of the SAF-m emulsion can be achieved when operating the Microfluidizer at higher internal pressures (20,000 psi, this feature is model-dependent). The higher-pressure equipment produces emulsions with a reduced amount of the larger droplets. Particle size analysis showed that the population of larger particles was reduced with each pass through the Microfluidizer. These larger particles, although few in number, were very likely responsible for plugging a 0.22-μm filter membrane, thus preventing sterile filtration. As these larger particles are reduced in size, sterile filtration became possible (Lidgate *et al.*, 1992). The ability to sterile filter SAF-m allows for a less cumbersome manufacturing process and provides a preferred method of ensuring sterility of the final product.

Most of our biological testing was done using a twofold concentrated emulsion, which was mixed gently with an equal volume of a twofold concentrated antigen and threonyl-MDP solution to prepare the vaccine used for immunization. For large-scale manufacturing, two presentations were considered: (1) a two-vial system as described above or (2) a three-vial system using threefold concentrations of emulsion, threonyl-MDP, and antigen. Expected storage conditions and antigen stability at the pH optimal for threonyl-MDP would be factors to consider in making a final choice of system for vaccine preparation.

7. FINAL PRODUCT

SAF-m emulsion maintains excellent physical stability when stored at or below 30°C. Over time, a small degree of creaming may occur. With minimal shaking, the emulsion appears homogeneous. After 6 years at ambient room temperature, SAF-m remains physically stable. While elevated temperatures were detrimental to the physical stability of the emulsion, very cold (freezing, −20°C) temperatures were found to be acceptable (no emulsion cracking or phase separation occurred on thawing).

The smaller particle size produced by the Microfluidizer contributes to greater physical stability to the emulsion. Aliquots of the emulsion were extensively centrifuged and the amount of creaming was determined (see Table III). An emulsion sample cycled ten times through the manufacturing equipment proved to be the most robust.

A number of variations on the original SAF formulations were tested. For example, we replaced the Pluronic® L121 with Tetronic® 1501 (a tetrafunctional block copolymer, with an HLB in the range of 1–7). We also evaluated reducing the amount of Pluronic® L121 and compared emulsion mixing methods (vortex mixing and Greerco Homogenizer mixing). Tables IV and V show some of the data obtained in these comparative studies. While all emulsion mixing methods produced biologically active emulsions, most of the other emulsions were not physically stable on long-term storage. Storage temperatures of −20 and 5°C (for 5 months) had no effect on physical stability or efficacy of the Microfluidizer-processed emulsion (see Table V). The ability to freeze a vaccine made with SAF-m and threonyl-MDP may be of practical advantage in storing vaccines.

Experiments were also done using synthetic squalane (Robane® SXL) or synthetic water-soluble squalane (Robane® SWS; 10,15-bis-[hydroxypolyoxyethylene]-2,6,10,15, 19,23-hexamethyltetracosane) to prepare the SAF-m emulsion. Neither of these forms of squalane is currently commercially available. Synthetic squalane was at least 99% pure and exhibited the same physical characteristics as its naturally derived counterpart. Synthetic water-soluble squalane was a white, waxy solid. Table VI shows a comparison of these emulsions using the hemagglutinin of influenza B virus (Yamagata strain) to immunize mice. The emulsions made with synthetic and natural squalanes induced essentially the same antibody response, while the emulsion with water-soluble squalane was only somewhat less efficacious.

Table III
Emulsion Creaming as a Function of Cycles through a Microfluidizer[a] and Time of Centrifugation[b]

Cycles through microfluidizer	% emulsion creaming (v/v) after time at centrifugation		
	20 min	40 min	60 min
1	10	15	20
4	2	4	8
10	0	2	3

[a]One liter of SAF-m was prepared with a Microfluidizer M110T having an internal operating pressure of 8000–10,000 psi.
[b]A tabletop centrifuge was used at approximately $4500 \times g$.

Table IV

Antibody Titers and Cell Mediated Responses of Guinea Pigs[a] Vaccinated with Ovalbumin in SAF Prepared by Different Methods

Preparation	Antibody levels, week 6		Skin tests, week 6	
	Titer ± SE[d]	Dilution[e]	Diam. ± SE (mm)	Inf. score[f]
Vortexed[b]	7.0 ± 0.3	1280	18.1 ± 0.3	1.7
Microfluidizer processed	6.9 ± 0.3	1178	19.4 ± 1.1	1.7
Tetronic® 1501, Microfluidizer processed[c]	7.1 ± 0.1	1410	16.8 ± 0.6	1.5
1.25% Pluronic® L121	6.5 ± 0.2	905	18.1 ± 0.7	1.8
Greerco Homogenizer processed	6.6 ± 0.3	990	17.3 ± 0.9	1.8

[a]Groups of 7 or 8 guinea pigs.

[b]Original mixing method.

[c]Tetronic® 1501 (2.5%) replaced the Pluronic® L121.

[d]Titer determined by the passive hemagglutination method, using twofold dilutions. Titer is expressed as $\log_2$ or serum dilution at the end point.

[e]Actual serum dilution at the end point.

[f]Infiltration score on a scale of 1 = no infiltration to 4 = maximum infiltration.

Table V

Comparisons of Different Storage Methods, and Different Preparations of SAF Emulsions, Used to Vaccinate Guinea Pigs[a] with Ovalbumin

	Preparation	Antibody levels (6 weeks)		Skin tests (6 weeks) Diameter ± SE (mm)
		Titer ± SE	Dilution[d]	
Experiment 1[b]	Vortexed	7.8 ± 0.2	2,153	18.4 ± 1.3
	Vortexed, then autoclaved	7.8 ± 0.2	2,153	15.8 ± 0.8
	Tetronic, vortexed[c]	8.8 ± 0.3	4,305	17.4 ± 1.0
Experiment 2[e]	Microfluidizer processed	9.0 ± 0.3	18,837	14.3 ± 0.7
	Microfluidizer processed, then frozen	8.9 ± 0.4	17,830	13.3 ± 2.3
	Microfluidizer processed, 4°C storage for 5 months	9.1 ± 0.4	21,729	13.3 ± 0.9

[a]Groups of 7 or 8 guinea pigs.

[b]Antibody titers determined by the passive hemagglutination method, using twofold dilutions. Titer is expressed as $\log_2$ or serum dilution at the end point.

[c]Tetronic® 1501 (2.5%) instead of Pluronic® L121.

[d]Actual serum dilution at end point.

[e]Antibody titers determined by the ELISA technique, using a threefold serum dilution. Titer is expressed as $\log_3$ of the serum dilution giving an optical density reading of 0.5 absorbance unit.

Table VI

Antibody Titers[a] of Mice[b] Immunized with Influenza B Hemagglutinin
in SAF-m Comparing Variants of Squalane

Type of squalane in SAF	Antibody levels		
	Week 3[c]	Week 5[c]	Week 9[d]
Squalane, NF	8.4	9.4	8.9 ± 0.7
Synthetic squalane	8.7	9.5	8.6 ± 0.9
Water-soluble squalane[e]	7.8	8.4	8.3 ± 0.6

[a]ELISA titer is expressed as $\log_3$ of the serum dilution giving an optical density reading of 0.5 absorbance unit.
[b]Mice were given a single injection of 1 μg of influenza B hemagglutinin in an SAF-m emulsion.
[c]Values were determined from pooled sera of the groups of immunized mice. Hence, no standard error is reported.
[d]Groups of 7, 8, and 8 mice, respectively.
[e]Robane® SWS (10,15-bis-[hydroxypolyoxyethylene]-2,6,10,15,19,23-hexamethyltetracosane).

8. MECHANISM OF ACTION

Rather than a water-in-oil emulsion like Freund's adjuvant, SAF forms an oil-in-water emulsion. We suggest that the oil droplets have Pluronic® L121 on the surface, and that the antigen is retained on the surface of the droplets, in part because of the amphipathic nature of the Pluronic® L121 and the antigens, and in part because of hydrogen bonding to the polyoxyethylene (Allison and Byars, 1990). Because the antigen is added to the preformed SAF emulsion, it is not subject to the mixing and shearing forces encountered during the emulsification process. The antigen can therefore be expected to retain its native structure. Antibodies, elicited following immunization with SAF, primarily recognize native determinants (Kenney et al., 1989). The gentle mixing of antigen–MDP solution with the preformed SAF-m emulsion differs from the method needed to make a Freund's-type emulsion, where the antigen is added to the oil phase prior to the emulsification process. As a result of using Freund's emulsion, high titers of antibodies recognizing internal determinants (exposed by antigen denaturation) are found (Kenney et al., 1989). We propose that the antigen-coated particles are targeted to follicular dendritic cells. This, in part, is a consequence of activation of complement components, present in tissue fluids, which are bound by the particles. This leads to the presence of activated C3b on the surface of the particles which then bind to the C3b receptors as the follicular dendritic cells. The dendritic cells endocytose the antigen(s), then reexpress antigenic determinants on the cell surface in association with major histocompatibility complex molecules for presentation to lymphocytes with the appropriate antigen receptors.

9. STUDIES UTILIZING SAF EMULSION WITH THREONYL-MDP

We tested SAF emulsion with a number of antigens in a variety of species. The response of mice to influenza hemagglutinins was significantly enhanced by use of the SAF emulsion with threonyl-MDP (Byars et al., 1990). Especially notable was the excellent response of aged mice to influenza hemagglutinins. The response to the presently available influenza vaccines of people over 65 years, who are especially vulnerable to morbidity and mortality related to influenza, is unsatisfactory (Arden *et al.*, 1986). Thus, a vaccine that enhances the response of older people to immunization would be valuable. We have also shown increased antibody response to hepatitis B vaccine (Byars *et al.*, 1991a) in guinea pigs and mice, including a genetic nonresponder strain of mice. Guinea pigs immunized with gD-2t of herpes simplex type 2 virus in SAF had excellent anti-gD-2t antibody titers, as well as enhanced cell-mediated response to the gD-2t as shown in vitro by the blastogenic response to gD-2t. More importantly, the guinea pigs vaccinated with gD-2t in SAF were better protected than controls against challenge with live virus (Byars *et al.*, 1994). Experiments with tumor antigens suggest that vaccines made using SAF-m could be useful therapeutic agents for melanoma (Chattopadhyay *et al.*, 1991) and B lymphoma (Campbell *et al.*, 1990). Other antigens for which SAF has proved efficacious include EBV in cotton top tamarins (Morgan *et al.*, 1989), SIV in monkeys (Murphy-Corb *et al.*, 1989), gp120 of HIV-1 in guinea pigs and monkeys (Byars *et al.*, 1991b), and HIV antigens in chimpanzees (Girard *et al.*, 1991).

10. CONCLUSION

Careful and rational selection of a MDP analogue, combined with an understanding of the functionality of each vehicle excipient, contributed to the development of an adjuvant that is both safe and effective. Understanding the chemistry of threonyl-MDP and the physical factors involved in emulsion preparation, facilitates reproducible manufacture of a commercially stable formulation. These elements of product development will enable the progress of vaccine development for both animal and human use.

REFERENCES

Allison, A. C., and Byars, N. E., 1986, An adjuvant formulation that selectively elicits the formation of antibodies of protective isotype and of cell-mediated immunity, *J. Immunol. Methods* **95**:157–168.

Allison, A. C., and Byars, N. E., 1990, Adjuvant formulations and their mode of action, *Semin. Immunol.* **2**:369–374.

Allison, A. C., and Byars, N. E., 1992, Syntex Adjuvant Formulation, *Res. Immunol.* **143**:519–525.

Arden, N. H., Patriarca, P. A., and Kendal, A. P., 1986, Experiences in the use and efficacy of inactivated influenza vaccine in nursing homes, in: *Options for Control of Influenza* (A. P. Kendal and P. A. Patriarca, eds.), Liss, New York, pp. 155–168.

Avallone, H. L., 1985, Control aspects of aseptically produced products, *J. Parenteral Sci. Technol.* **39**:75–79.

Boyd, J., Parkinson, C., and Sherman, P., 1972, Factors affecting emulsion stability, and the HLB concept, *J. Colloid Interface Sci.* **41**:359–370.

Byars, N. E., Allison, A. C., Harmon, M. W., and Kendal, A. P., 1990, Enhancement of antibody responses to influenza B virus hemagglutinin by use of a new adjuvant formulation, *Vaccine* **8**:49–56.

Byars, N. E., Nakano, G., Welch, M., Lehman, D., and Allison, A. C., 1991a, Improvement of hepatitis B vaccine by the use of a new adjuvant, *Vaccine* **9**:309–318.

Byars, N. E., Nakano, G., Welch M., and Allison, A. C., 1991b, Use of Syntex adjuvant formulation to enhance immune responses to viral antigens, in: *Vaccines* (G. Gregoriadis, A. C. Allison, and G. Poste, eds.), Plenum Press, New York, pp. 33–42.

Byars, N. E., Fraser-Smith, E. B., Pecyk, R. A., Welch, M., Nakano, G., Burke, R. L., Hayward, A. R., and Allison, A. C., 1994, Vaccinating guinea pigs with recombinant glycoprotein D of herpes simplex virus in an efficacious adjuvant formulation elicits protection against vaginal infection, *Vaccine* **12**:200–209.

Campbell, M. J., Esserman, L., Byars, N. E., Allison, A. C., and Levy, R., 1990, Idiotype vaccination against murine B cell lymphoma. Humoral and cellular requirements for the full expression of antitumor immunity, *J. Immunol.* **145**:1029–1036.

Chan, T. W., and Becker, A., 1988, Formulation of vaccine adjuvant muramyldipeptides (MDP). 1. Characterization of amorphous and crystalline forms of a muramyldipeptide analogue, *Pharm. Res.* **5**:523–527.

Chattopadhyay, P., Kaveri, S.-V., Byars, N. E., Starkey, J., Ferrone, S., and Raychauduri, S., 1991, Human high molecular weight melanoma associated antigen mimicry by an anti-idiotypic antibody: Characterization of the immunogenicity and the immune response to the mouse monoclonal antibody I Mel-1, *Cancer Res.* **51**:6045–6051.

Ellouz, F., Adams, A., Ciorbaru, R., and Lederer, E., 1974, Minimal structural requirements for adjuvant activity of bacterial peptidoglycan derivatives, *Biochem. Biophys. Res. Commun.* **59**:1317–1325.

Fraser-Smith, E. B., Waters, R. V., and Matthews, T. R., 1982, Correlation between in vivo anti-pseudomonas and anti-candida activities and clearance of carbon by the reticuloendothelial system for various muramyl dipeptide analogues, using normal and immunosuppressed mice, *Infect. Immun.* **35**:105–110.

Girard, M., Kieny, M.-P., Pinter, A., Barre-Sinoussi, F., Nara, P., Kolbe, H., Kusumi, K., Chaput, A., Reinhardt, T., Muchmore, E., Ronco, J., Kaczorek, M., Gomard, E., Gluckman, J.-C., and Fultz, P. N., 1991, Immunization of chimpanzees confers protection against challenge with human immunodeficiency virus, *Proc. Natl. Acad. Sci. USA* **88**:542–546.

Hunter, R. L., and Bennett, B., 1984, The adjuvant activity of nonionic block polymer surfactants. II. Antibody formation and inflammation related to the structure of triblock and octablock copolymers, *J. Immunol.* **133**:3167–3175.

Hunter, R. L., and Bennett, B., 1986, The adjuvant activity of nonionic block polymer surfactants. III. Characterization of selected biologically active surfaces, *Scand. J. Immunol.* **23**:287–300.

Hunter, R., Strickland, F., and Kedzy, F., 1981, The adjuvant activity of nonionic block polymer surfactants. 1. Role of hydrophile–lipophile balance, *J. Immunol.* **127**:1244–1250.

Hunter, R., Olsen, M., and Buynitzky, S., 1991, Adjuvant activity of nonionic block copolymers. IV. Effect of molecular weight and formulation on titer and isotype of antibody, *Vaccine* **9**:250–256.

Kenney, J. S., Hughes, B. W., Masada, M. P., and Allison, A. C., 1989, Influence of adjuvants on the quantity, affinity, isotype, and epitope specificity of murine antibodies, *J. Immunol. Methods* **121**:157–166.

Lidgate, D. M., Fu, R. C., Byars, N. E., Foster, L. C., and Fleitman, J. S., 1989a, Formulation of vaccine adjuvant muramyldipeptides. III. Processing optimization, characterization, and bioactivity of an emulsion vehicle, *Pharm Res.* **6**:748–752.

Lidgate, D. M., Fu, R. C., and Fleitman, J. S., 1989b, Using a Microfluidizer to manufacture parenteral emulsions, *Biopharm* **2**:28 33.

Lidgate, D. M., Trattner, T., Shultz, R. M., and Maskiewicz, R., 1992, Sterile filtration of a parenteral emulsion, *Pharm. Res.* **9**:860–863.

Morgan, A. J., Allison, A. C., Finerty, S., Scullion, F. T., Byars, N. E., and Epstein, M. A., 1989, Validation of a first generation Epstein–Barr virus vaccine preparation suitable for human use, *J. Med. Virol.* **24**:74–78.

Murphy-Corb, M., Martin, L. N., Davison-Fairburn, B., Montclaro, R. C., Miller, M., West, M., Ohkawa, S., Baskin, G. B., Zhang, J.-Y., Allison, A. C., and Eppstein, D. A., 1989, A formalin-inactivated whole SIV vaccine confers protection in macaques, *Science* **246**:1293–1297.

Murray, R., Cohen, P., and Hardegree, M. C., 1972, Mineral oil adjuvants: Biological and chemical studies, *Ann. Allergy* **30**:146–151.

Potter, M., and Boyce, C. R., 1962, Induction of plasma cell neoplasms in strain BALB/c mice with mineral oil and mineral oil adjuvants, *Nature* **193**:1086–1087.

Powell, M. F., Foster, L. C., Becker, A. R., and Lee, W., 1988, Formulation of vaccine adjuvant muramyldipeptides (MDP). 2. The thermal reactivity and pH of maximum stability of MDP compounds in aqueous solution, *Pharm. Res.* **5**:528–532.

Prince, L., 1967, A theory of aqueous emulsions. I. Negative interfacial tension at the oil/water interface, *J. Colloid Interface Sci.* **23**:165–173.

Prince, L., 1969, A theory of aqueous emulsion. II. Mechanism of film curvature at the oil/water interface, *J. Colloid Interface Sci.* **29**:216–221.

Waters, R. V., Terrell, T. G., and Jones, G. H., 1986, Uveitis induction in the rabbit by muramyl dipeptides, *Infect. Immun.* **51**:816–825.

Woodard, L. F., and Jasman, R. L., 1985, Stable oil-in-water emulsions: Preparation and use as vaccine vehicles for lipophilic adjuvants, *Vaccine* **3**:137–144.

Chapter 13

Liposomal Presentation of Antigens for Human Vaccines

Reinhard Glück

1. INTRODUCTION

The increasing use of liposomes in biology and medicine has prompted a rigorous characterization of both classical multilamellar vesicle and novel liposome preparations. Drug delivery applications of liposomes or liposomes as immunological adjuvants have necessitated the production of large quantities of defined phospholipids of high purity, prompting a similar intensification of research. The growing interest in liposomes can be attributed to three major perspectives: (1) physicists and physical chemists take an interest in liposomes as a system in which forces between amphiphilic molecules can be studied; (2) biochemists, biophysicists, and scientists in related areas consider the liposome to be an appropriate model for biological membranes; (3) scientists in other disciplines including pharmaceutical and agricultural industries are interested in the potential use of liposomes as carriers (vehicles) for the application of drugs, vaccines, insecticides, fertilizers, and genetic materials. The growing interest of industries has promoted the production of specific instrumentation for the scaleup of liposome production.

Since no single technique can meet all of these needs, a large number of techniques have been developed, and this trend is likely to continue. This growing interest in the potential of liposomes has led many people with no expertise in "liposomology" to make use of liposomes as tools. However, to make appropriate use of liposomes, one has to recognize both their potentials and limitations, and it is necessary to be aware of various possible pitfalls. Adopting this approach will make it possible to select the most suitable liposomes in terms of size, structure, and composition for a specific use. This chapter presents the practical use of liposomes in vaccinology. It details the benefit of liposomes

Reinhard Glück • Department of Virology, Swiss Serum and Vaccine Institute Bern, CH-3001 Bern, Switzerland.

Vaccine Design: The Subunit and Adjuvant Approach, edited by Michael F. Powell and Mark J. Newman. Plenum Press, New York, 1995.

in the field of vaccinology from the industrial point of view as well as from a regulatory viewpoint.

2. HISTORY OF LIPOSOMES

The formation of artificial lipid vesicles by allowing phospholipids to swell in aqueous media was first described by Bangham *et al.* (1965). Comprised of concentric bilayers that alternate with aqueous compartments, these vesicles (liposomes) entrapped ions in the aqueous phase between the lipid bilayers and had permeability properties resembling those of biological membranes. They were initially used as models of lipid bilayers (Bangham, 1968) to study ion transport across cell membranes, and those early experiments set the stage for a series of studies in membrane biophysics (Bangham *et al.*, 1974). Since their introduction, the use of liposomes as a research tool has undergone an impressive evolution. Liposomes have become the preferred system for studying the reconstitution of membrane transport proteins and enzymes, the mode of action of ionophoric peptides and a variety of anesthetics and other drugs (Brotherus *et al.*, 1981). Thus, liposomes have played an essential role in developing our current understanding of the structure and function of biological membranes in areas such as membrane fusion (Duzzqunes and Papahadjopoulos, 1983; Lüscher-Mattli and Glück, 1990; Tsurudome *et al.*, 1992; Lüscher-Mattli *et al.*, 1993), antigen–antibody interactions (Honegger *et al.*, 1980; Hafeman *et al.*, 1980), the complement system (Müller-Eberhard, 1988), blood coagulation (Bangham, 1961; Papahadjopoulos *et al.*, 1962), and arteriosclerosis (Papahadjopoulos, 1974; Small and Shipley, 1974). During the early 1970s, liposome research went beyond basic membrane physics and into the area of therapeutic application, as a vector system for altering the tissue disposition of various macromolecules in vitro (Gregoriadis and Leathwood, 1971), and for introducing foreign macromolecules into cells in vitro (Papahadjopoulos *et al.*, 1974). With these two new developments, liposome research bridges three different fields: biophysics, cell biology, and medicine. Their potentials as "magic bullets" caught the imagination of many researchers but yielded little success. However, in recent years there has been a greater appreciation of the limitation of liposomes as a drug delivery and targeting system and a realization of the enormous difficulties of in vivo administration. The early unrealistic expectations produced disappointments, but an alert scientific interest in liposomes has survived. In the past 25 years, investigators have contributed more than 20,000 scientific articles on liposomes in fields as diverse as gene transfer and mutation, and more than 200 patents have been issued covering their formation, structure, manufacture, and use (Dean, 1993).

To date, the most successful examples of liposomal pharmaceutical products are those with doxorubicin (an antineoplastic drug) (Treat *et al.*, 1990; Wälti and Glück, 1993), amphotericin (an antifungal drug) (Lopez-Berestein, 1989; Davidson *et al.*, 1991), and vaccines [hepatitis A vaccine (Glück *et al.*, 1992a)]. Liposomal amphotericin (1992) and liposomal hepatitis A vaccine (1994) are the first formulations of liposomes to become licensed for clinical use.

3. LIPOSOMES AS ADJUVANTS

An adjuvant can be defined as any agent that increases an immune response to a specific antigen. This includes aluminum hydroxide (alum), killed mycobacteria in mineral oil (complete Freund's adjuvant), lipopolysaccharide, and many others. Of these mentioned, only alum is included in licensed products in the United States for use in humans, even though alum has some disadvantages. Concerted efforts are in progress to develop a safe and effective adjuvant. Many studies have now shown that liposomes can serve as effective adjuvants for inducing humoral and cellular immunity to a number of antigens (Gregoriadis, 1990; Thérien *et al.*, 1990; Garçon and Six, 1991; Glück, 1992b; Alving *et al.*, 1992; Buiting *et al.*, 1992). The toxicity of antigens can be reduced or eliminated by their inclusion in liposomes (Glück *et al.*, 1992b). Both hydrophobic and hydrophilic antigens can be reconstituted in liposomes and a longer duration of antigenic activity can be obtained. The adjuvancy of liposomes has now been shown for different types of immune responses including lymphocyte cytotoxicity, lymphoproliferation, bacterial cytotoxicity of macrophages, production of soluble mediators, and antibody production (Shahum and Thérien, 1988).

Perhaps the most interesting application of liposomes is the use as vehicles for vaccines since almost all liposomes home to reticular-endothelial cells. Macrophages, and in particular Kupffer cells, are major sites for antigen processing. As discussed elsewhere (see Chapter 14) there are many aspects of liposomes in immunology. Different parameters such as liposomal size, surface charge, liquid and lipid–peptide composition, and the position of antigens can influence the degree of the eventual immunological response. For example, liposomal adjuvanticity was enhanced by spiking liposomes with fusogenic peptides or with T-cell epitopes (Goodman-Snitkoff *et al.*, 1991; Glück *et al.*, 1992b). Furthermore, it has been observed that unilamellar liposomes generate a stronger response than do multilamellar liposomes (Shek and Heath, 1983) and that the antibody response is low or absent when liposomes are made of lipids with a high transition temperature (Gregoriadis *et al.*, 1987). Because of the large experience and enormous knowledge about liposomes as adjuvants and because of the general absence of toxicity, liposomes may be the first candidates to replace alum as the classical adjuvant.

4. APPROACHES WITH LIPOSOMAL VACCINES

Antigens can be associated with liposomes in two ways. The antigenic determinant is masked (encapsulated within the internal aqueous spaces of the liposomes) or exposed (attached to the outer surface or reconstituted within the lipid bilayer of the liposomes). Surface exposure of antigen on the liposomes can be achieved by different methods of covalent binding of the antigen to the phospholipids used for preparation of the liposomes, or by nonspecific adsorption of hydrophobic antigens to the liposome surface directly (Mengiardi, 1994).

The adjuvanticity of liposomes depends on the number of layers (Shek *et al.*, 1983), charge (Allison and Gregoriadis, 1974), composition (Heath *et al.*, 1976; Tyrrel *et al.*, 1976), and method of liposome preparation (Van Rooijen and van Nieuwmegen, 1983a; Thérien *et al.*, 1990). In addition, both humoral and cell-mediated immunity are augmented

Table I
Examples of Liposomes as Immunoadjuvants

Immunogen	Reference
Diphtheria toxoid	Allison and Gregoriadis (1974)
Tetanus toxoid	Gregoriadis *et al.* (1987)
Streptococcus mutans	Wachsmann *et al.* (1986)
Streptococcus sobrinus	Gregory *et al.* (1986)
Bacillus subtilis	Antimisiaris *et al.* (1993)
Plasmodium falciparum	Alving and Richards (1990)
Hepatitis A	Glück (1992)
Hepatitis B	Manesis *et al.* (1979)
Influenza A and B	Glück *et al.* (1994)
Herpes simplex virus	Lawman *et al.* (1981)
Adenovirus	Kramp *et al.* (1982)
Rabies virus	Perrin *et al.* (1984)
Rubella virus	Trudel *et al.* (1982)
Measles virus	Garnier *et al.* (1991)
Semliki Forest virus	Morein *et al.* (1978)
Sendai virus	Goodman-Snitkoff *et al.* (1991)
Synthetic peptides	Lifshitz *et al.* (1981), Friede *et al.* (1993)

by liposomes, and they act as adjuvants with both protein and carbohydrate antigens (Allison and Gregoriadis, 1974; Sanchez *et al.*, 1980; Lawman *et al.*, 1981; Sarkar *et al.*, 1982; Garçon and Six, 1991). There are several reasons for liposome adjuvanticity. Perhaps the most likely reason is that the clearance of antigen incorporated into liposomes is markedly prolonged. Further, liposomal presentation of antigen ensures that a certain amount of antigen is made available to a single antigen-presenting cell (APC) at a time following phagocytosis of the liposomes. There are suggestions that liposomes increase antigen presentation to macrophages (Shek and Sabiston, 1982; Van Rooijen and van Nieuwmegen, 1983b). Adjuvants like LPS, lipid A, or muramyl dipeptide (MDP), when incorporated into liposomes, showed increased adjuvanticity (Gupta *et al.*, 1993). Recently, monophosphoryl lipid A (MPL-A), when incorporated into liposomes with recombinant antigens of *Plasmodium falciparum* and then mixed with alum, stimulated a high antibody response to the antigen with no pyrogenicity or toxicity in humans (Fries *et al.*, 1992). Liposomes incorporating IL-2 produced an elevated antibody response to LPS which was similar to that obtained with complete Freund's adjuvant (Mayoral *et al.*, 1990). Alpar *et al.* (1992) suggest that liposomes may be used as a mucosal adjuvant. Oral administration of antigens as liposomes resulted in an augmented mucosal response compared with the response obtained with oral antigen alone (Alpar *et al.*, 1992).

The immunoadjuvant action of liposomes has been demonstrated for a wide range of antigens relevant to human and animal immunization programs (for review see Gregoriadis, 1990, and Buiting *et al.*, 1992). Antigens include diphtheria and tetanus toxoids,

Streptococcus mutans, cell-wall antigens, *Streptococcus pneumoniae, Salmonella typhimurium* lipopolysaccharide, cholera toxin, adenovirus type 5 hexon, herpes simplex virus, hepatitis A and B antigens, Epstein–Barr virus glycoprotein, influenza and Sendai virus hemagglutinin, measles and rubella viral membrane antigens, HIV-1 glycoprotein, and various recombinant or synthetic antigens from a wide range of infective agents. Table I is a representative list of approaches with liposomal vaccines. In several experiments, protection of animal models was achieved by immunization with the relevant liposome-incorporated antigens. In one vaccination study in humans the protectivity of a liposomal hepatitis A vaccine was demonstrated (Poovorawan *et al.*, 1994).

5. TECHNOLOGIES FOR LIPOSOMAL VACCINES

A variety of liposome preparation techniques have been described. All methods involve a lipid hydration step. The presence of charge-inducing agents and the molecular geometry of the lipids (cone, cylinder, or inverse cone) have a strong impact on the morphology of the structures that will be formed (Israelachvili *et al.*, 1980). It is generally accepted that five basic principles can be combined in preparation protocols to achieve desired vesicle characteristics: (1) mechanical methods, (2) methods based on replacement of organic solvents by aqueous media, (3) methods based on detergent removal, (4) methods based on size transformation and fusion, and (5) methods based on pH adjustment. Batch-to-batch and interlaboratory variation can be minimized only if a specific preparation procedure is followed in precise detail. Some pharmaceutically relevant features of these methods include the following: If organic solvents or detergents are used during the preparation of liposome dispersions for parenteral use, regulatory authorities require the careful removal of traces of organic solvent or detergent. For methods based on pH adjustment, dispersion of the phospholipid in an aqueous phase is a prerequisite. This is generally accomplished either by mechanical forces or by the use of an organic solvent or detergent. The same applies to the methods based on size transformation, which at present usually involves freeze–thaw cycles (Ohsawa *et al.*, 1985).

The following classification system of liposomes according to size and properties is accepted today: multilamellar vesicles (MLV), oligolamellar vesicles (OLV), small unilamellar vesicles (SUV), large unilamellar vesicles (LUV), and giant unilamellar vesicles (GUV) [cell size vesicles with diameters > 1 μm]. The characterization parameters of these liposome groups most frequently used are: number of lamellae (NMR spectroscopy), liposome size and size distribution (microscopy methods, Coulter counter for particles larger than 1 μm, molecular sieve chromatography, analytical ultracentrifugation, light scattering, or NMR spectroscopy), liposome compositional heterogeneity (density gradient centrifugation, ion-exchange chromatography, or differential scanning colorimetry), trapped volume and osmotic activity (use of purified 6-carboxyfluorescein or radiolabeled glucose), structural and motional behavior of lipids in the liposome bilayer (freeze-fracture electron microscopy or ^{31}P-NMR), electrical surface potential (microelectrophoresis or electron spin resonance spectroscopy), and distribution of lipid components in the bilayer (differential scanning colorimetry or ^{31}P-NMR).

As stated above, the immunostimulatory effect of liposome-associated antigens on humoral and cellular response is now a widely recognized phenomenon. Although the mechanism by which the potentiation occurs is not totally elucidated at present, it is thought to require a physical association between antigen and liposomes, and to involve the targeting of this antigen to macrophages of the reticuloendothelial system by the liposomal vehicle, leading to a more efficient presentation to immunocompetent cells (Glück, 1992b). Despite the general agreement that a physical link between antigen and liposomes is required for the potentiation to be observed, the consensus as to which type of association is the most efficient at promoting the potentiation, especially in the case of soluble antigens that could be either encapsulated or surface linked, has not been as clearly established (Lifshitz et al., 1981; Shek and Sabiston, 1982; Shek and Heath, 1983; Van Rooijen and van Nieuwmegen, 1983a; Gregoriadis et al., 1987; Shahum and Thérien, 1988; Latif and Bachhavat, 1988; Vannier and Snyder, 1988; Thérien et al., 1990). Even though the differences in published data might partly reflect the behavioral characteristics of the different antigens tested with the liposomal systems, other reasons might also be involved, as conflicting data have also been published in studies using albumin of different origins (Shek and Sabiston, 1982; Shek and Heath, 1983; Van Rooijen and van Nieuwmegen, 1983b; Shahum and Thérien, 1988; Vannier and Snyder, 1988). Among these reasons, the characteristics of the liposomal preparations such as size and vesicle properties, lipid composition or protein:lipid ratio, and the classic immunogenicity factors such as dose administered or route of administration, all appear to be important. However, as the antigens could be expected to activate the immune system through different pathways depending on its mode of association with the liposomal vehicle, the particular aspect of the immunological response that is examined and the exact timing postimmunization at which the immunostimulating potential of liposomes is evaluated might also be important factors to consider.

Different interactions of phospholipids with antigens have been described in the literature. The interactions are classified according to the hydrophobic, hydrophilic, or mixed character of the interactive forces. Other described methods are the covalent attachment of antigens to liposomes. Examples of hydrophobic interactions have been described by several authors (Wieslander and Seltsam, 1987; Rietjens et al., 1989; Brunner, 1989): For instance, Harter et al. have found that the interaction of the bromelain-solubilized ectodomain of influenza virus hemagglutinin with egg lecithin liposomes is of hydrophobic character. The NH_2-terminal 21-amino-acid residue segment is rarely responsible for the hydrophobic interaction (Harter et al., 1989). Noncovalent association occurs between glycoprotein IIb heavy chain (GP II b/H) and the amino-terminus of glycoprotein IIIa (GP III a), thus forming a globular head. The tail regions correspond to GP III a, which contain the hydrophobic segments for insertion into the lipid bilayer. The globular head of the complex binds to Arg-Gly-Asp peptides (Lam et al., 1989). Bacterial outer membrane proteins (Wetzler et al., 1992) and viral envelope glycoproteins (Trudel et al., 1982; Garnier et al., 1991; Glück et al., 1994) are examples where such interactions lead to new and potent liposome vaccine designs. Manifold hydrophilic interactions were observed between proteins and phospholipids. They include the fusion of phospholipid vesicles and the insertion and/or total embedding of protein molecule into the phospholipid layers (Cserkáti and Szögyi, 1991). Examples of nonspecific interactions are the phospholipid–protein association of the hepatitis A virion particle with liposomes (Seganti et al., 1989; Glück et al., 1992b) or the binding of monoclonal antibodies to phospholipids and liposomes (Fogler *et al.*, 1987). Antigens that do not show any natural interaction with the phospholipid vesicles can be covalently coupled to the liposomal surface. Protein-conjugated liposomes have recently attracted a great deal of interest and several authors demonstrated a high immunostimulating efficacy of this approach (Thérien *et al.*, 1990; Goodman-Snitkoff *et al.*, 1991; Friede *et al.*, 1993; Glück, 1993). Coupling usually occurs via so-called cross-linker molecules such as sulfo-SMPB [sulfo-succinimidyl-4-(*p*-maleimidophenylbutyrate)] (Martin *et al.*, 1981), or SPDP [*N*-succinimidyl-3-(2-pyridyldithio) propionate] and derivatives (Martin and Papahadjopoulos, 1982).

Conjugation of proteins to liposomes with or without cross-linker first requires the synthesis of an activated phospholipid derivative [mostly phosphatidylethanolamine (PE)] (Martin and Papahadjopoulos, 1982). Cross-linkers spontaneously react with activated PE. Such activated phospholipids are then used to prepare the liposomal vesicles. The reduced antigens (e.g., with 20 mM dithiothreitol) are given to the activated liposomes for covalent attachment (Bredehorst *et al.*, 1986).

Another possible way to produce liposomal vaccines is the entrapment of water-soluble antigens in such vesicles. A common method is the so-called dehydration–rehydration procedure (Kirby and Gregoriadis, 1984), which produces multilamellar liposomes (Gregoriadis *et al.*, 1993b). Small unilamellar vesicles are mixed with the antigen. The mixture is freeze-dried and then rehydrated with water under controlled conditions (Kirby and Gregoriadis, 1984; Gregoriadis *et al.*, 1987). The resulting antigen-containing dehydration–rehydration vesicles are centrifuged and the pellet is washed twice in a buffer solution before being resuspended in PBS. Antigens presented to the immune system in such a way proved to be more immunogenic than in the soluble form (Alving and Richards, 1990; Thérien *et al.*, 1990; Fries *et al.*, 1992; Phillips and Emili, 1992; Gregoriadis *et al.*, 1993b).

Further strategies have been developed to additionally enhance the immunogenicity of liposomal vaccines: Liposomal preparations have been mixed with Al(OH)3 (Fries *et al.*, 1992), lipid A has been added to the phospholipid mixture (Alving and Richards, 1990), or specific T-cell epitopes have been covalently linked to the surface of the peptide–phospholipid complexes (Garçon and Six, 1991; Goodman-Snitkoff *et al.*, 1991). A highly promising approach is the immunopotentiating reconstituted influenza virosomes, which are discussed in detail in the following sections.

6. IMMUNOPOTENTIATING RECONSTITUTED INFLUENZA VIROSOMES (IRIV)

IRIVs are spherical, unilamellar vesicles with a mean diameter of ~ 150 nm. They show short surface projections of 10–15 nm (Fig. 1). IRIVs are prepared by detergent removal from influenza surface glycoproteins and a mixture of natural and synthetic phospholipids containing 70% egg yolk phosphatidylcholine (EYPC), 20% PE, and 10% envelope phospholipids originating from H1N1 influenza virus [A/Singapore/6/86] (Glück *et al.*, 1992b). The production of IRIVs is described in Figs. 2 and 3 (Glück *et al.*, 1992b). In our approach, we combined several components that are known to contribute to immunostimulating effects and that are harmless for parenteral use in humans. EYPC is known to be well tolerated in man and is an important constituent in commercial solutions

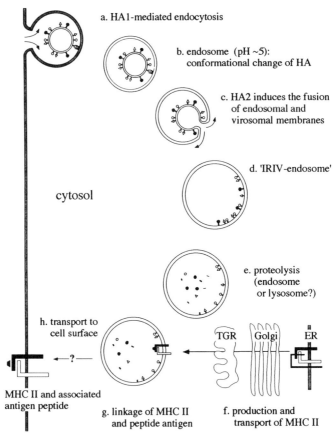

a. HA1-mediated endocytosis

b. endosome (pH ~5):
   conformational change of HA

c. HA2 induces the fusion
   of endosomal and
   virosomal membranes

d. 'IRIV-endosome'

cytosol

e. proteolysis
   (endosome
   or lysosome?)

h. transport to
   cell surface

TGR   Golgi   ER

MHC II and associated
antigen peptide

g. linkage of MHC II   f. production and
   and peptide antigen   transport of MHC II

Figure 1. Immunological basis of immunostimulation of IRIV-based vaccines. Detailed description in the text.

for i.v. applications in undernourished persons. PE was chosen for two reasons. First, it is known that hepatitis A virus (HAV) attachment to host cells occurs via binding to PE regions of the cell membrane (Seganti *et al.*, 1989). Furthermore, it has been shown that liposomes containing PE are able to directly stimulate B cells to produce antibodies without any T-cell determinant being present (Garçon and Six, 1991). The main reason for including influenza virus envelope phospholipids was to obtain vesicles that are stabilized (unpublished data). The hemagglutinin (HA) membrane glycoprotein of influenza virus plays a key role in the mode of action of the IRIVs. HA is the major antigen of influenza virus, containing epitopes on both HA1 and HA2 polypeptides, and is responsible for fusion of the virus with the endosomal membrane (Tsurudome *et al.*, 1992). The HA1 globular head groups contain the sialic acid site for HA and it is therefore expected that the IRIVs bind to such receptors of macrophages and immunocompetent cells, initiating a successful immune response. The entry of influenza viruses into cells occurs through HA-receptor-mediated endocytosis (Matlin *et al.*, 1981). It is likely that this mechanism also functions

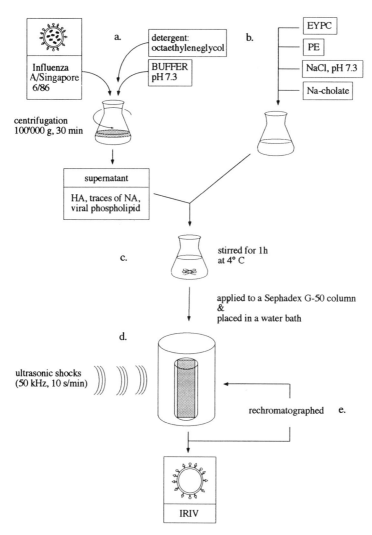

Figure 2. Production scheme for IRIVs. EYPC, egg yolk phosphatidylcholine; PE, phosphatidylethanolamine; HA, hemagglutinin; NA, neuraminidase; IRIV, immunopotentiating reconstituted influenza virosome.

with the IRIV particles. The HA2 subunit of HA mediates the fusion of viral and endosomal membranes, which is required in order to initiate infection of cells. At the low pH of the host cell endosome (~ pH 5), a conformational change occurs in HA that is a prerequisite for fusion to occur. Thus, the essential feature of the IRIVs is that they carry on their surface, beside an antigen, the fusion-inducing component HA. We expect that this mediates the rapid release of the transported antigen into the membranes of the target cells. Figure 1 summarizes in a simplified schedule the mode of efficacy of an IRIV-conjugated hepatitis

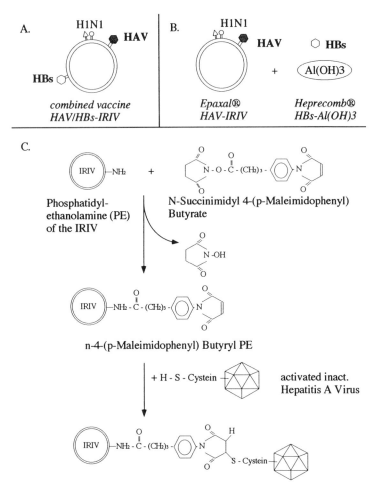

Figure 3. Coupling scheme with viral antigens. (A) Hepatitis A virus antigen (HAV) and hepatitis B surface antigen (HBs). (B) Two commercial vaccines: Epaxal Berna (IRIV-HAV) and Heprecomb Berna (alum-adsorbed HBs). (C) Covalent coupling of HAV–antigen onto IRIV using a chemical cross-linker.

A antigen (Mengiardi, 1994; lowercase letters indicate position on Fig. 1): (a) After a direct binding to the HA1 receptor (e.g., of a macrophage), endocytosis is induced (Matlin *et al.*, 1981). (b) The pH of ~5 prevailing in the endosome results in a change in conformation of the HA, so that the HA2 subunit interacts with the endosomal membrane (Wiley and Skehel, 1987). (c) This interaction leads to fusion of the IRIV membrane with the endosomal membrane. (d) The result is a slightly larger endosome—an "IRIV endosome." However, if the IRIV (including antigens) is bound and taken up by preexisting antibodies to HA, the IRIV can, in theory, only actively fuse with the endosomal membrane if the HA comes into contact with this membrane. The remainder of the procedure, after uptake by endocytes, corresponds to the now familiar procedure of antigen processing. (e) The first stage of antigen presentation is the degradation or proteolysis of the foreign proteins/antigens to peptides. The location of this process, the coupling of these peptides to the MHC class II molecule is not yet fully understood and there have been reports of so-called early and/or late endosomes (Pieters *et al.*, 1991), and also of lysosomes (Harding *et al.*, 1991; Peters *et al.*, 1991). (f) The MHC class II molecule consists initially of an alpha, a beta, and a third, constant, chain. These three constituents are produced and linked together in the endoplasmic reticulum (ER). [Since the constant chain no longer appears on the cell surface and it can be shown that peptides only bind to the MHC class II molecule after removal of the constant chain (Roche and Cresswell, 1990), the function of the constant chain is to prevent premature binding of peptides in the ER.] The MHC class II trimeric molecule is then transported via the Golgi apparatus to the *trans*-Golgi reticulum, and then funneled into the endocytotic pathway (Neefjes *et al.*, 1990). (g) In a late-type endocytotic compartment with lysosomal characteristics, the constant chain is broken down by proteases (Blum and Cresswell, 1988). This frees the binding site for the antigen peptide (Neefjes and Ploegh, 1992) and coupling with the MHC class II molecule occurs (alpha and beta chain). (h) This MHC II peptide complex is then transported to the cell surface, the antigen peptide is presented together with the MHC class II molecule to a $CD4^+$ cell, and the specific humoral immune response comes into play.

The second influenza glycoprotein exposed on the IRIV surface, the enzyme neuraminidase (NA), is a tetramer composed of four equal, spherical subunits that are hydrophobically embedded in the membrane by a central stalk. The entire enzymatic activity takes place in the region of the head. NA catalyzes the cleavage of *N*-acetylneuraminic acid (sialic acid) from bound sugar residues (Air and Laver, 1989). In the mucus, this process leads to a decrease in viscosity and allows the influenza virus easier access to epithelial cells. In the area of the cell membrane, the same process leads to destruction of the HA receptor. The consequence of this is, first, that newly formed virus particles do not adhere to the host cell membrane after budding, and second, that aggregation of the viruses is prevented. NA therefore allows the influenza virus to retain its mobility. In terms of the IRIV, these characteristics of NA can, in theory, be utilized in that, after coupling with HA, IRIVs not taken up by phagocytoses could be cleaved off again and would therefore not be lost. Also, the reduction in viscosity of the mucus could be useful in connection with the development of a nasal IRIV vaccine.

7. EXAMPLES OF IRIV-BASED VACCINES

The excellent characteristics of IRIVs as adjuvants have been demonstrated in several systems. IRIVs were first utilized in the manufacture of a hepatitis A vaccine. This contains formalin-inactivated and highly purified hepatitis A viruses (HAV) of strain RG-SB, cultured on human diploid cells, which are electrostatically coupled to the IRIV vesicle (Glück *et al.*, 1992b). A further use of IRIVs was found in the manufacture of a new liposomal influenza vaccine (Glück *et al.*, 1994). The surface spikes (HA and NA) of three currently circulating influenza strains were jointly inserted in the vesicle membrane of the IRIVs and successfully tested clinically. A combined hepatitis A–hepatitis B vaccine was also produced, based on IRIVs. The highly purified, inactivated hepatitis A virions and the HBs antigens genetically engineered in yeast were together covalently coupled to the surface of the IRIVs (Mengiardi, 1994). Finally, combination vaccines were developed, for example, a combined diphtheria–tetanus–hepatitis A vaccine. For this, the diphtheria toxoid, the alpha-tetanus toxoid, the beta-tetanus toxoid, and the inactivated hepatitis A virion were covalently bound via cross-linker molecules to the IRIV surface. Finally, a "supercombined" vaccine based on IRIV was developed, containing covalently bound HAV, HBs, diphtheria, alpha- and beta-tetanus as well as HA and NA from three different influenza strains (Glück, 1993; Just, 1993).

8. PRECLINICAL EVALUATIONS OF IRIV-BASED VACCINES

A manufacturer's primary goal in conducting preclinical studies is to obtain data necessary to initiate clinical trials. These data provide the scientific basis for the development of clinical monitoring parameters and the rational selection of a route of administration and schedule of vaccination. Therefore, preclinical studies have been designed to answer specific questions of safety and efficacy. Additional studies were designed to help discern the product's mechanism of action and to establish or to promote a marketing advantage.

In the case of IRIV-based vaccines, the common safety and efficacy tests, recommended by WHO, the European Pharmacopoeia, or the FDA, were performed. Since no special guidelines exist for liposomal vaccines, the so-called "case by case (creative)" tests were established. For instance, extended immunological studies in animals had to show that the employed phospholipids did not provoke any immunological responses (Alving, 1992) or any pathological reactions. Another test series should demonstrate the physiological and chemical consistency of the IRIV structure over a certain period. In vitro tests and in vivo studies in animals had to demonstrate the mode of action of IRIV-based vaccines in the immune system. Specific fusion tests with "nude" liposomes should show the intact biological activity of the produced IRIV vaccine (Lüscher-Mattli and Glück, 1990). Finally, an important question was the future stability of such a novel product: During a period of 2 years the vaccine had to be consistent in biophysical, biochemical, and immunological characteristics, a difficult goal to achieve with liposomal products.

9. CLINICAL EVALUATION OF IRIV-BASED VACCINES

The clinical evaluation program for IRIV-based vaccines, as for other new vaccines, was based on the international regulations governing Good Clinical Practice and Standard Ethical Guidelines. A clinical trial must comprise Phases I through III. Two IRIV products have so far been fully tested under this procedure: a hepatitis A vaccine and a trivalent influenza vaccine.

In Phase I trials, the hepatitis A vaccine was tested to determine the ideal vaccination regime, the correct dosage, and safety (Glück et al., 1992a). In addition, comparative trials with aluminum-adsorbed preparations and with a nonadjuvanted vaccine were conducted to demonstrate the superiority of the IRIV vaccine (Glück et al., 1992b; Just et al., 1992; Eng et al., 1993). Trials with freshly prepared vaccines and vaccines stored for 3 years showed that the IRIV vaccines were highly stable with regard to efficacy (Wegmann *et al.*, 1994).

In Phase II clinical trials, well over 1000 volunteers—from children to the elderly—were entered in the trial to test safety and efficacy (Just, 1993; Althaus and Glück, 1993; Loutan *et al.*, 1994; Frösner *et al.*, 1994, 1995; Holzer *et al.*, 1994). A single dose of the IRIV vaccine showed protective antibody titers in over 90% of immunized subjects, after only 2 weeks in the case of hepatitis A. After 4 weeks, the seroconversion rate was 98–100%. An interesting phenomenon in connection with the IRIV-based hepatitis A vaccine relates to the kinetics of the antibody titer. These have a tendency to increase still further between 4 and 26 weeks after vaccination (Glück *et al.*, 1992b). The fall in the anti-HAV titer is very slow, so that the seroconversion rate is still almost 100% at 1 year (Glück *et al.*, 1992b; Loutan *et al.*, 1994). A booster injection after 1 year showed a very high increase in titer, which in view of the very slow decrease in titer suggests that the protective effect will last for several decades (Loutan *et al.*, 1994). In addition, it was possible to show that there is no development of epitope suppression associated with the HAV IRIV vaccine. A particularly impressive feature was the outstanding tolerability of the vaccine. This was always significantly better than that of comparable products whether adsorbed to aluminum or administered without adjuvants (Glück *et al.*, 1992b; Just *et al.*, 1992; Holzer *et al.*, 1994; Loutan *et al.*, 1994). Further clinical trials showed that in urgent cases, where immediate protection from hepatitis A was required, the IRIV HAV vaccine could be administered at the same time as anti-HAV gammaglobulins without impairing immunogenicity (Althaus and Glück, 1993). In Phase III clinical investigations that included field studies, excellent tolerability was documented in thousands of vaccinated subjects and, in exposed populations (children), efficacy was statistically confirmed (Poovorawan *et al.*, 1994; Frösner *et al.*, personal communication).

The influenza IRIV vaccine was subjected to similar clinical testing, but efficacy was not determined. Comparable tests with whole-virus and subunit vaccines demonstrated the significant superiority of the IRIV vaccine over the conventional influenza vaccine (Glück *et al.*, 1994). The antibody titer in the hemagglutination inhibition test showed the highest increase in the group of subjects vaccinated with the virosomal vaccine (see Table II). Again, this type of vaccine showed excellent results with regard to tolerability and side effects.

Clinical trials with the combination vaccines are still at the Phase I stage. For the combined IRIV hepatitis A–hepatitis B vaccine, the effect was again superior to that of commercial monovalent products adsorbed to aluminum (Glück, 1993). Very interesting results were obtained in a series of clinical trials with a combined IRIV hepatitis A + BDT vaccine. After exclusion of epitope-specific suppression by the individual components, it was evident that particularly the diphtheria and tetanus constituents exerted "antigenic competition" on the HAV antigen and possibly also on the HBs antigen (Mengiardi, 1994). By reducing the diphtheria and tetanus toxoid molecules per IRIV particle, it was possible not only to increase significantly the immune response to these antigens but also to remove completely the antigenic competition on the HAV and HBs antigens. Once the optimum composition of the vaccine had been achieved (careful dosing of antigens per IRIV particle), an immunological effect clearly superior to that of comparable, aluminum-adsorbed products was obtained (Table III).

Table II
Immune Response following Vaccination with Various Influenza Vaccine Preparations

| | Geometric mean anti-HA titer (range) | | | | | | No. ≥ four-fold rise/total (%) | | |
| | H1N1 Singapore | | H3N2 Beijing | | B/Yamagata | | H1N1 Singapore | H3N2 Beijing | B/Yamagata |
Vaccine	Pre	Post	Pre	Post	Pre	Post			
Whole virus	2.9 (0–80)	29.1* (0–320)	25.2 (0–160)	130* (10–640)	3.4 (0–20)	16.3* (0–640)	19/32 (59) $p < 0.01$	19/32 (59) $p < 0.05$	14/32 (44) $p < 0.05$
Virosome	2.4 (0–80)	44.2* (0–640)	20.6 (0–320)	142* (20–2560)	2.4 (0–40)	17.5* (0–320)	52/63 (83) $p < 0.01$	50/63 (79) $p < 0.01$	42/63 (67) $p < 0.01$
Subunit	1.8 (0–40)	14* (0–320)	26.4 (0–160)	121* (10–5120)	2.9 (0–40)	11.4* (0–160)	14/31 (45)	16/32 (52)	10/32 (32)

*Denotes values that are significant ($p < 0.01$) relative to baseline values.

Table III
IRIV-Combination Vaccine versus Single Alum Vaccines

Immunogen	Adjuvant	Day 0 GMT[a]	p	Day 28 GMT[a]	p
Alpha DT	Alum	0.4 IU/mL	0.4	0.7 IU/mL	0.00007
	IRIV	0.8 IU/mL		3.2 IU/mL	
Alpha TT	Alum	4.3 IU/mL	0.07	13.1 IU/mL	0.00002
	IRIV	6.6 IU/mL		45.2 IU/mL	
HBs	Alum	292 IU/mL	0.4	6373 IU/mL	0.002
	IRIV	343 IU/mL		13,204 IU/mL	
HAV	Alum	8.0 mIU/mL	0.6	252 mIU/mL	0.08
	IRIV	7.0 mIU/mL		361 mIU/mL	

[a]Geometric mean titers (alum $n = 26$, IRIV $n = 27$) for diphtheria, tetanus, hepatitis B, and hepatitis A.

10. PATENT PROTECTION AND PRODUCT LICENSING OF IRIV-DESIGNED VACCINES

The technology for the manufacturing of vaccines based on IRIV has been patented worldwide by the Swiss Serum and Vaccine Institute Berne. A preliminary patent search revealed that hundreds of liposomal vaccine patents already exist, and some are products similar to IRIV. These so-called "reconstituted influenza virosomes" which are used as antigen carriers, differ particularly in the method of manufacture and in the biological activity of the fusion peptide, which is inserted in the hemagglutinin. Comparative fusion studies with IRIV-like virosomes indicated that fusion activities varied considerably depending on the method of preparation. In fusion assay (Lüscher-Mattli and Glück, 1990), IRIVs showed the highest fusogenic activity, which was even higher than that of live influenza viruses. This IRIV preparation was more immunogenic in man than the inactivated whole virus influenza preparation (Glück et al., 1994). A subunit preparation with little fusogenic activity showed the lowest immune response.

The IRIV-based hepatitis A vaccine, Epaxal Berna, was licensed in Switzerland in the spring of 1994. This was the first product license for a liposomal vaccine to be issued by a national authority anywhere in the world, and is an important step toward safe vaccines with few side effects. The license is valid for a period of 18 months, which is longer than for conventional vaccines. Since this is a completely new vaccine design, the authorities had no recommendations or guidelines for marketing authorization of such products on which to base their decision. These had to be prepared by the authorities in meticulous detail. They therefore based their work on discussions with the manufacturing company and with experts throughout the world. These recommendations will certainly be of great importance in the development of international guidelines for liposomal vaccines. In the future, applications for marketing authorization will certainly be submitted for further vaccines based on IRIV technology. Moreover, the countless scientific publications on liposomal vaccines will also lead to new, commercial liposomal products which will have to meet the standards for marketing authorization. The national authorities and international organizations (WHO, European Pharmacopoeia, FDA) will therefore have to set up guidelines shortly to regulate the marketing authorization on these products. The experience of the Swiss health authorities will certainly play a useful part in this process.

11. PROSPECTS FOR THE FUTURE

The development of adjuvant and carrier systems that are effective and safe in humans is critical to the development of vaccines using small antigens, nonimmunogenic proteins, or synthetic peptides. The liposome systems described herein indicate that peptide immunogenicity can be improved without using components that are toxic for humans. Experience with the liposome system indicates that the immunogenicity of such antigens can be significantly influenced by seemingly "minor" variations in the antigen such as lengthening the peptide or hydrophobic anchor, changes in the orientation of the linkage or in the composition of the carrier system such as phospholipid composition, vesicle structure or stabilization, and spiking with specific transmembrane proteins. The biophysical, cellular, and immunological bases for these effects—specifically, the extent to which these factors influence complex stability or antigen processing and presentation—have been previously discussed in this and in other chapters.

Because it is not clear which (if any) animal species or strain correlates with human immunity (Lowell, 1990), products that show promise in an animal system need to be tested in humans for both safety and immunogenicity. Liposomes have been extensively given to humans of all ages in the context of pharmaceutical preparations or vaccine formulations. Therefore, such efforts should prove exciting for the successful application of the molecular approach to new and improved vaccines.

There are several ways to increase adjuvant activity over that observed with alum, the only adjuvant in approved products licensed by the FDA (Eng *et al.*, 1993) and which is far from ideal: (1) by developing an adjuvant vaccine formulation that is more dispersable, therefore improving transfer of antigens to draining lymph nodes; (2) by using immunostimulants that help to trap and activate appropriate cells within these lymph nodes; (3) by providing for a physical or chemical association of these immunostimulants with vaccine antigens so that both are delivered simultaneously to lymphoid tissues; and (4) by using substances and molecules selected on the basis of prior documented safety when parenterally administered to humans. Liposomal preparations and specially IRIV-designed vaccines and similar formulations seem to do all four and therefore hold promise as immunopotentiating delivery systems for whichever vaccine is approved next.

12. SUMMARY

Liposomes are considered prime candidates to improve the immunogenicity of both antigens with hydrophobic anchor sequences and soluble, nonmembrane proteins or synthetic peptides. During the 20 years since liposomes were first demonstrated to have adjuvant potential, studies have shown that variation in liposomal size, lipid composition, surface charge, membrane fluidity, lipid–protein composition, anchor molecules, and fusogenicity can significantly influence results. In addition, antigen location (e.g., whether it is adsorbed or covalently coupled to the liposome surface or encapsulated in liposomal aqueous compartments) may also be important. Analysis of these variables as well as a comparison of the various techniques used to ensure the efficacy, stability, homogeneity, and safety of liposomal vaccine have been discussed.

ACKNOWLEDGMENT

Preparation of the figures by Bernard Mengiardi is kindly acknowledged.

REFERENCES

Air, G. M., and Laver, W. G., 1989, The neuraminidase of influenza virus, *Proteins* **6**:341–356.

Allison, A.C., and Gregoriadis, G., 1974, Liposomes as immunological adjuvants, *Nature* **252**:252–255.

Alpar, H. O., Bowen, J. C., and Brown, M. R. W., 1992, Effectiveness of liposomes as adjuvants of orally and nasally administered tetanus toxoid, *Int. J. Pharmacol.* **88**:335–344.

Althaus, B., and Glück, R., 1993, Clinical experience with the first liposomal hepatitis A vaccine, Abstract, in: *International Symposium on Viral Hepatitis and Liver Disease*, Tokyo.

Alving, C. R., 1992, Immunologic aspects of liposomes, Presentation and processing of liposomal protein and phospholipid antigens, *Biochim. Biophys. Acta,* **1113**:307–322.

Alving, C. R., and Richards, R. L., 1990, Liposomes containing lipid A: A potent nontoxic adjuvant for a human malaria sporozoite vaccine, *Immunol. Lett.* **25**:275–280.

Alving, G. R., Wassef, N. M., Verma, J. N., Richard, R. L., Atkinson, C. T., and Aikawa, M., 1992, Liposomes as vehicles for vaccines—Intracellular fate of liposomal antigen in macrophages, *Biochim. Biophys. Acta* **1113**:307–322.

Antimisiaris, S. G., Jayasekera, P., and Gregoriadis, G., 1993, Liposomes as vaccine carriers—Incorporation of soluble and particulate antigens in giant vesicles, *J. Immunol. Methods* **166**:271–280.

Ashley, H., and Ovary, Z., 1965, Effect of bovine gamma globulin on subsequent immunization with dinitrophenylated bovine gamma globulin, *Proc. Soc. Exp. Biol. Med.* **119**:311–314.

Bangham, A. D., 1961, A correlation between surface charge and coagulant action of phospholipids, *Nature* **192**:1197–1198.

Bangham, A. D., 1968, Membrane models with phospholipids, *Prog. Biophys. Mol. Biol.* **18**:29–37.

Bangham, A. D., Standish, M. M., and Watkins, J. C., 1965, Diffusion of univalent ions across the lamellae of swollen phospholipids, *J. Mol. Biol.* **13**:238–252.

Bangham, A. D., Hill, M. W., and Miller, N. G. A., 1974, Preparation and use of liposomes as models of biological membranes, in: *Methods in Membrane Biology* (E. D. Korn, ed.), Plenum Press, New York, pp. 1–23.

Blum, J. S., and Cresswell, P., 1988, Role for intracellular proteases in the processing and transport of class II HLA antigens, *Proc. Natl. Acad. Sci. USA*, **85**:3975–3979.

Bredehorst, R., Ligler, F. S., Kusterbeck, A. W., Chang, E. L., Gaber, B. P., and Vogel, L.-W., 1986, Effect of covalent attachment of immunoglobulin fragments on liposomal integrity, *Biochemistry* **25**:5693–5699.

Brotherus, J. R., Griffith, O. H., and Brotherus, M. O., 1981, Lipid–protein multiple binding equilibria, *Biochemistry* **20**:5261–5267.

Brunner, J., 1989, Testing topological models for the membrane penetration of the fusion peptide of influenza virus hemagglutinin, *FEBS Lett.* **57**:369–372.

Buiting, A. M. J., van Rooijen, N., and Claassen, E., 1992, Liposomes as antigen carriers and adjuvants in vivo, *Res. Immunol.* **143**:541–548.

Cserkáti, T., and Szögyi, M., 1991, Interaction of phospholipids with proteins, peptides and amino acids. New advances 1987–1989, *Int. J. Biochem.* **23**:131–145.

Davidson, R. N., Croft, S. L., and Scott, A., 1991, Liposomal amphotericin B in drug resistant visceral leishmaniasis, *Lancet* **337**:1061–1062.

Dean, T., 1993, Liposomes in allergy and immunology, *Clin. Exp. Allergy* **23**:557–563.

Duzzqunes, N., and Papahadjopoulos, D., 1983, Ionotropic effects on phospholipid membranes: Calcium/magnesium specificity in binding, fluidity and fusion, in: *Membrane Fluidity in Biology* (R. C. Aloia, ed.), Academic Press, New York, pp. 187–197.

Eng, R. S., Pomerantz, R. J., and Friedman, L. S., 1993, Hepatitis A vaccines: Past, present, and future, *Gastroenterology* **105**:943–945.

Fogler, W. E., Schwartz, G. M., Jr., and Alving, C. R., 1987, Antibodies to phospholipids and liposomes, *Biochim. Biophys. Acta* **903**:265–272.

Friede, M., Muller, S., Briand, J.-P., Van Regenmortel, M. H. V., and Schuber, F., 1993, Induction of immune response against a short synthetic peptide antigen coupled to small neutral liposomes containing monophosphoryl lipid A, *Mol. Immunol.* **30**:539–547.

Fries, L. F., Gordon, D. M., Richards, R. L., Egan, J. E., Hollingdale, M. R., Gross, M., Silverman, C., and Alving, C. R., 1992, Liposomal malaria vaccine in humans: A safe and potent adjuvant strategy, *Proc. Natl. Acad. Sci. USA* **89**:358–362.

Frösner, G. G., Dathe, O., Althaus, B., Glück, R., Erhardt, F., Eisenburg, J., Phillip, J., Heun, M., and Fröhlich, C., 1994, Hohe Immunogenität und geringe Nebenwirkungen eines neuartigen Liposomenimpfstoffes gegen Hepatitis A, in: *Virushepatitis A bis E* (G. Maass, and B. Stück, eds.), Kilian Verlag, pp. 222–224.

Frösner, G. G., Herzog, C., and Glück, R., 1995, Efficacy of an inactivated virosome hepatitis A vaccine in children in a highly endemic country (in preparation).

Garçon, N. M., and Six, H. R., 1991, Universal vaccine carrier. Liposomes that provide T-dependent help to weak antigen, *J. Immunol.* **146**:3697–3702.

Garnier, F., Forquet, F., Bertolino, P., and Gerlier, D., 1991, Enhancement of in vivo and in vitro T-cell response against measles virus hemagglutinin after its incorporation into liposomes: Effect of the phospholipid composition, *Vaccine* **9**:340–345.

Glück, R., 1992, Immunopotentiating reconstituted influenza virosomes (IRIVs) and other adjuvants for improved presentation of small antigens, *Vaccine* **10**:915–919.

Glück, R., 1993, Towards a universal IRIV traveller vaccine, in: *Third Conference on International Travel Medicine*, Paris (April, 1993), Abstract No. 259.

Glück, R., Althaus, B., Berger, R., Just, M., and Cryz, S. J., 1992a, Development, safety and immunogenicity of new inactivated hepatitis A vaccines: Effect of adjuvants, in: *Travel Medicine 2* (H. O. Lobel, R. Steffen, and P. E. Kozarsky, eds.), International Society of Travel Medicine, pp. 135–136.

Glück, R., Mischler, R., Brantschen, S., Just, M., Althaus, B., and Cryz, S. J., Jr., 1992b, Immunopotentiating reconstituted influenza virosome (IRIV) vaccine delivery system for immunization against hepatitis A, *J. Clin. Invest.* **90**:2491–2495.

Glück, R., Mischler, R., Finkel, B., Que, J. U., Scarpa, B., and Cryz, S. J., Jr., 1994, Immunogenicity of new virosome influenza vaccine in elderly people, *Lancet* **344**:160–163.

Goodman-Snitkoff, G., Good, M. F., Berzofsky, J. A., and Mannino, R. J., 1991, Role of intrastructural/intermolecular help in immunization with peptide–phospholipid complexes, *J. Immunol.* **147**:410–415.

Gregoriadis, G., 1990, Immunological adjuvants: A role for liposomes, *Immunol. Today* **11**:89–97.

Gregoriadis, G., and Leathwood, P. D., 1971, Enzyme entrapment in liposomes, *FEBS Lett.* **14**:95–99.

Gregoriadis, G., Davis, J., and Davis, A., 1987, Liposomes as immunological adjuvants. Antigen incorporation studies, *Vaccine* **5**:145–151.

Gregoriadis, G., Wang, Z., Barenholz, Y., and Francis, M. J., 1993a, Liposome-entrapped T-cell peptide provides help for a co-entrapped B-cell peptide to overcome genetic restriction in mice and induce immunological memory, *Immunology* **80**:535–540.

Gregoriadis, G., Garçon, N., Da Silva, H., and Sternberg, B., 1993b, Coupling of ligands to liposomes independently of solute entrapment: Observations on the formed vesicles, *Biochim. Biophys. Acta* **1147**:185–190.

Gregory, R. L., Michalek, S. M., Richardson, G., Harmon, C., Hilton, T., and McThee, J. R., 1986, Characterization of immune response to oral administration of Streptococcus sobrium ribosomal preparation in liposomes, *Infect. Immun.* **54**:780–786.

Gupta, R. K., Relyveld, E. H., Lindblad, E. B., Bizzini, B., Ben-Efraim, S., and Kanta Gupta, C., 1993, Adjuvants—A balance between toxicity and adjuvanticity, *Vaccine* **11**:293–306.

Hafeman, D. G., Lewis, T. J., and McConnel, H. M., 1980, Triggering of the macrophage and neutrophil respiratory burst by antibody bound to a spin-label phospholipid hapten in model lipid bilayer membranes, *Biochemistry* **19**:5387–5394.

Harding, C. V., Collins, D. S., Slot, J. W., Geuze, H. J., and Unanue, E. R., 1991, Liposome-encapsulated antigens are processed in lysosomes, recycled, and presented to T cells, *Cell* **64**:393–401.

Harter, C., James, P., Bachi, T., Semenza, G., and Brunner, J., 1989, Hydrophobic binding of the ectodomain of influenza hemagglutinin to membranes occurs through the "fusion peptide," *J. Biol. Chem.* **264**:6459–6464.

Heath, T. D., Edwards, D. L., and Ryman, B. E., 1976, The adjuvant properties of liposomes, *Biochem. Soc. Trans.* **4**:129–138.

Holzer, B. R., Hatz, C., Smith, D., Sissolak, R., Glück, R., and Egger, M., 1994, Immunogenicity and side effects of IRIV versus Al(OH)3 hepatitis A vaccine: A randomized controlled trial, Abstract, in: *Assemblée annuelle commune de la Société Suisse de Médecine Intensive et de la Société Suisse d'Infectiologie*, Lausanne, September 8–9, 1994.

Honegger, J. L., Isakron, P. C., and Kinsky, S. C., 1980, Murine immunogenicity of N-substituted phosphatidylethanolamine derivatives in liposomes: Response to the hapten phosphocholine, *J. Immunol.* **124**:669–675.

Israelachvili, J. N., Marcelja, S., and Horn, R. G., 1980, Physical principles of membrane organization, *Q. Rev. Biophys.* **13**:121–200.

Just, M., 1993, Experience with IRIV as carrier for hepatitis A and other antigens, Abstract No. 277, in: *Third Conference on International Travel Medicine*, Paris (April, 1993).

Just, M., Berger, R., Drechsler, H., Brantschen, S., and Glück, R., 1992, A single vaccination with an inactivated hepatitis A liposome vaccine induces protective antibodies after only two weeks, *Vaccine* **10/11**:737–739.

Kirby, C., and Gregoriadis, G., 1984, Dehydration–rehydration vesicles (DRV): A new method for high yield drug entrapment in liposomes, *Biotechnology* **2**:979–984.

Kramp, W. J., Six, H. R., and Kasel, J. A., 1982, Post-immunization clearance of liposome-entrapped adenovirus type 5 hexon, *Proc. Soc. Exp. Biol. Med.* **169**:135–139.

Lam, S. C. T., Plow, E. F., and Ginsberg, M. H., 1989, Platelet membrane glycoprotein II h heavy chain forms a complex with glycoprotein III a that binds Arg-Gly-Asp peptides, *Blood* **73**:1513–1518.

Latif, N. A., and Bachhavat, B. K., 1988, The effect of surface-coupled antigen of liposomes in immunopotentiation, *Immunol. Lett.* **15**:45–51.

Lawman, M. J. P., Naylar, P. T., Huang, L., Courtney, R. J., and Rouse, B. T., 1981, Cell-mediated immunity to herpes simplex virus: Induction of cytotoxic T-lymphocyte response by viral antigens incorporated into liposomes, *J. Immunol.* **126**:304–308.

Lifshitz, R., Gitler, C., and Mozes, E., 1981, Liposomes as immunological adjuvants in eliciting antibodies specific to the synthetic polypeptide poly (L-Tyr, L-Glu)–poly (DL-Ala)–poly (L-Lys) with high frequency of site-associated idiotypic determinants, *Eur. J. Immunol.* **11**:398–410.

Lopez-Berestein, G., 1989, Treatment of systemic fungal infections with liposomal amphotericin B, in: *Liposomes in the Therapy of Infectious Diseases and Cancer* (G. Lopez-Berestein and I. J. Fidler, eds.), Liss, New York, pp. 317–327.

Loutan, L., Bovier, P., Althaus, B., and Glück, R., 1994, Inactivated virosome hepatitis A vaccine, *Lancet* **343**:322–324.

Lowell, G. H., 1990, Proteosomes, hydrophobic anchors, iscoms and liposomes for improved presentation of peptide and protein vaccines, in: *New Generation Vaccines* (G. C. Woodrow and M. M. Levine, eds.), Dekker, New York, pp. 141–160.

Lüscher-Mattli, M., and Glück, R., 1990, Dextran sulfate inhibits the fusion of influenza virus with model membranes, and suppresses influenza virus replication in vivo, *Antiviral Res.* **14**:39–50.

Lüscher-Mattli, M., Glück, R., Kempf, C., and Zanoni-Grassi, M., 1993, A comparative study of the effect of dextran sulfate on the fusion and the in vitro replication of influenza A and B, Semliki Forest, vesicular stomatitis, rabies, Sendai and mumps virus, *Arch. Virol.* **130**:317–326.

Manesis, E. K., Cameron, C. H., and Gregoriadis, G., 1979, Hepatitis B surface antigen-containing liposomes enhance humoral and cell-mediated immunity to the antigen, *FEBS Lett.* **102**:107–111.

Martin, F. J., and Papahadjopoulos, D., 1982, Irreversible coupling of immunoglobulin fragments to preformed vesicles: An improved method for liposome targeting, *J. Biol. Chem.* **257**:286–288.

Martin, F. J., Hubbell, W. L., and Papahadjopoulos, D., 1981, Immunospecific targeting of liposomes to cells, *Biochemistry* **20**:4229–4238.

Matlin, K. S., Reggio, H., Helenius, A., and Simmons, K., 1981, Infection entry pathway of influenza virus in a canine kidney cell line, *J. Cell. Biol.* **91**:601–613.

Mayoral, J. L., Loeffler, C. M., Ochoa, A., and Dunn, D. L., 1990, Liposomal interleukin-2 (IL-2) a potential clinical vaccine adjuvant, in: *Abstracts of the First Congress of the International Endotoxin Society*, San Diego (May 1990), p. 67.

Mengiardi, B., 1994, Virosomen als Träger von Kombinationsimpfstoffen. Inauguraldissertation, Universitätskinderklinik Basel, Mediz. Fakultät der Universität Basel.

Morein, B., Helenius, A., Simons, K., Petterson, R., Kääriäinen, L., and Schirrmacher, V., 1978, Effective subunit vaccines against an enveloped virus, *Nature* **276**:715–718.

Müller-Eberhard, H. J., 1988, Molecular organization and function of the complement system, *Annu. Rev. Biochem.* **57**:321–347.

Neefjes, J. J., and Ploegh, H. L., 1992, Inhibition of endosomal proteolytic activity by leupeptin blocks surface expression of MHC class II molecules and their conversion to SDS resistant alpha/beta heterodimers in endosomes, *EMBO J.* **11**:411–416.

Neefjes, J. J., Stoollorz, V., Peters, P. J., Geuze, H. J., and Ploegh, H. L., 1990, The biosynthetic pathway of MHC class II but not class I molecules intersects the endocytotic route, *Cell* **61**:171–183.

Ohsawa, T., Miura, H., and Harada, K., 1985, Evaluation of a new liposome preparation technique, the freeze-thawing method, using L-asparaginase as a model drug, *Chem. Pharm. Bull.* **33**:2916–2923.

Papahadjopoulos, D., 1974, Cholesterol and cell membrane functions: A hypothesis concerning the etiology of arteriosclerosis, *J. Theor. Biol.* **43**:329–337.

Papahadjopoulos, D., Hougie, C., and Hanacham, D. J., 1962, Influence of surface charge of phospholipids on their clot-promoting activity, *Proc. Soc. Exp. Biol. Med.* **111**:412–416.

Papahadjopoulos, D., Maykew, E., Poste, G., Smith, S., and Vail, W. J., 1974, Incorporation of lipid vesicles by mammalian cells provides a potential method for modifying cell behavior, *Nature* **252**:163–165.

Perrin, P., Thibodeau, L., Dauguet, C., Fritsch, A., and Sureau, P., 1984, Amplification des propriétés immunogènes de la glycoprotéine rabique par ancrage sur des liposomes préformés, *Ann. Virol. (Inst. Pasteur)* **135E**:183–199.

Peters, P. J., Neefjes, J. J., Oorschot, V., Ploegh, H. J., and Geuze, H. J., 1991, Segregation of MHC class II molecules from MHC class I molecules in the Golgi complex for transport to lysosomal compartments, *Nature* **115**:1213–1223.

Phillips, N. C., and Emili, A., 1992, Enhanced antibody response to liposome-associated protein antigens: Preferential stimulation of IgG 2a/b production, *Vaccine* **10**:151–158.

Pieters, J., Horstmann, H., Bakke, O., Griffiths, G., and Lipp, J., 1991, Intracellular transport and localization of major histocompatibility complex class II molecules and associated invariant chain, *J. Cell Biol.* **115**:1213–1223.

Poovorawan, Y., Tieamboonlers, A., Chundermpadetsuk, S., Glück, R., and Cryz, S. J., 1994, Control of a hepatitis A outbreak by active immunization of high-risk susceptible subjects, *J. Infect. Dis.* **169**:228–229.

Rietjens, I. M. C. M., Anchor, L. J., and Veager, C., 1989, On the role of phospholipids in the reconstituted cytochrome P-450 system. A model study using dilaureyl and distearoyl glycerophosphocholine, *Eur. J. Biochem.* **181**:309–316.

Roche, P. A., and Cresswell, P., 1990, Invariant chain association with HLA-DR molecules inhibits immunogenic peptide binding, *Nature* **348**:36–44.

Sanchez, Y., Ionescu-Matiu, J., Dreesman, G. R., Kramp, W., Six, H. R., Hollinger, F. B., and Melnick, J. L., 1980, Humoral and cellular immunity to hepatitis B virus-derived antigens: Comparative activity of Freund complete adjuvant, alum and liposomes, *Infect. Immun.* **30**:728–733.

Sarkar, D. P., Das, P. K., Bachhawat, B. K., and Das, M. K., 1982, The adjuvant effect of liposomes in eliciting anti-galactosyl antibodies, *Immunol. Commun.* **11**:175–179.

Seganti, L., Superti, F., Orsini, N., Gabrielli, R., Divizia, M., and Panà, A., 1989, Membrane lipid components interacting with hepatitis A virus, *Microbiologica* **12**:225–230.

Shahum, E., and Thérien, H.-M., 1988, Immunopotentiation of the humoral response by liposomes: Encapsulation versus covalent linkage, *Immunology* **65**:315–317.

Shek, P. N., and Heath, T. D., 1983, Immune response mediated by liposome-associated protein antigens, *Immunology* **50**:101–107.

Shek, P. N., and Sabiston, B. H., 1982, Immune response mediated by liposome-associated protein antigens. II. Comparison of the effectiveness of vesicle-entrapped and surface-associated antigen in immunopotentiation, *Immunology* **47**:627–631.

Shek, P. N., Yung, B. Y. K., and Stanacev, N. Z., 1983, Comparison between multilamellar and unilamellar liposomes in enhancing antibody formation, *Immunology* **49**:37–42.

Small, D. M., and Shipley, G. G., 1974, Physical-chemical basis of the lipid deposition in arteriosclerosis, *Science* **185**:222–229.

Thérien, H.-M., Lair, D., and Shahum, E., 1990, Liposomal vaccine: Influence of antigen association on the kinetics of the humoral response, *Vaccine* **8**:558–562.

Treat, J., Greenspan, A., and Trost, D., 1990, Antitumour activity of liposome-encapsulated doxorubicin in advanced breast cancer: Phase II study, *J. Natl. Cancer Inst.* **82**:1706–1710.

Trudel, M., Nadon, F., Comtois, R., Ravacarinoro, M., and Payment, P., 1982, Antibody response to rubella virus proteins in different physical forms, *Antiviral Res.* **2**:347–352.

Tsurudome, M., Glück, R., Graf, R., Falchetto, R., Schaller, U., and Brunner, J., 1992, Lipid interactions of the hemagglutinin HA2NH2-terminal segment during influenza virus-induced membrane fusion, *J. Biol. Chem.* **267**:20225–20232.

Tyrrel, D. A., Heath, T. D., Celley, C. M., and Ryman, B. E., 1976, New aspects of liposomes, *Biochim. Biophys. Acta* **457**:229–235.

Vannier, W. E., and Snyder, S. L., 1988, Antibody response to liposome associated antigen, *Immunol. Lett.* **19**:59–67.

Van Rooijen, N., and van Nieuwmegen, R., 1983a, Use of liposomes as biodegradable and harmless adjuvants, *Methods Enzymol.* **93**:83–89.

Van Rooijen, N., and van Nieuwmegen, R., 1983b, Association of an albumin antigen with phosphatidyl-choline liposomes alters the nature of immunoglobulins produced during the immune response against the antigen, *Biochim. Biophys. Acta* **755**:434–440.

Wachsmann, D., Klein, J. P., Schaller, M., Ogier, J., Ackermann, F., and Frank, R. M., 1986, Serum and salivary antibody response in rats orally immunized with Streptococcus mutans carbohydrate protein conjugate associated with liposomes, *Infect. Immun.* **52**:408–413.

Wälti, E., and Glück, R., 1993, Virosomes: A new specific drug delivery system for cancer therapy, *J. Mol. Recogn.* **6(1)**:21.

Wegmann, A., Zellmeyer, M., Glück, R., Finkel, B., Flückiger, A., Berger, R., and Just, M., 1994, Immunogenicity and stability of an alumfree liposomal hepatitis A vaccine, *Schweiz. Med. Wochenschr.* **124**:2053–2056.

Wetzler, L. M., Blake, M. S., Barry, K., and Gotschlich, E. C., 1992, Gonococcal porin vaccine evaluation: Comparison of Por proteosomes, liposomes and blebs isolated from rmp depletion mutants, *J. Infect. Dis.* **166**:551–555.

Wieslander, A., and Seltsam, E., 1987, Acyl-chain-dependent incorporation of chlorophyll and cholesterol in membranes of Acholeplasma laidlawii, *Biochim. Biophys. Acta* **901**:250–254.

Wiley, D. C., and Skehel, J. J., 1987, The structure and function of the hemagglutinin membrane glycoprotein of influenza virus, *Annu. Rev. Biochem.* **56**:365–394.

Chapter 14

Liposome Design and Vaccine Development

Patricia J. Freda Pietrobon

1. INTRODUCTION

Highly purified subunit vaccines are available for use worldwide. These vaccines are both safe and effective in adult and infant populations. Examples include vaccines against hepatitis B (Emini *et al.,* 1986; Andre and Safary, 1988), viral influenza (see Recommendations of the ACIP, 1993), and bacterial pathogens such as acellular *Bordetella pertussis* formulated in combination with purified toxoids that are effective against diphtheria and tetanus (Kallings *et al.,* 1988; Storsaeter and Olin, 1992). Clinical trials are also ongoing to investigate the safety and efficacy of recombinant protein antigens from the human immunodeficiency virus (HIV-1) (Koff and Hoth, 1988; Wintsh *et al.,* 1991), pertussis toxoid (Burnette, 1992; Nencioni *et al.,* 1990), and malaria (Gordon, 1993; Fries *et al.,* 1992; Richards *et al.,* 1988). A common thread in the composition of many of these subunit vaccines is the inclusion of an adjuvant.

Among the most effective adjuvants used in laboratory animals are complete Freund's (CFA) and incomplete Freund's adjuvants (IFA), lipopolysaccharide (LPS), and adjuvants containing bacterial products (e.g., wax D, trehalose dimycolate, lipid A) (Warren *et al.,* 1986; Gall, 1966; Stewart-Tull, 1985; Bomford, 1980). The immune enhancing characteristics of these adjuvants on humoral and cell-mediated immune responses may be related to their lipoidal nature. Although several have been clinically evaluated (Gupta *et al.,* 1993; Davenport, 1968), these adjuvants are not licensed for human use because of associated toxic properties.

Only aluminum-based compounds, generically referred to as "alum" (Edelman, 1980), are presently incorporated in licensed products for human use in the United States. These compounds have a history of safety in humans, but adverse reactions in animals have been reported (Wilson, 1967; White *et al.,* 1955; Turk and Parker, 1977). Whereas all alums are composed of aluminum, the final precipitated products may possess differences

Patricia J. Freda Pietrobon • Connaught Laboratories, Inc., Swiftwater, Pennsylvania 18370.

Vaccine Design: The Subunit and Adjuvant Approach, edited by Michael F. Powell and Mark J. Newman. Plenum Press, New York, 1995.

from one another. Such formulation differences can have profound effects on antigen adsorption, vaccine stability, pharmacokinetics, and adjuvanticity (Shirodkar *et al.,* 1990; Callahan *et al.,* 1991; Bomford, 1987). (An in-depth discussion of aluminum-based adjuvants is presented in Chapters 8 and 9.) In addition, the effectiveness of alum-precipitated adjuvants varies with the antigen type and final vaccine formulation. For these and other reasons, vaccinologists are developing alternative human vaccine adjuvants.

Liposomes have been viewed as a substitute to aluminum-based adjuvants in human vaccine development. The flexibility and versatility of liposomal formulation methods make liposomes an ideal system for probing immunological responses. Liposomes are composed of biological compounds that are biocompatible and biodegradable. Phospholipid-based liposomes are not associated with significant local or systemic reactions and have not been linked with significant antigen accumulation in blood or internal organs of animals or humans (Kramp *et al.,* 1982; Eichler *et al.,* 1988). In addition, practical large-scale methods are now available for preparing liposomes for use in clinical studies (Schwender, 1993; Amselem *et al.,* 1993; Barenholz and Amselem, 1993).

Liposomes have been clinically evaluated as delivery vehicles for therapeutic drugs. Recently, clinical studies investigating liposomes as vaccine adjuvants have also been conducted (Fries *et al.,* 1992; Glück *et al.,* 1992). In all cases liposomes were found to be safe with varying degrees of effectiveness. Our laboratory has recently completed studies evaluating the adjuvant action of liposomes, and will be reported elsewhere. This chapter is intended to review current advances in liposome design and how process changes may affect the immune response to liposome-adjuvanted vaccines. The focus is on aspects of liposome design that influence the humoral and/or cell-mediated immune responses. The impact of these formulation changes on antibacterial, antiviral, and antiparasitic immunity is discussed.

2. GENERAL PROPERTIES OF LIPOSOMES

Liposomes are vesicular bilayer structures generally composed of phospholipids and cholesterol (see Tom, 1980; Alving, 1987; Gregoriadis, 1990, 1991, for reviews). The first report of liposomes as immunological adjuvants was made 20 years ago (Allison and Gregoriadis, 1974), and since then, numerous studies showing the adjuvant action of liposomes have been published. Applications for liposomes include haptens (Uemura *et al.,* 1975), hepatitis B-derived polypeptides (Sanchez *et al.,* 1980), subunit antigens from the influenza virus (Tan *et al.,* 1989; Burkhanov *et al.,* 1988), adenovirus type 5 hexon (Kramp *et al.,* 1982), allergens (McWilliam and Stewart, 1989), and polysaccharide–protein conjugates (Bruyere *et al.,* 1987), to name a few. Recently, several laboratories have studied liposomes made with detergent-extracted envelope glycoproteins from HIV-1 (Thibodeau *et al.,* 1989), and a synthetic peptide carrying a CTL epitope from the simian immunodeficiency virus gag protein (Miller *et al.,* 1992). As testament to the increased interest in liposome technology, 353 patents on liposomes and related topics were issued in the United States between 1975 and October, 1990 (Grove and Jensen, 1993), with most occurring in 1989–1990. Universities and individuals hold the largest share of patents (27%) filed during the 15-year period.

Table I
Nomenclature and Description of Various Liposomes[a]

Liposome type	Abbreviation	Size (nm)	Mode of preparation
Small unilamellar vesicles	SUV	25–50	Sonication
		30–100	Ethanol injection
		100–200	Detergent dialysis
Large unilamellar vesicles	LUV	150–250	Ether infusion
		200–1000	Calcium-induced fusion
LUV/reverse phase evaporation	REV	100–1000	Reverse phase evaporation
Large unilamellar vesicles by extrusion	LUVET	100–1000	Membrane extrusion
Multilamellar vesicles	MLV	25–100	French Press extrusion
		400–5000	Rotoevaporation
Freeze & thaw multilamellar vesicles	FT-MLV	100–500	Freeze & thaw MLV
Stable pluerilamellar vesicles	SPLV	100–1000	Ether infusion/osmotic buffers

[a]See Szoka and Papahadjopoulos (1980) for details.

Based on particle size and mode of preparation, liposomes can be separated into various types (see Table I). A detailed description of nomenclature and formulation processes has been given by Szoka and Papahadjopoulos (1980; and New, 1990, for reviews). Although the mechanism(s) responsible for enhanced immunogenicity by liposomes have not been defined, increased retention of antigen at the site of administration along with increased antigen delivery to macrophages are thought to be responsible for this phenomenon (Kramp et al., 1982; Verma et al., 1991). Immune enhancement by liposomes can be affected by liposome type, size, bilayer composition, lamellarity, net surface charge (Raz et al., 1981; Schroit and Fidler, 1982), and the need for a physical association between antigen and liposome (Therien and Shahum, 1989). Methods have been developed for the chemical coupling of antibodies (Martin and Papahadjopoulos, 1982; Shen et al., 1982; Huang et al., 1982; Leserman et al., 1983; Derksen and Scherphof, 1985; Chua et al., 1984; Bogdanov et al., 1988), antigens (Torchilin et al., 1978; van Rooijen and van Nieuwmegen, 1980a; Gregoriadis et al., 1987; Shahum and Therien, 1989; Dal Monte and Szoka, 1989b), and sugars (Weissig et al., 1989; Garcon et al., 1988) to liposomes. In addition, several groups have shown that phospholipid composition can affect the antibody IgG subclass response to viral antigens (Balkovic et al., 1987; Ben Ahmeida et al., 1993). Whatever the final liposome formulation, it seems clear that immune enhancement is linked to the physicochemical properties inherent in the *combined* antigen–liposome formulation.

3. LIPOSOMES AND ENHANCEMENT OF HUMORAL IMMUNE RESPONSES

3.1. Antibody Responses to Thymus-Independent Antigens

There are fundamental differences between immune responses mounted against protein antigens and certain antigens of bacterial origin, such as polysaccharides and LPS.

These differences have been attributed to the presence or absence of T-cell involvement in the immune response. The dogma for many years has been that thymus-independent (TI) antigens can stimulate an immune response in the absence of T cells while thymus-dependent (TD) antigens require cognate T-cell help in order to mount an effective immune response. The immune response to TI antigens is characterized by an IgM primary response and a lack of an anamnestic booster response of the IgG class. The multiple repeating antigenic determinants of polysaccharide antigens are capable of binding to and cross-linking sIg on B cells, leading to B-cell proliferation and production of antibodies in the relative absence of T cells. Recent studies in mice, however, have shown that IgG and IgA antibody responses can be produced in response to TI antigen stimulation. It is the murine IgG3 isotype that appears as the predominant immunoglobulin subclass and is generally a low-affinity antibody (see Moller *et al.,* 1991, for review).

TI antigens have been grouped into TI type 1 (TI-1) and TI type 2 (TI-2) antigens. This grouping is based on the immune response of the CBA/N mouse strain to certain TI antigens. Because of an X-linked defect, these mice are unable to respond to TI-2 antigens such as dextran, Ficoll, polyvinylpyrrolidone (PVP), and bacterial polysaccharides. These mice can, however, mount a normal immune response to TI-1 antigens (given high antigen doses) such as LPS, *Brucella abortus* bacteria, and lipoprotein. Using CBA/N mice, Mosier et al. (1977) have shown that their inability to respond to TI-2 antigens is related to the lack of appearance of certain subpopulations of B lymphocytes during ontogeny. Furthermore, from studies in defective and nondefective mice, Slack *et al.* (1980) concluded that TI-1 antigens stimulate two subpopulations of B lymphocytes—one subpopulation produces IgM and IgG2 and the other subpopulation produces IgM and IgG3. TD antigens stimulate a third subpopulation of B cells with subsequent IgM and IgG1 production. In contrast, TI-2 antigens may stimulate only one subpopulation of B cells and the synthesis of IgM and IgG3 antibodies only (Table II).

In humans, the ability to mount an effective immune response to TI-2 antigens from pathogenic bacteria is age-dependent. A direct link has not been made between the observed immune response of infants and the CBA/N mouse model to TI-2 antigens. Investigators, however, have speculated that the ineffective immune response of infants to polysaccharide antigens may be related to the absence of certain subpopulations of B lymphocytes at birth

Table II
Antibody Isotype Response to Thymus-Independent and Thymus-Dependent
Antigens[a]

Antigen type	Antigen	No. of major B-cell subpopulations	Ab isotype (murine)
TI-1	LPS, *Brucella abortus*, lipoproteins	2	IgM and IgG3 IgM and IgG2
TI-2	Dextran, Ficoll, PVP, polysaccharides	1	IgM and IgG3
TD	Proteins, pathogens, polysaccharide–protein conjugates	3	IgM and IgG1 IgM and IgG2 IgM and IgG3

[a]See Slack *et al.* (1980) for details.

and early months of life. As a result, the efficacy of purified polysaccharide-based vaccines in children less than 18 months of age is limited. This inability to mount an effective immune response to polysaccharide antigens has been successfully overcome, however, through the use of polysaccharide–protein conjugate vaccines (see Bixler and Pillai, 1989, for review).

Currently in the United States, there are four licensed conjugate vaccines effective against *Haemophilus influenzae* type b (Hib) disease in children and infants. The first of these was licensed in 1987 (Lepow *et al.*, 1985). These vaccines are composed of the purified capsular polysaccharide from the Hib bacterium linked in a controlled fashion to a protein carrier. These conjugates are effective in converting the human immune response from a TI-2 to a TD response.

Conjugate chemistry has also been used to enhance the immune response to peptide antigens. Targeted approaches utilizing monoclonal antibodies directed against histocompatibility antigens expressed on T-cell surfaces (Carayanniotis and Barber, 1990) as well as multiple antigen peptide (MAP) constructs (Tam, 1988, 1992, and see Chapter 36) have provided exciting preclinical results. Each of these methods, however, carries the potential to affect important protective epitopes on the antigen. In addition, there have been a limited number of reports suggesting that certain carrier proteins can induce carrier toxicity (Jacob *et al.*, 1985) or epitope suppression (Nussenzweig and Nussenzweig, 1989). For these reasons, alternate methods for enhancing the immune responses to TI and TD antigens are under development. As will be discussed below, adjuvants, especially liposomes, are a promising alternative to conjugate technology for enhancing the immune response to TI and TD antigens.

3.2. Liposome Stimulation of Thymus-Independent Type 1 and Thymus-Independent Type 2 Antibody Responses

LPS AND MPL

Studies in mice and guinea pigs have shown that liposomes can stimulate immune responses to TI antigens. Antihapten responses can be enhanced by incorporation of phospholipid–hapten derivatives into liposomes. In these studies, immune enhancement by haptenated liposomes was dependent on the fatty acid constituents of the phospholipids (Dancey *et al.*, 1978; Uemura *et al.*, 1974; Yasuda *et al.*, 1977a) contained within liposomes and the hapten epitope density (Yasuda *et al.*, 1977b). Dancey *et al.* (1979) further showed that the length of the spacer group between the hapten and phospholipid tail influenced the immune response. The inclusion of lipid A in haptenated liposomes was effective in converting the TI-2 antihapten response to a TI type 1 response (Tadakuma *et al.*, 1982). The usefulness of such an approach in the development of effective human vaccines may be in the generation of antibody responses to polysaccharide antigens in infants or in adults with deficient T-cell functions.

Another approach employing TI antigens to augment immune responses involves the use of *B. abortus* (BA). Golding *et al.* (1991) recently reported on an HIV-1 conjugate that was prepared by linking the intact HIV-1 virus to the TI-1 antigen, BA. Their results suggested that the BA carrier had the capacity to augment a TI-1 anti-HIV-1 specific response, rather than a TD response, against HIV-1 pathogens. In CD4$^+$ T-cell-depleted mice, results showed that the HIV–BA conjugate, but not HIV-1, stimulated an anti-HIV-1 antibody response that was neutralizing to HIV-1 specific syncytium formation. The authors speculated that a TI vaccine rather than a TD vaccine could be more efficacious in humans with T-cell deficiencies, such as HIV-infected patients. The authors are continuing these studies, replacing the whole BA pathogen with BA-LPS.

The above findings bring attention to the role of LPS and its derivatives in modulating immune responses to both TI-2 and TD antigens. LPS and its nontoxic derivative monophosphoryl lipid A (MPL) have been studied extensively as adjuvants in liposomal vaccines (van Rooijen and van Nieuwmegen, 1980b; see Alving, 1992, 1993, for reviews). The ability of MPL-bearing liposomes to modulate antipeptide responses was correlated with liposome size, liposome net surface charge, and the immunization schedule employed (Friede *et al.*, 1993). The authors linked the adjuvant effect of MPL to direct activation of B lymphocytes by liposomes, in the virtual absence of T-cell help.

A major concern with the use of LPS in vaccine development is its associated toxicity. This can be overcome by employing formulation methods that incorporate LPS into the liposomal bilayers. Dijkstra *et al.* (1987, 1988) reported that the efficient incorporation of LPS in liposomes led to a reduced ability of LPS to react in the LAL test and to activate macrophages. Further, Petrov *et al.* (1992) showed that the toxicity of *Neisseria meningitidis* LPS was significantly reduced while anti-OMP immunogenicity was increased by incorporation into liposomes.

The above findings demonstrate the usefulness of liposomes as adjuvants themselves, or as vehicles for the co-formulation of antigens and adjuvants such as LPS. Both liposomes and the LPS-bearing liposomes can have profound effects on augmenting the immune responses to TI antigens.

3.3. Liposomes That Provide T-Dependent Help to Weak (T-Independent) Antigens

3.3.1. THE UNIVERSAL CARRIER APPROACH

Stimulation of an IgG antibody response to peptide antigens in unprimed animals can be achieved by conjugating peptides to carrier proteins. The same is true for purified polysaccharide antigens in unprimed hosts. Recently, Garcon and Six (1991) reported on a potentially universal TD liposome carrier model able to induce T-cell help for weak TD or TI antigens. From studies with enveloped viruses, internal (nonexposed) proteins have been shown to provide cognate T-cell help for B-cell epitopes (Milich *et al.*, 1987, 1988). Hence, through the incorporation of both a TI hapten and a purified TD polypeptide in the same multilamellar liposome, Garcon and Six demonstrated the generation of a TD response to the hapten. Briefly, purified HA2 subunit polypeptide from influenza virus was used to provide T-cell epitopes for recruiting cognate TD help against the hapten, dinitrophenol (DNP). To ensure that the hapten was surface-exposed, the lipophilic derivative DNP–aminocaproyl phosphatidylethanolamine (DNP-CapPE) was used in MLV liposomes. Serological results from studies in outbred mice showed the generation of an anti-DNP specific antibody response, composed of the four murine IgG subclasses. Since the DNP molecules were covalently coupled to PE and exposed on the liposome's outer surface, the DNP was available for binding to sIg on B cells. This led to antigen processing and presentation by B cells to T cells, primarily Th2 clones (Rothermel *et al.*, 1991), and the observed predominant IgG1 subclass response. Liposomes lacking the HA2 polypeptide elicited a detectable IgM response only.

It was observed in this study that mice primed with hybrid DNP-CapPE/HA2 liposomes and then boosted with DNP-CapPE liposomes, elicited a better antibody response to DNP than mice boosted with hybrid liposomes. These findings demonstrated the ability of hybrid liposomes to prime mice and instill memory to the hapten. To expand on these initial observations, studies were subsequently carried out with the TI-1 antigen, LPS, incorporated into HA2 hybrid liposomes. Again, LPS/HA2 hybrid liposomes induced a TD response to the TI antigen LPS. The authors also presented methods for bioorganic synthesis of neo-LPS antigens useful in hybrid polysaccharide-bearing liposomes (Pietrobon *et al.*, 1994).

The usefulness of TI-1/ or TI-2/HA2 liposomes in human vaccine development remains to be proven. The advantages of such an adjuvant for polysaccharide antigens may lie in the ability to apply a single, noncovalently coupled protein carrier to polysaccharides that have been purified from multiple strains of pathogenic bacteria. Constraints associated with carrier protein selection, the potential for carrier-induced epitope suppression, and the potentially large "protein loads" that may arise as more and more conjugate vaccines are formulated into combination vaccines that are protective against several serotypes of the same pathogen or multiple pathogens, can be avoided with this liposomal formulation.

3.3.2. MULTIVALENT LIPOSOME COMPLEXES

Another approach utilizing liposomes as adjuvants was reported by Goodman-Snitkoff *et al.* (1988, 1990) and Mannino *et al.* (1993). Incorporation of peptides carrying both B- and T-cell epitopes into liposomes, resulted in significant enhancement in antipeptide specific antibody responses. The adjuvant properties of these liposomes were dependent on the covalent coupling of peptides to each other, each peptide carrying a B- and T-cell epitope. Peptide conjugates were subsequently derivatized with PE and incorporated into liposomes as lipopeptides. The authors linked the immune enhancing characteristics of these liposomes to the amphipathic nature of the lipopeptide–phospholipid complex. Further, the authors speculated that liposome-bearing lipopeptides composed of putative B- and T-cell epitopes created a multivalent array of antigens that mimicked the natural presentation of these antigens, as found on viral or bacterial cell surfaces. (A more detailed description of this work is presented in Chapter 15.)

3.4. Liposomes and Enhancement of Thymus-Dependent Antibody Responses

The first demonstration of liposomes as adjuvants utilized the TD antigen diphtheria toxoid. Since then, a myriad of TD antigens have been incorporated into liposomes. For hydrophilic antigens, incorporation is generally into the aqueous spaces between the lipid bilayers. For more hydrophobic antigens, incorporation can be accomplished through intercalation into lipid bilayers or through covalent coupling of antigens to phospholipids contained within the liposomal bilayers.

The topographical location of liposome-associated antigens may affect antigen processing and presentation to helper T lymphocytes. Dal Monte and Szoka (1989a,b), using an in vitro antigen presentation system, demonstrated that antigens exposed on external liposome surfaces were preferentially processed and presented by B cells. Non-surface-exposed (entrapped) antigens, however, were more effectively processed and presented by macrophages than by B cells. Therien *et al.* (1991) expanded these findings to an in vivo mouse model. Using BSA either entrapped within liposomes or covalently linked to the liposome surface, the authors demonstrated preferential immune responses. For surface-linked antigen, the synthesis of IgG3 and IgG2a antibodies increased at high and low protein-to-lipid ratios, respectively. The authors speculated that this shift in subclass response pattern was related to whether B cells or macrophages, respectively, served as the primary antigen-presenting cells (APCs). In the case of liposomes with surface-exposed antigen and at high protein-to-lipid ratios, B cells may have actually behaved in a TI fashion, leading to the predominant IgG3 subclass response. Therefore, it seems that presentation and processing by APCs may be influenced by the topographical location of liposome-associated antigen, by the protein-to-lipid ratio, and by epitope density.

4. LIPOSOMES AND CELL-MEDIATED IMMUNE RESPONSES

4.1. Liposomal Antigen Delivery and CTL Induction

The generation of a $CD8^+$ cytotoxic T-cell response against intracellular pathogens such as viruses and parasitic organisms can have profound effects on pathogen clearance and recovery from infection. Stimulation of a CTL response first requires antigen processing and presentation by APCs.

Generally, subunit and purified antigens are handled as exogenous antigens by the immune system. These antigens are processed by APCs through the endocytic pathway and presented in the context of major histocompatibility complex (MHC) class II proteins. In contrast to this, viruses and intracellular pathogens produce endogenous proteins, etc., that can be processed and presented with MHC class I proteins. Vaccines composed of purified subunit antigens readily induce a $CD4^+$ T-helper response while live virus vaccines can also induce a $CD8^+$ response.

Improvement in the efficacy of viral and parasitic vaccines may find success in adjuvants that induce a $CD8^+$ CTL response. Nair *et al.* (1992) demonstrated the induction of an in vitro primary CTL response to ovalbumin (OVA) using pH-sensitive liposomes. Dendritic cells were found to be the predominant APCs for these pH-sensitive liposomes. Previously, Brynestad *et al.* (1990) showed that standard liposomes bearing lipopeptide conjugates (prepared by derivatization of peptide with palmitate) enhanced murine humoral responses to the peptide. In these studies, liposome enhancement was further increased by inclusion of immunomodulators such as MTP-PE and MPL within liposomes. Inclusion of immunomodulators was needed in order to induce a cell-mediated immune response against peptides contained within these pH-insensitive liposomes.

Recent studies have expanded on these earlier reports. In these studies, both pH-sensitive and pH-insensitive liposomes successfully induced in vivo primary CTL responses against OVA (Reddy *et al.,* 1992). The authors speculated that for both liposome types, liposomes successfully delivered a portion of their antigen cargo to the cytosol of cells, leading to processing and presentation of peptide antigens with MHC class I molecules. Inclusion of the immunomodulator MPL in liposomes enhanced CTL responses at reduced OVA antigen concentrations, and through various injection routes (Zhou and Huang, 1993).

Another approach for the induction of a CTL response against peptide antigens is the derivatization of antigens with lipophilic compounds. This approach has previously been shown to enhance humoral as well as cell-mediated immune responses (see Pietrobon and Kanda, 1992, for review). Induction of a primary in vivo murine CTL response against a liposome-associated peptide from the glycoprotein B (gB) protein of herpes simplex virus (HSV) has recently been demonstrated (Nair *et al.,* 1993). Lipidation of the gB peptide by conjugation to the B-cell mitogen *S*-[2,3-bis-palmitoyloxy-(2*RS*)-propyl]-*N*-palmitoyl-(*R*)-cysteine (Pam3Cys) resulted in an enhanced CTL response to liposome-associated lipopeptide. Here, again, dendritic cells rather than macrophages were the primary APCs for liposome-associated peptide and lipopeptide.

One alternate approach to peptide lipidation with Pam3Cys includes derivatization with phospholipids. Using a phospholipid-derivatized synthetic peptide bearing a CTL epitope from the gag protein of SIV, Miller *et al.* (1992) have demonstrated in vivo CTL priming in a nonhuman primate model. These results are quite encouraging for peptide vaccine development and protection from diseases caused by viral and parasitic pathogens.

4.2. Liposomes and Their Effect on Antiviral and Antiparasitic Immunity

Several laboratories have reported on the successful application of liposome-adjuvanted vaccines in clinical studies. The first of these studies performed in the United States was effective in stimulating an antigen-specific antibody response to a synthetic malarial peptide (Fries *et al.,* 1992). The liposome vaccine also contained the immunomodulator MPL and an alum adjuvant. The vaccine was found to be safe following multiple injections in seronegative volunteers, and stimulated strong anti-NANP antibody responses. Although not tested, it would be interesting to determine whether these liposomes stimulated effective cell-mediated responses.

A recent study carried out in Switzerland also demonstrated the safety of a liposome viral vaccine (Glück and Mischler, 1992; Glück *et al.,* 1992). This hepatitis A virus (HAV) vaccine formulation contained proteins from the influenza virus and viral lipids within the liposome bilayer. Whole inactivated HAV was then adsorbed to the surface of preformed immunopotentiating reconstituted influenza virosomes (IRIV). Volunteers received 0.5 mL of the experimental IRIV-HAV liposome vaccine, fluid, or alum-adsorbed HAV vaccine. The IRIV-HAV vaccine was found to be safe and extremely effective in stimulating a "protective" anti-HAV specific antibody response. At all time points tested, the liposome vaccine stimulated a greater antibody response than the fluid or alum-adsorbed HAV vaccines. Additionally, the duration of the antibody response was greatest with the liposomal IRIV-HAV vaccine.

5. CONCLUSION

The past 10 years has brought forth a plethora of information on novel vaccine adjuvants. Acronyms such as ISCOMs, SAF-1, MF-59, QS-21, MPL, RIBI, MDP, MAP, Pam3Cys, Pluronic L121, and MLV are as commonplace in vaccine literature as is CFA. In animal models, each of these adjuvants and/or immunomodulators has demonstrated potentiation of antigen-specific immune responses. The degree of immune enhancement as well as the effects on humoral or cell-mediated immune response were clearly dependent on the combined antigen–adjuvant formulation.

Key aspects influencing the development of new and effective adjuvants for human vaccines are the safety, purity, and physicochemical characteristics of the final adjuvanted formulation. As reviewed herein, liposomes have been safely used clinically as vaccine adjuvants for parasitic and viral antigens. Thus, clinical-scale liposome manufacturing processes and quality-control release tests establishing purity, safety, and stability of liposomal vaccine have been confirmed. Such successes continue to support the rationale for incorporating liposomal adjuvants into the design of new human vaccines.

ACKNOWLEDGMENTS

I would like to thank Dr. Maurice Harmon and Dr. Dave Lamb for helpful discussion and manuscript review, and Mrs. Joyce Moynihan for clerical support.

REFERENCES

Allison, A. C., and Gregoriadis, G., 1974, Liposomes as immunological adjuvants, *Nature* **252**:252.
Alving, C. R., 1987, Liposomes as carriers for vaccines, in: *Liposomes from Biophysics to Therapeutics* (J. M. Ostro, ed.), Dekker, New York, pp. 195–218.
Alving, C. R., 1992, Lipid A and liposomes containing lipid A as adjuvants for vaccines, in: *Bacterial Endotoxic Lipopolysaccharides,* Vol. II (J. Ryan and D. C. Morrison, eds.), CRC Press, Boca Raton, pp. 429–443.
Alving, C. R., 1993, Lipopolysaccharide, lipid A, and liposomes containing lipid A as immunologic adjuvants, *Immunobiology* **187**:430–446.
Amselem, S., Babizon, A., and Barenholz, Y., 1993, A large-scale method for the preparation of sterile nonpyrogenic liposomal formulations of defined size distributions for clinical use, in: *Liposome Technology*, Vol. I, 2nd ed. (G. Gregoriadis, ed.), CRC Press, Boca Raton, pp. 501–525.
Andre, F. E., and Safary, A., 1988, Clinical experience with a yeast derived hepatitis B vaccine, in: *Viral Hepatitis and Liver Diseases* (A. J. Zuckerman, ed.), Liss, New York, pp. 1025–1030.
Balkovic, E. S., Florack, J. A., and Six, H. R., 1987, Immunoglobulin subclass antibody responses of mice to influenza virus antigens given in different forms, *Antiviral Res.* **8**:151–160.
Barenholz, Y., and Amselem, S., 1993, Quality control assays in the development and clinical use of liposome-based formulations, in: *Liposome Technology*, Vol. I, 2nd ed. (G. Gregoriadis, ed.), CRC Press, Boca Raton, pp. 527–616.
Ben Ahmeida, E. T. S., Jennings, R., Tan, L., Gregoriadis, G., and Potter, C. W., 1993, The subclass IgG response of mice to influenza surface proteins formulated into liposomes, *Antiviral Res.* **21**:217–231.
Bixler, G. S., and Pillai, S., 1989, The cellular basis for the immune response to conjugate vaccines, in: *Conjugate Vaccines* (J. M. Cruse and R. E. Lewis, eds.), Karger, Basel, pp. 18–47.
Bogdanov, A. A., Klibanov, A. L., and Torchilin, V. P., 1988, Protein immobilization on the surface of liposomes via carbodiimide activation in the presence of N-hydroxysulfosuccinimide, *Fed. Eur. Biochem. Soc.* **231**(2):381–384.

Bomford, R., 1980, The comparative selectivity of adjuvants for humoral and cell-mediated immunity, *Clin. Exp. Immunol.* **39**:435–441.

Bomford, R. H., 1987, The differential adjuvant activity of Al(OH)3 and saponin, in: *Progress in Leucocyte Biology: Immunopharmacology of Infectious Diseases* (J. A. Majde, ed.), Liss, New York, pp. 165–170.

Bruyere, T., Wachsmann, D., Klein, J.-P., Scholler, M., and Frank, R. M., 1987, Local response in rat to liposome-associated Streptococcus mutans polysaccharide–protein conjugate, *Vaccine* **5**:39–42.

Brynestad, K., Babbitt, B., Huang, L., and Rouse, B. T., 1990, Influence of peptide acylation, liposome incorporation, and synthetic immunomodulators on the immunogenicity of a 1-23 peptide glycoprotein D of herpes simplex virus: Implications for subunit vaccines, *J. Virol.* **64**:680–685.

Burkhanov, S. A., Mazhul, L. A., Torchilin, V. P., Ageyeva, O. N., Saatov, T. S., and Andzhanaridze, O. G., 1988, Protective action of influenza-virus surface antigens incorporated in liposomes in various methods of immunization, *Vop. Virusol* **33**:151–153.

Burnette, W. N., 1992, Perspectives in recombinant pertussis toxoid development, in: *Vaccine Research and Development* (W. C. Koff and H. R. Six, eds.), Dekker, New York, pp. 143–193.

Callahan, P. M., Shorter, A. L., and Hem, S. L., 1991, The importance of surface charge in the optimization of antigen–adjuvant interactions, *Pharm. Res.* **8**:851–858.

Carayanniotis, G., and Barber, B. H., 1990, Characterization of the adjuvant-free serological response to protein antigens coupled to antibodies specific for class II MHC determinants, *Vaccine* **8**:137–144.

Chua, M.-M., Fan, S.-T., and Karush, F., 1984, Attachment of immunoglobulin to liposomal membrane via protein carbohydrate, *Biochim. Biophys. Acta* **800**:291–300.

Dal Monte, P., and Szoka, F. C., 1989a, Effect of liposome encapsulation on antigen presentation in vitro, *J. Immunol.* **142**:1437–1443.

Dal Monte, P. R., and Szoka, F. C., 1989b, Antigen presentation by B cells and macrophages of cytochrome c and its antigenic fragment when conjugated to the surface of liposomes, *Vaccine* **7**:401–408.

Dancey, G. F., Yasuda, T., and Kinsky, S. C., 1978, Effect of liposomal model membrane composition on immunogenicity, *J. Immunol.* **120**:1109–1113.

Dancey, G. F., Isakson, P. C., and Kinsky, S. C., 1979, Immunogenicity of liposomal model membranes sensitized with dinitrophenylated phosphatidylethanolamine derivatives containing different length spacers, *J. Immunol.* **122**:638–642.

Davenport, F. M., 1968, Seventeen years' experience with mineral oil adjuvant-influenza virus vaccine, *Ann. Allergy* **26**:288–292.

Derksen, J. T. P., and Scherphof, G. L., 1985, An improved method for the covalent coupling of proteins to liposomes, *Biochim. Biophys. Acta* **814**:151–155.

Dijkstra, J., Mellors, J. W., Ryan, J. L., and Szoka, F. C., 1987, Modulation of the biological activity of bacterial endotoxin by incorporation into liposomes, *J. Immunol.* **138**:2663–2670.

Dijkstra, J., Ryan, J. L., and Szoka, F. C., 1988, A procedure for the efficient incorporation of wild-type lipopolysaccharide into liposomes for use in immunological studies, *J. Immunol. Methods* **114**:197–205.

Edelman, R., 1980, Vaccine adjuvants, *Rev. Infect. Dis.* **2**:370–383.

Eichler, H. G., Senior, J., Stadler, A., Pfundner, P., and Gregoriadis, G., 1988, Kinetics and disposition of fluorescein-labelled liposomes in healthy human subjects, *Eur. J. Clin. Pharmacol.* **34**:475–479.

Emini, E. A., Ellis, R. W., Miller, W. J., McAleer, W. L., Scolnick, E. M., and Gerety, R. J., 1986, Production and immunological analysis of recombinant hepatitis B vaccine, *J. Infect.* **13**(Suppl. A):3–9.

Friede, M., Muller, S., Briand, J.-P., Van Regenmortel, M. H. V., and Schuber, F., 1993, Induction of immune response against a short synthetic peptide antigen coupled to small neutral liposomes containing monophosphoryl lipid A, *Mol. Immunol.* **30**:539–547.

Fries, L. F., Gordon, D. M., Richards, R. L., Egan, J. E., Hollingdale, M. R., Gross, M., Silverman, C., and Alving, C. R., 1992, Liposomal malaria vaccine in humans: A safe and potent adjuvant strategy, *Proc. Natl. Acad. Sci. USA* **89**:358–362.

Gall, D., 1966, Observations on the properties of adjuvants, *Symp. Ser. Immunobiol. Stand.* **6**:39–48.

Garcon, N. M., and Six, H. R., 1991, Universal vaccine carrier: Liposomes that provide T-dependent help to weak antigens, *J. Immunol.* **146**:3697–3702.

Garcon, N., Gregoriadis, G., Taylor, M., and Summerfield, J., 1988, Mannose-mediated targeted immunoadjuvant action of liposomes, *Immunology* **64**:743–745.

Glück, R., and Mischler, R., 1992, Immunostimulating and immunopotentiating reconstituted influenza virosomes and vaccines containing them, WO 92/19267.

Glück, R., Mischler, R., Brantschen, S., Just, M., Althaus, B., and Cryz, S. J., 1992, Immunopotentiating reconstituted influenza virus virosome vaccine delivery system for immunization against hepatitis A, *J. Clin. Invest.* **90**:2491–2495.

Golding, B., Golding, H., Preston, S., Hernandez, D., Beining, P., Manischewitz, J., Harvath, L., Blackburn, R., Lizzio, E., and Hoffman, T., 1991, Production of a novel antigen by conjugation of HIV-1 to Brucella abortus: Studies of immunogenicity, isotype analysis, T-cell dependency, and syncytia inhibition, *AIDS Res. Hum. Retroviruses* **7**:435–446.

Goodman-Snitkoff, G., Heimer, E. P., Danho, W., Felix, A. M., and Mannino, R. J., 1988, Induction of antibody production to synthetic peptides via peptide–phospholipid complexes, in: *Technological Advances in Vaccine Development*, Liss, New York, pp. 335–344.

Goodman-Snitkoff, G., Eisele, L. E., Heimer, E. P., Felix, A. M., Andersen, T. T., Fuerst, T. R., and Mannino, R. J., 1990, Defining minimal requirements for antibody production to peptide antigens, *Vaccine* **8**:257–262.

Gordon, D. M., 1993, Use of novel adjuvants and delivery systems to improve the humoral and cellular immune responses to malaria vaccine candidate antigens, *Vaccine* **11**:591–593.

Gregoriadis, G., 1990, Immunological adjuvants: A role for liposomes, *Immunol. Today* **11**:89–97.

Gregoriadis, G., 1991, Overview of liposomes, *J. Antimicrob. Chemother.* **28(Suppl. B)**:39–48.

Gregoriadis, G., Davis, D., and Davies, A., 1987, Liposomes as immunological adjuvants: Antigen incorporation studies, *Vaccine* **5**:145–151.

Grove, C. F., and Jensen, M., 1993, Liposome-related U.S. patents, in: *Liposome Technology*, Vol. II, 2nd ed. (G. Gregoriadis, ed.), CRC Press, Boca Raton, pp. 487–500.

Gupta, R. K., Relyveld, E. H., Lindblad, E. B., Bizzini, B., Ben-Efraim, S., and Gupta, C. K., 1993, Adjuvants—A balance between toxicity and adjuvanticity, *Vaccine* **11**:293–306.

Huang, A., Ysao, Y. S., Kennel, S. J., and Huang, L., 1982, Characterization of antibody covalently coupled to liposomes, *Biochim. Biophys. Acta* **716**:140–150.

Jacob, C. O., Arnon, R., and Sela, M., 1985, Effect of carrier on the immunogenic capacity of synthetic cholera vaccine, *Mol. Immunol.* **22**:1333–1339.

Kallings, L. O., Olin, P., Storsaeter, J., and The Ad Hoc Group for the Study of Pertussis Vaccines, 1988, Placebo controlled trial of two acellular pertussis vaccines in Sweden—Protective efficacy and adverse events, *Lancet* **1**:955–960.

Koff, W. C., and Hoth, D. F., 1988, Development and testing of AIDS vaccines, *Science* **241**:426–432.

Kramp, W. J., Six, H. R., and Kasel, J. A. 1982, Postimmunization clearance of liposome entrapped adenovirus type 5 hexon, *Proc. Soc. Exp. Biol. Med.* **169**:135–139.

Lepow, M. J., Samuelson, J. S., and Gordon, L. K., 1985, Safety and immunogenicity of Haemophilus influenzae type b polysaccharide–diphtheria toxoid conjugate vaccine in infants 9 to 15 months of age, *J. Pediatr.* **106**:185–189.

Leserman, L. D., Machy, P., and Barbet, J., 1983, Covalent coupling of monoclonal antibodies and protein A to liposomes: Specific interaction with cells in vitro and in vivo, in: *Liposome Technology*, Vol. III (G. Gregoriadis, ed.), CRC Press, Boca Raton, pp. 29–40.

McWilliam, A. S., and Stewart, G. A., 1989, Production of multilamellar, small unilamellar and reverse-phase liposomes containing house dust mite allergens, *J. Immunol. Methods* **121**:53–69.

Mannino, R. J., Gould-Fogerite, S., and Goodman-Snitkoff, S., 1993, Liposomes as adjuvants for peptides: Preparation and use of immunogenic peptide–phospholipid complexes, in: *Liposome Technology*, Vol. II (G. Gregoriadis, ed.), CRC Press, Boca Raton, pp. 167–184.

Martin, F. J., and Papahadjopoulos, D., 1982, Irreversible coupling of immunoglobulin fragments to preformed vesicles, *J. Biol. Chem.* **257**:286–288.

Milich, D. R., McLachlan, A., Moriarty, A., and Thornton, G. B., 1987, Immune response to hepatitis B virus core antigen (HBcAg): Localization of T cell recognition sites within HBcAg/HBeAg, *J. Immunol.* **139**:1223–1231.

Milich, D. R., Hughes, J. L., McLachlan, A., Thornton, G. B., and Moriarty, A., 1988, Hepatitis B synthetic immunogen comprised of nucleocapsid T-cell sites and an envelope B-cell epitope, *Proc. Natl. Acad. Sci. USA* **85**:1610–1614.

Miller, M. D., Gould-Fogerite, S., Shen, L., Woods, R. M., Koenig, S., Mannino, R. J., and Letvin, N. L., 1992, Vaccination of rhesus monkeys with synthetic peptide in a fusogenic proteoliposome elicits simian immunodeficiency virus-specific CD8[+] cytotoxic T lymphocytes, *J. Exp. Med.* **176**:1739–1744.

Moller, G., Fernandez, C., and Alarcon-Riquelme, M., 1991, Thymus independent antigens, in: *T-Cell Dependent and Independent B-Cell Activation* (E. C. Snow, ed.), CRC Press, Boca Raton, pp. 65–74.

Mosier, D. E., Mond, J. J., and Goldings, E. A., 1977, The ontogeny of thymic independent antibody response in vitro in normal mice and mice with an X-linked B cell defect, *J. Immunol.* **119**:1874–1878.

Nair, S., Zhou, F., Reddy, R., Huang, L., and Rouse, B. T., 1992, Soluble proteins delivered to dendritic cells via pH-sensitive liposomes induce primary cytotoxic T lymphocyte responses in vitro, *J. Exp. Med.* **175**:609–612.

Nair, S., Babu, J. S., Dunham, R. G., Kanda, P., Burke, R. L., and Rouse, B.T., 1993, Induction of primary, antiviral cytotoxic, and proliferative responses with antigens administered via dendritic cells, *J. Virol.* **67**:4062–4069.

Nencioni, L., Pizza, M., Bugnoli, M., Bugnoli, M., De Magistris, T., Di Tommaso, A., Giovannoni, F., Manetti, R., Marsili, I., Matteucci, G., Nucci, D., Olivieri, R., Pileri, P., Presentini, R., Villa, L., Kreeftenberg, J. G., Silvestri, S., Tagliabue, A., and Rappuoli, R., 1990, Characterization of genetically inactivated pertussis toxin mutants: Candidates for a new vaccine against whooping cough, *Infect. Immun.* **58**:1308–1315.

New, R. R. C., 1990, Preparation of liposomes, in: *Liposomes: A Practical Approach* (R. R. C. New, ed.), Oxford University Press, London, pp. 33–104.

Nussenzweig, V., and Nussenzweig, R. S., 1989, Rationale for the development of an engineered sporozoite malaria vaccine, *Adv. Immunol.* **45**:283–334.

Petrov, A. B., Semenov, B. F., Vartanyan, Y. P., Zakirov, M. M., Torchilin, V. P., Trubetskoy, V. S., Koshkina, N. V., L'Vov, V. L., Verner, I. K., Lopyrev, I. V., and Dmitriev, B. A., 1992, Toxicity and immunogenicity of Neisseria meningitidis lipopolysaccharide incorporated into liposomes, *Infect. Immun.* **60**:3897–3903.

Pietrobon, P. J. Freda, and Kanda, P., 1992, Lipopeptides and their effects on the immune system, in: *Vaccine Research and Developments* (W. C. Koff and H. R. Six, eds.), Dekker, New York, pp. 3–42.

Pietrobon, P. J. Freda, Garcon, N., Lee, C. H., and Six, H. R., 1994, Liposomes that provide T-dependent help to weak antigens (T-independent antigens), *ImmunoMethods* **4**:236–243.

Raz, A., Bucana, C., Fogler, W. E., Poste, G., and Fidler, I. J., 1981, Biochemical, morphological, and ultrastructural studies on the uptake of liposomes by murine macrophages, *Can. J. Res.* **41**:487–494.

Recommendations of the Immunization Practices Advisory Committee (ACIP), 1993, Prevention and control of influenza: Part I, Vaccines, *MMWR* **42**: No. RR-6.

Reddy, R., Zhou, F., Nair, S., Huang, L., and Rouse, B. T., 1992, In vivo cytotoxic T lymphocyte induction with soluble proteins administered in liposomes, *J. Immunol.* **148**:1585–1589.

Richards, R. L., Hayre, M. D., Hockmeyer, W. T., and Alving, C. R., 1988, Liposomes, lipid A, and aluminum hydroxide enhance the immune response to a synthetic malaria sporozoite antigen, *Infect. Immun.* **56**:682–686.

Rothermel, A. L., Gilbert, K. M., and Weigle, W. O., 1991, Differential abilities of Th1 and Th2 to induce polyclonal B cell proliferation, *Cell. Immunol.* **135**:1–15.

Sanchez, Y., Ionescu-Matiu, I., Dreesman, G. R., Kramp, W., Six, H. R., Hollinger, F. B., and Melnick, J. L., 1980, Humoral and cellular immunity to hepatitis B virus-derived antigens: Comparative activity of Freund complete adjuvant, alum and liposomes, *Infect. Immun.* **30**:728–733.

Schroit, A. J., and Fidler, I. J., 1982, Effects of liposome structure and lipid composition on the activation of the tumoricidal properties of macrophages by liposomes containing muramyl dipeptide, *Can. J. Res.* **42**:161–167.

Schwender, R. A., 1993, The preparation of large volumes of sterile liposomes for clinical applications, in: *Liposome Technology*, Vol. I, 2nd ed. (G. Gregoriadis, ed.), CRC Press, Boca Raton, pp. 487–500.

Shahum, E., and Therien, H.-M., 1989, Comparative effect on humoral response of four different proteins covalently linked on BSA-containing liposomes, *Cell. Immunol.* **123**:36–43.

Shen, D.-F., Huang, A., and Huang, L., 1982, An improved method for covalent attachment of antibody to liposomes, *Biochim. Biophys. Acta* **689**:31–37.

Shirodkar, S., Hutchinson, R. L., Perry, D. L., White, J. L., and Hem, S. L., 1990, Aluminum compounds used as adjuvants in vaccines, *Pharm. Res.* **7**:1282–1288.

Slack, J., Der-Balian, G. P., Nahm, M., and Davie, J. M., 1980, Subclass restriction of murine antibodies. II. The IgG plaque-forming cell response to thymus-independent type 1 and type 2 antigens in normal mice and mice expressing an X-linked immunodeficiency, *J. Exp. Med.* **151**:853–862.

Stewart-Tull, D., 1985, Symposium on Immunological Adjuvants, *Vaccine* **3**:152–157.

Storsaeter, J., and Olin, P., 1992, Relative efficacy of two acellular pertussis vaccines during three years of passive surveillance, *Vaccine* **10**:142–144.

Szoka, F., and Papahadjopoulos, D., 1980, Comparative properties and methods of preparation of liposomes, *Annu. Rev. Biophys. Bioeng.* **9**:467–508.

Tadakuma, T., Yasuda, T., Saito, K., Tsumita, T., and Kinsky, S. C., 1982, Effect of lipid A incorporation on characterization of liposomal model membranes as thymus-independent type 1 or type 2 immunogens, *J. Immunol.* **128**:206–210.

Tam, J. P., 1988, Synthetic peptide vaccine design: Synthesis and properties of a high-density multiple antigen peptide system, *Proc. Natl. Acad. Sci. USA* **85**:5409–5413.

Tam, J. P., 1992, Chemically defined synthetic immunogens and vaccines by the multiple antigen peptide approach, in: *Vaccine Research and Development* (W. C. Koff and H. R. Six, eds.), Dekker, New York, pp. 51–87.

Tan, L., Loyter, A., and Gregoriadis, G., 1989, Incorporation of reconstituted influenza virus envelopes into liposomes: Studies of the immune response in mice, *Biochem. Soc. Trans.* **17**:129–130.

Therien, H.-M., and Shahum, E., 1989, Importance of physical association between antigen and liposomes in liposomes adjuvanticity, *Immunol. Lett.* **22**:253–258.

Therien, H.-M., Shahum, E., and Fortin, A., 1991, Liposome adjuvanticity: Influence of dose and protein:lipid ratio on the humoral response to encapsulated and surface-linked antigen, *Cell Immunol.* **136**:402–413.

Thibodeau, L., Chagnon, M., Flamand, L., Oth, D., Lachapelle, L., Tremblay, C., and Montagnier, L., 1989, Role of liposomes in the presentation of HIV envelope glycoprotein and the immune response in mice, *C. R. Acad. Sci.* **309**:741–747.

Tom, B. H., 1980, An overview: Liposomes and immunobiology—macrophages, liposomes, and tailored immunity, in: *Liposomes and Immunobiology* (B. H. Tom and H. R. Six, eds.), Elsevier North-Holland, Amsterdam, pp. 3–22.

Torchilin, V. P., Goldmacher, V. S., and Smirnov, V. N., 1978, Covalent studies on covalent and noncovalent immobilization of protein molecules on the surface of liposomes, *Biochem. Biophys. Res. Commun.* **85**:983–990.

Turk, J. L., and Parker, D., 1977, Granuloma formation in normal guinea pigs injected intradermally with aluminum and zirconium compounds, *J. Invest. Dermatol.* **68**:336–340.

Uemura, K., Nicolotti, R. A., Six, H. R., and Kinsky, S. C., 1974, Antibody formation in response to liposomal model membranes sensitized with N-substituted phosphatidylethanolamine derivatives, *Biochemistry* **13**:1572–1578.

Uemura, K.-I., Claflin, J. L., Davie, J. M., and Kinsky, S. C., 1975, Immune response to liposomal model membranes: Restricted IgM and IgG anti-dinitrophenyl antibodies produced in guinea pigs, *J. Immunol.* **114**:958–961.

Van Rooijen, N., and van Nieuwmegen, R., 1980a, Liposomes in immunology: Evidence that their adjuvant effect results from surface exposition of the antigen, *Cell. Immunol.* **149**:402–407.

Van Rooijen, N., and van Nieuwmegen, R., 1980b, Endotoxin enhanced adjuvant effect of liposomes, particularly when antigen and endotoxin are incorporated within the same liposome, *Immunol. Commun.* **9**:747–757.

Verma, J. N., Wassef, N. M., Wirtz, R. A., Atkinson, C. T., Aikawa, M., Loomis, L. D., and Alving, C. R., 1991, Phagocytosis of liposomes by macrophages: Intracellular fate of liposomal malaria antigen, *Biochim. Biophys. Acta* **1066**:229–238.

Warren, H. S., Vogel, F. R., and Chedid, L. A., 1986, Current status of immunological adjuvants, in: *Annual Review of Immunology*, Vol. 4 (W. E. Paul, ed.), Annual Reviews, Palo Alto, pp. 369–388.

Weissig, V., Lasch, J., and Gregoriadis, G., 1989, Covalent coupling of sugars to liposomes, *Biochim. Biophys. Acta* **1003**:54–57.

White, R. G., Coons, A. H., and Connally, J. M., 1955, Studies on antibody production. III. The alum granuloma, *J. Exp. Med.* **102**:73–82.

Wilson, G. S., 1967, *The Hazards of Immunization*, Athlone Press, London.

Wintsh, J., Chiagnut, C. L., Braun, D., Jeannet, M., Stadler, H., Abrignani, J., Montagna, D., Chavijo, F., Moret, P., Dayer, J. M., and Staehelin, T., 1991, Safety and immunogenicity of a genetically engineered human immunodeficiency virus vaccine, *J. Infect. Dis.* **163**:219–225.

Yasuda, T., Dancey, G. F., and Kinsky, S. C., 1977a, Immunogenicity of liposomal model membranes in mice: Dependence on phospholipid concentration, *Proc. Natl. Acad. Sci. USA* **74**:1234–1236.

Yasuda, T., Dancey, G. F., and Kinsky, S. C., 1977b, Immunogenic properties of liposomal model membranes in mice, *J. Immunol.* **119**:1863–1867.

Zhou, F., and Huang, L., 1993, Monophosphoryl lipid A enhances specific CTL induction by a soluble protein antigen entrapped in liposomes, *Vaccine* **11**:1139–1144.

Chapter 15

Lipid Matrix-Based Vaccines for Mucosal and Systemic Immunization

Raphael J. Mannino and Susan Gould-Fogerite

1. INTRODUCTION

Immunization is today the most effective defense mechanism against microbial infections. Although highly effective vaccines are currently available for a number of infectious diseases, vaccine formulations can still be improved in a number of important areas. The ability to induce antigen-specific humoral and cell-mediated immunity is crucial to the development of effective prophylactic and therapeutic vaccines. The approaches to the design of human vaccines currently include the use of live attenuated viruses and bacteria, inactivated micro-organisms (killed vaccines), live-recombinant vaccines, subunit vaccines, and, more recently, naked DNA.

The approach of our laboratories has been to design and test simple, highly defined antigen–lipid complexes that would stimulate antibody and cell-mediated immune responses in the absence of any nonspecific immunological activators such as Freund's, LPS, or alum. This chapter is comprised of three sections that describe distinct but related lipid matrix-based vaccine formulations developed in our laboratories.

In considering the structural components common to natural immunogens, we determined that the immune system most often encounters antigens in the context of a lipid matrix. Antibodies, T helper, T cytolytic, B cells, and other antigen-presenting cells react with proteins, peptides, and carbohydrates presented from the surfaces of biological membranes. The structural foundation of our reconstituted immunogens was, therefore, artificial lipid vesicles (liposomes) or other lipid-based matrices. Several laboratories had previously reported that proteins reconstituted into the bilayers of liposomes could be

Raphael J. Mannino and Susan Gould-Fogerite • Department of Laboratory Medicine and Pathology, University of Medicine and Dentistry of New Jersey, New Jersey Medical School, Newark, New Jersey 07103.

Vaccine Design: The Subunit and Adjuvant Approach, edited by Michael F. Powell and Mark J. Newman. Plenum Press, New York, 1995.

vigorous immunogens (reviewed in Gregoriadis, 1990, and see chapters 13 and 14, this volume). Our goal has been to elucidate the chemical and physical properties controlling this immunological phenomenon. We have utilized a classical biochemist's approach toward understanding the structure–function relationships between immunogens and the immune response (Goodman-Snitkoff *et al.,* 1990, 1991; Miller *et al.,* 1992). Complex, multicomponent biological systems are disassembled and the component parts are identified and purified or synthesized. Specific components are then systematically reassembled until biological function is reconstituted. This results in simple, well-defined, and fully functional macromolecular structures.

Our recent studies have focused on defining the parameters involved in the induction of mucosal immune responses and long-term immunological memory. Section 2 reports the development of a new type of subunit vaccine, the protein cochleate, which is highly effective when given orally or intramuscularly (Gould-Fogerite *et al.,* 1994a, 1994b; Kheiri *et al.,* 1994; Edghill-Smith *et al.,* 1994a, 1994b). In Section 3 we describe methods for the preparation of fusogenic proteoliposomes and their utilization to stimulate CD8$^+$ cytolytic responses against proteins or peptides associated with the lipid bilayer, and against peptides, proteins, and whole fixed viruses encapsulated within them. Using these formulations, we have elucidated structure–function relationships in peptide vaccines which affect induction of CD8$^+$ cytolytic cell responses (Gould-Fogerite and Mannino, 1992; Canki *et al.,* 1994; Gould-Fogerite *et al.,* 1994a). Section 4 summarizes our earlier work with unique covalent peptide–lipid complexes designed to stimulate humoral and T helper cell responses. In those studies we demonstrated that strong antibody responses could be generated to peptides without the use of carrier proteins or Freund's adjuvant. The minimal structures required for the induction of antibody responses consist of a T- and B-cell epitope (in the same or separate peptides), covalently cross-linked to a phospholipid, and multivalent presentation in the context of a lipid bilayer (Goodman-Snitkoff *et al.,* 1988; Mannino *et al.,* 1992).

Information gained by utilizing this type of structure–function approach facilitates the elucidation of parameters regulating the induction of immune responses, the mechanisms of pathogenesis, and the correlates of protective immunity. It also makes possible the production of custom-designed vaccines that elicit desired immune responses to specific parts of the pathogen that are relevant to protection. Harmful or competitive responses can be minimized or avoided. In addition to preventing disease, as a consequence of their specificity and flexibility, custom-designed lipid matrix-based subunit vaccines hold great promise as therapeutic vaccines for the treatment of chronic viral, parasitic, or autoimmune diseases and cancer.

2. PROTEIN COCHLEATE VACCINES

A new type of subunit vaccine, the protein cochleate, has been developed in our laboratories. Oral administration of these vaccines (simply by drinking) leads to strong, long-lasting circulating and mucosal antibody responses, and long-term immunological memory to influenza and parainfluenza type I virus glycoproteins. Cell-mediated immune responses, including proliferative and cytolytic activities, are also generated. Protection from replication of virus in the trachea and lungs following intranasal challenge with live influenza virus is obtained (Gould-Fogerite *et al.,* 1994; Kheiri *et al.,* 1994; Edghill-Smith *et al.,* 1994a). In contrast to most other subunit or to killed vaccines, priming or boosting by another route, or inclusion of extraneous, problematic, mucosal adjuvants such as cholera toxin (CT) or heat-labile toxin of enterotoxigenic *E. coli* (LT) are not necessary for these activities.

Protein cochleates are also highly effective immunogens when administered intramuscularly. Intramuscular immunization stimulates strong circulating and mucosal antibody, proliferative, and cytolytic responses to viral glycoproteins, including recombinant gp160 from HIV-1 (Edghill-Smith *et al.,* 1994b). Recent data indicate that intranasal immunization stimulates strong circulating antibody titers (other immune responses have not yet been characterized). Peptides are also strongly immunogenic when formulated as protein cochleates and given perorally or intramuscularly (Edghill-Smith *et al.,* 1994b). Long-term persistence of immune responses (in many cases increasing over a period of several months) indicates a high probability of slow-release characteristics for protein cochleate formulations which would be consistent with their solid multilayered structure.

2.1. Structure

Protein cochleates are stable protein–phospholipid–calcium precipitates that are structurally distinct from liposomes. They have a unique structure consisting of a large, continuous, *solid*, lipid bilayer sheet rolled up in a spiral, with *no internal aqueous space*. The calcium ion maintains the cochleate in its rolled up form, bridging between successive layers. One of its positive charges interacts with a single negative charge on a phospholipid head group in one bilayer, and the other with a phospholipid in the opposing bilayer. Cochleates may be stored in calcium-containing buffer, or lyophilized to a powder, stored at room temperature, and reconstituted with liquid prior to administration. Removal of the calcium ion, by chelating agents or diffusion in a low-calcium environment, allows the cochleate to unroll and form large, mainly unilamellar liposomes. Membrane proteins, such as the surface glycoproteins of enveloped viruses, can be integrated into the lipid bilayers of the cochleates, and exist as integral membrane proteins in the end product liposomes (Fig. 1 and see Section 3). When protein cochleates are used as vaccines we hypothesize that they slowly unroll, and that proteoliposomes thus produced may be a major structure interacting with cells of the immune system.

While appropriately formulated liposome-based vaccines are highly effective immunogens when given parenterally, they do not have the structural properties necessary to efficiently survive the harsh acid and degradative environments encountered on peroral administration. In contrast, the solid rolled up precipitate structure of the cochleates apparently survives the stomach, protecting the proteins within, to be taken up by the Peyer's patches of the small intestine. Protein cochleates given orally stimulate strong mucosal and systemic antibody, proliferative, and cytotoxic responses. Protection from infection with virus introduced on a mucosal surface is also achieved.

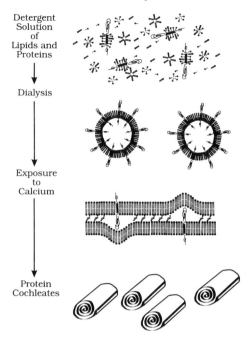

Figure 1. Preparation of protein cochleates. (1) Proteins or peptides containing hydrophobic domains are solubilized with the detergent B-D Octylglucopyranoside in high-salt buffer. (2) This solution is added to dried phosphatidylserine and cholesterol. (3) The detergent is removed by dialysis resulting in the formation of small proteoliposomes. (4) The addition of calcium results in the formation of long sheets of calcium-chelated phospholipid bilayers. (5) The sheets roll up to form cochleate cylinders which are insoluble precipitates containing no internal aqueous space.

2.2 Formulation

We have introduced methods for the incorporation of proteins or peptides into protein–phospholipid–calcium precipitates known as protein cochleates (Gould-Fogerite and Mannino, 1985; Gould-Fogerite *et al.*, 1987). These unique structures may be used as vaccines directly, or converted to proteoliposome vaccines and/or delivery vehicles by addition of EDTA (Section 3 and Miller *et al.*, 1992; Gould-Fogerite *et al.*, 1994; Kheiri *et al.*, 1994; Edghill-Smith *et al.*, 1994a,b; Canki *et al.*, 1994). These methods have been described in detail elsewhere (Gould-Fogerite and Mannino, 1992). Very briefly, Sendai (parainfluenza type 1) and influenza (A/PR8/34) viruses were propagated in the allantoic sac of embryonated chicken eggs. Virus was purified from allantoic fluid by differential centrifugation. Sterile technique and materials were used throughout virus inoculation, isolation, and purification. The viral envelope glycoproteins and lipids were extracted using octylglucoside in a high-salt buffer and separated from the nucleocapsids by centrifugation. The extracted viral envelope, recombinant protein, and/or lipid-linked peptide are added to dried phosphatidylserine and cholesterol, vortexed, incubated on ice, then dialyzed to remove detergent. This is followed by dialysis against buffer containing calcium to form protein cochleates.

2.3. Oral Immunization and the Common Mucosal Immune System

Mucous membranes are the primary routes of entry for a large number and wide variety of human disease-causing agents, including those that are inhaled, ingested, or sexually transmitted. Intramuscular or subcutaneous administration of vaccines often does not lead to optimal or long-lasting protection against these infectious agents (Formal et al., 1967; American Academy of Pediatrics, 1991). In contrast, the oral route of delivery can stimulate strong protective responses on mucous membranes and in the circulation (Mestecky and McGhee, 1989; Horre and Hackett, 1989; Faden et al., 1990; Holmgren, 1991; Cui et al., 1991). The oral route has been chosen by the WHO Children's Vaccine Initiative because of ease of administration, low cost, safety, and the opportunity to prime mucosal as well as circulating immune responses. Also, combining antigens from a variety of pathogens to form effective "multicomponent vaccines" is one of the challenges of modern vaccine research. A potential problem for multicomponent vaccines is limitations on the volume of material that can be injected, particularly in infants. Oral administration may circumvent this problem, as well as avoid many of the adverse effects seen when vaccines are administered parenterally. In addition, peroral vaccination may be an effective strategy for immunizing infants who contain circulating maternal antibodies.

Antigens or invading pathogens that can survive the harsh acid and degradative environments encountered following oral entry may be taken up by the specialized microfold or "M" cells of the small intestine. These cells can take up antigens, including whole bacteria, and transport them to the follicle beneath known as a Peyer's patch. The induction of T- and B-cell responses to the antigen occurs here and is followed by migration of the immune cells to the mesenteric lymph nodes. They then travel via the efferent lymphatics to the thoracic duct, where they enter the circulation. Later, cells migrate to various effector sites in the gastrointestinal, respiratory, and genitourinary tracts. This is known as the common mucosal immune system (reviewed in Mestecky and McGhee, 1989; Bradtzaeg, 1989; Holmgren, 1991; McGhee et al., 1992). IgA plasma cells initially stimulated by cognate B and T cell interactions in gut-associated lymphoid tissue (GALT) secrete local antibody that is specifically taken up by epithelial cells, transported to the mucosal surface, and released with a part of the receptor as secretory IgA (Bergmann and Waldman, 1988; Dahlgren et al., 1989). Secretory IgA can protect against pathogens that replicate on or enter via mucosal surfaces (Michetti et al., 1992; Walker et al., 1992). IgG which may be either locally secreted or appear as a result of transudation from the serum can also play a role in protection (Dahlgren et al., 1989; Robbins et al., 1992). Hyperimmunization parenterally can therefore sometimes lead to protection on mucosal surfaces, but such protection is usually short lived (American Academy of Pediatrics, 1991; Conner et al., 1994). For optimal mucosal protection, induction of immune responses via mucosal routes is probably required (Formal et al., 1967; Horre and Hackett, 1989; McGhee et al., 1992; Treanor et al., 1992).

Despite the attractiveness of the oral route for vaccine administration, little success has been achieved in this area. Positive results have mainly been limited to viruses and bacteria that have evolved to infect via the oral route of entry, to eventually replicate in the gut (e.g., poliovirus, salmonella, cholera bacteria). The only currently licensed oral live attenuated vaccines are polio and *Salmonella typhi* Ty 21a (Faden *et al.,* 1990). Live attenuated vaccines pose risks of reversion to wild type or pathogenicity in immunocompromised individuals (a category that can include malnourished children). It is often difficult to maintain protective immunogenicity without associated pathogenicity even in immunocompetent individuals (e.g., live shigella vaccines). Live vaccines also lose much of their advantage over subunit vaccines when they need to be given multiple times in large doses (e.g., *S. typhi* 21a).

The ability to construct immunogenic preparations that are safe, efficacious, stable, cost-effective, and able to induce humoral and cell-mediated immune responses to antigens from a variety of pathogens following oral administration is one of the major goals of contemporary vaccine research and development. Protein cochleates represent a promising new approach toward achieving this goal.

2.4. Influenza: Immune Response to Cochleate Vaccines

2.4.1. INFLUENZA: STRUCTURE, PATHOGENESIS, AND CURRENT VACCINE STATUS

Influenza is a myxovirus that causes acute infection of the respiratory tract and resultant serious morbidity and significant mortality worldwide among the young, old, and immunocompromised on an annual basis (Webster and Rott, 1987; Wilson and Cox, 1990). In addition, infection of the remainder of the population is responsible for considerable discomfort and inconvenience, as well as decreased productivity related to lost work hours. Vaccines currently in use are fixed whole virus or detergent extracted, preparations which are given intramuscularly. The systemic IgG responses they generate reduce the incidence of pneumonia and death. Very little mucosal immunity or cytotoxic T-cell responses are induced by these vaccines and protocols (Treanor *et al.,* 1992). Protective humoral (antibody) responses are directed mainly against the receptor binding portion of the hemagglutinin (HA) surface glycoprotein (Wiluz *et al.,* 1981; Webster and Rott, 1987; Wilson and Cox, 1990). Cytotoxic T-cell responses against the HA glycoprotein and the nucleocapsid protein (NP) have been shown to be protective from lethal infection in animal models, cross-react between strains, and appear to play a major role in clearance of virally infected cells, limiting virus spread and contributing to recovery (Yap *et al.,* 1978; Wells *et al.,* 1981; McMichael *et al.,* 1983). The presence of significant mucosal humoral and cell-mediated immune responses might diminish or protect individuals from clinical symptoms. Widespread usage of an oral vaccine that could stimulate long-lasting mucosal and systemic immunity might have a major positive impact on epidemic spread and associated morbidity as well as mortality. Such a vaccine would represent a major step forward in the prophylaxis of this disease.

2.4.2. ORAL IMMUNIZATION: CIRCULATING ANTIBODY RESPONSES

Cochleate vaccines containing the glycoproteins and lipids from the envelope of influenza virus plus phosphatidylserine and cholesterol were given to mice by gradually

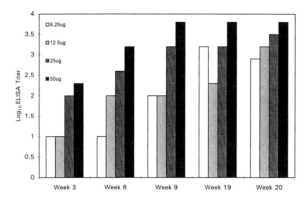

Figure 2. Serum antibody titers in mice following oral administration of influenza protein cochleates. Initial vaccine doses of 50, 25, 12.5, or 6.25 μg were administered orally at 0 and 3 weeks. The third and fourth immunizations, given at 6 and 19 weeks, were at one-fourth the dose used for the initial two immunizations.

dispensing 0.1 mL liquid into the mouth and allowing it to be comfortably swallowed. Figure 2 shows resulting total circulating antibody levels specific for influenza glycoproteins, as determined by ELISA. The data demonstrate that high circulating antibody titers can be achieved by simply drinking cochleate vaccines containing influenza virus glycoproteins. The response is boosted by repeated administration, and is dose related to the amount of glycoprotein used. Hemagglutination inhibition titers ranged from 28 to 160 (increasing with larger doses), indicating maintenance of the native viral glycoprotein conformation following formulation and oral administration.

These observations were confirmed and extended in a second study (Gould-Fogerite *et al.*, 1994). Vaccine was given at 0, 3, and 15 weeks, with the third immunization at one fourth the dose of the initial two. Circulating influenza glycoprotein-specific responses were detectable after a single administration for the top five doses, and for all groups (3.1 μg–100 μg dose range) after two feedings. All of the mice given the four highest doses, and four of five mice in the groups that received either 6- or 3-μg doses responded to the vaccine with circulating antibody titers ranging from 100 to 102,400. Control mice, which received no vaccine, had titers less than 50 for all mice at all time points. The antibody responses were long-lived. Titers remained the same or within one dilution for at least 13 weeks after the first or second boost (see Section 4).

2.4.3. ORAL IMMUNIZATION: PROTECTION FROM INTRANASAL CHALLENGE

In order to determine whether oral administration of this subunit vaccine affords protective immunity in the respiratory tract, mice were immunized with cochleates and then were challenged by intranasal application (while awake) of 2.5×10^9 particles of influenza virus at 1 week after the final boost. Three days after viral challenge, mice were sacrificed, and lungs (first experiment) or lungs and trachea (second experiment) were obtained. The entire lung or trachea was triturated and sonicated, and aliquots were injected into embryonated chicken eggs to allow amplification of any virus present. After 3 days at 37°C, allantoic fluid was obtained from individual eggs, and hemagglutination (HA) titers were performed. All five of the unvaccinated mice had sufficient virus in the trachea to infect the embryonated chicken eggs. In contrast, the oral vaccine provided a high degree of protection from viral replication in the trachea. Of the mice that received the five highest doses (100μg to 6.5μg), 22 out of 25 had no culturable virus in the trachea (Gould-Fogerite *et al.*, 1994). In the 3-μg dose group, 4 out of 5 were infected. The oral protein cochleate vaccine also provided protection against viral replication in the lungs. In the first experiment, 20 out of the 25 vaccinated mice were negative for virus when lung suspensions were cultured in embryonated chicken eggs. In the second experiment, all 20 mice that received the four highest doses of vaccine were negative for virus on culture (Gould-Fogerite *et al.*, 1994). The 3- and 6-μg dose groups had reduced viral burdens in the lungs when compared to the controls.

In contrast to these results, analogous experiments utilizing influenza polylactide polyglycolide microspheres required intramuscular priming to obtain significant circulating or mucosal responses, and resulted in reduction of viral burdens in the respiratory tract rather than protection from infection (Moldoveanu *et al.*, 1993). Hemagglutination inhibition titers generated by microspheres are also significantly lower, while corresponding ELISA titers were high. This probably indicates a loss of native HA glycoprotein conformation on exposure to the organic solvents involved in their formulation (Moldoveanu *et al.*, 1993). The physiologically gentle conditions and lack of antigen exposure to organic solvents are one of the advantages of cochleate vaccine formulation.

2.4.4. SINGLE ORAL OR INTRAMUSCULAR ADMINISTRATION: ANTIBODY AND PROLIFERATIVE RESPONSES

We have begun to investigate the role of route of administration and number of vaccinations on the kinetics, magnitude, and types of attendant humoral and cellular immune responses. A single peroral (drinking) or i.m. immunization containing 50 μg influenza glycoprotein cochleates was given to BALB/c mice. Antibody titers climbed over the following 5 months and consisted mostly of IgG (ELISA titer of 800 at 20 weeks). Comparable IgM, higher IgG levels (ELISA titer 3200 at 20 weeks), and a small amount of IgA at 20 weeks were also obtained following the single i.m. injection. These data demonstrate the potency and applicability of cochleate formulations to parenteral routes of immunization as well as oral (Kheiri *et al.*, 1994). Influenza-specific proliferative responses 2 weeks after a single oral or i.m. administration were also measured. Stimulation indexes of two- to threefold, when compared to a naive mouse, were obtained (Kheiri *et al.*, 1994).

2.4.5. SEVERAL IMMUNIZATIONS BY THE SAME ROUTE: ANTIBODY ISOTYPES AND CELL-MEDIATED RESPONSES

Mice were given three high-dose immunizations orally or intramuscularly at 0, 3, and 13 weeks (50, 50, and 12.5 μg of glycoproteins, respectively) (Table I). The oral route gave very strong circulating IgG titers (25,600 at 14 weeks). Intramuscular introduction gave higher circulating IgG levels at all time points (e.g., 204,800 at week 14). Three low-dose immunizations (6 μg at 0 and 3 weeks, 1.25 μg at 13 weeks) resulted in *higher* circulating

Table I

Serum Ig Isotypes in Mice following Immunization with Influenza Cochleates

Route of immunization	IgM	IgG	IgA
IM–low dose	1600	100,000	10
Oral–low dose	<100	800	40
IM–high dose	1600	204,800	10
Oral–high dose	400	25,600	640

antibody levels than the higher dose when given intramuscularly (102,400 and 51,200 respectively at week 20). In contrast, higher doses given orally gave higher circulating IgM, IgG, and IgA levels. Very significantly, and consistent with induction of immune responses at mucosal surfaces, the circulating IgA levels were much higher for oral than parenteral immunization (titer of 640 versus 10 at 14 weeks). Subtype analysis of serum from intramuscularly or orally immunized animals demonstrates the production of both IgG1 and IgG2a (Kheiri *et al.*, 1994).

Studies are in progress to determine the levels of IgG and IgA in saliva following single and multiple administrations of influenza cochleates by various routes. In initial studies, mice were boosted with 12.5 μg of glycoproteins in cochleates 1 year after a 50-μg priming immunization. Oral immunization with influenza glycoprotein cochleates lead to antigen-specific IgA in the saliva. In contrast, i.m. immunization resulted in the appearance of only IgG in the saliva, probably as a result of transudation from the circulation.

Antigen-specific proliferative responses in the spleen were quantitated from some mice at week 14 (Fig. 3). Very high stimulation indexes (up to 25-fold) were obtained with either oral or i.m. administration. Splenic cytolytic responses are also induced following i.m. or oral administration of influenza glycoprotein cochleates (Gould-Fogerite *et al.*, 1994).

2.4.6. EFFECTS OF ALTERNATE ROUTES OF PRIMING AND BOOSTING

In most vaccination systems studied, a combination of routes leads to superior immune responses and protection (Treanor *et al.*, 1992). In contrast to most subunit vaccines,

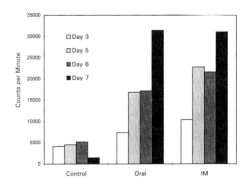

Figure 3. Splenocyte proliferation in mice following administration of influenza protein cochleates. Mice were immunized at weeks 0 and 3 with 50 μg of influenza protein cochleates. At week 13 they received 12.5 μg, and were sacrificed at week 14. Splenocytes were incubated in vitro with 16 μg/mL UV-inactivated influenza virus. Proliferation was determined by measuring the uptake of [^{3}H]-TdR into DNA.

cochleates containing glycoproteins from influenza (and parainfluenza type 1) do not require priming parenterally (Moldoveanu *et al.*, 1993). However, it is of interest to determine the effects of combining alternate routes of antigen presentation for considerations of basic understanding of the parameters regulating immune response induction as well as optimizing protective immunity. In parallel studies to the ones just described, mice were primed either orally or intramuscularly and then boosted twice by the alternate route. Three oral immunizations were superior to an i.m. prime followed by oral boosts, both in terms of antibody and proliferative responses. In contrast, an oral prime with i.m. boosts gave comparable circulating IgG titers and somewhat higher cellular responses than obtained with three i.m. doses. The amount of circulating IgA obtained was proportional to the number of oral immunizations given (Kheiri *et al.*, 1994).

It should be noted that no evidence of systemic tolerance following oral administration has been demonstrated using influenza cochleates. Indeed, slowly climbing antibody levels following single immunizations, higher responses with larger doses, and boosting of circulating antibody and proliferative responses following subsequent administrations (including oral prime with i.m. boosts) indicate that tolerance is not occurring with these antigenic formulations, at least at these doses and immunization regimens. In addition, while 50 μg was chosen for this particular series of studies, oral administration of 12.5 μg two times, followed by a 3-μg boost gave high circulating antibody responses and complete protection from influenza infection in the trachea and lungs following intranasal challenge (Fig. 2 and Sections 2.4.2 and 2.4.3 above). Regimens that induce oral tolerance usually require chronic dosing of larger quantities of antigen (Mestecky and McGhee, 1989; McGhee *et al.*, 1992). The particulate nature of cochleates and proteoliposomes may also favor immune response over induction of tolerance.

2.5. Parainfluenza Type 1: Immune Response to Cochleate Vaccines

2.5.1. PARAINFLUENZA TYPE 1: STRUCTURE, PATHOGENESIS, AND CURRENT VACCINE STATUS

Human parainfluenza virus type 1 (hPIV-1) is a major lower respiratory tract pathogen (Lyn *et al.*, 1991; Komoda *et al.*, 1992; Henrickson and Savatski, 1992). Its most severe clinical effects occur in infants and small children, with many cases resulting in hospitalization. There is currently no licensed vaccine available for hPIV-1. Sendai virus is the murine counterpart to hPIV-1, belonging to the same group within the paramyxovirus genus. Analysis of the nucleotide sequences of both viruses has revealed considerable amino acid similarities between them (HN 72%, F 68%, NP 81.3%, P 53%). hPIV-1 and Sendai have been reported to be antigenically similar as shown by cross-reactivity to polyclonal antisera (for references see Komoda *et al.*, 1992) although monoclonal antibody analysis suggests that they have a more limited antigenic similarity.

Sendai virus infections of mice have provided important insights into the pathogenesis of parainfluenza virus type 1 infections as well as into the correlates of protective immunity. Humoral responses to the envelope proteins, HN and F, and cytotoxic T-lymphocyte responses, especially to epitopes derived from NP, have been shown to interfere with the development of clinical symptoms. An evaluation of the immune response in mice to

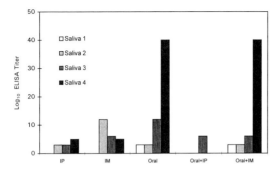

Figure 4. Sendai-specific salivary IgA induced by oral administration of Sendai protein cochleates. Mice were immunized as described in the text. Antibody titers were determined by ELISA against detergent-extracted Sendai envelopes.

Sendai antigens formulated into cochleate structures should provide important information toward the development of a subunit vaccine effective against hPIV-1 infections.

Using parainfluenza virus type 1 (Sendai) glycoproteins formulated as protein cochleates, results similar to our influenza virus studies have been obtained. These include the priming and boosting of the systemic and mucosal antibody responses, antibody isotypes induced, the induction of antigen-specific splenocyte proliferation, cytolytic activity, and long-term immunological memory.

2.5.2. ORAL IMMUNIZATION: MUCOSAL ANTIBODY RESPONSES

BALB/c mice were given Sendai glycoprotein-containing cochleates (50-μg dose) by a single route or two routes simultaneously. They were boosted using the same immunization protocol at 3 weeks. Saliva one was 1 week after the first immunization. Salivas two and three were 1 and 3 weeks after the second immunization, respectively. All mice were given cochleates by oral administration at 24 weeks. Saliva four was taken 1 week later. As can be seen in Fig. 4, the oral route and oral plus i.m. routes generated the highest Sendai glycoprotein-specific salivary IgA titers. The establishment of long-term immunological memory, with boosting to high mucosal antibody titers following oral immunization is of considerable significance and highly desired for protection against organisms invading through mucosal surfaces.

2.5.3. ORAL IMMUNIZATION: PEYER'S PATCH CELL PROLIFERATION AND ANTIBODY SECRETION

The ability to stimulate mucosal humoral and cell-mediated responses is crucial to a successful oral vaccine. Peyer's patch cells were obtained from cochleate-immunized mice (Fig. 5). It can be seen that, consistent with the mitogenic activity of Sendai virus glycoproteins, cells from a naive (unimmunized) mouse proliferate to some degree in response to UV-inactivated Sendai virus. The immunized animal, however, proliferated to a much greater degree. Also, Peyer's patches are larger and more plentiful in animals given protein cochleates orally than those seen in unimmunized animals. This indicates that the

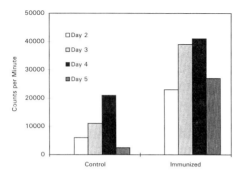

Figure 5. Peyer's patch lymphocyte proliferation in mice following oral administration of Sendai protein cochleates. Mice cochleates containing 50 μg of Sendai envelope proteins. They were sacrificed 2 weeks after the immunization and the Peyer's patches were obtained by cutting the surface of the small intestine. Isolated cells were incubated in vitro with UV-inactivated Sendai virus. Proliferation was determined by measuring the uptake of [^{3}H]-TdR into DNA.

protein cochleates survived the stomach to be taken up by the microfold (M) cells overlaying the Peyer's patches in the small intestine, were processed by antigen-presenting cells, and stimulated resident immune cells. Antigen-specific ELISpot assays of Peyer's patch cells indicate stimulation of large numbers of IgG and IgA Sendai-specific antibody-secreting cells following oral administration of Sendai cochleates (Edghill-Smith *et al.*, 1994a).

2.6. Human Immunodeficiency Virus: Immune Response to Cochleate Vaccines

2.6.1. HIV: IMMUNE RESPONSE, PATHOGENESIS, AND CURRENT VACCINE STATUS

The immune response to HIV has been studied extensively and intensively since the recognition of its association with the disease process known as AIDS. The interactions of HIV with the components of the immune system are extremely complex. Essentially all aspects of the immune system are affected, with eventual changes in hematopoiesis, immune reactivity, cytokines, immunoglobulin levels, and the hallmark of the disease, significant decreases in circulating CD4$^+$ T cells. Long-term infection generally leads to a profound immune suppression, accompanied by susceptibility to opportunistic infections and death. The antigen-specific immune responses against HIV include antibodies and T help and cytolytic activities directed against internal and external proteins. There is evidence for both humoral and cell-mediated responses contributing to control of the virus and having the potential for preventive or therapeutic effects. Neutralizing antibodies may be at least limiting viral replication and exerting selective pressure on the virus. There appears to be some correlation between the presence of high-titer neutralizing antibodies to the envelope glycoprotein of HIV and protection from infection with homologous free or cell-associated virus and reduction of virus load in chimpanzees (Berman *et al.*, 1990; Mannhalter *et al.*, 1991; Fultz *et al.*, 1992; Emmini *et al.*, 1992; Bruck *et al.*, 1994).

Cytolytic T-cell responses play an important role in control and recovery from many viral infections (Wells *et al.*, 1981; McMichael *et al.*, 1983). The evidence suggests this is also the case with HIV infection. The CD8$^+$ response precedes the specific antibody response and correlates temporally with the control of viremia in primary HIV-1 syndrome (Koup *et al.*, 1991, 1994). This is also the case with SIV infection of rhesus monkeys.

Anti-HIV activity of CD8$^+$ cells has also been correlated with the clinical state of the infected individual (Mackewicz *et al.,* 1991). The capability to stimulate CD8$^+$ responses to appropriate epitopes is probably an important requirement for optimal HIV prophylactic or therapeutic vaccines. The ability of our fusogenic lipid matrix-based vaccines to stimulate CD8$^+$ responses to peptides, glycoproteins, and even whole fixed viruses makes them attractive candidates for diseases where clearance of infected cells is important in protection and recovery. The current pandemic of HIV infection is spreading mainly via mucosal surfaces through sexual contact. Cellular and humoral mucosal immune responses have the potential to reduce the spread of HIV by contributing to the protection of HIV-negative individuals, and by reducing the amount of free and cell-associated virus present on mucosal surfaces and in secretions of infected individuals.

2.6.2. PEPTIDE COCHLEATES: ANTIBODY RESPONSES FOLLOWING ORAL OR INTRAMUSCULAR IMMUNIZATION

A peptide from the envelope glycoprotein of HIV-1 was covalently cross-linked to a phospholipid and incorporated into cochleates with or without Sendai glycoproteins (Table II). Following three oral administrations with cochleates containing only peptide, low levels of circulating antipeptide antibodies could be detected. However, antibodies to the peptide were much higher when the peptide was formulated with Sendai virus envelope proteins. This could be related to the ability of Sendai glycoproteins to bind to M cells and/or their adjuvanting effect on antigen presentation and processing. In more recent studies, humoral responses to the V3 loop of HIV gp160 have been obtained by formulation in cochleates and oral or i.m. administration (Edghill-Smith *et al.,* 1994b). The ability to stimulate circulating antibody responses to a peptide given orally represents a significant achievement for this new class of vaccines.

2.6.3. gp160 COCHLEATES: ANTIBODY, PROLIFERATIVE, AND CYTOTOXIC RESPONSES

We have begun to investigate the properties of cochleates containing vaccinia-expressed gp160. Our initial experiment involving a single i.m. administration of cochleates containing 35 µg of gp160 stimulated strong humoral (ELISA titer 1600 at 8 weeks), proliferative (stimulation index of 4 at 17 weeks), and cytolytic (60 to 70% specific kill at 17 weeks)

Table II
Serum Antibody Responses following Oral Administration of Cochleates Containing HIV gp120 Peptide 487-511 + Sendai Envelopes

Antigen	Naïve	487–511	Sendai	487–511 + Sendai
		Immunogen		
487–511	50^a	100	50	800
Sendai	50	50	3200	2400

^{a}ELISA titers.

responses. These responses are equivalent to or better than those obtained with a single administration of other subunit or live vector vaccines containing gp160.

In addition, protein cochleates containing both HIV gp160 and Sendai glycoproteins have been given orally to mice. Proliferative responses to Sendai and gp160 were obtained (stimulation indexes of four- to eightfold). Preliminary data indicate that cytolytic responses against the Sendai and gp160 were also generated.

3. FUSOGENIC PROTEOLIPOSOMES

3.1. Introduction

Current concepts regarding the mechanisms through which peptide epitopes are presented to CD8[+], MHC class I-restricted cytotoxic T lymphocytes indicate that a crucial aspect of this process is the capacity to introduce antigen into the cytoplasm (but not endosomes) of antigen-presenting cells (Allen, 1987). This phenomenon explains, at least in part, the success of live-attenuated and live-vector vaccines for stimulating cell-mediated immune responses. Our approach to investigating the structure–function relationship

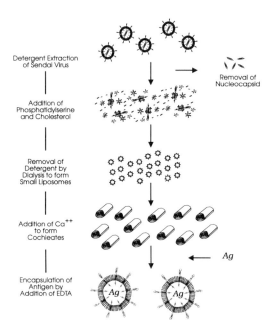

Figure 6. Encapsulation of antigen in fusogenic proteoliposomes. Protein cochleates are produced as described in Fig. 1. Removal of calcium (usually through chelation with EDTA) results in the unrolling of the cochleates and the spontaneous formation of large unilamellar vesicles. Material (such as antigen) present in the aqueous environment during the vesicle formation step is encapsulated within the aqueous interior of the proteoliposome.

between immunogens and their in vivo ability to elicit cytotoxic T-lymphocyte responses has been to formulate simple, well-defined structures that vary in their ability to introduce associated antigens directly into the cytoplasms of antigen-presenting cells.

3.2. Sendai Fusogenic Proteoliposomes

We have introduced methods for integrating biologically active membrane proteins into the lipid bilayer of large, mainly unilamellar liposomes (Gould-Fogerite and Mannino, 1985). These methods involve the formation of protein cochleates as precursor structures that are converted to proteoliposomes by addition of EDTA (Fig. 6). We have previously demonstrated that the glycoproteins of influenza and parainfluenza type 1 (Sendai) viruses maintain their biological activities of receptor binding and membrane fusion when reconstituted into protein lipid vesicles (proteoliposomes) using these methods (Gould-Fogerite et al., 1987, 1989). In addition, water-soluble materials can be encapsulated within the aqueous interior of the vesicles at high efficiency. We have also shown that these vesicles act as effective delivery vehicles for encapsulated drugs, proteins, and DNA. They were used to achieve the first stable gene transfer in animals via a liposome-based system (Gould-Fogerite et al., 1987, 1989).

Proteoliposomes produced by these methods are also highly effective immunogens in mice, rabbits, and monkeys (Miller et al., 1992; Canki et al., 1994). This includes the ability to stimulate strong $CD8^+$ cytotoxic T-cell responses (CTL) to lipid bilayer-integrated glycoproteins as well as encapsulated peptides, proteins, and whole formalin-fixed viruses (Miller et al., 1992; Canki et al., 1994; NIH comparative adjuvant study, unpublished). This ability probably arises from their membrane attachment and fusion activity which facilitates introduction into the cytoplasm and access to an MHC class I presentation pathway (Allen, 1987). The characteristics of physiologically gentle conditions of preparation, efficient protein reconstitution, maintenance of biological activity, and high encapsulation efficiency and capacity, make this a unique and attractive method for the preparation of protein lipid vesicles and vaccines.

3.2.1. FORMULATION

Methods for the formation of proteoliposomes from protein cochleates have been described in detail elsewhere (Gould-Fogerite and Mannino, 1992). Briefly, plain lipid or protein cochleates were pelleted by high-speed centrifugation. If material was to be encapsulated (e.g., peptides, proteins, or whole fixed viruses), it was added in a small volume of buffer to the dry pellet. Cochleates were converted to liposomes by addition of buffered EDTA. Alternatively, rotary dialysis or agarose plug diffusion may be used (Gould-Fogerite and Mannino, 1992).

3.2.2. SIV: INDUCTION OF $CD8^+$ CTLs

In our initial studies performed in collaboration with Drs. Michael Miller and Norman Letvin, a 12-amino-acid peptide (11C) representing a CTL epitope from the SIV gag protein was encapsulated within nonfusogenic phosphatidylserine–cholesterol liposomes. No detectable cytolytic responses were generated following three i.m. immunizations of rhesus

Table III
CTL-Inducing Activity of Peptides

Peptide	Membrane-perturbing activity	CTL induction[a]	
		Lipid	Lipid + Sendai
SIV gag 11C	–	5%	30%
10-mer	–	10%	70%
15-mer	–	7%	65%
GG-15-mer	+	32%	63%
V3 loop	+	43%	59%

[a] % specific lysis at a 100:1 effector-to-target ratio.

monkeys. Subsequently, when the peptide was encapsulated within fusogenic Sendai proteoliposomes, the monkeys developed a strong CD8$^+$ cell-mediated, MHC class I-restricted CTL response after a single i.m. immunization (Table III and Miller *et al.*, 1992). In a separate study, as part of an NIH-sponsored comparative adjuvant trial, formalin-fixed SIV was encapsulated within Sendai proteoliposomes and given to eight rhesus monkeys by i.m. immunization. No negative local or systemic side effects were observed. Strong proliferative and cytoxic T-cell responses, and low-titer neutralizing antibodies were obtained.

3.2.3. HIV: INDUCTION OF CD8$^+$ CYTOLYTIC RESPONSES

In more recent studies, performed in our laboratory, peptides from regions of the V3 loop of HIV III B have been formulated into either plain lipid-based complexes or lipid complexes containing Sendai virus surface glycoproteins (F and HN). The results of these studies demonstrate strong antigen-specific CTL responses which are MHC class I-restricted and are CD8$^+$. All CTL responses were specific to peptide-pulsed targets, as well as 3T3 cells transfected with a plasmid expressing gp160. Induction of helper T lymphocytes was also demonstrated as indicated by proliferative responses (Canki *et al.*, 1994).

Some peptide–lipid complexes were less immunogenic, however. We attribute this to the properties of the peptides. Peptides that are not disruptive to the membrane bilayer of the liposome do not induce CD8$^+$ CTLs when formulated in plain liposomes. These peptides can be enhanced to optimal levels, however, by the addition of Sendai virus envelope binding and fusion proteins to the formulation (Table III).

3.2.4. PARAMETERS REGULATING CYTOLYTIC RESPONSE INDUCTION

Our laboratory's hypothesis that immunogens that contain membrane-perturbing characteristics, related to the presence either of viral fusion proteins, or of amphipathic (detergentlike) peptides, is substantiated by the work of others. Comparing the physical and chemical nature of our formulations with those from other laboratories that have reported the use of subunit preparations to induce CD8$^+$ CTLs, leads us to propose that a

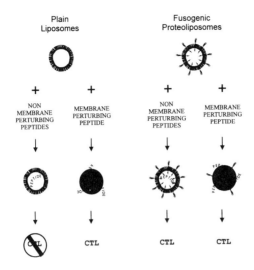

Figure 7. Properties of peptide–lipid complexes that induce CD8$^+$, MHC class I-restricted cytotoxic T lymphocytes. (Left) Plain liposomes are capable of inducing CTL responses only if the peptide/CTL epitope has membrane-perturbing characteristics. Non-membrane-perturbing epitopes are efficiently encapsulated but do not elicit CD8$^+$ CTL responses. (Right) Integration of fusogenic viral glycoproteins (e.g., Sendai virus F and HN proteins) onto plain liposomes induces strong CTL responses to otherwise nonimmunogenic peptides (non-membrane-perturbing) as well as immunogenic peptides (membrane-perturbing).

minimal immunogenic formulation capable of eliciting CD8$^+$, MHC class I-restricted CTLs includes: (1) a peptide that represents a MHC class I epitope, (2) a component that enhances the affinity of the immunogen for MHC class I-positive antigen-presenting cells, and (3) properties that can compromise the integrity of a lipid bilayer, facilitating delivery of the antigen directly into the cytoplasm and the class I presentation pathway. This hypothesis is illustrated in Fig. 7.

4. UNIQUE COVALENT PEPTIDE–PHOSPHOLIPID COMPLEXES

4.1. Introduction

The most significant impediment to the use of synthetic peptides as vaccines has been that they are only weakly or nonimmunogenic when injected by themselves into animals (Morein and Simons, 1985; Muller *et al.,* 1982). This property has necessitated the use of carriers, usually large, highly "immunogenic" proteins, to which the peptides are covalently coupled. These carriers, although helpful in producing an initial antibody response, have no relationship to the pathogen against which the vaccine is designed and therefore do not elicit pathogen-specific T-cell help. Therefore, when an individual who has been vaccinated with a peptide–carrier complex is challenged with the pathogen, a primary, rather than a secondary (faster, stronger), response results. Also, boosting immunizations often lead to a larger antibody response to the carrier and a diminishing one to the peptide. In addition, these peptide–carrier complexes must usually be combined with other adjuvants (e.g., Freund's) to enhance the response to the peptide. These adjuvants frequently induce undesirable side effects that make them unacceptable for use in humans.

We hypothesized that anchorage of a peptide in the liposomal bilayer might mimic the normal presentation of antigen on an infectious agent (i.e., multivalent and projecting outward from an anchor on the surface of the cell) and thereby potentiate the immune response to the peptide. To test this hypothesis, peptides were covalently linked to a phospholipid, providing a hydrophobic anchorage into the phospholipid bilayer.

We found that when molecules capable of stimulating helper T cells (either viral envelope proteins or peptides representing Th cell epitopes) are integrated into the same phospholipid matrix as a B-cell epitope, a highly efficient immunogen is produced. Sequences that are not recognized by T helper cells do not elicit antibody responses even when formulated into peptide–phospholipid complexes. Antibody production is observed solely through inoculation of peptides conjugated to phospholipids. No carrier proteins or additional adjuvants are required to stimulate antibody production. Furthermore, we have observed no immune response directed against the phospholipids (Goodman-Snitkoff *et al.*, 1988, 1990, 1991).

4.2. Formulation

The procedure for covalently coupling peptides to phosphatidylethanolamine is summarized in Fig. 8 and described in detail elsewhere (Mannino *et al.*, 1992). All peptides are synthesized with either an N-terminal or C-terminal cysteine.

4.3. Stimulation of an Immune Response to Hydrophilic B-Cell Determinants through an Association with Putative Th-Cell Determinants

4.3.1. EFFECT OF ADDITION OF NONCOVALENTLY LINKED Th-CELL EPITOPES

Humoral responses to a B-cell epitope were determined for complexes containing Th- and B-cell determinants not covalently linked, but placed in the same lipid matrix (Table IV). In these studies we used the B-cell epitope $(NANP)_n$ from the circumsporozoite of *Plasmodium falciparum*. To stimulate T-helper cells we used either the highly immunogenic envelope glycoproteins of Sendai virus, or the malaria Th-cell epitope Th2R, which was identified by the AMPHI computer program (Good *et al.*, 1987) and its role as a Th-cell epitope confirmed experimentally (Good *et al.*, 1987, 1988).

Using different immunizing procedures, other workers have shown that the response of mice to $NP(NANP)_5NA$ is under genetic control (Del Giudice *et al.*, 1986; Togna *et al.*, 1986; Good *et al.*, 1986). Immunization with our peptide–phospholipid complexes (in the absence of additional carrier proteins or adjuvants) results in the same genetic restriction observed by others. C57.Bl (H-2b) mice mount a significant antibody response, whereas B10.BR (H-2K) and B10.D2 (H-2d) mice do not make antibodies to $NP(NANP)_5NA$ when it is inoculated alone.

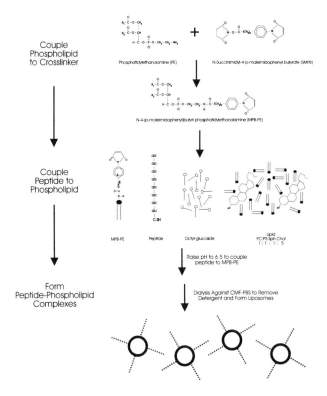

Figure 8. Outline of the procedure for the preparation of covalent peptide–phospholipid complexes. A heterobifunctional cross-linking reagent [in this protocol succinimidyl-4-(*p*-maleimidophenyl) butyrate is used] is coupled to phosphatidylethanolamine (PE), producing MPE-PE. A peptide containing a reduced cysteine is mixed with MPB-PE and additional lipids solubilized in octylglucoside-containing buffer at pH 4.5. The pH is raised to 6.5 and the solution reacts overnight at room temperature. The solution is dialyzed, resulting in the loss of detergent and the spontaneous formation of peptide–lipid complexes.

Table IV
T-Helper-Cell Epitopes Are Required for Induction of Antipeptide B-Cell Responses

	Mouse strain		
Antigen	B10.BR	B10.D2	C57.Bl
NANP	<100[a]	<100	51,200
NANP + Sendai	25,600	1600	12,800
NANP + Th2R	12,800	6400	3,200

[a]ELISA titer.

4.3.1.1. Sendai Glycoproteins as Adjuvants

Exogenous T-cell help was added to NP(NANP)₅NA by incorporating trace amounts of Sendai virus glycoproteins into the peptide–phospholipid complex. Sendai virus glycoproteins are highly immunogenic and can stimulate both B and Th lymphocytes (El Guink *et al.,* 1989; Edghill-Smith *et al.,* 1994a, 1994b). These glycoproteins, included at 1/200th of their concentration in the viral envelope, could enhance the antibody production to NP(NANP)₅ NA in B10.BR and B10.D2 mice, but did not enhance the antibody response of C57.Bl mice. Thus, Sendai envelopes can induce T-cell help resulting in antibody production to NP(NANP)₅NA in mouse strains in which NP(NANP)₅NA is not immunogenic on its own. We have also utilized Sendai glycoproteins to enhance antibody, T help, and cytolytic responses to other peptides, proteins, and even whole fixed viruses.

4.3.1.2. Use of Endogenous T-Helper Peptides

When immunized with NP(NANP)₅NA-PE and Th2R-PE in the same peptide–phospholipid complex, all of the mouse strains tested made antibodies to both epitopes. In B10.BR and B10.D2 mice the antibody response to NP(NANP)₅NA was significantly greater than that in mice immunized only with NP(NANP)₅NA. In contrast, when C57.Bl mice are immunized with NP(NANP)₅NA and Th2R together, the response to NP(NANP)₅NA is less and the response to Th2R is greater than when either is inoculated alone. It appears that in B10.BR and B10D2 mice the Th2R acts as a Th epitope for the production of antibodies to NP(NANP)₅NA, while in C57.Bl mice the NP(NANP)₅NA acts as a Th epitope to enhance the production of antibodies to Th2R.

4.3.2. EFFECT OF CONTIGUOUS SYNTHESIS OF NONIMMUNOGENIC PEPTIDE WITH IMMUNOGENIC PEPTIDES

To test whether high levels of antibody may be obtained when putative B- and Th-cell determinants are present in the same peptide, a single peptide was synthesized that consisted of the nonimmunogenic peptides HIV 476-492 and/or 507-518 together with HIV 494-506, a putative T-helper epitope. The peptides were then cross-linked to PE, complexed with additional phospholipids, and used to immunize mice as described above. Antisera were produced by immunizing mice with HIV 494-518 peptide–phospholipid complexes or HIV 476-518 peptide–phospholipid complexes. Antibodies were identified (by ELISA) that were reactive with peptides describing HIV 476-492, 476-518, 494-518, and 507-518. In contrast, when mice were immunized with HIV 476-492 peptide–phospholipid complexes or HIV 507-518 peptide–phospholipid complexes, no antibodies were detected. It appears that antibodies to the nonimmunogenic peptides could be produced when T-cell help was supplied by the HIV 494-506 region (Goodman-Snitkoff *et al.,* 1988, 1990, 1991).

5. SUMMARY

For more than a decade our laboratories have been combining concepts in biochemistry, virology, and immunology in order to develop a conceptual basis for vaccine design.

Our long-term goals have been to construct simple and well-defined immunogens that would stimulate specific immune responses in vivo. Using this approach, we hypothesized that it should be possible to define the structural and biochemical parameters of an immunogen that are necessary and sufficient to stimulate designated effector arms of the immune system.

Through the use of covalently coupled peptide complexes, we have been able to define minimal requirements for the induction of humoral immune responses (Mannino *et al.,* 1992). This represents a significant advance in eliciting an immune response to peptides, because it requires only peptides and phospholipids in the absence of additional adjuvants. It is different from the previous use of peptides and liposomes since here the peptides are covalently linked to a hydrophobic anchor and integrated into the phospholipid complex, rather than passively adsorbed or encapsulated. The presentation of peptide as part of a peptide–phospholipid complex (in contrast to encapsulation or nonspecific absorption) may be more similar to the natural presentation of an epitope in the context of an in vivo antigenic challenge. This technology also allows us to incorporate B and Th epitopes in a number of forms—as a single peptide, as two peptides in the same liposome, or as a peptide with viral glycoproteins in the same liposome. These data also demonstrate that Th epitopes do not have to be covalently linked to the B-cell epitope in order to provide help for that epitope. The implications of the data reported here are significant for both basic science and applied technologies. In basic science, the peptide–phospholipid complexes are potentially useful for analyzing the cooperative effects of B- and T-cell epitopes in the in vivo immune response. Since the peptide–phospholipid complexes are totally synthetic and highly immunogenic, they may be constructed in any formulation required to answer questions on the roles of B and T cells in promoting an immune response. Furthermore, since the number of antigenic sites is limited only by the number of peptides included in the peptide–phospholipid complexes, these constructs may be useful in producing antisera or monoclonal antibodies to weakly antigenic regions of a large protein, since the lack of antigenic competition should enhance the immunogenicity of these regions. Clinically, this technology will expand the potential for subunit vaccines. The use of T- and B-cell epitopes from a single pathogen in a highly immunogenic peptide–phospholipid complex will bypass the requirement for carrier proteins which lack homology with the pathogen. Additionally, since these constructs contain B and Th epitopes from the infectious pathogen, they will prime the organism for a secondary response to the pathogen, rather than simply provide immunity for a single encounter.

Minimal requirements for the induction of $CD8^+$, MHC class I-restricted CTLs have been defined through the use of fusogenic proteoliposomes and simple peptide–lipid complexes (Miller *et al.,* 1992; Canki *et al.,* 1994). Using these concepts we have been able to formulate safe and highly efficacious subunit vaccine preparations that elicit vigorous helper and cytolytic immune responses in the absence of other adjuvants or immunopotentiating agents. These structures have great promise in contributing toward the search for effective preventive and therapeutic human vaccines.

Finally, we have described a unique, highly stable, lyophilizable, lipid-based vaccine carrier and delivery formulation called protein cochleates. Oral immunization with cochleates containing only viral glycoproteins and pure nontoxic, noninflammatory phospholipids stimulates strong, long-lasting circulating and mucosal antibody responses. A single oral dose of protein cochleates results in slowly increasing circulating antibody titers over several months. High salivary IgA levels are detected, and high circulating antibody titers including IgM, IgG (IgG1 and IgG2a), and IgA are maintained for many months following two or three oral administrations. These data indicate the possibility of persistence and slow release of antigen. Strong proliferative responses in Peyer's patches and spleen, and cytolytic responses (spleen) are also generated following one and boosted by several doses. In the mouse model for influenza, these vaccines protect against infection following mucosal challenge. Intramuscular immunizations have resulted in strong, long-lasting, antibody, proliferative, and cytotoxic responses in a number of systems. Protein cochleates are safe, highly defined, and flexible in terms of antigenic content. They can be utilized as tools to understand pathogenesis and immune response induction. They also hold great promise for use as preventative and therapeutic vaccines. In mouse models for HIV, influenza, and parainfluenza virus type 1, cochleate-based vaccines have proven to be safe and highly efficacious. Their unique structural properties make cochleates far more stable than standard liposome formulations. This includes the ability to be lyophilized and stored at room temperature for months and be reconstituted by the addition of liquid prior to use. The ability of cochleates to prime and boost immune responses following oral administration adds significantly to their potential utility as human vaccines. Efforts have been initiated to test safety and immunogenicity of protein cochleates in human clinical trials.

Using more classical liposome-based systems, we have made substantial progress toward understanding how the structural and biochemical properties of immunogens are related to their in vivo immune responses. In parallel studies, we have demonstrated the extraordinary properties of an insoluble, stable, nonliposome, lipid matrix-based antigen carrier and delivery system, the protein cochleate. Our current focus is to combine these concepts and structures to the preparation of subunit vaccines for humans.

ACKNOWLEDGMENTS

We gratefully acknowledge the theoretical and technical contributions of Mario Canki, Kumud Das, Yvette Edghill-Smith, Leslie Eisele, Dr. Eleanora Feketeova, Dr. Gail Goodman-Snitkoff, Masoumeh Kheiri, and Zheng Wang. This work has been supported in part by grants from the NIH, Division of AIDS, and IGI, Inc.

REFERENCES

Allen, P. M., 1987, Antigen processing at the molecular level, *Immunol. Today* **8**:270–273.
American Academy of Pediatrics, 1991, Cholera. Report of the Committee on Infectious Diseases, American Academy of Pediatrics, Elk Grove Village, IL, p. 170–177.
Bergmann, K.-C., and Waldman, R. H., 1988, Stimulation of secretory antibody following oral administration of antigen, *Rev. Infect. Dis.* **10**:939–950.
Berman, P. W., Gregory, T. J., Riddle, L., Nakamura, G. R., Champo, M. A., Porter, J. P., Wurm, F., Hershberg, R. D., Cobbs, E. K., and Eichberg, J. W., 1990. Protection of chimpanzees from infection by HIV-1 after vaccination with recombinant glycoprotein gp120 but not gp160, *Nature* **345**:622–625.
Brandtzaeg, P., 1989, Overview of the mucosal immune system, *Curr. Top. Microbiol. Immunol.* **146**:13–25.

Bruck, C., Thiriart, C., Fabry, L., Fracotte, M., Pala, P., van Opstal, D., Culp, J., Rosenberg, M., DeWild, M., Heidt, P., 1994, HIV-1 neutralizing antibody titers induced by vaccination correlate with protection from infection and decreased virus load in chimpanzees (abstract), *Vaccine* **12**:1141–1148.

Canki, M., Gould-Fogerite, S., and Mannino, R. J., 1994, Induction of HIV specific CD8[+] cytolytic T cells with peptide subunit vaccines, *J. Exp. Med.* (submitted).

Conner, M. E., Crawford, S. E., Barone, C., and Estes, M. K., 1993, Rotavirus vaccine administered parenterally induces protective immunity, *J. Virol.* **67**:6633–6641.

Cui, Z.-D., Tristram, D., LaScolea, L. J., Kwiatkowski, T., Jr., Kospti, S., and Ogra, P. L., 1991, Induction to antibody response to Chlamydia trachomatis in the genital tract by oral administration, *Infect. Immun.* **59**:1465–1469.

Dahlgren, U., Carlsson, B., Jalil, F., MacDonald, R., Mascart-Lemone, F., Nilsson, K., Robertson, D., Sennhauser, F., Wold, A., and Hanson, L. A., 1989, Induction of the mucosal immune response, *Curr. Top. Microbiol. Immunol.* **146**:155–160.

Del Giudice, G., Cooper, J. A., Merino, J., Verdini, A. S., Pessi, A., Togna, A. R., Engers, H. D., Corradin, G., and Lambert, P. H., 1986, The antibody response in mice to carrier-free synthetic polymers of Plasmodium falciparum circumsporozoite repetitive epitope is 1-Ab-restricted: Possible implications for malaria vaccines, *J. Immunol.* **137**:2952–2955.

Edghill-Smith,Y., Feketeova, E., Wang, Z., Mannino, R. J., and Gould-Fogerite, S., 1994a, A new type of subunit vaccine induces mucosal and systemic responses to parainfluenza type I virus, *J. Inf. Dis.* (submitted).

Edghill-Smith, Y., Gould-Fogerite, S., and Mannino, R. J., 1994b, HIV subunit protein and peptide cochleate vaccines, *Science* (submitted).

El Guink, N., Kris, R., Goodman-Snitkoff, G. W., Small, P. A., and Mannino, R. J., 1989, Intranasal immunization with proteoliposomes protects against influenza, *Vaccine* **7**:147–151.

Emmini, E. A., Schleif, W. A., Nunberg, J. H., Conlay, A. J., Eda, Y., Tokiyoshi, S., Putney, S. D., Matsushita, S., Cobb, K. E., Jett, C. M., Eichberg, J. W., and Murthy, K. K., 1992, Prevention of HIV-1 infection in chimpanzees by gp120 V3 domain-specific monoclonal antibody, *Nature* **355**:728–730.

Faden, H., Modlin, J. F., Thomas, M. L., McBean, A. M., Ferdon, M. B., and Ogra, P. L., 1990, Comparative evaluation of immunization with live attenuated and enhanced-potency inactivated trivalent poliovirus vaccines in childhood: Systemic and local immune responses, *J. Infect. Dis.* **162**:1291–1297.

Formal, S. B., Maenza, R. M., Austin, S., and LaBrec, E. H., 1967, Failure of parenteral vaccines to protect monkeys against experimental shigellosis, *Proc. Soc. Exp. Biol. Med.* **125**:347–349.

Fultz, P. N., Nara, P. Barre-Sinoussi, F. Chaput, A., Greenberg, M. L., Muchmore, E., Kieny, M. P., and Girard, M., 1992, Vaccine protection of chimpanzees challenged with HIV-1 infected peripheral blood mononuclear cells, *Science* **256**:1687–1690.

Good, M. F., Berzofsky, J. A., Maloy, W. L., Hayashi, Y., Fujii, N., Hockmeyer, W. T., and Miller, L. H., 1986, Genetic control of the immune response in mice to a Plasmodium falciparum sporozoite vaccine. Widespread nonresponsiveness to a single malaria T epitope in highly repetitive vaccine, *J. Exp. Med.* **164**:655–660.

Good, M. F., Malloy, W. L., Lunde, M. N., Margalit, H., Cornette, J. L., Smith, G. L., Moss, B., Miller, L. H., and Berzofsky, J. A., 1987, Construction of synthetic immunogen: Use of new T-helper epitope on malaria circumsporozoite protein, *Science* **235**:1059–1062.

Good, M. F. B., Berzofsky, J. A., and Miller, L. H., 1988, The T cell response to the malaria circumsporozoite protein: An immunological approach to vaccine development, *Annu. Rev. Immunol.* **6**:663–688.

Goodman-Snitkoff, G., Heimer, E., Danho, W., Felix, A., and Mannino, R. J., 1988, Induction of antibody production to synthetic peptides via peptide–phospholipid complexes, in: *Technological Advances in Vaccine Development*, Liss, New York, pp. 335–344.

Goodman-Snitkoff, G., Eisele, L. E., Heimer, E. P., Felix, A. M., Andersen, T. T., Fuerst, T. R., and Mannino, R. J., 1990, Defining minimal requirements for antibody production to peptide antigens, *Vaccine* **8**:257–262.

Goodman-Snitkoff, G., Good, M., Berzofsky, J., and Mannino, R. J., 1991, Role of intrastructural/intermolecular help in immunization with peptide–phospholipid complexes, *J. Immunol.* **147**:410–415.

Gould-Fogerite, S., Edghill-Smith, Y., Kheiri, M., Wang, Z., Das, K., Fedeteova, E., Canki, M., and Mannino, R. J., 1994a, Lipid matrix-based subunit vaccines: A structure-function approach to oral and parenteral immunization, *AIDS Res. Hum. Retroviruses* **10**, (suppl. 2): pp. 99–103.

Gould-Fogerite, S., and Mannino, R. J., 1985, Rotary dialysis: Its application to the production of large liposomes and large proteoliposomes (protein–lipid vesicles) with high encapsulation efficiency and efficient reconstitution of membrane proteins, *Anal. Biochem.* **148**:15–25.

Gould-Fogerite, S., and Mannino, R. J., 1992, Targeted fusogenic liposomes: Functional reconstitution of membrane proteins into large unilamellar vesicles via protein-cochleate intermediates, in: *Liposome Technology*, 2nd ed., Vol. III (G. Gregoriadis, ed.), CRC Press, Boca Raton, pp. 262–275.

Gould-Fogerite, S., Mazurkiewicz, J. E., Bhisitkul, D., and Mannino, R. J., 1987, The reconstitution of biologically active glycoproteins into large liposomes: Use as a delivery vehicle to animal cells, in: *Advances in Membrane Biochemistry and Bioenergetics* (C. H. Kim, T. Tedeschi, J. J. Diwan, and J.C. Salerno, eds.), Plenum Press, New York, pp. 569–586.

Gould-Fogerite, S., Mazurkiewicz, J., Lehman, J., Raska, K., Jr., Voelkerding, K., and Mannino, R. J., 1989, Chimerasome-mediated gene transfer in vitro and in vivo, *Gene* **84**:429–438.

Gould-Fogerite, S., Kheiri, M., Edghill-Smith, Y., Das, K. D., Wang, Z., Feketeova, E., and Mannino, R. J., 1994, Orally delivered protein cochleate vaccines stimulate mucosal and circulating immunity and protection from mucosal challenge with live influenza virus, *Science* (submitted).

Gregoriadis, G., 1990, Immunological adjuvants: A role for liposomes, *Immunol. Today* **11**:89–97.

Henrickson, K. J., and Savatski, L. L., 1992, Genetic variation and evolution of human parainfluenza virus type 1 hemagglutinin neuraminidase: Analysis of 12 clinical isolates, *J. Infect. Dis.* **166**:995–1005.

Holmgren, J., 1991, Mucosal immunity and vaccination, *FEMS Microbiol. Immunol.* **4**:1–18.

Horre, D., and Hackett, J., 1989, Vaccination against enteric bacterial diseases, *Rev. Infect. Dis.* **11**:853–877.

Kheiri, M., Feketeova, E., Mannino, R. J., and Gould-Fogerite, S., 1994, Mucosal and systemic responses to influenza glycoproteins in protein cochleates, *J. Immunol.* (submitted).

Komoda, H., Kusagawa, S., Orvell, C., Tsurudome, M., Nishio, M., Bando, H., Kawano, M., Norby, E., and Ito, Y., 1992, Antigenic diversity of human parainfluenza type 1 isolates and their immunological relationship with Sendai virus revealed by using monoclonal antibodies, *J. Gen. Virol.* **73**:875–884.

Koup, R. A., Pikora, C. A., Mazzara, G., Panicati, D., and Sullivan, J. L., 1991, Broadly reactive antibody-dependent cellular cytotoxic response to HIV-1 envelope glycoproteins precedes broad neutralizing response in human infection, *Viral Immunol.* **4**:215–223.

Lyn, D., Gill, D. S., Scroggs, R. A., and Portner, A., 1991, The nucleoproteins of human parainfluenza virus type 1 and Sendai virus share amino acid sequences and antigenic and structural determinants, *J. Gen. Virol.* **72**:983–987.

McGhee, J. R., Mestecky, J., Dertzbaugh, M. T., Eldridge, J. H., Hirasawa, M., and Kiyono, H., 1992, The mucosal immune system: From fundamental concepts to vaccine development, *Vaccine* **10**:75–88.

Mackewicz, C. E., Ortega, H. W., and Levy, J. A., 1991, $CD8^+$ cell anti-HIV activity correlates with the clinical state of the infected individual, *J. Clin. Invest.* **87**:1462–1466.

McMichael, A. J., Gotch, F. M., Noble, G. R., and Beare, P. A. S., 1983, Cytotoxic T-cell immunity to influenza, *N. Engl. J. Med.* **309**:13–17.

Mannhalter, J. W., Pum, M., Wolf, H. M., Kupcu, Z., Barrett, N., Dorner, F., Eder, G., and Eibl, M. M., 1991, Immunization of chimpanzees with the HIV-1 glycoprotein gp 160 induces long-lasting T-cell memory, *AIDS Res. Hum. Retroviruses* **7**:485–493.

Mannino, R. J., and Gould-Fogerite, S., 1988, Liposome mediated gene transfer, *Biotechniques* **6**:682–690.

Mannino, R. J., Gould-Fogerite, S., and Goodman-Snitkoff, G., 1992, Liposomes as adjuvants for peptides: Preparation and use of immunogenic peptide–phospholipid complexes, in: *Liposome Technology*, 2nd ed., Vol. II (G. Gregoriadis, ed.), CRC Press, Boca Raton, pp. 168–183.

Mestecky, J., and McGhee, J. R., 1989, Oral immunization: Past and present, *Curr. Top. Microbiol. Immunol.* **146**:3–11.

Michetti, P., Mahan, M. J., Slauch, J. M., Mekalanos, J. J., and Neutra, M. R., 1992, Monoclonal secretory immunoglobulin A protects mice against oral challenge with the invasive pathogen Salmonella typhimurium, *Infect. Immun.* **60**:1786–1792.

Miller, M. D., Gould-Fogerite, S., Shen, L., Woods, R. M., Koenig, S., Mannino, R. J., and Letvin, N., 1992, Vaccination of rhesus monkeys with synthetic peptide in a fusogenic proteoliposome elicits simian immunodeficiency virus-specific CD8[+] cytotoxic T lymphocytes, *J. Exp. Med.* **176**:1739–1744.

Moldoveanu, Z., Novak, M., Huang, W.-Q., Gilley, R. M., Staas, J. K., Schafter, D., Compans, R. W., and Mestecky, J., 1993, Oral immunization with influenza virus in biodegradable microspheres, *J. Infect. Dis.* **167**:84–90.

Morein, B., and Simons, K., 1985, Subunit vaccines against enveloped viruses: Virosomes, micelles and other protein complexes, *Vaccine* **3**:83–94.

Muller, G. M., Shapira, M., and Arnon, R., 1982, Anti-influenza response achieved by immunization with a synthetic conjugate, *Proc. Natl. Acad. Sci. USA* **79**:569–573.

Robbins, J. B., Chu, C., and Schneerson, R., 1992, Hypothesis for vaccine development: Protective immunity to enteric diseases caused by non-typhoidal salmonellae and shigellae may be conferred by serum IgG antibodies to the O-specific polysaccharide of their lipopolysaccharrides, *Clin. Infect. Dis.* **15**:346–361.

Safrit, J. T., Andrews, C. A., Zhu, T., Ho, D. D., and Koup, R. A., 1994, Characterization of human immunodeficiency virus type 1-specific cytotozic T lymphocyte clones isolated during acute seroconversion: Recognition of autologous virus sequences within a conserved immunodominant epitope, *J. Exp. Med.* **179**:463–472.

Togna, A. R., Del Giudice, G., Verdini, A. S., Bonelli, F., Pessi, A., Engers, H. D., and Corradin, G., 1986, Synthetic Plasmodium falciparum circumsporozoite peptides elicit heterogenous L3T4[+] T cell proliferative responses in H-2b mice, *J. Immunol.* **137**:2956–2960.

Treanor, J. J., Mattison, H. R., Dumyati, G., Yinnon, A., Erb, S., O'Brien, D., Dolin, R., Betts, R., and Betts, R. F., 1992, Protective efficacy of combined live intranasal and inactivated influenza A virus vaccines in the elderly, *Ann. Intern. Med.* **117**:625–633.

Walker, M. J., Rohde, M., Timmis, K. N., and Guzman, C. A., 1992, Specific lung mucosal and systemic immune responses after oral immunization of mice with Salmonella typhimurium aro A, Salmonella typhi Ty21a, and invasive Escherichia coli expressing recombinant pertussis toxin S1 subunit, *Infect. Immun.* **60**:4260–4268.

Webster, R. G., and Rott, R., 1987, Influenza virus A pathogenicity: The pivotal role of hemagglutinin, *Cell* **50**:665–666.

Wells, M. A., Ennis, F. A., and Albrecht, P., 1981, Recovery from a viral respiratory tract infection. II. Passive transfer of immune spleen cells to mice with influenza pneumonia, *J. Immunol.* **126**:1042–1046.

Wilson, J. A., and Cox, N. J., 1990, Structural basis of immune recognition of influenza virus hemagglutinin, *Annu. Rev. Immunol.* **8**:737–771.

Wiluz, D. L., Wilson, J. A., and Skehel, J. J., 1981, Structural identification of the antibody binding sites of Hong Kong influenza virus hemagglutinin and their involvement in antigenic variation, *Nature* **289**:373–378.

Yap, K. L., Ada, G. L., and McKenzie, I. P. C., 1978, Transfer of specific cytotoxic T lymphocytes protect mice inoculated with influenza virus, *Nature* **273**:238–239.

Chapter 16

Polymer Microspheres for Vaccine Delivery

Justin Hanes, Masatoshi Chiba, and Robert Langer

1. INTRODUCTION

Every year millions of people, particularly children, die of diseases for which a vaccine exists (Walsh, 1988; Warren, 1989). Countless others are left blinded, mentally retarded, or severely crippled. The problem is most significant in developing countries where access to health care is poor. In these countries, it is estimated that more than half of the children who receive primary vaccinations do not complete their required booster immunization schedule (Aguado, 1993; Bloom, 1989). These children are left unprotected, accounting for the enormous number of reported deaths.

Because of the complexities of developing safe whole-killed or attenuated vaccines, and because of advances in biotechnology, many future vaccines will likely be peptide or protein subunits made by chemical synthesis or recombinant DNA technology. Subunit vaccines are chemically well-defined, compared to classical vaccines, resulting in safe and reproducible vaccination. However, subunit vaccines are often poorly immunogenic, and therefore require several boosters in order to fully protect the vaccinated individual. As a result, in order to make mass immunization programs effective and economically feasible, stronger adjuvants are needed to reduce the number of shots required for effective immunization.

Controlled release antigen delivery systems offer an exciting addition to existing adjuvants for vaccination (Bloom, 1989; Gibbons, 1992; Langer, 1990). In fact, the investigation of controlled release formulations for vaccine delivery is a top priority of the World Health Organization because of their potential for reducing the number of injections required for successful vaccination. These systems slowly leak antigen into the tissues of a vaccinated individual while simultaneously serving as a repository for unreleased antigen, a phenomenon known as the depot theory of adjuvant action (Freund, 1956; Glenny *et al.*, 1931). Although the modes of action of adjuvants are not completely

Justin Hanes, Masatoshi Chiba, and Robert Langer • Department of Chemical Engineering, Massachusetts Institute of Technology, Cambridge, Massachusetts 02139: Present address of M. C.: Pharmaceutical Development Laboratory, Mitsubishi Kasei Corporation, Kashima-gun, Ibaraki 314-02, Japan.

Vaccine Design: The Subunit and Adjuvant Approach, edited by Michael F. Powell and Mark J. Newman. Plenum Press, New York, 1995.

understood, according to the depot theory, subsequently released antigen behaves as a secondary stimulus to the sensitizing action of the antigen released earlier, often leading to a dramatic increase in protective antibody production (Edelman, 1980).

Controlled release systems are already used in humans as "depots" to deliver an array of drugs and hormones (Langer, 1990). Such systems may have a tremendous impact on immunization programs since they can be designed to deliver controlled amounts of antigen continuously or in spaced pulses at predetermined rates (Cohen *et al.*, 1991b; Eldridge *et al.*, 1991a; Gander *et al.*, 1993), while simultaneously protecting undelivered antigen from rapid degradation in vivo. Controlled release microspheres have also shown considerable potential for oral immunization (Edelman *et al.*, 1993; Eldridge *et al.*, 1990; McQueen *et al.*, 1993; Moldoveanu *et al.*, 1989; O'Hagan *et al.*, 1993b; Reid *et al.*, 1993). Other potential advantages of polymeric controlled release systems include: lower dosage requirements, leading to a decreased probability of unwanted side effects and decreased cost; localized or targeted delivery of antigen to antigen-presenting cells or the lymphatic system; more than one antigen may be encapsulated, facilitating the design of a formulation that can immunize an individual against more than one disease, or against several epitopes of a given pathogen in a single injection; and improved patient compliance. In addition, controlled release systems may eventually reduce the number of vaccine doses required for successful vaccination to a single injection, thus reducing the cost of immunization programs while increasing coverage.

2. POLYMER MICROSPHERES FOR VACCINE DELIVERY

2.1. Parenteral Immunization

The effectiveness of polymeric controlled release technology for immunization was first demonstrated in 1979, in studies in which mice were immunized with bovine serum albumin (BSA) entrapped in a nondegradable ethylene-vinyl acetate (EVAc) copolymer matrix (Preis and Langer, 1979). These controlled release vehicles induced antibody responses for more than 6 months at levels comparable to the antibody levels obtained after two injections of the same total amount of BSA emulsified in complete Freund's adjuvant (Fig. 1). Similar responses were obtained with other antigens of widely varying molecular weights (Langer, 1981; Preis and Langer, 1979). The sustained immune responses from a single polymer implant were of the IgG class, and tolerance was not induced.

In order to develop a more convenient method for immunizing humans, polymeric controlled release antigen delivery has focused on the use of biodegradable polymer microspheres as vaccine carriers. Microspheres less than about 100 μm in diameter can be easily administered by injection through standard-sized needles (i.e., 22 gauge or smaller), thus obviating the need for surgical implantation.

Microspheres may be particularly suited as controlled release vaccine carriers for two reasons: (1) particles greater than 10 μm in diameter are capable of providing a long-term persistence of antigen at the site of injection which may be necessary for a sustained high-level humoral immune response and (2) microparticles in the size range of 1–10 μm

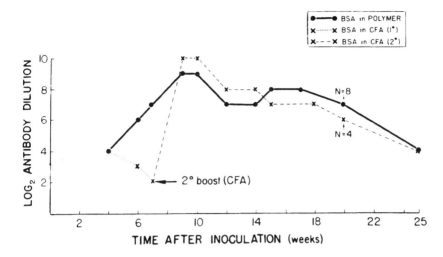

Figure 1. IgG antibody levels in mice following the implantation of bovine serum albumin (BSA) entrapped in a single controlled release device made of ethylene-vinyl acetate copolymer or following injection of two doses of BSA emulsified in complete Freund's adjuvant (CFA). Reproduced from Preis and Langer (1979) with kind permission from Elsevier Science.

are readily phagocytosed by macrophages (Eldridge *et al.*, 1989; Tabata and Ikada, 1988a,b), leading to direct intracellular delivery of antigen to antigen-presenting cells. Rapid intracellular delivery of antigen may protect the antigen from neutralization by maternal antibodies, and thus allow immunization of children shortly after birth. In addition, antigen-presenting cells such as macrophages play a fundamental role in the production of T-cell-dependent humoral immunity. Thus, the targeting of vaccines to macrophages by utilizing microspheres of the appropriate size may be expected to lead to enhanced antibody responses and to a decrease in the required antigen dose for immunization. In fact, at least two groups have shown that the injection of antigen in microspheres less than 10 μm in diameter leads to a substantially higher level of adjuvanticity than when microspheres of a size that precludes their uptake by phagocytosis are used (Eldridge *et al.*, 1991b; O'Hagan *et al.*, 1993a) (Fig. 2). Consistent with this possibility is the observation that the immune response to T-cell-independent antigens, such as bacterial carbohydrates, is generally not enhanced through delivery in small-diameter microspheres (Eldridge *et al.*, 1991a). However, caution should be used in interpreting these results. Small microspheres, which are phagocytosed by macrophages, and large microspheres, which are not phagocytosed, are certain to have different antigen release kinetics in vivo which may be partly responsible for the higher "adjuvanticity" seen with microspheres in the size range 1–10 μm.

It may also be possible to increase microsphere phagocytosis by macrophages by altering their surface characteristics. Microspheres with hydrophobic surfaces are generally more readily phagocytosed than those with hydrophilic surfaces (Tabata and Ikada, 1988a, 1990). These results are not surprising since it has been established that an increase in

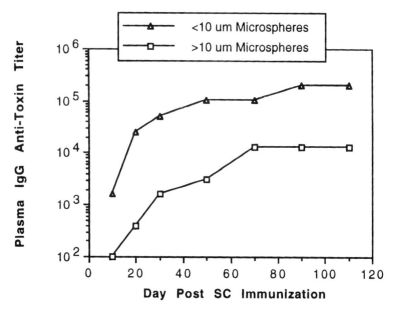

Figure 2. IgG antitoxin titer to SEB toxin in the plasma of mice induced by subcutaneous (SC) immunization with 10 μg of SEB toxoid encapsulated in 1- to 10-μm (< 10 μm, 0.65% w/w SEB) or 10- to 110-μm (> 10 μm, 1.03% w/w SEB) D,L-PLGA 85:15 microspheres. Reproduced from Eldridge *et al.* (1991b) with kind permission from the American Society for Microbiology.

particle uptake by macrophages is seen with an increase in surface hydrophobicity (Carr, 1973; Evans and Alexander, 1972; Fidler *et al.*, 1976; Hibbs *et al.*, 1977). Precoating of microspheres with various molecules, including opsonins such as gelatin, can also result in a dramatic increase in macrophage phagocytosis of microspheres (Tabata and Ikada, 1988b; 1989a).

In addition to the propensity of small microspheres (1–10 μm) to be taken up by macrophages, larger microspheres are capable of providing the long-term delivery of antigen often regarded as crucial to the success of a single-injection subunit vaccine formulation. However, little is known regarding the vaccine release kinetics that would maximize the humoral response to a given antigen, and most importantly, that will induce long-term immune protection.

Recently it was suggested that the ideal vaccine release pattern should mimic the profile of antigen concentration seen during the course of natural infection, namely, a high dose of antigen within a few days followed by a period of delivering decreasing amounts of antigen (Ada, 1991). The initial high load of antigen is expected to influence the extent of memory T-cell formation, while the subsequent steady decrease in antigen load would be expected to enhance the development of antibody affinity maturation. According to this theory, a pulsatile release system may be particularly well-suited for vaccine delivery since release from these systems is characterized by discrete bursts of antigen, followed by a period of decreasing rates of antigen release. However, a constant release pattern has also been suggested as appropriate for vaccine delivery (Alonso *et al.*, 1993, 1994; Preis and Langer, 1979).

Among the advantages of using polymer microspheres for vaccine delivery is the ability to control the time following administration at which the antigen is released. This capability allows the fabrication of a single-injection formulation that releases multiple "pulses" of vaccine at predetermined times following administration (Gilley *et al.*, 1992). Antigen release kinetics from polymer microspheres can be controlled to a great extent by the simple manipulation of such variables as: polymer composition and molecular weight, the weight ratio of vaccine to polymer used (i.e., the vaccine loading), and microsphere size (Hanes and Langer, 1995). Using the polyesters of lactic and glycolic acid as an example, the onset of antigen release may usually be delayed and/or the duration of antigen release extended by using: (1) a higher percentage of the more hydrophobic monomer lactic acid [poly(lactic co-glycolic acid) (PLGA) with a 50:50 lactide/glycolide ratio is the fastest degrading copolymer; from there, an increase in the lactide content leads to slower degradation and prolonged release]; (2) a higher-molecular-weight polymer; (3) a lower vaccine loading; and/or (4) microspheres greater than 10 μm in diameter (versus those less than 10 μm; microspheres less than 10 μm in diameter are often phagocytosed by macrophages, where they are subjected to enhanced degradation rates compared to particles of a size that precludes their uptake by macrophages). For example, by simply changing polymer molecular weight and/or co-monomer ratio of PLGA, vaccine release may be varied from as short as 1 week to over 1 year (Cohen *et al.*, 1994). In addition, microspheres that release antigen continuously or in discrete pulses have been formulated using the same polymer simply by varying fabrication conditions during encapsulation (Cohen *et al.*, 1991b). In another approach, Eldridge *et al.* (1991a) used a combination of copolymer ratios and microsphere sizes to achieve four discrete releases of antigen over a 120-day period. In fact, an endless array of release profiles may be obtained by using combinations of: (1) microspheres of different sizes and vaccine loadings; (2) polymers of different compositions and molecular weights; (3) monolithic and reservoir-type microspheres; or (4) microspheres made from completely different polymers (Hanes and Langer, in press; Lewis, 1990). In addition, self- or externally-regulated systems currently in the early stages of development may be able to produce preprogrammed or "on demand" pulses of antigen in the future (Kost and Langer, 1992).

The remarkable control over release profiles that can be obtained using controlled release from polymer microspheres may eventually help define the optimal release pattern for effective immunization against a variety of infectious diseases. However, to date there have been a limited number of reports on the effect of various antigen release patterns and formulations on the quality and duration of the resultant immune response. The remainder of this section reviews the experiences of a few groups who have tested various vaccine formulations for their ability to produce high and long-lasting humoral immune responses.

Using staphylococcal enterotoxin B (SEB) toxoid antigen, Eldridge and co-workers showed that vaccine formulations that contain a combination of both small (1–10 μm) and larger (20–50 μm) microspheres may produce higher and longer-lasting antibody levels compared to the administration of vaccine encapsulated in microspheres with diameters of exclusively 1–10 or 20–50 μm (Eldridge *et al.*, 1991a) (Fig. 3). Mice immunized intraperitoneally with SEB toxoid in 1- to 10-μm microspheres produced a plasma IgG

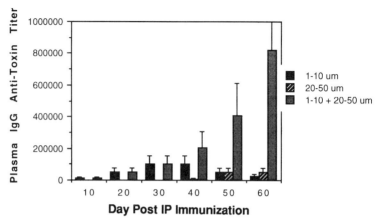

Figure 3. IgG antitoxin titer to SEB toxin in the plasma of mice induced by intraperitoneal immunization with SEB toxoid in 50:50 D,L-PLGA microspheres of diameter 1–10 μm, 20–50 μm, or a mixture of 1–10 and 20–50 μm. Reproduced from Eldridge *et al.* (1991a) with kind permission from Elsevier Science.

antitoxin response detected on day 10, which reached a maximal titer of 102,400 between days 30 and 40, followed by a decrease to 25,600 by day 60. On the other hand, the response to the toxoid administered in larger microspheres (greater than 20 μm) was not detected until day 30, and thereafter approached a maximal titer between days 50 and 60 that was approximately half the maximal titer seen with the smaller microsphere formulation. However, the coadministration of SEB toxoid in microspheres 1–10 and 20–50 μm in diameter led to an IgG response that was essentially the same as that stimulated by the 1- to 10-μm microspheres administered alone for the first 30 days. Thereafter, however, the titer rose to a level of 819,200 on day 60 (the last day of the study), a level far higher than the additive amount of the responses induced by the two size ranges administered alone. One explanation for this phenomenon may be that a large number of particles with diameters less than 10 μm enter macrophages, where they release their vaccine at a substantially accelerated rate, leading to the stimulation of helper T cells and the subsequent formation of a pool of memory B cells. The larger microspheres, which are unable to be phagocytosed, subsequently provide an initial booster effect followed by a subsequent long-term persistence of antigen necessary for the production of a high-level sustained antibody response.

Tetanus vaccines have also received a great deal of attention since they have been targeted by the World Health Organization as the first controlled release single-shot vaccine formulation. In one study, tetanus toxoid (TT)-containing microspheres were tailored to produce a strong priming antigen dose released over the first few days after injection followed by two "boosting" doses released after 1 and 3 months, respectively, in order to mimic conventional vaccination schedules (Gander *et al.*, 1993). The pulsatile release pattern was achieved by using fast-releasing particles (i.e., PLGA 50:50) of a size in which many particles are susceptible to macrophage phagocytosis (1–15 μm) and which contain a relatively high TT loading (14.2 μg/mg microspheres), combined with larger (10–60 μm) microspheres made up of slower-degrading PLGA 75:25 with a relatively low TT loading

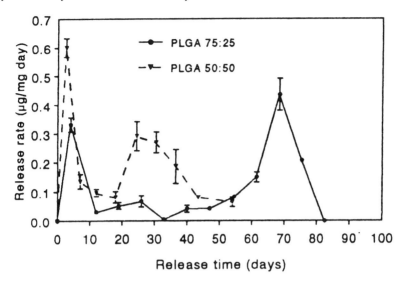

Figure 4. In vitro tetanus toxoid (TT) release from PLGA 50:50 (1–15 μm in diameter, 14.2 μg TT/mg microspheres) and PLGA 75:25 (10–60 μm in diameter, 3.1 μg TT/mg microspheres) microspheres. Reproduced from Gander *et al.* (1993) with kind permission from the Controlled Release Society.

(3.1 μg/mg). In vitro release studies (Fig. 4) revealed that the primary dose results from the burst release of both the PLGA 50:50 and PLGA 75:25 microspheres. The first "booster" (second release phase), which came 3 to 5 weeks later, was the result of release from the fast-releasing PLGA 50:50 microspheres. The second booster was provided by the larger PLGA 75:25 microspheres and occurred between approximately weeks 9 and 11. Antibody titers in mice were higher and lasted longer when a combination of the 1- to 15-μm PLGA 50:50 and 10- to 60-μm 75:25 microspheres were administered together than when either the 50:50 or 75:25 microsphere formulations were administered alone.

Others have investigated the use of a continuous antigen release pattern for TT from PLA or PLGA microspheres (Alonso *et al.*, 1993, 1994; Gupta *et al.*, 1993). In each of these studies, mice immunized with microencapsulated TT produced greatly enhanced antitoxin neutralizing antibody titers compared to mice immunized with soluble TT for over 24 weeks. However, perhaps the most important result was that the neutralizing IgG antibody titers (evaluated by the toxin neutralization assay) increased with time, while total antitoxin IgG (evaluated by ELISA) remained approximately constant or decreased with time. The difference in the in vivo responses obtained by ELISA and neutralization tests was explained in terms of a progressive affinity maturation of the tetanus antibodies. This phenomenon correlates, again, with in vitro release studies, which show a decreasing TT release rate over time (Alonso *et al.*, 1993, 1994). Furthermore, in one of these studies (Alonso *et al.*, 1993), two microsphere formulations were tested: (1) TT microspheres made of PLA (molecular weight 3000) with a small size and rapid release kinetics in vitro (average size 9 μm, and 50% released within 10 days) and (2) TT microspheres made of PLGA (50:50, molecular weight 100,000) with a larger size and slow release kinetics in vitro (average size 50 μm, and 30% released at day 30). Mice receiving TT in the fast-releasing PLA formulation produced higher toxin neutralizing antibody titers at earlier times (e.g., 4 weeks) than mice receiving the slow-releasing PLGA formulation. This behavior correlates with the faster initial in vitro release kinetics from these formulations, and the theoretical provision of the early high antigen load in vivo. However, a combination of fast- and slow-releasing microspheres was not evaluated.

Birth control vaccines, seeking to intercept fertility at one or more points in the reproductive process, have also been investigated extensively (Mitchison, 1990; Talwar and Raghupathy, 1989). The most advanced antifertility vaccines are based on raising antibodies against human chorionic gonadotropin (hCG), a hormone necessary for the establishment of pregnancy. Stevens *et al.* (1992) have encapsulated an hCG peptide, conjugated to either diphtheria toxoid or TT for T-cell help, in various PLGA microsphere formulations and have shown that a mixture of slow-, medium-, and fast-releasing microspheres results in higher and longer-lasting anti-hCG antibody titers than an injection of any of the formulations singly. The adjuvant compound *N*-acetyl-nor-muramyl-L-alanyl-D-isoglutamine (nor-MDP) was encapsulated and co-released, and microspheres were suspended in "appropriate" vehicles to attract lymphoid cells to the site of injection. The vehicles used consist of a mixture of oils or water-in-oil emulsions (Stevens *et al.*, 1992). Rapid release of vaccine components was accomplished either by using PLGA polymers with a 50:50 lactide/glycolide ratio, or by using small D,L-PLA microspheres with component loads of 10% or more. With fast-degrading formulations, anti-hCG levels of 100 nanomol/L or higher were maintained from 4 to 20 weeks of immunization (Fig. 5). When slow-releasing PLA formulations were tested, antibody levels took longer to rise and were generally lower than when using the more rapidly degrading polymers (Fig. 6). However, when a combination of fast-, intermediate-, and slow-degrading microspheres was used for immunization, antibody levels rose quickly to higher levels (greater than 1000 nanomol/L) than with any formulation given singly, and were sustained well over 100 nanomol/L for over 45 weeks.

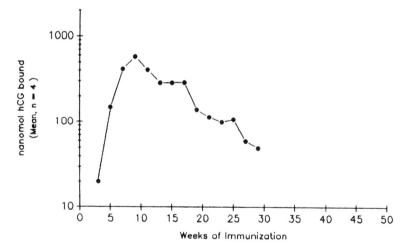

Figure 5. Mean antibody levels reactive with hCG in rabbits following a single injection of fast-release PLGA copolymer microspheres containing an hCG peptide immunogen and nor-MDP adjuvant. Reproduced from Stevens (1993) with kind permission from Munksgaard.

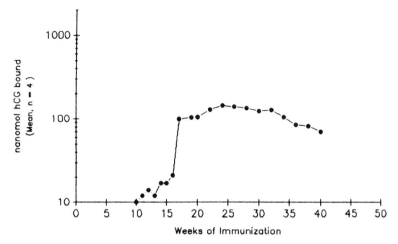

Figure 6. Mean antibody levels reactive with hCG in rabbits following a single injection of slow-release polylactide microspheres containing an hCG peptide immunogen and nor-MDP adjuvant. Reproduced from Stevens (1993) with kind permission from Munksgaard.

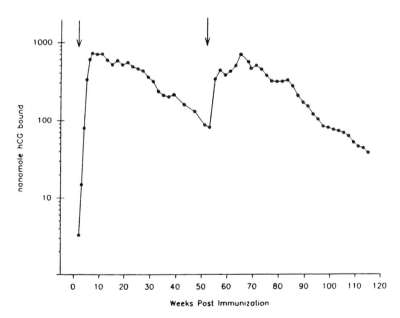

Figure 7. Mean antibody levels reactive with hCG in rabbits following immunizations with an hCG peptide immunogen and nor-MDP adjuvant entrapped in a blend of fast-, intermediate-, and slow-release lactide/glycolide microspheres at weeks 0 and 52. Reproduced from Stevens (1993) with kind permission from Munksgaard.

Furthermore, a repeat of the first immunization at week 52 resulted in a significant boost to antibody production which was sustained for another year (Fig. 7).

2.2. Mucosal Immunization

The mucosal surfaces, including the lungs, nose, vagina, and lining of the GI tract, are the site of entry of most pathogens into the body. For this reason, the ability to induce high titers of secretory IgA (sIgA) may be important for protection against challenge by many infectious agents. Parenteral injections of antigen are usually ineffective at stimulating production of sIgA, which is most effectively elicited by immunization of mucosal surfaces (e.g., oral or intratracheal administration). Oral administration of vaccines often leads to the induction of sIgA antibody production not only in the mucosa of the gut, but also in the other mucosal surfaces of the body, including the genitourinary and respiratory tracts. Furthermore, oral immunization offers the advantages of convenience and reduced cost of administration, and greater patient acceptance.

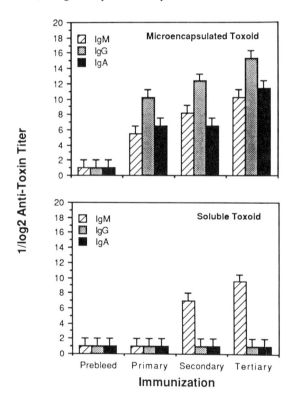

Figure 8. Plasma anti-SEB toxin antibody levels of the IgM and IgG isotypes induced following primary, secondary, and tertiary oral immunizations in mice with 100-µg doses of microencapsulated or soluble SEB toxoid. The microencapsulated form induced the appearance of high levels of IgG antibodies in contrast to the free vaccine, which was only effective at stimulating antitoxin antibodies of the IgM class. Reproduced from Eldridge *et al.* (1990) with kind permission from Elsevier Science.

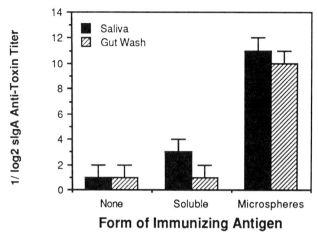

Figure 9. IgA anti-SEB toxin antibody levels in the saliva and gut wash of mice obtained 20 days following a tertiary oral immunization with microencapsulated or free SEB toxoid vaccine. Reproduced from Eldridge *et al.* (1990) with kind permission from Elsevier Science.

Since microspheres are taken up from the intestine by the Peyer's patches, they have considerable potential as carriers for oral immunization (Eldridge *et al.*, 1989; O'Hagan, 1990). The polymer wall of microspheres is expected to protect encapsulated vaccine from degradation by the low pH of the stomach and from proteolysis in the gut. Recent studies by Eldridge *et al.* (1990) have shown that orally administered microspheres containing SEB toxoid induced not only circulating IgM, IgG, and IgA antitoxin antibody, but also a disseminated mucosal IgA response in mice. In contrast, oral immunization with the same amount of fluid antigen resulted in minimal to absent antibody titers of all classes (Figs. 8 and 9).

Eldridge and co-workers have also reported on the role that microsphere size plays in determining the type and quality of the immune response to oral immunization. They showed that orally administered microspheres less than 10 μm in diameter are preferentially absorbed by the Peyer's patches in the GI tract and passed to the immune inductive environment of both the Peyer's patches and systemic lymphoid organs (Eldridge *et al.*, 1990). Time-course studies on the fate of the microspheres within the gut-associated lymphoid tissue showed that the majority of microspheres less than 5 μm in diameter were transported through the efferent lymphatics within macrophages, while the majority of those more than 5 μm in diameter remained in the Peyer's patches for up to 35 days (Eldridge *et al.*, 1990) (Fig. 10). This pattern of absorption and redistribution suggests that particle size may be a determinant in the type of immune response (i.e., circulating versus mucosal) elicited by oral vaccination with antigen-containing microspheres. Microspheres with diameters less than 5 μm would be predicted to induce primarily a circulating immune response because of their propensity to disseminate into the systemic lymphoid tissues, while microspheres with diameters more than 5 μm would be expected to induce primarily a mucosal response because they remain in the IgA inductive environment of the Peyer's patches.

The extent of microsphere uptake by the Peyer's patches also seems to correlate with the effective hydrophobicity of the polymer used. Microspheres composed of polystyrene,

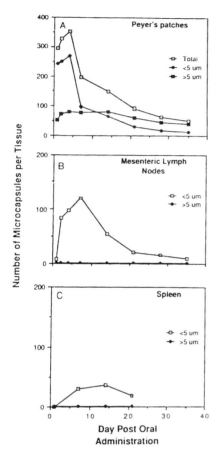

Figure 10. Absorption of 50:50 D,L-PLGA microspheres into the Peyer's patches and their tissue redistribution as a function of time. (A) The total microsphere number within three representative Peyer's patches was seen to rise through day 4 and then fall as the <5-μm particles extravasated. (B) The peak number of microspheres within the first mesenteric lymph node proximal to the appendix was observed on day 7 and consisted entirely of <5-μm particles. (C) Microspheres observed in the spleen were most abundant on day 14 and were all <5-μm in diameter. Reproduced from Eldridge *et al.* (1990) with kind permission from Elsevier Science.

polymethyl methacrylate, poly(hydroxybutyrate), poly(DL-lactide), poly(L-lactide), and of poly(DL-lactide-co-glycolide) with various ratios of lactide to glycolide were all shown to be absorbed into the Peyer's patches (Eldridge *et al.*, 1990). However, the polymers with the greatest relative hydrophobicity (polystyrene, polymethyl methacrylate, and polyhydroxybutyrate) were absorbed most readily, while similar-sized microspheres made of the relatively less hydrophobic polymers [poly(DL-lactide), poly(L-lactide), and poly(DL-lactide-co-glycolide)] were also absorbed, but in lower numbers. In contrast, very few or no microspheres made of ethyl cellulose, cellulose triacetate, or cellulose acetate hydrogen phthalate were taken up by the Peyer's patches (Table I).

Influenza virus proteins have also been encapsulated into microspheres and delivered orally in animals (Moldoveanu *et al.*, 1989, 1993; Santiago *et al.*, 1992). Mice given microencapsulated influenza A virus vaccine orally produced higher salivary IgA antibody titers which lasted longer (up to 4 months) than titers in mice given equivalent doses of free antigen (Moldoveanu *et al.*, 1989). Subsequently, it was shown that orally delivered microencapsulated influenza virus provided protection against viral challenge, and that the

Table I

Targeted Absorption of 1- to 10-μm Microspheres with Various Excipients by the Peyer's Patches of the Gut-Associated Lymphoid Tissues following Oral Administration[a]

Microsphere type	Biodegradable	Absorption by the Peyer's patches[b]
Polystyrene	No	Very good[c]
Polymethyl methacrylate	No	Very good
Polyhydroxybutyrate	Yes	Very good
Poly(DL-lactide)	Yes	Good
Poly(L-lactide)	Yes	Good
85:15 poly(DL-lactide-co-glycolide)	Yes	Good
50:50 poly(DL-lactide-co-glycolide)	Yes	Good
Cellulose acetate hydrogen phthalate	No	None
Cellulose triacetate	No	None
Ethyl cellulose	No	None

[a]Reproduced from Eldridge et al. (1990) with kind permission from Elsevier Science.

[b]Mice were administered 0.5 mL of a suspension containing 20 mg of coumarin-containing microspheres into the stomach by syringe gavage. After 48 h, three representative Peyers patches per animal were removed, sectioned at 5-μm intervals, and examined for microsphere uptake by fluorescence microscopy.

[c]The results indicate the efficiency of absorption by the Peyer's patches of the microspheres composed of various excipients where very good = 1000 to 1500, good = 200 to 1000, and none = < 10 microspheres observed when all sections from the three Peyer's patches were viewed with a fluorescence microscope.

oral route boosted antibody titers which resulted from primary oral or systemic immunization (Moldoveanu et al., 1993).

Microencapsulated oral vaccines designed to protect against diarrhea induced by enterotoxigenic E. coli are also currently in the early stages of development. Encapsulation of a pilus protein (colonization factor antigen) in microspheres has been shown to preserve its immunogenicity on oral administration and, subsequently, protection of rabbits from pathogen challenge has been demonstrated (Edelman et al., 1993; McQueen et al., 1993; Reid et al., 1993). Systemic IgG and local mucosal IgA responses were elicited in animals following both intragastric and intraduodenal immunization.

Mucosal immunization has also shown a great deal of potential as a means of boosting the immune response to achieve a high level of local mucosal IgA antibody. For example, oral or intratracheal (i.t.) boosting of mice that received intraperitoneal (i.p.) primary immunizations with microencapsulated SEB toxoid was as effective at inducing disseminated mucosal IgA antitoxin antibodies as three oral doses in microspheres. On the other hand, soluble toxoid was ineffective for boosting (Eldridge et al., 1991a) (Fig. 11). In a subsequent study, rhesus macaques that received two intramuscular (i.m.) primary immunizations, followed by i.t. boosting, were protected against aerosol challenge with lethal doses of SEB (Staas et al., 1993). Monkeys receiving i.t. immunizations developed bronchial–alveolar wash anti-SEB toxin titers that were superior to those achieved by oral or i.m. boosting. This study also showed that i.m. priming with microencapsulated simian immunodeficiency virus (SIV), followed by either oral or i.t. boosting in microspheres,

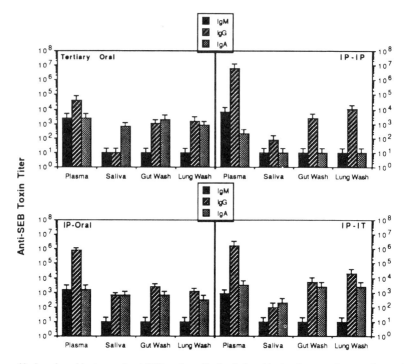

Figure 11. Levels and isotypes of anti-SEB toxin antibodies induced in the plasma and mucosal secretions of mice immunized by various protocols with SEB toxoid in 1- to 10-μm 50:50 D,L-PLGA microspheres (IP, intraperitoneal; IT, intratracheal). Reproduced from Eldridge *et al.* (1991a) with kind permission from Elsevier Science.

was capable of protecting four out of six monkeys from two vaginal challenges with 2 LD_{50} of $SIV_{mac}251$.

Oral and i.t. administration of microspheres have shown potential in the production of secretory and, to a somewhat lesser degree, circulating antibody. However, experience with these routes of administration has been brief and no long-term studies have been done to determine the quality of protection that can be achieved. In the very least, both oral and i.t. administration may ultimately find use as methods of boosting the immune response to a previously parenterally administered vaccine formulation (Eldridge *et al.*, 1991a).

3. POLYMERS FOR VACCINE MICROENCAPSULATION

3.1. Lactide/Glycolide Polyesters

The most widely used polymers for vaccine microencapsulation have been the polyesters based on lactic and glycolic acid. These polymers have several advantages, including extensive data on their in vitro and in vivo degradation rates (Lewis, 1990; Tice and Tabibi, 1992), and FDA approval for a number of clinical applications in humans such as surgical sutures (Gilding and Reed, 1979; Schneider, 1972) and a 30-day microsphere-based controlled delivery system for leuprolide acetate (Lupron Depot) used in the treatment of prostate cancer and endometriosis (Okada *et al.*, 1991). The future of these polymers for the delivery of conventional pharmaceuticals looks promising as several products are already moving through the regulatory process in the United States, Europe, and Japan. It is clear, however, that there are limitations on their use for vaccine delivery. For example, it is possible that an acidic environment is created locally as these polymers degrade. A lowered pH may cause stability problems with pH-sensitive vaccines such as TT (Schwendeman, personal communication). Other macromolecules have also been shown to be incompatible with lactide/glycolides (Lewis, 1990). As with other polymeric excipients, lactide/glycolides will serve some but not all applications.

3.2. Polymers with Built-in Adjuvanticity

There are several interesting alternatives to the lactide/glycolide polyesters for vaccine delivery. For example, some biodegradable polymers degrade to give molecules with adjuvant properties, and may prove particularly useful as carriers of weakly immunogenic antigens. Because of the known adjuvanticity of L-tyrosine derivatives (Wheeler *et al.*, 1982, 1984), a polymer based on a dityrosine derivative was synthesized (Kohn and Langer, 1987) and studied using the model antigen BSA (Kohn *et al.*, 1986). Biodegradable poly(CTTH iminocarbonate) was selected since its primary degradation product, *N*-benzyloxycarbonyl-L-tyrosyl-L-tyrosine hexyl ester (CTTH) (Fig. 12), was found to be as potent an adjuvant as CFA and MDP when measuring the serum antibody response to BSA in mice over 1 year. BSA released from implanted poly(CTTH iminocarbonate) antigen delivery devices resulted in significantly higher antibody responses than BSA released from poly(bisphenol A iminocarbonate) (a polymer that does not contain a tyrosine derivative), or from two injections of the antigen over 1 year. Since the two types of implants were made in the same way, contained an identical dose of antigen, were shown to have comparable release profiles in vitro (Kohn and Langer, 1986), and share the same iminocarbonate backbone structure, Kohn and co-workers suggested that the observed

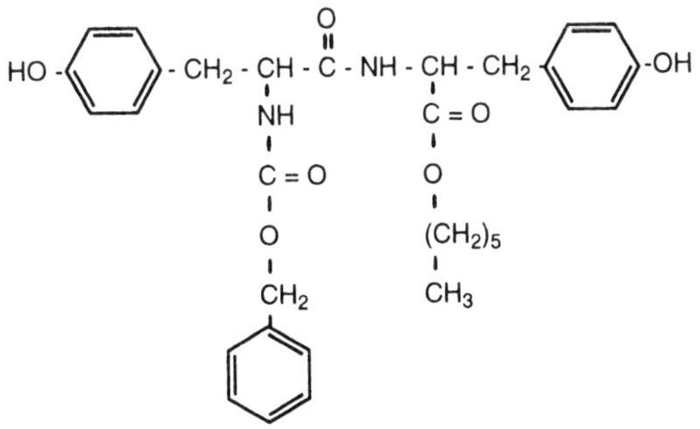

Figure 12. Chemical structure of *N*-benzyloxycarbonyl-L-tyrosyl-L-tyrosine hexyl ester (CTTH).

higher antibody titers obtained for poly(CTTH iminocarbonate) might be attributed to an intrinsic adjuvanticity of CTTH, its monomeric repeat unit.

3.3. Gelatin

Because of its inherent propensity to be phagocytosed by macrophages (Tabata and Ikada, 1986) and its extensive use in pharmaceutical and medical applications, gelatin has also been used as a polymer for vaccine microencapsulation (Tabata *et al.*, 1993). Tabata and co-workers have shown that mice immunized with cross-linked gelatin microspheres containing human gamma globulin (hGG) produced antibody levels approximately three times higher at their highest levels than those induced by hGG emulsified in incomplete Freund's adjuvant (IFA). However, antibody levels fell to the level of hGG-in-IFA titers only a few days after reaching their peak levels. This may be related to the rapid destruction of vaccine within the macrophage, resulting in the lack of antigen persistence necessary for sustained high-level antibody titers. Cell-mediated immunity, measured by delayed-type hypersensitivity (DTH) reaction to injection of hGG in the footpad, was also enhanced by the gelatin microsphere formulation.

Gelatin microspheres have also been used to encapsulate immunostimulators, such as MDP and interferon-α (Tabata and Ikada, 1987, 1989b). MDP encapsulated in gelatin microspheres was shown to potentiate the tumor growth inhibitory activity of macrophages (Tabata and Ikada, 1987). Microsphere-encapsulated MDP activated macrophages in much shorter periods than with free MDP, and inhibited growth of tumor cells at concentrations approximately 2000 times lower. A combination of MDP and vaccine-containing gelatin microspheres may yield a very potent vaccine formulation.

3.4. Polyphosphazene Gels

Poly[bis(carboxylatophenoxy)phosphazene] (PCPP) is a synthetic polymer that can encapsulate proteins at room temperature without the need for potentially denaturing organic solvents (Cohen *et al.*, 1990), the only solvents for lactide/glycolide polyesters. This facilitates the mild encapsulation of vaccines with fragile three-dimensional structures, which are often subject to denaturation or aggregation in the presence of organic solvents. Water-soluble vaccines may be encapsulated into PCPP microspheres at room temperature by the addition of an aqueous solution of antigen and PCPP to calcium chloride solution via a droplet-forming apparatus (see Chapter 20 and Payne, *et al.*, 1994). Calcium ions presumably form salt bridges between carboxylate groups of adjacent polymer chains, creating an ionically cross-linked matrix (Allcock and Kwon, 1989). PCPP microspheres may then be coated with polymer (e.g., poly-L-lysine) for an additional layer of protection (Cohen *et al.*, 1990).

A potential problem with PCPP is that it is not bioerodible. To overcome this problem, hydrolysis-sensitive glycinato side groups were used to make poly(glycinato phosphazene) copolymers. These copolymers have been designed to erode from within a few days to longer than 20 days (Andrianov *et al.*, 1994). The erosion rates of these polymers can be manipulated by controlling their initial molecular weight, monomer composition, or by coating with poly-L-lysine polymer.

3.5. Microencapsulated Liposomes (MELs)

An interesting challenge for controlled release immunization is the improvement of liposomal preparations for vaccine administration. Liposomes are often unstable in vivo, most likely because of their rapid destruction by macrophages and high-density lipoproteins (Schreier *et al.*, 1987), and therefore provide only a brief antigen depot effect when injected subcutaneously or intramuscularly (Eppstein *et al.*, 1985; Weiner *et al.*, 1985).

One approach to extending the in vivo lifetime of liposomes was demonstrated by Cohen *et al.* (1991a) who used alginate polymers to encapsulate vaccine-containing liposomes into microspheres, thereby protecting them from rapid destruction in vivo. Fifty days after injection into rats, almost 50% of the model vaccine was recovered when the liposomal formulation had been microencapsulated before injection. On the other hand, no radiolabeled BSA was detected at the injection site after 50 days when liposomes alone were used as the carrier. The increased antigen retention time correlated with the higher and longer-lasting anti-BSA antibody titers seen with the MEL formulation. Antibody titers were two to three times higher at their maximal levels with MELs than with nonencapsulated liposomes (Fig. 13). Enzymatically activated MELs that are capable of providing pulsatile vaccine release kinetics have also been prepared (Kibat *et al.*, 1990). MELs are also expected to show increased stability as a carrier for oral vaccine administration.

4. THE ROLE OF IMMUNOSTIMULANTS

The induction of neutralizing antibody titers is one hallmark of an efficacious vaccine for the prevention of disease. Indeed, many of the currently available vaccines against human diseases exert their protective effect by circulating neutralizing antibody (Bomford *et al.*, 1991). For subunit vaccines, which are often weak immunogens, it may be difficult to elicit a vigorous humoral response with a controlled release system alone (Stevens, 1993). In this case, the use of an immunostimulant with an optimal controlled release system may be vital to the success of the vaccine. In addition, many existing or contemplated vaccines against viral or parasitic diseases would benefit greatly if cell-mediated immunity (CMI) was engaged as well. It is, therefore, an interesting prospect to incorporate into controlled release systems an immunostimulant that is known to induce a CMI response.

The use of an immunostimulant seems particularly attractive for use in controlled release vaccine formulations, since a major problem in therapeutic trials of immunostimulators is often the high dose of immunostimulant required. This high dosage often invokes unwanted reactions, such as pyrogenicity (Tabata and Ikada, 1987). However, incorporation of an immunostimulant in a controlled release device may lead to a dramatic decrease in its required dose. Tabata and Ikada (1987) have shown that encapsulation of a lipophilic derivative of MDP (MDP-B30) allowed the use of a dose approximately 2000-fold lower than free MDP-B30 to enhance the tumor growth inhibitory activity of macrophages.

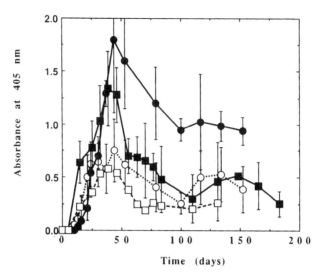

Figure 13. Humoral immune response to bovine serum albumin. Rats were immunized subcutaneously with antigen in saline (□), complete Freund's adjuvant (■), liposomes (○), or microencapsulated liposomes (●). Reproduced from Cohen *et al.* (1991a).

Further, they showed that macrophage activity correlated with extent of MDP-B30-containing microsphere phagocytosis and that macrophage activity was found to increase with an enhancement in the phagocytosis. Microsphere phagocytosis could be readily regulated by changing the microsphere size and by coating the microspheres with various water-soluble macromolecules, including proteins (Tabata and Ikada, 1988b).

5. MICROSPHERE PRODUCTION

A variety of methods may be used to prepare vaccine-loaded polymer microspheres that are capable of a wide range of release patterns and durations. The method of choice usually is determined by the relative compatibility of the process conditions with the antigen (e.g., the method that results in the least loss of vaccine immunogenicity) and the polymer excipient used, combined with the ability of the method to produce appropriately sized microspheres.

Solvent evaporation techniques are very popular for vaccine encapsulation because of their relative ease of preparation, amenability to scaleup, and because high encapsulation efficiencies can be attained. Of particular importance for vaccines that are sensitive to organic solvents may be the multiple emulsion technique (Cohen *et al.*, 1991b), in which antigen is first dissolved in water before being emulsified into a polymer/organic solvent solution to create the first inner emulsion (water-in-oil). This suspension is then emulsified again in a second aqueous phase, containing polyvinyl alcohol as an emulsion stabilizer, to produce a double emulsion [(water-in-oil)-in water]. The solvent is allowed to evaporate or is extracted (Alonso *et al.*, 1993), leaving behind solid microspheres. Subsequently, the water and any residual solvent are removed by freeze-drying. The result is a free-flowing powder, consisting of antigen that is homogeneously dispersed throughout a monolithic polymer matrix. This method has been used to encapsulate model proteins such as horseradish peroxidase, and several candidate antigens, including TT and a synthetic malarial peptide, with encapsulation efficiencies in excess of 90% (Cohen *et al.*, 1991b, 1992). More importantly, these antigens were shown to retain their solubility, activity, and immunogenicity following microencapsulation.

Spray drying and film casting techniques have also been used to prepare monolithic polymer microspheres. In the spray drying procedure, antigen is dissolved or suspended in a polymer/organic solvent solution and aerosolized via a nozzle to create microdroplets. The solvent is removed as the microdroplets enter a heated chamber, leaving behind hardened microspheres containing antigen. Polymer concentration, knowledge of suspension rheology, and nozzle design may be used to control microsphere size and shape. In the film casting procedure, antigen is dissolved or suspended in a solution of polymer and organic solvent and cast into thin films. The film is then converted into microparticles by pulverization, shredding, or cryogenic grinding.

Another type of microparticle that is not often used for vaccine delivery, but which may provide an additional means of achieving pulsatile release, are microcapsules. Microcapsules consist of a vaccine-loaded core surrounded by a thin polymer membrane and, as a result, are often referred to as "reservoir" systems.

Phase separation is a commonly used method to produce microcapsules. In this process, molecules or antigens are typically dissolved in water and emulsified with a polymer/organic solvent solution to form a water-in-oil emulsion. To this, a nonsolvent such as silicone oil, or an incompatible second polymer, is added causing the polymer to phase separate and collect on the surface of the antigen/water microdroplets, forming a microcapsule containing a reservoir of vaccine (Donbrow, 1992; Fong, 1979).

6. CONSIDERATION OF VACCINE FORMULATION STABILITY

Although a great deal of progress toward the development of polymeric controlled release systems as vaccine carriers has been made, several challenges remain. A primary concern is the issue of carrier and vaccine stability during device development, storage, and in vivo depoting. Many antigens are proteins with fragile three-dimensional structures vital to the immunogenicity of the vaccine. This three-dimensional structure may be compromised or lost as the antigen denatures or aggregates. Exposure to organic solvents, rehydration after lyophilization on exposure to moisture, or complex chemical interactions with the polymer excipient or other chemicals in the preparation of the controlled release device may result in loss or reduction of immunogenicity of protein-based vaccines. For these reasons, studies being performed on stabilizing complex antigens (Arakawa *et al.*, 1993; Liu *et al.*, 1991; Volkin and Klibanov, 1989) will be important for the future success of most controlled release vaccine systems.

An advantage of polymer microsphere formulations is that many polymers are stable at room temperature for extended periods of time if they are kept dry. For example, lactide/glycolide polyesters have been reported to be stable if kept dry and below about 40°C (Aguado and Lambert, 1992). In addition, vaccine can be stored in the dry state within

microsphere formulations, an important advantage considering many proteins are susceptible to moisture-induced aggregation (Liu *et al.*, 1991).

7. REGULATORY ISSUES

The final microsphere/vaccine product requires sterilization testing, in addition to
assessment of residual solvent levels. Organic solvents such as methylene chloride, a
commonly used solvent for microsphere preparation, are carcinogenic and thus should be
completely removed from the final product. Orally administered pharmaceuticals generally are not required to be sterile; however, sterilization may be necessary for orally
administered microsphere preparations because of the propensity of microspheres to be
taken up from the GI tract into the Peyer's patches. Sterilization may be achieved by using
aseptic processing conditions throughout formulation, or via the use of gamma irradiation
at the end of the process. However, gamma irradiation may lead to polymer or antigen
degradation leading to reduced vaccine immunogenicity. The preparation of microspheres
under good manufacturing practices (GMP) conditions has been reported to result in a
product with acceptable levels of nonpathogenic bacteria and solvents (Reid *et al.*, 1993).

Once sterile microspheres are produced, they should be evaluated extensively to
demonstrate the reproducibility of the method, and clinical safety and efficacy. In order to
adequately demonstrate reproducibility, microsphere size, surface characteristics, and
antigen loading should be consistent for each batch. Vaccine stability should also be
assessed immediately following encapsulation, as well as at various points during the
release process to confirm that immunogenic antigen is being released at all times. Finally,
the reproducibility of the release performances in vitro and in vivo should be established,
along with a correlation between the two.

In order to demonstrate safety and efficacy, evidence should be provided to show that
the delivery system: (1) leads to an acceptably low level of side effects, (2) is immunologically inert (i.e., does not induce an immune response by itself), (3) provides long-term
protection using fewer injections than is typically necessary with standard adjuvants (e.g.,
alum), and (4) induces effective immunity in most, if not all, target populations (Cohen *et
al.*, 1994).

8. CONCLUSIONS

Because of their unique properties, microspheres show promise in achieving the lofty
goals of single-step immunization with a heat-stable, nontoxic vaccine formulation that
can be administered by injection to protect against a number of childhood diseases. In
addition, by administering vaccines in microspheres of a size readily taken up by macrophages, it may be possible to evade antigen neutralization by maternal antibody (see
Chapter 1). This would theoretically allow children to be vaccinated at a much earlier age,
which is of particular importance in developing countries where hundreds of thousands of
children are infected before they are old enough to receive their first immunization.

The fact that very little is known regarding the optimal release kinetics for controlled
release vaccination shows that this field is still in the early stages of development. However,

controlled release systems are capable of providing a wide range of release patterns and durations and, thus, may ultimately play an important role in determining the most appropriate vaccine release kinetics for a given antigen.

The polyesters based on lactic and glycolic acid are likely to be the first polymers approved as vaccine vehicles. However, polymers designed specifically to deliver vaccines, such as those with "built-in adjuvanticity," may ultimately be better suited for the delivery of poorly immunogenic subunit vaccines.

The role of oral administration at this point appears to be primarily as a booster to a previously administered parenteral immunization. Boosting orally with microspheres has been shown to produce a high level of mucosal-specific IgA antibody, which may act as an important initial barrier against infection. However, strategies being developed to increase the uptake of vaccine-containing microspheres in the GI tract may eventually lead to the reality of single-step vaccination that is given via the oral route (Kraehenbuhl and Neutra, 1992; Neutra and Kraehenbuhl, 1992).

ACKNOWLEDGMENTS

This work has been supported by NIH grant number HD 29129.

REFERENCES

Ada, G., 1991, Strategies for exploiting the immune system in the design of vaccines, *Mol. Immunol.* **28(3)**:225–230.

Aguado, M. T., 1993, Future approaches to vaccine development: Single-dose vaccines using controlled-release delivery systems, *Vaccine* **11(5)**:596–597.

Aguado, M. T., and Lambert, P.-H., 1992, Controlled-release vaccines—Biodegradable polylactide/polyglycolide (PL/PG) microspheres as antigen vehicles, *Immunobiology* **184**:113–125.

Allcock, H. R., and Kwon, S., 1989, An ionically cross-linkable polyphosphazene: Poly[bis(carboxylatophenoxy)phosphazene] and its hydrogels and membranes, *Macromolecules* **22**:75–79.

Alonso, M. J., Cohen, S., Park, T. G., Gupta, R. K., Siber, G. R., and Langer, R., 1993, Determinants of release rate of tetanus vaccine from polyester microspheres, *Pharm. Res.* **10(7)**:945–953.

Alonso, M. J., Gupta, R. K., Min, C., Siber, G. R., and Langer, R., 1994, Biodegradable microspheres as controlled release tetanus toxoid delivery systems, *Vaccine* **12(4)**:299–306.

Andrianov, A. K., Payne, L. G., Visscher, K. B., Allcock, H. R., and Langer, R., Hydrolytic degradation of ionically cross-linked polyphosphazene microspheres, *J. Appl. Polym. Sci.* **53**:1573–1578.

Arakawa, T., Prestrelski, S. J., Kenney, W. C., and Carpenter, J. F., 1993, Factors affecting short-term and long-term stabilities of proteins, *Adv. Drug Deliv. Rev.* **10**:1–28.

Bloom, B. R., 1989, Vaccines for the third world, *Nature* **342**:115–120.

Bomford, R., Stapleton, M., and Winsor, S., 1991, Immunomodulation by adjuvants, in: *Vaccines* (G. Gregoriadis, A. C. Allison, and G. Poste, eds.), Plenum Press, New York, pp. 25–32.

Carr, I., 1973, *The Macrophage: A Review of Ultrastructure and Function*, Academic Press, New York.

Cohen, S., Baño, M. C., Visscher, K. B., Chow, M., Allcock, H. R., and Langer, R., 1990, Ionically cross-linkable polyphosphazene: A novel polymer for microencapsulation, *J. Am. Chem. Soc.* **112**:7832–7833.

Cohen, S., Bernstein, H., Hewes, C., Chow, M., and Langer, R., 1991a, The pharmacokinetics of, and humoral responses to, antigen delivered by microencapsulated liposomes, *Proc. Natl. Acad. Sci. USA* **88**:10440–10444.

Cohen, S., Yoshioka, T., Lucarelli, M., Hwang, L. H., and Langer, R., 1991b, Controlled delivery systems for proteins based on poly(lactic/glycolic acid) microspheres, *Pharm. Res.* **8(6)**:713–720.

Cohen, S., Cochrane, A., Nardin, E., and Langer, R., 1992, Poly(lactic/glycolic acid) microspheres—Immunization vehicles for synthetic peptide vaccines, *Polym. Mater. Sci. Eng.* **66**:91–92.

Cohen, S., Alonso, M. J., and Langer, R., 1994, Novel approaches to controlled release antigen delivery, in: *Int. J. Tech. Assess. Health Care* (A. Robbins and P. Freeman, eds.), Cambridge University Press, London, pp. 121–130.

Donbrow, M., 1992, Developments in phase separation methods, aggregation control, and mechanisms of microencapsulation, in: *Microcapsules and Nanoparticles in Medicine and Pharmacy* (M. Donbrow, ed.), CRC Press, Boca Raton, pp. 17–45

Edelman, R., 1980, Vaccine adjuvants, *Rev. Infect. Dis.* **2(3)**:370–383.

Edelman, R., Russell, R. G., Losonsky, G., Tall, B. D., Tacket, C. O., Levine, M. M., and Lewis, D. H., 1993, Immunization of rabbits with enterotoxigenic *E. coli* colonization factor antigen (CFA/I) encapsulated in biodegradable microspheres of poly(lactide-*co*-glycolide), *Vaccine* **11(2)**:155–158.

Eldridge, J. H., Meulbroek, J. A., Staas, J. K., Tice, T. R., and Gilley, R.M., 1989, Vaccine-containing biodegradable microspheres specifically enter the gut-associated lymphoid tissue following oral administration and induce a disseminated mucosal immune response, *Adv. Exp. Med. Biol.* **251**:192–202.

Eldridge, J. H., Hammond, C. J., and Meulbroek, J. A., 1990, Controlled vaccine release in the gut-associated lymphoid tissues. I. Orally administered biodegradable microspheres target the Peyer's patches, *J. Control. Rel.* **11**:205–214.

Eldridge, J. H., Staas, J. K., Meulbroek, J. A., McGhee, J. R., Tice, T. R., and Gilley, R. M., 1991a, Biodegradable microspheres as a vaccine delivery system, *Mol. Immunol.* **28(3)**:287–294.

Eldridge, J. H., Staas, J. K., Meulbroek, J. A., Tice, T. R., and Gilley, R. M., 1991b, Biodegradable and biocompatible poly(DL-lactide-co-glycolide) microspheres as an adjuvant for staphylococcal enterotoxin B toxoid which enhances the level of toxin-neutralizing antibodies, *Infect. Immun.* **59**:2978–2986.

Eppstein, D. A., Marsh, Y. V., van der Pas, M. A., Felgner, P. L., and Schreiber, A. B., 1985, Biological activity of liposome-encapsulated murine interferon gamma is mediated by a cell membrane receptor, *Proc. Natl. Acad. Sci. USA* **82**:3688–3692.

Evans, R., and Alexander, P., 1972, Mechanism of immunologically specific killing of tumor cells by macrophages, *Nature* **236**:168–170.

Fidler, I. J., Darnell, J. H., and Budmen, M. B., 1976, Tumoricidal properties of mouse macrophages activated with mediators from rat lymphocytes stimulated with concanavalin A, *Cancer Res.* **36**:3608–3615.

Fong, J. W., 1979, Processes for preparation of microspheres, U.S. Patent 4,166,800.

Freund, J., 1956, The mode of action of immunological adjuvants, *Adv. Tuberc. Res.* **7**:130–148.

Gander, B., Thomasin, C., Merkle, H. P., Men, Y., and Corradin, G., 1993, Pulsed tetanus toxoid release from PLGA-microspheres and its relevance for immunogenicity in mice, in: *Proc. Int. Symp. Control. Rel. Bioact. Mater.*, Controlled Release Society, Washington, DC, pp. 65–66.

Gibbons, A., 1992, A booster shot for children's vaccines, *Science* **255**:1351.

Gilding, D. K., and Reed, A. M., 1979, Biodegradable polymers for use in surgery: Polyglycolic/poly(lactic acid) homo- and copolymers: 1, *Polymer* **20**:1459–1464.

Gilley, R. M., Staas, J. K., Tice, T. R., Morgan, J. D., and Eldridge, J. H., 1992, Microencapsulation and its application to vaccine development, in: *Proc. Int. Symp. Control. Rel. Bioact. Mater.*, Controlled Release Society, Orlando, pp. 110–111.

Glenny, A. T., Buttle, G. A. H., and Stevens, M. F., 1931, Rate of disappearance of diphtheria toxoid injected into rabbits and guinea-pigs: Toxoid precipitated with alum, *J. Pathol. Bacteriol.* **34**:267–275.

Gupta, R. K., Siber, G. R., Alonso, M. J., and Langer, R., 1993, Development of a single dose tetanus toxoid based on controlled release from biodegradable and biocompatible polyester microspheres, in: *Vaccines 93* (F. Brown, R. Chenock, H. Ginsberg, and R. Lerner, eds.), Cold Spring Harbor Laboratory Press, Cold Spring Harbor, NY. pp. 391–396.

Hanes, J., and Langer, R., 1995, Polymeric controlled release vaccine delivery systems, in: *Reproductive Immunology* (R. Bronson, N. Alexander, D. Anderson, D. W. Branch, and W. H. Kutteh, eds.), Blackwell, Oxford (in press).

Hibbs, J. B. Jr., Taintor, R. R., Chapman, H. A. Jr., and Weinberg, J. B., 1977, Macrophage tumor killing: Influence of the local environment, *Science* **197**:279–282.

Kibat, P. G., Igari, Y., Wheatley, M. A., Eisen, H. N., and Langer, R., 1990, Enzymatically activated microencapsulated liposomes can provide pulsatile drug release, *FASEB J.* **4**:2533–2539.

Kohn, J., and Langer, R., 1986, Poly(iminocarbonates) as potential biomaterials, *Biomaterials* **7**:176–182.

Kohn, J., and Langer, R., 1987, Polymerization reactions involving the side chains of alpha-L-amino acids, *J. Am. Chem. Soc.* **109**:817–820.

Kohn, J., Niemi, S. M., Albert, E. C., Murphy, J. C., Langer, R., and Fox, J. G., 1986, Single-step immunization using a controlled release, biodegradable polymer with sustained adjuvant activity, *J. Immunol. Methods* **95**:31–38.

Kost, J., and Langer, R., 1992, Responsive polymer systems for controlled delivery of therapeutics, *Trends Biotechnol.* **10(4)**:127–131.

Kraehenbuhl, J.-P., and Neutra, M. R., 1992, Transepithelial transport and mucosal defence II: Secretion of IgA, *Trends Cell Biol.* **2**:170–174.

Langer, R., 1981, Polymers for the sustained release of macromolecules: Their use in a single-step method of immunization, *Methods Enzymol.* **73**:57–75.

Langer, R., 1990, New methods of drug delivery, *Science* **249**:1527–1533.

Lewis, D. H., 1990, Controlled release of bioactive agents from lactide/glycolide polymers, in: *Biodegradable Polymers as Drug Delivery Systems* (M. Chasin and R. Langer, eds.), Dekker, New York, pp. 1–41.

Liu, R., Langer, R., and Klibanov, A. M., 1991, Moisture-induced aggregation of lyophilized proteins in the solid state, *Biotechnol. Bioeng.* **37**:177–184.

McQueen, C. E., Boedeker, E. C., Reid, R., Jarboe, D., Wolf, M., Le, M., and Brown, W. R., 1993, Pili in microspheres protect rabbits from diarrhoea induced by *E. coli* strain RDEC-1, *Vaccine* **11(2)**:201–206.

Mitchison, N.A., 1990, Gonadotrophin vaccines, *Curr. Opin. Immunol.* **2**:725–727.

Moldoveanu, Z., Staas, J. K., Gilley, R. M., Ray, R., Compans, R. W., Eldridge, J. H., Tice, T. R., and Mestecky, J., 1989, Immune responses to influenza virus in orally and systemically immunized mice, *Curr. Top. Microbiol. Immunol.* **146**:91–99.

Moldoveanu, Z., Novak, M., Huang, W. Q., Gilley, R. M., Staas, J. K., Schafer, D., Compans, R. W., and Mestecky, J., 1993, Oral immunization with influenza virus in biodegradable microspheres, *J. Infect. Dis.* **167(1)**:84–90.

Neutra, M. R., and Kraehenbuhl, J.-P., 1992, Transepithelial transport and mucosal defence I: The role of M cells, *Trends Cell Biol.* **2**:134–138.

O'Hagan, D. T., 1990, Intestinal translocation of particulates—Implications for drug and antigen delivery, *Adv. Drug Deliv. Rev.* **5**:265–285.

O'Hagan, D. T., Jeffery, H., and Davis, S. S., 1993a, Long-term antibody responses in mice following subcutaneous immunization with ovalbumin entrapped in biodegradable microparticles, *Vaccine* **11(9)**:965–969.

O'Hagan, D. T., McGee, J. P., Holmgren, J., Mowat, A. M., Donachie, A. M., Mills, K. H. G., Gaisford, W., Rahman, D., and Challacombe, S. J., 1993b, Biodegradable microparticles for oral immunization, *Vaccine* **11**:149–154.

Okada, H., Inoue, Y., Heya, T., Ueno, H., Ogawa, Y., and Toguchi, H., 1991, Pharmacokinetics of once-a-month injectable microspheres of leuprolide acetate, *Pharm. Res.* **8**:787–791.

Payne, L. G., Jenkins, S. A., Andrianov, A., Langer, R., and Roberts, B. E., 1995, Xenobiotic polymers as vaccine vehicles, in: *Advances in Experimental Medicine and Biology* (J. R. McGee and J. Mestecky, eds.), Plenum Press, New York (in press).

Preis, I., and Langer, R., 1979, A single-step immunization by sustained antigen release, *J. Immunol. Methods.* **28**:193–197.

Reid, R. H., Boedeker, E. C., McQueen, C. E., Davis, D., Tseng, L.-Y., Kodak, J., Sau, K., Wilhelmsen, C. L., Nellore, R., Dalal, P., and Bhagat, H. R., 1993, Preclinical evaluation of microencapsulated CFA/II oral vaccine against enterotoxigenic *E. coli, Vaccine* **11(2)**:159–167.

Santiago, N., Milstein, S. J., Rivera, T., Garcia, E., Chang, T. C., Baughman, R. A., and Bucher, D., 1992, Oral immunization of rats with influenza virus M protein (M1) microspheres, in: *Proc. Int. Symp. Control. Rel. Bioact. Mater.*, Controlled Release Society, Orlando, pp. 116–117.

Schneider, A. K., 1972, Polylactide sutures, U.S. Patent 3,636,956.

Schreier, H., Levy, M., and Milhalko, P., 1987, Sustained release of liposome-encapsulated gentamicin and fate of phospholipid following intramuscular injection in mice, *J. Control. Rel.* **5**:187–192.

Staas, J. K., Hunt, R. E., Marx, P. A., Compans, R. W., Smith, J. F., Eldridge, J. H., Gibson, J. W., Tice, T. R., and Gilley, R. M., 1993, Mucosal immunization using microsphere delivery systems, in: *Proc. Int. Symp. Control. Rel. Bioact. Mater.*, Controlled Release Society, Washington, DC, pp. 63–64.

Stevens, V. C., 1993, Vaccine delivery systems: Potential methods for use in antifertility vaccines, *Am. J. Reprod. Immunol.* **29**:176–188.

Stevens, V. C., Powell, J. E., Lee, A. E., Kaumaya, P. T. P., Lewis, D. H., Rickey, M., and Atkins, T. J., 1992, Development of a delivery system for a birth control vaccine using biodegradable microspheres, in: *Proc. Int. Symp. Control. Rel. Bioact. Mater.*, Controlled Release Society, Orlando, pp. 112–113.

Tabata, Y., and Ikada, Y., 1986, Phagocytosis of bioactive microspheres, *J. Bioact. Compat. Polym.* **1**:32–46.

Tabata, Y., and Ikada, Y., 1987, Macrophage activation through phagocytosis of muramyl dipeptide encapsulated in gelatin microspheres, *J. Pharm. Pharmacol.* **39**:698–704.

Tabata, Y., and Ikada, Y., 1988a, Effect of the size and surface charge of polymer microspheres on their phagocytosis by macrophage, *Biomaterials* **9(4)**:356–362.

Tabata, Y., and Ikada, Y., 1988b, Macrophage phagocytosis of biodegradable microspheres composed of L-lactic/glycolic acid homo- and copolymers, *J. Biomed. Mater. Res.* **22**:837–858.

Tabata, Y., and Ikada, Y., 1989a, Protein precoating of polylactide microspheres containing a lipophilic immunopotentiator for enhancement of macrophage phagocytosis and activation, *Pharm. Res.* **6(4)**:296–301.

Tabata, Y., and Ikada, Y., 1989b, Synthesis of gelatin microspheres containing interferon, *Pharm. Res.* **6(5)**:422–427.

Tabata, Y., and Ikada, Y., 1990, Drug delivery systems for antitumor activation of macrophages, *Crit. Rev. Ther. Drug Carrier Syst.* **7(2)**:121–148.

Tabata, Y., Nakaoka, R., and Ikada, Y., 1993, Potentiality of gelatin microspheres as an immunological adjuvant, in: *Proc. Int. Symp. Control. Rel. Bioact. Mater.*, Controlled Release Society, Washington, DC, pp. 392–393.

Talwar, G. P., and Raghupathy, R., 1989, Anti-fertility vaccines, *Vaccine* **7**:97–101.

Tice, T. R., and Tabibi, S. E., 1992, Parenteral drug delivery: Injectables, in: *Treatise on Controlled Drug Delivery* (A. Kydonieus, ed.), Dekker, New York, pp. 315–339.

Volkin, D. B., and Klibanov, A. M., 1989, Minimizing protein inactivation, in: *Protein Function: A Practical Approach* (T. E. Creighton, ed.), IRL Press, Oxford, pp. 1–24.

Walsh, J. A., 1988, Establishing health priorities in the developing world, United Nations Development Programme, Report.

Warren, K. S., 1989, The biotechnology and children's revolutions, in: *Immunization* (R. K. Root, K. S. Warren, J. Griffiss, and M. A. Sande, eds.), Churchill Livingstone, Edinburgh, pp. 1–9.

Weiner, A. L., Carpenter-Green, S. S., Soehngen, E. C., Lenk, R. P., and Popescu, M. C., 1985, Liposome–collagen gel matrix: A novel sustained drug delivery system, *J. Pharm. Sci.* **74(9)**:922–925.

Wheeler, A. W., Moran, D. M., Robins, B. E., and Driscoll, A., 1982, L-Tyrosine as an immunological adjuvant, *Int. Arch. Allergy Appl. Immun.* **69**:113–119.

Wheeler, A. W., Whittall, N., Spackman, V., and Moran, D. M., 1984, Adjuvant properties of hydrophobic derivatives prepared from L-tyrosine, *Int. Arch. Allergy Appl. Immunol.* **75**:294–299.

Chapter 17

Vehicles for Oral Immunization

Noemi Santiago, Susan Haas, and
Robert A. Baughman

1. ORAL DELIVERY OF ANTIGENS

1.1. Introduction

New approaches to vaccine development have become possible since a common mucosal defense system was recognized whereby an antigen interacting with localized lymphoid tissue could stimulate IgA precursor cells that may then migrate to other mucosal surfaces (Craig and Cebra, 1971). Several oral vaccines have been shown to induce IgA responses at mucosal sites distal from that of the immunization, suggesting the feasibility of developing oral vaccines for protection against pathogens that gain entry through other mucosal routes (Table I). Mucosal surfaces represent the largest like-tissue type in vertebrates, providing an important anatomical, mechanical, and chemical barrier to the diverse environmental antigens of microbial and food origin, including pathogenic microorganisms, that are encountered daily. It is not surprising then that it is the most common portal of entry of ubiquitous viral, bacterial, and parasitic infectious agents. Oral immunization, by stimulating the gut-associated lymphoid tissue (GALT), presents a promising approach for protecting many secretory surfaces against a variety of infectious diseases. Not only are more lymphocytes found in the gut than in any organ in the body, but IgA is produced in twice the quantity of IgG, and more IgA is poured into the bowel each day than the combined IgG synthesized and released into the blood.

An enteric mucosal IgA response is probably best stimulated by locally administered antigen. Immature B cells that are precommitted to synthesis of IgA are especially numerous in gut-associated lymphoreticular tissue (Gearhart and Cebra, 1979) and are efficiently exposed to luminal antigens by a specialized mucosal antigen sampling mecha-

Noemi Santiago, Susan Haas, and Robert A. Baughman • Emisphere Technologies, Inc., Hawthorne, New York 10532.

Vaccine Design: The Subunit and Adjuvant Approach, edited by Michael F. Powell and Mark J. Newman. Plenum Press, New York, 1995.

nism (Owen, 1977; Owen *et al.*, 1986). By contrast, parenteral immunization is usually inefficient at evoking mucosal secretory IgA (sIgA) responses, and may actually suppress them (Pierce and Koster, 1980). It has been shown that mucosal lymphoid tissue differs from that of the systemic immune system in its lack of an age-associated decline in primary immune responsiveness (Szewczuk and Wade, 1983; Chen and Quinnan, 1989b). If the secretory antibody failed as the body's "first line of defense," the lack of serum antibody might allow pathogenesis. Thus, it would be advantageous to develop a system with a sequence of immunizations that would induce both a strong secretory antibody response as well as efficient humoral and cellular immune responses.

Immunizing via the oral route to stimulate the mucosal immune system offers several advantages over parenteral vaccination: (1) Ease and economics of preparation. Oral vaccines need not be highly purified, which would greatly simplify preparation. Larger amounts of material would probably be needed because of higher doses, but this could be offset by the less stringent requirements for manufacturing an oral formulation. In addition, preliminary studies indicate that some oral formulations may be lyophilized, thus reducing the need for refrigerated storage. (2) Ease and economics of dosing. These are probably the greater advantages. Oral formulations promote better patient compliance. The need to train in parenteral dosing is eliminated. Oral dosing enables home administration and facilitates mass vaccination. Intranasal immunization, although shown to be more efficient than oral immunization in several systems, has less acceptance by patients. In addition, appropriate inhalation delivery requires a critical level of cooperation and coordination not usually possible in young children. (3) Safety. Side effects (such as fever, diarrhea, flulike symptoms, malaise, erythema, and edema) associated with parenteral vaccines may be reduced or absent. For example, bacterial lipopolysaccharide contaminants are far less reactogenic by the oral route. These are important considerations, especially when vaccinating the chronically ill, children, and the elderly. (4) Efficacy. Effective stimulation of the mucosal immune system may improve vaccines that offer incomplete protection by parenteral immunization. Efficacy could also be improved in the elderly, since mucosal-associated lymphoid tissue appears not to undergo age-associated dysfunction. In addition, oral immunity may not be affected by maternal antibodies.

In addition, oral immunization may be more effective in controlling the spread of disease, facilitating eradication of diseases that persist through asymptomatic colonization of mucosal surfaces. An additional advantage is the potential of administering greater volumes of vaccine antigens used in combination vaccine strategies.

Several important barriers, however, must be overcome in order to efficiently immunize by the oral route: the obvious practical difficulties of avoiding degradation by the low pH and proteases in the GI tract, the short exposure to immune induction sites resulting from normal GI transit, and the very limited permeability that large molecules have through the GI tract. In addition, various tolerance mechanisms must be overcome in order to effectively immunize via the oral route. In that the gut is in constant contact with a large amount and variety of proteinaceous material, effective regulation mechanisms have been developed. Thus, mucosal immunosuppressant mechanisms have evolved to minimize the immune response to fed antigens (Genco *et al.*, 1983). Prior mucosal contact of antigen may not only suppress the induction of serum antibody, it may also reduce the subsequent absorption of antigen. This is a function of intestinal antibodies and is known as immune exclusion (Ogra and Karzon, 1970). Enteric administration of antigen to unprimed animals can blunt the immune response to that antigen following subsequent parenteral challenge, i.e., systemic tolerance (Wells, 1911; Wells and Osborne, 1911). Such systemic hyporesponsiveness is antigen-specific and will not develop if the animal has received prior systemic exposure to that antigen. Hyporesponsiveness appears to occur via a suppressor circuit initiated in the GALT on antigen exposure, and is time and dose dependent (Mattingly and Waksman, 1978).

Increasing clinical and experimental data have shown that small amounts of antigenically active proteins and macromolecules penetrate the adult intestinal epithelium. The extent of their absorption is dependent on the physical characteristics of the molecules, such as molecular weight, charge, configuration, and structure (O'Hagan *et al.*, 1987). Both soluble and particulate antigens have been used extensively for the induction of secretory immune responses in several animal models and humans (Emmings *et al.*, 1975; Kawanishi *et al.*, 1983; McDonald, 1993). Although some glycoprotein antigens such as bacterial pili, flagella, and enterotoxins, viral hemagglutinins, and other antigens have induced both secretory and mucosal responses when dosed orally (Pierce and Gowans, 1975; De Aizpurua and Russell-Jones, 1988), it is generally accepted that much higher and more frequent oral doses are necessary than with systemic immunization (McGhee *et al.*, 1992). Response to orally administered antigens will thus depend on antigen type, dose, frequency of exposure, and prior immune status. The simultaneous production of secretory antibodies and systemic tolerance, or enhanced antigen exclusion at the same time as the systemic tolerance, has been observed (Challacombe and Tomasi, 1980; Swarbrick *et al.*, 1979). Mattingly and Waksman (1980) have suggested that the sIgA response may be achieved most effectively by parenteral immunization followed by oral immunization with the appropriate antigen.

1.2. Approaches for Oral Immunization

Many groups have developed technologies for oral immunization that overcome several of the physiological and immunological barriers described above. Most involve carrier molecules either covalently bonded to or mixed with antigen, entrapment in vesicles, micro- or nanospheres of different types, or expression of antigen genes in bacterial and viral strains that are made avirulent but retain the ability to colonize the GI tract. General approaches that have been used are summarized below; references for each are found in Table I.

1.2.1. PROTECTION FROM PROTEASES

The ability to protect the antigen from degradation in the gut is of utmost importance in order to maintain doses at a level that provides efficacy. Ideally, a system should be able to protect from both gastric and intestinal proteases in the lumen and the membrane. Initial approaches to protect from gastrointestinal proteases involved the coadministration of large doses of bicarbonate to increase the pH of the stomach, rendering pepsin inactive (Mestecky, 1987). Other groups have pretreated animals with cimetidine for the ablation of gastric secretions (Klipstein *et al.*, 1983). Currently, protection of antigens in the GI

Table I
Adjuvants and Vehicles Used for Oral Immunization: Recent Developments[a]

Antigen delivery system	Antigen	Animal model	Responses monitored	Comments	References
Surfactant based					
Liposomes	*S. mutans* cell wall antigen	Rats	IgG and IgA in serum, IgA in saliva	IgA in serum and saliva IgG lower than IgA	Wachsmann *et al.* (1985)
	S. mutans	Rats	IgA in saliva	IgA and protection vs. challenge	Michalek *et al.* (1989)
ISCOMs	OVA	Mice	IgG, DTH, CTL	Low IgG, strong primary DTH (nothing with oral OVA alone)	Mowat *et al.* (1991)
Cochleates	Influenza envelope antigens	Mice	IgA in saliva, IgG in serum	Long-lasting titers	Mannino *et al.* (1993)
Emulsions			IgA in intestine, IgG in serum	Significant titers of both	Olsen and Hunter (1992)
Microorganism based					
Attenuated *Salmonella typhimurium*	Circumsporozoite protein	Mice	DTH	CMI response Protection without specific Ab	Sadoff *et al.* (1988)
Staph. xylosus	Heterologous receptors expressed on cell surface	Mice	Serum Ab	Receptor-specific humoral response	Nguyen *et al.* (1993)
Adenovirus	Hepatitis B	Chimpanzees	Anti-HBs antigen response	Antibodies + protection	Lubeck *et al.* (1989)
	Hepatitis B	Dogs	Anti-HBs antigen response	Oral response not comparable to i.t.	Chengalvala *et al.* (1991)
	HIV Env and Gag subunits	Chimpanzees	Anti-HIV IgG serum and IgA in nasal secretions Cell proliferation	Anti-Env Ab + CMI Gag boosted humoral + CMI to Gag antigen Env boosted CMI but not humoral response	Natuck *et al.* (1993)
Baculovirus	Rabies virus glycoprotein	Racoons	Neutralizing Ab in serum	Ab + protection vs. rabies virus	Fu *et al.* (1993)

Vehicle	Antigen	Animal	Immune response	Comments	Reference
Proteosomes	Neisseria meningitidis outer membrane protein; Shigella flexneri 2a or Shigella sonnei LPS	Mice, guinea pigs	IgG and IgA in intestinal and respiratory secretions and in sera	Anti-LPS Ab in mice. Oral followed by i.n. gave protection	Orr et al. (1993)
Microspheres					
PLGA	OVA	Mice	Serum and secretory IgG and IgA	IgG and IgA higher than with soluble OVA. High proliferative T-cell and CTL	O'Hagan et al. (1993), Challacombe et al. (1992)
	SEB	Mice	Serum IgG, IgM, IgA; IgA in saliva, gut, and lung	Injected + oral or i.t. induced mucosal IgA. Soluble gave no response	Eldridge et al. (1991)
	Simian immunodeficiency virus	Macaques	Serum IgG	i.m. + oral or i.m. + i.t. gave systemic and mucosal immunity + protection vs. vaginal challenge. Oral alone did not protect	Marx et al. (1993)
	Influenza virus A/H3N2	Mice	IgA in saliva	Higher salivary IgA with oral boost than with systemic. Serum IgG and protection comparable to systemic immunization	Moldoveanu et al. (1993)
Poly(butyl-2-cyanoacrylate)	OVA	Rats	IgG and IgA in serum and saliva	Significant secretory response	O'Hagan et al. (1989b)
Polyacrylamide	OVA	Rats	sIgA in saliva, IgG in serum	i.p. + oral boost induced IgG and IgA	O'Hagan et al. (1989a)
Proteinoids	Influenza M1, HA–NA; OVA/CT	Rats, mice	Serum IgG; IgA in intestinal secretions	Enhanced serum IgG and intestinal IgA titers	Santiago et al. (1993a, this chapter)

Table I

(continued)

Antigen delivery system	Antigen	Animal model	Responses monitored	Comments	References
Cholera toxin-based oral adjuvants					
CT+ CTB	Sendai virus	Mice	IgG and IgA in gut, nasal, and lung washes	Free toxoid (CTB) more effective in conjugated form than in mixture	Nedrud et al. (1989)
CTB	Influenza vaccine	Mice	IgG and IgA in serum and gut washings; HI Ab in serum	Oral induced low IgG, no HI; i.n. gave higher IgA than did oral	Hirabayashi et al. (1990)
	E. coli (ETEC) vaccine (CFA and LT)	Human	IgA in intestinal washings, IgG and IgA in serum	IgG and IgA response to toxin	Ahren et al. (1993)
	Strep. mutans I/II covalently coupled	Mice	Ab-secreting cells (ELISPOT) in salivary glands, mesenteric lymph nodes and spleen; Circulating IgG, IgA, IgM	Mucosal and serum IgA and IgG; Large number of Ab-secreting cells; Requires CT in addition to conjugated CTB	Czerkinsky et al. (1989), Russell and Wu (1991)
CT	S. mutans	Mice	IgM, IgG, IgA in serum and intestinal, vaginal, and lung washings	With or without CT, i.n. immunization was effective	Wu and Russell (1993)
	Trichinella spiralis	Mice	IgA, IgG, IgM in serum, bile, intestinal washings; Total muscle larvae recovery	T.s. antigen + CT gave protection	DeVos and Dick (1993)
	Helicobacter felis	Germfree mice	IgA and IgG	Elevated serum, gastric, and intestinal IgA + protection	Czinn et al. (1993)
	H. pylori	Mice, ferrets	IgG and IgA in serum and gastric and intestinal secretions	CT enhanced IgA and IgG in GI secretions and sera	Czinn and Nedrud (1991)

CT or CTB	*Toxoplasma gondii*	Mice	T-cell proliferation	CT gave enhanced splenic T-cell proliferation CTB alone did not	Bourguin *et al.* (1993)
	OVA	Mice	Serum IgA, IgG1, IgG2, IgG3	Oral (25 mg OVA + CT) + subcutaneous boost (100 μg OVA/CFA) gave strong response *vs.* OVA fed alone	Pierre *et al.* (1992)
	KLH	Mice		KLH + CT induced long-term memory KLH alone or with CTB did not	Vajdy and Lycke (1992)
CTB (conjugated) + CT adjuvant	KLH	Rats	IgA, IgG, IgM in secretions ELISPOT for IgA- and IgG-secreting cells	High IgA and IgG in mucosal washings after local immunization in genital tract or after combined oral and local immunization	Menge *et al.* (1993)
Others					
Chicken red blood cells	Influenza A vaccine	Mice	IgG and IgA in serum and secretions	High IgG and protection as compared to virus or chicken RBC alone	Pang *et al.* (1992)
pH-sensitive enteric coating	LT	Rats	Serum IgG; sIgA in intestinal washings	IgG and IgA + protection	Klipstein *et al.* (1983)

[a]ISCOMs: immune-stimulating complexes; OVA: ovalbumin; DTH: delayed-type hypersensitivity; CTL: cytotoxic T lymphocytes; CMI: cell-mediated immunity; Ab: antibody; i.t.: intratracheal; LPS: lipopolysaccharde; i.m.: intramuscular; i.n.: intranasal; i.p.: intraperitoneal; CT: cholera toxin; CTB: cholera toxin B-subunit; CFA: complete Freund's adjuvant; LT: *E. coli* labile toxin; HA: hemagglutinin; NA: neuraminidase; HI: hemagglutination inhibition; KLH: keyhole limpet hemocyanin; SEB: staphylococcal enterotoxin B.

tract has been achieved to varying degrees of success with entrapment or encapsulation of antigens in vesicles and microspheres of different types (Table I).

1.2.2. TARGETING TO IgA INDUCTIVE SITES

It is generally agreed that antigen administered orally is taken up in the Peyer's patches by modified epithelial cells (M cells) and is transported to the lymphoid tissue of the Peyer's patches, where the initial mucosal immune response occurs. Antigen-presenting cells in this site include macrophages, dendritic cells, and B cells. After antigen-induced proliferation and partial differentiation, both T and B cells enter the regional mesenteric nodes and, after further differentiation, are transported through the thoracic duct into the circulatory system (reviewed by Butcher, 1986). Eberson and Molinari (1978) demonstrated that oral immunization with particulate antigens induced higher salivary antibody levels than the corresponding soluble antigens. Cox and Taubman (1982, 1984) have also demonstrated from gastric intubation studies that particulate antigens generally lead to a higher salivary antibody response than an equivalent dose of that same antigen in solution. This may be related to a greater ability of particulate material to gain access to the tissue of the Peyer's patches (O'Hagan *et al.*, 1987). Studies done with labeled PLGA microspheres have demonstrated that these microspheres are taken up in Peyer's patches if they are within a particle size range of 1–10 μm (Eldridge *et al.*, 1989). It has been suggested that surface properties, as well as particle size, govern accumulation in Peyer's patches, with penetration of the Peyer's patch epithelium being more easily achieved by particles with hydrophobic surfaces (LeFevre *et al.*, 1985). Soluble antigen, when injected systemically, is more effective at priming for a secretory antibody response than is an equivalent dose of particulate antigen (Cox and Taubman, 1984). This is probably because the particulate antigen is more likely to be filtered from the circulatory system by secondary lymphoid tissues (Waldman *et al.*, 1970; Ebersole and Molinari, 1978; Cox and Taubman, 1984).

Another approach used to target antigens to epithelial cells is to administer them with adhesins or lectins, molecules that are usually of bacterial origin and that bind to cell surface molecules or receptors. These molecules are, in fact, good oral immunogens by themselves. Examples of these are viral HA antigens, bacterial adhesins, bacterial toxins (or subunits of these), and lipopolysaccharide and pokeweed mitogens (De Aizpurua and Russell-Jones, 1988; Shahin *et al.*, 1992).

1.2.3. MUCOSAL ADJUVANTS

Oral adjuvants have been used to abrogate tolerance and immunopotentiate the immune response, thus reducing the dose required. Compounds such as detergents, lipid-conjugates, streptomycin, and vitamin A have been used as oral adjuvants (reviewed by Holmgren *et al.*, 1992). These agents may influence the structural and/or functional integrity of mucosal surfaces. Cholera toxin is by far the most potent and well-characterized oral adjuvant, and has been mixed with or linked to a wide variety of viral, bacterial, and parasitic antigens, as well as several well-characterized model antigens. This work is summarized in Table I and in Section 2.2.

1.2.4. OTHER APPROACHES TO INDUCE MUCOSAL IMMUNITY

Recently, novel approaches have been used in order to induce a potent secretory immune response by circumventing the need for oral administration of antigens. One of these approaches is the use of isotype stimulation of IgA by monoclonal antibodies (mAbs) specific to the extracellular segment of the membrane anchor peptide of membrane-bound IgA (mIgA). These mAbs bind to mIgA on B cells but not to soluble IgA, and are being studied as potential agents for isotype-specific regulation of IgA-expressing B cells (Chang, 1993a,b).

The concept of biomimesis has also been used for this purpose. The microenvironmental influences that exist within mucosal draining lymphoid tissues have been mimicked in peripheral lymph nodes. Humoral and common mucosal immune responses are induced when this technique is linked to subcutaneous vaccination afferent to the manipulated lymphoid organ (Daynes and Areneo, 1992).

2. NOVEL ADJUVANTS AND VEHICLES FOR ORAL IMMUNIZATION

Recent years have seen a flurry of research activity focused toward the development of adjuvants and vehicles for oral immunization that better protect vaccine integrity and provide more efficient targeting and immunopotentiation. Several excellent reviews have been published that summarize the work conducted with live oral vaccines and well-known antigen delivery systems such as cholera toxin, liposomes, attenuated bacterial strains, and biodegradable polymer microspheres (Mestecky and McGhee, 1989; Mestecky, 1987; Holmgren et al., 1992; McGhee et al., 1992; O'Hagan et al., 1987). This section groups and discusses these approaches, emphasizes the work done during the past 5 years, and includes various novel adjuvants and vehicles that have been developed during this period. For ease of reference, Table I summarizes the more recent efforts.

2.1. Surfactant-Based Vehicles

Several vesicle or particulate lipid-based vehicles have been developed and used for oral immunization with varying degrees of success. Liposomes (Genco et al., 1983) are probably the best known and have been used by a number of groups as carriers or vehicles for drugs and adjuvants. It has been suggested that binding of the antigen's hydrophobic regions to the liposome surface provides a critical epitope density. The liposome–antigen complex may attach to the gut epithelial cells, and be taken up in a more immunogenic manner.

Genco et al. (1983) have appreciably augmented the IgA response in saliva with orally administered lecithin–cholesterol liposomes that incorporate BSA with and without MDP as adjuvant. Immunized animals were found to have IgA anti-BSA antibodies in their saliva at 21, 35, and 49 days, while IgG and IgM responses in serum were virtually absent. Rats immunized by the intragastric route with liposome-associated soluble antigen extracted from S. mutans cell wall showed significantly higher IgA (and IgG) responses than did rats that were injected with the soluble antigen alone (Wachsmann et al., 1985). These results are in agreement with Morisaki et al. (1983) who found that oral immunization of rats with

S. mutans cell wall and MDP elicited a strong salivary IgA response. Work done by this same group (Michalek *et al.*, 1989) showed that while purified *S. mutans* antigen did not induce a salivary response or protection, oral administration in liposomes induced a good salivary response and a reduction in caries activity. Incorporation of MDP augmented both the salivary response and the protection observed. More recent studies have been done with purified fimbriae of *Porphyromonas gingivalis* orally dosed in liposomes to BALB/c mice (Hamada *et al.*, 1992; Kusumoto *et al.*, 1993). Not only were enhanced fimbria-specific salivary IgA responses observed, but significant numbers of fimbria-specific IgA spot-forming cells (SFCs) were found in the intestinal lamina propia, mesenteric lymph nodes, and the parotid and submandibular glands.

ISCOMs are cagelike micelles formed by the spontaneous coalescence of phosphatidylcholine and cholesterol in the presence of Quil A (saponin). They have been widely used as parenteral adjuvants, and are reviewed in Chapter 23. ISCOMs containing 100μg of ovalbumin induced, in BALB/c mice, serum IgG titers 21 days after oral immunization, although levels were generally low. Oral dosing of 100μg of soluble OVA produced no systemic DTH or antibody response. The required dose for oral immunization with ISCOMs was 10-fold higher (100μg) than that needed for parenteral immunization, but 100-fold less than that needed to induce a response by OVA alone (Mowat *et al.*, 1991).

Recent reports describe the use of cochleates—rolled-up phospholipid precipitates that entrap antigens—in oral immunization (Mannino *et al.*, 1993; see Chapter 15). A single oral dose of cochleates with influenza virus envelope glycoproteins resulted in slowly increasing antibody titers (IgA, IgG) in mice. Higher titers were obtained with two oral doses, and the response obtained was shown to be protective from challenge with virus.

Other groups have found multiple phase vaccines containing high-molecular-weight polymers to be highly efficient in the delivery of native antigens past the stomach and upper gastrointestinal tract (Brey, 1993, see Chapter 11). This formulation appeared to be stable in an acid environment and to be taken up in Peyer's patches, as evidenced by induction of circulating IgG and intestinal IgA. Antibody to intranasal, intragastric, or intramuscular immunization with a particulate (influenza HA) and a soluble (rHSV2 glycoprotein D) antigen in low-oil emulsions were compared. Intranasal immunization did not require parenteral priming if MF59 was present (Barchfeld, 1993).

2.2. Microorganism-Based Delivery

The ability of attenuated *Salmonella typhi* or *S. typhimirium* to invade, persist, and proliferate in the human or murine GALT and induce a protective immune response, without causing clinical symptoms, has been known for many years (Curtiss *et al.*, 1989). Several systems of attenuated bacteria have been successfully tested and used in large-scale immunization (Sabin, 1976; Clements *et al.*, 1986; Cardenas and Clement, 1992). Concomitant appearance of secretory and serum IgA, IgG, and IgM is a result of the colonization within the GI tract of orally administered *Salmonella*. These findings have prompted many investigators to introduce coding genes for other antigens into modified strains of *Salmonella*, thus using them as vectors for the selective delivery of antigen to the GALT (see Table I). Auxotrophic mutants, which are avirulent but still immunogenic (Curtiss *et al.*, 1989), are capable of expressing virulent antigens from other pathogens and are less dangerous. Other bacteria and viruses have also been used as live vectors: *E. coli* (Hale, 1991; Ahren *et al.*, 1993), *Yersinia enterolitica* (Sory and Cornelis, 1990), *Staphylococcus xylosus* (Nguyen *et al.*, 1993), lactobacilli (Gerritse *et al.*, 1990), or BCG (Barletta *et al.*, 1990). A prototype vaccine containing enterotoxigenic *E. coli* (formalin inactivated) expressing Cf/I and CFA/II mixed with CTB was tested in Swedish volunteers (Ahren *et al.*, 1993). Three doses were given at 2-week intervals. A rise in IgA in intestinal lavages was obtained at levels comparable to those found in patients with severe enterotoxigenic *E. coli* diarrhea.

Viruses that infect the GI tract such as baculovirus and adenovirus (Chengalvala *et al.*, 1991; Fu *et al.*, 1993; Natuk *et al.*, 1993) are also being considered as potential vectors for expressing antigens of other viruses. A complicating factor in microorganism-based delivery, which may limit its utility to a single immunization protocol, is the immune response to both the carrier and the antigen. The anticarrier response will prevent colonization of the GALT following a second immunization. However, given adequate time for the anticarrier response to decrease, subsequent doses may be effective. This has been experimentally demonstrated by Pierce *et al.* (1987).

In addition, purified *Neisseria* outer membrane protein preparations noncovalently complexed to antigens (proteosomes) can be dosed intranasally or orally and induce respiratory and intestinal IgA as well as serum IgG (Orr *et al.*, 1993). Protection has also been demonstrated in models of shigellosis or staphylococcal enterotoxin intoxication (Lowell, 1993).

2.2.1. CELL ADHESION MOLECULES

Antigens dosed orally, even in milligram doses, are inefficient in inducing a strong immune response and, in fact, can induce a state of tolerance. Molecules that possess lectin-like qualities, however, have been shown to elicit both secretory and systemic immune responses. Oral administration of various bacterial adhesive molecules, such as pili, flagella, *E. coli* LTB, viral HA, and LPS, were found to induce a vigorous immune response, while molecules that do not possess this binding activity (e.g., BSA) did not elicit significant responses at the doses tested (De Aizpurua and Russell-Jones, 1988). LT-OA is an *E. coli* heat-labile enterotoxin that has been shown to induce immunity in the intestine and the lung when mixed with peptides or microbial vaccines dosed orally. LT-OA induced high levels of systemic antibody and generated protective and long-lasting immunity to *Campylobacter* (Bourgeois, 1993), influenza (Majde, 1994; Katz, 1993), and other unrelated protein antigens (Clements *et al.*, 1988). Purified *Bordetella pertussis* filamentous hemagglutinin (FHA) dosed intranasally or orally was found to protect from *B. pertussis* infection as measured by the reduction in the recovery of bacteria from the lungs and the trachea of BALB/c mice (Shahin *et al.*, 1992). This major adhesin generates a specific immune response in the respiratory tract. The response to many of these lectin-like molecules is abolished by co-feeding sugars that are homologous to the terminal sugars of GM1 and GM2 gangliosides, to which these molecules are known to bind (De Aizpurua and Russell-Jones, 1988). It appears that these antigens bind to glycolipids and glycoproteins on the intestinal mucosa and stimulate these cells to transport the proteins into the circulatory system, thereby eliciting a systemic immune response.

2.2.2. CHOLERA TOXIN

Cholera toxin (CT) is one of the most potent oral immunogens identified (Pierce and Gowans, 1975). CT is composed of A and B subunits. The toxicogenic A subunit is involved in the ADP-ribosylation of the adenylate cyclase regulatory protein Gs. This modification increases cAMP levels and causes intestinal secretion, resulting in the diarrhea and fluid loss observed in patients with cholera. The B subunit (CTB) is composed of five identical noncovalently associated subunits that serve as the carrier for the A and bind to the monosialoganglioside GM1 (Cuatrecasas, 1973), which is abundant on the surface of intestinal cells. From a practical standpoint, CT cannot be used in humans because of its potential toxicity; thus, many studies have focused on using CTB, which retains the binding capabilities but does not have the toxic activity. Chemical coupling appears to be more efficient; conjugated horseradish peroxidase (HRP)–CT induced higher antibody levels in the gut and in serum than those obtained with HRP alone or coadministered with CT (Lycke and Holmgren, 1986). In other systems, coadministration worked only when small amounts of holotoxin were added (McKenzie and Halsey, 1984).

CT and CTB do not induce oral tolerance. CT and CTB dosed orally also result in prolonged memory responses in the intestinal lamina propria and, presumably, other mucosal effector sites. Elson and Ealding (1984) demonstrated the ability of CT to abrogate oral tolerance to keyhole limpet hemocyanin (KLH) when mice were fed with both proteins together; an intestinal IgA response was obtained with the co-feeding but not with KLH alone. CT does not fit the classical definition of an adjuvant because it stimulates an immune response to itself. It has, however, been successfully used with a variety of antigens as an oral adjuvant (Elson and Ealding, 1984; McKenzie and Halsey, 1984; Liang *et al.*, 1988; Czerkinsky *et al.*, 1989).

Lycke and Holmgren (1986) have also shown CT to be a potent adjuvant of enteric mucosal immune responses to KLH, and effective in both priming and boosting. Elicitation of a secondary-type response did not require CT and could result from reencounter with specific bacterial or viral antigens (Vajdy and Lycke, 1992). They have examined its adjuvant activity and found the required adjuvant dose (100–500 ng) lower than the required immunogenic dose (2 μg), and much below the dose that elicits fluid secretion increases in mouse intestine. Activity was found to be dose-dependent and required coadministration. High numbers of specific antibody-producing cells, as well as mucosal memory in the lamina propria, were obtained when CT was included in the oral booster. Menge *et al.* (1993) also dosed KLH/CT orally and found IgA titers in salivary glands and gut, but not in vaginal secretions. A vigorous local immune response in the vagina was only achieved when an oral dose was boosted with intravaginal dosing.

Oral immunization with an intranasal booster has been shown to induce immunity to Sendai viruses (Nedrud *et al.*, 1989). Cholera toxoid is equally effective at enhancing IgA viral antibodies when covalently linked to or mixed with Sendai virus. *Helicobacter felis* has been coadministered with CT orally in order to immunize against *H. pylori* (Czinn and Nedrud, 1991). A protective response was obtained, accompanied by gastric, intestinal, and serum antibodies; proliferative responses of spleen cells to bacterial antigens were also observed. Antigen-specific antibodies in the gastric secretions coincided with oral immunization and protection of the stomach from infection with the pathogen. Optimal immunization of murine mucosa-associated lymphoid tissue was achieved by intragastrically immunizing mice four times over a 4-week period (1 mg *H. pylori*).

Intranasal immunization also was optimal for influenza virus vaccine coadministered with CTB. Oral vaccination induced low levels of antiviral serum IgG but no detectable serum hemagglutination inhibition titers, while parenteral immunization failed to induce IgA in intestinal secretions (Hirabayashi *et al.*, 1990). Mice dosed with soluble, particulate, or soluble plus particulate *Trichinella spiralis* antigen plus CT at days 0, 14, and 21 yielded significant reductions in adult worm fecundity and size and mean number of total muscle larvae. The response was also enhanced in the particulate, but not in soluble or soluble/particulate antigen treatments without CT (DeVos and Dick, 1993). *Toxoplasma gondii* sonicates have also been dosed with CT (Bourgin *et al.*, 1993). Increased proliferation of specific splenic T lymphocytes, increased IL-2 and gamma interferon, and significant protection was obtained with CT, but not with CTB.

Russell and Wu (1991) demonstrated that microgram amounts of *S. mutans* protein ag I/II covalently coupled to the B subunit of CT elicit vigorous mucosal, as well as extramucosal, IgA and IgG antistreptococcal antibody responses in mice, as manifested by large numbers of antibody-secreting cells in salivary glands, mesenteric lymph nodes, and spleens, and high levels of circulating antibodies (Czerkinsky *et al.*, 1989). A subclinical dose of free CT was necessary for the generation of optimal antibody responses; purified CTB was not able to fulfill this adjuvant role by itself. Cells actively secreting IgA against *S. mutans* protein ag I/II but not against CT were detected in salivary glands. Two to three intragastric doses of 15 μg or more were needed and the response persisted for 5 to 6 months. Intranasal immunization induced stronger initial antibody responses in both serum and saliva than intragastric, but the response did not increase after a booster at 3 months. Free CTB was able to replace CT as an adjuvant by the intranasal route. Recently, significant IgA titers were obtained in fecal extracts of mice receiving two oral doses of tetanus toxoid dosed orally with CT (Jackson *et al.*, 1993).

There are indications that the mechanism of CT adjuvanticity involves multiple aspects of mucosal immune induction, including increased uptake of antigen into mucosal follicles [mediated by its ability to bind ganglioside receptors on intestinal epithelium and/or submucosal lymphoid cells (Pierce, 1978)], enhancement of IL-1 production by APCs, altered regulation of T cells (especially inhibition of $CD8^+$ suppressor cells), stimulation of B cell switching to IgA and IgG, and possibly enhancement of B-cell clonal expansion (reviewed by McGhee *et al.*, 1992). A combination of these signals may result in altering the regulatory environment of the GALT from one of suppression to one of responsiveness. CT has to be administered simultaneously and by the same route, suggesting that the mucosal tissue is altered in a way that favors responsiveness to the antigens presented to it.

Although some studies have failed to show an enhancing effect of CT on the mucosal immune response to a "bystander antigen" (Pierce, 1978), CT or substances that use similar adjuvant mechanisms may substantially increase the mucosal immunogenicity and efficacy of most nonreplicating oral vaccines.

2.3. Microspheres

One oral delivery system for antigens that has been more widely used is the PLGA microsphere system, which is made out of the biocompatible and biodegradable polymer PLGA. This material has a history of safe application in humans and has been shown to have adjuvant properties following parenteral administration. It also has been used for the oral delivery of a number of antigens (Table I). Microspheres less than 10 μm have been shown to be taken up by the M cells in the Peyer's patches throughout the GI tract and are carried within macrophages to the mesenteric lymph nodes and spleen. This process allows these vehicles to be effective not only in protecting the antigens throughout the GI tract, but also in targeting the appropriate induction sites (Eldridge *et al.*,1989). Three oral doses of *Staphylococcus* toxoid microspheres stimulated circulating IgM, IgG, and IgA antitoxin antibodies and a concurrent mucosal IgA response in saliva, gut, and lung washings (Eldridge *et al.*, 1991). However, neither free nor encapsulated toxoid induced a detectable mucosal IgA response following systemic injection. Systemic immunization with toxoid microspheres primed for the induction of disseminated mucosal IgA responses by subsequent oral and intratracheal boosting in microspheres. while soluble boosting was ineffective. More recently, Marx *et al.* (1993) showed protection against vaginal challenge with SIV in macaques immunized intramuscularly with formalinized SIV in PLGA microspheres followed with an oral booster.

Antigenicity of *E. coli* heat-labile enterotoxin was not protected against the adverse effect of gastric acidity when the toxin was given together with bicarbonate for oral immunization to rats (Klipstein *et al.*, 1983). Immunization with the heat-labile enterotoxin encapsulated in microspheres with pH-dependent dissolution properties induced the same serum and mucosal antitoxin responses and protection against challenge infection achieved by oral immunization after ablation of gastric secretions by pretreatment with cimetidine.

Polyacrylamide microparticles (O'Hagan *et al.*, 1989b) have been used to encapsulate ovalbumin. Mice were primed i.p. and given four consecutive oral doses 2 weeks later. The memory IgA antibody response (day 65) to the microparticle-incorporated antigen group was significantly higher relative to the soluble antigen control group response following administration of a booster dose of soluble antigen to both groups. Finally, water-soluble phosphazene polymers have been used for mucosal immunization with tetanus and influenza antigens (see Chapter 20).

3. PROTEINOID-BASED ORAL ANTIGEN DELIVERY

3.1. Review of the Technology

Proteinoid-based oral delivery stems from the finding that condensation polymers of mixed natural amino acids, with a stoichiometric excess of acidic amino acids, form microspheres when subjected to acid pH (Fox, 1977). In our search for an oral delivery system that protects antigens from degradation by the acids and enzymes of the GI tract, proteinoid microspheres were shown to effectively protect and deliver a variety of agents, including heparin and insulin (Steiner and Rosen, 1990). The proteinoids, initially evaluated for oral drug delivery, were relatively low-molecular-weight (< 1500) polymers with linear and/or branched chain structures, derived from a combination of acidic and aromatic amino acids (e.g., tyrosine and aspartic acid). Typically, a stirred mixture of amino acids was heated for varying lengths under nitrogen to 160–190°C and the evolution of water was monitored. After a defined reaction time, the mixture was brought to room temperature, and extracted into water (process described in Steiner and Rosen,1990). The final product was dried and ground to a powder. Subsequent evaluation of the condensation process indicated that greater yields could be achieved with the sequential addition of the amino acids and the use of inert solubilizers. Microsphere-forming material could be produced with as few as two or three amino acids. However, the final product of any given condensation reaction remained a mixture of proteinoids, with little control over the distribution of the various components. Microspheres are prepared by dissolving the synthesized proteinoid in water and mixing with the protein cargo that is dissolved in a mild organic acid. Preparation of microspheres does not expose antigens to organic solvents or extremes of pH or temperature.

Spectral analysis of the thermal condensation products suggested that a series of small peptides (and their analogues) were responsible for microsphere formation. These second-generation products were then synthesized as discrete chemical entities via solution and solid-phase chemistry, and subjected to in-depth in vitro and in vivo testing with active agents that ranged in size from 500 to 150,000 Da. These data, correlating a physicochemical parameter (or parameters) to a biological response, were then used to create families of carriers. Individual carriers were then altered to increase or decrease a given parameter (e.g., lipophilicity) with a series of modifying agents selected for that purpose. These third-generation compounds, now produced via simple, defined synthetic processes, are those compounds now being developed for the oral delivery of macromolecules. Agents that have elicited therapeutic responses following proteinoid oral delivery include salmon calcitonin (Sarubbi *et al.*, 1994), low-molecular-weight heparin (Milstein *et al.*, 1993a), and heparin (Santiago *et al.*, 1992, 1993b). Since we had already achieved the more difficult task of delivering peptides and macromolecules to the circulatory system (Sarubbi *et al.*, 1994; Milstein *et al.*, 1993b; Santiago *et al.*, 1992, 1993b) we decided to study these vehicles for the oral delivery of antigens. This work is described in the sections below.

3.2. Oral Immunization with Flu Antigens

Immunity to influenza induced by parenteral or intranasal immunization has been extensively studied (Schvartsman and Zycov, 1976; Clements and Murphy,1986; Ray *et al.*, 1988; Moldoveanu *et al.*, 1989). Oral immunization of mice with inactivated influenza virus has been shown to induce hemagglutinin-specific IgA in the lung and IgG isotype antibodies in the serum (Chen *et al.*, 1987: Bergmann and Waldman, 1989). This immune response resulted in protection against challenge with a lethal dose of the virus. Moldoveanu *et al.* (1989, 1993) have immunized mice with influenza virus by oral and systemic routes using PLGA microspheres as the delivery system. They found that microencapsulated vaccine given by the oral route induced higher antibody titers than a similar dose of nonencapsulated antigen. In contrast to mice immunized with free antigen, influenza-specific IgA and IgG antibodies remained elevated in mice that were orally immunized with microencapsulated material. Most of these responses were only observed after the mice were boosted by additional oral doses of microencapsulated antigen. Two oral doses induced significant priming, but neither antibody titer nor protection was comparable to that obtained with two systemic doses of either microencapsulated or free antigen. In saliva, higher levels of specific antibodies were observed in orally boosted versus systemically boosted animals.

We have successfully manufactured proteinoid microspheres with both HA–NA and M1 antigens of influenza virus type A (Santiago *et al.*, 1992). These microspheres, when examined by scanning electron microscopy, were found to be fenestrated structures of about 0.1 to 10 μm diameter (Fig. 1). The proteinoid microspheres used in this study were stable when incubated in simulated gastric fluid; but disassembled rapidly and released their contents when exposed to a pH greater than 5 in in vitro tests. Additional studies have shown that disassembly can be influenced by ionic concentration, degree of dilution, and the type of material being encapsulated.

We have been able to induce a significant primary antibody response to M1 antigen from influenza type A virus with a single enteric dose of M1 entrapped in proteinoid microspheres (Table II). A vigorous response, but in a lower percentage of animals, was also generated with HA–NA spheres (Table III). These titers were obtained with a single

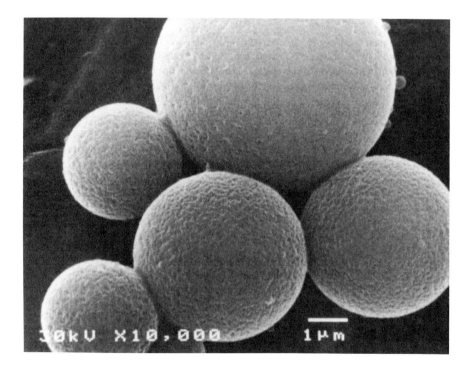

Figure 1. Scanning electron micrograph of proteinoid microspheres.

Table II
Dosing of Rats with Encapsulated Influenza Type A M_1 Protein:
Mean Anti-M_1 Protein Serum IgG Titers

Dosing formulation	Day 14	Day 28	Day 42
Oral M_1 protein: unencapsulated 1 mg/rat	<30	<30	36 ± 5
M_1 protein microspheres 1 mg/rat	760 ± 388	630 ± 338	1890 ± 985
Empty microspheres	<30	<30	69 ± 7

oral microsphere dose and were increasing up to 6 weeks postdose, at which time the experiment was terminated. Unencapsulated HA–NA did induce a moderate serum IgG response, while unencapsulated M1 did not. The techniques used for the preparation and purification of HA–NA allow it to retain its lectin properties and thus bind to mucosal cells, possibly facilitating its transport and allowing it to induce a systemic IgG response. It has been demonstrated that antigens with lectinlike properties can induce a response on their own when dosed orally (De Aizpurua and Russell-Jones, 1988). M1, being an internal component and lacking these properties, should not be transported by this mechanism. Thus, M1 was able to induce an IgG response only when dosed in microspheres. Two of the five animals dosed with M1 microspheres failed to show a significant increase in antibody titers, as did four of the rats dosed with HA–NA microspheres. This may reflect interanimal variability in the response or variability in physiologic factors such as gastric emptying time and/or intestinal pH and motility.

3.3. Ovalbumin as a Model Antigen

Various laboratories have used OVA as a model antigen to examine immune responses to orally administered antigens encapsulated in biodegradable microspheres and other vehicles. Poly(butyl-2-cyanoacrylate) particles with adsorbed OVA have been dosed orally to rats previously primed by intraperitoneal injection (O'Hagan et al., 1989a). Salivary IgA was significantly increased in animals receiving the adsorbed OVA versus a control group receiving soluble antigen. This group also used polyacrylamide microspheres to orally dose encapsulated OVA (O'Hagan et al., 1989b). These microspheres were dosed orally on four consecutive days to rats primed 14 days earlier by intraperitoneal injection.

Table III
Dosing of Rats with Encapsulated HA–NA Antigen: Mean Anti-HA Serum IgG Titers

Dosing formulation[a]	Day 7	Day 14	Day 28	Day 42	Day 56
Oral HA–NA control	<30	640 ± 258	2460 ± 720	5080 ± 3360	5180 ± 3100
	(N=7)	(N=7)	(N=5)	(N=5)	(N=5)
Oral HA–NA	85 ± 55	460 ± 331	4000 ± 2900	$12,280 \pm 10,100$	$22,170 \pm 21,740$
microspheres	(N=6)	(N=6)	(N=6)	(N=6)	(N=3)

[a]Antigen was dosed alone (control) or in microspheres at days 0 and 42.

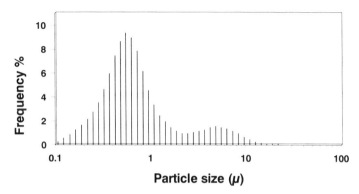

Figure 2. Laser particle size distribution analysis of proteinoid microspheres prepared by combining an aqueous solution of proteinoid EMI119 with an acidic solution of ovalbumin and cholera toxin (pH 3). Microsphere sample was diluted in citric acid (0.4 mL in 7.0 mL) for analysis. Measurements were done in a Horiba LA-500 Laser Particle Size Distribution Analyzer.

Again, salivary IgA was found to be enhanced by microencapsulation of the OVA. Oral administration of OVA encapsulated in PLGA microspheres to mice also showed much higher salivary IgA responses than those mice receiving soluble antigen. However, these differences were only observed after two series of intragastric immunizations (Challacombe *et al.*, 1992). Serum IgG levels were also significantly higher in the group receiving microspheres (O'Hagan *et al.*, 1993). Finally, a single dose of OVA encapsulated in ISCOMs has been shown to induce low levels of serum IgG and a strong DTH response (Mowat *et al.*, 1991).

A secondary immunization with OVA induces a stronger response in mice primed with unencapsulated OVA plus CT than in mice primed with OVA alone or with saline (Pierre *et al.*, 1992). In order to examine whether proteinoid microspheres would be efficacious in inducing a strong mucosal response as well as serum antibodies, we coencapsulated OVA and CT, the latter as a mucosal adjuvant. OVA and CT were encapsulated in microspheres made with "third-generation" proteinoids, which are low-molecular-weight peptides made by synthetic methods that do not require thermal condensation. Microspheres were made as described above. The resulting microspheres were examined by microscopy and laser particle size distribution analysis (Fig. 2). OVA/CT spheres exhibited properties similar to those observed with regular proteinoid microspheres in terms of particle size distribution and solubility profile. Approximately 90% of the OVA in the dosing preparation was entrapped in the microspheres.

BALB/c mice received either a single dose of OVA/CT spheres or were primed i.p. or s.c. with soluble OVA/CT and received an oral booster dose with microspheres 11 days later. The i.p. and s.c. doses consisted of 10 μg OVA and 10 μg CT; oral doses consisted of 100 μg OVA and 10 μg CT. Control groups that received a single oral dose or those receiving primary and booster immunizations received OVA/CT in soluble form only. Serum samples we collected after immunization, and intestinal secretions were collected by administering a hypertonic solution (Elson *et al.*, 1984).

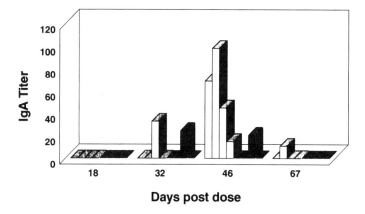

Figure 3. Kinetics of anti-OVA IgA response in individual animal to a single oral dose of OVA/CT microspheres (white bars) or soluble OVA/CT control (black bars).

Administration of single doses of OVA/CT in microspheres resulted in significant IgA titers in intestinal secretions, peaking at 46 days postimmunization (Fig. 3). Significant IgG titers were also obtained. IgA and IgG titers were much lower in response to dosing with OVA/CT in soluble form (Figs. 3 and 4). Mice primed with soluble OVA/CT by the i.p. and s.c. route and then boosted with OVA/CT microspheres had IgA titers similar to those obtained in mice receiving a single oral dose of microspheres. Preliminary data suggest, however, that priming parenterally appears to make the secretory response of greater duration (data not shown). IgG responses were greatly increased in the animals primed parenterally before receiving the oral boost with microspheres. The IgG titers in

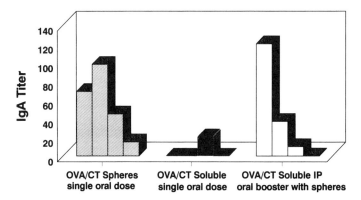

Figure 4. Peak anti-OVA IgA titers in intestinal secretions (46 days after primary immunization) in mice given a single oral dose of microspheres (hatched bars) versus a single oral dose of soluble OVA/CT (black bar) versus an intraperitoneal primary dose followed by an oral boost with microspheres (white bars).

both the single oral dose and the primed animals have continued to increase up to 9 weeks postimmunization.

Recent investigations with our microsphere technology have yielded further evidence of efficacy in inducing immune responses in various animal models. In studies performed in collaboration with Dr. Fidel Zavala (New York University), significant stimulation of specific helper T cells (CD4+) was measured in mice immunized with OVA encapsulated in microspheres (0.1 mg per mouse). Three different dosing schedules were tried, and all induced OVA-dependent proliferation of CD4+ T cells. In addition, preliminary studies with a poultry vaccine encapsulated in microspheres show protection against challenge after three consecutive oral doses in 19 out of 19 chickens.

These results confirm that the lymphoid tissues of the gut have a high potential to initiate immune responses against antigens that are effectively delivered. They also indicate that the microspheres may be able to provide protection and/or immunopotentiation by either appropriate targeting or facilitation of transport to the bloodstream. Experiments with oral dosing of parenterally primed animals versus oral dosing alone confirm oral exposure is more effective in inducing secretory immunity. The serum IgG response observed when orally dosing antigens in proteinoid microspheres may be the result of uptake of antigen-loaded microspheres into Peyer's patches and eventual delivery of antigen into the circulation. The microspheres thus not only protect the antigen through the GI tract but may, in addition, target the antigen to mucosally associated lymphoid tissues; microspheres this size have been demonstrated to be taken up at these sites (Eldridge *et al.*,1989). This may not, however, be the only mechanism by which proteinoid microspheres facilitate transport of proteins to the bloodstream. Both proteinoid microspheres, as well as the soluble carriers based on this technology, have been shown to facilitate the delivery of macromolecules dosed orally. Sarubbi *et al.* (1994) have demonstrated the oral delivery of calcitonin in rats and primates, while collaborative studies (Milstein *et al.*, 1993b) show oral delivery of a monoclonal antibody. Recent work done by Leipold and collaborators (personal communication) confirms the oral delivery of interferon α. Thus, the proteinoid microspheres may be acting in three different ways: protecting the antigen in the GI tract, targeting the antigen to the Peyer's patches, and facilitating transport of native antigen to the bloodstream.

Most studies with oral microsphere administration induced a significant immune response only after repeated exposures over a period of weeks or as a booster after parenteral immunization. These microspheres and other vehicles require antigen doses in the milligram range. For example, studies conducted with microencapsulated OVA (discussed previously) used up to 60 times the amount of antigen that was dosed with the proteinoid microspheres. The studies with OVA and CT in soluble form used 250-fold greater antigen dose than in the proteinoid microspheres. Microspheres made with proteinoid carriers allow antigens to survive acidic and proteolytic conditions of the GI tract, and because of their size range may target the antigen effectively to the Peyer's patches. These microspheres offer the additional advantage of being able to entrap antigens of different molecular weights and characteristics, including co-encapsulation of antigens and adjuvants, without exposure to organic solvents. In addition, the proteinoid may provide additional immune stimulation by facilitating the transport of the antigen to the bloodstream.

REFERENCES

Ahren, C., Wenneras, C., Holmgren, J., and Svennerholm, A. M., 1993, Intestinal antibody response after oral immunization with a prototype cholera B subunit-colonization factor antigen enterotoxigenic *Escherichia coli* vaccine, *Vaccine* **11**:929–934.

Barchfeld, G., 1993, Serum and mucosal antibody responses to parenteral or mucosal subunit vaccines in animal models, International Business Communications Symposium on Novel Vaccine Strategies (Mucosal Immunization, Adjuvants, and Genetic Approaches), Bethesda, MD.

Barleta, R. G., Snapper, B., Cirillo, J. D., Cornell, N. D., Kim, D. D., Jacobs, W. R., and Bloom, B. R., 1990, Recombinant BCG as a candidate oral vaccine vector, *Res. Microbiol.* **141**:931.

Bergmann, K. C., and Waldman, R. H., 1989, Oral immunization with influenza virus: Experimental and clinical studies, *Curr. Top. Microbiol. Immunol.* **146**:83–89.

Bougeois, A. L., 1993, Evaluation of *E. coli* LT as a mucosal adjuvant for oral killed *Campylobacter* vaccine, International Business Communications Symposium on Novel Vaccine Strategies (Mucosal Immunization, Adjuvants, and Genetic Approaches), Bethesda, MD.

Bourguin, I., Chardes, T., and Bout, D., 1993, Oral immunization with *Toxoplasma gondii* antigens in association with cholera toxin induces enhanced protection and cell mediated immunity in mice, *Infect. Immun.* **61**:2082–2088.

Brey, R. N., 1993, Multiple emulsions: New vehicles for oral immunization, International Business Communications Symposium on Novel Vaccine Strategies (Mucosal Immunization, Adjuvants, and Genetic Approaches), Bethesda, MD.

Butcher, E. C., 1986, The regulation of lymphocyte traffic, *Curr. Top. Microbiol. Immunol.* **128**:85.

Cardenas, L., and Clement, J. D., 1992, Oral immunization using live attenuated *Salmonella* species as carriers of foreign antigens, *Clin. Microbiol. Rev.* **5**:328–342.

Challacombe, S. J., and Tomasi, T. B., 1980, Systemic tolerance and secretory immunity after oral immunization, *J. Exp. Med.* **152**:1459.

Challacombe, S. J., Rahman, H., Jeffery, H., Davis, S. S., and O'Hagan, D. T., 1992, Enhanced secretory IgA and systemic IgG antibody responses after oral immunization with biodegradable microparticles containing antigens, *Immunology* **76**:164–168.

Chang, T. W., 1993a, An approach for enhancing mucosal immunity: Isotype-specific stimulation of IgA, International Business Communications Symposium on Novel Vaccine Strategies (Mucosal Immunization, Adjuvants, and Genetic Approaches), Bethesda, MD.

Chang, T.W., 1993b, Enhancing mucosal immunity by isotype-specific stimulation of IgA, Cambridge Healthtech Institute Symposium on Vaccines: New Technology and Applications, Washington, DC.

Chen, K. S., and Quinnan, G. V., 1989a, Efficacy of inactivated influenza vaccine delivered by oral administration, *Curr. Top. Microbiol. Immunol.* **146**:101.

Chen, K. S., and Quinnan, G. V., 1989b, Secretory immunoglobulin A antibody response is conserved in aged mice following oral immunization with influenza virus vaccine, *J. Gen. Virol.* **70**:3291–3296.

Chen, K. S., Burlington, D. B., and Quinnan, G. V., 1987, Active synthesis of hemagglutinin-specific immunoglobulin A by lung cells of mice that were immunized intragastrically with inactivated influenza virus vaccine, *J. Virol.* **61**:2150–2154.

Chengalvala, M., Lubeck, M. D., Davis, A. R., Mizutani, S., Molnar-Kimber, K., Morin, J., and Hung, P. P., 1991, Evaluation of adenovirus type 7 recombinant hepatitis B vaccine in dogs, *Vaccine* **9**:485–490.

Clements, J. D., Sack, D. A., Harris, J. R., Chakraborty, J., Khan, M. R., Stanton, B. F., Kay, B. A., Khan, M. U., Yunus, M., Atkinson, W., Svennerholm, A. M., and Holmgren, J., 1986, Field trial of oral cholera vaccines in Bangladesh, *Lancet* **2**:124–127.

Clements, J. D., Hartzog, N. M., and Lyon, F. L., 1988, Adjuvant activity of *Escherichia coli* heat-labile enterotoxin and effect on the induction of oral tolerance in mice to unrelated protein antigens, *Vaccine* **6**:269–273.

Clements, M. L., and Murphy, B. R., 1986, Development and persistence of local and systemic antibody responses in adults given live attenuated or inactivated influenza A virus vaccine, *J. Clin. Microbiol.* **23**:66–72.

Cox, D. S., and Taubman, M. A., 1982, Systemic priming of the secretory antibody response with soluble and particulate antigens and carriers, *J. Immunol.* **128**:1844.

Cox, D. S., and Taubman, M. A., 1984, Oral induction and systemic priming of the secretory antibody response by soluble and particulate antigens, *Int. Arch. Allergy Appl. Immunol.* **75**:126.

Craig, S. W., and Cebra, J. J., 1971, Peyer's patches: An enriched source of precursors for IgA-producing immunocytes in the rabbit, *J. Exp. Med.* **134**:188–200.

Cuatrecasas, P., 1973, Gangliosides and membrane receptors for cholera toxin, *Biochemistry* **12**:3558.

Curtiss, R., III, Kelly, S. M., Gulig, P. A., and Nakayama, K., 1989, Selective delivery of antigens by recombinant vaccine, *Curr. Top. Microbiol. Immunol.* **146**:35.

Czerkinsky, C., Russell, M. W., Lycke, N., Lindbland, M., and Holmgren, J., 1989, Oral administration of a streptococcal antigen coupled to cholera toxin B subunit evokes strong antibody responses in salivary glands and extramucosal tissues, *Infect. Immun.* **57**:1072.

Czinn, S. J., and Nedrud, J. G., 1991, Oral immunization against *Helicobacter pylori*, *Infect. Immun.* **59**:2359–2363.

Czinn, S. J., Cai, A., and Nedrud, J. G., 1993, Protection of germ-free mice from infection by *Helicobacter felis* after active oral or passive IgA immunization, *Vaccine* **11**:637–642.

Daynes, R. A., and Araneo, B. G., 1992, Programming of lymphocytes responses to activation: Extrinsic factors, provided microenvironmentally, confer flexibility and compartmentalization to T-cell function, in: *Regulation and Functional Significance of T-cell Subsets,* Vol. 54 (R.L. Coffman, ed.), Karger, Basel, pp. 1–20.

De Aizpurua, H. J., and Russell-Jones, G. J., 1988, Oral vaccination. Identification of classes of proteins that provoke an immune response upon oral feeding, *J. Exp. Med.* **167**:440–451.

De Vos, T., and Dick, T. A., 1993, *Trichinella spiralis*: The effect of oral immunization and the adjuvancy of cholera toxin on the mucosal and systemic immune response of mice, *Exp. Parasitol.* **76**:182–191.

Ebersole, J. L., and Molinari, J. A., 1978, The induction of salivary antibodies by topical sensitization with particulate and soluble bacterial immunogens, *Immunology* **34**:969.

Eldridge, J. H., Staas, J. K., Meulbroek, J. A., McGhee, J. R., Tice, T. R., and Gilley, R. M., 1989, Vaccine containing biodegradable microspheres specifically enter the gut-associated lymphoid tissue following oral administration and induce a disseminated mucosal immune response, *Adv. Exp. Med. Biol.* **251**:191–202.

Eldridge, J. H., Staas, J. K., Meulbroek, J. A., McGhee, J. R., Tice, T. R., and Gilley, R. M., 1991, Biodegradable microspheres as a vaccine delivery system, *Mol. Immunol.* **28**:287–294.

Elson, C. O., and Ealding, W., 1984, Cholera toxin feeding did not induce oral tolerance in mice and abrogated oral tolerance to an unrelated protein antigen, *J. Immunol.* **133**:2892.

Elson, C. O., Ealding, L. O., and Lefkowitz, J., 1984, A lavage technique allowing repeated measurements of IgA antibodies in mouse intestinal secretions, *J. Immunol. Methods* **67**:101–108.

Emmings, F. G., Evans, R. T., and Genco, R. J., 1975, Antibody response in the parotid fluid and serum of irus monkeys (Macaca fascicularis) after local immunization with *Streptococcus mutans, Infect. Immun.* **12**:281.

Fox, S. W., 1977, Coacervate droplets, proteinoid microspheres, and the genetic apparatus, in: *Molecular Evolution and the Origin of Life* (S. W. Fox and K. Dose, eds.), Dekker, New York, pp. 119–132.

Fu, Z. F., Ruppretch, C. E., Dietzschold, B., Saikuman, P., Niu, H. S., Babka, I., Wummer, W. H., and Koprowski, H., 1993, Oral vaccination of raccoons (*Procyon lotor*) with baculovirus-expressed rabies virus glycoprotein, *Vaccine* **11**:925–928.

Gearhart, P. J., and Cebra, J. J., 1979, Differentiated B lymphocytes potential to express particular antibody variable and constant regions depends on site of lymphoid tissue and antigen load, *J. Exp. Med.* **149**:216–227.

Genco, R., Linzer, R., and Evans, R. T., 1983, Effect of adjuvants on orally administered antigens, *Ann. N.Y. Acad. Sci.* **409**:650–667.

Gerritse, K., Posno, M., Schelleken, M. M., Boersma, W. J. A., and Classen, E., 1990, Oral administration of TNP-*Lactobacillus* conjugates in mice. A model for evaluation of mucosal and systemic immune responses and memory formation elicited by transformed *Lactobacilli, Res. Microbiol.* **141**:955.

Hale, T. L., 1991, Hybrid vaccines using *Escherichia coli* as an antigen carrier, *Res. Microbiol.* **141**:913.

Hamada, S., Ogawa, T., Shimauchi, H., and Kusumoto, Y., 1992, Induction of mucosal and serum immune responses to a specific antigen of periodontal bacteria, *Adv. Exp. Med. Biol.* **327**:71–78.

Hirabayashi, Y., Kurata, H., Funati, H., Nagamine, T., Aizawa, C., Lamura, S., Shimada, K., and Kurata, T., 1990, Comparison of intranasal inoculation of influenza HA vaccine combined with cholera toxin B subunit with oral or parenteral vaccination, *Vaccine* **8**:243–248.

Holmgren, J., Czerkinsky, C., Lycke, N., and Svennerholm, A., 1992, Mucosal immunity: Implications for vaccine development, *Immunobiology* **184**:157–179.

Jackson, R. J., Fujihashi, K., Xu-Amano, J., Kiyono, H., Elson, C. O., and McGhee, J. R., 1993, Optimizing oral vaccines: Induction of systemic and mucosal B-cell and antibody responses to tetanus toxoid by use of cholera toxin as an adjuvant, *Infect. Immun.* **61**:4272–4279.

Katz, J. M., 1993, Use of enterotoxin LT from *E. coli* as a mucosal adjuvant for oral immunization with inactivated influenza vaccine, International Business Communications Symposium on Novel Vaccine Strategies (Mucosal Immunization, Adjuvants, and Genetic Approaches), Bethesda, MD.

Kawanishi, H., Salzman, L. E., and Strober, W., 1983, Mechanisms relating immununoglobulin A specific immunoglobulin production in murine gut associated lymphoid tissues. I. T. cells derived from Peyer's patches that switch surface immunoglobulin M cells to surface immunoglobulin A B cells *in vitro*, *J. Exp. Med.* **157**:433.

Klipstein, F. A., Engert, R. F., and Sherman, W. T., 1983, Peroral immunization of rats with *Escherichia coli* heat labile enterotoxin delivered by microspheres, *Infect. Immun.* **39**:1000–1003.

Kusumoto, Y., Ogawa, T., and Hamada, S., 1993, Generation of specific antibody-secreting cells in salivary glands of BALB/c mice following parenteral or oral immunization with *Porphyromonas gingivalis* fimbriae, *Arch. Oral Biol.* **38**:361–367.

LeFevre, M. E., Warren, J. B., and Joel, D. D., 1985, Particles and macrophages in murine Peyer's patches, *Exp. Cell Biol.* **53**:121.

Liang, X., Lamm, M., and Nedrud, J., 1988, Oral administration of cholera toxin Sendai virus conjugates potentiates gut and respiratory immunity against Sendai virus, *J. Immunol.* **141**:1495.

Lowell, G. H., 1993, The proteosome vaccine delivery system: Intranasal or oral immunization induces respiratory, intestinal and systemic antibodies and protection, International Business Communications Symposium on Novel Vaccine Strategies (Mucosal Immunization, Adjuvants, and Genetic Approaches). Bethesda, MD.

Lubeck, M. D., Davis, A. R., Chengalvala, M., Natuck, R. J., Morin, J. E., Molnar-Kimberg, K., Mason, B. B., Bhat, B. M., Mizurani, S., and Hung, P. P., 1989, Immunogenicity and efficacy testing in chimpanzees of an oral hepatitis B vaccine based on live recombinant adenovirus, *Proc. Natl. Acad. USA* **86**:6763–6767.

Lycke, N., and Holmgren, J., 1986. Intestinal mucosal memory and presence of memory cells in lamina propria and Peyer's patches in mice two years after oral immunization with cholera toxin, *Scand. J. Immunol.* **23**:611.

McDonald, T. J., 1993, Immunosuppression caused by antigen feeding. II. Suppressor T cells mask Peyer's patch B cell priming to orally administered antigens, *Eur. J. Immunol.* **13**:138.

McGhee, J. R., and Curtis, R., III, 1989, Liposomes as oral adjuvants, *Curr. Top. Microbiol.* **146**:51–57.

McGhee, J. R., Mestecky, J., Dertzbaugh, M. T., Eldridge, J. H., Hirapawa, M., and Kiyono, H., 1992, The mucosal immune system: From fundamental concepts to vaccine development, *Vaccine* **10**:75.

McKenzie, S., and Halsey, J.,1984, Cholera toxin B subunit as a carrier protein to stimulate a mucosal immune response, *J. Immunol.* **133**:1818.

Majde, J. A., 1994, LT-OA, a candidate oral adjuvant for mucosal and systemic immunization, Cambridge Healthtech Institute Symposium on Vaccines: New Technology and Applications, Alexandria, VA.

Mannino, R. J., Gould-Fogerite, S., and Goodman-Snitkoff, S. G., 1993, Targeted fusogenic proteo-liposomes: Functional reconstitution of membrane proteins through protein-cochleate intermediates, in: *Liposome Technology*, 2nd ed., Vol. III (G. Gregoriadis, ed.) CRC Press, Boca Raton, pp. 261–276.

Marx, P. A., Compans, R. W., Gettie, A., Staas, J. K., Gilley, R. M., Mulligan, M. J., Yamchikov, G. V., Chen, D., and Eldridge, J. H., 1993, Protection against vaginal SIV transmission with microencapsulated vaccine, *Science* **260**:1323–1327.

Mattingly, J. A., and Waksman, B. H., 1978, Immunologic suppression after oral administration of antigen. I. Specific suppressor cells formed in rat Peyer's patches after oral administration of sheep erythrocytes and their systemic migration, *J. Immunol.* **121**:1878–1883.

Mattingly, J. A., and Waksman, B. H., 1980, Immunologic suppression after oral administration of antigen. II. Antigen-specific helper and suppressor factors produced by spleen cells of rats fed sheep erythrocytes, *J. Immunol.* **125**:1044.

Menge, A. C., Michalek, S. M., Russell, M. W., and Mestecky, J., 1993, Immune response of the female rat genital tract after oral and local immunization with keyhole limpet hemocyanin conjugated to the cholera toxin B subunit, *Infect. Immun.* **61**:2162–2171.

Mestecky, J.,1987, The common mucosal immune system and current strategies for induction of immune responses in external secretions, *J. Clin. Immunol.* **7**:265–276.

Mestecky, J., and McGhee, J. R., 1989, Oral immunization: Past and present, *Curr. Top. Microbiol. Immunol.* **146**:3–11.

Michalek, S. M., Childers, N. K., Kak, N. K., Denys, F. R., Berry, A. K., Eldridge, J. H., McGhee, J. R., and Curtiss, R., 1989, Liposomes as oral adjuvants, *Curr. Top. Microbiol. Immun.* **146**:51.

Milstein, S., Baughman, R., Santiago, N., Rivera, T., Falzarano, L., Dewland, P., and Welch, S., 1993a, Initial clinical assessment of the oral administration of low molecular weight heparin (LMWH) using the proteinoid oral delivery system, Symposia Abstracts—American Association of Pharmaceutical Scientists Annual Meeting, San Antonio, TX, p. 35.

Milstein, S., Baughman, R. A., Kuhn, L., Santiago, N., Lyons, A., Meyer, E., Saragovi, U., and Greene, M., 1993b, Efficient oral delivery of monoclonal antibodies by proteinoid encapsulation, *Proc. Miami Biotech. Winter Symp.* **3**:116.

Moldoveanu, S., Staas, J. K., Gilley, R., Ray, R., Compans, R. W., Eldridge, J. H., Tice, T. R., and Mestecky, J., 1989, Immune responses to influenza virus in orally and systemically immunized mice, *Curr. Top. Microbiol.* **146**:91–99.

Moldoveanu, Z., Novak, M., Huang, W., Gilley, R. M., Staas, J. K., Schafer, D., Compans, R. W., and Mestecky, J., 1993, Oral immunization with influenza virus in biodegradable microspheres, *J. Infect. Dis.* **167**:84–90.

Morisaki, I., Michalek, S. M., Harmon, C. C., Torii, M., Hamada, S., and McGhee, J. R., 1983, Effective immunity to dental caries: Enhancement of salivary anti-*Streptococcus mutans* antibody responses with oral adjuvants, *Infect. Immun.* **40**:577.

Mowat, A. McI., Donachie, A. M., Reid, G., and Jarrett, O., 1991, Immunostimulating complexes containing Quil A and protein antigen prime class I MHC-restricted T lymphocytes *in vivo* are immunogenic by the oral route, *Immunology* **72**:317–322.

Natuck, R. J., Lubeck, M. D., Chanad, P. K., Chengalvala, M., Wade, M. S., Murthy, S. C. S., Wilhelm, J., Vernon, S. K., Dheer, S. K., Mizutani, S., Lee, S. J., Murthy, K. K., Eichberg, J. W., Davis, A. R., and Hung, P. P., 1993, Immunogenicity of recombinant human adenovirus–human immune deficiency virus vaccine in chimpanzees, *AIDS Res. Hum. Retroviruses* **9**:395–404.

Nedrud, J. G., Liang, X. P., and Lamm, M. E., 1989, Oral immunization with Sendai virus in mice, *Curr. Top. Microbiol. Immunol.* **146**:117–122.

Nguyen, T. N., Hansonn, M., Stahl, S., Bachi, T., Robert, A., Domzig, W., Bing, H., and Uhlen, M., 1993, Cell surface display of heterologous epitopes on *Staphylococcus xylosus* as a potential delivery system for oral vaccination, *Gene* **128**:89–94.

Ogra, P. L., and Karzon, D. T., 1970, The role of immunoglobulins in the mechanisms of mucosal immunity to viral infection, *Pediatr. Clin. North Am.* **17**:385.

O' Hagan, D. T., Palin, K. J., and Davis, S. S., 1987, Intestinal absorption of proteins and macromolecules and the immunological response, *CRC Crit. Rev. Ther. Drug Carrier Syst.* **4**: 197–220.

O'Hagan, D. T., Palin, K. J., and Davis, S. S., 1989a, Poly(butyl-2-cyanoacrylate) particles as adjuvants for oral immunization, *Vaccine* **7**:213–216.

O'Hagan, D. T., Palin, K., Artursson, P., Davis, S. S., and Sjöholm, I., 1989b, Microparticles as potentially orally active immunological adjuvants, *Vaccine* **7**:421–424.

O'Hagan, D. T., McGhee, J. P., Holmgren, J., Mowat, A. McI., Donaehie, A. M., Mills, K. H. G., Gaisford, W., Rahman, D., and Challacombe, S. J., 1993, Biodegradable microparticles for oral immunization, *Vaccine* **11**:149–154.

Olsen, M. R., and Hunter, R. L., 1992, Induction of mucosal IgΛ by oral immunization with multiple emulsions, *FASEB J.* **6**:A1229.

Orr, N., Robin, G., Cohen, D., Arnon, R., and Lowell, G. H., 1993, Immunogenicity and efficacy of oral or intranasal *Shigella flexneri 2a* and *Shigella sonnei* proteosome–lipopolysaccharide vaccines in animal models, *Infect. Immun.* **61**:2390–2395.

Owen, R. L., 1977, Sequential uptake of horseradish peroxidase by lymphoid follicle epithelium of Peyer's patches in the normal unobstructed mouse intestine: An ultrastructural study, *Gastroenterology* **72**:440–451.

Owen, R. L., Pierce, N. F., Apple, R. T., and Cray, W. C., Jr. 1986, M cell transport of *Vibrio cholera* from the intestinal lumen into Peyer's patches: A mechanism for antigen sampling and for microbial transepithelial migration, *J. Infect. Dis.* **153**:1108–1118.

Pang, G. T., Clancy, R. L., O'Reilly, S. E., and Cripps, A. W., 1992, A novel particulate influenza vaccine induces long-term and broad-based immunity in mice after oral immunization, *J. Virol.* **66**:1162–1170.

Pierce, N. F., 1978, The role of antigen form and function in the primary and secondary intestinal immune responses to cholera toxin and toxoid in rats, *J. Exp. Med.* **148**:195–206.

Pierce, N. F., and Gowans, J., 1975, Cellular kinetics of the intestinal immune response to cholera toxin in rats, *J. Exp. Med.* **142**:1550.

Pierce, N. F., and Koster, F. T., 1980, Priming and suppression of the intestinal immune response to cholera toxoid/toxin by parenteral toxoid in rats, *J. Immunol.* **124**:307–311.

Pierce, N. F., Kaper, J. B., Mekalanos, J. J., Cray, W. C., and Richardson, K., 1987, Determinants of the immunogenicity of live virulent and mutant *Vibrio cholera* 01 in rabbit intestine, *Infect. Immun.* **55**:477–481.

Pierre, P., Denis, O., Bazin, H., Mbongolo Mbella, E., and Vaerman, J. P., 1992, Modulation of oral tolerance to ovalbumin by cholera toxin and its B subunit, *Eur. J. Immunol.* **22**:3179–3182.

Ray, R., Glaze, B. J., Moldoveanu, Z., and Compans, R. W., 1988, Intranasal immunization of hamster with envelope glycoproteins of human parainfluenza virus type 3, *J. Infect. Dis.* **157**:648–654.

Russell, M. W., and Wu, H. Y., 1991, Distribution, persistence, and recall of serum and salivary antibody responses to peroral immunization with protein antigen I/II of *Streptococcus mutans* coupled to the cholera toxin B subunit, *Infect. Immun.* **59**:4061–4070.

Sabin, A. B., 1976, Vaccination at the portal of entry of infectious agents, *Dev. Biol. Stand.* **33**:3–9.

Sadoff, J. C., Ballou, W. R., Baron, L. S., Majariau, W. R., Brey, R. N., Hockmeyer, W. T., Young, J. F., Cryz, S. J., Ou, J., Lowell, G. H., and Chulay, J. D., 1988, Oral *Salmonella typhimurium*: Vaccine expressing circumsporozoite protein protects against malaria, *Science* **240**:336–338.

Santiago, N., Rivera, T., Mayer, E., and Milstein, S., 1992, Proteinoid microspheres for the oral delivery of heparin, *Proc. Int. Symp. Control. Rel. Bioact. Mater.* **19**:514.

Santiago, N., Milstein, S., Rivera, T., Garcia, E., Zaidi, T., Hong, H., and Bucher, D., 1993a, Oral immunization of rats with proteinoid microspheres encapsulating influenza virus antigens, *Pharm. Res.* **10**:1243–1247.

Santiago, N., Rivera, T., Wang, N.F., Maher, J., and Baughman, R. A., 1993b, Initial studies in the assessment of proteinoid microsphere activity, *Proc. Int. Symp. Control. Rel. Bioact. Mater.* **20**:300.

Sarubbi, D., Variano, B., Haas, S., Maher, J., Falzarano, L., Burnett, B., Fuller, G., Santiago, N., Milstein, S., and Baughman, R.A., 1994, Oral delivery of calcitonin in rats and primates using proteinoid microspheres, *Proc. Int. Symp. Control. Rel. Bioact. Mater.* **21**:288–289.

Schvartsman, Y. A. S., and Zycov, M. P., 1976, Secretory anti influenza immunity, *Adv. Immunol.* **22**:291–330.

Shahin, R. D., Amsbaugh, D. F., and Leef, M. F., 1992, Mucosal immunization with filamentous hemagglutinin protects against *Bordetella pertussis* respiratory infection, *Infect. Immun.* **60**:1482–1488.

Sory, M. P., and Cornelis, G. R., 1990, Delivery of the cholera toxin-B subunit by using a recombinant *Yersinia enterocolitica* strain as a live oral carrier, *Res. Microbiol.* **141**:921.

Steiner, S., and Rosen, R., 1990, Delivery Systems for Pharmacological Agents Encapsulated with Proteinoids, U.S. Patent 4,925,673, May 15.

Swarbrick, E. T., Stokes, C. R., and Soothill, J. F., 1979, Absorption of antigens after oral immunization and simultaneous induction of specific systemic tolerance, *Gut* **20**:121.

Szewczuk, M. R., and Wade, A. W., 1983, Aging and the mucosal-associated lymphoid system, *Ann. N.Y. Acad. Sci.* **409**:333.

Vajdy, M., and Lycke, N.Y., 1992, Cholera toxin adjuvant promotes long-term immunological memory in the gut mucosa to unrelated immunogens after oral immunization, *Immunology* **75**:488–492.

Wachsmann, D., Klein, J. P., Scholler, M., and Frank, R. M., 1985, Local and systemic immune response to orally administered liposome-associated soluble *S. mutans* cell wall antigen, *Immunology* **54**:189–193.

Waldman, R. H., Wood, S. H., Torres, E. J., and Small, P. A., 1970, Influenza antibody response following aerosol administration of inactivated virus, *Am. J. Epidemiol.* **91**:575.

Wells, H. G., 1911, Studies on the chemistry of anaphylaxis. III. Experiments with isolated proteins, especially those of the hen's egg, *J. Infect. Dis.* **9**:147–151.

Wells, H. G., and Osborne, T. B., 1911, The biological reactions of the vegetable proteins I. Anaphylaxis, *J. Infect. Dis.* **8**:66–70.

Wu, H. Y., and Russell, M. W., 1993, Induction of mucosal immunity by intranasal application of a streptococcal surface protein antigen with the cholera toxin B subunit, *Infect. Immun.* **61**:314–322.

Chapter 18

Design and Production of Single-Immunization Vaccines Using Polylactide Polyglycolide Microsphere Systems

Jeffrey L. Cleland

1. INTRODUCTION

1.1. Rationale for Single-Immunization Vaccines

Over the past several years, many new adjuvant formulations have been developed to elicit both humoral and cell-mediated responses to antigens. Each of these new formulations must be given in repeated immunizations to yield antibody titers that result in protection. Typically, a minimum of three immunizations is required to invoke antibody titers or cellular responses that are sufficient to neutralize an infection. In addition, the patient may be required to return several years after the last immunization for a final booster immunization to again establish a neutralizing response. These repeated immunizations in developed countries may require repeated visits to the physician and increase the cost of health care. In developing countries and large urban areas, clinics are responsible for immunization of the children against many potentially fatal childhood diseases. Unfortunately, these clinics may have difficulty with repeated immunizations, since the patient population is transient or patients do not understand the necessity for additional shots. Thus, vaccine preparations requiring repeated immunizations are generally inefficient and may not always be successful in preventing disease because of poor patient compliance.

Jeffrey L. Cleland • Pharmaceutical Research & Development, Genentech, Inc., South San Francisco, California 94080.

Vaccine Design: The Subunit and Adjuvant Approach, edited by Michael F. Powell and Mark J. Newman. Plenum Press, New York, 1995.

439

1.2. Potential Single-Immunization Vaccine Formulations

A controlled-release formulation such as a single-immunization vaccine would eliminate or reduce the need for patients to receive repeated immunizations. Also, it is possible
that these formulations may generate a greater neutralizing response than the multiple-dose
formulations. A controlled-release formulation could be developed to mimic a continuous
or pulsatile release of antigen. The dosing schedule of the antigen may then be optimized
to provide the best immune response. For example, a formulation may be designed to
release the antigen at predetermined times after injection and, therefore, it would mimic
repeated immunizations. As discussed in a recent review, there are several potential
technologies for the development of a single-shot vaccine (Khan *et al.*, 1994). However,
only systems that provide an in vivo depot for the antigen can yield a single-shot vaccine.
Two systems, lipids and polymers, have been used as depots for the controlled delivery of
antigens. Unfortunately, many lipid formulations have not been tested in humans and their
ability to reproducibly deliver antigens in vivo has not been assessed in most studies. One
of the first studies to demonstrate the concept of single-shot immunization was performed
by Preis and Langer in 1979 using a nondegradable polymer, polyethylene-vinyl acetate.
A major disadvantage of the nonbiodegradable polymers is that they must be surgically
removed after the antigen has been released. The long-term effects of these polymers have
not been determined and they can have potential adverse side effects as observed in the
recent reports on silicone breast implants, a system previously considered safe and
biocompatible (Kessler, 1992). On the other hand, biodegradable polymers do not require
surgical removal and the long-term side effects can be minimized since these polymers
degrade with time. Many biodegradable polymers have been synthesized for use in
biomedical applications (Langer, 1993; Heller, 1993; Kalpana and Park, 1993). Most of
these polymers contain a labile moiety such as an ester which is hydrolyzed over time to
yield acidic monomers. There are three general classes of these polymers: polyanhydrides
(Langer, 1993), polyortho esters (Heller, 1993), and polyesters (Heller, 1993). Although
each system offers specific advantages, only one class of polyesters, polylactides and
copolymers of lactide and glycolide, have been approved for use in humans. Polylactides
[polylactic acid (PLA), polylactic coglycolic acid (PLGA), and polyglycolic acid (PGA)]
degrade to form lactic and glycolic acid. These polymers have been used for over 20 years
in resorbable sutures. In addition, luteinizing hormone-releasing hormone (LHRH) agonist
PLGA microsphere formulations were approved by the U.S. FDA several years ago for
prostate cancer, endometriosis, and precocious puberty in children (Okada *et al.*, 1991;
Ogawa *et al.*, 1988a,b,c; Furr and Hutchinson, 1992). These formulations were developed
as 1-month depot systems that continuously released an LHRH agonist (leuprolide acetate,
Lupron Depot®; goserelin acetate, Zoladex®; triptorelin, Decapeptyl®). Overall, the polylactides have a long and well-established safety and toxicology record as well as detailed
Drug Master Files at the FDA. These polymers have also been extensively studied for the
delivery of proteins and peptides (Cleland and Langer, 1994). These polymers have
physical and mechanical properties that allow their fabrication into different forms such
as implants or injectable microspheres. Considering their advantages in safety, toxicity,
and characterization, the polylactides are well suited for use in vaccine formulations, if
they can be designed to provide either a continuous or pulsatile delivery of antigen.

Several recent studies have investigated the potential application of polylactides in vaccine formulations. As illustrated in Table I, these vaccines were prepared from different polymers and produced by different methods of encapsulation. The methods of preparation include solvent evaporation or solvent extraction (coacervation). The polylactides are insoluble in water and must be dissolved in an organic solvent such as ethyl acetate or methylene chloride (oil phase). The solid or liquid antigen is then dispersed in the oil phase to form a fine suspension or emulsion. This emulsion is used to produce the microspheres. For solvent evaporation, the emulsion is typically added to a water phase containing an emulsifying agent such as polyvinyl alcohol. By mixing the antigen/oil phase with the water phase, microspheres are formed by precipitation of the polylactide, resulting in encapsulation of the antigen. The organic solvent is removed by the addition of excess water followed by drying (e.g., lyophilization) of the microspheres. If the aqueous antigen droplets are dispersed in the oil phase, the preparation is a water-in-oil-in-water emulsion (double emulsion; see Fig. 1). For coacervation, the antigen/oil phase is emulsified in a nonsolvent, which extracts the organic solvent. This method has been extensively reviewed by Lewis (1990). As the antigen/oil phase is added to silicone oil, it forms an antigen-in-oil-in-oil emulsion. The silicone oil and remaining organic solvent are then extracted with another nonsolvent (e.g., heptane; see Fig. 2). By varying the process conditions in each method, the physical properties of the microspheres can be altered to yield the desired size and amount of encapsulated antigen.

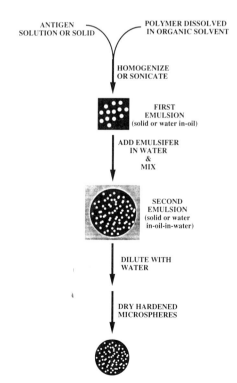

Figure 1. Solvent evaporation method for production of polylactide microspheres. The polymer (PLGA or PLA) is dissolved in organic solvent (e.g., methylene chloride or ethyl acetate). The aqueous or solid antigen is then added and the solution is mixed by sonication or homogenization to form the first emulsion (solid or water in-oil). This emulsion is then transferred to water containing an emulsifying agent (e.g., PVA). Mixing of the first emulsion in the water phase produces the microspheres resulting in a second emulsion (solid or water in-oil-in-water). The final emulsion is diluted with excess water to facilitate removal of the organic solvent in the oil phase. The microspheres are then dried.

Table I

Recent Examples of Polylactide Microsphere Vaccines—Encapsulation and in Vitro Properties

Antigen	Polymer[a]	Encapsulation[b]	Size (μm)	Release profile[c]	Reference
Colonizing factor antigen (*E. coli*)	PLGA (0.73 dL/g)	Coacervaton (solid-in-oil)	1–10 (5–10)	30% initial burst, continuous release	Reid *et al.* (1993)
Cholera toxin B	PLA (2 kDa)	N.A.[e]	0.3–3.5	Protein adsorbed	Almeidia *et al.* (1992)
Diphtheria toxoid formalin treated	PLA (49 kDa)	Solvent evaporation (double emulsion)	5–85 (40–50)	Continuous release; small burst: 30–40 days	Singh *et al.* (1992)
MN rgp120 (± QS21)	PLGA	Solvent evaporation (double emulsion)	N.A.	Pulsatile release at 0 and 1,2,3, or 4 months	Cleland *et al.* (1994)
Ovalbumin	50:50 PLGA (22 kDa) 85:15 PLGA (53 kDa)	Solvent evaporation (double emulsion)	1.5, 73	Continuous release	O'Hagen *et al.* (1993)
Salmonella enteritidis	PLA (58.3 kDa) 50:50 PLGA (72 kDa) 65:35 PLGA (62.3 kDa)	Coacervation (water–oil–oil)	N.A.	Continuous release	Hazrati *et al.* (1993)
Simian immuno-deficiency virus formalin treated	54:46 PLGA	Solvent evaporation (double emulsion)	1–10	N.A.	Marx *et al.* (1993)
Staphylococcal enterotoxin B toxoid	PLGA	Solvent evaporation (double emulsion)	1–10, 20–50	Continuous release	Eldridge *et al.* (1991a,b)
Tetanus toxoid	50:50 PLGA (100 kDa) PLA (3 & 50 kDa)	Solvent evaporation (double emulsion)	6–70[d]	Continuous release	Alonso *et al.* (1993)

[a]X:Y PLGA indicates the mole fraction (%) of lactide (X) and glycolide (Y) in the copolymer. The polymer size is reported as either molecular mass in kilodaltons (kDa) or intrinsic viscosity in decaliters/gram.

[b]Synthesis of the drug-loaded microspheres was performed by emulsifying either aqueous or solid drug in the organic phase (oil; polymer/solvent). This emulsion was then added to a non-solvent (water or silcone oil) and residual solvent removed by extraction (coacervation: heptane) or evaporation (excess water and drying).

[c]Release of the antigen from the microspheres was measured in vitro under physiological conditions.

[d]Several preparations were made and each batch of microspheres had a distinct size distribution with a mean size between 6 and 70 μm.

[e]N.A., not available.

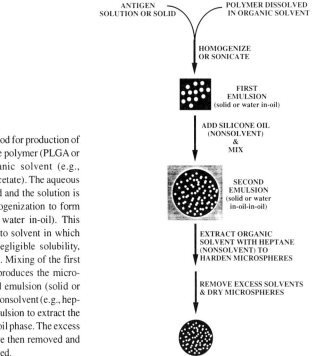

Figure 2. Coacervation method for production of polylactide microspheres. The polymer (PLGA or PLA) is dissolved in organic solvent (e.g., methylene chloride or ethyl acetate). The aqueous or solid antigen is then added and the solution is mixed by sonication or homogenization to form the first emulsion (solid or water in-oil). This emulsion is then transferred to solvent in which the polymer has a low or negligible solubility, nonsolvent (e.g., silicone oil). Mixing of the first emulsion in the nonsolvent produces the microspheres resulting in a second emulsion (solid or water in-oil-in-oil). Another nonsolvent (e.g., heptane) is added to the final emulsion to extract the organic solvent from the first oil phase. The excess solvents in the supernatant are then removed and the final microspheres are dried.

For the studies listed in Table I, the microspheres used in a particular vaccine were either small (<10 μm) or large (>20 μm). The larger microspheres (>20 μm) were not effective for oral vaccination since they would not be efficiently delivered to Peyer's patches in the duodenum (Eldridge *et al.*, 1991a,b). The smaller microspheres (<10 μm) might be phagocytosed and antigen would then be directed to the draining lymph nodes (Eldridge *et al.*, 1991a). In addition, the concept of mixing small microspheres for macrophage uptake and large microspheres for sustained delivery was patented by Eldridge and co-workers using staphylococcal enterotoxin B toxoid as the model antigen (Tice *et al.*, 1991). However, the utility of this patent has not been demonstrated with other antigens. Thus, a systematic study should be performed with each antigen to determine the best method of preparation and the appropriate size to invoke the desired immune response.

As shown in Table II, the encapsulated antigen vaccines were tested in different animals to assess the immune response. The single-immunization potential of these systems was demonstrated for diphtheria toxoid (Singh *et al.*, 1992), tetanus toxoid (Alonso *et al.*, 1993), and MN rgp120 for human immunodeficiency virus type 1 (HIV-1) (Cleland *et al.*, 1994). A single immunization with encapsulated diphtheria toxoid (75 Lf units) yielded antibody titers equivalent to three immunizations of alum-formulated diphtheria toxoid (25 Lf units/dose) given at 0, 1, and 2 months and these titers were comparable at every time point analyzed (Singh *et al.*, 1993). For tetanus toxoid, a single immunization of the encapsulated form yielded an early and persistent neutralizing antibody response

Table II

Recent Examples of Polylactide Microsphere Vaccines—Administration and in Vivo Results[a]

Antigen	Administration[b]	Animal model	Summary of study results
Colonizing factor antigen (E. coli)	Oral (intraduodenal) (0, 1, 2 weeks)	Rabbits	Lymphocyte proliferation (Peyer's patch cells) greater and B-cell response higher for encapsulated antigen.
Cholera toxin B	Oral (1, 2, 3, 28 days)	Mice	Demonstrated higher humoral response than soluble which was given at 40-fold higher antigen dose.
Diphtheria toxoid formalin treated	i.m. (0 or 0, 1, 2 months)[c]	Balb/c mice	Single immunization yielded equal antibody titers to three immunizations with alum-formulated antigen.
MN rgp120 (± QS21)	s.c. (0 or 0, 2 months)	Guinea pigs	Single immunization demonstrated in vivo autoboost, and invoked equal or greater neutralizing antibody titers to two or three soluble immunizations.
Ovalbumin	s.c. (day 0)	Balb/c mice	Response greater than alum formulated at early time-points (< 10 weeks). Slightly higher titers for smaller microspheres.
Salmonella enteritidis	i.m. (0, 97, 196 days)	Chickens	Microspheres provided better priming and higher immune response. Antigen released intact.
Simian immunodeficiency virus formalin treated	Oral/i.m./i.t. (various schedules)	Macaques	Animals immunized by i.m./oral, i.m./i.m., or i.m./i.t. were protected from one challenge. i.m./oral protected 2/3 animals after second challenge.
Staphylococcal enterotoxin B toxoid	Oral/i.p./s.c./i.t. (various schedules)	Mice	s.c.: IgG titers were 30- to 60-fold higher for encapsulated. Best response from mixture of 1–10 and 20–50 μm microspheres. Oral: Invoke IgG, IgM, and IgA response.
Tetanus toxoid	s.c. (day 0)	CD-1 mice	Single immunization with encapsulated (3-kDa PLA) provided neutralizing antibody titers greater than soluble.

[a]References are listed in Table I.
[b]Route of vaccine administration: i.m. = intramuscular, i.p. = intraperitoneal, i.t. = intratracheal, s.c. = subcutaneous.
[c]Microspheres dosed once (day 0) and alum-formulated antigen dosed three times (0,1,2 months).

while the soluble form was ineffective after one immunization (Alonso *et al.*, 1993). Microencapsulated MN rgp120 given in a single immunization invoked an initial immune response equivalent to a bolus injection and the immune response increased dramatically after the remaining antigen was released from the microspheres at 8 to 10 weeks (Cleland *et al.*, 1994). This study with a subunit antigen indicated the potential to mimic bolus injections with a single immunization by achieving an in vivo autoboost. In addition, a single immunization with MN rgp120 and QS-21 in microspheres provided higher neutralizing antibody titers than two or three doses of the soluble form that was administered at a significantly greater QS-21 and MN rgp120 dose (Cleland *et al.*, 1994). Repeated dosing by injections or oral administration indicated that microsphere formulations also provided enhanced priming of the immune response (Almeidia *et al.*, 1992; Hazrati *et al.*, 1993). For oral administration, many vaccines may be ineffective because of degradation in the stomach. Encapsulation may protect the antigen from degradation. Recent studies have shown that PLGA microspheres are transcytosed by M cells in the intestine and, thus, can also generate a systemic immune response (Jepson *et al.*, 1993). For colonizing factor antigens that facilitated infection by enterotoxigenic *E. coli*, encapsulation protected the antigen and resulted in mucosal (IgA) and systemic (B and T cell responses) immune responses (Reid *et al.*, 1993). The combination of oral administration with intramuscular injections yielded both systemic and mucosal immunity and protection against vaginal challenge with whole inactivated simian immunodeficiency virus in macaques (Marx *et al.*, 1993). Thus, microsphere vaccine formulations may provide a method for generating a humoral response that is sufficient to neutralize both systemic and mucosal challenges.

2. PREDEVELOPMENT STUDIES FOR DESIGN OF IN VIVO RELEASE PROFILE

To develop a single-immunization vaccine, the optimum schedule and dose of the antigen must be determined. Several of the current human vaccines have been studied with regard to antigen dose and schedule dependence of the immune response. In the case of the hepatitis B subunit vaccine, an accelerated immunization schedule (e.g., 0, 1, 2 months) induced higher initial antibody titers than a slower immunization schedule (e.g., 0, 1, 6 months), but the accelerated schedule requires an additional booster immunization at a later time (e.g., 12 months) (Hess *et al.*, 1992). An accelerated schedule requiring an additional immunization can, however, reduce the efficacy of the vaccine as a result of poor patient compliance for the final immunization (Hess *et al.*, 1992). Two or three immunizations are typically required to achieve efficacy of vaccines currently approved for use in humans. For the diphtheria–tetanus–pertussis (DTP) vaccine, three immunizations are required to invoke sufficient antibody responses (Barkin *et al.*, 1985) and the immune response is not significantly different for either a 0, 1, 2 or 0, 2, 4 month immunization schedule (Just *et al.*, 1991). Often, a single-immunization vaccine is effective in producing antibody titers sufficient to neutralize an infection, but these vaccines may require a booster immunization several years later to assure long-lasting protection (measles, mumps, rubella: Christenson and Bottinger, 1991; hepatitis A: Just *et al.*, 1992). The time interval between immunizations may also be a function of the vaccine potency. This effect was observed for rabies vaccines where an accelerated schedule yielded a better immune response for a low-potency vaccine (Cabasso *et al.*, 1978) and a longer duration between immunizations provided a greater and longer-lasting immune response for a more potent vaccine (Serufo *et al.*, 1987). The delay time between immunizations may also affect the extent of the subsequent response (secondary or tertiary). For example, rgp120, which is significantly less immunogenic in baboons than hepatitis B surface antigen, was most potent (best immune response and neutralizing antibody titers) when the delay between the second and third immunizations was extended to 20 weeks (0, 4, 24 week schedule) (Anderson *et al.*, 1989). Thus, the schedule and dose of a vaccine will vary depending on the required response, potency, and duration of the response. Although the response of animals to schedule and dose may be quite different from the response observed in humans, each vaccine should be thoroughly tested, if possible, in animal models prior to clinical trials.

   Additional complexity in dosing and schedules is involved in oral vaccinations and parenteral–oral immunizations. Currently, the only vaccine administered orally in humans in the United States is the polio vaccine. The use of three or four doses of a trivalent (types 1, 2, and 3) vaccine provides a sufficient neutralizing response to resist infection (Hardy *et al.*, 1970). One difficulty with oral vaccination is the delivery of the antigen to the immune cells of the intestine and the systemic circulation. Many vaccines are not stable in the harsh environment of the gastrointestinal system and the few vaccines that may be stable may not be efficiently transported to the systemic immune cells or may not interact with M cells lining the intestinal wall. In the case of cholera toxin B subunit whole-cell vaccine, the addition of a stabilizing agent, bicarbonate powder, facilitated its use as an oral vaccine formulation and invoked both IgA and IgG titers against the toxin (Jertborn *et al.*, 1993). Again, the schedule had an impact on the extent of the immune response. A delay time of less than 7 days between the two immunizations resulted in lower antibody titers (Jertborn *et al.*, 1993). It is likely that oral vaccinations would also require extensive studies to optimize the schedule and dose. In addition, if both mucosal (IgA) and systemic (IgG) antibody titers are desired at high levels, a combination regime of oral and parenteral immunizations may be required. The order of these immunizations can also affect the immune response. For example, parenteral immunization (intraperitoneal) suppressed the IgA response to subsequent oral immunizations with the cholera toxoid (Pierce, 1984). Thus, the use of different routes of immunization (parenteral versus mucosal) affects the type and extent of the immune response. The requirements for a localized immune response (e.g., intestinal mucosa) must be determined prior to the development of the vaccine.

   For both oral and parenteral delivery of vaccines, the dose is administered as a bolus. An exhaustive literature search did not reveal any studies investigating the immune response to a continuous infusion of antigen as compared to bolus injections. Most of the vaccine preparations listed in Tables I and II continuously release antigen when incubated at 37°C in physiological buffer. These vaccines are completely different from the bolus injections currently used in human vaccines. One concern of a constant infusion of antigen may be the ability to invoke a low-dose tolerance where the antibody titers are low and do not neutralize. However, the results of the studies described in Table II would suggest that this effect has not been observed. On the other hand, the MN rgp120 PLGA formulations demonstrate that a pulsatile release of antigen that simulates repeated bolus injections can be achieved (Cleland *et al.*, 1994). To properly design and develop a polymeric vaccine formulation, feasibility studies should be performed to assess the possible regimes required to invoke the desired immune response. For the continuous delivery polymer systems, studies should be performed with implantable pumps (e.g., Alzet® minipumps) to determine the best schedule and dose for a continuous infusion of antigen. The immune response from this type of administration should then be compared to repeated bolus injections. If bolus administration of the vaccine in repeated doses provides the optimum immune response, the polymer formulation must be modified to deliver the antigen in a pulsatile manner. Once the optimum schedule and dose are determined from the feasibility studies, a polylactide delivery system can be designed by choosing the appropriate formulation.

3. RELATIONSHIP BETWEEN POLYMER PROPERTIES AND VACCINE DESIGN

The polylactide chosen for use in the vaccine formulation will directly determine the characteristics of the formulation. The release of the antigen from polylactide formulations is controlled by two major mechanisms: diffusion of the antigen out of the device and erosion of the polymer. Antigen is released initially from polylactide microspheres by diffusion. Antigen that is at or near the surface of the microspheres diffuses into the surrounding media within minutes to hours after contact with an aqueous environment. The continued diffusion of the antigen out of the polylactide microspheres is dependent on the porosity of the microspheres. The number of channels available for the antigen to diffuse out of the microspheres will affect the rate of antigen release into the surrounding environment. In many cases, the initial diffusive phase will only last a few hours and little or no additional antigen will be released for several days (see Fig. 3). This lag period is controlled by the erosion of the polymer. Significant bulk erosion of the polymer may be necessary to allow new channels to form for diffusion of the antigen out of the microspheres. This type of release profile is often referred to as triphasic release: initial diffusion, erosion, and final diffusion, as demonstrated in Fig. 3. If the release of antigen is limited during the erosion phase, the overall release is analogous to repeated immunizations except that the final diffusive phase may last several weeks, unlike a single bolus administration. A triphasic release profile is effective as a single immunization vaccine as demonstrated for the subunit vaccine, MN rgp120/PLGA (Cleland *et al.*, 1994). In contrast, if the microspheres are sufficiently porous to allow continuous diffusion, the diffusive phase can occur simultaneously with the erosion of the polymer (Fig. 3). The continuous diffusion of antigen results in a continuous release formulation. Most of the formulations shown in Table I continuously release antigen.

The duration of antigen release from the microspheres is dependent on the rate of diffusion of the antigen and the degradation of the polymer. If the antigen is able to rapidly diffuse out of the microsphere, the antigen will be completely released before the complete degradation of the polymer is achieved. For triphasic release, the length of the lag period between the initial and final diffusive phases is dependent on the time required to achieve bulk erosion of the polymer. Bulk erosion is generally a complete loss of the microsphere's structural integrity resulting in an opening of large pores or channels for diffusion of the

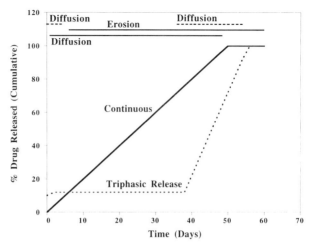

Figure 3. Illustration of the two primary types of release patterns for materials encapsulated in polylactides. Continuous release of the drug may be achieved by the continuous diffusion of the drug out of the polymer matrix. In this case, the rate of drug release is primarily controlled by the diffusivity of the drug. The triphasic release of drug is, however, dependent on the erosion of the polymer matrix. This type of release (also referred to as the S release pattern) is characterized by an initial diffusion of drug at or near the microsphere surface. After the initial diffusive phase, a lag phase occurs until the polymer achieves bulk erosion resulting in a significant increase in pores or channels for diffusion of the drug. The remaining drug may then diffuse out of the more porous polymer matrix. The time scale listed for each type of release is directly dependent on the processing conditions, polymer characteristics, and drug properties as discussed in the text.

entrapped antigen. The amount of time required for the polymer to achieve bulk erosion and complete degradation is dependent on the polymer molecular weight, composition, and the degree of crystallinity. Previous studies in rats assessed the degradation rate for several polymers and observed some general trends (Miller *et al.*, 1977). As the polymer molecular weight increases, the duration of the erosion phase increases since more extensive hydrolysis is required to achieve complete degradation (see Fig. 4). The relative proportion of lactide and glycolide monomers in the polymer can also affect the degradation rate. A polymer with high lactide or glycolide content (e.g., 85:15 lactide:glycolide PLGA) will degrade more slowly than a polymer with an equal mole ratio of lactide and glycolide (50:50 lactide:glycolide PLGA). This difference is partially attributed to the differences in the degree of crystallinity of the polymers. A more crystalline polymer will hydrate more slowly and, thus, have a longer degradation time. A block copolymer (segments of lactide and glycolide) synthesized from lactide and glycolide monomers may form crystalline phases, thereby reducing the degradation rate. However, a polymer produced from the cyclic monomer of lactide-coglycolide will not form crystalline phases since it will have contiguous lactide/glycolide repeating segments. To develop a polylactide vaccine formulation, the appropriate polymer must then be chosen to match the desired schedule for delivery of the antigen.

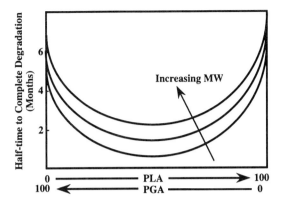

Figure 4. A modified version of the in vivo degradation profile for polylactides in rats as described by Miller *et al.* (1977). As the relative amount of either monomer, glycolide or lactide, increases, the degradation time increases because of the differences in the hydrophobicity and crystallinity of the polymer. Experimental data from Miller *et al.* (1977):

Polymer composition (lactide:glycolide)	Mass (kDa)	Half-time to complete degradation (months)	Crystallinity
PLA	85	6.1	Moderate
75:25 PLGA	50	0.6	Low/moderate
50:50 PLGA	46	0.24	Low
25:75 PLGA	N.A.[a]	0.55	Moderate
PGA (slow cured)	N.A.	5.0	N.A.

[a]N.A., not available.

4. STABILITY CONSTRAINTS ON SUBUNIT VACCINES IN POLYLACTIDE MICROSPHERES

While one can design formulations that release antigen for several months or years, the antigen released from the microspheres after incubation at 37°C under physiological conditions must maintain its ability to invoke the desired immune response. Subunit antigens are often lipid-associated proteins that are present on the infectious bacterial or viral surface. If the whole protein is used for the vaccine, the lipid-soluble portion of the protein may cause self-association or irreversible aggregation resulting in a loss of epitopes. The lipid-soluble portion of the protein is often extremely hydrophobic and will not maintain its conformation without lipids to stabilize the hydrophobic surfaces. Alternatively, a soluble protein consisting of the whole protein without the lipid-associated domain may be used for the vaccine. Although a soluble protein may also have greater physical stability at 37°C than the self-associated whole protein, it can still degrade by several pathways (see Cleland and Langer, 1994, and Cleland *et al.*, 1993, for reviews of protein degradation pathways). Recent studies have demonstrated that significant degradation of proteins occurs under conditions that mimic the environment of the protein in the microspheres after administration (Hageman *et al.*, 1992; Costantino *et al.*, 1994). The chemical degradation pathways may result in small changes in the antigen such as oxidation of a methionine residue or deamidation of an asparagine residue. If these changes do not alter the conformation of the protein antigen or disrupt the neutralizing epitope, they will not adversely affect the immunogenicity of the vaccine. However, physical denaturation including aggregation of the antigen can have detrimental effects on the potency of the vaccine. The addition of stabilizing agents such as sugars or surfactants may provide some protection if they can be retained within the polymer matrix with the protein. To avoid the aggregation of the antigen, the antigen concentration used in the first emulsion phase should be minimized since this concentration should be comparable to the concentration within the individual droplets in the final microspheres (see Section 1.2). By reducing the antigen concentration in the pores, aggregation will probably be reduced and the amount of antigen loaded in the microspheres may also be reduced unless the volume of aqueous antigen is increased. In some cases such as hepatitis B surface antigen, the antigen may be most immunogenic as an aggregate (~20-nm particles) and it may be more stable to physical denaturation during incubation at physiological conditions. For whole inactivated or killed viral or cellular vaccines, similar degradation issues exist and the overall stability of these antigens can be more difficult to achieve since the noninfectious virus or cell may not retain its structure after incubation at physiological conditions. In general, the development of a vaccine formulation to provide stability of the antigen for several months at physiological conditions is often more difficult than the development of a liquid or solid formulation because the stabilizing components (e.g., various excipients) may diffuse out of the microspheres at a greater rate than the antigen. Thus, preliminary screening studies must be carefully designed to assess the stability of candidate antigens and formulations.

   In addition to stabilizing the antigen at 37°C during its residence in the microspheres after administration, the antigen must be stabilized during the encapsulation process since it contacts organic solvents and is eventually dried. Denaturation during processing for delivery applications has been observed for several proteins and delivery systems (Jones *et al.*, 1994). Stabilization of the antigen during processing must be achieved to assure release of antigen that will invoke a neutralizing immune response. A few studies have analyzed the conformational integrity of the antigen after processing. For example, ovalbumin (O'Hagen *et al.*, 1993), MN rgp120 (Cleland *et al.*, 1994), *Salmonella enteritidis* (Hazrati *et al.*, 1993), and tetanus toxoid (Alonso *et al.*, 1993) were observed to maintain their antigenic epitopes and aggregation was not observed. However, the overall conformational state of the protein was not assessed for most of these antigens. The conformation of MN rgp120 was analyzed by several chromatographic methods, ELISAs, CD4 (receptor for MN rgp120) binding, and circular dichroism. All of these assays indicated that MN rgp120 was released from PLGA in its intact native state (Cleland *et al.*, 1994). In many cases, the intact native structure is necessary to invoke a neutralizing immune response. For HIV-1, the subunit antigen, gp120, must be administered in its native state to generate neutralizing antibodies (Haigwood *et al.*, 1992). The generation of neutralizing antibodies after several months in vivo was achieved for the MN rgp120 (Cleland *et al.*, 1994) and tetanus toxoid (Alonso *et al.*, 1993) formulations. Overall, a successful single-immunization vaccine must release antigen in its intact native form both initially and after incubation at 37°C for weeks or months.

5. MANUFACTURING HURDLES FOR POLYLACTIDE MICROSPHERE-BASED VACCINES

While developing vaccine preparations that are resistant to denaturation by organic solvents, drying, and incubation at 37°C, the microencapsulation process design should also be considered. If the schedule and dose are known from feasibility experiments (see Section 2), then the appropriate polymer and amount of antigen can be chosen for the initial studies (see Section 3). Prior to designing the microencapsulation process, one must evaluate the potential patent issues involved in polylactide delivery systems. Several patents cover the controlled or continuous release of biological agents from biodegradable polymers (Ludwig and Ose, 1981; Ludwig and Bosvenue, 1982; Folkman and Langer, 1983; Okada et al., 1987; Hutchinson, 1988; Eppstein and Schryver, 1990). Each of these patents is very similar in its basic composition, but has subtle differences in the claims or definitions. The unclear definitions and broad claims in these patents make their interpretation difficult. To further complicate the legal issues in developing these formulations, patents have been issued on the use of polymeric matrices and microspheres as vaccine formulations (Beck, 1990; Tice et al., 1991). The development, manufacture, and eventual sale of polylactide vaccines must account for these patents and appropriate contractual agreements may be required in some cases.

Once any necessary contracts and licenses are established, a manufacturing process can be designed to produce sufficient quantities of material for Phase I human clinical trials. As mentioned in Section 1.2, there are two traditional approaches to the production of microspheres. Each method, solvent evaporation or coacervation, should be evaluated for its effect on the antigen as well as the quality of the final product. Both methods require the use of an organic solvent to dissolve the polymer (see Figs. 1 and 2). The coacervation method also utilizes silicone oil and a nonsolvent such as heptane, both of which may cause safety concerns as discussed below. The solvent evaporation process does not require any additional organic solvents and the emulsifying agent, polyvinyl alcohol, is considered safe and nontoxic. However, the encapsulation efficiency, the amount of entrapped antigen relative to the amount added, may often be greater for the coacervation method. In addition, the coacervation method prevents the antigen from contacting water prior to its final use. Many antigens may be more susceptible to denaturation in the presence of water and organic solvents because of the interfacial interactions and the solubility of some antigens in aqueous environments. Again, the best process method will depend on the individual antigen and the process requirements.

5.1. Aseptic Manufacturing and Terminal Sterilization

After the method of production is chosen, an overall manufacturing scheme is constructed from the basic unit operations. A simplified manufacturing process diagram for the solvent evaporation method is shown in Fig. 5. The first emulsion is formed by homogenization of the antigen in the organic solvent in a tank (all equipment and plumbing should be pharmaceutical grade, e.g., 316L electropolished stainless steel). The emulsion is then transferred to a second larger tank containing the emulsifying agent, polyvinyl alcohol (PVA), in water (approximately 20- to 100-fold the volume of the first emulsion).

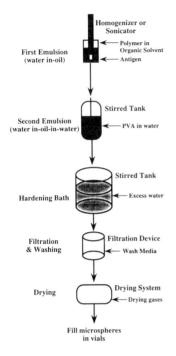

Figure 5. Simplified process diagram for production of polylactide microspheres using the solvent evaporation method. The items listed next to arrows on the right-hand side of the process diagram indicate the materials that must be added by sterile filtration. The first emulsion may be performed by homogenization or sonication in a sealed sterile vessel. The emulsion is then transferred to a stirred tank containing the emulsifying agent in water to form the second emulsion. After mixing, the second emulsion is added to a large excess of water in a stirred tank (hardening bath). The hardening bath step may require incubation and ventilation with nitrogen sparging to facilitate removal of the organic solvent. Filtration and washing of the hardened microspheres is then performed to remove the emulsifying agent, small particulates, and large agglomerates. The final microspheres are then dried (e.g., lyophilization or vacuum drying) to produce a free flowing powder. Each addition of components as well as the connections between unit operations may compromise the sterility of the system and will require thorough testing for an aseptic process. The process variables for each step are listed in Table III.

This second tank is continuously stirred to produce the microspheres. The rate of agitation in this tank as well as the process conditions (polymer composition and concentration, PVA concentration, temperature, etc.) determine the size of the final microspheres. The microsphere suspension is then transferred to a third tank containing excess water (approximately 3- to 10-fold the volume of the microsphere solution) to facilitate removal of the organic solvent. The final suspension may then be sieved to remove large particles (> 100 μm), or filtered to remove fine particulates (< 1 μm). The microspheres are washed to remove excess solvent or emulsifying agents. Finally, a drying step such as lyophilization is performed and the final powder is filled into vials.

There are several potential steps in the overall manufacturing process that could compromise the sterility of the final product (see Fig. 5). Since the final product has a particle size of 1–100 μm, it cannot be filtered with 0.22-μm filters to remove contaminants such as bacterial spores prior to final filling into vials. Thus, it is crucial to develop an aseptic manufacturing process or investigate methods to terminally sterilize the final product.

For an aseptic manufacturing process, the major difficulties are encountered in the beginning and end of the process stream. The addition of sterile materials such as the polymer, antigen, emulsifying agent, and water to the beginning of the process is often difficult. The optimum conditions for polymer, antigen, and emulsifying concentration as determined at the laboratory scale can result in solutions that are difficult to sterile filter on addition to the processing tanks. After addition of all of the materials, the overall manufacturing process stream must be tested for sterility. One sterility test method involves the addition of bacterial spores (e.g., bacillus) to the individual units prior to steam sterilization. A nutrient broth is then added by the same method as the antigen to the process stream. The final solution is cultured for several days and assessed for bacterial growth. The next difficult sterile procedure is the handling of the microspheres prior to the drying step. If a uniform suspension is obtained, the microspheres are filled and dried in the vials. Alternatively, the microsphere suspension is often transferred to a containment device for final drying. If the drying process is performed prior to vial filling, then the dry powder must be handled and filled into vials. Dry powder handling is usually very complex. The flow properties of the final material and the filling requirements must be considered prior to design of the aseptic process. For dry powder handling, a Class 100 air handling system is required along with special gowning procedures. The overall aseptic process is performed under Class 1000 air handling units to reduce the potential for contamination. Both the air handling system and the process require extensive validation. In addition, the final process must be operated under Good Manufacturing Practice (GMP) guidelines with appropriate documentation for Standard Operating Procedures (SOPs). Prior to the production of material for toxicology testing and clinical trials, the documentation on validation of the aseptic GMP process must be ready for eventual review by the FDA.

If the complex problems in aseptic manufacturing cannot be resolved, a possible alternative may be terminal sterilization of the vaccine. Terminal sterilization usually involves the use of either electron beam or gamma irradiation. A radiation dose of 2.5 Mrad is usually considered sufficient for sterilization of medical devices and drugs. Although lower doses (e.g., 1 Mrad) may be effective in sterilizing the final product, each dose must be thoroughly tested by biological challenge, i.e., the addition of microorganisms prior to sterilization as per U.S. Pharmacopoeia guidelines. Radiation can degrade the polymer and denature the antigen. The polymer molecular weight decreases on radiation treatment as a result of the formation of free radicals (Horacek and Kudlacek, 1993; Birkinshaw et al., 1992). The release properties of the microspheres are then altered, as observed previously (Hartas et al., 1992; Spenlehauer et al., 1989). For subunit antigens (e.g., proteins), the generation of free radicals by radiation treatment may result in oxidation, denaturation, and aggregation of the protein (see Haskill and Hunt, 1967a,b). In general, terminal irradiation may cause significant degradation of the polymer and antigen resulting in major changes in the performance characteristics of the microspheres. These changes are usually reduced by increasing the polymer molecular weight and adding free radical scavengers to protect the antigen. The radiation effects on the vaccine formulation should be determined at an early stage of development to assess the potential for terminal sterilization of the product.

5.2. Scaleup, Process Integration, and Solvent Handling Concerns

The overall process conditions greatly influence the antigen encapsulation efficiency and its subsequent release from the microspheres. Each individual process step as detailed in Fig. 5 is thoroughly studied and optimized both alone and in combination with the other unit operations. Once the optimum process conditions are determined for a given antigen/polylactide formulation, the scaleup parameters are then assessed to develop a process that will meet the requirements for the initial clinical trials. The main process parameters

Table III
Main Process Variables for Double Emulsion Method in Production of Polylactide Vaccine[a]

Process step	Variables
First emulsion	Polymer concentration in organic solvent
	Polymer composition and molecular weight
	Organic solvent (e.g., methylene chloride or ethyl acetate)
	Oil phase volume
	Concentration of antigen in aqueous solution
	Antigen solution volume
	Mixing rate
	Mixing device (e.g., homogenization or sonication)
	Rate of antigen addition to oil phase
	Duration of mixing
	Temperature and pressure
Second emulsion	Water phase volume
	Concentration of emulsifying agent in water phase
	Rate of oil phase addition to water phase
	Mixing rate
	Mixing device (e.g., stirred tank)
	Duration of mixing
	Temperature and pressure
Hardening bath	Water volume
	Presence of additives or stabilizers
	Incubation time
	Mixing rate
	Mixing device (e.g., stirred tank)
	Temperature and pressure
Filtration & washing	Filtration device (e.g., stirred cell)
	Rate of filtration
	Filtration mesh size
	Wash volume
	Wash composition
	Temperature and pressure
Drying	Method of drying (e.g., lyophilization)
	Facilitated mass transfer (e.g., fluidized bed)
	Drying time
	Amount of residual moisture
	Addition of excipients

[a]See Fig. 5 for process diagram.

are listed in Table III. Although there are a large number of variables, only a few of them dramatically impact the final product characteristics and process yield. The viscosity of the first emulsion (polymer concentration, molecular weight, and composition, and temperature) and the amount of antigen added to the emulsion have the greatest impact on the efficiency of encapsulation (e.g., antigen in microspheres/antigen added to first emulsion) assuming that the antigen is well dispersed in the emulsion. The extent and rate of solvent removal during the second emulsion and hardening bath stages will also affect the encapsulation efficiency as well as the initial release of antigen. A large amount of antigen is released initially if the microspheres were hardened slowly allowing the antigen to migrate to the surface. While many of the process steps involve similar variables, each variable has a direct impact on the individual process step as well as the overall process. It is also essential to consider the interaction between each process step. For example, the amount of oil phase used in the first emulsion often has a dramatic impact on the amount of water phase used in the second emulsion. The water solubility of the organic solvent (e.g., ~10% for ethyl acetate and ~2% for methylene chloride) and the water phase volume determine the rate of solvent removal from the oil phase and formation of the microspheres. As the volume ratio of water phase to oil phase increases, the rate of microsphere formation also increases since the organic solvent partitions into a larger excess of water. Also, the water phase volume in the second emulsion and the oil phase volume in the first emulsion affect the volume of water used in the hardening bath. The hardening bath further reduces the amount of organic solvent in the oil phase, resulting in more stable microspheres that do not allow rapid release of antigen through diffusion. From the first emulsion to the hardening bath stage, the antigen may diffuse out of the oil phase or droplets of the antigen may move to the microsphere surface and contact the second water phase. Thus, the yield of encapsulated antigen and the amount of initial antigen released are directly affected by the emulsion steps and the final hardening process. A systematic analysis of each process step and integration of the unit operations is required prior to optimization and process scaleup.

In addition to process design considerations, the solvent handling issues must be addressed. Both the solvent evaporation and coacervation methods involve the use of organic solvents to dissolve the polymer. These solvents are usually volatile and flammable. Special solvent handling procedures are then required to comply with Environmental Protection Agency (EPA) and Occupational Safety and Hazards Association (OSHA) requirements. Depending on the process scale, a special containment facility may be required for the process stream waste and the overall manufacturing process may require a facility that meets regulatory guidelines for solvent handling.

6. REGULATORY AND TOXICOLOGY ISSUES

The FDA not only reviews the overall manufacturing process, but also assesses the final product. Each batch of the antigen/polylactide formulation must meet predetermined specifications for release as a final product. The reproducibility of the manufacturing process must be demonstrated and the quality of the final product must meet several strict guidelines. While these issues are similar for every new vaccine, a polylactide vaccine preparation may encounter additional difficulties. For example, the characterization of a polylactide vaccine that releases antigen at 0, 1, and 6 months would require a real-time in vitro incubation of the vaccine preparation for 6 months before the final product could be released. However, if an accelerated release method was developed and validated, the analysis time could be greatly reduced, thereby decreasing the delay before release of the final vaccine product. Unfortunately, the FDA usually requires real-time data for final approval of the product. The quality of the released antigen must also be thoroughly assessed for each preparation since denaturation of the antigen could reduce the potency of the vaccine. The in vitro analysis methods include the assumption that the solvent conditions (e.g., buffer species, ionic strength) are representative of the vaccine performance in vivo. Depending on the regulatory agency's requirements, the manufacturer may need to test the vaccine with an in vivo potency assay. These assays usually involve the administration of small vaccine doses to a small animal (e.g., mouse or guinea pig). The production of antibodies in the animal is then measured as an indication of vaccine potency. The in vivo potency assay usually delays the release of the final product for clinical or commercial use.

Other assays of the final product may include sterility, endotoxin burden, fill consistency, and content uniformity. The sterility of the final product must be assessed by CFR guidelines, and the FDA Center for Drug Evaluation and Review (CDER) has previously used surface testing of microspheres as an acceptable test for sterility based on the current commercial PLGA products (Lupron Depot® and Zoladex®). The endotoxin levels in the polylactide formulation can be determined by incubation of the microspheres in physiological buffer to facilitate release of any surface-associated endotoxins. The supernatant from this incubation is then assayed for endotoxin content. The vial fill consistency and content uniformity require random sampling of vials. Vials should be analyzed for fill volume, product quality (e.g., flow properties, color), and the amount of antigen should be determined by extraction methods (e.g., 1 N sodium hydroxide or organic solvent). Once these issues have been addressed, the final product meets many of the necessary regulatory standards.

6.1. Residual Solvent Concerns

In addition to quality and potency concerns, the regulatory agency defines the acceptable level of residual solvent in the final vaccine product. The production of polylactide formulations often requires the use of organic solvents, and in these cases, the amount of residual organic solvent and its toxicity must be determined. The two most commonly used organic solvents for microencapsulation, methylene chloride and ethyl acetate, are very different in their toxicity. As shown in Table IV, methylene chloride is much more toxic in the final product and in the manufacturing process than ethyl acetate. Further, low concentrations of ethyl acetate are often used in foods as a flavor enhancer (apple flavor). Unfortunately, the solubility of many polylactides, particularly 50:50 lactide:glycolide PLGA, is much lower in ethyl acetate than methylene chloride. If the solubility of the required polylactide in ethyl acetate makes manufacturing difficult or impossible, methylene chloride must be used and the amount of residual solvent must be dramatically reduced (e.g., < 50 ppm/dose for Lupron Depot®) to assure safety. In contrast, the residual solvent levels that are acceptable for ethyl acetate may be much higher since it is not considered a carcinogen. In each case, the FDA requires extensive toxicology to assure that the final product is safe. Excess solvent is often removed by extended drying times, but this processing can increase the vaccine manufacturing cost and alter the properties of the final product. The excess residual solvent is bound to the polymer and the amount bound depends on drying process and the type of polylactide (more hydrophobic, more bound solvent). To remove the bound solvent, high temperatures (>20°C) and a vacuum may be required. Regulatory agencies require justification for any residual solvent

Table IV
Toxicity Data for Methylene Chloride and Ethyl Acetate [a]

Component	Toxicity[b]
Methylene chloride	Rat LD_{50} 1.6 g/kg (oral)
	Human LDLo 357 mg/kg (oral)—Narcotic effect
	Suspected carcinogen and mutagen
	Damage to liver and kidneys
	Metabolized to carbon monoxide
	Nervous system disorders
	Skin irritation
	Therapeutic category: Pharmaceutical aid (solvent)[c]
Ethyl acetate	Mouse LD_{50} 709 mg/kg (i.p.)
	LD_{50} 4.1 g/kg (oral)
	Rat LD_{50} 5.62 g/kg (oral)
	LD_{50} 5.0 g/kg (s.c.)
	Rabbit LD_{50} 4.9 g/kg (oral)
	Cat LD_{50} 3.0 g/kg (s.c.)
	Skin and eye irritation
	Target organs: Liver, kidneys, central nervous system, and blood
	Therapeutic category: Pharmaceutical aid (flavor)[c]

[a]Material safety data sheets—Sigma and Aldrich corporations.
[b]The toxicity results are reported as a lethal dose that causes 50% of the treated animals to die (LD_{50}). For humans, the lethal dose resulting in a few deaths is referred to as LDLo.
[c]Merck Index M. Windholz, S. Budavari, R. F. Blumetti, and E. S. Otterbein, eds.), 1983, 10th ed., Merck & Co., Rahway, NJ, pp. 545 and 869.

and, therefore, manufacturers should attempt to remove as much solvent as possible without compromising the quality of the final vaccine product.

Other processing materials may also contaminate the final product. For the solvent evaporation method, residual PVA or wash components (e.g., filtration aids) can be found in the final product. More toxic components (e.g., mutagens or carcinogens) such as silicone oil and heptane are often difficult to remove when used in the coacervation method. The acceptable safe levels should be determined for each of these individual components by testing in animal toxicology studies. Often, extensive toxicology studies are required to validate the safety of the final vaccine product. The FDA evaluates these studies and works with the manufacturer to determine the amount of residual processing materials that may be safely included in the final product.

6.2. Histology Studies of Polylactide Formulations

Along with overall toxicity, injection site inflammation and other side effects must be minimized to assure safety. The tissue at the injection site of a polylactide microsphere preparation usually experiences a minimal initial acute inflammation (Visscher et al., 1987). This response includes the infiltration of immune cells and a minimal foreign body response including some small foreign body giant cells (Visscher et al., 1985, 1987). Little or no fibrous tissue forms around the injection site as a part of the foreign body response

(Visscher *et al.*, 1985). Eventually, the tissue at the injection site returns to normal after the polymer has completely degraded (Visscher *et al.*, 1987). The time course for the polymer degradation and resolution of the injection site depends on the polymer molecular weight and composition as discussed above (Section 3, Miller *et al.*, 1977). A minimal tissue response to polylactides has also been observed when used in surgical applications such as sutures and embolic material (Grandfils *et al.*, 1992). In general, the administration of polylactides is well tolerated with no reported adverse events.

In addition to histological examination at the site of injection, safety assessment of the vaccine includes a minimum requirement of toxicology studies in two different species (e.g., mice and primates). This study would include observation of injection sites, notation of adverse side effects, screening for uveitis, clinical pathology, and other medical assessments of the animals. Any negative results (e.g., positive uveitis test) limit the use of the vaccine product or prevent its commercialization. Many of these studies are performed at an early stage of the vaccine development to assess the potential for toxicity. Early and intensive assessment of toxicity-related events greatly reduces the probability of encountering unexpected side effects in human clinical trials.

7. OVERVIEW OF MAJOR ISSUES IN DESIGN OF POLYLACTIDE VACCINE FORMULATIONS

The design and production of single-immunization vaccines using polylactide systems is a complex process requiring a well-planned strategy for successful commercialization. Animal testing and formulation studies should be performed initially. Animal studies should be designed to assess the optimum schedule and dose required to achieve the maximum immune response. Initial assessments of immunogenicity may be made by testing the antigen in small animal models (e.g., mice or guinea pigs). Additional studies in primates (e.g., monkeys or baboons) are usually required since their immune systems are the most comparable to humans. While determining the optimal schedule and dose of the antigen in animals, formulations must be developed to stabilize the antigen against denaturation by the organic solvents used in the process and during incubation of the antigen in vivo at 37°C. Once the antigen dose, schedule, and formulation have been developed, the polymer characteristics are then chosen. For a longer release period or delay time in triphasic release, polylactides with a higher molecular weight and lactide content are used for erosion controlled release. The polymer characteristics as well as the antigen stability affect the choice of microencapsulation methods, solvent evaporation or coacervation. After choosing the method, a lab-scale process system is designed to produce small quantities of material for animal experiments. The lab-scale system serves as a platform for evaluation of system parameters. Design for aseptic manufacturing and scaleup of the process is then performed with the knowledge of each system parameter's influence on the overall process. With an aseptic GMP pilot-scale process in place, vaccine preparations are then prepared for toxicological testing and immunogenicity evaluation in primates. Final processing steps are also optimized to remove the maximum amount of residual solvents from the vaccine product. After all of these complex issues are addressed, the polylactide vaccine formulation is ready for testing in human Phase I clinical trials.

8. FUTURE DIRECTIONS IN THE DEVELOPMENT OF SINGLE-SHOT SUBUNIT VACCINES

If the major hurdles in polylactide formulations are overcome, it is possible, in theory, to develop single-immunization vaccines for many currently FDA-approved vaccine products, assuming that the polymer formulation can be designed to deliver the appropriate schedule and dose. The manufacturing hurdles are surmounted by aseptic production in specialized facilities. Stability issues for the antigen both during processing and under physiological conditions are resolved by development of new formulations. The innovative development of unique methods for stabilizing antigens in these devices at physiological conditions for long periods (e.g., months) may determine the future success of the technology.

Several subunit antigens are likely candidates for this type of delivery system. In particular, diphtheria toxoid (Singh *et al.*, 1992) and tetanus toxoid (Alonso *et al.*, 1993) encapsulation in polylactides may yield a single-immunization vaccine to replace the current DT formulation. Other vaccine formulations such as hepatitis B surface antigen may also be suitable for use in a polylactide delivery system. In each case, the vaccine will require development of a stable antigen formulation for use in the final polylactide product formulation.

Another advantage of polylactides beyond their single-immunization potential is their stability at room temperature. Most polylactides have a glass transition temperature of greater than $25\,°C$ (e.g., $MW_n > 20$ kDa). Thus, if the microsphere release characteristics are not altered by storage at room temperature, these formulations may also eliminate the need to refrigerate the vaccine, assuming that the dried antigen is also stable. Ultimately, these formulations may then lead to single-immunization vaccines that are stable at moderate temperatures. Thus, the refrigeration requirements for vaccines would be eliminated, increasing their availability. This advantage of polylactide vaccines has not been previously addressed and long-term stability (e.g., >2 years) of both the polymer and antigen must be thoroughly investigated. If these formulations are stable at room temperature, these vaccines would then be used extensively in underdeveloped countries and urban clinics, saving thousands or millions of lives.

ACKNOWLEDGMENTS

The author thanks Dr. Tue Nguyen for his thorough review of the manuscript and suggestions. In addition, the author is very grateful for the support of this work by Drs. Michael F. Powell, Andrew J. S. Jones, and Rodney Pearlman. The continued efforts and support of this work by Amy Lim, Lorena Barrón, Robert Perry Weissburg, and Katrina Brabham are also greatly appreciated.

REFERENCES

Almeidia, A. J., Alpar, H. O., Williamson, D., and Brown, M. R., 1992, Poly(lactic acid) microspheres as immunological adjuvants for orally delivered cholera toxin B subunit, *Biochem. Soc. Trans.* **20**:316S.
Alonso, M. J., Cohen, S., Park, T. G., Gupta, R. K., Siber, G. R., and Langer, R., 1993, Determinants of release rate of tetanus vaccine from polyester microspheres, *Pharm. Res.* **10**:945–953.

Anderson, K. P., Lucas, C., Hanson, C. V., Londe, H. F., Izu, A., Gregory, T., Ammann, A., Berman, P. W., and Eichberg, J. W., 1989, Effect of dose and immunization schedule on immune response of baboons to recombinant glycoprotein 120 of HIV-1, *J. Infect. Dis.* **160**:960–969.

Barkin, R. M., Samuelson, J. S., Gotlin, L. P., and Barkin, S. Z., 1985, Primary immunization with diphtheria–tetanus toxoids vaccine and diphtheria–tetanus toxoids–pertussis vaccine adsorbed: Comparison of schedules, *Pediatr. Infect. Dis.* **4**:168–171.

Beck, L. R., 1990, Mammal immunization, U.S. Patent 4,919,929.

Birkinshaw, C., Buggy, M., Henn, G. G., and Jones, E., 1992, Irradiation of poly(D,L-lactide), *Polym. Degrad. Stab.* **38**:249–253.

Cabasso, V. J., Louie, R. E., Lo, B., and Dobkin, M. B., 1978, Antibody levels following W138 rabies vaccine, *Dev. Biol. Stand.* **40**:231–235.

Christenson, B., and Bottinger, M., 1991, Changes of the immunological patterns against measles, mumps, and rubella: A vaccination program studied 3 to 7 years after the introduction of a two-dose schedule, *Vaccine* **9**:326–329.

Cleland, J. L., and Langer, R., 1994, Formulation and delivery of proteins and peptides: Design and development strategies, in: *Protein Formulations and Delivery* (J. L. Cleland and R. Langer, eds.), ACS Books, New York, pp. 1–21.

Cleland, J. L., Powell, M. F., and Shire, S. J., 1993, Development of stable protein formulations: A close look at protein aggregation, deamidation, and oxidation, *CRC Crit. Rev. Ther. Drug Carrier Syst.* **10**:307–377.

Cleland, J. L., Powell, M. F., Lim, A., Barrón, L., Berman, P. W., Eastman, D. J., Nunberg, J. H., Wrin, T., and Vennari, J. C., 1994, Development of a single-shot subunit vaccine for HIV-1, *AIDS Res. Hum. Retroviruses* **10**:s21–s26.

Costantino, W. R., Langer, R., and Klibanov, A., 1994, Moisture-induced aggregation of lyophilized insulin, *Pharm. Res.* **11**:21–29.

Eldridge, J. H., Staas, J. K., Meulbroek, J. A., Tice, T. R., and Gilley, R. M., 1991a, Biodegradable and biocompatible poly(DL-lactide-co-glycolide) microspheres as an adjuvant for staphylococcal enterotoxin B toxoid which enhances the level of toxin-neutralizing antibodies, *Infect. Immun.* **59**:2978–2986.

Eldridge, J. H., Staas, J. K., Meulbroek, J. A., McGhee, J. R., Tice, T. R., and Gilley, R. M., 1991b, Biodegradable microspheres as a vaccine delivery, *Mol. Immunol.* **28**:287–294.

Eppstein, D. A., and Schryver, B. B., 1990, Controlled release of macromolecular polypeptides, U.S. Patent 4,962,091.

Folkman, M. J., and Langer, R. S., 1983, Systems for the controlled release of macromolecules, U.S. Patent 4,391,797.

Furr, B. J. A., and Hutchinson, F. G., 1992, A biodegradable delivery system for peptides: Preclinical experience with the gonadotropin-release hormone agonist Zoladex[®], *J. Control. Rel.* **21**:117–128.

Grandfils, C., Flandroy, P., Nuhant, N., Barbette, S., Jérome, R., Teyssié, P., and Thibaut, A., 1992, Preparation of poly (D,L) lactide microspheres by emulsion-solvent evaporation, and their clinical applications as a convenient embolic material, *J. Biomed. Mater. Res.* **26**:467–479.

Hageman, M. J., Bauer, J. M., Possert, P. L., and Darrington, R. T., 1992, Preformulation studies oriented toward sustained delivery of recombinant somatotropins, *J. Agric. Food Chem.* **40**:348–355.

Haigwood, N. L., Nara, P. L., Brooks, E., Van Nest, G. A., Ott, G., Higgins, K. W., Dunlop, N., Scandella, C. J., Eichberg, J. W., and Steimer, K. S., 1992, Native but not denatured recombinant human immunodeficiency virus type 1 gp120 generates broad-spectrum neutralizing antibodies in baboons, *J. Virol.* **66**:172–182.

Hardy, G. E., Hopkins, C. C., Linnemann, C. C., Hatch, M. H., Chambers, J. C., and Witte, J. J., 1970, Trivalent oral poliovirus vaccine: A comparison of two infant immunization schedules, *Pediatrics* **45**:444–448.

Hartas, S. R., Collett, J. H., and Booth, C., 1992, The influence of gamma-irradiation on the release of melatonin from poly(lactide-coglycolide) microspheres, *Proc. Int. Symp. Control. Rel. Bioact. Mater.* **19**:321–322.

Haskill, J. S., and Hunt, J. W., 1967a, Radiation damage to crystalline ribonuclease: Identification of polypeptide chain breakage in the denatured and aggregated products, *Radiat. Res.* **32**:827–848.

Haskill, J. S., and Hunt, J. W., 1967b, Radiation damage to crystalline ribonuclease: Importance of free radicals in the formation of denatured and aggregated products, *Radiat. Res.* **32**:606–624.

Hazrati, A. M., Lewis, D. H., Atkins, T. J., Stohrer, R. C., McPhillips, C. A., and Little, J. E., 1993, *Salmonella enteritidis* vaccine utilizing biodegradable microspheres, *Proc. Int. Symp. Control. Rel. Bioact. Mater.* **20**:101–102.

Heller, J., 1993, Polymers for controlled parenteral delivery of peptides and proteins, *Adv. Drug Deliv. Rev.* **10**:163–204.

Hess, G., Hingst, V., Cseke, J., Bock, H. L., and Clemens, R., 1992, Influence of vaccination schedules and host factors on antibody response following hepatitis B vaccination, *Eur. J. Clin. Microbiol. Infect. Dis.* **11**:334–340.

Horacek, I., and Kudlacek, L., 1993, Influence of molecular weight on the resistance of polylactide fibers by radiation sterilization, *J. Appl. Polym. Sci.* **50**:1–5.

Hutchinson, F. G., 1988, Continuous release pharmaceutical compositions, U.S. Patent 4,767,628.

Jepson, M. A., Simmons, N. L., O'Hagen, D. T., and Hirst, B. H., 1994, Comparison of poly(DL-lactide-co-glycolide) and polystyrene microsphere targeting to intestinal M cells, *J. Drug Target.* **1**:245–249.

Jertborn, M., Svennerholm, A.-M., and Holmgren, J., 1993, Evaluation of different immunization schedules for oral cholera B subunit-whole cell vaccine in Swedish volunteers, *Vaccine* **11**:1007–1012.

Jones, A. J. S., Nguyen, T. H., Cleland, J. L., and Pearlman, R., 1994, New delivery systems for recombinant proteins—practical issues from proof of concept to clinic, in: *Trends and Future Perspectives in Peptide and Protein Drug Delivery* (V. H. L. Lee, M. Hashida, and Y. Mizushima, eds.), Harwood Academic, Amsterdam (in press).

Just, M., Kanra, G., Bogaerts, H., Berger, R., Ceyhan, M., and Petre, J., 1991, Two trials of an acellular DTP vaccine in comparison with a whole-cell DTP vaccine in infants: Evaluation of two PT doses and two vaccination schedules, *Dev. Biol. Stand.* **73**:275–283.

Just, M., Berger, R., Drechsler, H., Brantschen, S., and Glück, R., 1992, A single vaccination with an inactivated hepatitis A liposome vaccine induces protective antibodies after only two weeks, *Vaccine* **10**:737–739.

Kalpana, K. R., and Park, K., 1993, Biodegradable hydrogels in drug delivery, *Adv. Drug Deliv. Rev.* **11**:59–84.

Kessler, D. A., 1992, The basis of the FDA's decision on breast implants, *N. Engl. J. Med.* **326**:1713–1715.

Khan, M. Z. I., Opdebeeck, J. P., and Tucker, I. G., 1994, Immunopotentiation and delivery systems for antigens for single-step immunization: Recent trends and progress, *Pharm. Res.* **11**:2–11.

Langer, R., 1993, Polymer-controlled drug delivery systems, *Acc. Chem. Res.* **26**:537–542.

Lewis, D. H., 1990, Controlled release of bioactive agents from lactide glycolide polymers, in: *Drugs and the Pharmaceutical Sciences* (M. Chasin and R. Langer, eds.), Vol. 45, Dekker, New York, pp. 1–42.

Ludwig, N. H., and Bosvcnuc, R. J., 1982, Controlled release parasitic formulations and method, U.S. Patent 4,331,652.

Ludwig, N. H., and Ose, E. E., 1981, Controlled release formulations and method of treatment, U.S. Patent 4,293,539.

Marx, P. A., Compans, R. W., Gettie, A., Staas, J. K., Gilley, R. M., Mulligan, M. J., Yamshchikov, G. V., Chen, D., and Eldridge, J. H., 1993, Protection against vaginal SIV transmission with microencapsulated vaccine, *Science* **260**:1323–1327.

Miller, R. A., Brady, J. M., and Cutright, D. E., 1977, Degradation rates of oral resorbable implants (polylactates and polyglycolates): Rate modification with changes in PLA/PGA copolymer ratios, *J. Biomed. Mater. Res.* **11**:711–719.

Ogawa, Y., Yamamoto, M., Okada, H., Yashiki, T., and Shimamoto, T., 1988a, A new technique to efficiently entrap leuprolide acetate into microcapsules of polylactic acid or copoly(lactic/glycolic) acid, *Chem. Pharm. Bull.* **36**:1095–1103.

Ogawa, Y., Yamamoto, M., Okada, H., Yashiki, T., and Shimamoto, T., 1988b, Controlled-release of leuprolide acetate from polylactic acid or copoly(lactic/glycolic) acid microcapsules: Influence of molecular weight and copolymer ratio of polymer, *Chem. Pharm. Bull.* **36**:1502–1507.

Ogawa, Y., Yamamoto, M., Okada, H., Yashiki, T., and Shimamoto, T., 1988c, In vivo release profiles of leuprolide acetate from microcapsules prepared with polylactic acids or copoly(lactic/glycolic) acids and in vivo degradation of these polymers, *Chem. Pharm. Bull.* **36**:2576–2581.

O'Hagen, D. T., Jeffery, H., and Davis, S. S., 1993, Poly(lactide-co-glycolide) microparticles as controlled release vaccines, *Proc. Int. Symp. Control. Rel. Bioact. Mater.* **20**:59–60.

Okada, H., Ogawa, Y., and Yashiki, T., 1987, Prolonged release microcapsule and its production, U.S. Patent 4,652,441.

Okada, H., Inoue, Y., Heya, T., Ueno, H., Ogawa, Y., and Toguchi, H., 1991, Pharmacokinetics of once-a-month injectable microspheres of leuprolide acetate, *Pharm. Res.* **8**:787–791.

Pierce, N. F., 1984, Induction of optimal mucosal antibody responses: Effects of age, immunization route(s), and dosing schedule in rats, *Infect. Immun.* **43**:341–346.

Preis, I., and Langer, R. S., 1979, A single-step immunization by sustained antigen release, *J. Immunol. Methods* **28**:193–197.

Reid, R. H., Boedeker, E. C., McQueen, C. E., Davis, D., Tseng, L. Y., Kodak, J., and Sau, K., 1993, Preclinical evaluation of microencapsulated CFA/II oral vaccine against enterotoxigenic *E. coli*, *Vaccine* **11**:159–167.

Serufo, J. C., Lima, M. G., Ribeiro, M. F. B., and Santos, J. L. D., 1987, Comparative study of schemes of preexposure vaccination against human rabies: Importance of the interval between doses and laboratory control, *Cienc. Cult. (Sao Paulo)* **39**:193–197.

Singh, M., Singh, O., Singh, A., and Talwar, G. P., 1992, Immunogenicity studies on diphtheria toxoid loaded biodegradable microspheres, *Int. J. Pharm.* **85**:R5–R8.

Spenlehauer, G., Vert, M., Benoit, J. P., and Boddaert, A., 1989, In vitro and in vivo degradation of poly (D,L-lactide/glycolide) type microspheres made by solvent evaporation method, *Biomaterials* **10**:557–563.

Tice, T. R., Gilley, R. M., Eldridge, J. H., Staas, J. K., Hollingshead, M. G., and Shannon, W. M., 1991, Method of potentiating an immune response, U.S. Patent 5,075,109.

Visscher, G. E., Robinson, R. L., Maulding, H. V., Fong, J. W., Pearson, J. E., and Argentieri, G. J., 1985, Biodegradation of and tissue reaction to 50:50 poly(DL-lactide-co-glycolide) microcapsules, *J. Biomed. Mater. Res.* **19**:349–365.

Visscher, G. E., Robinson, R. L., and Argentieri, G. J., 1987, Tissue response to biodegradable injectable microcapsules, *J. Biomater. Appl.* **2**:118–131.

Chapter 19

Nanoparticles as Adjuvants for Vaccines

Jörg Kreuter

1. INTRODUCTION

Many immunogens used in vaccine formulations, especially split (or subunit) virus preparations or proteins manufactured by genetic engineering, require the use of adjuvants to boost the immune response. Classical adjuvants include different kinds of emulsions, as well as aluminum derivatives such as aluminum hydroxide (Hem and White, 1984; and Chapter 9), aluminum phosphate (Hennessy *et al.*, 1971), and aluminum oxide (Grafe and Kuhn, 1962a,b). Aluminum hydroxide adjuvants have been used most widely because of their reputation for safety in humans. Further, aluminum-based ("alum") adjuvants are the only adjuvants currently included in vaccines licensed by the Food and Drug Administration (Hem and White, 1984). Despite alum's common use, variations in alum quality frequently occur between different batches of the same aluminum hydroxide-adjuvanted vaccine. This inconsistent response is understandable in view of the structure of aluminum hydroxide (see Chapter 9). The structure and physicochemical properties of aluminum adjuvants change significantly with slight alterations in production conditions and with aging (Kreuter and Haenzel, 1978; Feldkamp *et al.*, 1982; Nail *et al.*, 1976a,b). With emulsions, the degree of dispersions defined as the particle size distribution of the inner-phase droplets, may vary from preparation to preparation and may also change after injection. For example, the droplet size may be decreased by frictional forces during injection into tight muscular tissues whereas injection into fatty tissues may result in a coalescence of the emulsion droplets, leading to a larger droplet (particle) size.

Polymeric particles offer the advantage that they can be manufactured in a reproducible manner and that their composition and particle size can be monitored within narrow limits. Submicron, nanometer-sized polymeric carrier particles for drugs or antigens are called nanoparticles (Kreuter, 1983a). Drugs or vaccine immunogens may be incorporated into these particles by polymerization in the presence of these compounds or, in the case of smaller molecules, by absorption into previously polymerized particles. Alternatively,

Jörg Kreuter • Institute for Pharmaceutical Technology, Johann Wolfgang Goethe University, D-60439 Frankfurt am Main, Germany.

Vaccine Design: The Subunit and Adjuvant Approach, edited by Michael F. Powell and Mark J. Newman. Plenum Press, New York, 1995.

drugs or antigens may be bound to the nanoparticles by adsorption to the surface of these particles by chemical bonding. As will be shown in this chapter, polymethyl methacrylate (PMMA) is the material of choice for nanoparticle adjuvants.

2. PRODUCTION OF NANOPARTICLES

Vaccine immunogens may be incorporated into the nanoparticles or may be adsorbed to the surface. Large molecules such as immunogens cannot be expected to diffuse into the polymers used thus far for the preparation of nanoparticulate adjuvants. Consequently, nanoparticles with incorporated immunogens must be manufactured by polymerization in the presence of the immunogen. This requires the use of a polymerization method that does not destroy the antigenicity or conformational properties of the immunogen. For this reason, heat-induced polymerization is not applicable with most immunogens. Since gamma irradiation, UV irradiation, or light irradiation does not destroy the antigenicity of most protein immunogens (Birrenbach and Speiser, 1976; Kreuter and Zehnder, 1978), these methods are usually employed for the initiation of polymerization.

2.1. Polymerization in the Presence of the Immunogen

For the production of nanoparticles in the presence of the immunogen, the monomer—in most cases methyl methacrylate—is dissolved at 0.1–2.0% (v/v) in the immunogen suspension. For encapsulation of most immunogens tested thus far, the optimal monomer concentration was 0.5% (v/v) (Kreuter and Speiser, 1976b; Kreuter and Liehl, 1978, 1981). By adding the monomer directly to the immunogen suspension, the immunogen is incorporated at a known final concentration in its optimal buffer system. This preparation is then polymerized with gamma irradiation at a temperature of 2–10 °C. The optimal irradiation conditions for the immunogens tested thus far were doses of 0.5 Mrad at a rate of 2 krad/min (Kreuter and Zehnder, 1978).

2.2. Polymerization in the Absence of the Immunogen

Empty nanoparticles may also be produced be gamma irradiation as described in the previous paragraph (Kreuter and Speiser, 1976a,b). Alternatively, heat polymerization may be used with empty nanoparticles for their production (Berg *et al.*, 1986). In this case, the monomer is added to distilled water and heated to 65–85°C for 2 h. At approximately 40°C a polymerization initiator, potassium peroxodisulfate or ammonium peroxodisulfate, is added. The particle size of the resulting nanoparticles and the molecular weight of the polymer can be controlled by the amounts of monomer and initiator used (Table I).

Nanoparticles made by both polymerization methods, gamma irradiation or heat-induced polymerization, can either be stored in a liquid suspension, or may be stored in dry form after lyophilization. In the latter case, PMMA nanoparticles can be stored for over 20 years without any alteration. The liquid or dried nanoparticles are then added to the antigen suspension in the appropriate amounts to obtain the desired antigen and adjuvant concentration.

Table I

Influence of Monomer Concentration, Initiator Concentration, and Temperature on Particle Size and Molecular Weight of Polymethyl Methacrylate Nanoparticles[a]

Potassium peroxodisul- fate concen- tration (mmol)	Particle size (nm)								Molecular weight		
	Methyl methacrylate concentration (mmol) at two temperatures										
	10		33.75		80		156.25		80		156
	65°C	85°C	65°C	85°C	65°C	85°C	65°C	85°C	65°C	85°C	85°C
0.3	85	72	129	128	181	170	256	262	—	434,000	—
1.65	98	88	151	169	212	193	248	248	—	—	—
3.0	92	72	135	149	223	177	250	258	289,000	220,500	400,000

[a]Adapted from Berg, U., 1979, Immunostimulation durch hochdisperse Polymersuspensionen, Diss. ETH Zürich No. 6481, pp. 34 and 67. Reproduced from Kreuter, J., (ed.), 1994, *Controlled Drug Delivery Systems*, Dekker, New York, p. 224, with permission of the copyright holder.

2.3. Nanoparticles Produced in an Organic Phase

Nanoparticles with incorporated proteins also may be produced in an organic phase (Birrenbach and Speiser, 1976). In this case the aqueous antigen suspension is solubilized in an organic phase, usually *n*-hexane. This method requires surfactant(s). A useful surfactant combination is bis(2-ethylhexyl) sodium sulfosuccinate and polyoxyethylene-4-lauryl ether in a ratio of 2:1. The solubilization requires large amounts of surfactants, ~30% (v/v organic phase). Thereafter the water-soluble monomers, acrylamide, and the cross-linker *N,N'*-bis-acrylamide are added and also solubilized in the aqueous phase. Polymerization and nanoparticle formation then is carried out by irradiation with gamma rays, UV light, or after a sensitizer such as riboflavin 5'-sodium phosphate is added with visible light. The organic phase is then replaced first by methanol and subsequently by the appropriate aqueous buffer employing ultrafiltration or ultracentrifugation. The resulting nanoparticles with incorporated immunogen are stored in liquid form or may be stored in lyophilized form if the immunogenicity of the protein is not destroyed by this process.

3. CHARACTERIZATION OF NANOPARTICLES

Methods for the characterization of nanoparticles are described by Kreuter (1983b, 1992) and by Magenheim and Benita (1991). From an immunological viewpoint, the most important feature of nanoparticles is their size. Particle size determination can be done by photon correlation spectroscopy or by electron microscopy (Kreuter, 1983b). Photon correlation spectroscopy has the advantage that it is a rapid method, whereas the microscopic methods are more laborious, but allow the visualization of the nanoparticle surface and interior. Transmission electron microscopy after freeze-fracture is especially useful for the investigation of the particle's interior. Simple transmission electron microscopy may lead to a coalescence of polymer particles with a low melting point or transition temperature because of the high energy of the electron beam (Kreuter, 1983b). Often with scanning electron microscopy, the metallic coating of the particles, which is necessary for the visualization of organic surfaces, yields erroneous information concerning the surface morphology and particle size (Kreuter, 1983b). Another method that is routinely used for the characterization of nanoparticles is the determination of molecular weight (Bentele *et al.*, 1983). Here the method of choice is gel permeation chromatography after dissolution of the nanoparticle polymer in an appropriate organic solvent.

An additional important in vitro characterization parameter is the determination of the adsorption behavior of immunogens on the nanoparticle adjuvant, although the importance of the quantitative and qualitative aspects of adsorption for the immune response presently is not fully understood. A number of reports in the literature (Pyl, 1953; Kreuter and Speiser, 1976a; Kreuter and Liehl, 1981) indicate that no overall correlation seems to exist between the amount of immunogen adsorbed and the antibody response or the protection against infection. Nevertheless, the quantitation of immunogen adsorption remains an important question that cannot be answered easily. Immunogens may be adsorbed not only by particulate adjuvants, but also by the container materials. Because of this adsorption problem, the determination of immunogen in the supernatant after centrifugation of the particulate adjuvants may not be sufficient for the quantification of immunogen adsorption to the nanoparticles. Instead, radiolabeled antigens are required for rigorous adsorption experiments. In addition, a single homogeneous protein, e.g., gp120, should be used for these experiments. Since mixtures of immunogens are used for many vaccines, the different proteins, glycoproteins, and lipids contained therein may influence their respective adsorption behavior differently at different concentrations. Moreover, it should be remembered that when large molecules are used, head-on, tail-on, or side-on adsorption can occur. This in turn is dependent on the concentration of the immunogen and on the presence of other substances including buffer salts, cryoprotectants, and other immunogens. This type of adsorption, however, may be very important for the quantity and quality of the immune response in that the immunogen conformations presented to the immunocompetent cells might be different.

4. INFLUENCE OF PARTICLE SIZE AND HYDROPHOBICITY ON THE ADJUVANT EFFECT OF NANOPARTICLES

The particle size and the hydrophobicity of nanoparticles may be monitored by the choice of monomers and by the polymerization conditions. As shown in Fig. 1 and in a number of investigations (Kreuter and Haenzel, 1978; Kreuter *et al.*, 1986, 1988; Stieneker *et al.*, 1994), a decrease in particle size and an increase in hydrophobicity of nanoparticles increased the antibody responses after immunization against influenza whole and split virus, bovine serum albumin (BSA), and HIV-2 split virus. These higher levels of antibodies were correlated with a higher protection after immunization with influenza vaccines containing PMMA nanoparticles and challenge with live influenza virus. It is not known if the optimal particle size is approximately 100 nm, or if smaller particles lead to higher antibody responses. The reason for the enhanced immune response by the increase in the hydrophobicity of the nanoparticle carrier is not fully understood. This effect is also

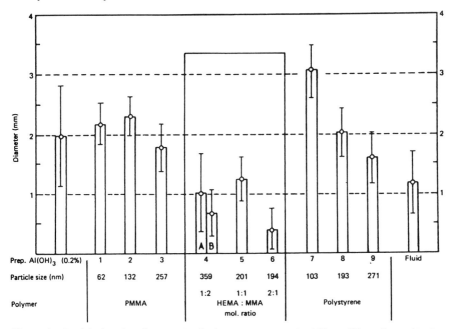

Figure 1. Precipitation ring diameters (antibody response; mean ± ~95% confidence intervals) after immunization of mice with different bovine serum albumin vaccines. The variables shown are size of the adjuvant particles, and copolymer composition: PMMA, polymethyl methacrylate; HEMA/MMA, 2-hydroxyethyl methacrylate/methyl methacrylate copolymer. The standard deviations of the polymer particle sizes are: preparation 1, 9 nm; preparation 2, 12 nm; preparation 3, 12 nm; preparation 4, 83 nm; preparation 5, 12 nm; preparation 6, 17 nm; preparation 7, 35 nm; preparation 8, 2 nm; and preparation 9, 6 nm. Reproduced from Kreuter *et al.* 1988, *Vaccine* **6**:255, by permission of the publishers, Butterworth Heinemann Ltd.

dependent on the immunogen. It seems to be likely that with some immunogens, the interaction with the carrier particles leads to a favorable presentation of the immunogen to the immunocompetent cells.

PMMA is less hydrophobic than polystyrene and, as a result, augmented antibody responses to a lesser degree (Fig. 1). However, since information is available about the biocompatibility of PMMA in contrast to polystyrene, and since it has been routinely used in surgery for over 40 years, PMMA seems to be the material of choice for nanoparticle adjuvants.

5. ANTIBODY RESPONSE AND PROTECTION INDUCED WITH VACCINES CONTAINING PMMA NANOPARTICLES

PMMA nanoparticles exhibited an optimal adjuvant response and an optimal protection against challenge with live mouse-adapted virus after s.c. immunization with whole virus and subunit vaccines at a polymer concentration of 0.5% (Kreuter and Speiser, 1976b; Kreuter *et al.*, 1976; Kreuter and Liehl, 1978, 1981). This optimum was observed using

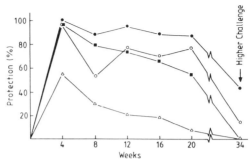

Figure 2. Protection of mice against infection with a dose of 50 LD$_{50}$ of infectious mice-adapted influenza virus after s.c. immunization with 20 IU of A$_0$PR 8 whole virus using the following adjuvants: ●, incorporation into 0.5% PMMA; ○, adsorption onto 0.5% PMMA; ■, adsorption onto 0.2% aluminum hydroxide; △, fluid vaccine without adjuvant. Higher challenge = 250 LD$_{50}$. Reproduced from Kreuter, 1988, *J. Microencapsul.* **5**:116, by permission of the publishers, Taylor & Francis.

immunogen incorporated into particles or adsorbed, although the adjuvant effect was more pronounced with the incorporated immunogens. Similar results were obtained in mice and guinea pigs. Incorporation of influenza immunogen into particles using higher amounts (2.0%) of PMMA nanoparticles was less effective and resulted in lower antibody responses than a corresponding fluid vaccine 4 weeks after s.c. immunization. Longer time periods and boosting led to a decrease of the differences in the immune responses between different nanoparticle concentrations. At the optimal polymer concentration of 0.5%, nanoparticles achieved a better antibody response and a better protection than 0.2% aluminum hydroxide, which in turn was better than a fluid vaccine (Kreuter and Liehl, 1981). This effect was more pronounced at longer time periods after immunization (Fig. 2). Dilution of the nanoparticle concentration to low levels decreased the adjuvant effect considerably (Kreuter and Liehl, 1978). Similar results as with influenza were obtained after immunization of mice with BSA (Kreuter *et al.*, 1986, 1988).

Both nanoparticle preparations, containing incorporated or adsorbed immunogen, stabilized influenza antigens against inactivation by storage at elevated temperatures (40°C) for up to 240 h (Kreuter and Liehl, 1981).

With HIV-1 and HIV-2 split virus, produced by Tween$^®$/ether splitting, the ELISA-antibody responses after s.c. immunization of mice using PMMA nanoparticles were even more pronounced than was observed with influenza and BSA compared to aluminum hydroxide and to the use of soluble HIV-2 proteins. With both HIV preparations, HIV-1 and HIV-2, the maximum antibody titers were observed after about 10 weeks with a single injection (Stieneker *et al.*, 1991, 1993). The delay in antibody response compared with that seen with other immunogens was extremely pronounced, and significant titers were observed after 4 weeks and only with the PMMA preparation. PMMA nanoparticles induced 20- to 100-fold higher antibody titers against HIV-2 immunogens and about 10- to 20-fold higher titers against HIV-1 immunogens, compared to aluminum hydroxide. Aluminum hydroxide, in turn, was significantly superior to the soluble vaccine (Stieneker *et al.*, 1993). Antibody titers generally disappeared 40 weeks after vaccination with the fluid- and the aluminum hydroxide-containing vaccines. The antibody titers of the PMMA-containing vaccine decreased to levels of about 1:1000 to 1:2000 after this time. Recently,

Figure 3. Serum antibody titers against HIV-2 inactivated split whole virus in mice immunized with 5 μg viral proteins in combination with different adjuvants. Mice immunized with ISCOMs received 0.5 μg protein. PMMA, polymethyl methacrylate nanoparticles; Alum HC, aluminum hydroxycarbonate (produced by S. L. Hem, Purdue University); FCA, complete Freund's adjuvant; FIA, incomplete Freund's adjuvant; MLV, multilamellar large vesicles, incorporated antigen; SUV, bilayer, small unilamellar vesicles, protein integrated into the bilayer; SUV, adsorbed, small unilamellar vesicles, protein adsorbed onto the surface; MDP, N-acetyl-muramyl-L-alanyl-D-isoglutamine; SAF-l, Syntex Adjuvant Formulation-1; PHCA, polyhexylcyanoacrylate nanoparticles; PBCA, polybutylcyanoacrylate nanoparticles; ISCOMs, immunostimulating complexes; Alphos/Ll2l, combination of aluminum phosphate and Synperonic PE Ll2l; PMMA/Ll2l, combination of PMMA and Synperonic PE L121; PMMA/F68, combination of PMMA and Pluronic F68. Reproduced by permission of the publisher, Butterworth Heinemann Ltd. (Steineker *et al.*, 1995).

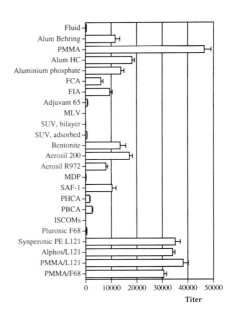

Stieneker *et al.* (1995) compared 24 different adjuvants and carriers using HIV-2 split vaccines with an antigen content of 5 μg/0.5 mL in mice (Fig. 3). In addition to the ELISA-antibody titers, the specificity of antibodies was determined using Western blots. All sera were tested 10 weeks after a single immunization. Again, PMMA particles augmented the immune responses by far the most. However, they failed to induce significant antibodies against gp120 as detected by the Western blot. Only aluminum hydroxide, aluminum phosphate, Aerosil 200, Aerosil R972, Freund's complete (FCA) and incomplete (FIA) adjuvants were able to induce significant antibody responses to gp120. This antigen is very hydrophilic and it appears that in an immunogen mixture as was used in the split virus vaccine, the gp120 was not able to interact with the very hydrophobic PMMA nanoparticles and, therefore, was unable to induce antibodies in significant amounts. This observation demonstrates that the choice of an optimal adjuvant or carrier depends on the physicochemical and biochemical properties of the immunogen. A combination of two or more different carriers or adjuvants may be necessary to induce the optimal immune response.

6. BODY DISTRIBUTION, ELIMINATION, AND TOXICOLOGICAL REACTIVITY OF PMMA ADJUVANTS

PMMA is a material that has been used in surgery for over 40 years in humans (Charnley, 1970; Cabanela *et al.*, 1972). It is today's workhorse in artificial bone replacements. Particles of this material similar in size to nanoparticles that we prepared are frequently present in the patient's body as the result of such bone replacement implants. These particles originate from mechanic abrasions of the implants and from interaction with the body's cells. The body burden from these implants is much greater than is necessary for use in a vaccine formulation.

PMMA nanoparticles labeled with polymethyl [1-^{14}C]methacrylate were used to determine biodistribution. In mice and rats, unexcreted radioactivity remained at the injection site for 287 days (Kreuter *et al.*, 1979, 1983). Less than 1% of the remaining dose at a given time point was distributed to tissues of the residual body. The initial urinary and fecal excretion amounted to about 1% of the administered dose per day. However, the elimination rate dropped rapidly within a few days to very low levels of about 0.0005% per day in the urine and 0.005% per day in the feces within 70 days. After 200 days, the rate of the fecal elimination started to increase exponentially until a >100-fold increase was observed after 287 days. Simultaneously, the radioactivity in all organs and tissues increased about 100-fold in comparison to the organ activities determined at earlier times. The ratio of organ to blood activity, on the other hand, remained unaltered. The residual radioactivity at the injection site after 287 days amounted to 55–71%.

These findings combined with the observation of a lag period of 27 weeks for excretion point to the following scenario, which is similar to other polymers (Kreuter *et al.*, 1983; Schindler *et al.*, 1977). The degradation of the polymer may have started much earlier than the observed increase in excretion. As with other polymers, the removal of material, however, seems to have occurred only after a lower molecular weight was reached. In any case, these results show that PMMA is slowly biodegradable. This slow biodegradation rate very likely is beneficial if the attainment of a prolonged immunostimulation is desired.

Histological examinations of the tissue at the injection site 1 year after intramuscular injection of a PMMA nanoparticle-containing influenza vaccine in seven guinea pigs showed no abnormalities (Kreuter *et al.*, 1976). Histological reactions such as the appearance of giant cells and eosinophils were the same as with the soluble vaccine control.

7. SUMMARY

PMMA nanoparticle adjuvants can be manufactured in a physicochemically reproducible manner. Their particle size can be controlled within narrow limits. Immunogens may be either incorporated or adsorbed to these nanoparticles. PMMA nanoparticles induced significantly higher and more prolonged antibody responses against a variety of immunogens, including influenza virions and subunit vaccines, BSA, and HIV-1 and HIV-2 split vaccines. In addition, a protective immune response against challenge with live influenza virus was induced and a better stability of the immunogen was observed after incorporation or adsorption of influenza virions or subunits to PMMA nanoparticles. The observation that PMMA did not induce antibodies against gp120 contained in the HIV-2 split vaccine demonstrates that different adjuvants or carriers may be required for different antigens. A combination of two or more different adjuvants or carriers may be necessary to induce the optimal immune response against antigen mixtures as present in most vaccine preparations. PMMA seems to be a safe adjuvant material. It is very slowly biodegradable and has been used in surgery in humans for over 40 years, and now warrants continued investigation as a vaccine adjuvant.

REFERENCES

Bentele, V., Berg, U. E., and Kreuter, J., 1983, Molecular weights of poly(methyl methacrylate) nanoparticles, *Int. J. Pharm.* **13**:109–113.

Berg, U. E., Kreuter, J., Speiser, P. P., and Soliva, M., 1986, Herstellung und In-Vitro-Prufung von polymeren Adjuvantien fur Impfstoffe, *Pharm. Ind.* **48**:75–79.

Birrenbach, G., and Speiser, P. P., 1976, Polymerized micelles and their use as adjuvants in immunology, *J. Pharm. Sci.* **65**:1763–1766.

Cabanela, M. E., Coventry, M. B., MacCarty, C. S., and Miller, W. E., 1972, The fate of patients with methyl methacrylate cranioplasty, *J. Bone Joint Surg.* **54**:278–281.

Charnley, J., 1970, *Acrylic Cement in Orthopaedic Surgery*, Livingstone, Edinburgh.

Feldkamp, J. R., White, J. L., and Hem, S. L., 1982, Effect of surface charge and particle size on gel structure of aluminum hydroxycarbonate gel, *J. Pharm. Sci.* **71**:43–46.

Grafe, A., and Kuhn, R. B., 1962a, Die Potenzierung von Impfstoffen durch Al_2O_3-Adsorption. 1. Mitteilung: Al_2O_3-Polio-Impfstoff, *Arzneim. Forsch.* **12**:33–37.

Grafe, A., and Kuhn, R. B., 1962b, Die Potenzierung von Impfstoffen durch Al_2O_3-Adsorption. 2. Mitteilung: Al_2O_3-Oliomyelitis-Diphtherie-Tetanus-Impfstoffe, *Arzneim. Forsch.* **12**:392–395.

Hem, S. L., and White, J. L., 1984, Characterization of aluminum hydroxide for use as an adjuvant in parenteral vaccines, *J. Parenteral Sci. Technol.* **38**:2–10.

Hennessy, A. V., Patno, M. E., and Davenport, F. M., 1971, Effect of $AlPO_4$ on antibody response, *Proc. Soc. Exp. Biol. Med.* **138**:396–398.

Kreuter, J., 1983a, Evaluation of nanoparticles as drug delivery systems. I: Preparation methods, *Pharm. Acta Helv.* **58**:196–209.

Kreuter, J., 1983b, Physicochemical characterization of polyacrylic nanoparticles, *Int. J. Pharm.* **14**:43–58.

Kreuter, J., 1992, Physicochemical characterization of nanoparticles and their potential for vaccine preparation, *Vaccine Res.* **1**:93–98.

Kreuter, J., and Haenzel, I., 1978, Mode of action of immunological adjuvants: Some physicochemical factors influencing the effectivity of polyacrylic adjuvants, *Infect. Immun.* **19**:667–675.

Kreuter, J., and Liehl, E., 1978, Protection induced by inactivated influenza virus vaccines with polymethyl-methacrylate adjuvants, *Med. Microbiol. Immunol.* **165**:111–117.

Kreuter, J., and Liehl, E., 1981, Long-term studies of microencapsulated and adsorbed influenza vaccine nanoparticles, *J. Pharm. Sci.* **70**:367–371.

Kreuter, J., and Speiser, P. P., 1976a, In vitro studies of poly(methyl methacrylate) adjuvants, *J. Pharm. Sci.* **65**:1624–1627.

Kreuter, J., and Speiser, P. P., 1976b, New adjuvants on a polymethylmethacrylate base, *Infect. Immun.* **13**:204–210.

Kreuter, J., and Zehnder, H. J., 1978, The use of Co-γ-irradiation for the production of vaccines, *Radiat. Effects* **35**:161–166.

Kreuter, J., Mauler, R., Gruschkau, H., and Speiser, P. P., 1976, The use of new polymethylmethacrylate adjuvants for split influenza vaccines, *Exp. Cell Biol.* **44**:12–19.

Kreuter, J., Tauber, U., and Illi, V., 1979, Distribution and elimination of poly(methyl-2-^{14}C-methacrylate) nanoparticle radioactivity after injection in rats and mice, *J. Pharm. Sci.* **68**:1443–1447.

Kreuter, J., Nefzger, M., Liehl, E., Czok, R., and Voges, R., 1983, Distribution and elimination of poly(methyl methacrylate) nanoparticles after subcutaneous administration to rats, *J. Pharm. Sci.* **72**:1146–1149.

Kreuter, J., Berg, U., Liehl, E., Soliva, M., and Speiser, P. P., 1986, Influence of the particle size on the adjuvant effect of particulate polymeric adjuvants, *Vaccine* **4**:125–129.

Kreuter, J., Berg, U., Liehl, E., Soliva, M., and Speiser, P. P., 1988, Influence of the hydrophobicity on the adjuvant effect of particulate polymeric adjuvants, *Vaccine* **6**:253–256.

Magenheim, B., and Benita, S., 1991, Nanoparticle characterization: A comprehensive physicochemical approach, *S.T.P. Pharma Sci.* **1**:221–241.

Nail, S. L., White, J. L., and Hem, S. L., 1976a, Structure of aluminum hydroxide gel. I: Initial precipitate, *J. Pharm. Sci.* **65**:1188–1191.

Nail, S. L., White, J. L., and Hem, S. L.., 1976b, Structure of aluminum hydroxide gel. II: Aging mechanism, *J. Pharm. Sci.* **65**:1192–1195.

Pyl, G., 1953, Die Prufung von Aluminium hydroxid auf seine Eignung fur die Maul- und Klauen-seuchevakzine, *Arch. Exp. Veterinärmed.* **7**:9–17.

Schindler, A., Jeffcoat, R., Kimmel, G. L., Pitt, C. G., Wall, M. E., and Zweidinger, R., 1977, Biodegradable polymers for sustained drug delivery, in: *Contemporary Topics in Polymer Science*, Vol. 2 (E. M. Pearce and J. R. Schaefgen, eds.), Plenum Press, New York, pp. 251–289.

Stieneker, F., Kreuter, J., and Lower, J., 1991, High antibody titres in mice with polymethylmethacrylate nanoparticles as adjuvant for HIV vaccines, *AIDS* **5**:431–435.

Stieneker, F., Lower, J., and Kreuter, J., 1993, Different kinetics of the humoral immune response to inactivated HIV-1 and HIV-2 in mice: Modulation by PMMA nanoparticle adjuvant, *Vaccine Res.* **2**:111–118.

Stieneker, F., Kersten, G., van Bloois, L., Crommelin, D. J. A., Hem, S. L., Lower, J., and Kreuter, J., 1995, Comparison of 24 different adjuvants for inactivated HIV-2 split whole virus as antigen in mice: Induction of titres of antibodies and toxicity of the formulations, *Vaccine* (in press).

Chapter 20

Water-Soluble Phosphazene Polymers for Parenteral and Mucosal Vaccine Delivery

Lendon G. Payne, Sharon A. Jenkins,
Alexander Andrianov, and Bryan E. Roberts

1. INTRODUCTION

The advent of modern molecular biology has provided us with a means of producing antigens with unprecedented ease and precision. It is ironic that these new methodologies generate purified antigens that do not generally induce a strong immune response in the absence of an effective adjuvant. The development of improved vaccine adjuvants for use in humans has therefore become a priority area of research. Nevertheless, research on adjuvants has lagged seriously behind the work done on antigens. For decades the only adjuvant widely used in humans has been alum. Saponin and its purified component Quil A, complete Freund's adjuvant (CFA) and other adjuvants used in research and veterinary applications have toxicities that limit their potential use in human vaccines. New chemically defined preparations such as QS-21, muramyl dipeptide, and monophosphoryl lipid A are being studied.

The traditional view on how adjuvants exert their effect is that adjuvants such as mineral oil emulsions or aluminum hydroxide form an antigen depot at the site of injection that slowly releases antigen. However, excision of the injection site after only 3 days had little effect on immune responses (White, 1976). Recent studies indicate that adjuvants enhance the immune response by stimulating specific and sometimes very narrow arms of the immune response by the release of cytokines (Allison and Byars, 1992).

There is considerable interest in the development of controlled release vaccines, since the major disadvantage of several currently available vaccines is the need for repeated administrations. Controlled release vaccines could obviate the need for booster immunizations and would be particularly advantageous in developing countries, where repeated

Lendon G. Payne, Sharon A. Jenkins, Alexander Andrianov, and Bryan E. Roberts • Virus Research Institute, Inc., Cambridge, Massachusetts 02138.

Vaccine Design: The Subunit and Adjuvant Approach, edited by Michael F. Powell and Mark J. Newman. Plenum Press, New York, 1995.

contact between the healthcare worker and the vaccine recipient is often difficult to achieve.

There is a growing body of evidence to suggest that antigen persisting on the external membrane of follicular dendritic cells and lymph node organs is involved in the recruitment of B memory cells to form antibody-secreting cells (Gray, 1993). The continual release of circulating antibodies suggests this recruitment happens continually. As the level of antigen decreases, affinity maturation of antibody occurs. This concept of antigen persistence has an important implication in vaccine development. Ideally, it would be advantageous to be able to formulate vaccines in a way such that antigen is presented to the immune system and in particular the follicular dendritic cells over an extended period of time.

An area of adjuvant research that has developed over the last few years is the utilization of synthetic polymers in formulating vaccines to effect the controlled release of antigens. The nonionic block copolymer surfactants (Hunter, 1991) with molecular weights below approximately 10,000 have a simple structure composed of two blocks of hydrophilic polyoxyethylene (POE) flanking a single block of hydrophobic polyoxypropylene (POP). They are considered to be among the least toxic of surfactants and are widely used in foods, drugs, and cosmetics. Some of the large hydrophobic copolymers are effective adjuvants, whereas closely related preparations are not. There is a correlation between the adjuvant activity of these copolymers with differences in the chain links of the POE and POP. Currently, these adjuvants are used in an oil and water emulsion.

A wide range of polyelectrolytes of various molecular weights have been shown to have adjuvant activity (Petrov *et al.*, 1992). Macromolecules bearing either positive or negative charges have displayed a similar immunostimulatory activity. The polyelectrolytes form complexes with antigens through electrostatic and hydrophobic bonds. On the other hand, neutral and uncharged polymers had no effect on the immune response unless the uncharged polymers were conjugated to the protein antigens.

Polymers have also been used to entrap antigens. An early example of this was the polymerization of methyl methacrylate into spheres having diameters less than 1 μm to form so-called nanoparticles (Kreuter, 1992; Chapter 19 this volume). The antibody response as well as the protection against infection with influenza virus was significantly better than influenza that was adjuvanted with aluminum hydroxide. Experiments with other particles demonstrated that the adjuvant effect of these polymers depends on particle size and hydrophobicity.

Microencapsulation has been applied to the injection of pharmaceuticals to give a controlled release. A frequent choice of a carrier for pharmaceuticals is poly D,L-lactide-co-glycolide (PLGA). This is a biodegradable polyester that has a long history of medical use in erodible sutures, bone plates, and other temporary prostheses. This widespread use of PLGA was achieved without any toxicity. The use of a biodegradable microencapsulation system that permits controlled release of antigens certainly presents a very attractive approach to mucosal immunization. In the last few years, a body of data has accumulated on the adaptation of PLGA for the controlled release of antigen (Eldridge *et al.*, 1989, 1991). The entrapment of antigens in PLGA microspheres of 1 to 10 μm in diameter has been shown to have a remarkable adjuvant effect. The disadvantage of the PLGA system is that the use of organic solvents and long preparation times for the microencapsulation

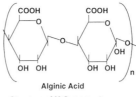

Alginic Acid
Structure of M-G segment

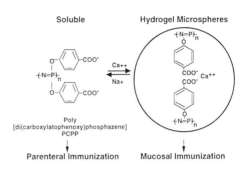

Figure 1. Ionically cross-linked polymers. The chemical structures for alginic acid and PCPP are shown in their un-ionized states. Ionic cross-linking is exemplified for the polyphosphazenes. The addition of heavy metal ions (e.g., Ca^{2+}) to the soluble polymer initiates cross-linking of polymer strands via the divalent cation, resulting in the formation of a hydrogel.

of the antigens may alter antigen conformation required for a functional or efficacious immune response.

The elucidation of a new class of ion cross-linkable water-soluble polyphosphazenes (PCPP) (Fig. 1) (Allcock and Kwon, 1989) has made it possible to generate microspheres in an aqueous environment (Cohen *et al.,* 1990; Payne *et al.,* 1994). The model for the development of the polyphosphazenes was the naturally occurring alginates prepared from brown algae and used in food stuffs. Gelation by ionic cross-linking of an aqueous-based polymer solution at room temperature eliminates the long exposure of antigens to organic solvents, elevated temperatures, and drying required by polymers dissolved in organic solvents. These characteristics make polyphosphazene microspheres an interesting potential vaccine delivery vehicle. Since anionic and cationic polymers have previously been shown to have immunoadjuvant activity, we were also interested in investigating the immunoadjuvant properties of the phosphazene and alginate polymers in the absence of ionic cross-linking. Thus, polyphosphazene can be combined with antigens in two different ways to potentially effect immunopotentiation. Antigens can be mixed with the soluble polyphosphazene and injected directly into an animal for parenteral immunization. Alternatively, the water-soluble polyphosphazene and antigen solution can be formulated into hydrogel microspheres by ionically cross-linking the carboxyl groups with divalent cations, and then used for parenteral or mucosal immunization.

Since the polyphosphazenes do represent a new class of polymers, it was of interest to determine the toxicity of this class of polymers. Cell culture dishes were coated with polyphosphazene and chicken embryo fibroblasts were seeded onto the coated petri dish. Three days after seeding, the cells had become flattened and spindlelike, and under contrast microscopy we could see mitotic figures. We have also encapsulated hybridoma cells in polyphosphazene microspheres having a diameter between 150 and 200 μm. The encapsulated hybridoma cells were able to undergo cell divisions, and by 10 days after encapsulation the microspheres were essentially filled with living cells (Bano *et al.*, 1991). This demonstrated the innocuous nature of the polyphosphazenes in cell culture.

In vivo acute toxicity of alginate and polyphosphazene has been evaluated in 6- to 8-week-old Sprague–Dawley rats. The study consisted of four groups of five male rats/group. Following an overnight fast, each animal in each group received a single oral dose of 5000 mg/kg (in water) via gavage. The dose volume was 20 mL/kg. Group one rats were the control and received water. Group two animals received alginate microspheres. Group three rats received alginate microspheres coated with poly-L-lysine (PLL; 68 kDa) (Sigma, St. Louis, MO). Group four animals received polyphosphazene microspheres. The animals were clinically observed for 7 days. Body weights were recorded on day 1 prior to immunization and at euthanasia. Blood samples were obtained by puncture of the retroorbital sinus after anesthetization with CO_2 at euthanasia. Animals were fasted overnight prior to blood collection. Tissues were examined and saved at necropsy. There were no significant differences in body weight gain between the rats that received microspheres and the rats in the control group. The results of hematology and clinical chemistry were normal for all rats in each group. There were no treatment-related abnormalities observed in any organ at necropsy. This study demonstrated that an oral dose of 5000 mg/kg of polyphosphazene or alginate microspheres was not acutely toxic.

2. MICROSPHERE FORMULATION AND CHARACTERIZATION

2.1. Microsphere Generation

Poly[di(carboxylatophenoxy)phosphazene] (PCPP) solutions were prepared by dissolving the appropriate amount of PCPP in one part 3% Na_2CO_3 while stirring, then slowly adding three parts phosphate buffer pH 7.4. The antigen solution was then slowly added to the polymer solution so that the final concentration of PCPP was 2.5%. Sodium alginate solutions were prepared by dissolving the appropriate amount of polymer in deionized water. The antigen was then slowly added to the alginate solution so that the final concentration of alginate is 1.25%. Constant stirring, as well as the slow addition of the antigen to the polymer, was necessary in order to obtain a homogeneous solution.

Protein molecular weight markers (Amersham) and FITC-labeled bovine serum albumin (BSA) (Sigma) have been microencapsulated to study release kinetics of soluble proteins. The release kinetics of 24-nm polystyrene beads (Duke Scientific) were also studied. Tetanus toxoid (TT) (Connaught Laboratories) and influenza virus were encapsulated for antigenicity studies. Influenza was grown in eggs according to standard methods and quantitated by protein, hemagglutination, and plaque assays. Influenza was inactivated by formalin by the addition of a 38% formaldehyde solution at a final dilution of 1:4000. Virus infectivity was also inactivated by exposure to gamma irradiation from a ^{60}Co source to 1.2×10^6 rad.

Previous work has shown that uptake of particulate material by Peyer's patch M-cells and subepithelial macrophages is limited to particles having diameters of 10 μm or less (Eldridge *et al.*, 1991). We therefore developed a process for generating microspheres in the size range of 1–10 μm (Fig. 2). The key component of our current encapsulation

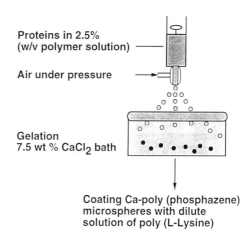

Figure 2. Microencapsulation process and size distribution. Cells or protein antigens are dispersed in an appropriate concentration of polymer to give a homogeneous solution. The solution is pumped into a Sonimist nozzle and forced through a 0.3-mm orifice by pressurized air, resulting in the generation of a microdroplet spray that impacts a calcium chloride bath. The polymer in the microdroplets is cross-linked (gelation) by the calcium ions to form microspheres. The microspheres can then be coated with other polymers.

procedure is an ultrasonic spray nozzle (Medsonic, Inc., Farmingdale, NY) that forces a polymer solution containing dispersed antigens through a small orifice under approximately 40 pounds per square inch of sterile air. The configuration of the nozzle results in the generation of a spray cloud containing microdroplets of polymer solution and antigen that impact a calcium chloride bath where the microdroplets begin to gel into microspheres. The microspheres are then collected and used as they are or can subsequently be coated with various other polymers such as PLL. Approximately 95% of alginate and PCPP microspheres generated under these conditions have diameters in the 1–10 μm range (Fig. 3). Ionically cross-linked microspheres were stored in buffers that are conducive to the maintenance of their integrity. Conditions were defined that maintain the integrity of the microspheres as well as the antigens entrapped within the polymer matrix. Microspheres containing antigen were stable for 7 days if stored at 4°C in sterile deionized water. Standard buffers such as phosphate-buffered saline (PBS) were not used because the replacement of calcium ions with sodium leads to the liquification of the matrix. Coating the microspheres with PLL allowed storage in PBS.

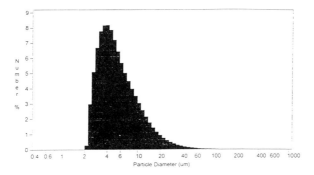

Figure 3. The size of the microspheres was analyzed by a Coulter LS 100 Particle Sizer. The graph shows the percentage of microspheres as a function of diameter.

2.2. Characterization of Microspheres

For immunogenicity studies, the protein content of microspheres was determined both directly after generation of the microspheres to assess the percent incorporation and also immediately before injection into animals to ensure delivery of known antigen quantities. The protein content of the microspheres could not be assessed by the Bio-Rad protein assay. Although the protein can be released from the microspheres by chelating the Ca^{2+} responsible for forming the hydrogel, the addition of the Bio-Rad reagent that contains divalent cations causes the polymer to re-cross-link rendering the antigen unavailable to the dye reagent. The quantitation of protein antigens encapsulated in ionically cross-linked microspheres was determined by electrophoresis of a known quantity of intact microspheres in SDS-PAGE. During electrophoresis, the proteins migrated out of the microsphere matrix and into the polyacrylamide gel. The protein concentration was determined by comparison to known quantities of the encapsulated protein electrophoresed in parallel to the microsphere preparation.

A body of data accumulated on the adaptation of PLGA for controlled antigen release has shown that the entrapment of antigens in 1- to 10-μm microspheres has a remarkable adjuvant effect (Eldridge *et al.*, 1991). The size of alginate and PCPP microspheres was measured utilizing a Coulter LS100 Particle Sizer. The size is reported as % number in the size range 1–10 μm.

2.3. Antigen Release

In order for the microencapsulated antigens to elicit an immune response, the antigen must be released from the microspheres. Antigen is released from a microsphere through the two different but not mutually exclusive processes of diffusion and erosion (Fig. 4). If the hydrogel is permeable to the dispersed antigens, then the antigens can simply diffuse out of the microspheres following the water phase that fills the matrix of the microsphere. Release of antigen is, therefore, an indication of the permeability of the microsphere matrix

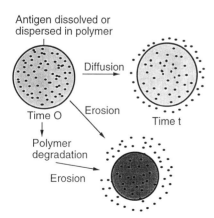

Figure 4. Release mechanisms of microencapsulated antigens. Polydispersed antigen can be released by simple diffusion or erosion. Erosion can occur through the redissolving of the polymer or by polymer degradation.

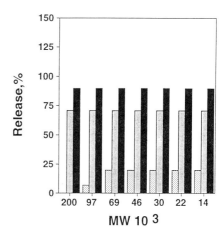

Figure 5. Permeability of polyphosphazene microspheres. Rainbow protein markers were microencapsulated in three concentrations of PCPP and incubated in HEPES buffer pH 7.4 at room temperature for 24 h before the amount of protein in the supernatant was spectrophotometrically measured.

to the antigen. Conversely, adsorption of the antigens to the polymer matrix will serve to either reduce or eliminate the diffusion of the antigen out of the microsphere.

The permeability of the PCPP microspheres was investigated by encapsulating the rainbow protein molecular weight markers (Amersham) that are commonly used in polyacrylamide gel electrophoresis (Fig. 5) (Andrianov *et al.*, 1993a). Release of the proteins was assayed by spectrophotometric measurements of the supernatant. The permeability of a particular protein such as the 14.3 kDa lysozyme was affected by the concentration of the polymer in the gel. As the polymer concentration rises from 1.5% to 3.3% there is a marked decrease in the diffusion of the protein out of the microsphere matrix. Similarly, as the molecular weight of the protein increases, diffusion of the protein out of the matrix is retarded. For example, the 200-kDa myoglobin protein was unable to diffuse out in a period of 24 h from a 3.3% PCPP matrix.

The second mechanism by which the antigens can be released from microspheres is through the erosion of the polymer matrix that makes up the microsphere (Fig. 4). Erosion occurs through the reversal of the gelation reaction, thus resulting in the solubilization of polymer molecules and their return to the surrounding aqueous environment. Degradation of PCPP microspheres was studied in saline solution (pH 7.4) by monitoring mass loss, molecular weights of polymer matrices and formation of soluble products. Erosion profiles for PCPP microspheres of varied molecular weights are shown in Fig. 6 (Andrianov *et al.*, 1993b, 1994). No detectable mass loss was observed during 180 days' incubation of high-molecular-weight PCPP microspheres in solution. However, gel permeation chromatography (GPC) showed significant decrease in polymer molecular weight during the same period of time (Fig. 7a). The mechanism of degradation apparently involves intramolecular carboxylic group catalysis. Use of low-molecular-weight PCPP for microsphere preparation leads to significant erosion of the hydrogel during the first 10 days and a decrease in molecular weight of polymer (Fig. 7b). Water-soluble polymeric products of practically the same molecular weight as in the matrix were detected. The data indicate that there is a molecular weight threshold of approximately 200 kDa in the release of PCPP from the matrix into the solution in this system. However, it is obvious that polymer solubility also

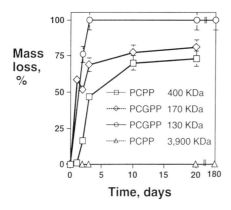

Figure 6. The effect of polymer side chains and molecular weight on microsphere erosion rates. Microspheres composed of PCPP and PCGPP were incubated in HEPES buffer pH 7.4 at 37°C. At various times, the dry weight of the microcapsules was assayed and expressed as the percent mass loss.

depends on the amount of calcium ions held by the matrix and the ionization degree of macromolecules.

Polyphosphazenes can be efficiently tailored by incorporating appropriate side groups to provide a controllable set of properties, including hydrolytic degradability. It was anticipated that introduction of a hydrolysis-sensitive pendant group, such as a glycinato group (Fig. 8), would result in an increased degradation rate in an aqueous environment. Cleavage of an external P–N bond occurring in neutral media in these aminophosphazenes to yield hydroxy derivative produces hydrolytic instability in the polymer. Poly[(carboxylatophenoxy)(glycinato) phosphazene] (PCGPP) containing 10% of glycinato groups was used for the preparation of microspheres and degradation studies. Erosion rates for these polymer hydrogels also depend on the molecular weight of PCPPs. PCGPP of weight

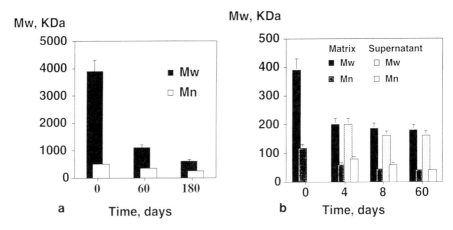

Figure 7. Molecular weight degradation profiles for PCPP hydrogel microspheres formed by ionic cross-linking of PCPP of 3900 kDa (a) and 400 kDa (b). Microspheres were incubated in HEPES-buffered saline (pH 7.4). Weight average and number average molecular weights of water-soluble degradation products in supernatant were determined. Matrix samples were isolated and then dissolved to measure weight average and number average molecular weights.

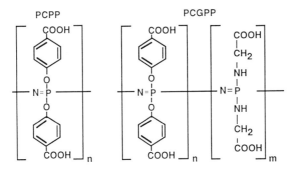

Figure 8. Chemical structures of PCPP and PCGPP. The ratio of the two side chains in PCGPP determines the rate of degradation.

average 130 kDa has a 100% mass loss within 3 days (Fig. 6). GPC analysis of matrix and soluble products (Fig. 9) showed that incubation for 240 days in an aqueous environment results in breakdown of the polymer backbone leading to fragments of less than 1 kDa and inorganic phosphate. Coating hydrogel microspheres with PLL (62 kDa) to yield a polyelectrolyte-complex membrane significantly decreases the erosion rate by 2.5 times because of steric hindrance. This appears to provide an additional approach to control the degradation and stability of PCPP microspheres. These results indicate the potential for specific regulation of the degradation kinetics and, therefore, release kinetics of encapsulated antigens. It is not known if this in vitro degradation mimics the in vivo situation, or if there is also enzymatically driven degradation.

The third means by which we have been able to regulate the release of antigen from microspheres is by coating the PCPP microspheres with PLL to form a semipermeable membrane on the outside of the microspheres (Fig. 10). The microsphere core can then be liquefied by the addition of chelating agents such as EDTA, which reverses the gelation process and results in the solubilization of the PCPP matrix. The degree of permeability can be regulated by the size of the PLL that is used in the coating process. We have used PLLs ranging from 12 to 295 kDa (Fig. 11). As the molecular weight of the PLL increases,

Figure 9. Molecular weight degradation profiles for PCGPP hydrogel microspheres formed by ionic cross-linking of PCGPP of 130 kDa. Weight average and number average molecular weights of water-soluble degradation products in supernatant were determined. Matrix samples were isolated and then dissolved to measure weight average and number average molecular weights.

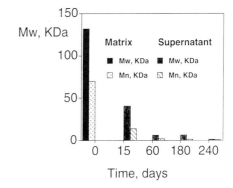

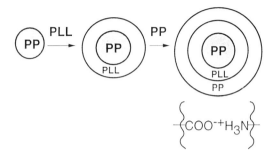

Figure 10. Coating of microspheres. Microspheres can be sequentially coated with polyanions. The positively charged poly-L-lysine (PLL) builds ionic linkages to the surface of the negatively charged polyphosphazene (PP) microspheres. Subsequently, another polymer coat can be added by reacting the PLL surface with negatively charged PP. In this way the surface charge and hydrophilicity of the microspheres can be regulated.

the permeability of the coating increases, resulting in an increased release of 24-nm polystyrene beads from the microsphere.

3. IMMUNOGENICITY STUDIES

3.1. Parenteral Immunization

Traditionally, most injected nonreplicating vaccines have required multiple doses to achieve protective serum antibody titers. For obvious reasons, it would be much more desirable to achieve protection with a single inoculation. Therefore, the effect of PCPP on the immunogenicity of antigens was examined in mice that were immunized subcutaneously with a single dose. Antigen formulated in water, alum, and CFA was included in many experiments for comparison.

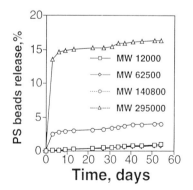

Figure 11. Release from microspheres coated with poly-L-lysines of different molecular weights. Fluorescent polystyrene (PS) beads measuring 20 nm in diameter were encapsulated in polymer 1 and then coated with poly-L-lysines of different molecular weights. The coated beads were incubated in HEPES buffer pH 7.4 at room temperature. Polystyrene beads released into the supernatant were measured by quantitative fluorimetry and expressed as a percent of the initially encapsulated beads.

Antigen was precipitated onto alum by adding dropwise 1.0 mL of a 10% solution of Al(K)(SO$_4$)$_2$·12H$_2$O (Sigma) to 2.5 mL of antigen solution with stirring, and adjusting the pH to 6.5 with approximately 0.65 mL of 1 N NaOH. After 30 min at room temperature, the suspension was centrifuged at 1000g at 5°C for 10 min. The amount of antigen adsorbed was determined by analyzing the amount of antigen in the supernatant and subtracting this amount from the total. The pellet was resuspended in sterile deionized water and adjusted to the proper concentration for injection. Antigens are also formulated into CFA (Sigma) by preparing an emulsion made with a 1:1 mixture of CFA and antigen in sterile deionized water.

Female 7- to 8-week-old BALB/c mice were randomized into groups. Mice were inoculated subcutaneously with a sample volume of 0.2 mL with a 25-gauge needle in the loose skin over the neck. Blood samples were taken from the retroorbital sinus of CO$_2$-anesthetized mice. Mice were euthanized with CO$_2$ in an inhalation chamber. It should be noted that all of the data reported here result from single dose immunizations.

Antibodies specific to TT in mouse serum were determined by a horseradish peroxidase ELISA in 96-well microtiter plates coated with 1 μg/mL TT. The end-point titers are the reciprocal of the greatest sample dilution producing a signal twofold greater than that of an antibody-negative sample at the same dilution. The ELISA for influenza antibody substitutes 10 μg/mL of influenza-infected MDCK cell lysate for TT in the coating step. The IgG1, 2a, 2b, and 3 isotypes of the ELISA-reactive TT and influenza-specific antibodies were determined by the detection of murine antibodies bound to the antigens. Influenza-specific functional antibodies were measured by 50% plaque reduction and hemagglutination inhibition assays (HAI). The HAI titers are expressed as the reciprocal of the highest dilution that completely inhibits hemagglutination of erythrocytes.

3.1.1. PCPP MICROSPHERES

The immunogenicity of TT antigen formulated in polymeric microspheres composed of alginate or PCPP was compared to soluble TT and TT in alum and CFA (Table I). Groups of five mice were immunized by the subcutaneous route with 20 μg of TT. The antibody response to TT was assayed by ELISA. Soluble TT antigen and alginate-microencapsulated TT induced a maximum titer of 512 by week 13. PCPP microspheres containing TT induced higher antibody titers at early times postimmunization than alum- or CFA-adjuvanted TT. Furthermore, PCPP microspheres containing TT induced antibody titers that were still rising at 13 weeks postimmunization. At this late time point, TT in PCPP microspheres had elicited a titer of 65,536, which was approximately 100-fold higher than seen for soluble TT and 2- to 4-fold higher than was seen for alum and CFA. PCPP microspheres were clearly superior to alginate microspheres in the induction of antibodies to TT.

The dose-dependent effect of immunization with TT was examined by immunizing mice with varying amounts of TT formulated into PCPP microspheres or CFA (Table II). The immunogenicity of TT in PCPP microspheres compared very favorably with TT formulated with CFA. At all time points and TT doses, the ELISA titers for the two formulations were within a fourfold dilution of each other.

Table I

Effect of Adjuvants on the Antibody Response to Tetanus Toxoid as Measured by ELISA[a]

	TT-specific titer at week				
	3	5	7	9	13
TT in water	<256	256	256	256	512
TT in alginate MS	256	512	512	512	512
TT in alum	2048	8192	16,384	32,768	32,768
TT in CFA	2048	16,384	16,384	32,768	16,384
TT in polyphosphazene MS	8192	16,384	32,768	32,768	65,536

[a]Mice were immunized s.c. with 20 μg of tetanus toxoid (TT).

3.1.2. SOLUBLE PCPP

The ability of PCPP microspheres to dramatically potentiate the immune response to TT raised the possibility that the polymer could be acting as an immunoadjuvant, rather than as a simple vaccine vehicle. To examine this possibility, TT was mixed in an aqueous solution of PCPP but the antigen polymer solution was not formulated into microspheres (Table III). The antigen polymer solution elicited, in a dose-dependent manner, antibodies to TT. PCPP at 0.5% enhanced the immune response to TT more than 100-fold compared to the response to TT in water. PCPP at 0.05 and 0.005% concentrations also elicited higher antibody titers than TT in water, although not as high as what was obtained with 0.5% PCPP. Furthermore, the 0.5% PCPP concentration was as strong an adjuvant as CFA.

We next compared the effect of various TT antigen doses formulated in 0.1% PCPP solutions with 25 μg TT formulated in either water or CFA (Table IV). As expected, there was a clear antigen dose-dependent response at all time points using soluble PCPP. The 25 μg TT dose formulated into 0.1% PCPP elicited antibody titers that were dramatically higher than the same amount of immunogen in water, and compared very favorably with 25 μg of TT in CFA. It should be noted that at the 5, 1, and 0.2 μg immunogen dose levels

Table II

Effect of Encapsulated Tetanus Toxoid Dose on the Antibody Response to Tetanus Toxoid as Measured by ELISA

	TT-specific titer at week							
	PCPP microspheres				CFA			
TT (μg)	3	5	7	9	3	5	7	9
25	32,768	65,536	131,072	131,072	16,384	131,072	262,144	262,144
5	8192	32,768	65,536	65,536	4096[a]	16,384[a]	32,768[a]	16,384[a]
1	4096	16,384	65,636	65,536	16,384	32,768	32,768	32,768
0.2	2048	4096	8192	8192	1024	4096	4096	4096
0.04	<256	<256	256	256	<256	<256	<256	<256

[a]Mice were immunized s.c. with 2.5 μg tetanus toxoid (TT).

Table III
Effect of PCPP Concentration on the Antibody Response to
Tetanus Toxoid as Measured by ELISA[a]

	TT-specific titer at week			
	3	5	7	9
TT in water	1024	2048	2048	4096
TT/0.5% PCPP	65,536	262,144	524,288	524,288
TT/0.05% PCPP	16,384	32,768	32,768	65,636
TT/0.005% PCPP	4096	8192	32,768	32,768
TT/CFA	16,384	131,072	262,144	262,144

[a]Mice were immunized s.c. with 25 μg of tetanus toxoid (TT).

in PCPP, the antibody titers were still rising at week 25, whereas with the CFA formulation the ELISA titers had peaked earlier.

Mice were also immunized with 5 μg of formalin-inactivated influenza virus particles formulated in polymeric microspheres, alum, and CFA to determine if the relative efficiencies of the formulations would be the same for an enveloped virus as they were for TT (Table V). Again, PCPP microspheres were as efficient as CFA but much more efficient than water, alum, or alginate microspheres at inducing a very high titer anti-influenza immune response. In contrast to the TT results, alum-adjuvanted influenza was no better than soluble influenza and alginate-microencapsulated influenza in eliciting a rather low titer anti-influenza response. Taken together, these results demonstrate that PCPP microspheres containing an immunogen provoke an antibody response equal in magnitude to immunogens formulated with CFA.

The mouse sera were also tested for the presence of functional antibodies by hemagglutination inhibition (Table VI) and neutralization assays (data not shown). As measured by the HAI assay, the PCPP microspheres containing influenza elicited an antibody titer of 1280 by week 7. Influenza formulated in water, alum, CFA, and alginate microspheres elicited either no detectable or very low HAI titers. Antibodies that neutralize influenza

Table IV
Effect of PCPP-Adjuvanted Tetanus Toxoid Dose on the Antibody Response as
Measured by ELISA[a]

	TT-specific titer at week				
	3	6	9	17	25
25 μg TT/0.1% PCPP	16,384	65,536	131,072	>524,288	262,144
5 μg TT/0.1% PCPP	4096	16,384	32,768	65,536	131,072
1 μg TT/0.1% PCPP	2048	16,384	16,384	32,768	65,536
0.2 μg TT/0.1% PCPP	512	1024	1024	2048	4096
25 μg TT in water	2048	2048	8192	8192	16,384
25 μg TT in CFA	16,384	131,072	262,144	131,072	131,072

[a]Mice were immunized s.c.

Table V

Effect of Adjuvants on the Antibody Response to Influenza as Measured by ELISA[a]

	Flu-specific titer at week				
	3	5	7	9	13
Flu in water	256	1024	1024	512	512
Flu in alginate MS	512	1024	2048	2048	2048
Flu in alum	<256	512	1024	2048	2048
Flu in CFA	8192	16,384	32,768	32,768	16,384
Flu in polyphosphazene MS	8192	32,768	32,768	8192	16,384

[a]Mice were immunized with 5 μg of whole formalin-inactivated influenza virus particles.

infectivity were assayed in a 50% plaque reduction assay. Influenza in PCPP microspheres induced a detectable titer of 800 by week 13, whereas influenza in water and CFA did not elicit detectable neutralizing antibody titers. This result was very encouraging since the HAI and neutralization assays are sensitive functional antibody assays for influenza.

The IgG isotypes of the antibodies induced by these formulations were determined by an ELISA assay (Table VII). Alum-adjuvanted influenza elicited a purely IgG1 response as was expected. Influenza formulated in CFA induced mostly an IgG1 response that peaked by week 7 and waned by week 13. Influenza formulated in alginate and PCPP microspheres also induced largely an IgG1 response that by week 7 was higher than influenza formulated in alum. Again, PCPP microsphere-formulated antigen induced titers that compared very favorably with those induced by CFA-formulated antigen. PCPP microspheres, like CFA, were able to induce significant levels of IgG2a and IgG2b antibodies. A significant difference in the immune response was found in the level of activity detected in the IgG3 isotype. PCPP microspheres were the only formulation able to induce a significant IgG3 antibody titer.

Table VI

Effect of Adjuvants on the Antibody Response to Flu Proteins as Measured by the Influenza Hemagglutination Inhibition Assay[a]

	HAI titer at week				
	3	5	7	9	13
Flu in water	neg	neg	neg	40	neg
Flu in alginate MS	neg	neg	40	40	40
Flu in alum	neg	neg	neg	neg	neg
Flu in CFA	neg	neg	neg	40	neg
Flu in polyphosphazene MS	320	640	1280	1280	1280
Water[b]	neg	neg	neg	neg	neg

[a]Mice were immunized s.c. with 5 μg of whole formalin-inactivated influenza virus particles.
[b]Negative control had a titer of 20 because of nonspecific serum hemagglutination inhibitors. Neg ≤ 20.

Table VII

Effect of Adjuvants on the Antibody Isotype Response to Influenza as Measured by ELISA[a]

Adjuvant Used	Antibody isotype titer at week															
	3				7				13			
	IgG1	IgG2a	IgG2b	IgG3	IgG1	IgG2a	IgG2b	IgG3	IgG1	IgG2a	IgG2b	IgG3
Flu in alginate MS	1024	<256	256	<256	65,536	1024	512	<256	8192	512	<256	<256
Flu in PCPP MS	8192	4096	512	512	131,072	16,384	1024	4096	16,384	16,384	2048	1024
Flu in alum	512	<256	<256	<256	16,384	<256	<256	<256	8192	<256	<256	<256
Flu in CFA	8192	1024	4096	<256	>524,288	8192	4096	<256	32,768	2048	2048	<256
Flu in water	256	512	256	<256	2048	1024	256	<256	1024	512	<256	<256

[a]Mice were immunized with 5 μg of whole inactivated influenza virus particles.

Table VIII

Effect of PCPP-Adjuvanted Influenza Dose on the Antibody Response to Influenza as Measured by ELISA[a]

	Flu-specific titer at week					
	3	6	9	17	25	37
5 μg flu/0.1% PCPP	2048	16,384	16,384	32,768	65,536	16,384
1 μg flu/0.1% PCPP	4096	16,384	16,384	21,768	131,072	16,384
0.2 μg flu/0.1% PCPP	<256	4096	4096	16,384	65,536	8192
0.04 μg flu/0.1% PCPP	<256	<256	<256	<256	4096	1024
5 μg flu in water	256	256	256	<256	<256	<256
5 μg flu in CFA	512	4096	4096	2048	1024	2048

[a]Mice were immunized s.c.

The successful immunopotentiation of the influenza-specific immune response with immunogen formulated in PCPP microspheres prompted us to examine the possibility that influenza could also be adjuvanted with soluble PCPP. Mice were inoculated subcutaneously with varying influenza doses formulated in 0.1% PCPP or 5 μg of influenza in water or CFA (Table VIII). As expected, there was a dose-dependent immune response at all time points after inoculation with the 0.1% PCPP-formulated influenza antigen. In this experiment, 5 μg of influenza in 0.1% PCPP induced a dramatically higher influenza-specific response than 5 μg of influenza in CFA. Furthermore, all antigen doses in the PCPP formulation elicited an immune response that was still rising at week 25 whereas the CFA formulation induced peak titers at earlier time points. This was similar to the results seen in the TT experiments. It is particularly noteworthy that the 0.04 μg dose in PCPP did not induce detectable antibody levels until week 25. This can be interpreted as evidence for sustained release of antigen. The ability of 0.1% PCPP solution to induce functional antibodies was assayed in HAI (Table IX) and neutralization (Table X) assays. Once again, the PCPP formulation induced very high antibody activities in the hemagglutination and

Table IX

Effect of Influenza Dose on the Antibody Response to Flu Proteins as Measured by the Influenza Hemagglutination Inhibition Assay[a]

	HAI titer at week					
	3	6	9	17	25	37
5 μg PCPP	160	1280	1280	2560	640	1280
1 μg flu/0.1% PCPP	320	1280	1280	2560	2560	1280
0.2 μg flu/0.1% PCPP	40	640	640	2560	1280	1280
0.04 μg flu/0.1% PCPP	neg	40	80	160	160	160
5 μg flu in water	neg	neg	20	neg	neg	neg
5 μg flu in CFA	neg	80	40	40	40	40

[a]Mice were immunized s.c.

Table X

Effect of PCPP Concentration on the Antibody Response to Flu Proteins Measured by the Influenza Neutralization Assay[a]

	50% plaque reduction titer at week					
	3	6	9	17	25	37
5 μg flu/0.1% PCPP	200	400	400	200	400	1600
1 μg flu/0.1% PCPP	400	—	200	400	400	400
0.2 μg flu/0.1% PCPP	<100	—	100	100	400	400
0.04 μg flu/0.1% PCPP	<100	—	<100	<100	—	<100
5 μg flu in water	<100	<100	<100	<100	—	<100
5 μg flu in CFA	<100	<100	<100	<100	—	<100

[a]Mice were immunized s.c.

neutralization assays whereas there was little or no activity detectable in these assays in CFA formulations.

The influenza vaccine is administered to humans without alum because alum has little positive effect on the immune response. In a mouse potency test, an antigen dose that induces HAI antibody titers ≥ 40 units is predictive of protection in a human. Thus, 0.04 μg of total influenza antigen in 0.1% PCPP was able to induce protective levels of antibody that were not achieved with 5 μg of unadjuvanted antigen.

The antibody isotypes engendered in this response were also assayed (Table XI). Although the PCPP-formulated influenza antigen induced largely an IgG1 response, significant IgG2a and IgG2b responses were also detected. The level of this response was greater than that observed for influenza antigens formulated in CFA. In contrast to the results observed in Table VII, no IgG3 antibodies were detectable in this experiment. It should be noted, although not overinterpreted, that the IgG3 antibody responses were observed with influenza antigen formulated into PCPP microspheres but not in soluble PCPP solutions. Further experimentation must be conducted in order to confirm these results.

Table XI

Effect of PCPP-Adjuvanted Influenza Dose on the Antibody Isotype Response to Influenza as Measured by ELISA[a]

	Antibody isotype titer at week								
	3			6			9		
	IgG1	IgG2a	IgG2b	IgG1	IgG2a	IgG2b	IgG1	IgG2a	IgG2b
5 μg flu/0.1% PCPP	8192	<256	<256	131,072	<256	256	131,072	256	1024
1 μg flu/0.1% PCPP	8192	<256	<256	65,536	256	1024	65,536	1024	4096
0.2 μg flu/0.1% PCPP	256	<256	<256	16,384	1024	2048	16,384	1024	1024
5 μg flu/water	<256	1024	<256	256	1024	<256	256	512	<256
5 μg flu/CFA	2048	<256	<256	16,384	1024	512	16,384	1024	256

[a]All samples had IgG3 antibody titers <256.

All of the above experiments have been conducted using PCPP having only a phenoxycarboxy side chain, or PCPP. More recent experimentation has been done to examine the immunopotentiation effect of PCGPP (data not shown). In addition to the phenoxycarboxy side chain, PCGPP has a glycine side chain at a 10% frequency. PCGPP immunopotentiates the immune response to influenza virus compared to influenza in water, but is unable to increase the immune response to the level achieved with antigen formulated in PCPP. We are currently trying to determine the molecular basis for this difference in immunopotentiation.

3.2. Mucosal Immunization

An alternative to the use of injectable vaccines is the mucosal administration of a live attenuated virus. Such a vaccine induces both a strong oral and systemic immunity mimicking the immune response induced by natural infection with the wild-type virus. This constellation of immune responses eliminates not only the systemic spread of virus but also viral replication in the mucosa. Thus, the immune response elicited by a replicating oral vaccine is superior to that induced by injectable vaccines, either live or inactivated. The best example of this type of vaccine is the live attenuated oral poliovirus vaccine. Unfortunately the use of this vaccine is associated with reversion to neurovirulence and the development of paralytic polio in a few vaccinees and their contacts. The increasing appreciation of the importance of mucosal immunity in protection has spawned in recent years efforts to induce both the mucosal and systemic immunity by the delivery of nonreplicating viral antigens to mucosal surfaces.

Vaccines formulated into microspheres can be used to deliver antigen to the respiratory tract in the form of an aerosol or intranasal droplets. This delivery mode induces a mucosal response in lymphoid tissue located in the nasal pharynx and bronchial mucosa. Microsphere vaccines can also be formulated into a tablet or solution format that can be swallowed. This delivery mode induces a mucosal response in lymphoid tissue located in the pharynx and intestinal mucosa. Regardless of which site is the target for initiating the mucosal response, the existence of the common mucosal system results in specific IgA secretion at all mucosal sites.

The most studied ion-cross-linkable polymer is the naturally occurring alginate that is prepared from brown algae for use in foodstuffs. Although we use alginates in our microencapsulation of immunogens, most of the present in vitro data pertain to the synthetic ion-cross-linkable PCPPs. Alginates and PCPPs are cross-linked by di- and trivalent metallic ions to form hydrogels. The extent of cross-linking and, therefore, the rigidity of the prepared microspheres is influenced by polymer molecular weight, concentration, and cation concentration.

Microencapsulated antigens were prepared and quantitated as described above. The antigen concentration in alginate and PCPP microspheres as determined by SDS-PAGE was adjusted with sterile deionized water before immunization. Female 7- to 8-week-old BALB/c mice were randomized into groups and immunized by intranasal instillation with 48 μL of the antigen formulations. Blood samples were taken from the retroorbital sinus of CO_2-anesthetized mice. The blood was centrifuged and sera collected and stored at $-70°C$ until it was analyzed.

Table XII

Effect of Adjuvants on the Antibody Response to Tetanus Toxoid after a Single Intranasal Immunization[a]

Mouse No.	Antigen formulation	Serum TT-specific titer at week						
		2	4	8	13	17	21	28
1	TT in water	256	<256	256	<256	<256	<256	<256
2	TT in water	<256	<256	<256	512	<256	<256	<256
3	TT in water	<256	<256	<256	256	<256	<256	<256
4	TT in Alg MS	<256	<256	<256	<256	<256	<256	<256
5	TT in Alg MS	<256	<256	<256	<256	<256	<256	<256
6	TT in Alg MS	<256	<256	<256	<256	<256	<256	<256
7	TT in PCPP MS	1024	1024	1024	2048	256	1024	1024
8	TT in PCPP MS	1024	1024	4096	4096	2048	8192	16,384
9	TT in PCPP MS	512	1024	2048	1024	1024	2048	2048
10	TT in Alg/5% PCPP MS	2048	8192	32,768	16,384	4096	8192	31,768
11	TT in Alg/5% PCPP MS	2048	4096	8192	16,384	4096	32,768	65,536
12	TT in Alg/5% PCPP MS	1024	2048	4096	4096	4096	2048	8192

[a]Mice were immunized by the intranasal instillation of a single dose of 50 μg tetanus toxoid (TT) in 48 μL.

The immunogenicity of a single 50 μg dose of TT (Table XII) was tested in four different formulations; (1) in water, (2) in alginate microspheres, (3) in PCPP microspheres, and (4) in microspheres composed of 95% alginate and 5% PCPP. Water-based formulations and alginate microspheres were unable to elicit serum IgG responses after intranasal instillation of mice. On the other hand, PCPP microspheres and alginate/PCPP microspheres induced very strong long-lived serum IgG responses to TT. Mucosal IgA specific for TT was not detected at any time point in the bronchial and lung washes of any mice. There was, however, a distinct, albeit transient, appearance of TT-specific IgA in the serum between weeks 2 and 8 postimmunization (data not shown). In a dose–response experiment, a 50 μg dose in microspheres composed of 95% alginate and 5% PCPP elicited a serum IgG response whereas a 5 μg dose did not (data not shown).

3.3. The Role of Polyphosphazene in Vaccine Delivery

Polyphosphazene is a water-based ionically cross-linkable polymer that can be used to generate polymeric hydrogel microspheres. Encapsulation conditions often play an important role in maintaining immunogenic integrity of labile antigens. Because there are no organic solvents involved in the encapsulation procedure, labile immunological epitopes are most likely preserved. Mild encapsulation conditions, hydrophobic surface properties, ability to alter the side chains on the polymer and formulate microspheres that will release antigens with pulsatile and/or sustained release kinetics make this polymer system a strong candidate for developing single-dose parenteral and mucosal vaccines.

Polyphosphazene microspheres have three desirable properties. Microspheres have the size and physical characteristics that facilitate uptake in the mucosal lymphoid tissue to stimulate an immune response. The microspheres are formulated under very mild conditions so that antigenic integrity is maintained. The hydrogel properties of these microspheres allow a sustained antigen release to maximally stimulate the immune response over a long period. The microsphere technology has demonstrated great utility in the microencapsulation of a diverse spectrum of biological materials.

The immunogenicity of influenza and TT is dramatically enhanced in the presence of PCPP as either microencapsulated or soluble PCPP formulations. The results of these experiments clearly demonstrate that soluble PCPPs at very low concentrations are as efficient as PCPP microencapsulation and CFA at inducing high serum IgG responses. Furthermore, influenza admixed with soluble PCPPs or encapsulated in PCPP microspheres elicited HAI and neutralization antibody titers that were much higher than what was observed for alum and CFA.

Polyphosphazene, in either its soluble state or as microspheres, has two important characteristics in its interaction with antigens: sustained antigen release and the maintenance of antigenic integrity. Sustained antigen release has the benefit of potentially inducing longer-lasting immunity and the conversion of nonresponders. The data also suggest that smaller immunogen doses are required with this adjuvant, which lowers production costs. The antigenic integrity is evident in the induction of high titers of functional antibodies. Sustained antigen release and maintenance of antigenic integrity are characteristics of an immunoadjuvant that may have the greatest effect on antigens that are poorly immunogenic. Polyphosphazene has, thus, been proven to be a versatile molecule with both adjuvant and antigen depot characteristics.

4. SUMMARY

PCPP can be used in two different ways to potentiate an immune response. The soluble form of the polymer has been found to have immunoadjuvant activity. A single subcutaneous injection of polymer/influenza dramatically increases the ELISA, neutralizing, and HI antibodies to influenza virus compared to CFA. The polymer has also succeeded in dramatically increasing the amount of ELISA antibodies to TT. The antibody response elicited was predominantly of the IgG1 isotype. PCPP has also been used to generate micron-sized hydrogel microspheres through a process of divalent ion cross-linking of the polymer strands. These microspheres can induce significantly higher anti-TT serum IgG titers after a single intranasal immunization than TT alone.

ACKNOWLEDGMENTS

We thank Eric M. Grund, J. Michael Roos, and Angela L. Woods for expert technical assistance and Joanie Slyne for graphic design.

REFERENCES

Allcock, H. R., and Kwon, S., 1989, An ionically cross-linkable polyphosphazene: Poly[bis(carboxylato-phenoxy)phosphazene] and its hydrogels and membranes, *Macromolecules* **22**:75–79.

Allison, A. C., and Byars, N. E., 1992, Immunological adjuvants and their mode of action, in *Vaccines: New Approaches to Immunological Problems* (R. W. Ellis, ed.), Butterworth–Heinemann, Oxford, pp. 431–448.

Andrianov, A. K., Cohen, S., Visscher, K. B., Payne, L. G., Allcock, H. R., and Langer, R., 1993a, Controlled release using ionotropic polyphosphazene hydrogels, *J. Controlled Rel.* **27**:69–77.

Andrianov, A. K., Payne, L. G., Visscher, K. B., Allcock, H. R., and Langer, R., 1993b, Hydrolytic degradation of polyphosphazene hydrogels, *Polym. Prepr.* **34**:233–234.

Andrianov, A. K., Payne, L. G., Visscher, K. B., Allcock, H. R., and Langer, R., 1994, Hydrolytic degradation of ionically cross-linked polyphosphazene microspheres, *J. Appl. Polym. Sci.* **53**:1573–1578.

Bano, M. C., Cohen, S., Visscher, K. B., Allcock, H. R., and Langer, R., 1991, A novel synthetic method for hybridoma cell encapsulation, *Bio/Technol.* **9**:468–471.

Cohen, S., Bano, M. C., Visscher, K. B., Chow, M., Allcock, H. R., and Langer, R., 1990, Ionically cross-linkable polyphosphazene: A novel polymer for microencapsulation, *J. Am. Chem. Soc.* **112**:7832–7833.

Eldridge, J. H., Gilley, R. M., Staas, J. K., Moldoveanu, Z., Meulbroek, J. A., and Tice, T. R., 1989, Biodegradable microspheres: Vaccine delivery system for oral immunization, *Curr. Top. Microbiol. Immunol.* **146**:59–66.

Eldridge, J. H., Staas, J. K., Meulbroek, J. A., Tice, T. R., and Gilley, R. M., 1991, Biodegradable and biocompatible poly(DL-lactide-co-glycolide) microspheres as an adjuvant for staphylococcal enterotoxin B toxoid which enhances the level of toxin-neutralizing antibodies, *Infect. Immun.* **59**:2978–2986.

Gray, D., 1993, Immunological memory, *Annu. Rev. Immunol.* **11**:49–77.

Hunter, R. L., 1991, Nonionic block copolymers: New preparations and review of the mechanism of action, in: *Topics in Vaccine Adjuvant Research* (D. R. Spriggs and W. C. Koff, eds.), CRC Press, Boca Raton, pp. 89–97.

Kreuter, J., 1992, Microcapsules and nanoparticles, in: *Medicine and Pharmacology* (M. Donbrow, ed.), CRC Press, Boca Raton, pp. 125–148.

Payne, L. G., Jenkins, S. A., Andrianov, A., Langer, R., and Roberts, B. E., 1995, Xenobiotic polymers as vaccine vehicles, *Adv. Exp. Med. Biol.* (in press).

Petrov, R., Mustafaev, M., and Norimov, A., 1992, Physico-chemical criteria for the construction of artificial immunomodulators and immunogens on the basis of polyelectrolyte complexes, *Sov. Med. Rev. Sect. D Immunol.* **4**:1–113.

White, R. G., 1976, Adjuvant effect of microbial products in the immune response, *Annu. Rev. Microbiol.* **30**:579–600.

Chapter 21

Monophosphoryl Lipid A as an Adjuvant

Past Experiences and New Directions

J. Terry Ulrich and Kent R. Myers

1. INTRODUCTION

The increasing threat to the human population posed by new or resurgent infectious diseases, coupled with an alarming rise in the incidence of antibiotic-resistant microbes, has created a tremendous need for new vaccines. A critical element in the development of these new vaccines is the ability, via adjuvants, to potentiate and focus the immune response to the vaccine in beneficial ways so that optimal protection can be achieved. One promising candidate adjuvant in this regard is MPL® immunostimulant, a monophosphoryl lipid A preparation derived from the lipopolysaccharide (LPS) of *Salmonella minnesota* R595. MPL® is being considered as an adjuvant for a number of human vaccines, and experience to date has shown that it is safe, well tolerated, and able to provide a heightened immune response to coadministered antigens. In this chapter, various topics related to the preparation, formulation, and use of MPL® as an adjuvant will be discussed. In addition, our current knowledge of the mechanisms of action of MPL® will be reviewed.

1.1. Historical Perspective

The emergence of MPL® as a promising adjuvant for human vaccines is the result of efforts that can be traced back to the seminal studies of Johnson *et al.* (1956). Those studies showed that LPS was a potent adjuvant for protein antigens, and, furthermore, that it possessed the unusual property of acting as an adjuvant even if administered at a different site and at a different time than the antigen (Munoz, 1964; Johnson, 1964). This property set LPS apart from other adjuvants in use at that time, such as alum or complete Freund's

J. Terry Ulrich and Kent R. Myers • Ribi ImmunoChem Research, Inc., Hamilton, Montana 59840.

Vaccine Design: The Subunit and Adjuvant Approach, edited by Michael F. Powell and Mark J. Newman. Plenum Press, New York, 1995.

adjuvant (CFA), since these materials had to be directly associated with the antigen in order to be effective.

The discovery that LPS was a potent and unique adjuvant could not be translated into practical application until a method could be found to attenuate its extreme toxicity while leaving its beneficial immunostimulating properties intact. A significant step toward this goal occurred when Ribi *et al.* (1979) found that exposure of LPS to mild acid hydrolytic conditions reduced its endotoxic activities without altering its ability to regress tumors. It was subsequently shown that, following treatment of LPS from the heptose-less mutant *S. typhimurium* G30/C21 with sodium acetate, pH 4.5, at 100°C, a minor fraction could be isolated by ion-exchange chromatography that was as active as the starting LPS with respect to antitumor activity, and yet was nonpyrogenic and nonlethal in 11-day-old chick embryos at the doses tested (Takayama *et al.*, 1981). A method of producing this nonendotoxic material in almost quantitative yield, i.e., by treatment of LPS with 0.1 N HCl at 100°C for 30 min, was subsequently reported (Ribi *et al.,* 1982). The acid hydrolysate was soon shown to be the 4′-monophosphoryl derivative of the lipid A moiety (Qureshi *et al.,* 1982). Numerous biological studies confirmed that this 4′-monophosphoryl lipid A derivative was a potent immunostimulant and yet seemed to lack many of the toxic properties of the parent LPS (Ribi, 1984). It was later found that mild alkaline treatment caused specific removal of one fatty acid from monophosphoryl lipid A, resulting in further attenuation of toxicity with no change in immunostimulating activity (Myers *et al.*, 1990). These observations eventually led to the creation of the product now referred to as MPL®.

1.2. Rationale for Using MPL® as an Adjuvant

The mammalian immune system evolved under continual selective pressure from pathogenic bacteria and other disease-causing microorganisms. Therefore, it is not surprising that the immune system should be able to detect the presence of bacteria with exquisite sensitivity and to respond in a rapid and vigorous fashion when bacteria are "perceived" (Rook, 1993). The immune system recognizes molecules or substructures of bacteria, and all of the immune responses elicited by a bacterial infection can be reproduced by exposure to these bacterial signal molecules. One of the most active immunological signals is the LPS present in the outer membranes of gram-negative bacteria. Submicrogram amounts of LPS induce high levels of proinflammatory cytokines and other mediators in humans (Michie *et al.*, 1988; Engelhardt *et al.*, 1990; Martich *et al.,* 1991).

Against this backdrop, MPL® emerges as an interesting choice for use as an immunological adjuvant in humans. As described earlier, MPL® is obtained by exposing the LPS of *S. minnesota* R595 to hydrolytic conditions sufficient to cause the loss of certain chemical groups. MPL® retains many of the activities associated with the parent LPS structure, but at reduced potencies. Significantly, the toxic activities of LPS are attenuated to a greater extent by the hydrolytic treatments than are the immunostimulatory activities, allowing MPL® to be used safely in humans at doses that provide beneficial levels of immune stimulation (Ribi, 1986).

2. CHARACTERISTICS OF MPL$^{®}$ AS A PRODUCT

2.1. Manufacturing, Chemistry, and Quality Control

2.1.1. THE MANUFACTURE OF MPL$^{®}$ FOR CLINICAL USE

The process used for the production of MPL$^{®}$ is summarized in Fig. 1. The starting point in this process is the growth of *S. minnesota* R595 cells in culture conditions that provide for optimal biosynthetic production of LPS. Initial lots of MPL$^{®}$ were prepared from cells grown in static, "sparged" cultures, but considerations of scale and demand have necessitated a switch to a fermentor-based process. The conditions of cell growth used in this step are important, since culture conditions are known to influence LPS biosynthesis (e.g., Marr and Ingraham, 1962; Batley *et al.*, 1985).

Following harvesting and drying, the cell mass is subjected to a solvent extraction step in which the LPS is obtained in soluble form. The solvent is removed, and the dry LPS residue is solubilized in aqueous solution followed by brief exposure to 0.1 N HC1 at reflux. This treatment primarily causes the loss of the glycosidic phosphate at the 1 position and the inner core residues attached via the 6′ position, thus generating 4′-mono-phosphoryl lipid A (MLA; see Fig. 1). The MLA is next dissolved in organic solvents and exposed to very mild alkaline treatment, which removes the base-labile fatty acyl residue attached to the 3 position, yielding 3-*O*-desacyl-4′ monophosphoryl lipid A (3D-MLA; see Fig. 1). This crude product is then purified by liquid chromatography, and the resulting pure material is converted to the monobasic triethylammonium salt and lyophilized, yielding the bulk form of MPL$^{®}$. This form of MPL$^{®}$ is used for formulation in vaccines.

2.1.2. THE CHEMICAL COMPOSITION AND STRUCTURE OF MPL$^{®}$

2.1.2a. The Heterogeneous Nature of MPL$^{®}$

The manner in which MPL$^{®}$ is manufactured gives rise to two levels of heterogeneity. The first level relates to the potential presence of components other than monophosphoryl lipid A in MPL$^{®}$ that may result from the bacterial extraction. Possible impurities include phospholipids, fatty acids, nucleic acids, and proteins that can coextract with LPS. However, these materials are efficiently removed by purification processes employed in the production of MPL$^{®}$, and so they do not contribute significantly to the composition of the final product.

The second level of heterogeneity reflects an inherent property of MPL$^{®}$, namely that this product is a mixture of closely related 3-*O*-desacyl-4′-monophosphoryl lipid A species that differ with respect to the number and location of ester-linked fatty acids they contain. This structural heterogeneity is readily apparent by thin-layer chromatography (TLC) on silica gel, which reveals a ladderlike pattern of closely spaced bands. The bands in the pattern arise from 4′-monophosphoryl lipid A species with different numbers of fatty acyl groups (Fig. 2).

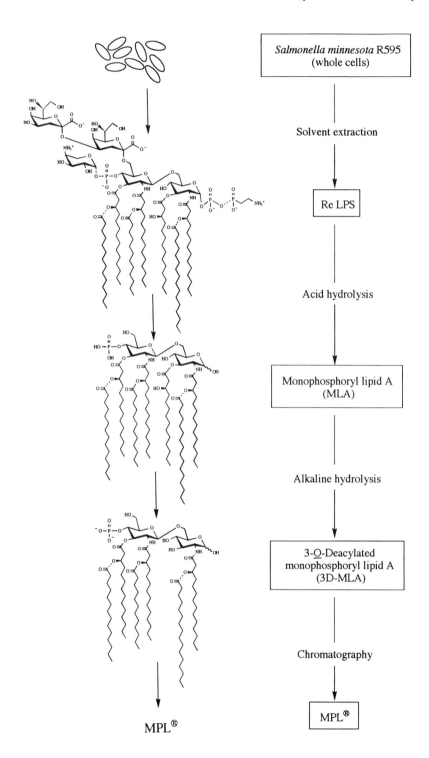

Salmonella minnesota R595 (whole cells)

Solvent extraction

Re LPS

Acid hydrolysis

Monophosphoryl lipid A (MLA)

Alkaline hydrolysis

3-<u>O</u>-Deacylated monophosphoryl lipid A (3D-MLA)

Chromatography

MPL®

MPL®

Figure 1. A schematic representation of the production process for MPL®. The structures shown are the most highly substituted forms that are observed at each step. Dashed lines are used for bonds to groups that occur in nonstoichiometric amounts. The structure for MPL® corresponds to that shown for 3D-MLA.

2.1.2b. The Detailed Structure of MPL®

The detailed structure of MPL®-immunostimulant has been studied by combined use of TLC, HPLC, and fast-atom bombardment mass spectroscopy (Myers and Snyder, 1992). The six major species of 3-*O*-desacyl-4′-monophosphoryl lipid A present in MPL® were isolated and their structures were determined (Fig. 2). Of these species, one contained six fatty acids, three contained five fatty acids, and two contained four fatty acids. Several features were common to all of these species: they all had (1) a backbone consisting of β-1′,6-diglucosamine, monophosphorylated at the nonreducing end; (2) fatty acyl groups at the 2, 2′, and 3′ positions, with (*R*)-3′-dodecanoyloxytetradecanoyl always present at the 2′ position; and (3) a free hydroxyl group at the 3 position of the diglucosamine backbone. The species differed with respect to whether or not they contained (1) (*R*)-3-hydroxytetradecanoyl or (*R*)-3-hexadecanoyloxytetradecanoyl at the 2 position and (2) (*R*)-3-hydroxytetradecanoyl, (R)-3-tetradecanoyloxytetradecanoyl, or tetradecenoyl at the 3′ position.

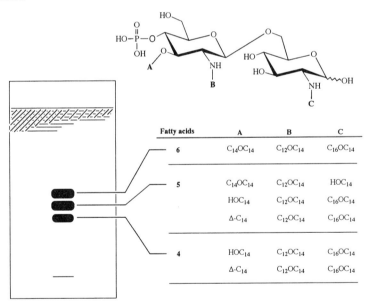

Fatty acids	A	B	C
6	$C_{14}OC_{14}$	$C_{12}OC_{14}$	$C_{16}OC_{14}$
5	$C_{14}OC_{14}$	$C_{12}OC_{14}$	HOC_{14}
	HOC_{14}	$C_{12}OC_{14}$	$C_{16}OC_{14}$
	Δ-C_{14}	$C_{12}OC_{14}$	$C_{16}OC_{14}$
4	HOC_{14}	$C_{12}OC_{14}$	$C_{16}OC_{14}$
	Δ-C_{14}	$C_{12}OC_{14}$	$C_{16}OC_{14}$

Figure 2. Tentative structural assignments for the major species present in MPL® (Myers and Snyder, 1992). A production lot of MPL® was separated into pure TLC bands, individual species were isolated from each band as the dimethyl derivatives by HPLC, and the resulting pure compounds were analyzed by fast-atom bombardment mass spectroscopy. Structures were postulated based on the *m/z* values for the parent ion and the nonreducing end oxonium fragment ion for each compound (Qureshi *et al.*, 1986). HOC_{14}, (*R*)-3-hydroxytetradecanoyl; $C_{12}OC_{14}$, (*R*)-3-dodecanoyloxytetradecanoyl; $C_{14}OC_{14}$, (*R*)-3-tetradecanoyloxytetradecanoyl; $C_{16}OC_{14}$, (*R*)-3-hexadecanoyloxytetradecanoyl; Δ-C_{14}, tetradecenoyl.

2.1.2c. The Origins of Structural Heterogeneity in MPL®

The heterogeneity in the monophosphoryl lipid A species found in MPL® is attributable to two sources: (1) biosynthetic variability in the assembly of the lipid A moiety and (2) loss of fatty acids from the lipid A backbone during manufacture. The biosynthetic contribution to heterogeneity in MPL® is evident by TLC analysis of *S. minnesota* R595 LPS, which reveals that this LPS is a mixture of several species (Chen *et al.*, 1973). The species present in *S. minnesota* R595 LPS differ in terms of the degree of substitution of the lipid A phosphates by 4-amino-4-deoxy-arabinose and phosphoethanolamine and, significantly, in the fatty acid content of the lipid A moiety (Rietschel *et al.*, 1984; Caroff *et al.*, 1991). The variability in fatty acid content reflects incomplete or variable incorporation of ester-linked normal fatty acids in the lipid A structure during biosynthesis. Some of this variability presumably occurs because of nonabsolute substrate specificity of the acyltransferases involved in the terminal steps of lipid A biosynthesis (Brozek and Raetz, 1990).

The other cause of heterogeneity in MPL® is loss of esterlinked fatty acids during the hydrolytic steps in the production process. This has been demonstrated by exposing a synthetic hexaacyl 3-*O*-desacyl-4′-monophosphoryl lipid A derivative, corresponding to the most highly acylated component in MPL®, to the acid and alkaline hydrolytic conditions used in the preparation of natural MPL® (Myers, personal communication). It was found that exposure of this single component to the acid hydrolytic conditions yielded a material with an HPLC pattern that was remarkably similar to that of natural MPL®, suggesting that much of the heterogeneity in MPL® may arise from this step. The alkaline hydrolytic conditions, on the other hand, caused much less degradation of the 3-*O*-desacyl starting material.

2.1.2d. Contributions of Individual Species in MPL® to Overall Activity

The different 3-*O*-desacyl-4′-monophosphoryl lipid A species present in MPL® may contribute differently to the biological activity of this material. These species differ with respect to their fatty acid content and distribution, and the activity of lipid A is known to be highly dependent on such differences (reviewed in Kotani and Takada, 1989). For example, the hexaacyl lipid A produced by *Escherichia coli* is considered to represent the optimal structure for full endotoxic activity, and species with more (i.e., seven) or fewer (i.e., five, four, or three) fatty acids tend to be much less active. This same overall relationship between activity and fatty acid content has been observed with the 3-*O*-desacyl-4′-monophosphoryl lipid A species in MPL®, although the exact relationship varies with the particular activity under consideration. For example, several synthetic hexaacyl compounds were found to be up to 20-fold more active than a synthetic pentaacyl derivative in terms of their abilities to induce nitric oxide synthase in murine macrophages, and up to 40-fold more lethal in D-galactosamine-primed mice (Myers, personal communication). On the other hand, the hexaacyl compounds did not cause fever in rabbits even at doses of 10 μg/kg, whereas the pentaacyl derivative was highly pyrogenic at 2.5 μg/kg. No differences were observed between MPL® and the hexaacyl or pentaacyl derivatives with respect to their adjuvant activities for a peptide–tetanus toxoid conjugate, either in saline or oil-in-water emulsions (Ulrich, personal communication). These observations indicate that (1) the 3-O-desacyl-4'-monophosphoryl lipid A species in MPL® differ in their activities in various biological models and (2) the activity of MPL® in a given biological model will represent the cumulative contributions of each of its constituent species.

2.1.3. QUALITY CONTROL OF MPL®—FACTORS TO CONSIDER

MPL® is a biological product, and as such it falls under the regulatory authority of the Center for Biologics Evaluation and Research (CBER) branch of the Food and Drug Administration. This has important implications for the quality control of MPL®, since CBER recognizes that biological products will be regulated for purity and composition differently than will synthetically prepared materials. In general, specifications for impurity levels in biological products are largely determined by the manufacturer but are reviewed by CBER. Specifications for active components are derived from theoretical expectations arising from the known structure and/or activities of the product. Thus, the attributes of MPL® that are identified as important quality control release specifications include levels of potential impurities (e.g., protein, nucleic acid, phospholipids, free fatty acids, and 2-keto-3-deoxyoctulonate, as well as process-derived contaminants) and the presence of structural components (e.g., phosphate, glucosamine, and fatty acids). An additional specification, relating to the content of monophosphoryl lipid A species with different numbers of fatty acids, also applies to MPL®. This latter specification is based on the historical values obtained with repeated batches of MPL®, and reflects the consistency of the manufacturing process. Finally, the safety of each lot of bulk MPL® must be demonstrated. Currently, this is ascertained by measuring the LD_{50} in 11-day-old chick embryos and pyrogenic activity in rabbits. Both tests are sensitive indicators of the presence of unattenuated LPS species. The widely used *Limulus* amoebocyte lysate (LAL) test is inappropriate for determination of the safety of MPL® lots, since MPL® retains much of the activity of the parent LPS in this assay (Takayama *et al.*, 1984).

2.2. Stability of MPL®—Considerations for Formulation

A key consideration in the development of any vaccine is the effect of formulation on the stability of the active components. With respect to MPL® as an active component, two criteria of stability must be considered. The first criterion is the *chemical* stability of the individual molecular species present in MPL®. The fact that MPL® is prepared by a process that involves exposure to relatively harsh conditions indicates that it is fairly stable. Nonetheless, inappropriate formulation or storage conditions can lead to partial degradation of species within MPL®. By far the most facile chemical degradation process that MPL® undergoes in aqueous solution is loss of ester-linked fatty acyl groups resulting from acid- or base-catalyzed hydrolysis. This process is easily monitored with any reverse-phase HPLC method that is capable of resolving the various acylated species of monophosphoryl lipid A present in MPL® (e.g., Qureshi *et al.*, 1985). Exposure of MPL® to conditions that favor ester hydrolysis causes a decrease in the content of hexaacyl monophosphoryl lipid A species (four fatty esters), and a coincident increase in the amount of tetraacyl species (two fatty esters). The content of pentaacyl species remains relatively constant under these conditions, indicating that they are in a steady state. This degradation process is highly dependent on pH and formulation, although in general optimum stability occurs between pH 5 and 6. Based on accelerated stability studies, it appears that MPL® in appropriate aqueous solutions can be stored for over 2 years at 4°C with little change in chemical composition (Crane and Leesman, personal communication).

In practice, the biological activities of MPL® are not particularly sensitive to partial deacylation, and preparations that have been treated to cause almost complete loss of the hexaacyl component behave essentially like intact MPL® (Myers, personal communication). This indicates that the chemical stability of MPL® is not necessarily a critical attribute for maintenance of biological activity during long-term storage. Of greater functional importance is the second stability criterion that must be considered with MPL®, namely the stability of its *physical* state in aqueous solution. MPL® is a lipidic material, and as such it spontaneously associates with itself or other surfactants in aqueous solution. The degree of self-association of MPL® in aqueous solution plays an important role in determining its activity as an immunostimulant (Rudbach *et al.*, 1994). The formulation chosen for an MPL®-containing vaccine therefore must be one in which the state of aggregation of MPL® does not change significantly over time. The aggregation state can be assessed by physical methods such as dynamic light scattering, assuming that such methods are compatible with the vaccine formulation, or by biological evaluation. This consideration will be more or less important depending on the nature of the formulation. For example, MPL® in an oil-in-water emulsion will remain associated with the oil phase indefinitely and will therefore have a stable physical state over time (although the oil phase may itself tend to coalesce). On the other hand, MPL® dispersed in water may undergo a slow reaggregation over time, resulting in a gradual change in biological activity.

3. METHODS OF USING MPL® AS AN ADJUVANT

An important characteristic of MPL®'s action as an adjuvant is that, like LPS, it can enhance the generation of specific immunity without being directly associated with an antigen. This reflects the fact that the adjuvant activity of MPL® is related, at least in part, to its ability to induce the release of cytokines that promote the generation of specific immune responses (Gustafson and Rhodes, 1992a). These cytokines can be induced in the absence of antigen, and they can stimulate cells that are distal to the site of induction. This is in sharp contrast to the action of adjuvants such as oil-in-water emulsions and alum. Such depot-type adjuvants function by creating a reservoir of antigen at the site of injection, and therefore they must be intimately associated with antigen in order to be effective. Because of its mode of action, MPL® can be used either alone or in combination with these depot-type adjuvants. The choice of adjuvant formulation will depend on a number of factors, such as the nature of the antigen, the characteristics of the desired immune response, and the level of local reactogenicity that is tolerable. Some of the preferred methods for formulating MPL®-containing vaccines are reviewed briefly in this section. Throughout this section, and the rest of the chapter, the following terminology proposed by Edelman (1992) will be used: *adjuvant*—the component(s) in a vaccine that increases the specific immune response to the antigen; *carrier*—an immunogenic protein, capable of eliciting T-cell help, to which antigen can be bound; *vehicle*—the substrate in the vaccine for the antigen, adjuvant, and antigen–carrier complex; and *adjuvant formulation*—the combination of adjuvant plus vehicle.

3.1. Aqueous (Nonparticulate) Vehicles

The simplest adjuvant formulations consist of MPL® plus antigen in water, with appropriate solutes added to maintain isotonicity. MPL® in such solutions exists in aggregated form. This is because MPL®, as described earlier, is composed of a series of closely related monophosphoryl lipid A species that all possess well-defined hydrophobic and hydrophilic domains. As with all lipids, these highly amphipathic structures do not dissolve in water to yield a solution of fully solvated molecules, but instead form aggregated structures in which the hydrophobic regions are excluded from the aqueous milieu while the hydrophilic domains remain solvated. MPL® dispersed in dilute aqueous triethylamine (TEA) was shown by electron microscopy to form liposome-like suspensions (Ribi *et al.*, 1986).

Aqueous solutions of MPL® in saline can provide a strong adjuvant effect when combined with soluble protein antigens (Myers *et al.,* 1990; Schneerson *et al.*, 1991). The contribution of MPL® to the observed immune response is often more apparent in these simple preparations than in cases where the antigen is incorporated into a depot-type adjuvant, such as an oil-in-water emulsion. An advantage of these simple vaccine preparations, comprising only MPL® plus antigen in aqueous solution, is that they tend to be well tolerated and induce little or no local tissue reaction at the site of injection.

3.2. Particulate Vehicles

3.2.1. EMULSIONS

A large body of experimental work, reviewed in greater detail in Section 4.1, has demonstrated that oil and water emulsions are an effective way of using MPL® as an adjuvant. The effectiveness of such formulations can be rationalized in terms of the expected behavior of MPL® in an emulsion environment. A key attribute of emulsions in general is that they contain an insoluble (oil) phase into which antigen can be incorporated. The antigen thus becomes more particulate, and therefore more readily ingested by phagocytic antigen-presenting cells (APCs). In addition, the oil phase can also serve as a depot for antigen at the site of injection. When MPL® is added to such emulsions, its amphipathic nature predisposes it to localize largely at the oil/water interface. Antigen and MPL® will therefore be contained in the same particulate structures, allowing for more efficient delivery of antigenic and immunostimulatory signals to the same cells. MPL® may also serve as an opsonin for the oil droplets in an emulsion, thereby enhancing uptake by APCs.

In most cases, the emulsions used with MPL® have been of the oil-in-water (O/W) type, with 1–2% oil and a surfactant such as Tween 80 at a concentration of 0.1–0.2%. Commonly used oils include squalane, mineral oil, and squalene (the biodegradable precursor of squalane). The type of oil that is used is important, since it influences both the immunogenicity and the tissue reactogenicity of the preparation. Any of the usual methods for preparing emulsions can be used to make MPL®-containing formulations. Usually, the MPL® is first dissolved in the oil, and the oil is then dispersed into the water phase. The amount of antigen that is incorporated into the oil phase should be maximized. One method of achieving this is with a formulation and preparation method that results in a water-in-oil-in-water (W/O/W) emulsion, with antigen captured in the internal aqueous phase (Florence and Whitehill, 1982).

3.2.2. ALUMINUM SALTS

Precipitated aluminum salts, or alum, are the only adjuvants that are currently used in licensed human vaccines. Accordingly, much is known about the manufacture, efficacy, and safety of such adjuvants. Addition of MPL® to alum-based vaccine formulations therefore represents a more conservative departure from existing vaccine technology than do formulations in which MPL® is incorporated into emulsions or liposomes. Accordingly, vaccines containing MPL® in combination with alum may be easier to develop and introduce to the market than would other MPL®-containing vaccine formulations.

To date, there has been very little information available concerning the adjuvant activity of MPL® in combination with alum. Two recent reports are of note, however (Leroux-Roels et al., 1993; DeWilde, 1994). These studies, described in more detail in Sections 4.1 and 4.2, involved vaccine preparations in which a recombinant herpes simplex antigen, designated gD2, was adsorbed onto aluminum hydroxide with or without MPL®. It was found that the preparation with MPL® plus alum performed significantly better than did alum alone in mice (DeWilde, 1994) and in humans (Leroux-Roels et al., 1993). These results demonstrated that MPL® is able to further enhance the immunogenicity of an alum-adsorbed antigen, and that MPL® is therefore compatible with alum-based vaccine formulations.

Many of the considerations raised earlier regarding the use of MPL® in O/W emulsions probably also apply to MPL® in alum-based formulations. Thus, the efficacy of an alum-based vaccine should be enhanced by optimizing the association of both antigen and MPL® with the solid alum. The mechanism by which MPL® adsorbs onto alum is likely to be more complex, and therefore more sensitive to preparation and formulation methods, than in the case of MPL®'s association with the oil phase in O/W emulsions.

3.2.3. LIPOSOMES

Much attention has been focused on the use of liposomes as vehicles for vaccines (Gregoriadis, 1990). Liposomes are effective vehicles for antigens and lipophilic adjuvants (Alving, 1991), and liposomes exhibiting carrier activity for haptenic peptides have been prepared (Garcon and Six, 1991). Lipid A and MPL® are especially well suited for incorporation into liposomes, since the natural milieu for the lipid A domain of LPS is a phospholipid bilayer membrane. Several studies have demonstrated that formulations comprising lipid A or MPL® in liposomes are safe and effective as adjuvants for generation of humoral immunity against a variety of antigens (Alving, 1991; see also Sections 4.1 and 4.2). Recently, it was found that liposomes containing MPL® were also effective adjuvants for enhancing a cytotoxic T-cell response against an encapsulated protein antigen (Zhou and Huang, 1993) (see Section 4.1). The potential suitability of liposomal MPL®

as an adjuvant for human vaccines has been demonstrated in a recent clinical trial (Fries *et al.*, 1992) (see Section 4.2).

One of the attractive, and perhaps perplexing, features of liposomes as vehicles or carriers is that there is considerable flexibility with regards to composition and methodologies for preparation. Some of the factors that can be manipulated in liposomal formulations are: (1) mode of association of antigen (i.e., encapsulated, covalently anchored, or intercalated), (2) lipid composition, (3) liposome size and type (e.g., small unilamellar vesicles or multilamellar vesicles), (4) presence of other immunostimulants and/or targeting structures, and (5) relative amounts of antigen, lipid, MPL$^{®}$, and other components. While a discussion of these factors is well beyond the scope of this review, the point should be made that there is enormous potential for tailoring the characteristics of a liposomal formulation to match the requirements of a particular application.

The flexibility that one has in formulating and preparing liposomes can also be a source of potential difficulties in the manufacturing setting. For example, the lipids used to prepare the liposomes are critical and potentially expensive raw materials. Appropriate sources of these materials must be located, and methods of testing to assure quality must be in place. In addition, consistency of manufacture and stability during storage may be more difficult to achieve and to verify than with other less complex formulations. In view of the other options available for formulation of MPL$^{®}$, the question of whether or not to use liposomes must first be addressed by determining if a simpler formulation will perform adequately.

4. PAST EXPERIENCES—THE EFFECTIVENESS OF MPL$^{®}$ AS AN ADJUVANT

4.1. Preclinical Experience

4.1.1. BIOLOGICAL CHARACTERIZATION OF MPL$^{®}$

The potential use of MPL$^{®}$ as an adjuvant for vaccines is based on the consequences of its interaction with cells of the immune system. These have been assessed by: (1) its potential to activate macrophages, (2) its ability to enhance nonspecific resistance to microbial infections, and (3) its ability to induce the synthesis of certain cytokines and lymphokines.

Cells of the monocyte/macrophage lineage have been the subject of several investigations with MPL$^{®}$. An early study (Masihi *et al.*, 1986) demonstrated that MPL$^{®}$ induced an increase in luminol-dependent, zymosan-stimulated chemiluminescence in mouse peritoneal macrophages. This respiratory burst was apparent in a dose-dependent manner and was paralleled by a fivefold increase in the phagocytic index of the cells. In another study, Pohle *et al.* (1990) showed that treatment of mice with HIV synthetic peptides, p24 and gp120, suppressed the respiratory burst of spleen cells tested in vitro. MPL$^{®}$ added to the spleen cell cultures from these mice significantly restored their chemiluminescence.

Enhancement of nonspecific resistance to microbial challenges by MPL$^{®}$ treatment has been well documented (Ulrich *et al.*, 1988; Chase *et al.*, 1986). MPL$^{®}$ in saline or formulated in 2% O/W emulsions has been shown to effectively protect mice from subsequent lethal challenges with *E. coli*, *Staphylococcus epidermidis*, *Salmonella enteritidis*, *Listeria monocytogenes*, or *Toxoplasma gondii*. The duration of the protection following MPL® pretreatment in these models varied with the formulation used. A 2- to 4-day window of protection was seen in mice pretreated with MPL® solubilized in saline, while protective windows of 14 days were seen when MPL® in O/W emulsions were given as pretreatments. This enhancement of nonspecific resistance induced by MPL® is regarded to be caused primarily by a direct activation of macrophages resulting in enhanced phagocytosis and microbicidal activities. Additionally, the ability of MPL® to induce TNF-α and IFN-γ is important for activating and sustaining the macrophages in a bacteriocidal state. Indeed, the work of Havell (1989) established the importance of TNF-α-activated macrophages in resistance to *L. monocytogenes* by showing that treatment of mice with anti-TNF-α exacerbated sublethal infections of both T-cell-intact mice and T-cell-deficient (athymic) nude mice.

The release of local cytokines in response to antigen and/or adjuvant is prerequisite to the initiation of immune responses. Several cytokines have been studied in association with macrophage activation by MPL®. In vitro, MPL® has been shown to induce interleukin 1 (IL-1) in cell cultures of a mouse macrophage cell line, RAW 264.7 (Dijkstra *et al.*, 1987), human peritoneal macrophages (Carozzi *et al.*, 1989), and human peripheral blood monocytes (Ribi *et al.*, 1986).

The studies of Carozzi *et al.* (1989) are particularly informative about the biological activity of MPL® on peritoneal cell populations recovered from dialysis fluids of uremic patients undergoing continuous ambulatory peritoneal dialysis. Previous studies showed that these peritoneal dialysis patients have suboptimal cellular and humoral defenses and exhibit high infection rates (Keane and Peterson, 1984; Lamperi et al., 1985). Peritoneal cells were recovered from the dialysis fluids of patients selected from a cohort with a high incidence of peritonitis. Control cell populations were obtained from dialysis patients with a low incidence of peritonitis or from healthy women undergoing laparoscopy for diagnostic evaluation. MPL® induced a dose-dependent increase in production of IFN-γ and IL-2 in cultures of the hyporesponsive peritoneal lymphocytes obtained from these high-incidence peritonitis patients. At a concentration of 5 μg/mL, MPL® stimulated the production of IFN-γ to within 70% and IL-2 to 100% of the levels seen with the control cell population. The IL-1 levels stimulated by MPL® in the adherent peritoneal macrophages were equivalent to those of the control cell populations. Also, Fc receptor density and bactericidal activities of the macrophages were induced by MPL® to within 80% of control cell population levels. These results indicate that the immunopotentiating nature of MPL® is associated with its capacity to induce cytokine synthesis.

4.1.2. ADJUVANT STUDIES WITH CAPSULAR POLYSACCHARIDE ANTIGENS

Infants and young children fail to make adequate immune responses to capsular polysaccharides, and this is considered a major factor in the high incidence of various bacterial infections in this population (Klein, 1981; Peltola *et al.*, 1984). Likewise, aged adults mount poor responses to pneumococcal vaccines (Roghmann *et al.*, 1987), hence the increased incidence of bacterial pneumonia in this population (Verghese and Berk, 1983). In the past, vaccines composed of purified polysaccharide antigens have generally met with only limited success.

The antibody response to capsular polysaccharides is the hallmark of the host defense against many virulent microorganisms. Capsular polysaccharides, consisting of high-molecular-weight polymers with simple repeating subunits, can directly stimulate responses in B cells by cross-linking surface antigen receptors without the assistance of antigen-specific T-helper cells. Such antigens are termed T-cell (or thymus)-independent (TI) antigens in contrast to thymus-dependent (TD) antigens, which require T-helper cells to activate B-cells. TI antigens can be further subdivided into TI type 1 (TI-1) and TI type 2 (TI-2) antigens based on the observations that TI-1 antigens are mitogenic, induce polyclonal B-cell activation, and induce an immune response in neonates; whereas immune responses to TI-2 antigens develop late in ontogeny, have no memory response and no isotype restrictions (Mosier *et al.*, 1977). Capsular polysaccharides are considered TI-2 antigens (Mosier and Subbarao, 1982).

Although T-cells are not essential for an antibody response to TI-2 antigens, they can influence the magnitude of the response in mice (Baker and Prescott, 1979) and humans (Griffioen *et al.*, 1991, 1992). Baker (1990) has reviewed a large body of findings relating to studies of the pneumococcal polysaccharide type 3 (PPS-3) response in mice. In this model, suppressor T-cells (Ts) play a major role in limiting antibody responses, presumably by recognizing idiotypic determinants on antigen-activated B cells. To counterbalance this, amplifier T-cells (Ta) appear to drive a clonal expansion through stimulation of antigen-specific B-cells. In the neonatal mouse, Ts functional activity predominates, suggesting a plausible explanation for the poor immune responses to polysaccharides observed in newborns. Mice treated with subimmunogenic doses of PPS-3 become unresponsive to subsequent injections of immunogenic doses of PPS-3 as a result of the accumulation of Ts, a phenomenon termed low-dose paralysis.

The adjuvant effect of MPL$^{®}$ on the immune response to PPS-3 in mice has been studied extensively. Treatment of mice with MPL$^{®}$ inactivates Ts activity, as evidenced by a decrease in low-dose paralysis and an increase in the magnitude of the antibody response to PPS-3 (Baker *et al.*, 1988a). The optimal effect on the immune response was observed when MPL$^{®}$ was given 48 h after either a subimmunogenic or optimal dose of PPS-3; this is when antigen-specific Ts activity was maximal. In a related study (Baker *et al.*, 1988b), MPL$^{®}$ was shown to augment the PPS-3 response in young mice. Treatment of 2- to 3-week-old mice with MPL$^{®}$ 48 h after PPS-3 immunization resulted in significant enhancement of IgM- and IgG3-secreting PPS-3-specific plaque-forming cells. A possible mechanism of action of MPL$^{®}$ in enhancing the PPS-3 response has been described (Baker *et al.*, 1990). In these studies, spleen cells were removed from mice 48 h following priming with PPS-3. The cells were incubated in plastic dishes coated with MPL$^{®}$ and allowed to bind. The eluted cell population resulted in a 100- to 1000-fold enhancement of antigen-specific Ts activity when assayed by adoptive transfer studies. These results suggest an active binding of MPL$^{®}$ to Ts which subsequently interferes with their functional activity. Since the phenotype of PPS-3-specific Ts has been shown to be CD8^{+} (Baker, 1990), a phenotype of virus-specific cytotoxic T-cells (CTLs), the question was raised whether MPL$^{®}$ might interfere with virus-induced CD8^{+} CTLs. In these studies (Esquivel *et al.*, 1991), treatment with MPL$^{®}$ in a regimen shown to abolish the expression of CD8^{+} Ts activity to PPS-3, was shown to have no adverse effect on either the induction or expression of CD8^{+} CTL activity specific for influenza A antigens. Indeed, in vivo treatments with four MPL® treatments on days 1 and 2 and days 6 and 7 after 200 HAU of influenza A (PR/8/34) resulted in a marked increase in CTL activity specific for the influenza A target antigens.

Studies by Domer *et al.* (1989, 1993) have provided additional evidence that MPL® can interfere with T-cell-mediated suppression of immune responses to polysaccharide antigens. These investigations documented the development of delayed-type hypersensitivity (DTH) to a mannan epitope found on *Candida albicans* cell walls. It was shown that mice treated with purified mannan, prior to immunization with *C. albicans* blastoconidia, had suppressed DTH responses to mannan. However, treatment of mannan-injected mice with MPL® abrogated this suppression.

It is apparent from the above discussion that MPL® can exert adjuvant effects on both humoral and cellular responses by interfering with antigen-specific Ts cells. Future experiments should reveal whether these MPL® effects are associated with a downregulation of the functional activity of Ts cells, killing of these cells, or changes in T-cell trafficking within the host.

In recent years, another approach has been taken to circumvent the problem of the poor immunogenicity of polysaccharide vaccine antigens (Robbins and Schneerson, 1990). In this approach the TI polysaccharides have been converted to TD antigens by conjugation to various carrier proteins. The *Haemophilus influenzae* type b, conjugate vaccines, approved for use in young infants in 1990, are the first marketed conjugate vaccines, and it is clear that the rate of invasive *H. influenzae* infections in the United States has fallen dramatically as a result of this vaccine (Shapiro *et al.*, 1992).

At the preclinical level, MPL® has been evaluated as an adjuvant with several candidate polysaccharide-conjugate vaccine antigens (Schneerson *et al.*, 1991). Coinjection of MPL® in saline or as an O/W emulsion enhanced both the primary and secondary serum antibody response to the capsular polysaccharides of six conjugate vaccines. The capsular polysaccharides studied were: Hib, Pn6B, Pnl2F, Vi, *S. aureus* type 5 and type 8. Concurrent administration of MPL® in saline with five of the six unconjugated capsular polysaccharides did not significantly enhance the response. However, an O/W emulsion containing MPL® and Vi capsular polysaccharide significantly enhanced both the primary and secondary antibody response when compared to an O/W emulsion containing Vi only. These responses were further enhanced when trehalose dimycolate (TDM) from *Mycobacterium phlei* was added to the MPL®–Vi O/W emulsion. A somewhat related study (Devi *et al.*, 1991) evaluated the adjuvant effect of MPL® in saline on the murine antibody response to a tetanus toxoid (TT) conjugate (GXM-TT) of *Cryptococcus neoformans* capsular polysaccharide, glucuronoxylomannan (GXM). Of interest was the finding that when MPL® was used concurrently with GXM-TT, there was only a marginal increase in both the IgM- and IgG-specific response to GXM; however, when MPL® was administered 2 days after the GXM-TT, there was a significant increase in both the IgM and IgG antibody responses to GXM. This finding in the context of the extensive work with MPL® in the PPS-3 model cited above, strongly argues that the immune response to the polysaccharide component of these polysaccharide–protein conjugates was influenced by Ts cell regulation.

The practicality of using an immunization scheme that requires a delay in the administration of MPL® relative to antigen, especially in infants, is questionable. However, the adjuvant effect of MPL® with polysaccharides and polysaccharide–protein conjugates appears to be formulation-dependent. As mentioned above (Schneerson *et al.*, 1991), MPL® in an O/W emulsion was very effective when coadministered with polysaccharide conjugate vaccine antigens. Moreover, recent work (Garg and Subbarao, 1992) has demonstrated that O/W emulsions containing MPL® and TDM provided excellent antibody responses to a commercially available polyvalent pneumococcal polysaccharide vaccine, especially in a poor-responding aged-mouse population. These results suggest that incorporation of MPL® in suitable slow-release delivery systems provides a more durable adjuvant effect and circumvents the problem of timing and delayed administration.

Carcinoma-associated carbohydrate antigens, known as mucins, are potential target molecules for cancer immunotherapy. These carcinoma-associated mucins often have shortened carbohydrate side chains exposing normally cryptic *O*-linked core carbohydrate determinants such as Tn, sialyl Tn (STn), and the Thomsen–Friedenreich (TF) determinant (Springer, 1984). The murine mammary adenocarcinoma cell line, TA3-Ha, syngeneic in CAF1/J mice, produces a mucin called epiglycanin, which is composed of 75–80% carbohydrate containing repeating TF and Tn determinants (Codington *et al.*, 1975). A synthetic TF-conjugate vaccine was combined with the adjuvant system MPL® + TDM and tested for efficacy in generating antitumor immunity in mice challenged with the TA3-Ha tumor cell line (Fung *et al.,* 1990; Fung and Longenecker, 1991). The results showed that a protocol of low-dose cyclophosphamide in tumor-bearing mice, followed by an immunization series using the TF-conjugate/MPL® + TDM vaccine resulted in 90% long-term survival, with strong antigen-specific DTH and high-titered IgG antibody responses in the survivors. The authors pointed out that the adjuvant was essential for an effective vaccine and suggested that the adjuvant molecules served not only to heighten the antitumor immunity, but might also help to restore immune cell populations removed by the cyclophosphamide treatment. These preclinical results provided the rationale for the initiation of clinical studies as will be discussed below.

4.1.3. ADJUVANT STUDIES WITH PROTEIN AND PEPTIDE ANTIGENS

The modern era of vaccine development, nurtured by recent developments in molecular biology, chemistry, and immunology, has moved away from killed, whole organism vaccines. Unfortunately, it has also become clear that most recombinant DNA- or synthetic-derived peptides, while providing specific and appropriate epitopes for immune recognition, are intrinsically poor immunogens. Therefore, appropriate adjuvants and delivery systems are viewed as critical for augmenting the immunogenicity of these peptide-based vaccines.

The following discussion highlights preclinical adjuvant work with MPL® used alone or in combination with TDM or with cell wall skeleton (CWS) of *M. phlei* delivered in aqueous admixtures, in 1–2% O/W emulsions, or in liposomal vehicles. For the most part, the discussion will focus on potentially clinically relevant peptides.

Altman and Dixon (1989) have used a model antigen, a conjugate of the peptide 72 (p72), a synthetic 28 amino acid peptide corresponding to residues 110-137 of the surface glycoprotein of hepatitis B virus, to examine the respective roles of carriers, vehicles, and adjuvants in generating immune responses. The effect of a combination of MPL® and TDM in a 1% O/W emulsion on the primary and secondary anti-p72 responses in mice and rabbits was evaluated. The addition of these adjuvants to the primary vaccine resulted in a secondary response similar in magnitude and duration to the vaccine formulated in incomplete Freund's adjuvant (IFA). The authors suggest that these results imply that vaccine formulations potentially acceptable for human use, i.e., 1–2% O/W emulsions of a biodegradable oil, or perhaps alum supplemented with defined adjuvants like MPL® and TDM, might be adequate replacements for IFA. Of particular importance was the observation that these formulations stimulated B-cell memory, as evidenced by potent secondary responses.

The synergistic effects on the specific antibody response of mice to a variety of peptide and subunit antigens by combinations of MPL® and TDM in 2% O/W emulsions have been described (Rudbach et al., 1990). These studies used TT or keyhole limpet hemocyanin (KLH) conjugates of p72 or a subunit structure of *Brucella abortus*, and ELISA titers between 1 and 5×10^5 were achieved 14 days after a booster immunization using the combination adjuvant formulation. In another study (Myers and Ulrich, 1993), MPL® and TDM were dispersed by sonication in 0.2% Tween 80 in saline and mixed with TT; clear synergy of the adjuvant combination was observed in the anti-TT response.

The potency of the MPL® and TDM adjuvant formulation was recently described in a mouse study evaluating the immune response to candidate antigens that could be used in vaccines to block transmission of malaria (Rawlings and Kaslow, 1992). This study showed an adjuvant dependency of immune responses in major histocompatibility complex (MHC)-disparate congenic mouse strains immunized with sexual stage malarial parasites or purified recombinant proteins. When immunized with newly emerged *Plasmodium falciparum* gametes in CFA, the mice produced limited antibody responses. However, all five congenic mouse strains responded to the transmission-blocking vaccine antigens when the parasites were emulsified in 2% O/W emulsion containing MPL® and TDM. The humoral response was Th dependent, as evident by boosting of the antibody response after a second immunization. If a purified recombinant protein antigen was used, the immune response was not MHC class II restricted in mice immunized with the MPL® + TDM adjuvant formulation.

The IgG2a and to some extent the IgG2b immunoglobulin isotypes of the mouse have been considered as a measure of the protective quality of the immune response to a specific antigen. Specific antibodies of these isotypes provide immunity in many viral and bacterial infections (Kenney et al., 1989; Hocart et al., 1989). It has been reported that LPS can increase IgG2 responses in mice (Hadjipetrou-Kourounakis and Moller, 1984; Izui et al., 1981). Recent studies (Takayama et al., 1991) evaluated the effects of various adjuvants on the mouse IgG isotype response to trinitrophenyl-conjugated hen egg albumin (TNP-HEA). MPL® and LPS were added to the TNP-HEA antigen and formulated into O/W emulsions with or without the block copolymer, L141, or TDM. Of interest is that MPL® alone, like LPS, induced an increased IgG2a concentration, moderately increased the IgG2b concentration, and had no effect on the IgG1 concentration of anti-TNP-specific antibody in the mouse sera. A combination of L141 with MPL® produced higher concentrations of all subclasses, especially the IgG2a, than did MPL® and TDM combined. However, a combination of all three adjuvants produced large increases in the IgG2a and IgG2b concentrations, with little or no effect on the IgG1. It was also reported (Myers and Ulrich, 1993) that MPL® formulated in saline or as a 1% O/W emulsion with p72–TT induced high concentrations, 125 and 250 μg/mL, respectively, of anti-p72 IgG2a antibody, whereas the IgG1 concentrations induced were only 20 and 34 μg/mL, respectively.

In a recent study (DeWilde, 1994) it was shown that mice immunized with 5 μg HA equivalents of a detergent-split vaccine of influenza A/Singapore (H1N1) containing MPL® produced hemagglutinin (HA) inhibition titers approximately 2.5-fold higher than those mice immunized with 5 μg HA equivalents of split virus alone. Of interest was the 5-fold increase of both IgG2a and IgG2b titers, and the coincident 3-fold decrease in IgG1 titer in the MPL® group. These data support the concept that MPL® used alone or in combinations with other adjuvant materials promotes either cytokine and/or cellular activities that are responsible for protective isotype selection.

A demonstration of cellular immunity is an important consideration in adjuvant selection for certain vaccines. In the guinea pig, it has been shown that adjuvant formulations of MPL® combined with TDM and/or CWS in 1–2% O/W emulsions, provoke strong DTH to a variety of antigens (Ulrich, personal communication). A limiting dilution assay for enumerating T-cells reactive to *M. tuberculosis* and specific for the 64-kDa protein has been used to evaluate the cellular immune response to this antigen (Kaufmann *et al.*, 1987). Immunization of mice with the 64-kDa recombinant protein in CFA failed to induce significant T-cell responses. However, when the antigen was administered in 2% O/W emulsions containing MPL® + TDM or MPL® + TDM + CWS, high numbers of *M. tuberculosis*-reactive T-cells were identified, ranging in frequency between 1/2000 and 1/3000. These T-cell numbers were comparable to those seen after immunization with whole *M. tuberculosis* organisms.

In the process of generating specific T-cell responses, soluble proteins are usually processed by the host APCs as exogenous antigens in the endocytic pathway for MHC class II-restricted presentation. This is in contrast to endogenously synthesized viral proteins, which are processed in the cytosol and presented in the context of class I molecules for CTL induction (Townsend and Bodmer, 1989). Several approaches have been used to introduce exogenous soluble antigens into the class I-restricted pathway. These approaches have employed presentation of antigen by liposomes (Collins *et al.*, 1992), ISCOMs (Takahashi *et al.*, 1990), or as conjugates of antigens with lipid molecules (Deres *et al.*, 1989). Recently, the MPL® mediated enhancement of liposomal antigen induction for CTL responses was characterized (Zhou and Huang, 1993). Using ovalbumin (OVA) entrapped in liposomes to induce CTLs, the authors showed that incorporation of 1–2% by weight of MPL® into the liposomes provided significant adjuvant activity. Moreover, the presence of MPL® provided good CTL priming by the liposomes when given by the intraperitoneal, subcutaneous, or intramuscular routes, whereas liposomes without MPL® did not induce CTLs by any route other than intravenous. In addition, it was shown that free MPL® and liposomal OVA injected at the same site gave enhanced CTL responses. The authors speculate that the adjuvant activity of MPL® could be related to the activation of macrophages to serve as better CTL antigen-presenting cells.

Another example of the ability of MPL® to engender T-cell responses in mice was recently shown (DeWilde, 1994). In this work, a recombinant antigen of herpesvirus type 2, gD2t, was adjuvanted with alum alone or with alum plus MPL®. The cell-mediated immune responses of mice were evaluated in spleen cell cultures by measuring lymphoproliferation and IL-2 and IFN-γ production in response to antigen. The stimulation index of spleen cells of mice receiving the vaccine with alum and MPL® was tenfold higher than the vaccine with alum alone. Likewise, IL-2 measured in culture supernatants was 650 and 111 pg/mL, respectively, and IFN-γ measured was 1661 and <50 pg/mL, respectively, for the MPL® plus alum versus alum alone groups.

The most useful preclinical test of the activity of a vaccine is a protection study, using the infectious organisms as the challenge. Animal models are not always available, so the previously discussed correlates of protective immunity have to be used. There are, however, a few studies demonstrating that MPL® alone or in combination with TDM provides an adjuvant effect in models of protective immunity. An early study (Rudbach *et al.*, 1988) showed that a single immunization of mice with 1 HA unit of an inactivated influenza A virus preparation containing MPL® and TDM gave excellent protection (88% survival) against a lethal intranasal challenge with virus given 14 days later. Control animals immunized with up to 8 HA units of inactivated virus without adjuvant were not protected. The 1 HA unit of inactivated influenza was calculated to contain 25 ng of viral protein.

The pertussis toxin subunit, S1, was produced in *Bacillus subtilis* as a secretory protein, partially purified, and used to immunize mice in combination with various adjuvants (Olander *et al.*, 1991). Of the four adjuvants tested, alum was ineffective, whereas IFA, Klebsiella 03:KN, LPS, and a 2% O/W emulsion containing MPL® + TDM all resulted in protective antibody production. Protection was tested by passive administration of the immune sera into naive mice followed by intranasal challenge with 10^7 virulent *Bordetella pertussis* organisms.

Guinea pigs have been documented to be a good model for anthrax vaccine research and investigations of *Bacillus anthracis* pathogenesis (Ivins *et al.*, 1986). The existing, licensed, human anthrax vaccine consists of aluminum hydroxide-adsorbed protective antigen (PA) from the supernatant fluids of fermentor cultures of *B. anthracis* (Puziss *et al.*, 1963). Subcutaneous injection of the commercial vaccine occasionally causes local pain, and six immunizations initially are required within 18 months, with yearly boosters in order to generate and to maintain protection (Brachman *et al.*, 1962). A recent study examined PA combined with various adjuvants to elicit protective immunity in guinea pigs challenged i.m. with spores of *B. anthracis*, Ames (Ivins *et al.*, 1992). Statistical analysis of the survival data indicated that vaccines containing PA plus MPL® and CWS, or PA plus MPL® and TDM and CWS in 2% O/W emulsions were more effective than the currently licensed vaccine, or even O/W emulsions containing the lipid-amine, CP20,961, or threonyl-muramyl dipeptide as adjuvants. In a follow-up study, it was shown that either one dose of PA–MPL® plus CWS or two doses of PA–MPL® protected 75% of the guinea pigs given a more stringent aerosol challenge of *B. anthracis* spores, whereas two immunizations of PA adsorbed to alum protected less than 40% of the guinea pigs (Ivins *et al.*, 1993).

The envelope protein of Friend murine leukemic helper virus (F-MuLV) has been shown to induce protective immunity against Friend virus leukemia (Hunsmann *et al.*, 1981). Ishihara *et al.* (1992) showed that a single injection of inactivated F-MuLV particles combined with MPL® and TDM gave protection comparable to CFA in mice. Protection was scored on the basis of the mice showing splenomegaly or death 50–60 days after intravenous challenge with Friend virus B. The authors concluded that immune protection was associated with T-cell priming by the MPL®+TDM-adjuvanted vaccine, since neutralizing antibodies appeared in the mice only after challenge.

Lastly, recent work has demonstrated that a split influenza A vaccine containing MPL® protects mice against a heterosubtypic challenge (DeWilde, 1994). Mice were immunized on day 0 and day 21 with 5 μg HA equivalents of influenza A/Singapore (H1N1); on day 49 the mice were challenged with 10^7 TCID$_{50}$ of influenza A/PR8. Virus was recovered from the turbinates, trachea, and lungs of the challenged mice on successive days following challenge. The results showed a rapid clearance of virus from the turbinates, with the recoverable virus reaching a log TCID$_{50}$ of 0 by day 5 in the trachea and lungs of mice immunized with MPL® and split virus. The kinetics of viral clearance were similar to those seen in the group of A/PR8-challenged mice that had recovered from an A/PR8 infection.

In summary, the preclinical studies discussed above are evidence that MPL® alone and in combination with other immunomodulators and vehicles provides appropriate adjuvant activities for a variety of potential vaccine antigens.

4.2. Clinical Experiences

Over the past 6 years clinical experience has accumulated with MPL® and the MPL® and CWS formulation, DETOX™, as adjuvants for human vaccines.

The most widespread use of the DETOX™ adjuvant formulation has been in the development of therapeutic vaccines for cancer. Mitchell *et al.* (1988) have reported on a Phase I trial of active specific immunity in disseminated malignant melanoma patients using a lysate of two allogeneic melanoma cell lines combined with DETOX™. The 22-patient trial was designed to measure toxicity and immunological effects of the vaccine. Other than soreness at the injection sites, no other toxicities were noted. A rise in the frequency of peripheral blood precursors of CTLs (pCTLs) was found in 12 of the 22 patients. Antibody titers, measured by ELISA using one of the vaccine cell lines as solid-phase antigen, were increased in 5 of the 22 patients. Three patients became DTH positive to the lysate after treatment.

A second clinical study confirmed that active specific immunotherapy with the melanoma cell line lysate plus DETOX™ induced immune responses to melanoma antigens (Mitchell *et al.*, 1990). Indeed, 59% of the treated patients became CTL positive and objective clinical responses were seen in 16% of the patients. There appeared to be a positive relationship between a rise in CTLs in these treated patients with extended survivorship.

An additional Phase II multicenter clinical trial using the melanoma cell line lysate and DETOX™ has been reported (Elliott *et al.*, 1993). Approximately 50% of the patients treated in this study had an increase in CTLs. Once again, extended survival times were observed in the CTL-positive patients.

A synthetic TF glycoconjugate antigen combined with DETOX™ has been tested in a Phase I trial of ovarian carcinoma patients with metastatic disease (MacLean *et al.*, 1992). Most of the immunized patients exhibited a "classical" anti-TF hapten response with an increase in IgM titer followed by increases in IgG and IgA titers. The humoral response to the TF hapten was specific as demonstrated by antibody binding to solid-phase synthetic and natural TF antigens, by complement-mediated cytotoxicity assays, and by hapten-inhibition experiments. The authors concluded that KLH is an acceptable carrier for TF haptens in the human and that DETOX™ is an appropriate adjuvant for the generation of high-titer specific anticarbohydrate responses in human cancer patients.

A small Phase I trial using synthetic sialyl Tn (STn) hapten conjugated to KLH with DETOX™ has been conducted in 12 patients with metastatic breast cancer (MacLean *et al.*, 1993). The results of this study showed toxicity was minimal and restricted to local cutaneous reactions. All patients developed IgM and IgG antibodies specific for the STn hapten, with increased titers of complement-mediated cytotoxic antibodies; these were partially inhibited by STn hapten, but not by TF hapten. The STn glycoconjugate vaccine with the DETOX™ adjuvant is undergoing a Phase II multicenter clinical study in breast cancer patients in order to test clinical activity.

Adjuvant effects of MPL® and MPL® plus CWS with certain prophylactic vaccine antigens for infectious disease have been evaluated in several studies. The DETOX™ adjuvant, formulated at a fivefold lesser concentration of MPL® and CWS than is used in the cancer vaccines, was formulated with a malaria circumsporozoite candidate antigen, $R32NS1_{81}$, and tested in normal volunteers (Rickman *et al.*, 1991). In this study, five volunteers received the vaccine at 0, 2, 4, and 6 months. The geometric mean titer measured by ELISA of anticircumsporozoite protein antibody progressively increased after each immunization, reaching a concentration of 25.4 μg/mL 2 weeks after the last booster. Archived sera from historical controls immunized with $R32NS1_{81}$ in alum had a geometric mean titer of 2.0 μg/mL after the last boost. This difference in titers was also shown by the indirect immunofluorescent antibody test and by the capacity of the serum to inhibit sporozoite invasion of hepatoma cells. Although the vaccine was reasonably well tolerated, some local reactogenicity was observed. All five volunteers had pain at the injection site within 48 h after each dose. Other signs at the injection site included warmth, erythema, and swelling after about one-half the doses given. One volunteer had a large, red, indurated injection site area after the third dose. However, none of the volunteers declined further participation because of side effects.

Rationale for the use of liposomes as an antigen/adjuvant delivery vehicle has been established (Alving, 1991, 1992). In a human study, the safety and activity of liposome-encapsulated malaria recombinant protein ($R32NS1_{81}$) and MPL® have been reported (Fries *et al.*, 1992). A single formulation containing 1260 μg/mL $R32NS1_{81}$, 4400 μg/mL MPL®, encapsulated in phosphatidylcholine-, phosphatidylglycerol-, and cholesterol-containing liposomes, was prepared. Actual vaccine doses were made at the time of vaccination by mixing an undiluted sample, a 1:2, 1:4, 1:10, or 1:100 dilution with an equal volume of aluminum hydroxide. This resulted in five vaccine dose levels with constant ratios of liposome components and a decreasing liposome-to-alum ratio. Thirty malaria-naive normal volunteers were randomized into the five dose groups, six volunteers per group. The vaccine was generally well tolerated and objective local reactions were limited to erythema or induration observed after 11 of the 88 administered doses. All vaccine doses were highly immunogenic. At 8 weeks after the third dose of vaccine, the five individuals receiving the most dilute preparation (6.3 μg $R32NS1_{81}$ and 22 μg MPL®) had a geometric mean antibody level of 22.7 μg/mL. Increasing the amount of $R32NS1_{81}$ and MPL® to 630 and 2200 μg/mL, respectively, resulted in an increase in the geometric mean antibody level to 33 μg/mL. Of all the individual sera tested for inhibition of sporozoite invasion in hepatoma cells, at least 88% inhibition was observed.

Phase I safety studies using the recombinant truncated type 2 glycoprotein D (gD2t) of herpesvirus, type 2, formulated with MPL® in alum have been reported (Leroux-Roels *et al.*, 1993; DeWilde, 1994). Twenty micrograms of gD2t adsorbed to aluminum hydroxide with or without 50 μg MPL® was administered to 40 HSV seronegative and 40 seropositive individuals. Twenty individuals in each group received the vaccine containing MPL® and 20 individuals in each group received the vaccine without MPL® according to a 0, 1, 6 month schedule. Headache, malaise, and fatigue were reported in 10–35% of the subjects; however, they were always mild and there was little difference between the groups with and without MPL®. Local reactions (soreness, itching, erythema, induration) were rare and mild, except that local soreness was more frequent in the seropositive group. In the seropositive group, after two doses of either vaccine, all individuals had at least fourfold increases in their preexisting antibody titers to gD2t and developed neutralizing antibody to HSV. In the seronegative group, the MPL®-containing vaccine induced significantly higher neutralizing antibody titers to HSV after two doses than did the vaccine without MPL®. Cell-mediated immunity was evaluated in vitro by lymphoproliferation, IL-2 production, and IFN-γ production after stimulation of peripheral blood cell cultures by gD2t. The MPL®–alum gD2t vaccine group had a significantly higher lymphoproliferation stimulation index, and significantly larger amounts of IL-2 and IFN-γ in the culture supernatants. DTH was measured by skin testing with gD2t and again significantly more hypersensitivity was recorded in the MPL®-containing vaccine groups. The authors concluded that the addition of MPL® to the gD2t vaccine was well tolerated and induced a more vigorous neutralizing antibody response and cellular immunity in the seronegative vaccines.

A Phase I safety trial of the adjuvant effect of MPL® on an existing recombinant vaccine for hepatitis B (recombinant HBsAg) was studied (Van Damme *et al.*, 1993; Thoelen *et al.*, 1993). In the first trial, 27 individuals were immunized at 0, 1, and 6 months with 20 μg recombinant HBsAg combined with 50 μg MPL®. Concurrently, 27 individuals received the vaccine without MPL®. No differences were observed between the two groups in tissue reactogenicity to the vaccines. One week after the second dose of vaccine, the MPL® group had an anti-HBs seroprotection rate ($\geq$ 10 mIU/mL) of 80%, compared to 58% for the group receiving the vaccine without MPL®. This seroprotection increased to 100% in the MPL® group at 2 months after the second dose, compared to 58% for the group receiving vaccine without MPL®. Thus, the vaccine with MPL® was judged to be well tolerated and induced a faster seroprotective conversion in the recipients.

In a second trial, individuals were administered HBsAg with and without MPL® in a two-dose schedule at 0 and 2 months. As was observed above, 1 month after the second dose of vaccine, 96% of the MPL® group had seroprotective titers, whereas only 73% of the vaccine-alone control group had seroconverted. The volunteers receiving HBsAg plus MPL® had a significantly higher geometric mean titer than did the HBsAg-alone group (214 versus 72 mIU/mL). No differences in reactogenicity were observed between the two vaccine groups.

At this time, over 700 vaccinations using recombinant antigens with MPL® have been administered to human subjects without significant adverse effects. The immune responses measured in these individuals suggest that MPL® provides a clinically useful adjuvant effect to these new-generation vaccines.

4.3. Modes of Action of MPL® as an Adjuvant

The differential production of cytokines by the helper T-cell population during an immune response has important regulatory effects on the nature of the response. A paradigm exists in that production of IFN-γ leads to expression of a Th1 phenotype, orchestrating DTH and the appearance of the IgG2a immunoglobulin isotype, whereas production of IL-4 and IL-5 leads to expression of the Th2 phenotype and the appearance of IgG1 and IgE isotypes (reviewed by Finkelman et al., 1990). Several factors have been proposed to explain the selection of the Th phenotypes, including the intrinsic properties of antigens, dose of antigen, site of exposure, and the ongoing immune response in the host. Romagnani (1992) presented evidence to indicate a determining role for the "natural" immune response, including NK cells, and cells of the mast cell/basophil lineage, in the subsequent selection of Th phenotype. In response to this paper, Rook (1993) expanded this concept by pointing out that a large number of microbial components are recognized by cell receptors that are phylogenetically ancient, and unrelated to the later-evolving antigen-specific receptors of T and B lymphocytes. These microbial components include LPS, lipoteichoic acids, peptidoglycans, polyanions, mannans, muramic acid derivatives, double-stranded RNA, and, undoubtedly, many others that are yet to be defined. Recognition of these microbial components rapidly can provide the host with useful information about the invading organism and it can be postulated that the pattern of response set in motion by a given combination of these microbial components is genetically programmed to be appropriate and protective to the host (Rook, 1991). Conceptually, microbial components that are recognized by mechanisms other than antigen receptors of T and B cells can be envisioned as adjuvants. Within the scope of the foregoing, the mode of action of MPL® as an adjuvant can be addressed.

An early measurable activity of MPL® after injection is its capacity to interact with and induce local macrophages to synthesize TNF-α, IL-1, and other cytokines. Recent experiments show that MPL® induces IL-12 mRNA expression in mouse macrophages (Salkowski and Vogel, personal communication). The chemotactic activities of these cytokines lead to a migration of cells into the local site. Within this population of cells are natural killer (NK) cells which are induced by cytokines to synthesize IFN-γ (Wherry et al., 1991; Gustafson and Rhodes, 1992a, 1994). Local IFN-γ next primes macrophages to process antigen and to serve as APCs. These APCs and the production of a high local concentration of IFN-γ by NK cells lead to the selection of the Th1 phenotype for the specific immune response. As has been previously mentioned, the hallmarks of Th1-type help are antigen-specific DTH and the predominance of an IgG2a immunoglobulin isotype, particularly following secondary responses. The role of MPL® in promoting these markers of Th1 response has been documented previously by Gustafson and Rhodes (1992b).

It can be postulated that for most of the new-generation vaccines for infectious disease, the addition of MPL® will provide a sufficient and safe adjuvant activity for enhancing the appropriate protective immune response. However, in consideration of the appropriate adjuvant formulation for active specific immunotherapy of cancer using tumor antigens, a combination of MPL® with either CWS, or TDM in O/W vehicles will likely be required, in order to force a predominantly cell-mediated response.

5. NEW DIRECTIONS

A goal of this review has been to bring together information relating to the potential usefulness and suitability of MPL® as an adjuvant for human vaccines. Hopefully, it has become clear that MPL® is a reasonable choice for use in vaccines that require a more potent adjuvant than alum. While MPL® stands as a choice that is available for use at this time, it can also be regarded as a starting point in the development of the next generation of LPS-derived adjuvants. Some of the areas in which further innovation can be envisioned are discussed in this section.

The vehicle component of an adjuvant formulation plays a key role in controlling the presentation of the adjuvant and associated antigen to the immune system, and this in turn influences the nature and magnitude of the observed immune response. At the present time, MPL® has been used successfully with vehicles consisting of water, O/W emulsions, alum, and liposomes in preclinical and clinical vaccine studies. A number of other materials are currently being developed as potential vehicles for vaccines, and combinations of MPL® with some of these new vehicles may have advantages over current formulations. It is also possible that combinations of MPL® with other immunostimulants that exhibit complementary immunostimulatory activities will lead to formulations with unique activities. Several examples of such synergistic combinations were discussed in Section 4.

Considerable effort is being focused on the development of new antigenic constructs in which two or more immunological "messages" are combined in the same molecule or particulate assembly. Examples of such chimeric structures include peptides that contain both a helper T-cell and a B-cell epitope (e.g., Good et al., 1987), and conjugates of peptide haptens and immunostimulants (e.g., Bessler and Jung, 1992). Potential advantages of these novel antigenic structures are that they can be designed to elicit only the desired immune response, and yet they can be relatively simple and well-defined compounds. The preparation of antigenic constructs involving MPL® is an attractive possibility. Support for this approach was provided recently by a paper in which it was reported that liposomes containing MPL® could act as carriers for a lipid-anchored peptide hapten (Friede et al., 1993). The authors found that MPL® had to be present in the same liposomes as the hapten in order to be effective, suggesting that codelivery of MPL® and hapten to the same cellular target was necessary for the carrier effect to be manifested. This indicates that direct covalent conjugation of MPL® to the hapten may represent an effective approach. Recently, a method of incorporating a free amino group into MPL® was reported, thereby providing a potentially useful derivative for the preparation of MLA–antigen constructs (Myers et al., 1992).

New synthetic lipid A analogues that exhibit improved therapeutic indices are continually being sought in many laboratories around the world. Such an effort is under way in our laboratory, using the chemical structures present in MPL® as inspiration for the design of new compounds with improved properties. A major goal of this effort is to identify the structural features in MPL® that are essential for biological activity, and then to use this information to design simplified compounds that retain or exceed MPL®'s biological activity and yet are amenable to synthesis on commercial scales.

6. SUMMARY AND CONCLUSIONS

The current era of vaccinology has resulted in antigens produced by synthetic chemistry and by genetic engineering techniques; these may provide more effective and safe vaccines. Many of these antigens can be produced in large quantities and in relatively pure form. However, inherent in their simplified, defined structures is a lack of immunogenicity and they require an immunostimulant or adjuvant to elicit appropriate immunity. It has been the purpose of this chapter to document the potential use of MPL® as a vaccine adjuvant. In this regard, it has been demonstrated that (1) MPL® has retained the useful immunostimulating activities of the parent LPS molecule, but has greatly attenuated toxicity; (2) MPL® produces diverse effects on the cellular elements of the immune system, including macrophage activation and T and B cell interaction, with concomitant cytokine and lymphokine release; (3) MPL® has proven adjuvant activity, in both the cellular and humoral effector arms of immunity; (4) MPL® has adjuvant activity when used alone, or in combination with other immunostimulants and delivery vehicles; and (5) MPL® has been administered safely to humans in various clinical vaccine trials. Thus, MPL® is emerging as a promising new adjuvant for use in human vaccines.

ACKNOWLEDGMENTS

The authors wish to thank Drs. Baldridge, Cantrell, Gustafson, and Rudbach for their critical reading of the manuscript and for their valuable editorial advice. In addition, the excellent assistance of Ms. Nancy Pollman in preparing the manuscript and Ms. Christie Loch in preparing the figures is gratefully acknowledged.

REFERENCES

Altman, A., and Dixon, F. J., 1989, Immunomodifiers in vaccines, *Adv. Vet. Sci. Comp. Med.* **33**:301–343.
Alving, C. R., 1991, Liposomes as carriers of antigens and adjuvants, *J. Immunol. Methods* **140**:1–13.
Alving, C. R., 1992, Lipid A and liposomes containing lipid A as adjuvants for vaccines, in: *Bacterial Endotoxic Lipopolysaccharides*, Vol. 2 (J. L. Ryan and D. C. Morrison, eds.), CRC Press, Boca Raton, pp. 430–443.
Baker, P. J., 1990, Regulation of magnitude of antibody response to bacterial polysaccharide antigens by thymus-derived lymphocytes, *Infect. Immun.* **58**:3465–3468.
Baker, P. J., and Prescott, B., 1979, Regulation of the antibody response to pneumococcal polysaccharides by thymus-derived (T) cells: Mode of action of suppressor and amplifier T cells, in: *Immunology of Bacterial Polysaccharides* (J. A. Rudbach and P. J. Baker, eds.), Elsevier/North-Holland, Amsterdam, pp. 67–105.
Baker, P. J., Hiernaux, J. R., Fauntleroy, M. B., Stashak, P. W., Prescott, B., Cantrell, J. L., and Rudbach, J. A., 1988a, Inactivation of suppressor T-cell activity by nontoxic monophosphoryl lipid A, *Infect. Immun.* **56**:1076–1083.
Baker, P. J., Hiernaux, J. R., Fauntleroy, M. B., Prescott, B., Cantrell, J. L., and Rudbach, J. A., 1988b, Ability of monophosphoryl lipid A to augment the antibody response of young mice, *Infect. Immun.* **56**:3064–3066.

Baker, P. J., Haslov, K. R., Fauntleroy, M. B., Stashak, P. W., Myers, K., and Ulrich, J. T., 1990, Enrichment of suppressor T cells by means of binding to monophosphoryl lipid A, *Infect. Immun.* **58**:726–731.

Batley, M., Packer, N. H., and Redmond, J. W., 1985, Analytical studies of lipopolysaccharide and its derivatives from *Salmonella minnesota* R595. I. Phosphorous magnetic resonance spectra, *Biochim. Biophys. Acta* **821**:179–194.

Bessler, W. G., and Jung, G., 1992, Synthetic lipopeptides as novel adjuvants, *Res. Immunol.* **5**:548–553.

Brachman, P. S., Gold, H., Plotkin, S. A., Fekety, F. R., Werrin, M., and Ingraham, N. R., 1962, Field evaluation of a human anthrax vaccine, *Am. J. Public Health* **52**:632–645.

Brozek, K. A., and Raetz, C. R. H., 1990, Biosynthesis of lipid A in *Escherichia coli*. Acyl carrier protein-dependent incorporation of laurate and myristate, *J. Biol. Chem.* **265**:15410–15417.

Caroff, M., Deprun, C., Karibian, D., and Szabó, L., 1991, Analysis of unmodified endotoxin preparations by ^{252}Cf plasma desorption mass spectrometry. Determination of molecular masses of the constituent native lipopolysaccharides, *J. Biol. Chem.* **266**:18543–18549.

Carozzi, S., Salit, M., Cantaluppi, A., Nasini, M. G., Barocci, S., Cantarella, S., and Lamperi, S., 1989, Effect of monophosphoryl lipid A on the in vitro function of peritoneal leukocytes from uremic patients on continuous ambulatory peritoneal dialysis, *J. Clin. Microbiol.* **27**:1748–1753.

Chase, J. J., Kubey, W., Dulek, M. H., Holmes, C. J., Salit, M. G., Pearson, F. C., III, and Ribi, E., 1986, Effect of monophosphoryl lipid A on host resistance to bacterial infection, *Infect. Immun.* **53**:711–712.

Chen, C. H., Johnson, A. G., Kasai, N., Key, B. A., Levin, J., and Nowotny, A., 1973, Heterogeneity and biological activity of endotoxic glycolipid from *Salmonella minnesota* R595, *J. Infect. Dis.* **128**(Suppl):43–51.

Codington, J. F., Linsley, K. B., and Jeanlot, R. W., 1975, Immunochemical and chemical investigations of the structure of glycoprotein fragments obtained from epiglycanin, a glycoprotein at the surface of the TA3-Ha cancer cell, *Carbohydr. Res.* **40**:171–182.

Collins, D. S., Findlay, K., and Harding, C. V., 1992, Processing of exogenous liposome-encapsulated antigen in vivo generates class I MHC-restricted T cell responses, *J. Immunol.* **148**:3336–3341.

Deres, K., Schild, H., Wiesmuller, K.-H., Jung, G., and Rammensee, H. G., 1989, *In vivo* priming of virus-specific cytotoxic T lymphocytes with synthetic lipopeptide vaccine, *Nature* **342**:561–564.

Devi, S. J. N., Schneerson, R., Egan, W., Ulrich, J. T., Bryla, D., Robbins, J. B., and Bennett, J. E., 1991, *Cryptococcus neoformans* serotype A glucuronoxylomannan–protein conjugate vaccines: Synthesis, characterization, and immunogenicity, *Infect. Immun.* **59**:3700–3707.

DeWilde, M., 1994, Preclinical and clinical experience with MPL and QS21 adjuvanted recombinant subunit vaccines, in: *Novel Vaccine Strategies*, IBC Conference, February, Bethesda, Maryland.

Dijkstra, J., Mellors, J. W., Ryan, J. L., and Szoka, F. C., 1987, Modulation of the biological activity of bacterial endotoxin by incorporation into liposomes, *J. Immunol.* **138**:2663–2670.

Domer, J. E., Garner, R. E., and Befidi-Mengue, R. N., 1989, Mannan as an antigen in cell-mediated immunity (CMI) assays and as a modulator of mannan-specific CMI, *Infect. Immun.* **57**:693–700.

Domer, J. E., Human, L. G., Andersen, G. B., Rudbach, J. A., and Asherson, G. L., 1993, Abrogation of suppression of delayed hypersensitivity induced by *Candida albicans*-derived mannan by treatment with monophosphoryl lipid A, *Infect. Immun.* **61**:2122–2130.

Edelman, R., 1992, An update on vaccine adjuvants in clinical trial, *AIDS Res. Hum. Retroviruses* **8**:1409–1411.

Elliott, G. T., McLeod, R. A., Perez, J., and Von Eschen, K. B., 1993, Interim results of a Phase II multicenter clinical trial evaluating the activity of a therapeutic allogeneic melanoma vaccine (Theraccine) in the treatment of disseminated malignant melanoma, *Semin. Surg. Oncol.* **9**:264–272.

Engelhardt, R., Mackensen, A., Galanos, C., and Andreesen, R., 1990, Biological response to intravenously administered endotoxin in patients with advanced cancer, *J. Biol. Response Mod.* **9**:480–491.

Esquivel, F., Taylor, C. E., and Baker, P. J., 1991, Differential sensitivity of CD8+ suppressor and cytotoxic T lymphocyte activity to bacterial monophosphoryl lipid A, *Infect. Immun.* **59**:2994–2998.

Finkelman, F. D., Holmes, J., Katona, I. M., Urban, J. F., Jr., Beckmann, M. P., Park, L. S., Schooley, K. A., Coffman, R. L., Mosmann, T. R., and Paul, W. E., 1990, Lymphokine control of in vivo immunoglobulin isotype selection, *Annu. Rev. Immunol.* **8**:303–333.

Florence, A. T., and Whitehill, D., 1982, The formulation and stability of multiple emulsions, *Int. J. Pharm.* **11**:277–308.

Friede, M., Muller, S., Briand, J.-P., Van Regenmortel, M. H. V., and Schuber, F., 1993, Induction of immune response against a short synthetic peptide antigen coupled to small neutral liposomes containing monophosphoryl lipid A, *Mol. Immunol.* **30**:539–547.

Fries, L. F., Gordon, D. M., Richards, R. L., Egan, J. E., Hollingdale, M. R., Gross, M., Silverman, C., and Alving, C. R., 1992, Liposomal malaria vaccine in humans: A safe and potent adjuvant strategy, *Proc. Natl. Acad. Sci. USA* **89**:358–362.

Fung, P. Y. S., and Longenecker, B. M., 1991, Specific immunosuppressive activity of epiglycanin, a mucin-like glycoprotein secreted by a murine mammary adenocarcinoma (TA3-HA), *Cancer Res.* **51**:1170–1176.

Fung, P. Y. S., Madej, M., Koganty, R. R., and Longenecker, B. M., 1990, Active specific immunotherapy of a murine mammary adenocarcinoma using a synthetic tumor-associated glycoconjugate, *Cancer Res.* **50**:4308–4314.

Garcon, N. M. J., and Six, H. R., 1991, Universal vaccine carrier. Liposomes that provide T-dependent help to weak antigens, *J. Immunol.* **146**:3697–3702.

Garg, M., and Subbarao, B., 1992, Immune responses of systemic and mucosal lymphoid organs to Pnu-Imune vaccine as a function of age and the efficacy of monophosphoryl lipid A as an adjuvant, *Infect. Immun.* **60**:2329–2336.

Good, M. F., Maloy, W. L., Lunde, M. N., Margalit, H., Corvette, J. L., Smith, G. L., Moss, B., Miller, L. H., and Berzofsky, J. A., 1987, Construction of synthetic immunogen: Use of new T-helper epitope on malaria circumsporozoite protein, *Science* **235**:1059–1062.

Gregoriadis, G., 1990, Immunological adjuvants: A role for liposomes, *Immunol. Today* **11**:89–97.

Griffioen, A. W., Rijkers, G. T., Toebes, E. A. H., and Zegers, B. J. M., 1991, The human *in vitro* anti-type 4 pneumococcal polysaccharide antibody response is regulated by suppressor T cells, *Scand. J. Immunol.* **34**:229–236.

Griffioen, A. W., Toebes, E. A., Rijkers, G. T., Claas, F. H., Datema, G., and Zegers, B. J. M., 1992, The amplifier role of T cells in the human in vitro B cell response to type 4 pneumococcal polysaccharide, *Immunol. Lett.* **32**:265–272.

Gustafson, G. L., and Rhodes, M. J., 1992a, A rationale for the prophylactic use of monophosphoryl lipid A in sepsis and septic shock, *Biochem. Biophys. Res. Commun.* **182**:269–275.

Gustafson, G. L., and Rhodes, M. J., 1992b, Bacterial cell wall products as adjuvants: Early interferon gamma as a marker for adjuvants that enhance protective immunity, *Res. Immunol.* **143**:483–488.

Gustafson, G. L., and Rhodes, M. J., 1994, Effects of tumor necrosis factor and dexamethasone on the regulation of interferon-γ induction by monophosphoryl lipid A, *J. Immunother.* **15**:129–133.

Hadjipetrou-Kourounakis, L., and Moller, E., 1984, Adjuvants influence the immunoglobin subclass distribution of immune responses *in vivo, Scand. J. Immunol.* **19**:219–225.

Havell, E. A., 1989, Evidence that tumor necrosis factor has an important role in antibacterial resistance, *J. Immunol.* **143**:2894–2899.

Hocart, M. J., MacKenzie, J. S., and Stewart, G. A., 1989, The immunoglobulin G subclass responses of mice to influenza A virus: The effect of mouse strain, and the neutralizing abilities of individual protein A-purified subclass antibodies, *J. Gen. Virol.* **70**:2439–2448.

Hunsmann, G., Schneider, J., and Schulz, A., 1981, Immunoprevention of Friend virus-induced erythroleukemia by vaccination with viral envelope glycoprotein complexes, *Virology* **113**:602–612.

Ishihara, C., Miyazawa, M., Nishio, J., Azuma, I., and Chesebro, B., 1992, Use of low toxicity adjuvants and killed virus to induce protective immunity against the Friend murine leukaemia retrovirus-induced disease, *Vaccine* **10**:353–356.

Ivins, B. E., Ezzell, J. W., Jr., Jemski, J., Hedlund, K. W., Ristroph, J. D., and Leppla, S. H., 1986, Immunization studies with attenuated strains of *Bacillus anthracis, Infect. Immun.* **52**:454–458.

Ivins, B. E., Welkos, S. L., Little, S. F., Crumine, M. H., and Nelson, G. O., 1992, Immunization against anthrax with *Bacillus anthracis* protective antigen combined with adjuvants, *Infect. Immun.* **60**:662–668.

Ivins, B. E., Fellows, P. F., Welkos, S. L., and Pitt, M. L., 1993, Experimental anthrax vaccines: Efficacy studies in guinea pigs, Abstr. E-104, Am. Soc. Microbiol. Annu. Meet., May, p. 160.

Izui, S., Eisenberg, R. A., and Dixon, F. J., 1981, Subclass-restricted IgG polyclonal antibody production in mice injected with lipid A-rich lipopolysaccharides, *J. Exp. Med.* **153**:324–338.

Johnson, A. G., 1964, Adjuvant action of bacterial endotoxins on the primary antibody response, in: *Bacterial Endotoxins* (M. Landy and W. Braun, eds.), Rutgers University Press, New Brunswick, pp. 252–262.

Johnson, A. G., Gains, S., and Landy, M., 1956, Studies on the O antigen of *Salmonella typhosa*. V. Enhancement of antibody responses to protein antigens by the purified lipopolysaccharide, *J. Exp. Med.* **103**:225–246.

Kaufmann, S. H. E., Vath, U., Thole, J. E. R., Van Embden, J. D. A., and Emmrich, F., 1987, Enumeration of T cells reactive with *Mycobacterium tuberculosis* organisms and specific for the recombinant mycobacterial 64-KDa protein, *Eur. J. Immunol.* **17**:351–357.

Keane, W. F., and Peterson, P. K., 1984, Host defense mechanisms of peritoneal cavity and continuous ambulatory peritoneal dialysis, *Peritoneal Dial. Bull.* **4**:122–127.

Kenney, J. S., Hughes, B. W., Masada, M. P., and Allison, A. C., 1989, Influence of adjuvants on the quantity, affinity, isotype, and epitope specificity of murine antibodies, *J. Immunol. Methods* **121**:157–166.

Klein, J. O., 1981, The epidemiology of pneumococcal disease in infants and children, *Rev. Infect. Dis.* **3**:246–253.

Kotani, S., and Takada, H., 1989, Structural requirements of lipid A for endotoxicity and other biological activities—An overview, *Crit. Rev. Microbiol.* **16**:477–523.

Lamperi, S., Carozzi, S., Icardi, A., and Nasini, M. G., 1985, Peritoneal membrane defense mechanism in CAPD, *Trans. Am. Soc. Artif. Intern. Organs* **31**:33–37.

Leroux-Roels, G., Moreux, E., Verhasselt, B., Biernaux, S., Brulein, V., Francotte, M., Pala, P., Slaoui, M., and Vandepapeliere, P., 1993, Immunogenicity and reactogenicity of a recombinant HSV-2 glycoprotein D vaccine with or without monophosphoryl lipid A in HSV seronegative and seropositive subjects, Abstr. 1209, 33rd Intersci. Conf. Antimicrob. Agents Chemother., p. 341.

MacLean, G. D., Bowen-Yacyshyn, M. B., Samuel, J., Meikle, A., Stuart, G., Nation, J., Poppema, S., Jerry, M., Koganty, R., Wong, T., and Longenecker, B. M., 1992, Active immunization of human ovarian cancer patients against a common carcinoma (Thomsen–Friedenreich) determinant using a synthetic carbohydrate antigen, *J. Immunother.* **11**:292–305.

MacLean, G. D., Reddish, M., Koganty, R. R., Wong, T., Gandhi, S., Smolenski, M., Samuel, J., Nabholtz, J. M., and Longenecker, B. M., 1993, Immunization of breast cancer patients using a synthetic sialyl-Tn glycoconjugate plus Detox adjuvant, *Cancer Immunol. Immunother.* **36**:215–222.

Marr, A. G., and Ingraham, J. L., 1962, Effect of temperature on the composition of fatty acids in *Escherichia coli, J. Bacteriol.* **84**:1260–1267.

Martich, G. D., Danner, R. L., Ceska, M., and Suffredini, A. F., 1991, Detection of interleukin 8 and tumor necrosis factor in normal humans after intravenous endotoxin: The effect of antiinflammatory agents, *J. Exp. Med.* **173**:1021–1024.

Masihi, K. N., Lange, W., Johnson, A. G., and Ribi, E., 1986, Enhancement of chemiluminescence and phagocytic activities by nontoxic and toxic forms of lipid A, *J. Biol. Response Mod.* **5**:462–469.

Michie, H. R., Manogue, K. R., Spriggs, D. R., Revhaug, A., O'Dwyer, S., Dinarello, C. A., Cerami, A., Wolff, S. M., and Wilmore, D. W., 1988, Detection of circulating tumor necrosis factor after endotoxin administration, *N. Engl. J. Med.* **318**:1481–1486.

Mitchell, M. S., Kan-Mitchell, J., Kempf, R. A., Harel, W., Shau, H. Y., and Lind, S., 1988, Active specific immunotherapy for melanoma: Phase I trial of allogeneic lysates and a novel adjuvant, *Cancer Res.* **48**:5883–5893.

Mitchell, M. S., Harel, W., Kempf, R. A., Hu, E., Kan-Mitchell, J., Boswell, W. D., Dean, G., and Stevenson, L., 1990, Active-specific immunotherapy for melanoma, *J. Clin. Oncol.* **8**:856–869.

Mosier, D. E., and Subbarao, B., 1982, Thymus-independent antigens: Complexity of B lymphocyte activation revealed, *Immunol. Today* **3**:217–222.

Mosier, D. E., Zaldivar, N. M., Goldings, E., Mond, J., Scher, I., and Paul, W. E., 1977, Formation of antibody in the newborn mouse: Study of T-cell-independent antibody response, *J. Infect. Dis.* **136** (Suppl.):S14–S19.

Munoz, J., 1964, Effects of bacteria and bacterial products on antibody response, in: *Advances in Immunology* (F. J. Dixon and H. G. Kunkel, eds.), Academic Press, New York, pp. 397–440.

Myers, K. R., and Snyder, D. S., 1992, Detailed composition of natural MPL®-immunostimulant, *J. Cell. Biochem.*, Abstr. Suppl. 16C, abstract CB112.

Myers, K. R., and Ulrich, J. T., 1993, Effective use of monophosphoryl lipid A as an adjuvant, in: *Novel Vaccine Strategies*, IBC Conference, October, Bethesda.

Myers, K. R., Truchot, A. T., Ward, J., Hudson, Y., and Ulrich, J. T., 1990, A critical determinant of lipid A endotoxic activity, in: *Cellular and Molecular Aspects of Endotoxin Reactions* (A. Nowotny, J. J. Spitzer, and E. J. Ziegler, eds.), Elsevier, Amsterdam, pp. 145–156.

Myers, K. R., Ulrich, J. T., Qureshi, N., Takayama, K., Wang, R., Chen, L., Emary, W. B., and Cotter, R. J., 1992, Preparation and characterization of biologically active 6'-O-(6-aminocaproyl)-4'-O-monophosphoryl lipid A and its conjugated derivative, *Bioconjugate Chem.* **3**:540–548.

Olander, R.-M., Muotiala, A., Himanen, J.-P., Karvonen, M., Airaksinen, U., and Runeberg-Nyman, K., 1991, Immunogenicity and protective efficacy of pertussis toxin subunit S1 produced by *Bacillus subtilis, Microb. Pathog.* **10**:159–164.

Peltola, H., Kayhty, H., Virtanen, M., and Makela, P. H., 1984, Prevention of *Haemophilus influenzae* type B bacteremic infections with the capsular polysaccharide vaccine, *N. Engl. J. Med.* **310**:1561–1566.

Pohle, C., Rohde-Schultz, B., and Masihi, K. N., 1990, Effects of synthetic HIV peptides, cytokines, and monophosphoryl lipid A on chemiluminescence response, in: *Immunotherapeutic Disease* (K. N. Masihi and W. Lange, eds.), Springer-Verlag, Berlin, pp. 143–149.

Puziss, M., Manning, L. C., Lynch, L. W., Barclay, E., Abelow, I., and Wright, G. G., 1963, Large-scale production of protective antigen of *Bacillus anthracis* anaerobic cultures, *Appl. Microbiol.* **11**:330–334.

Qureshi, N., Takayama, K., and Ribi, E., 1982, Purification and structural determination of nontoxic lipid A obtained from lipopolysaccharide of *Salmonella typhimurium, J. Biol. Chem.* **257**:11808–11815.

Qureshi, N., Mascagni, P., Ribi, E., and Takayama, K., 1985, Monophosphoryl lipid A obtained from lipopolysaccharides of *Salmonella minnesota* R595: Purification of the dimethyl derivative by high performance liquid chromatography and complete structural determination, *J. Biol. Chem.* **260**:5271–5278.

Qureshi, N., Cotter, R. J., and Takayama, K., 1986, Application of fast atom bombardment mass spectrometry and nuclear magnetic resonance on the structural analysis of purified lipid A, *J. Microbiol. Methods* **5**:65–77.

Rawlings, D. J., and Kaslow, D. C., 1992, Adjuvant-dependent immune response to malarial transmission-blocking vaccine candidate antigens, *J. Exp. Med.* **176**:1483–1487.

Ribi, E., 1984, Beneficial modification of the endotoxin molecule, *J. Biol. Response Mod.* **3**:1–9.

Ribi, E., 1986, Structure–function relationship of bacterial adjuvants, in: *Advances in Carriers and Adjuvants for Veterinary Biologics* (R. M. Nervig, P. M. Gough, M. L. Kaeberle, and C. A. Whetstone, eds.), Iowa State University Press, Ames, pp. 35–49.

Ribi, E., Parker, R., Strain, S. M., Mizuno, Y., Nowotny, A., Von Eschen, K. B., Cantrell, J. L., McLaughlin, C. A., Hwang, K. M., and Goren, M. B., 1979, Peptides as requirement for immunotherapy of the guinea-pig Line 10 tumor with endotoxins, *Cancer Immunol. Immunother.* **7**:43–58.

Ribi, E., Amano, K., Cantrell, J., Schwartzman, S., Parker, R., and Takayama, K., 1982, Preparation and antitumor activity of nontoxic lipid A, *Cancer Immunol. Immunother.* **12**:91–96.

Ribi, E., Cantrell, J. L., Takayama, K., Ribi, H. O., Myers, K. R., and Qureshi, N., 1986, Modulation of humoral and cell-mediated immune responses by a structurally established nontoxic lipid A, in: *Immunobiology and Immunopharmacology of Bacterial Endotoxins* (A. Szentivanyi and H. Friedman, eds.), Plenum Press, New York, pp. 407–420.

Rickman, L. S., Gordon, D. M., Wistar, R. Jr., Krzych, U., Gross, M., Hollingdale, M. R., Egan, J. E., Chulay, J. D., and Hoffman, S. L., 1991, Use of adjuvant containing mycobacterial cell-wall skeleton, monophosphoryl lipid A, and squalane in malaria circumsporozoite protein vaccine, *Lancet* **337**:998–1001.

Rietschel, E. T., Wollenweber, H.-W., Russa, R., Brade, H., and Zähringer, U., 1984, Concepts of the chemical structure of lipid A, *Rev. Infect. Dis.* **6**:432–438.

Robbins, J. B., and Schneerson, R., 1990, Polysaccharides–protein conjugates: A new generation of vaccines, *J. Infect. Dis.* **161**:821–832.

Roghmann, K. J., Tabloski, P. A., Bentley, D. W., and Schiffman, G., 1987, Immune response of elderly adults to pneumococcus: Variation by age, sex, and functional impairment, *J. Gerontol.* **42**:265–270.

Romagnani, S., 1992, Induction of TH1 and TH2 responses: A key role for the "natural" immune response? *Immunol. Today* **13**:379–381.

Rook, G. A., 1991, Mobilizing the appropriate T-cell subset: The immune response as taxonomist? *Tubercle* **72**:253–254.

Rook, G. A. W., 1993, New meanings for an old word: Adjuvanticity, cytokines and T cells, *Immunol. Today* **14**:95–96.

Rudbach, J. A., Cantrell, J. L., and Ulrich, J. T., 1988, Molecularly engineered microbial immunostimulators, in: *Technological Advances in Vaccine Development* (L. Lasky, ed.), Liss, New York, pp. 443–454.

Rudbach, J. A., Cantrell, J. L., Ulrich, J. T., and Mitchell, M. S., 1990, Immunotherapy with bacterial endotoxins, in: *Endotoxin* (H. Friedman, T. W. Klein, M. Nakano, and A. Nowotny, eds.), Plenum Press, New York, pp. 665–676.

Rudbach, J. A., Myers, K. R., Rechtman, D. J., and Ulrich, J. T., 1994, Prophylactic use of monophosphoryl lipid A in patients at risk for sepsis, in: *Bacterial Endotoxins: Basic Science to Anti-Sepsis Strategies* (J. Levin, S. J. H. Van Deventer, A. Sturk, and T. Van Der Poll, eds.), Wiley, New York, pp. 107–124.

Schneerson, R., Fattom, A., Szu, S. C., Bryla, D., Ulrich, J. T., Rudbach, J. A., Schiffman, G., and Robbins, J. B., 1991, Evaluation of monophosphoryl lipid A (MPL) as an adjuvant. Enhancement of serum antibody response in mice to polysaccharide–protein conjugates by concurrent injection with MPL, *J. Immunol.* **147**:2136–2140.

Shapiro, E. D., Wald, E. R., Margolis, A. G., and Ortenzo, M. E., 1992, The decreasing incidence of Hemophilus influenza type B (Hib) disease in both Connecticut and Greater Pittsburgh, PA., *Pediatr. Res.* **31**:100A.

Springer, G. F., 1984, T and Tn, general carcinoma autoantigens, *Science* **224**:1198–1206.

Takahashi, H., Takeshita, T., Morein, B., Putney, S., Germain, R. N., and Berzofsky, J. A., 1990, Induction of CD8[+] cytotoxic T cells by immunization with purified HIV-1 envelope proteins in ISCOMs, *Nature* **344**:873–875.

Takayama, K., Ribi, E., and Cantrell, J. L., 1981, Isolation of a nontoxic lipid A fraction containing tumor regression activity, *Cancer Res.* **41**:2654–2657.

Takayama, K., Qureshi, N., Raetz, C. R. H., Ribi, E., Peterson, J., Cantrell, J. L., Pearson, F. C., Wiggins, J., and Johnson, A. G., 1984, Influence of fine structure of lipid A on *Limulus* amebocyte lysate clotting and toxic activities, *Infect. Immun.* **45**:350–355.

Takayama, K., Olsen, M., Datta, P., and Hunter, R. L., 1991, Adjuvant activity of non-ionic block copolymers. V. Modulation of antibody isotype by lipopolysaccharides, lipid A, and precursors, *Vaccine* **9**:257–265.

Thoelen, S., Van Damme, P., Meeus, A., Collard, F., Slaoui, M., and Vandepapeliere, P., 1993, Immunogenicity of a recombinant hepatitis B vaccine with monophosphoryl lipid A administered following various two-dose schedules, Abstr. 340, 33rd Intersci. Conf. Antimicrob. Agents Chemother., p. 182.

Townsend, A., and Bodmer, H., 1989, Antigen recognition by class I-restricted T lymphocytes, *Annu. Rev. Immunol.* **7**:601–624.

Ulrich, J. T., Masihi, K. N., and Lange, W., 1988, Mechanisms of nonspecific resistance to microbial infections induced by trehalose dimycolate (TDM) and monophosphoryl lipid A (MPL), *Adv. Biosci.* **68**:167–178.

Van Damme, P., Thoelen, S., Van Passchen, M., Leroux-Roels, G., Meeus, A., Slaoui, M., and Vandepapeliere, P., 1993, Safety, humoral and cellular immunity of a recombinant hepatitis B vaccine with monophosphoryl lipid A in healthy volunteers, Abstr. 667, 33rd Intersci. Conf. Antimicrob. Agents Chemother., p. 241.

Verghese, A., and Berk, S. L., 1983, Bacterial pneumonia in the elderly, *Medicine* (*Baltimore*) **62**:271–285.

Wherry, J. C., Schreiber, R. D., and Unanue, E. R., 1991, Regulation of gamma interferon production by natural killer cells in SCID mice: Roles of tumor necrosis factor and bacterial stimuli, *Infect. Immun.* **59**:1709–1715.

Zhou, F., and Huang, L., 1993, Monophosphoryl lipid A enhances specific CTL induction by a soluble protein antigen entrapped in liposomes, *Vaccine* **11**:1139–1144.

Chapter 22

Structural and Immunological Characterization of the Vaccine Adjuvant QS-21

Charlotte Read Kensil, Jia-Yan Wu, and Sean Soltysik

1. INTRODUCTION

1.1. Historical Use of *Quillaja* Saponins as Adjuvants

QS-21 is a triterpene glycoside "saponin" isolated from the bark of the *Quillaja saponaria* Molina tree, a species native to South America. The bark of this tree, particularly the saponin fraction present in the bark, has long been known as a source of immune stimulators that can be used as vaccine adjuvants. Espinet (1951) noted the adjuvant activity of plant saponins to enhance the potency of foot-and-mouth disease vaccines. A number of commercially available complex saponin extracts were developed for adjuvant use. Not all of these extracts were effective as adjuvants. Dalsgaard (1970) showed that a correlation exists between adjuvant activity and the source of the saponin, and that the most adjuvant-active extracts were derived from the tree *Quillaja saponaria*. The use of *Quillaja* saponins as adjuvants has been reviewed by Campbell and Peerbaye (1992).

Crude *Quillaja saponaria* extracts caused local reactions when used in vaccines. Dalsgaard (1974) was able to partially purify the adjuvant activity through dialysis, ion-exchange, and gel filtration chromatography to produce a saponin fraction known as Quil A, which gave reduced local reactions and an increased potency on a weight basis. Quil A represented a significant improvement over crude extracts and has found widespread use as an adjuvant in veterinary vaccines. It has also been tested extensively as part of

---

Charlotte Read Kensil, Jia-Yan Wu, and Sean Soltysik • Cambridge Biotech Corporation, Worcester, Massachusetts 01605.

Vaccine Design: The Subunit and Adjuvant Approach, edited by Michael F. Powell and Mark J. Newman. Plenum Press, New York, 1995.

immune-stimulating complexes known as ISCOMs, consisting of antigen, lipid, and saponin (Morein *et al.*, 1984; see Chapter 23).

1.2. Discovery of Diversity of *Quillaja Saponaria* Adjuvants

Analysis via high-pressure liquid chromatography (HPLC) showed that saponin extracts such as Quil A were in fact heterogeneous mixtures of structurally related compounds. Kersten *et al.* (1988) analyzed Quil A via HPLC and noted at least 24 peaks, and the same heterogeneity was found in a separate study (Kensil *et al.*, 1991a,b). In the latter study, it was observed that not all saponins were active as adjuvants. However, the four most predominant saponins (designated QS-7, QS-17, QS-18, and QS-21 based on the HPLC elution profile) were found to be adjuvant-active, although differing in biologic activities such as hemolysis and toxicity in mice. For example, QS-18, the most predominant saponin in all crude extracts from *Quillaja saponaria*, was found to be particularly toxic to mice whereas QS-21 and QS-7 were less toxic.

1.3. Stimulon™ QS-21 Adjuvant

The ideal immunological adjuvant candidate should combine potent adjuvant activity with low toxicity and be available in reasonable abundance. The saponin designated QS-21 met these criteria (Kensil and Marciani, 1991). QS-21 is present in the bark of the *Quillaja saponaria* tree at levels that enable routine purification from this source. This chapter reviews the preclinical and clinical experience with QS-21 ("Stimulon") adjuvant as well as studies to determine its mechanism of action.

2. CHEMICAL AND PHYSICAL PROPERTIES

2.1. Structure

QS-21 is a complex triterpene glycoside of quillaic acid (Fig. 1). This structure was derived from mass spectral and carbohydrate analysis of QS-21 and fragments (Kensil *et al.*, 1992) and comparison to another closely related saponin from *Quillaja saponaria* (Higuchi *et al.*, 1988). Further, the assigned structure has been confirmed by 2-D NMR analysis. QS-21 is glycosylated at triterpene carbon 3, triterpene carbon 28, and carbon 5 of the second fatty acyl unit in a fatty acid domain. QS-21 is anionic at physiologic pH because of the glucuronic acid moiety.

Two structural features that distinguish *Quillaja saponaria* saponins from those of most other plant species are a fatty acid domain and a triterpene aldehyde at position 4. Higuchi *et al.* (1988) noted the presence of a 3,5-dihydroxy-6-methyl octanoic acid domain in purified saponins from *Quillaja*. This domain is also present in QS-21 (Kensil, unpublished data).

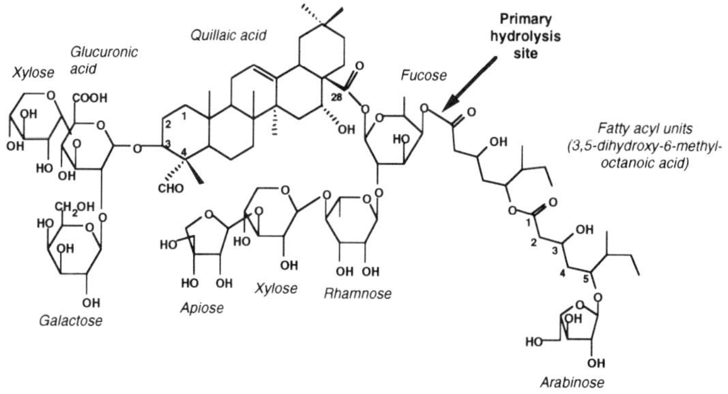

Figure 1. Proposed structure of QS-21. The primary degradation site in aqueous solution is noted.

2.2. Amphipathic Character

QS-21 is an amphipathic molecule because of the presence of both hydrophobic domains (triterpene and fatty acids) and hydrophilic domains (glycosides). It forms micelles in PBS at concentrations greater than 26 μM (Kensil et al.,1993). The Stokes' radius of the QS-21 micelle was determined by gel filtration to be approximately 35 Å (Kensil and Marciani, 1991). The shape and aggregation number of QS-21 micelles are unknown.

The propensity of QS-21 to form micelles raises the question of whether the adjuvant-active form of QS-21 is monomeric or micellar. In a QS-21 dose–response study in mice, it was shown that QS-21 was adjuvant active at concentrations well below the critical micellar concentration, suggesting that the monomer form is active (Kensil et al., 1993).

3. MANUFACTURING

3.1. Manufacturing and Quality Control

QS-21 is one of many structurally distinct triterpene glycosides ("saponins") that can be isolated from the bark of *Quillaja saponaria* Molina. These saponins are water soluble and can be readily extracted from chipped bark with water. The primary contaminants are tannins and polyphenolic compounds, which are also readily extracted with water. Although the saponins are small compounds, they form micelles in aqueous solution because of their amphipathic natures. Mixed saponin micelles can be separated from lower-molecular-weight tannins and polyphenolics by either dialysis (Dalsgaard, 1974), diafiltration (Kensil et al., 1991a), or gel filtration through Sephadex G-100 (Strobbe et al., 1974). These processes produce an enriched saponin fraction that represents a heterogeneous distribution of the saponins from *Quillaja saponaria*.

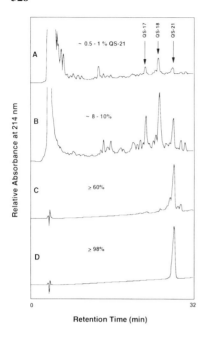

Figure 2. Purity at different stages of QS-21 purification. Analysis was carried out by RP-HPLC on Vydac C4 (4.6 mm internal diameter × 25 cm length, 300 Å pore size, 5 μm particle size) using a linear gradient of 30 to 40% acetonitrile containing 0.15% trifluoroacetic acid over 30 min at a 1 mL/min flow rate. (A) Aqueous *Quillaja saponaria* bark extract; (B) retentate after diafiltration; (C) partially purified QS-21 after chromatography on silica; (D) final product after preparative reverse phase chromatography. Approximate purity of QS-21 at each step is shown.

Purification of individual saponins requires the use of either normal phase or reverse phase chromatography (RP-HPLC) in the presence of an organic solvent or mixed organic solvent to disperse the mixed micelles that are formed by closely related saponins (Kensil *et al.,* 1991a; Kersten *et al.,* 1988). QS-21 can be purified either by a combination of adsorption chromatography on silica followed by RP-HPLC or by RP-HPLC alone (Kensil *et al.,* 1991a). The final product is lyophilized to produce a white powder that is resolubilized in buffer for use in vaccine formulations. Figure 2 outlines the purity of QS-21 at the different stages in the purification process.

The purification process has been scaled up to produce sufficient QS-21 for several clinical trials, and appropriate quality control procedures have been developed. Identity of the final product as QS-21 is determined by fast atom bombardment mass spectroscopy and infrared spectroscopy, and purity is assessed by RP-HPLC ($\geq$ 98%). Additional specifications include limits on residual moisture ($\leq$ 5%), endotoxin ($\leq$ 10 units/mg), bioburden ($\leq$ 10 CFU/mg, prior to formulation and sterile filtration), and residual solvents ($\leq$ 50 ppm each).

3.2. Formulation

Most adjuvants fall into two broad classes: those that are immunostimulants, such as muramyl dipeptide and monophosphoryl lipid A, and those that serve as antigen depot vehicles such as emulsions, block copolymers, mineral salts, or polylactide polyglycolide microspheres. In general, most adjuvant formulations are combinations of immunostimulants and vehicles. A classic example is complete Freund's adjuvant, consisting of a

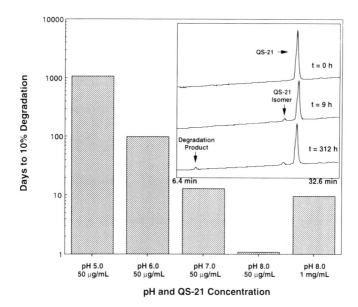

Figure 3. Stability of QS-21 in aqueous solution. Solutions of QS-21 (at 50 μg/mL and 1.0 mg/mL) were prepared at pH 5 through 8 in 20 mM buffer (sodium citrate for pH 5, sodium phosphate for pH 6, 7, and 8). Stability at 22°C was monitored via HPLC. An example of the assay on 200 μg/mL QS-21 at pH 7.0 is shown in the inset. An adjuvant-active equilibrium isomer (representing migration of fatty acid from position 4 to position 3 of fucose) of QS-21 appears first. This is followed by the appearance of the triterpene glycoside degradation product resulting from hydrolysis at the site noted in Fig. 1. Degradation rates were determined from the disappearance of the major and minor QS-21 equilibrium isomers.

mycobacterial muramyl dipeptide immunostimulant in a water-in-oil emulsion vehicle (Freund, 1956). Another example is the Ribi Detox™ formulation, consisting of monophosphoryl lipid A and cell wall skeleton immunostimulants in a squalene emulsion (Mitchell *et al.,* 1988). QS-21 is best defined as an immunostimulant rather than as a vehicle. In contrast to other adjuvant systems, it is typically used in absence of a carrier vehicle, and is effective in aqueous solution. QS-21 is water soluble (up to 30 mg/mL in PBS), and so does not require emulsification (Kensil *et al.,* 1991a). It has also been noted, however, that QS-21 is equally effective when added to aluminum hydroxide-absorbed antigens (Wu *et al.,* 1992).

3.3. Stability

In the solid state, QS-21 is stable for many years, even with storage at ambient temperature. Stability is lower in aqueous solution (Kensil *et al.,* 1995). The primary degradation reaction is an alkaline-catalyzed hydrolysis of the ester bond between fucose and the fatty acid domain (Fig. 1), generating two by-products that do not have adjuvant activity. Stability of QS-21 solutions is monitored by HPLC (Fig. 3). QS-21 can be stabilized by the use of lower pH and higher QS-21 concentration in formulations (Fig. 3), factors to consider when formulating vaccine that might be used in countries where access to refrigeration is limited. A reversible acyl migration of the fatty acid domain from position 4 of fucose to position 3 of fucose has also been noted in aqueous solution, with the 4 position being favored; both of these isomeric forms of QS-21 are adjuvant active.

4. ADJUVANT ACTIVITY

4.1. Antibody Response

4.1.1. ENHANCEMENT OF ANTIBODY RESPONSES TO T-DEPENDENT ANTIGENS

QS-21 has potent activity for induction of antibody to soluble T-dependent antigens. Indeed, QS-21 was first identified as an adjuvant by the demonstration that this saponin markedly increased the antigen-specific IgG response to bovine serum albumin (BSA) administered intradermally in mice (Kensil *et al.,* 1991a). The adjuvant effect, which increased the total IgG titer to BSA more than 1000-fold after two immunizations, was maximal at 5 μg of QS-21 and did not increase with increasing dose up to 80 μg. A QS-21 dose–response study carried out in C57BL/6 mice with the antigen ovalbumin (OVA) confirmed that the adjuvant effect of QS-21 in mice nears its peak response (approximately 100-fold increase in IgG to OVA) at a minimum QS-21 dose of 5 μg and a minimum OVA dose of 5 μg (Kensil *et al.,* 1993). Higher doses of QS-21 did not decrease the IgG titers. In that study, it was noted that 1 μg of OVA adjuvanted with 5 μg of QS-21 elicited superior titers than that elicited by 125 μg of OVA without adjuvant.

QS-21 can act as co-adjuvant with aluminum hydroxide (alum)-absorbed antigens, thereby stimulating higher antibody titers than those induced by alum alone. This was demonstrated in mice with a recombinant feline leukemia virus (FeLV) subunit vaccine based on the viral envelope protein gp70 (Kensil *et al.,* 1991b). A vaccine formulation consisting of gp70 absorbed to aluminum hydroxide elicited lower titers both to gp70 and to FeLV than the same formulation with added QS-21. QS-21 was also used to adjuvant recombinant HIV-1$_{IIIB}$ gp160 absorbed to alum (Wu *et al.,* 1992). The recombinant gp160/QS-21/alum combination induced titers in BALB/c mice that were 25- to 125-fold higher than those induced by the gp160/alum formulation alone.

Side-by-side comparisons of aluminum hydroxide-absorbed antigen/QS-21 formulations with soluble antigen/QS-21 formulations were not tested in either the FeLV or HIV studies. However, a direct comparison of anti-OVA IgG titers elicited by soluble OVA/QS-21 to those elicited by alum-absorbed OVA/QS-21 in C57BL/6 mice suggested that QS-21 alone was as effective an adjuvant as a combination of alum/QS-21 (Kensil *et al.,* 1993).

QS-21 has been compared to other adjuvants for induction of antigen-specific antibody. Kensil *et al.* (1991a) showed that 20 μg of QS-21 induced antibody titers to beef liver cytochrome b$_5$ that were equivalent to those induced by complete Freund's adjuvant, incomplete Freund's adjuvant, and a mixture of monophosphoryl lipid A/trehalose dimycolate in a squalene emulsion. Table I details four additional adjuvant comparison studies. Two of these studies showed the adjuvant effect with hapten-carrier antigens. For the

Table I

Comparison of QS-21 with Other Adjuvants

Antigen	Adjuvant	IgG titer	Reference
OVA[a]	None	<10	Kensil *et al.* (1993)
	Alum	70	"
	QS-21 (20 μg)	630	"
gp70[b]	Alum	40	Kensil and Marciani (1991)
	Alum + QS-21 (10 μg)	1,000	"
Hgp30–KLH[c]	Alum	400 (hapten)	Kirkley *et al.* (1992)
		400 (carrier)	
	QS-21 (20 μg)	6,400 (hapten)	"
		6,400 (carrier)	
TF–KLH[d]	None	20 (hapten)	Livingston *et al.* (1992)
		160 (carrier)	
	CFA	40 (hapten)	"
		640 (carrier)	
	Detox	40 (hapten)	"
		320 (carrier)	
	SAF-m	>10,000 (hapten)	"
		10,240 (carrier)	
	QS-21 (10 μg)	>10,000 (hapten)	"
		10,240 (carrier)	

[a] C57BL/6 mice (ten per group) were immunized s.c. at 0 and 2 weeks with OVA (25 μg) and indicated adjuvant. Antigen-specific IgG titers were determined at 4 weeks. Alum = 250 μg aluminum hydroxide (Superfos s/a).

[b] CD-1 mice (five per group) were immunized once i.d. with FeLV rgp70 (15 μg) and indicated adjuvant. Antigen-specific IgG titers (at cutoff of 0.25 absorbance) were determined at 4 weeks. Alum = 500 μg aluminum hydroxide (Superfos s/a).

[c] BALB/c mice (nine to ten per group) were immunized once s.c. with Hgp30–KLH conjugate (25 μg) and indicated adjuvant. Antigen-specific IgG titers were determined at 8 weeks. Hgp30 = synthetic peptide representing amino acids 85 to 114 of HIV-1 p17 gag protein. KLH carrier = keyhole limpet hemocyanin. Alum = 75 μg aluminum hydroxide (Superfos s/a).

[d] BALB/c–C57BL/6 F_1 mice (five per group) were immunized s.c. with TF–KLH conjugate (25 μg) at 0, 2, and 4 weeks. Antigen-specific IgG titers were determined at 6 weeks. TF = Thomsen–Friedenreich antigen (Galβ1-3GalNAcα-O-serine/threonine). Detox = 2.5 μg monophosphoryl lipid A and 25 μg bacillus Calmette–Guérin cell wall skeleton obtained from Ribi ImmunoChem (Hamilton, MT). SAF-m = Syntex Adjuvant Formulation consisting of threonyl MDP, squalane, Pluronic L121 block polymer, and Tween 80.

peptide hapten Hgp30 coupled to the carrier KLH (Hgp30–KLH), QS-21 improved titers to both hapten and KLH over those induced by alum (Kirkley *et al.*, 1992). For the polysaccharide hapten TF coupled to KLH, QS-21 induced higher titers to hapten and carrier than complete Freund's adjuvant and Ribi Detox and that were equivalent to titers induced by SAF-m (Livingston *et al.*, 1992).

Recently, it has become clear that adjuvants can influence the IgG subclass profile (Allison and Byars, 1986). It has been noted in murine studies that aluminum hydroxide promotes primarily the formation of IgG1, whereas the adjuvant SAF-1 also promotes the formation of IgG2b and IgG2a (Allison and Byars, 1986), mouse IgG subclasses that are typically involved in antibody-dependent cellular cytotoxicity and complement fixation via the classic pathway (Klaus *et al.*, 1979). The profile of mouse IgG subclass after vaccination has been correlated with the subset of Th cells produced, with predominant IgG1 responses being associated with a Th2-predominant response, and IgG2a responses being associated with a Th1-predominant response (Stevens *et al.*, 1988). QS-21 is noted for shifting predominant IgG1 responses to a profile that includes significant IgG2b and IgG2a responses. This has been noted for cytochrome b_5 (Kensil *et al.*, 1991a), recombinant *Borrelia burgdorferi* OspA and OspB (Ma *et al.*, 1994), and OVA (Kensil *et al.*, 1993). The addition of QS-21 to an aluminum hydroxide-associated antigen [recombinant FeLV gp70 (Kensil *et al.*, 1991b) or OVA (Kensil *et al.*, 1993)] clearly shifts the isotype profile from the typical response invoked by alum alone (predominantly IgG1) to a subclass response that is more typically associated with a QS-21-adjuvanted vaccine. This suggests that QS-21 actively sets up a Th1-predominant response.

The QS-21-mediated increase in IgG2a and IgG2b titers, which are noted as complement-fixing antibody isotypes in mice, was correlated with bactericidal activity in sera induced with experimental Lyme vaccine formulations. An OspA formulation adjuvanted with QS-21 induced a titer for complement-mediated lysis of spirochetes that was 16-fold higher than that induced by the same antigen adjuvanted with aluminum hydroxide (Ma *et al.*, 1994) when tested in C3H/Hej mice.

The activity of QS-21 for enhancing antigen-specific proliferative responses was assessed with an experimental HIV-1 recombinant gp160 vaccine in BALB/c mice (Wu *et al.*, 1992). Proliferative responses of splenic mononuclear cells harvested after three subcutaneous immunizations were determined. Antigen-specific proliferative responses were observed only at high in vitro antigen concentration if aluminum hydroxide was utilized as the adjuvant. However, proliferative responses were also observed at low in vitro antigen concentration if 10 μg of QS-21 was added to the recombinant antigen/aluminum hydroxide formulations.

4.1.2. ENHANCEMENT OF ANTIBODY RESPONSES TO T-INDEPENDENT ANTIGENS

Enhancement of immune responses to T-independent antigens such as bacterial polysaccharides has typically required the conjugation of these antigens to a carrier such as diphtheria toxoid or KLH in order to provide T-cell help to the polysaccharide. However, QS-21 was shown to adjuvant an unconjugated polysaccharide (PS) isolated by acid hydrolysis of phenol-extracted *E. coli* 055:B5 and shown to be free of contaminating LPS and lipid A (White *et al.*, 1991). The total antibody response to PS antigen, administered intradermally to CD-1 mice on days 0 and 14, was enhanced tenfold by the addition of 15 μg of QS-21. Adjuvant responses were observed in the IgM, IgG3, and particularly the IgG2b and IgG2a subclasses. The inclusion of an oil/water emulsion in the QS-21/PS formulation neither suppressed nor enhanced the immune response.

QS-21 also enhanced LPS-specific IgG2a response of mice to a vaccine consisting of a free PS isolated from the enterotoxigenic *E. coli* strain 018 (Coughlin *et al.*, 1994). The immunogenicity of the vaccine was further increased by conjugation of PS to diphtheria toxoid. QS-21 enhanced antibody response both to the PS and to the carrier.

4.2. Cell-Mediated Immune Response

An important effector mechanism of cell-mediated immunity (CMI) is the development of $CD8^+$ cytotoxic T lymphocytes. This occurs typically as a sequela to viral infection
as a result of endogenous viral antigen expression and is not a typical response to
exogenously added antigen (as with a subunit vaccine). Adjuvants or delivery systems that
direct subunit antigens into the cytoplasm of APCs (MHC class I pathway of antigen
presentation) rather than into the endosomal compartment (MHC class II pathway of
antigen presentation) will influence the immune response to give a CTL response. These
delivery systems include incorporating antigen into membrane fusogenic liposomes
(Miller *et al.*, 1992), conjugating antigen to lipopeptides that facilitate attachment to plasma
membranes (Deres *et al.*, 1989), presenting antigen in ISCOMs (Takahashi *et al.*, 1990),
and other strategies.

QS-21 is a potent stimulator of $CD8^+$ CTL responses to subunit antigens. Wu *et al.*
(1992) noted that a formulation consisting of 10 μg QS-21, 25 μg of a recombinant
truncated HIV-1_{IIIB} gp160, and aluminum hydroxide induced a splenic mononuclear cell
population (after three immunizations of BALB/c mice) that lysed p815 target cells that
were infected with gp120 vaccinia, but not those infected with control vaccinia. This
response was not observed with the protein/aluminum hydroxide formulation without
QS-21. Maturation of the effector CTLs by in vitro stimulation with P18(IIIB) peptide
was required for the observation of the lytic activity.

Newman *et al.* (1992a) confirmed QS-21-mediated induction of CTLs to subunit
antigen using OVA as immunogen and E.G7-OVA cells for targets. CTLs were induced in
a QS-21 dose-dependent manner, with as little as 2.5 μg QS-21 inducing a significant CTL
response to native OVA after three immunizations. The effector cell population was
confirmed as $CD8^+$ via depletion of either $CD4^+$ or $CD8^+$ cells after antigen stimulation
and prior to the CTL assay. As with the HIV-1 study, CTL activity was observed only after
in vitro antigen stimulation either with processed antigen or with soluble, unprocessed
antigen. In contrast to other formulations that have been tested to induce CTLs, the
formulations used to set up the responses reported in this study consisted simply of soluble
QS-21 and soluble OVA antigen.

HIV-1 peptide/QS-21 formulations have also been observed to induce CTLs (Shirai
et al., 1994). QS-21-adjuvanted formulations consisting of various synthetic peptides that
contained the gp160 immunodominant CTL epitope P18 and multideterminant Th epitopes
were administered subcutaneously to BALB/c mice and were shown to induce strong CTL
responses against P18 peptide-pulsed target cells at effector-to-target ratios as low as 7:1.
In the absence of QS-21, little CTL induction was observed.

4.3. Adjuvant Effect in Other Species

Most preclinical QS-21 evaluation studies have been carried out in mice. It has been
noted for other adjuvants that the adjuvant effect in small animals such as rodents is not
necessarily predictive of the adjuvant effect in large animal species such as goats and
baboons (Van Nest *et al.*, 1992). Interestingly, however, QS-21 has been shown to be
effective in several species, including nonhuman primates.

An example of adjuvant activity of QS-21 in dogs was shown with experimental Lyme vaccines. These vaccines, consisting of 25 μg each of *Borrelia burgdorferi* outer surface proteins OspA and OspB with and without 50 μg of QS-21, were tested by the subcutaneous route in beagles (see Chapter 32). The QS-21 vaccine induced IgG1 and IgG2 titers that were enhanced three- and fivefold, respectively, compared to the vaccine without QS-21.

Significant adjuvant activity has also been demonstrated in nonhuman primates. A dose of 50 μg was used to adjuvant an experimental recombinant HIV-1 gp160 vaccine in rhesus macaque (Newman *et al.*, 1992b). This vaccine induced considerably higher antibody titers than gp160 on alum. The administration of QS-21 did not alter preexisting immune responses to tetanus toxoid, suggesting that its adjuvant effect was limited to the vaccine antigen and that it did not act as a general immunostimulant. After vaccination, the macaques were rested for several months and were then inoculated with soluble, recombinant gp160. All animals (3/3) receiving the vaccine with QS-21 as adjuvant responded with a proliferative response to gp160 whereas none of the three animals receiving an alum-adjuvanted vaccine responded. Hence, QS-21 was demonstrated both to serve as an adjuvant in a nonhuman primate, and to invoke immunological memory. Powell *et al.* (1994) demonstrated that QS-21 significantly increased titers to HIV-1 gp120 in baboons when compared to alum. Interestingly, QS-21 also elicited earlier seroconversion. More recently, it has been demonstrated by Newman *et al.* (1994) that vaccination of rhesus macaques with a recombinant SIV gp120 adjuvanted with QS-21 sets up both CD4[+] and CD8[+] mediated CTL response (measured in PBL after in vitro stimulation with Con A, IL-2, and antigen).

5. MECHANISM OF ACTION

In contrast to other adjuvants such as MDP and LPS, the mechanism of action of QS-21 is poorly defined at the present. However, some recent studies have begun to address the mechanism of QS-21.

5.1. Effect of Accessory and Effector Cell Depletion on CTL and Antibody Response

Because it was observed earlier that alum-absorbed protein with added QS-21 could induce CTLs, it was proposed that phagocytic APCs, most likely macrophages, were the relevant APCs (Newman *et al.*, 1992a). The role of macrophages as APCs in the QS-21-mediated induction of CD8[+] CTLs was investigated by Wu *et al.* (1994). Phagocytic APCs were paralyzed by intraperitoneal injection of particulate silica or carrageenan prior to intraperitoneal immunization with OVA/QS-21. After a series of three silica treatments and immunizations, induction of precursor CTLs was assayed in splenocytes. Paralysis of macrophages by pretreatment with silica or carrageenan abrogated the CTL response (an example of the effect of silica treatment on CTL induction is shown in Fig. 4). In contrast, antigen-specific proliferative responses and specific antibody responses were largely unaffected. The CTL response in treated mice could be reconstituted by transfer of macrophages from naive mice prior to immunization. Phagocytic APCs were also shown to play a significant role in antigen processing and presentation for the in vitro CTL

Figure 4. Effect of in vivo immune deficiencies on QS-21-mediated induction of cytotoxic T-lymphocyte response. Mice were immunized s.c. with OVA (25 μg) and QS-21 at 0, 2, and 4 weeks. Splenic mononuclear cells were harvested at 6 weeks, were in vitro stimulated with mitomycin C-treated E.G7-OVA cells to induce CTL maturation, and used as effector cells for lysis of an OVA-expressing syngeneic cell line (^{51}Cr-labeled E.G7-OVA cells) as described in Wu et al. (1994). Data shown are from an effector-to-target ratio of 25: 1. Mouse strain used for the normal population was C57BL/6. APCs of C57BL/6 mice were paralyzed by preinjection with silica daily for the 2 days prior to each immunization. CD4[+] cell-deficient mice were C2D. CD8[+] cell-deficient mice were C1D. Both CD4[+] and CD8[+] mice were haplotype matched to C57BL/6. Data are adapted from Wu et al. (1994).

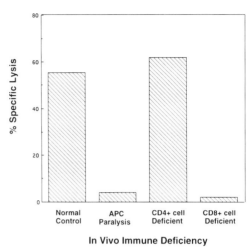

maturation step. Splenocytes depleted of macrophages did not process and present soluble antigen although they were still capable of presenting preprocessed antigen. Splenocytes depleted of dendritic cells were only marginally affected in their ability to process and present antigen, suggesting that macrophages play a critical role as APCs in QS-21-mediated CD8[+] CTL responses.

CD4[+] cells as accessory cells were expected to contribute to the CTL response by providing cytokine help (Wu et al., 1994). Elimination of CD4[+] cells as accessory cells via pretreatment with anti-CD4 rat monoclonal antibody GK1.5 did not affect the CTL response, although the antibody response was eliminated and antigen-specific proliferative response was reduced. This was confirmed in transgenic mice that were genetically deficient in CD4[+] cells as a result of a defect in MHC class II genes. Formulations consisting of OVA and QS-21 induced a CTL response in CD4[+] cell-deficient animals that was comparable to normal controls (Fig. 4), indicating that cytokines produced by CD8[+] cells and macrophages were sufficient to prime for the CTL response. The role of CD8[+] cells as the effectors of the CTL response was confirmed by immunization of transgenic mice that were deficient in CD8[+] cells; these mice did not produce detectable CTLs.

5.2. Cytokine Profile Induced by QS-21-Adjuvanted Vaccines

The regulatory functions of T cells and macrophages are in part mediated by Th cell-derived cytokines. The effects of QS-21 on induction of IgG2a antibody and on induction of CD8[+] CTLs (responses typically dependent on IL-2 and IFN-γ, cytokines produced by Th1 subset) suggest that QS-21 is activating cells that produce these cytokines. In order to understand the CTL mechanism of action of QS-21, the effect of QS-21 and other adjuvants on the cytokine secretion profile and resulting CTL response of splenocytes from immunized C57BL/6 mice was assessed (Pozzi, Wu, and Newman, unpublished data).

C57BL/6 mice were immunized subcutaneously with 25 μg/dose of OVA formulated with QS-21 (20 μg/dose), aluminum hydroxide (250 μg), or emulsified in CFA using a three-dose regimen at 0, 2, and 4 weeks. IFA was used in the booster shots in the Freund's adjuvant arm of the study. At week 6, splenic mononuclear cells were harvested, restimulated in vitro for 6 days with denatured OVA antigen to induce CTL maturation, and then assayed for CTL activity using E.G7-OVA cells. Cytokines IL-2 and IFN-γ are known to play a role in the maturation of CTL (Maraskovsky *et al.*, 1989). Hence, these were assayed in the spleen cell supernatants at daily intervals during the 6-day stimulation with antigen to induce CTL maturation (Fig. 5A,B), using separate culture wells for each time point. The highest levels of IL-2 and IFN-γ were observed in the splenocytes primed by immunization with OVA/QS-21. Considerably lower levels were produced by splenocytes primed by immunization with OVA/CFA or OVA/aluminum hydroxide. Significant IL-6

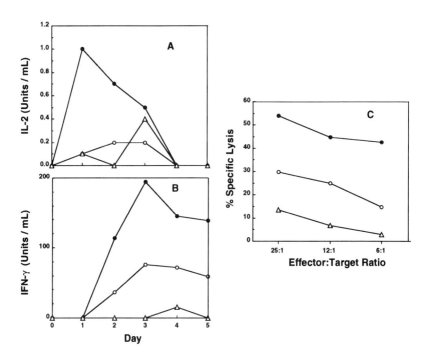

Figure 5. Effect of adjuvants on splenocyte secretion of cytokines IL-2 and IFN-γ during antigen stimulation and on CTL responses after antigen stimulation. Splenocytes were harvested from C57BL/6 mice 2 weeks after the last of three subcutaneous immunizations with OVA (25 μg) and either QS-21 (●), CFA/IFA (○), or aluminum hydroxide (Δ). Splenocytes were in vitro stimulated for 6 days with denatured OVA to induce antigen-specific CD8[+] CTLs. Panels A and B show the quantity of IL-2 and IFN-γ (units/mL) in the splenocyte supernatants at daily intervals during the CTL maturation step. At the end of the in vitro culture, splenocytes were assayed for lytic activity on ^{51}Cr-labeled E.G7-OVA cells. Panel C shows the CTL response after background subtraction of the lysis of a control cell line (EL4 cells).

was also noted in the QS-21-primed cells (data not shown). IL-6 is known to enhance the differentiation of CTLs in the presence of IL-2 and IFN-γ. The appearance of these three cytokines in culture after immunization with OVA/QS-21 suggests that the activation of Th1 cells by subunit antigen is enhanced by QS-21, and that this enhancement plays a role in the induction of CTLs to subunit antigens. This enhancement is reflected in the CTL response (Fig. 5C). Antigen-stimulated splenocytes from mice immunized with OVA/QS-21 had considerable CTL activity; lower-level CTL responses were induced after immunization with OVA/CFA and even lower responses after immunization with OVA/alum. A similar result on CTL induction was noted after immunization with the same three adjuvants with the human cytomegalovirus antigen gB in BALB/c mice (W. Britt, personal communication).

The effect of QS-21 on the isotype profile also suggests a predominant stimulation of Th1 cells. Immunization with QS-21 did not enhance the levels of the primary cytokines associated with Th2 cells (IL-4 and IL-5) over those induced by immunization with aluminum hydroxide (data not shown). These data, together with the data that immunization with OVA/QS-21 induces a population of splenocytes that produces IL-2 and IFN-γ in response to antigen, provide direct evidence that QS-21 primarily induces Th1-type cytokines. IFN-γ promotes the production of IgG2a and inhibits the action of IL-4 (Snapper and Paul, 1987), a response that correlates well with the observation that QS-21 is a potent stimulator of IgG2a antibody.

5.3. Structure/Function Studies

QS-21 is a complex triterpene glycoside. The structural heterogeneity of naturally occurring *Quillaja* saponins with adjuvant activity suggests that some of the glycoside moieties on QS-21 are unlikely to be important for adjuvant effect. QS-17, which differs from QS-21 primarily in glycosylation with a terminal glucose at the 3 position of rhamnose and with a terminal rhamnose on the fatty acid domain arabinose, is adjuvant-active for stimulation of antibody, suggesting that these regions of the molecule are not involved in stimulation of antibody response (Kensil *et al.*, 1992).

A derivative of QS-21 in which the fatty acid domain has been depleted has also been tested for stimulation of antibody. This derivative was shown to be inactive (Kensil *et al.*, 1992). The fatty acid domain was also shown to be inactive as an adjuvant (Kensil, unpublished data).

Additional sites have been modified in an attempt to further define critical sites. QS-21 was modified by conjugation of a small molecule, glycine, to the glucuronic acid via the carboxyl group on this sugar. This modification did not affect the charge of the QS-21 and increased the size by less than 5%. Despite this minimal change, the minimum dose of modified QS-21 for adjuvant activity was increased severalfold compared to intact QS-21 (Fig. 6). However, at sufficiently high doses, the same increase in antibody titers was observed. One possibility is that the glycyl modification sterically interferes with a nearby critical site. In contrast, modification of QS-21 by conjugation of ethylamine to the triterpene aldehyde eliminated the adjuvant effect over the range tested, suggesting that the aldehyde is critical for adjuvant effect. Studies are ongoing to assess whether the aldehyde is involved in binding to antigen or to a cellular target.

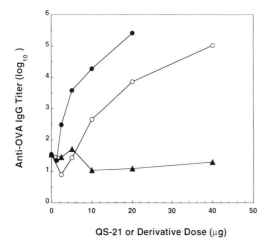

Figure 6. Effect of modification of glucuronic acid and triterpene aldehyde on adjuvant activity. IgG response to ovalbumin after two s.c. immunizations with ovalbumin ($25\,\mu g$) and the indicated doses of intact QS-21 (●), QS-21 conjugated to glycine at the glucuronic acid carboxyl group (○), and QS-21 conjugated to ethylamine through the triterpene aldehyde (▲). C57BL/6 mice (ten per group) were immunized at 0 and 2 weeks. Sera were collected at week 3 for analysis of ovalbumin-specific IgG by EIA.

6. CLINICAL EXPERIENCE WITH QS-21

Prior to clinical trials, QS-21 was tested extensively in preclinical animal trials. Studies in rhesus macaques showed that QS-21 was safely used at a s.c. dose of $50\,\mu g$ (Newman *et al.*, 1992b). Studies in New Zealand white rabbits showed that i.m. injection of QS-21 into the quadriceps muscle at doses up to $200\,\mu g$ was well tolerated, with no evidence of compound-related toxicity noted in clinical observations or serum chemistry. The majority of these injections were not associated with injection site reactogenicity. Where noted, these reactions were observed only on microscopic examination and consisted of moderate granulomatous inflammation and necrosis.

The first clinical experience with QS-21 was in experimental melanoma vaccines tested in patients with melanoma tumors at Memorial Sloan Kettering Cancer Center (1992). It was initially tested with the ganglioside melanoma antigen GM2 (which was coupled to a carrier, KLH). Despite coupling of this T-independent antigen to the KLH carrier to provide T-cell help, this antigen is typically ineffective in inducing IgG, inducing only low-level IgM responses with no IgG responses noted. The addition of $100\,\mu g$ of QS-21 to the vaccine resulted in six of six patients responding with IgG titers to GM2, some as high as 1280 after four immunizations (Livingston *et al.*, 1994). Some adjuvant effect was also observed at a QS-21 dose of $50\,\mu g$. The GM2-specific IgG response to GM2–KLH formulated with $100\,\mu g$ of QS-21 was higher than GM2–KLH formulated with other adjuvants (Livingston, 1993).

A dose-range study demonstrated that a 100-μg dose of QS-21 could be used safely without systemic effects (Livingston *et al.*, 1994). Moderate transient erythema with local tenderness (not requiring narcotic analgesics), attributed to QS-21, was noted after s.c. injections of $100\,\mu g$ QS-21 with GM2–KLH. These local reactions were observed for 2 to 4 days postimmunization. No ulceration, drainage, or nodules were noted. A higher dose of QS-21 ($200\,\mu g$) was associated with mild systemic effects [mild flu-like symptoms including low-grade fever (<38.5°C), headache, and myalgia lasting 8 to 24 h] after approximately 30% of the injections.

A Phase I AIDS vaccine trial comparing QS-21 and aluminum hydroxide as adjuvants for an HIV-1 gp120 vaccine is under way in healthy volunteers. To date, more than 100 healthy volunteers have received vaccine containing QS-21 without significant side effects; however, no immunogenicity data are yet available on these vaccine formulations. The current preclinical and clinical toxicology data on QS-21 suggest that it is acceptable for use in vaccines for healthy adults. Additional preclinical toxicology studies are under way to determine whether QS-21 is suitable for pediatric vaccines.

7. SUMMARY AND FUTURE DIRECTIONS

The properties of QS-21 adjuvant can be briefly summarized. It is a highly purified water-soluble triterpene glycoside that can be used in vaccines in the absence of emulsion-type formulations. Preliminary clinical testing suggests that QS-21 acts as an adjuvant in animals and humans, with an acceptable toxicological profile, and hence may have great utility as an adjuvant in commercial vaccines.

QS-21 adjuvant is novel in its induction of immune responses to subunit antigens that are more typically associated with an immune response to viral vectors, such as induction of IgG2a antibody and the induction of CD8$^+$ CTLs. Future studies will be directed toward determining the cellular events involved in the QS-21 adjuvant effect.

ACKNOWLEDGMENTS

We thank L. Pozzi and M. Newman (Vaxcel, Inc., Norcross, GA), A. Lim and N. Jacobsen (Genentech, Inc., South San Francisco, CA), W. Britt (University of Alabama, Birmingham), and D. Bedore (Cambridge Biotech Corp., Worcester, MA) for personal communication of unpublished data reported herein and J. Recchia and G. Beltz for helpful comments. A portion of the research reported here was supported by PHS-NIH grant AI33223 and was conducted according to the principles outlined in the "Guide for the Care and Use of Laboratory Animals," Institute of Laboratory Animals Resources, National Research Council.

REFERENCES

Allison, A. C., and Byars, N. E., 1986, An adjuvant formulation that selectively elicits the formation of antibodies of protective isotypes by cell-mediated immunity, *J. Immunol. Methods* **95**:157.
Campbell, J. B., and Peerbaye, Y. A., 1992, Saponin, *Res. Immunol.* **143**(5):526–530.
Coughlin, R. T., Chu, C., Fattom, A., White, A. C., and Winston, S., 1995, Adjuvant activity of QS-21 for experimental *E. coli* 018 polysaccharide vaccines, *Vaccine* **13**: 17–21.
Dalsgaard, K., 1970, Thin-layer chromatographic fingerprinting of commercially available saponins, *Dan. Tidsskr. Farm.* **44**:327–331.
Dalsgaard, K., 1974, Saponin adjuvants. III. Isolation of a substance from *Quillaja saponaria* Molina with adjuvant activity in foot-and-mouth disease vaccines, *Arch. Gesamte Virusforsch.* **44**:243–254.
Deres, K., Schild, H., Wiesmüller, K., Jung, G., and Rammensee, H., 1989, In vivo priming of cytotoxic T lymphocytes with synthetic lipopeptide vaccine, *Nature* **342**:561–564.

Espinet, R. G., 1951, Nouveau vaccin antiaphteux a complexe glucoviral, *Gac. Vet.* **13**:268.

Freund, J., 1956, The mode of action of immunological adjuvants, *Adv. Tuberc. Res.* **7**:130–148.

Higuchi, R., Tokimitsu, Y., and Komori, T., 1988, An acylated triterpenoid saponin from *Quillaja saponaria, Phytochemistry* **27**:1165–1168.

Kensil, C. R., and Marciani, D. J., 1991, Saponin adjuvant, U.S. Patent #5,057,540.

Kensil, C. R., Patel, U., Lennick, M., and Marciani, D., 1991a, Separation and characterization of saponins with adjuvant activity from *Quillaja saponaria* Molina cortex, *J. Immunol.* **146**:431–437.

Kensil, C. R., Barrett, C., Kushner, N., Beltz, G., Storey, J., Patel, U., Recchia, J., Aubert, A., and Marciani, D., 1991b, Development of a genetically engineered vaccine against feline leukemia virus infection, *J. Am. Vet. Med. Assoc.* **199**:1423–1427.

Kensil, C. R., Soltysik, S., Patel, U., and Marciani, D. J., 1992, Structure/function relationship in adjuvants from Quillaja saponaria Molina, in: *Vaccines 92* (F. Brown, R. M. Chanock, H. S. Ginsberg, and R. A. Lerner, eds.), Cold Spring Harbor Laboratory Press, Cold Spring Harbor, NY, pp. 35–40.

Kensil, C. R., Newman, M. J., Coughlin, R. T., Soltysik, S., Bedore, D., Recchia, J., Wu, J.-Y., and Marciani, D. J., 1993, The use of Stimulon adjuvant to boost vaccine response, *Vaccine Res.* **2**:273–281.

Kensil, C. R., Bedore, A., Cleland, J. L., Lim, A., Jacobsen, N., and Powell, M. F., 1995, Stability of QS-21 in aqueous solutions, (in preparation).

Kersten, G. F. A., Teerlink, T., Derks, H. J. G. M., Verkleij, A. J., van Wezel, T. L., Crommelin, D. J. A., and Beuvery, E. C., 1988, Incorporation of the major outer membrane protein of *Neisseria gonorrhoeae* in saponin–lipid complexes (Iscoms): Chemical analysis, some structural features, and comparison of their immunogenicity with three other antigen delivery systems, *Infect. Immun.* **56**:432–438.

Kirkley, J. E., Naylor, P. H., Marciani, D. J., Kensil, C. R., Newman, M. J., and Goldstein, A. L., 1992, QS-21 augments the antibody response to a synthetic peptide vaccine compared to alum, in: *Combination Therapies* (A. L. Goldstein and E. Garaci, eds.), Plenum Press, New York, pp. 231–236.

Klaus, G. G. B., Pepys, M. B., Kitajima, K., and Askonas, B. A., 1979, Activation of mouse complement by different classes of mouse antibody, *Immunology* **38**:687–695.

Livingston, P. O., 1993, Approaches to augmenting the IgG antibody response to melanoma ganglioside vaccines, *Ann. N.Y. Acad. Sci.* **690**:204–213.

Livingston, P. O., Koganty, R. B. M., Longenecker, B. M., Lloyd, K. O., and Calves, M., 1992, Studies on the immunogenicity of synthetic and natural Thomsen–Friedenreich (TF) antigens in mice: Augmentation of the response by Quil A and Saf-M adjuvants and analysis of the specificity of the responses, *Vaccine Res.* **1(2)**:99–109.

Livingston, P. O., Adluri, S., Helling, F., Yao, T.-J., Kensil, C. R., Newman, M. J., and Marciani, D., 1994, Phase I trial of immunological adjuvant QS-21 with a GM2 ganglioside–KLH conjugate vaccine in patients with malignant melanoma, *Vaccine* **12**:1275–1280.

Ma, J., Bulger, P. A., Davis, D.vR., Perilli-Palmer, B., Bedore, D. A., Kensil, C. R., Young, E. M., Hung, C. H., Seals, J. R., Pavia, C. S., and Coughlin, R. T., 1994, Impact of the saponin adjuvant QS-21 and aluminum hydroxide on the immunogenicity of recombinant OspA and OspB of *Borrelia burgdorferi, Vaccine* **12**:925–932.

Maraskovsky, E., Chen, W.-F., and Shortman, K., 1989, IL-2 and IFN-γ are two necessary lymphokines in the development of cytolytic T cells, *J. Immunol.* **143**:1210–1214.

Marciani, D. J., Kensil, C. R., Beltz, G. A., Hung, C.-H., Cronier, J., and Aubert, A., 1991, Genetically-engineered subunit vaccine against feline leukemia virus: protective immune response in cats, *Vaccine* **9**:89–96.

Miller, M. D., Gould-Fogerite, S., Shen, L., Woods, R. M., Koenig, S., Mannino, R. J., and Letvin, N. L., 1992, Vaccination of rhesus monkeys with synthetic peptide in a fusogenic proteoliposome elicits simian immunodeficiency virus-specific $CD8^+$ cytotoxic T lymphocytes, *J. Exp. Med.* **176**:1739–1744.

Mitchell, M. D., Kan-Mitchell, J., Kempf, R. A., Harel, W., Shan, H., and Lind, S., 1988, Active specific immunotherapy for melanoma: Phase I trial of allogeneic lysates and a novel adjuvant, *Cancer Res.* **48**:5883–5889.

Morein, B., Sundquist, B., Hoglund, S., Dalsgaard, K., and Osterhaus, A., 1984, Iscom, a novel structure for antigenic presentation of membrane proteins from enveloped viruses, *Nature* **308**:457–460.

Newman, M. J., Wu, J.-Y., Gardner, B. H., Munroe, K. J., Leombruno, D., Recchia, J., Kensil, C. R., and Coughlin, R. T., 1992a, Saponin adjuvant induction of ovalbumin-specific CD8$^+$ cytotoxic T lymphocyte responses, *J. Immunol.* **148**:2357–2362.

Newman, M. J., Wu, J.-Y., Coughlin, R. T., Murphy, C. I., Seals, J. R., Wyand, M. S., and Kensil, C. R., 1992b, Immunogenicity and toxicity testing of an experimental HIV-1 vaccine in nonhuman primates, *AIDS Res. Hum. Retroviruses* **8**:1413–1418.

Newman, M. J., Munroe, K. J., Anderson, C. A., Murphy, C. I., Panicali, D. L., Seals, J. R., Wu, J.-Y., Wyand, M. S., and Kensil, C. R., 1994, Induction of antigen-specific cytotoxic T lymphocytes using subunit SIV mac251 gag and env vaccines containing QS-21 saponin adjuvant, *AIDS Res. Hum. Retroviruses* **10(7)**:853–861.

Powell, M. F., Cleland, J. L., Murthy, K., Eastman, D. J., Lim, A., Newman, M. J., Nunberg, J. H., Weissburg, R. P., Vennari, J. C., Wrin, T., and Berman, P. W., 1994, Immunogenicity and HIV-1 virus neutralization of the MN rgp120/HIV-1 QS-21 vaccine in baboons, *AIDS Res. Hum. Retroviruses* **10(Suppl. 1)**:S85–S88.

Shirai, M., Pendleton, C. D., Ahlers, J., Takeshita, T., Newman, M., and Berzofsky, J. A., 1994, Helper-cytotoxic T lymphocyte (CTL) determinant linkage required for priming of anti-HIV CD8$^+$ CTL in vivo with peptide vaccine constructs, *J. Immunol.* **152**:549–556.

Snapper, C. M., and Paul, W. E., 1987, Interferon-γ and B cell stimulatory factor-1 reciprocally regulate Ig isotype production, *Science* **236**:944–947.

Stevens, T. L., Bossie, A., Sanders, V. M., Fernandez-Botran, R., Coffman, R. L., Mossman, T. R., and Vitetta, E. S., 1988, Regulation of antibody isotype secretion by subsets of antigen-specific helper T cells, *Nature* **334**:255–258.

Strobbe, R., Charlier, G., van Aert, A., Debecq, J., and Leunen, J., 1974, Studies about the adjuvant activity of saponin fractions in foot-and-mouth disease vaccine. II. Irritant and adjuvant activity of saponin fractions obtained by chromatography on Sephadex G100, *Arch. Exp. Vet. Med.* **28**:385–392.

Takahashi, H., Takeshita, T., Morein, B., Putney, S., Germain, R. N., and Berzofsky, J. A., 1990, Induction of CD8$^+$ cytotoxic T cells by immunization with purified HIV-1 envelope protein in ISCOMs, *Nature* **344**:873–875.

Van Nest, G. A., Steimer, K. S., Haigwood, N. L., Burke, R. L., and Ott, G., 1992, Advanced adjuvant formulations for use with recombinant subunit vaccines, in: *Vaccines 92: Modern Approaches to New Vaccines* (R. M. Chanock, R. A. Lerner, F. Brown, and H. Ginsburg, eds.), Cold Spring Harbor Laboratory Press, Cold Spring Harbor, NY, pp. 57–62.

White, A. C., Cloutier, P., and Coughlin, R. T., 1991, A purified saponin acts as an adjuvant for a T-independent antigen, in: *Immunobiology of Proteins and Peptides,* Vol. VI (M. Z. Atassi, ed.), Plenum Press, New York, pp. 207–210.

Wu, J.-Y., Gardner, B. H., Murphy, C. I., Seals, J. R., Kensil, C. R., Recchia, J., Beltz, G. A., Newman, G. W., and Newman, M. J., 1992, Saponin adjuvant enhancement of antigen-specific immune responses to an experimental HIV-1 vaccine, *J. Immunol.* **148**:1519–1525.

Wu, J.-Y., Gardner, B. H., Kushner, N. N., Pozzi, L. M., Kensil, C. R., Cloutier, P. A., Coughlin, R. T., and Newman, M. J., 1994, Accessory cell requirements for saponin adjuvant-induced class I MHC antigen-restricted cytotoxic T-lymphocytes, *Cell. Immunol.* **154**:393–406.

Chapter 23

A Novel Generation of Viral Vaccines Based on the ISCOM Matrix

G. F. Rimmelzwaan and A. D. M. E. Osterhaus

1. INTRODUCTION

The outcome of the immune response to subunit antigen preparations will depend largely on the physical form in which the immunogens are presented to the immune system. Vaccines based on individual viral proteins or subunits consisting of one or more B- and T-cell epitopes in a monomeric form are often weakly immunogenic compared to live attenuated or inactivated whole virus vaccines (Morein *et al.,* 1983; Morein and Simons, 1985). To enhance the immunogenicity of viral subunits, adjuvants are usually needed. Although most adjuvants facilitate a better induction of immunity than the antigen or subunit alone, resulting in higher titers of specific antibodies and T-helper (Th) cell responses, they may not induce cytotoxic T-cell (CTL) responses very efficiently.

In this chapter we describe the immune-stimulating complex (ISCOM) matrix as a highly effective antigen presentation form for viral antigens. This antigen presentation form is presently being studied in many laboratories involved in the development of novel generations of virus vaccines, since it was shown to be a potent inducer of both B- and T (Th and CTL)-cell responses leading to solid and long-lasting immunity against many viral infections.

2. THE ISCOM STRUCTURE

2.1. Components, Chemical and Physical Properties

The ISCOM is a cagelike structure with a diameter of 30–40 nm into which antigens can be incorporated (Morein *et al.,* 1984). It consists of glycosides of the adjuvant Quil A,

G. F. Rimmelzwaan and A. D. M. E. Osterhaus • Department of Virology, Erasmus University Rotterdam, 3000 DR Rotterdam, The Netherlands.

Vaccine Design: The Subunit and Adjuvant Approach, edited by Michael F. Powell and Mark J. Newman. Plenum Press, New York, 1995.

cholesterol, the antigen, and in most cases phospholipids, such as phosphatidylcholine or -ethanolamine. Quil A is a preparation from the bark of *Quillaja saponaria* Molina, consisting of a refined mixture of closely related saponins. Quil A has potent adjuvant activity and is widely used as an adjuvant in veterinary vaccines. The adjuvant activity is related to the triterpene glycosides (Dalsgaard, 1978). The typical cagelike structure is formed by Quil A–cholesterol micelles, which are held together through hydrophobic interactions. The ISCOM structure has been shown to be extremely stable, to resist repeated freezing and thawing, and to remain intact on lyophilization (Morein *et al.*, 1984). For the formation of the ISCOM structure, Quil A glycosides are indispensable constituents. In combination with cholesterol they may form so-called "empty ISCOMs" (Lövgren and Morein, 1988; Bomford *et al.*, 1992). The protein incorporated into the ISCOM matrix does not have a major influence on the size or morphology of the ISCOM structure. For the incorporation of certain proteins the addition of phospholipids is necessary to provide a certain flexibility of the ISCOM matrix, enabling the incorporation of these proteins into the structure (Lövgren and Morein, 1988).

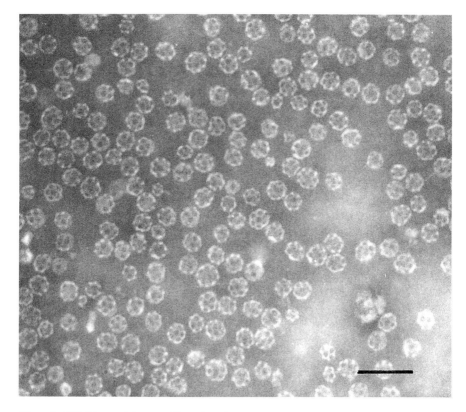

Figure 1. ISCOMs containing recombinant SIV glycoprotein after negative contrast electron microscopy. Bar = 100 nm. (Courtesy of E. Hulskotte for ISCOM preparation and K. Teppema for electron microscopy.)

2.2. Construction of ISCOMs

For the incorporation of viral membrane proteins into the ISCOM matrix, virus particles are usually solubilized by detergent to obtain them in noncomplexed monomeric forms. If necessary, the protein can be purified before ISCOMs are made. In the presence of cholesterol phospholipids and Quil A, ISCOMs will form spontaneously when the detergent is removed. The ratio of ISCOM components is critical. Generally, good results are obtained when cholesterol, aqueous protein solution, and Quil A are mixed together in a ratio of 1:1:5 (w/w/w), respectively. The detergent can be removed either by dialysis when dialyzable detergents such as octylglucoside or decanoyl-N-methyl glucamide (MEGA-10) are used, or by ultracentrifugation through sucrose gradients containing Quil A when nondialyzable detergents such as Triton X-100 are used. The formation of ISCOMs is usually demonstrated by negative contrast electron microscopy, revealing the typical cagelike morphology (Fig. 1). Most of the viral membrane proteins with their hydrophobic anchor sequences do not need special treatment prior to the formation of ISCOMs and are incorporated spontaneously (Rimmelzwaan *et al.,* 1994). Other proteins without hydrophobic transmembrane sequences can be incorporated into ISCOMs, but then pretreatment is required. To this end, the protein may be linked to hydrophobic carrier molecules such as palmitic acid (Mowat *et al.,* 1991; Reid, 1992) or bacterial lipopolysaccharide (Weiss *et al.,* 1990). Another approach uses treatment with low pH, by which hydrophobic stretches in the protein molecule that are normally hidden, are exposed (Morein *et al.,* 1990; Heeg *et al.,* 1991).

3. INDUCTION OF B- AND T-CELL RESPONSES BY ISCOMS

3.1. Induction of B-Cell Responses

Immunization with viral antigen incorporated into the ISCOM matrix generally results in the induction of high-titer virus-specific antibodies that persist for long periods of time. Examples of this efficient induction of B-cell responses can be found in a variety of viral systems, including feline leukemia virus (FeLV), human immunodeficiency virus, measles virus, and influenza virus (Osterhaus *et al.,* 1985; Pyle *et al.,* 1989; De Vries *et al.,* 1988b; Lövgren, 1988). Usually less antigen is required for the induction of the same antibody titers when incorporated into the ISCOM matrix as compared to soluble antigen with the adjuvant Quil A (Osterhaus *et al.,* 1989a). Several possible mechanisms may contribute to the efficient B-cell responses after immunization using ISCOMs. The multimeric presentation of antigen and the presence of an adjuvant in one structure has been shown to be essential for the induction of strong B-cell responses. The importance of multimeric presentation was demonstrated with different biotin/protein ratios. When three or more biotin molecules were coupled to preformed ISCOMs, the antibody response was ten times higher than when only one biotin molecule was coupled (Lövgren *et al.,* 1987). The high antibody responses implicate that Quil A incorporated into the ISCOM matrix retains its adjuvant activity. It has been suggested that the delayed release of antigen from the injection site (usually subcutaneous injection) to the immune system may be important for the efficient B-cell responses. Indeed, it has been demonstrated that ISCOMs and Quil A, like other oil/water emulsion adjuvants, can retain antigen at the site of injection (Watson *et al.,* 1989; Scott *et al.,* 1985). Using radioactively labeled antigen, the antigen could readily be demonstrated in the spleen after intraperitoneal injection when incorporated into ISCOMs but not when presented as micelles (Watson *et al.,* 1989). Furthermore it may be speculated that the effect is also largely related to the induction of a strong Th-cell response, resulting in the release of soluble factors that activate B cells.

3.2. Induction of T-Cell Responses

In addition to the induction of Th cells, the induction of CTLs has been shown to contribute to protection against disease in many virus systems (Van Binnendijk *et al.,* 1990; Kast *et al.,* 1986; Reddehase *et al.,* 1987; Cannon *et al.,* 1987). Thus, ideally, a vaccine induces both Th and CTL immunity. Two different routes, an exogenous and an endogenous pathway, have been identified for the processing and presentation to Th and CTLs, respectively. In the exogenous pathway, antigens are taken up into the endosomes where degradation of protein takes place, resulting in peptides that associate with MHC class II molecules and are subsequently recognized by CD4$^+$ T cells. In the endogenous pathway, protein predominantly derived from de novo synthesis is degraded in the cytosol and the resulting peptides are transported by transporter proteins (encoded by TAP transporter genes) into the endoplasmic reticulum, where they associate with MHC class I molecules. After reaching the cell surface, the complex is then recognized by CD8$^+$ T cells. In general, inactivated virus or subunit vaccines do not enter the endogenous pathway and are unable to activate specific CD8$^+$ T cells. Recently, however, it has been shown for several proteins that CD8$^+$ T cells can be stimulated both in vitro and in vivo when the antigen is incorporated into the ISCOM matrix. Antigen-specific CD8$^+$ CTLs were stimulated in vivo by ISCOMs into which proteins of influenza A virus, HIV-1, and respiratory syncytial virus, or the model protein ovalbumin were incorporated (Heeg *et al.,* 1991; Mowat *et al.,* 1991; Takahashi *et al.,* 1990; Jones *et al.,* 1988; Trudel *et al.,* 1992), and in certain cases even after oral immunization (Mowat and Donachie, 1991).

Several lines of evidence were provided by our laboratory that antigen presented by ISCOMs enters the endogenous pathway of antigen processing and presentation, resulting in the stimulation of CD8$^+$ T lymphocytes. First it was shown, with cloned CD4$^+$ and CD8$^+$ CTLs using MHC-matched antigen-presenting cells, that the fusion (F) protein of measles virus when incorporated into ISCOMs, could stimulate both CD4$^+$ and CD8$^+$ F protein-specific T lymphocytes. In contrast, inactivated measles virus or purified F protein could only stimulate CD4$^+$ T lymphocytes. Furthermore, it was shown that the stimulation of both CD4$^+$ and CD8$^+$ F protein-specific T cells by F protein-ISCOMs was insensitive to the action of chloroquine, which inhibits the exogenous pathway of processing by raising the pH of the endosomal compartment (Van Binnendijk *et al.,* 1992). In addition, the presentation of F protein by ISCOMs to CD8$^+$ T-cell clones, but not to CD4$^+$ T-cell clones, was abrogated when the TAP-negative mutant T2 cell line, transfected with HLA-B27, was used as antigen-presenting cells (Van Binnendijk *et al.,* 1992). Thus, the response elicited with ISCOMs, in which viral proteins have been incorporated, closely resembles the responses elicited by replicating virus, including antigen processing, presentation, and subsequent T-cell stimulation. These data suggest that ISCOMs can deliver proteins, probably after passing them through either the plasma or endosomal membranes, directly into the cytosolic compartment where proteolytic degradation of proteins takes place. The hydrophobic nature of the ISCOM structure and the inclusion of saponins that can insert into cholesterol membranes (Özel *et al.*, 1989), may explain its apparent capacity to pass antigen through membranes. Analysis of influenza virus-ISCOM-pulsed antigen-presenting cells by electron microscopy, showed that ISCOMs deliver antigen into the cytosolic compartment (Villacres-Eriksson, 1993).

4. VIRAL VACCINES BASED ON ISCOMS: EXAMPLES AND STATE OF THE ART

In several viral systems, immunization with ISCOMs has been proven to be highly effective in inducing protective immunity (Table I). Here some relevant examples are discussed.

4.1. Influenza Viruses

Influenza viruses are the causative agents of acute respiratory illness in many animal species, including humans. Immune response to the hemagglutinin (H) and neuraminidase (N) proteins of influenza virus are important for the induction of protective immunity. Unfortunately, the H protein shows considerable antigenic variation, resulting in the escape from virus-neutralizing antibodies (Both *et al.*, 1983; Yewdell *et al.*, 1979; Verhoeyen *et al.*, 1980).

Upon two intranasal immunizations with ISCOMs containing the H and N proteins of influenza virus, mice developed antibody titers that were comparable to those found after infection with influenza virus (Jones *et al.*, 1988; Lövgren, 1988; Ben Ahmeida *et al.*, 1992). Furthermore, cells secreting antibodies specific for influenza virus could be demonstrated in lavages of the respiratory tract. Since influenza viruses primarily infect the upper respiratory tract of different animals, the induction of local immunity may be important for protection. Influenza ISCOMs were shown to induce CTLs in the respiratory tract more efficiently than influenza virus micelles (Jones *et al.*, 1988). Complete protection of mice was induced against an intranasal challenge, by subcutaneous and intranasal immunization with ISCOMs containing both the H and N proteins (Sundquist *et al.*, 1988; Lövgren *et al.*, 1990; Ben Ahmeida *et al.*, 1992). In mice vaccinated with ISCOMs containing the influenza virus nucleoprotein (NP), NP-specific antibodies could be detected but apparently no virus-specific CTL responses. Protective immunity was induced in only 50% of these mice (Weiss *et al.*, 1990).

For the prevention of influenza in horses, an ISCOM-based vaccine has been developed that is highly effective in protecting horses from disease. This vaccine (Iscovac Equi F) has been registered and is the first commercially available ISCOM-based vaccine (Sundquist *et al.*, 1988).

Table I
Immune Response Induced by ISCOMs Containing Viral Antigens

Virus	Family	Route	Dose[a] (μg)	Species	Antibody response (VN)	T-cell response Th/CTL	Protection	Reference
Influenza virus	Orthomyxoviridae	s.c./i.n.	1–10	Mouse	+(*)	*/*	+	Lövgren (1988) Lövgren et al. (1990)
		i.n.	5	Mouse	+(*)	*/+	*	Jones et al. (1988)
		i.m.	0.25	Mouse	+(*)	*/*	+	Ben Ahmeida et al. (1992)
Measles virus	Paramyxoviridae	i.m.	2–20	Mouse	+(+)	+/*	+	De Vries et al. (1988b)
CDV		i.m.	7	Dog	+(+)	*/*	+	De Vries et al. (1988a)
		i.m.	?	Seal	+(+)	*/*	+	Visser et al. (1989)
BRSV		i.m.	100	Guinea pig	*(*)	*/*	*	Trudel et al. (1989)
HRSV		i.m./i.n.	3.5	Mouse	+(*)	+/+	*	Trudel et al. (1992)
HSV1	Herpesviridae	s.c.	1–15	Mouse	+(*)	*/*	+	Erturk et al. (1989, 1992)
BHV1		s.c.	5–50	Rabbit	+(+)	*/*	+	Trudel et al. (1987)
		i.m.	25–50	Calf	+(+)	*/*	+	Trudel et al. (1988a)
CMV		i.d.	15	Rhesus monkey	+(*)	+/*	*	Wahren et al. (1987)

Pseudorabies virus		i.m.	1	Mouse	+(+)	*/*	+	Tsuda et al. (1991)
		i.m.	170	Pig	+(+)	*/*	+	Tsuda et al. (1991)
EBV		s.c.	2–5	Tamarin	+(+)	+/*	+	Morgan et al. (1988)
Rabies virus	Rhabdoviridae	i.p.	0.360	Mouse	*(*)	*/*	+	Fekadu et al. (1992)
		i.m.	0.730	Dog	+(+)	*/*		Fekadu et al. (1992)
HBV	Hepadnaviridae	i.p.	1–5	Mouse	*(*)	*/*	*	Howard et al. (1987)
FeLV	Retroviridae	i.m.	3	Cat	+(+)	*/*	+	Osterhaus et al. (1985, 1989a)
BLV		s.c.	0.3–3	Mouse	+(*)	*/*	*	Merza et al. (1991a)
		s.c.	25–50	Calf	+/*	*/*	*	Merza et al. (1991a)
SIV		i.m.	1–5	Rhesus monkey	+(*)	*/*	+	Osterhaus et al. (1992a,b)
HIV		s.c.	1	Mouse	*/*	*/+	*	Takahashi et al. (1990)
		i.m.	0.5–5	Mouse	+(*)	*/*	*	Pyle et al. (1989)
		i.m.	5–20	Rhesus monkey	+(+)	*/*	*	Pyle et al. (1989)
Rubella virus	Togaviridae	i.m.	100	Rabbit	+(+)	*/*	*	Trudel et al. (1988b)
BVDV	Flaviviridae	s.c./i.m.	50	Sheep	+(+)	*/*	+	Carlson et al. (1991)

[a] Dose of antigen incorporated into ISCOMs

[b] +, induction of indicated response; –, no induction of indicated response; *, not determined.

4.2. Paramyxoviruses

Parainfluenza viruses, members of the genus *Paramyxovirus*, are important respiratory tract pathogens of infants and children. In animals, infection with these viruses has been associated with serious disease (Kingsbury *et al.*, 1978). Many of the early experiments with ISCOMs containing viral proteins were carried out with membrane proteins of parainfluenza viruses (Morein *et al.*, 1984). Recently a lot of work was carried out with ISCOMs that were prepared with morbillivirus antigens. Morbilliviruses are a group of viruses that have been associated with disease in both humans (measles virus) and animals (e.g., rinderpest, canine, and phocine distemper virus).

The evaluation of candidate subunit vaccines for morbilliviruses, based on the ISCOM matrix, has been the subject of investigation in our laboratory. It was shown that ISCOMs prepared from whole measles virus, containing predominantly the fusion (F) protein and minor amounts of the hemagglutinin (H), could induce virus-neutralizing, hemagglutination, and fusion-inhibiting antibodies. ISCOMs that contained immunoaffinity-purified F protein induced fusion inhibition but no virus-neutralizing antibodies. Both ISCOMs prepared with the F protein and the H protein induced protective immunity in BALB/c mice against an intracerebral challenge of rat brain-adapted CAM R/40 strain of measles virus after intramuscular immunization (Varsanyi *et al.*, 1987; De Vries *et al.*, 1988b). It was shown that immunization with F protein-containing ISCOMs resulted in cellular responses in mice and that from these mice, measles virus-specific $CD4^+$ T cell clones could be isolated (De Vries *et al.*, 1988b). The presence of passively transferred antibodies did not influence the induction of humoral responses in monkeys or cellular immune responses in mice by measles virus ISCOMs, indicating that ISCOM-based vaccines may also be efficacious in the presence of maternally derived antibodies (De Vries *et al.*, 1990). It was shown in vitro that F protein-containing ISCOMs, but not an inactivated whole virus preparation, could stimulate $CD8^+$ T-cell clones to cytotoxic activity, which have been shown to be important in the recovery from measles virus infections in children (Van Binnendijk *et al.*, 1990, 1992). For this stimulation to occur the physical incorporation of the F protein into the ISCOM matrix is necessary. Although dogs could not be fully protected against challenge with canine distemper virus (CDV) with ISCOMs prepared from measles virus, a morbillivirus closely related to CDV, dogs proved to be fully protected when ISCOMs prepared from CDV proteins were used. The CDV-based IS-COMs were also used successfully to vaccinate seals against phocid distemper virus (PDV), a morbillivirus that caused mass mortality in the seal population of the North Sea in 1988 (Osterhaus *et al.*, 1989b; Visser *et al.*, 1989). Vaccination of seals with CDV ISCOMs resulted in the induction of virus-neutralizing antibodies and protection against a lethal challenge with PDV (Visser *et al.*, 1989).

4.3. Herpesviruses

Successful results against different herpesviruses, which form an important family of pathogens for both humans and animals, have been obtained after immunization of ISCOMs containing viral membrane proteins. Mice developed high titers of virus-specific antibodies after a single subcutaneous immunization with ISCOMs prepared from herpes simplex virus 1 (HSV-1) and were protected against a lethal challenge with either HSV-1 or HSV-2 (Erturk *et al.,* 1989). ISCOMs also protected against skin and corneal challenges with HSV-1 (Ertuk *et al.,* 1992). ISCOMs prepared with pseudorabies virus (*H. suis*) glycoprotein gII, induced complement-dependent virus-neutralizing antibodies and partial protection in mice. In pigs, the natural host for pseudorabies virus, immunization with gII ISCOMs resulted in complete protection against a lethal challenge (Tsuda *et al.,* 1991).

ISCOMs containing bovine herpesvirus (BHV-1) glycoproteins induced virus-neutralizing antibodies in both rabbits and calves, the natural host species (Trudel *et al.,* 1987, 1988a). Calves proved to be protected against a challenge with BHV-1 after immunization with BHV-1 ISCOMs; vaccination with a commercial inactivated vaccine failed to protect against the same challenge (Merza *et al.,* 1991b).

Although protection was not studied, ISCOMs prepared with cytomegalovirus (CMV) proteins induced both a humoral and a cellular immune response in monkeys (Wahren *et al.,* 1987). For Epstein–Barr virus (EBV) it was shown that subcutaneous immunizations with ISCOMs containing the glycoprotein gp340 can prevent the formation of EBV-induced tumours in cottontop tamarin monkeys (*Saguinus oedipus*) (Morgan *et al.,* 1988). It was shown in vitro that gp340 ISCOMs stimulate CD4$^+$ T-cell clones from EBV-seropositive individuals (Ulaeto *et al.,* 1988).

4.4. Rhabdoviruses

Rabies virus, a member of the genus *Lyssavirus* of the Rhabdoviridae family, almost invariably causes fatal disease on infection in warm-blooded animals. For pre- and postexposure treatment, inactivated vaccines are commonly used. After immunization with ISCOMs that contained the rabies virus glycoprotein, both mice and dogs developed high titers of virus-neutralizing antibodies (Morein *et al.,* 1984). Furthermore, dogs immunized using ISCOMs were protected against a lethal challenge with street rabies virus (Fekadu *et al.,* 1992). When the ISCOMs were administered after exposure of mice to the challenge virus, almost complete protection was obtained, in contrast to postexposure vaccination with a widely used inactivated whole virus vaccine. The latter induced a fatal anaphylactic shock in mice when four doses were given as postexposure treatment. When ISCOMs were used, the postexposure treatment (four doses of 120 ng) was well tolerated and 94% of the mice were protected against a challenge with street rabies (Fekadu *et al.,* 1992).

4.5. Hepadnaviruses

Hepatitis B virus (HBV), a member of the Hepadnaviridae family, is a major human pathogen. HBV is a bloodborne virus that can cause chronic hepatitis or hepatocellular carcinoma. The first generation of HBV vaccines were hepatitis B surface antigen (HBsAg) particles derived from plasma from infected individuals. Currently licensed HBV vaccines are made of HBsAg particles produced in yeast cells, which carry recombinant yeast expression vectors (McAleer *et al.,* 1984). Immunization of mice with ISCOMs containing HBsAg resulted in high titers of virus-neutralizing serum antibodies (Howard *et al.,* 1987), indicating the potential of ISCOMs for the construction of new generations of HBV vaccines.

4.6. Retroviruses

One of the major challenges of the last decade is the development of a vaccine against human immunodeficiency virus (HIV-1), the causative agent of AIDS in humans. Probably the most important problem in the development of an HIV-1 vaccine is the variability of dominant neutralizing epitopes, notably the third variable region of the envelope protein gp120, resulting in escape from virus neutralization. Effective induction of both Th and CTL responses, which are not solely directed to the envelope protein but also to more conserved proteins like Gag and Nef (Van Baalen *et al.*, 1993), may contribute to protective immunity. Immunization experiments in mice showed that twofold higher antibody titers were induced using gp120-ISCOMs than gp120 with complete Freund's adjuvant, even when a tenfold higher dose of gp120 was used with CFA. Also, immunization of rhesus monkeys with HIV-1 gp120 ISCOMs resulted in tenfold higher titers of virus-neutralizing antibodies than with gp120 using alum as adjuvant (Pyle *et al.*, 1989). Additionally, with gp160 ISCOMs CD8$^+$ MHC class I-restricted CTLs were induced in mice (Takahashi *et al.*, 1990). The efficacy of candidate lentivirus ISCOM vaccines in nonhuman primates has been studied in our laboratory. After intramuscular immunization, both ISCOMs prepared from simian immunodeficiency virus (SIV) and an inactivated SIV preparation with muramyl dipeptide (MDP) protected rhesus monkeys against an intravenous challenge with 10 ID$_{50}$ doses of cell-free (homologous) SIV. The immunized animals remained aviremic during a follow-up period of 3 months after challenge. In a parallel experiment, 50% of the monkeys proved to be protected against an intravenous challenge with SIV-infected peripheral blood mononuclear cells (Osterhaus *et al.*, 1992a,b). ISCOMs prepared with HIV-2 proteins failed to protect cynomolgus monkeys against infection with HIV-2, which may be explained by the lack of incorporation of HIV-2 gp125 into the ISCOM preparation used (Putkonen *et al.*, 1991).

Immunization using ISCOMS has been successful in other retroviral systems. We showed that immunization with ISCOMs, prepared with the gp70/85 envelope proteins of FeLV, resulted in the protection of cats against FeLV infection. In ISCOM- vaccinated cats, 80% showed virus-neutralizing antibody responses to FeLV, whereas cats vaccinated with a commercial inactivated virus preparation showed less than 6% seroconversion of a virus-specific antibody response (Osterhaus *et al.*, 1985, 1989a; Akerblom *et al.*, 1989). In calves, virus-neutralizing antibodies were induced against bovine leukemia virus (BLV) after immunization with ISCOMs containing the gp51 envelope protein of BLV (Merza *et al.*, 1991a).

At present, the ISCOM adjuvant is being evaluated in our laboratory in a candidate vaccine for feline immunodeficiency virus infection in cats as a model for AIDS in humans.

5. GENERAL CONSIDERATIONS

5.1. Toxicological Aspects

Some components in Quil A have toxic effects, and this is especially relevant when ISCOMs are considered for use in candidate prophylactic vaccines in humans. However, no negative side effects have been observed with the use of a commercially available ISCOM-based equine influenza virus vaccine in horses (Sundquist *et al.*, 1988). Furthermore, Quil A is accepted in veterinary vaccine preparations for pigs and cows up to 100-mg doses, about 1000-fold higher than the Quil A content in ISCOM preparations. After intramuscular injection with an ISCOM dose containing 60 μg Quil A, only a moderate inflammatory reaction in one out of six rats was observed (Speijers *et al.*, 1987). Furthermore the hemolytic activity of free Quil A is 10-fold higher than Quil A incorporated into ISCOMs (Kersten, 1991). In order to study the hemolytic and adjuvant activity of the individual components of Quil A, these components have been separated using reverse phase HPLC (Kensil *et al.*, 1991; Kersten, 1991). In one study, four fractions were generated, of which all retained their adjuvant activity. Although not incorporated into ISCOMs, no direct lethal effect was observed in mice after injection of 500 μg with one of these fractions (QS-7) (Kensil *et al.*, 1991). In another study, 23 fractions were generated, all of which were tested for their capacity to form ISCOMs and for their hemolytic activity (Kersten, 1991). With one of the Quil A fractions (QA-3), ISCOMs were prepared containing protein I from *Neisseria gonorrhoeae*. This ISCOM preparation was as immunogenic as preparations made with unseparated Quil A, but was 17 times less toxic as measured by its hemolytic activity.

Thus, selection of the optimal saponin may result in the preparation of highly immunogenic ISCOMs that do not produce toxic side effects.

5.2. Mode of Administration

For the induction of systemic immunity, ISCOMs have been administered most commonly by the subcutaneous and intramuscular routes. Small doses (0.1–10 μg) of antigen incorporated into ISCOMs are usually sufficient to efficiently induce systemic immune responses in mice. Also, intraperitoneal injection with ISCOMs induces protective immunity in mice, for example against an intracerebral challenge with rabies virus (Fekadu *et al.*, 1992). Furthermore it has been shown that ISCOMs that contain the model protein ovalbumin administered by the oral route not only induced ovalbumin-specific serum antibodies (Mowat *et al.*, 1991), but also cellular immunity as measured by delayed-type hypersensitivity responses and the induction of MHC class I-restricted antigen-specific CTL responses. Soluble ovalbumin given by the oral route did not induce such responses. The required dose for oral immunization was ten times higher than for immunization by the intramuscular route. Local immunity against influenza in the lung could be induced by ISCOMs administered by the intranasal route. This route of administration also induced specific antibody responses of all immunoglobulin classes (Lövgren, 1988) including IgA and both NK and CTL responses in the lung (Jones *et al.*, 1988). After parenteral and intravaginal immunization with ISCOMs containing antigens of sheep red blood cells, secretory, vaginal immune responses were demonstrated in mice (Thapar *et al.*, 1991). Thus, ISCOMs can induce local immunity through either local or systemic administration. This may be of importance for the induction of protection against viruses that infect mucosal membranes.

6. CONCLUSIONS

We and others have shown that the ISCOM matrix has several properties that make it a promising antigen presentation form for viral antigens. ISCOMs containing viral proteins induce high titers of long-lasting biologically relevant antibodies, also in the presence of passively acquired antibodies. The ISCOM matrix has been shown to induce functional cell-mediated immune responses, including CD8$^+$, MHC class I-restricted, cytotoxic T-cell responses. Furthermore, local immunity has been induced after local and systemic administration with ISCOMs. These immune responses were shown to lead to solid protective immunity in many viral systems. The mechanisms, by which immunization using ISCOMs leads to enhanced immunogenicity of the viral proteins, are presently being unraveled. Attention is also being paid to the reduction of the toxicity of the respective components of the ISCOM preparations. Ultimately, the ISCOM approach may generate promising vaccines against viral infections, for which at present vaccines are not completely efficacious, unsafe, or for which the development of an efficacious vaccine has failed so far.

ACKNOWLEDGMENT

The authors wish to thank Ms. Conny Kruyssen for help in preparing the manuscript.

REFERENCES

Akerblom, L., Stromstedt, K., Höglund, S., Osterhaus, A. D. M. E., and Morein, B., 1989, Formation and characterization of FeLV iscoms, *Vaccine* **7**:142–146.

Ben Ahmeida, E. T. S., Jennings, R., Erturk, M., and Potter, C. W., 1992, The IqA and subclass IqG responses and protection in mice immunised with influenza antigens administered as iscomS, with FCA, ALH or as infectious virus, *Arch. Virol.* **125**:71–86.

Bomford, R., Stapleton, M., Winsor, J. E., Jessup, E. A., Price K. R., and Fenwick, G. R., 1992, Adjuvanticity and ISCOM formation by structurally diverse saponins, *Vaccine* **10**:572–577.

Both, G. W., Sleigh, M. J., Cox, N. J., and Kendal, A. P., 1983, Antigenic drift in influenza H3 hemagglutinin from 1968 to 1980: Multiple evolutionary pathways and sequential amino acid changes at key antigenic sites, *J. Virol.* **48**:52–60.

Cannon, J., Scott, E. J., Taylor, G., and Askonas, B. A., 1987, Clearance of persistent respiratory syncytial virus infection in immunodeficient mice following transfer of primed T cells, *Virology* **62**:133–183.

Carlson, U., Alenius, S., and Sundquist, B., 1991, Protective effect of an iscom bovine virus diarrhoea virus (BVDV) vaccine against an experimental BVDV infection in vaccinated and non-vaccinated pregnant ewes, *Vaccine* **9**:577–580.

Dalsgaard, K., 1978, A study of the isolation and characterization of the saponin Quil A. Evaluation of its adjuvant activity with special reference to the application in the vaccination of cattle against foot and mouth disease, *Acta Vet. Scand. Suppl.* **69**:1–40.

De Vries, P., UytdeHaag, F. G. C. M., and Osterhaus, A. D. M. E., 1988a, Canine distemper virus (CDV) immune-stimulating complexes (iscoms), but not measles virus iscoms, protect dogs against CDV infection, *J. Gen. Virol.* **69**:2071–2083.

De Vries, P., Van Binnendijk, R. S., Van der Marel, P., Van Wezel, A. L., Voorma, H. O., Sundquist, B., UytdeHaag, F. G. C. M., and Osterhaus, A. D. M. E, 1988b, Measles virus fusion protein presented in an immune stimulating complex (iscom) induces haemolysis-inhibiting and fusion inhibiting antibodies, virus-specific T cells and protection in mice, *J. Gen. Virol.* **69**:549–559.

De Vries, P., Visser, I. K. G., Groen, J., Broeders, H. W. J., UytdeHaag, F. G. C. M., and Osterhaus, A. D. M. E., 1990, Immunogenicity of measles virus iscoms in the presence of passively transferred MV-specific antibodies, in: *Vaccines 90: Proceedings of the Meeting "Modern Approaches to New Vaccines Including the Prevention of AIDS" 20–24 September 1989* (F. Brown, R. M. Chanock, H. S. Ginsberg, and R. A. Lerner, eds.), Cold Spring Harbor Laboratory Press, Cold Spring Harbor, NY, pp. 139–144.

Erturk, M., Jennings, R., Hockley, D., and Potter, C. W., 1989, Antibody responses and protection in mice immunized with herpes simplex virus type I antigen immunestimulating complex preparations, *J. Gen. Virol.* **70**:2149–2155.

Erturk, M., Hill, T. J., Shimeld, C., and Jennings, R., 1992, Acute and latent infection of mice immunized with HSV-1 iscom vaccine, *Arch. Virol.* **125**:87–101.

Fekadu, M., Shaddock, J. H., Ekström, J., Osterhaus, A. D. M. E., Sanderlin, D. W., Sundquist, B., and Morein, B., 1992, An immune stimulating complex subunit rabies virus vaccine protects mice and dogs against street rabies challenge, *Vaccine* **10**:192–197.

Heeg, K., Kuon, W., and Wagner, H., 1991, Vaccination of class I major histocompatibility complex (MHC) restricted murine CD8[+] T lymphocytes towards soluble antigens: Immune stimulating ovalbumin complexes enter the class I MHC antigen pathway and allow sensitization against the immunodominant peptide, *Eur. J. Immunol.* **21**:1523–1527.

Howard, C. R., Sundquist, B., Allan, J., Brown, S. E., Chen, S. H., and Morein, B., 1987, Preparation and properties of immune-stimulating complexes containing hepatitis B virus surface antigen, *J. Gen. Virol.* **68**:2281–2289.

Jones, P. D., Tha Hla, R., Morein, B., Lövgren, K., and Ada, G. L., 1988, Cellular immune responses in the murine lung to local immunization with influenza A virus glycoproteins in micelles and immunostimulatory complexes (iscoms), *Scand. J. Immunol.* **27**:645–652.

Kast, W. M., Bronkhorst, A. M., De Waal, L. P., and Melief, C. J. M., 1986, Cooperation between cytotoxic and helper T lymphocytes in protection against a lethal sendai virus infection, *J. Exp. Med.* **164**:723–738.

Kensil, C. R., Patel, U., Lennick, M., and Marciani, D., 1991, Separation and characterization of saponins with adjuvant activity from Quillaja saponaria Molina cortex, *J. Immunol.* **146**:431–437.

Kersten, G. F. A., 1991, Aspects of iscoms. Analytical, pharmaceutical and adjuvant properties, Thesis, State University, Utrecht, The Netherlands.

Kingsbury, D. W., Bratt, M. A., Choppin, P. W., Hanson R. P., Hosaka, Y., Termeulen, V., Norrby, E., Plowright, W., Rott, R., and Wunner, W. H., 1978, Paramyxoviridae, *Intervirology* **10**:137–152.

Lövgren, K., 1988, The serum antibody response distributed in subclasses and isotypes after intranasal and subcutaneous immunization with influenza virus immunostimulating complexes, *Scand. J. Immunol.* **27**:241–245.

Lövgren, K., and Morein, B., 1988, The requirement of lipids for the formation of immnuostimulating complexes (iscoms), *Biotech. Appl. Biochem.* **10**:161–172.

Lövgren, K., Lindmark, J., Pipkorn, R., and Morein, B., 1987, Antigenic presentation of small molecules and peptides conjugated to a preformed iscom as carrier, *J. Immunol. Methods* **98**:137–143.

Lövgren, K., Kaberg, H., and Morein, B., 1990, An experimental subunit vaccine (iscom) induced protective immunity to influenza virus infection in mice after a single intranasal administration, *Clin. Exp. Immunol.* **82**:435–439.

McAleer, W. J., Buynak, E. B., Maigetler, R. Z., Wampler, D. E., Miller, W. J., and Hilleman, M. R., 1984, Human hepatitis B vaccine from recombinant yeast derived surface antigen, *Nature* **307**:178–180.

Merza, M., Sober, J., Sundquist, B., Toots, I., and Morein, B., 1991a, Characterization of purified gp51 from bovine leukaemia virus integrated into iscom. Physicochemical properties and serum antibody response to the integrated gp51, *Arch. Virol.* **120**:219–231.

Merza, M., Tibor, S., Kucsera, L., Bognar, G., and Morein, B., 1991b, iscom of BHV-1 envelope glycoproteins protected calves against both disease and infection, *J. Vet. Med.* **38**:306–314.

Morein, B., and Simons, K., 1985, Subunit vaccines against enveloped viruses: Virosomes, micelles and other protein complexes, *Vaccine* **3**:83–89.

Morein, B., Sharp, M., Sundquist, B., and Simons, K., 1983, Protein subunit vaccines of parainfluenza type 3 virus: Immunogenic effect in lambs and mice, *J. Gen. Virol.* **64**:1557–1569.

Morein, B., Sundquist, B., Höglund, S., Dalsgaard, K., and Osterhaus, A. D. M. E., 1984, iscom, a novel structure for antigenic presentation of membrane proteins of enveloped viruses, *Nature* **308**:457–459.

Morein, B., Ekström, J., and Lövgren, K., 1990, Increased immunogenicity of a non-amphipathic protein (BSA) after inclusion into iscoms, *J. Immunol. Methods* **128**:177–181.

Morgan, A. J., Finerty, S., Lövgren, K., Scullion, F. T., and Morein, B., 1988, Prevention of Epstein–Barr (EB) virus-induced lymphoma in cottontop tamarins by vaccination with the EB virus envelope glycoprotein gp340 incorporated into immunestimulating complexes, *J. Gen. Virol.* **69**:2093–2096.

Mowat, A. M., and Donachie, A. M., 1991, iscoms–A novel strategy for mucosal immunization? *Immunol. Today* **12**:383–385.

Mowat, A. M., Donachie, A. M., Reid, G., and Jarret, O., 1991, Immune-stimulating complexes containing Quil A and protein antigen prime class I MHC restricted T lymphocytes in vivo and are immunogenic by the oral route, *Immunology* **72**:317–322.

Osterhaus, A. D. M. E., Weijer, K., UytdeHaag, F. G. C. M., Knell, P., Jarrett, O., Sundquist, B., and Morein, B., 1985, Induction of protective immune response in cats by vaccination with feline leukaemia virus iscoms, *J. Immunol.* **135**:591–596.

Osterhaus, A. D. M. E., Weijer, K., UytdeHaag, F. G. C. M., Knell, P., Jarrett, O., and Morein, B., 1989a, Serological responses in cats vaccinated with FeLV iscom and an inactivated FeLV vaccine, *Vaccine* **7**:137–141.

Osterhaus, A. D. M. E., UytdeHaag, F. G. C. M., Visser, I. K. G., Vedder, E. J., Reijnders, P. J. M., Kuiper, J., and Brugge, H. N., 1989b, Seal vaccination success, *Nature* **337**:21.

Osterhaus, A. D. M. E., De Vries, P., and Heeney, J., 1992a, AIDS vaccine developments, *Nature* **355**:684–685.

Osterhaus, A. D. M. E., De Vries, P., Morein, B., Akerblom, L., and Heeney, J., 1992b, Comparison of protection afforded by whole virus iscom versus MDP-adjuvanted formalin inactivated SIV vaccines from iv cell-free or cell associated homologous challenge, *AIDS Res. Hum. Retroviruses* **8**:1507–1510.

Özel, M., Höglund, S., Gelderblom, H. R., and Morein, B., 1989, Quaternary structure of the immunostimulating complex (iscom), *J. Ultrastruct. Mol. Struct. Res.* **102**:240–248.

Putkonen, P., Thorstensson, R., Walther, L., Albert, J., Akerblom, L., Granqist, O., Wadell, G., Norrby, E., and Biberfeld, G., 1991, Vaccine protection against HIV-2 infection in cynomolgus monkeys, *AIDS Res. Hum. Retroviruses* **7**:271–277.

Pyle, S. W., Morein, B., Bess, J. W. Jr., Akerblom, L., Nara, P. L., Nigida, S. M., Lerche, N. W., Robey, W. G., Fischinger, P. J., and Arthur, L. O., 1989, Immune response to immunestimulatory complexes (iscoms) prepared from human immunodeficiency virus type 1 (HIV-1) or the HIV-1 external envelope glycoprotein (gp120), *Vaccine* **7**:465–473.

Reddehase, M. J., Mutter, W., Munch, K., Buhring, H. J., and Koszinowski, U. H., 1987, CD8-positive T lymphocytes specific for murine cytomegalovirus immediate-early antigens mediate protective immunity, *J. Virol.* **61**:3102–3108.

Reid, G., 1992, Soluble proteins incorporate into iscoms after covalent attachment of fatty acid, *Vaccine* **10**:597–602.

Rimmelzwaan, G. F., Siebelink, K. H. J., Huisman, R. C., Moss, B., Francis, M. J., and Osterhaus, A. D. M. E., 1994, Removal of the cleavage site of recombinant FIV envelope protein facilitates incorporation of the surface glycoprotein in immune simulating complexes, *J. Gen. Virol.* **75**:2097–2102.

Scott, M. T., Goss-Sampson, M., and Bomford, R., 1985, Adjuvant activity of saponin: antigen localization studies, *Int. Arch. Allergy* **77**:409–412.

Speijers, G. J. A., Danse, L. H. J. C., Beuvery, E. C., Strik, J. J. T. W. A., and Vos, J. G., 1987, Local reactions of the saponin Quil A and a Quil A-containing iscom measles virus vaccine after intramuscular injection of rats: A comparison with the effect of DPT-polio vaccine, *Fundam. Appl. Toxicol.* **10**:425–430.

Sundquist, B., Lövgren, K., and Morein, B., 1988, Influenza virus iscoms: Antibody response in animals, *Vaccine* **6**:49–52.

Takahashi, H., Takeshita, T., Morein, B., Putney, S., Germain, R. N., and Berzofsky, J. A., 1990, Induction of CD8[+] cytotoxic T cells by immunization with purified HIV-1 envelope protein in iscoms, *Nature* **344**:873–875.

Thapar, M. A., Parr, E. J., Bozzola, J. J., and Parr, M. B., 1991, Secretory immune responses in the mouse vagina after parental or intravaginal immunization with an immunostimulating complex (iscom), *Vaccine* **9**:129–133.

Trudel, M., Nadon, F., Seguin, C., Boulay, G., and Lussier, G., 1987, Vaccination of rabbits with a bovine herpes type 1 subunit vaccine: Adjuvant effect of iscoms, *Vaccine* **5**:239–243.

Trudel, M., Boulay, G., Seguin, C., Nadon, F., and Lussier, G., 1988a, Control of infectious bovine rhinotracheitis in calves with a BHV-1 subunit iscom vaccine, *Vaccine* **5**:525–529.

Trudel, M., Nadon, F., Seguin, C., and Payment, P., 1988b, Neutralizing response of rabbits to an experimental rubella vaccine made from immunostimulating complexes, *Can. J. Microbiol.* **34**:1351–1354.

Trudel, M., Nadon, F., Seguin, C., Simard, C., and Lussier, G., 1989, Experimental polyvalent iscom subunit vaccine based on the fusion protein induces antibodies that neutralize human and bovine respiratory syncytial virus, *Vaccine* **7**:12–16.

Trudel, M., Nadon, F., Seguin, C., Brault, S., Lusignan, Y., and Lemieux, S., 1992, Initiation of cytotoxic T cell response and protection of BALB/c mice by vaccination with an experimental iscoms respiratory syncytial virus subunit vaccine, *Vaccine* **10**:107–127.

Tsuda, T., Sugimura, T., and Murakami, Y., 1991, Evaluation of glycoprotein gII iscoms subunit vaccine for pseudorabies in pig, *Vaccine* **9**:648–652.

Ulaeto, D., Wallace, L., Morgan, A., Morein, B., and Rickinson, A. B., 1988, *In vitro* T cell responses to a candidate Epstein Barr virus vaccine: Human CD4[+] T cell clones specific for the major envelope glycoprotein gp340, *Eur. J. Immunol.* **18**:1689–1697.

Van Baalen, C. A., Klein, M. R., Geretti, A. M., Keet, R. I. P. M., Miedema, F., Van Els, C. A. C. M., and Osterhaus, A. D. M. E., 1993, Selective *in vitro* expansion of HLA class I-restricted HIV-1 gaf-specific CD8[+] T cells: Cytotoxic T-lymphocyte epitopes and precursor frequencies, *AIDS* **7**:781–786.

Van Binnendijk, R. S., Poelen, M. C. M., Kuijpers, K. C., Osterhaus, A. D. M. E., and UytdeHaag, F. G. C. M., 1990, The predominance of CD8[+] cells after infection with measles virus suggests a role for CD8[+] class I MHC-restricted cytotoxic T lymphocytes (CTL) in recovery from measles virus, *J. Immunol.* **144**:2394–2399.

Van Binnendijk, R. S., Van Baalen, C. A., Poelen, M. C. M., De Vries, P., Boes, J., Cerundolo, V., Osterhaus, A. D. M. E., and UytdeHaag, F. G. C. M., 1992, Measles virus transmembrane fusion protein synthesized *de novo* or presented in iscom is endogenously processed for HLA class I and class II restricted cytotoxic T cell recognition, *J. Exp. Med.* **176**:119–128.

Varsanyi, T. M., Morein, B., Love, A., and Norrby, E., 1987, Protection against lethal measles virus infection in mice by immune-stimulating complexes containing the haemagglutinin or fusion protein, *J. Virol.* **61**:3896–3901.

Verhoeyen, M., Fang, R., Jou, W. M., Devos, R., Huylebro, D., Saman, E., and Fiers, W., 1980, Antigenic drift between the hemagglutinin of the Hong Kong influenza strains A/Aichi/2/68 and A/Victoria/3/75, *Nature* **286**:771–776.

Villacres-Eriksson, M., 1993, Induction of immune response by iscoms, Thesis, Swedish University of Agricultural Sciences, Uppsala.

Visser, I. K. G., Van de Bildt, M. W. G., Brugge, H. N., Reijnders, P. J. M., Vedder, E. J., Kuiper, J., De Vries, P., Groen, J., Walvoort, H. C., UytdeHaag, F. G. C. M., and Osterhaus, A. D. M. E., 1989, Vaccination of harbour seals (Phoca vitulina) against phocid distemper with two different inactivated canine distemper virus (CDV) vaccines, *Vaccine* **7**:521–526.

Wahren, B., Nordlund, S., Akesson, A., Sundqvist, V. A., and Morein, B., 1987, Monocyte and iscom enhancement of cell mediated response to cytomegalovirus, *Med. Microb. Immunol.* **176**:13–19.

Watson, D. L., Lövgren, K., Watson, N. A., Fossum, C., Morein, B., and Höglund, S., 1989, The inflammatory response and antigen localization following immunization with influenza virus iscoms, *Inflammation* **13**:641–649.

Weiss, H. P., Stitz, I., and Becht, H., 1990, Immunogenic properties of iscom prepared with influenza virus nucleoprotein, *Arch. Virol.* **114**:109–120.

Yewdell, J. W, Webster, R. G., and Gerhard, W., 1979, Antigenic variation in three distinct determinants of an influenza type A hemagglutinin molecule, *Nature* **279**:246–248.

Chapter 24

Vaccine Adjuvants Based on Gamma Inulin

Peter D. Cooper

1. INTRODUCTION

Vertebrates, and our particular concern the mammals, have obviously competed with microbes throughout their evolution and have tailor-made certain automatic defenses. Their leukocytes have evolved surface receptors specific for certain components of microbial cell walls such as β-glucan (Czop and Kay, 1991) and LPS (Lynn and Golenbock, 1992), ligation of which triggers particular *cellular* defenses. These are important in guarding against the targeted parasite. Several microbial components have been developed as vaccine adjuvants (Cox and Coulter, 1992), using the term in its original sense of "general helpers."

Mammals have also evolved a *humoral* defense, which acts as an immune surveillance system. This comprises the enzymatic cascade known as the alternative complement pathway (ACP) based on the multifunctional complement protein C3 (Müller-Eberhard, 1981; Lambris, 1988). The ACP detects and interacts with nonself surfaces, which activate the ACP (see Section 3). C3 is cleaved to pieces that tag or opsonize the surfaces to ligate specific receptors on many types of leukocytes (Ross and Medof, 1985). C3 pieces and Ig molecules are the major opsonins (Griffin, 1977). Substances that activate the ACP are highly effective and specific immune modulators (Cooper, 1993), usually with stimulant or upregulator effect.

The ACP has not been exploited for vaccine adjuvants before, although its parts and processes are well characterized (Müller-Eberhard and Schreiber, 1980; Müller-Eberhard, 1988; McAleer and Sim, 1993) and its many effects are of current research interest (Ross and Medof, 1985; Rosen and Law, 1990; Fearon and Ahearn, 1990; Erdei *et al.,* 1991; Lambris *et al.,* 1993). This chapter describes such a use, made possible by the serendipitous finding of gamma inulin (γ-IN), an insoluble polymorph of the polyfructose inulin that is 100-fold more active than the commercial inulin often used for complement studies.

Peter D. Cooper • Division of Cell Biology, John Curtin School of Medical Research, Australian National University, Canberra, ACT 2601, Australia.

Vaccine Design: The Subunit and Adjuvant Approach, edited by Michael F. Powell and Mark J. Newman. Plenum Press, New York, 1995.

2. THE NATURE OF EFFECTIVE VACCINE ADJUVANTS

In simple outline, the mammalian body's first immune reaction is to ligate exposed portions of an encountered immunogen (epitopes) to B-cell surface Ig that happens to be specific for that epitope. The B cell then internalizes the immunogen and degrades it into peptides, some of which are presented on its surface to T cells and ligate a TCR appropriate for each peptide. The specific T cells then stimulate clonal expansion of the specific B cell and are themselves stimulated with the same result. In time, by cooperative effort and with help from other T cells, large quantities of specific Ab are generated.

In practice, the immune response comprises a highly complex series of closely integrated reactions between many types of leukocytes. Such interactions increase the size and variety of the response, and improve its quality. At several stages during both primary and secondary responses immunogen specificity is selected and kept by recognition and ligation of peptide sequences related to the immunogen. Cells communicate via cell-surface molecules of many sorts and through release of and ligation with numerous types of soluble effector molecules (cytokines), which themselves exhibit pleiotropy and redundancy. The pattern of T-cell interactions falls into at least two main pathways, Th1 and Th2 (Mosmann and Coffman, 1989), fixed and typified by different cytokine patterns and T-cell functions. Several types of cell-mediated immunity are invoked. High-affinity memory B and T cells are clonally amplified and mature and the isotypes and subclasses of specific Ab and the types of specific cell-mediated immunity usually change during the process. The immune response is an amplification cascade network in which a small trigger eventually produces a large, varied (humoral and cell-mediated), and *remembered* response while keeping immunogen specificity.

In most natural infections, parasites invade via internal or external epithelia and their immunogens are initially presented as particles (e.g., bacterial, fungal, protozoan, or worm parasite cells, viruses, pollen grains, dust particles). These particles also contain or generate trigger substances such as LPS or double-stranded RNA that interact with various leukocytes to influence the size and type of response (Romagnani, 1992). Such triggers are immune modulators, of which we now know many. Some are related to natural immune modulators and some are derived from materials not normally met by the body.

Immune modulators or their effector products may intervene in various ways and at many points in the complex immune response and are likely to induce their own leukocyte-cytokine cascade(s). Their action is both quantitative and (usually) qualitative, enhancing humoral and cellular responses and selecting for or switching Ig isotype and cell type. These effects are of major importance for vaccines and probably result in part from changed cytokine patterns at critical steps. Immune modulators may also enhance or suppress expression of important cell surface molecules, such as MHC molecules or receptors for cytokines and Fc or complement moieties. The intracellular effect of immune signals may depend on receptor-mediated transduction involving G proteins (Gilman, 1987) or membrane phospholipases (Hamilton and Adams, 1987). Some examples such as muramyl peptides, aluminum hydroxide gel ("alum"), monophosphoryl lipid A, and saponins are reviewed elsewhere (Cooper, 1994).

The more effective vaccine adjuvants seem to mimic and possibly exaggerate the invasive process without harm, carrying and presenting immunogens naturally and triggering the correct leukocytes into appropriate cellular and cytokine responses. Such adjuvants carry immunogens on particles that also carry immune modulators. Focusing immunogen and immune modulator together in the draining lymph node gives best results, probably because cytokines act at short range and leukocyte activation is short-lived. A multimeric array of immunogen on particle surfaces may best mimic nature and can improve responses. The "particles" may be oil droplets suspended as water emulsions, liposomes, micelles or ISCOMs, or solid particles. In larger animals as opposed to rodents (Van Nest *et al.,* 1992), particles disperse and transfer more easily to lymph nodes if diameters are <1 μm.

3. INVOLVEMENT OF COMPLEMENT IN IMMUNE DEFENSES

The complement system comprises 20 plasma proteins operating in two converging enzymatic cascades, "classical" and "alternative" pathways (Fig. 1), both of which are well understood biochemically (Müller-Eberhard and Schreiber, 1980; Müller-Eberhard, 1988). Complement is crucial in coordinating the interactions of inflammatory cellular responses against invading nonself antigens (Müller-Eberhard, 1981; Lachmann, 1979), either via attached Ab complexes, activating the classical pathway, or by detection of nonself surfaces, primarily polysaccharide or glycoproteins, thus activating the ACP. The ACP plays a major role in the first line of defense, priming for lysis of bacteria and nucleated cells expressing nonself antigens. The terminal cascade of both classical and alternative pathways results in membrane attack complex formation, which mediates the lysis. Thus, the ACP is an effective humoral immune surveillance mechanism.

The ACP also enables certain leukocyte types to recognize nonself and initiate additional cellular responses. It does so through the interactions of complement products that bind specific cellular receptors. A pivotal component is complement protein C3, which is activated in both classical and alternative pathways through two different enzyme complexes with identical function (C3 convertases; Fig. 1). C3 is important in both primary and secondary immune responses (Bitter-Suermann and Burger, 1989).

C3 convertases proteolytically cleave protein C3 at residues 77–78 (Arg-Ser link) to create C3a and C3b, which then become prone to further cleavage by other serum proteases. The soluble C3 fragment C3e induces leukocytosis while C3a increases vascular permeability and suppresses Ab synthesis. C3a is an anaphylatoxin that is rapidly degraded by serum exopeptidases (Bokish and Müller-Eberhard, 1970). Other C3 pieces (C3b, iC3b, C3c, C3d, C3dg) contain a protected thioester bond that is exposed and destabilized by the initial cleavage, and this allows covalent binding of these proteins to other molecules or to biological surfaces. A crucial difference between classical and alternative pathways is that the ACP allows chain-reaction self-amplification (Fig. 2), producing a large local buildup of activation products. Chain reactions have a marked concentration dependence, and C3 activation is lost after a small (10- to 20-fold) dilution. This effect keeps the reaction localized.

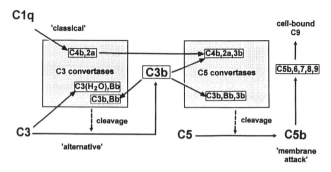

Figure 1. Summary of the relations between classical, alternative, and membrane attack pathways of complement. Broken lines indicate proteolytic cleavage activities.

3.1. Opsonic Effects of ACP Activation

The many facets of complement are all active during a normal infection. We consider here only a limited subset, namely those aspects involved in the mock infection represented by vaccination. These aspects contribute to immunological memory rather than immediate defense of the host and result from complement activators acting solely as immune modulators.

Let us first look in detail at the events following contact of an ACP activator such as γ-IN with plasma (Müller-Eberhard, 1988). In normal plasma, very few C3 molecules are hydrolyzed at the thioester bond but enough are present to form a trace of the fluid-phase "initial C3 convertase," $C3(H_2O)$, Bb, Mg^{2+}. This enzyme is unstable and is controlled by the specific enzymic regulators, factors H and I. The initial C3 convertase forms a small amount of C3b, in which the exposed thioester bond is very unstable ($t_{1/2} \sim 60\ \mu s$) and rapidly forms ester or amide covalent bonds with nearby nucleophilic groups such as hydroxyl or amino moieties. All form C3 convertases (C3b, Bb, Mg^{2+}), some of which are on the surface of cells or macromolecules such as Ig or Ag. The convertases form more C3b but are closely regulated by factors H and I. Subtle steric or conformational effects on C3b attached to *nonself* material, such as γ-IN, ensure that the bound C3b is not easily inactivated by factors H and I and this allows an active, autoamplifying enzyme to create more C3b in an explosive but localized chain reaction. Such nonself materials, usually on insoluble particles, are ACP activators. Self surfaces do not activate self ACP.

The local C3b excess produced by the mobile ACP-active centers can bond covalently with self or foreign material, such as vaccine Ag. C3b cleavage fragments (iC3b, C3d, C3dg) containing the thioester bond are also bound. With C3b they form the opsonins recognized and ligated by specific receptors on many types of leukocyte (Ross and Medof, 1985). Such ligation activates the leukocyte and so ACP activators are immune modulators in vivo.

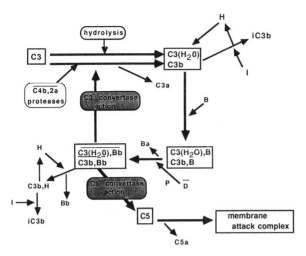

Figure 2. The alternative pathway of complement activation—a system for cyclic amplification of C3 convertase action. The outcome of particulate activation is determined by the nature of the surface that binds protein C3b. (Reprinted by permission of Kluwer Academic Publishers, from Cooper, 1993.)

3.2. Immune Modulator Effects of CR Ligation

There are five types of receptor (CR1-5) that recognize different sets of C3 pieces. The receptors promote binding and phagocytosis by neutrophils and monocytes and regulation of B- and T-cell functions. Their common designations and major roles are: CR1 (CD35, binding C3b), CR3 (CD11b, CD18, binding iC3b), and CR4 (CD11c, CD18, binding iC3b): phagocytosis; CR2 (CD21, binding C3b, iC3b, C3d): regulation of B-cell functions; CR5 (binding C3d, C3dg): ligation to neutrophils.

The C3 opsonins are direct and sometimes crucial primary immune system effectors that function via the CR in the acquired immune response (Erdei *et al.,* 1991). Cytokines are the secondary effectors in immune stimulation by ACP activation. C3 opsonins may be on the original activator particle, on adjacent Ab or Ag molecules, or on Ag-presenting, T- or B-cell surfaces. Nucleophilic groups on cell surfaces that can covalently bind C3 pieces, termed C3b-acceptor sites, are not available on all nucleated cells (Gergely *et al.,* 1984), and can interfere with or enhance certain FcγR functions (Erdei *et al.,* 1988).

C3 pieces function as bivalent adhesion molecules and exert many different effects. When specifically ligating CR on leukocyte surfaces they have many stimulatory effects. For example, DNA synthesis can be induced in the absence of macrophage-derived growth factors when CR2 is cross-linked with aggregated C3d (Melchers *et al.,* 1985). Chemical linking of C3b to tetanus toxoid targeted it to CR1 and CR2 of Ag-presenting B cells and enhanced specific proliferation and cytotoxic activities of responder T cells (Arvieux *et al.,* 1988). C3 complexes, such as aggregated C3 or C3b, further enhanced growth of T-helper cell clones stimulated by IL-2 (Erdei *et al.,* 1984). Binding of C3 to B cell CR2, and to some extent CR1, was shown to be necessary in the early stages of in vivo primary Ab responses to T-dependent and T-independent antigens but not for memory Ab responses

(Heyman *et al.,* 1990; Thyphronitis *et al.,* 1991; Wiersma *et al.,* 1991). Interestingly, soluble CR2 was itself immunosuppressive (Hebell *et al.,* 1991). C3 pieces linked by ester bonds to Ag-presenting macrophages influenced growth and differentiation of preactivated germinal center B cells into plasma cells (Erdei *et al.,* 1991). Similar actions of C3 pieces were found to be necessary for both Ag presentation and Ag-induced proliferation of responder T cells (Erdei *et al.,* 1992). The C3 pieces may react with CR1 and CR2 expressed on activated T cells (Lambris, 1988) and promote cell–cell adhesion. Follicular trapping of Ag was absolutely C3 dependent (Klaus and Humphrey, 1986).

4. COMPLEMENT ACTIVATORS AS IMMUNE MODULATORS

As expected, ACP activators have several immune modulator effects (Cooper, 1985) that are best studied using simple activators presenting only one or a very few immune

Table I

Comparison of Effects of Gamma Inulin, Yeast β-Glucan, and Lentinan
on Immune Responses[a]

Cell type	Property elicited	Cell contact with activator	Gamma inulin	Zymosan/yeast β-glucan	Lentinan
Whole body	Antitumor action with (before) antigen	Animal	+(+)	+(+)	+(+)
	Thymus dependence of activities	Animal	?	+	+
Macrophage	Superoxide release	Animal	– ("priming" only)	+	?
	Phagocytosis	Culture	?	+	–
	Phagocytosis	Animal	?	+	–
	Lysomal enzyme release	Culture	?	+	–
	Priming for LPS lethality/TNF release	Animal	–	+	?
	Cytotoxicity	Culture	?	+	–
	Cytotoxicity	Animal	+ (14 days)	+	+
	Il-1 production	Culture	–	?	+
	Increased response to MAF (IFN-γ)	Culture	?	+	+
	Pyrogenicity	Animal	–	?	–
Lymphocyte	Mitogenesis	Culture	–	?	–
	IL-2 production	Culture	+	?	+
	Enhanced DTH with (before) antigen	Animal	+(+)	?	+(+)
	Enhanced Ig with (before) antigen	Animal	+(+)	+(+)	+(+)
NK cells	Activation	Culture	?	+	–
	Activation	Animal	?	+	+

[a]Reprinted by permission of Kluwer Academic Publishers, from Cooper (1993).

signals, such as γ-IN, zymosan, and lentinan (Cooper, 1993). Their effects are similar (Table I), except that zymosan and lentinan (both β-polyglucoses) also ligate different β-glucan macrophage receptors that provide immune signals and effects other than ACP activation. C3 opsonins have macrophage activation factor (MAF) activity as they improve binding to monocytes, macrophages, or neutrophils (Czop *et al.*, 1978; Johnson *et al.*, 1984) but these cells need a second signal to be activated fully to phagocytosis. This signal is provided to macrophage receptors by the polyglucose of zymosan (Czop *et al.*, 1989; Czop and Kay, 1991) or lentinan but not by the polyfructose of γ-IN. Thus, γ-IN behaves as an MAF only (Section 6.3), while zymosan and lentinan both activate the macrophage fully. As the polyfructose of inulin lacks a secondary immune signal, it presents as an "immune monosignal."

All three substances have a local antitumor effect and a vaccine adjuvant effect that are active if given *before* as well as *with* or *after* the Ag. This is evidence that they are indeed immune modulators and not, say, vehicles or depots for other effectors. Both γ-IN and lentinan are nonpyrogenic and all three stimulate the lymphocyte compartment probably via their ACP activation. Lentinan differs from γ-IN and zymosan in that it also has a systemic antitumor effect that may be the result of its β-glucan macrophage and/or neutrophil activating capacity, with or without cooperation from its ACP-activating signal.

Two other, molecularly more simple, specific ACP activators are also immune modulators for leukocytes in culture or in vivo. These are the cobra venom factor (CVF) and the isolated protein C3b itself. They both have a local antitumor effect like that of γ-IN (Cooper and Sim, 1984), supporting the hypothesis that this effect is indeed the result of ACP activation.

5. INULIN AS COMPLEMENT ACTIVATOR

5.1. Chemistry of Inulin

"Inulin" is a family of neutral, linear (unbranched) β-D-$(2\rightarrow1)$ polyfructo-furanosyl α-D-glucose chains of simple and chemically well-known structure, of low molecular weight (3000–12,000) but having a range of degrees of polymerization. The single glucose terminal is joined by a sucroselike linkage to one end of the polyfructose. Methylation studies showed that the other end is fructose and that there is only one type of internal fructose (McDonald, 1946; Feingold and Avigad, 1956; Pollock *et al.*, 1979). There are no other components. Inulin is the storage carbohydrate of *Compositae* and is readily extracted in large yield from dahlia tubers. Working at the fructose end, the plant extends the chain in summer and fall and consumes it in the spring, so that chains are longest in early winter. A long chain is necessary for γ-IN formation (Section 5.2).

Inulin is very water-soluble yet "crystallizes" easily from water solutions, a property rare in a polysaccharide. Inulin suspensions and clear solutions can exist at the same temperature and concentration, and this makes purification in both solution and suspension phases easy and inexpensive. The particles dissolve on heating at a critical temperature related to the polymorphic "solubility form" of the inulin (Cooper and Steele, 1991): the more insoluble the particles the higher the critical temperature. The formation of quasicrystals probably derives from the unusual structure of inulin; the 2→1 linkage ensures that the chain backbone does not pass through the hydrophilic moiety but rather forms a polyoxyethylene-like (...C–C–O–C–C–O–...) hydrophobic backbone with hydrophilic side residues. The chains of most polysaccharides pass through the hydrophilic components, rendering the entire chain hydrophilic and difficult to purify in this way. Electron diffraction and X-ray studies of inulin pseudocrystals suggest that the chain is a helix with five residues per turn (Marchessault *et al.,* 1980). Space-filling atomic models (P. D. Cooper, unpublished) show there is room for two chains to interlock in the same sense to form a fairly rigid double helix, from which unattached tails could cross-link to adjacent helices forming an insoluble pseudocrystal with a fairly open structure.

5.2. Formation of Gamma Inulin

Inulin exists in many polymorphic solubility forms. There is a series starting with beta inulins (instantly soluble in cold water), through alpha inulins (decreasing solubility in water) to γ-IN (undetectably soluble at 37°C). The terms alpha and beta were used for inulins recrystallized from cold water and ethanol–water, respectively (McDonald, 1946; Phelps, 1965), which had different solubilities. Incubation of aqueous suspensions of alpha and beta inulins at 37°C transformed them to a form, termed γ-IN (Cooper and Carter, 1986a), whose turbidity did not clear in water at 37°C even in very dilute suspension.

Inulin suspensions progress along the series toward lesser solubility but are blocked at various stages according to the average chain length of the preparation; chains of lower molecular weight cannot form the more insoluble particles. The minimum size needed to form γ-IN is about 8000 (about 50 fructose residues), although lower-molecular-weight chains can cocrystallize. There is no chemical change and the physical changes are fully reversible when redissolved. The series is reentered at various points by, for example, adding ethanol, by freezing and thawing, or by changing the temperature. Such findings are compatible with an increasing interlocking of inulin chains, which becomes stronger with longer chain lengths. These ideas, together with structural data (Section 5.1) and its anisotropic ("swirly") appearance in suspension, support the concept that γ-IN forms rodlike microcrystals.

5.3. Inulin and Complement

Commercial samples of inulin have long been known to activate and destroy complement. They were shown to do so (Götze and Müller-Eberhard, 1971) by the ACP; inulin does not affect the classical pathway. Only particulate inulin activates the ACP; dissolved inulin is inactive. However, commercial inulin, which is a mixture of alpha and beta inulins, is not very active and impractically large doses in vivo would be needed. Fortunately, γ-IN is 100-fold more potent than commercial inulin (Cooper and Steele, 1991), and the anticomplementary action of alpha and beta inulins can be accounted for either by their gamma content or by creation of the gamma form during incubation at body heat (Cooper and Carter, 1986a). The gamma form is probably responsible for most complement activation by commercial inulin. Gamma inulin at low doses activates the complement of all mammalian species thus far tested (Cooper, 1993). This includes human, dog, horse, sheep, rabbit, guinea pig, and mouse.

6. GAMMA INULIN AS IMMUNE MODULATOR

Gamma inulin acts as an immune modulator by generating C3 pieces in vivo and these then act as effector molecules. Since local ACP activation by minor infections is a familiar experience for a normal individual, such modulator action is a desirable "natural" one with which the body has evolved mechanisms to cope well. Gamma inulin in vivo has antitumor actions (Cooper and Carter, 1986b, and unpublished studies) and effects on natural immunity (Chevis, 1990), but only its vaccine adjuvant action is reviewed here.

6.1. Gamma Inulin—The Product

Inulin was first purified in solution by adsorptive treatments, then crystallized, the particles washed and converted to the gamma form (Cooper and Carter, 1986a), as follows. The starting point was "inulin from dahlia tubers" (Sigma Corp., St. Louis, MO), a mixture of alpha and beta inulins with at least 40% of molecular weight >8000 and low in nitrogen, phosphorus, sulfur, and ash yet rapidly soluble in warm water. These impurities, together with endotoxin, some particulate matter, acidic caramelization products, and any trace anionic polysaccharides, were removed by filtration and treatment with aluminum hydroxide or DEAE-cellulose after dissolving in hot water (80°C) of pH >7. After crystallization, conversion to the gamma form at 37°C, and washing, the suspension was redissolved and Zetapor-filtered to sterilize it and remove residual endotoxin. Using endotoxin-free, sterile conditions, the inulin was recrystallized so as to give small crystals, reconverted to γ-IN, washed, heated (52°C) to elute low-molecular-weight inulins, washed again, and sterility- and endotoxin-tested. The γ-IN was finally formulated as a fine, milky suspension at 50 mg/mL in saline plus preservative (Cooper and Carter, 1986a) to form "γ-IN for injection," which can be used as is or in simple mixture with immunogen. Electron micrographs show translucent ovoids about 1 μm wide (Fig. 3). Such treatment for research purposes could no doubt be simplified commercially. Given a constant starting material the preparation is very reproducible. Yields were 40%.

Suggested doses are 100–500 μg (5–25 mg/kg) for mice and 5–25 mg (0.1–0.5 mg/kg) for humans or domestic animals. No change in properties was found after 8 years at 5°C and 4 years at room temperature (15–30°C). The particles do not aggregate, resuspension is rapid, and the suspension passes an intradermal (30 gauge) needle. The suspension will begin to dissolve above 45°C, and freezing and thawing changes gamma to an alpha inulin, which results in the loss of 80% activity. Storage at 2–8°C is recommended.

Purified inulin is characterized as containing no detectable material other than fructose and 1–2% glucose w/w, and the gamma form is characterized by negligible soluble material, a sharp 50% dissolving temperature in dilute water suspension of about 48°C (Cooper and Steele, 1991), insolubility at 37°C in water, particle size range of 0.5–3 μm, and ability to activate the ACP of undiluted human plasma at 37°C in comparison with a standard preparation of γ-IN, using a C3a-desarg RIA (Cooper and Steele, 1991). The

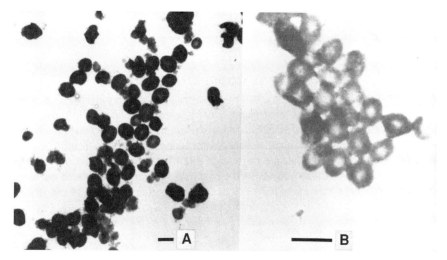

Figure 3. Electron micrographs of unstained (A) Algammulin and (B) gamma inulin particles at comparable photographic exposures. Bars = 2 μm. (Reprinted by permission of Butterworth–Heinemann Ltd., from Cooper and Steele, 1991.)

adjuvanticity of the preparation may be assayed reproducibly with a standard immunization test in mice (Cooper *et al.*, 1991a).

Gamma inulin itself, its manufacture and applications, are protected by patents (priority date October 31, 1985) Nos. 5,051,408 and 4,954,622 (USA), 589,233 (Australia), 1,300,612 (Canada), and accepted but not yet fully processed in Europe and Japan.

6.2. Vaccine Adjuvant Effects of Gamma Inulin

Minimal i.p. or s.c. doses of γ-IN that activate the ACP systemically (50–100 μg/mouse, 2.5–5 mg/kg) increase secondary IgG responses 5- to 28-fold ($p < 0.001$), based on experiments using keyhole limpet hemocyanin (KLH) as the immunogen (Cooper and Steele, 1988). The IgG2a, IgG2b, and IgG3 subclasses were boosted several hundredfold, IgG1 tenfold, and IgM and IgA four- to sixfold. The unusually large boost to IgG3 may be related (Greenspan and Cooper, 1992) to the highly multimeric and thus multivalent character of KLH, as for other antigens IgG3 was not much enhanced (unpublished). IgE was later (Cooper *et al.*, 1991a) shown to respond like IgA and IgM. The enhanced isotype and subclass ratios were similar to those of the naive animal. Immunological memory and memory recall at >80 days post primary injection were increased four- to tenfold.

Gamma inulin substantially enhanced specific IgG responses to KLH if given up to 9 days *before* Ag (Cooper *et al.*, 1993), and was indeed found to be optimally four- to sixfold more active if pretreatment was at 2 to 3 days. Specific IgG responses to KLH without adjuvant varied over a 61-fold range for different mouse strains, but were much more uniform (4.75-fold range, average 21-fold enhancement) with γ-IN as adjuvant (Fig 4). Such a reduction of individual variability is desirable in a vaccine. There was no relation

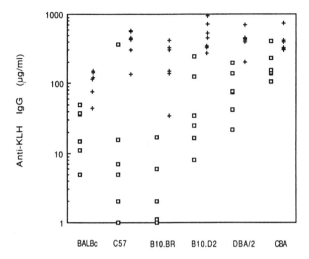

Figure 4. Responses of individual mice from six inbred strains to 10 μg keyhole limpet hemocyanin injected i.p. either alone (□) or with 100 μg gamma inulin (+). Mice were boosted at 14 days with the same dosages and bled for ELISA assay of specific serum IgG at 21 days. (E.J. Steele, unpublished.)

to H2 haplotype. The enhancement in responses and reduction in their diversity extended to immunological memory at 78 days and memory recall at 85 days for almost all of the mouse strains tested (data not shown). KLH-specific IgG responses were also enhanced by γ-IN in guinea pigs and rabbits (Steele and Cooper, unpublished).

Delayed-type hypersensitivity (DTH) reactions in mice to sheep RBCs were boosted by an amount equivalent to increasing RBC doses tenfold (Cooper and Steele, 1988), even if given up to 5 days before the immunogen, indicating that CD4$^+$ Th1 cell-mediated responses were substantially enhanced. In a live-influenza virus lethal-challenge model thought to reflect Th1 CD8$^+$ cytotoxic T-cell-mediated activity, γ-IN induced good heterotypic protection if given with the primary virus immunogen. Gamma inulin behaved as an enhancer of Th1 responses (Mosmann and Coffman, 1989) suggesting mainly involvement of the IFN-γ pathway, although some Th2 responses (IgA, IgE) were also boosted suggesting a lesser involvement of IL-4 pathways.

Studies in sheep have not provided results identical to those seen in mice. Vaccination with γ-IN did not much enhance IgG responses to a recombinant *Taenia ovis* antigen in sheep (H.S. Deol, D.G. Palmer, T. Dunsmore, and P.R. Carnegie, personal communication) but enhanced cellular responses (Section 6.3). Apparently the immune cascades induced by complement activation in sheep result in cell-mediated rather than humoral responses and suggest the use of γ-IN-based adjuvants in vaccines against sheep diseases needing cell-mediated defenses. Gamma inulin activates human and mouse complement equally well and so should be useful for human vaccines. Apart from an enhancement of specific IL-2 production in human PBLs in vitro (Section 6.3), the immune responses in humans have not yet been defined.

6.3. Effects of Gamma Inulin on Leukocyte–Cytokine Interactions

Human IL-2 secretion was enhanced 7- to 41-fold in response to γ-IN plus tetanus toxoid in PBL cultures in vitro (J. Hamilton, personal communication). Inoculation of sheep with a recombinant *Taenia ovis* Ag plus γ-IN (H. S. Deol, D. G. Palmer, T. Dunsmore, and P. R. Carnegie, personal communication) primed their PBLs for greater Ag-specific IL-2 and IFN-γ secretion and greater lymphocyte proliferation in vitro than did inoculation of CFA plus Ag.

Adherent PECs (monocytes/macrophages) were isolated from mice (D. George and M. J. Weidemann, personal communication) at intervals after a priming injection of 500 μg γ-IN i.p. Using a chemiluminescence assay, it was found that these cells did not produce a respiratory burst in vitro and thus were not fully activated. However, if phorbol ester was included in the culture medium, the PECs isolated 5 to 10 days after injection of γ-IN did produce a respiratory burst. This showed that these PECs were primed by γ-IN for full activation by the phorbol trigger. Injection of saline alone into control mice did not prime their PECs to respond to the phorbol trigger. Thus, γ-IN behaved as, or generated, a "priming" MAF in vivo rather than a fully activating "second signal," thus resembling the effect of C3 opsonins (Section 4). However, PEC macrophages developed cytotoxicity for L929 cells 15–20 days after receiving γ-IN i.p. provided the cells were adhered in culture for 1 h (G. S. Sraml and M. J. Weidemann, personal communication), which adherence presumably activated them fully. A differential count of fixed and stained PECs, isolated at intervals after injecting mice with 500 μg of γ-IN i.p. (Cooper, 1993), showed that the numbers of peritoneal macrophages were unchanged for at least 12 days, but lymphocyte numbers increased 8-fold ($p < 0.004$) by 5 days postinjection and neutrophils were massively (1000-fold) recruited by 5 h.

Since γ-IN is not pyrogenic, there is unlikely to be significant secretion in vivo of IL-1, tumor necrosis factor (TNF), or IFN-α, which are all products of fully activated macrophages that cause fever (Dinarello, 1987). If mice are primed with *C. parvum* their macrophages are fully activated, and the toxicity of subsequently given LPS is greatly enhanced as a result of copious release of TNF in vivo (Green *et al.*, 1977). Priming mice with γ-IN did not enhance the toxicity of LPS (Cooper, 1993), again showing that macrophages are not fully activated by γ-IN. These findings and the background studies of Section 3 make it likely that γ-IN, especially in its priming effect if given before Ag, results in polyclonal activation and proliferation of B and T cells. However, γ-IN, whether or not opsonized by normal mouse serum, was not mitogenic for mouse spleen cells in vitro (P. D. Cooper and A. Müllbacher, unpublished).

7. ALGAMMULIN—COMPOSITE OF ALUM AND GAMMA INULIN

When inulin is crystallized in a suspension of aluminum hydroxide gel ("alum"), the alum is included in the inulin particles. When the inulin is transformed to γ-IN, the composite particles can both activate complement and adsorb protein (Cooper and Steele, 1991). This creates a unique and highly effective adjuvant-active preparation termed Algammulin with some interesting properties.

7.1. Algammulin—The Product

A sterile, purified, and endotoxin-free solution of inulin prepared as for γ-IN (Cooper and Carter, 1986a) is mixed with Alhydrogel, a stable, neutral, safe, effective, and reproducible proprietary preparation of alum long used in vaccines and recommended as a standard (Stewart-Tull, 1989). The preparation is then crystallized and the inulin in the composite particles converted to the gamma form as for γ-IN. The particles are washed, sterility- and endotoxin-tested, and formulated to a fine milky suspension as for γ-IN (Cooper and Carter, 1986a). This forms "Algammulin for injection" (Cooper and Steele, 1991). Immunogen can then be mixed with stirring into Algammulin excess, and after a brief time for adsorption can be injected. Particles are ovoids of 2–3 μm resembling those of γ-IN but are electron-dense (Fig. 3). The alum-to-inulin ratio in the final product can be varied between 1:7 and 1:40 with effect on the response (Section 7.2). Since the adjuvant effect was found to be controlled more by the number of particles injected than by the total mass, while toxicity depended on mass alone, the toxicity-to-adjuvanticity ratio was improved by decreasing particle size, by ultrasonication. The optimal size and consequent Ag load, Ag molecules/particle, may depend on nature and dose of individual immunogens. As for γ-IN, preparation is very reproducible.

Suggested doses are 1–5 mg (50–250 mg/kg) for mice and 5–25 mg (0.1–0.5 mg/kg) for humans or domestic animals. No change in properties was found after at least 4 years at 5°C; since both components are stable separately no change is expected. The particles do not aggregate and resuspension is rapid. Temperatures should be kept below 45°C and above 0°C and storage at 2–8°C is recommended.

Algammulin is characterized with respect to both of its components (Cooper and Steele, 1991). The γ-IN component is monitored as is γ-IN alone (chemical composition, 50% dissolving temperature, insolubility at 37°C, particle size, and ACP activation, which are all identical to free γ-IN). The capacity of Algammulin to adsorb a standard protein (e.g., ^{125}I-labeled KLH) is measured, and the alum component is assayed after dissolving the inulin in hot water to obtain the alum-to-inulin ratio (Cooper and Steele, 1991). The adjuvanticity of Algammulin may be assayed reproducibly in a standard immunization test in mice (Cooper et al., 1991a). The ultrasonicated fine formulation is characterized for degree of dispersion by its optical density per milligram in dilute suspension (Cooper and Steele, 1991).

Algammulin itself, its manufacture and applications, are protected by patents (priority date August 18, 1988), No. 620149 (Australia) and others pending in the USA, Canada, Europe, and Japan.

7.2. Vaccine Adjuvant Effects of Algammulin

Algammulin was 10- to 20-fold more effective as an adjuvant than either of its components, alone or in simple mixture; levels similar to those from CFA could be obtained (Fig. 5). These tests used the moderately good Ag KLH, given at borderline seroconversion levels (1 μg/mouse) to mimic the effect of a poor Ag such as some commercial preparations. Use of "near self" materials such as albumin was avoided, since their poor antigenicity probably relates to a degree of self tolerance, interference with which is undesirable in a

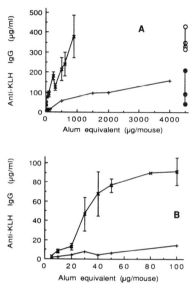

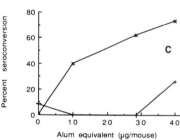

Figure 5. Comparison of secondary (21 day) specific serum IgG responses to 1 μg (A and B) or 0.1 μg (C) keyhole limpet hemocyanin i.p. per mouse, adsorbed either on Algammulin (X) or on alum (+). B is the low-dose portion of A; in C, seroconversion rates are responses greater than naive titers plus 2 SDs. ○, CFA; ●, IFA. (Reprinted by permission of Butterworth–Heinemann Ltd., from Cooper *et al.,* 1991a.)

vaccine. Most commercial immunogens will not have much homology with mammalian proteins.

Similar results were obtained with a malaria peptide–diphtheria toxoid conjugate as immunogen, directed against the malarial surface antigen MSA2 (Jones *et al.,* 1990). A protective response in mice against *Plasmodium chabaudi* challenge was obtained in this malaria model (Saul *et al.,* 1992); alum (a Th2 adjuvant), a high-alum Algammulin (a Th1/Th2 adjuvant), and CFA (a Th1 adjuvant) induced equally good immune protection correlated with Ab titer. Algammulin also induced four- to sixfold higher primary-response Ab titers in mice against HBsAg than did equivalent doses of alum (Cooper *et al.,* 1991b).

With Algammulin of a high alum/inulin ratio (1:10), the isotype profile against KLH was intermediate between those from alum and γ-IN, although IgG2a still predominated (Fig. 6). The IgE/IgG ratio was 50% that induced by alum, while IgA and total IgG were increased tenfold over alum values. When the Algammulin particle size was reduced by ultrasonication, its activity was increased fivefold w/w (Cooper *et al.,* 1991a). If the dose of Algammulin particles carrying a small constant Ag load (five molecules of KLH per

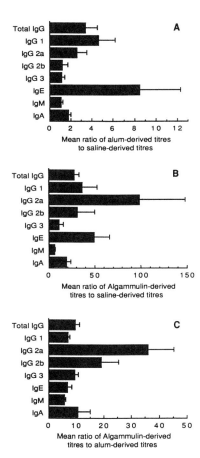

Figure 6. Secondary (21 day) specific isotype and IgG subclass responses to 1 μg keyhole limpet hemocyanin i.p. in saline or adsorbed to high-alum Algammulin (300–800 μg/mouse) or to equivalent doses of alum (30–100 μg/mouse). (Reprinted by permission of Butterworth–Heinemann Ltd., from Cooper *et al.,* 1991a.)

particle) was increased, the response was better than if the Ag load was increased equivalently on a constant dose of Algammulin particles; presumably it is more effective to increase the number of lymph node foci producing Ab than to increase the number of antigen molecules per focus. Immunological memory and memory recall were induced well by Algammulin, and seroconversion rates were increased from an average of 8% to an average of 57% at a sub-seroconversion dose (0.1 μg) of KLH (Fig. 5). Algammulin is both a Th2 and a strong Th1 adjuvant.

7.3. Effects of Algammulin on Leukocyte–Cytokine Interactions

Sheep were vaccinated either with KLH (Palmer *et al.,* 1990) or with a recombinant *Taenia ovis* protein (H. S. Deol, D. G. Palmer, T. Dunsmore, and P. R. Carnegie, personal communication), with or without Algammulin as adjuvant. When their PBLs were stimulated in vitro with the relevant immunogen, it was found that the use of Algammulin had greatly enhanced both immunogen-specific lymphocyte proliferation and immunogen-specific secretion of IL-2 and IFN-γ. Sheep IgG responses were unchanged; both of these effects resemble those of γ-IN. The cytokine responses from Algammulin equaled or exceeded those from CFA or Montanide ISA 50.

Alum is probably a Th2 immune modulator as well as an immunogen carrier (Cooper, 1994) as it changes the type of response (increasing especially IgE production). This effect may be related to signal proteins adsorbed on the alum surface in vivo such as Fc clusters from adsorbed Ig molecules. The inulin on the Algammulin particle surface decreases the number of alum adsorption sites, and so the Th2 character of Algammulin responses is decreased (with an increase in the Th1 character) at higher inulin contents (R. K. Gupta, personal communication). Thus, by adjusting the alum/inulin ratio the isotype response profile can be altered between that of alum (Th2, mostly IgG1 and IgE) and that of γ-IN (Th1, mostly IgG2a, IgG2b, and IgA). The Algammulin surface, like that of γ-IN, will carry a C3 complex, which, since it also includes Ag, will interact with B cell sIg to confer specificity on the proliferative response to C3. The C3 complex will also enhance follicular trapping of Ag carried on Algammulin particles (Klaus and Humphrey, 1986), and immunological memory will be promoted by the Ig complexes through Fc receptor interactions on leukocytes (Gray and Skarvall, 1988).

8. SAFETY PROFILE OF GAMMA INULIN-BASED VACCINE ADJUVANTS

8.1. Gamma Inulin

The essential effect of specific ACP activation in vivo is to dissect out a relatively harmless part of the inflammatory response. Results of that response undesirable for a vaccine such as fever, granuloma, and edema are avoided. Gamma inulin passes the British Pharmacopoeia pyrogenicity test at 10 mg/kg i.v. in rabbits, while projected human doses are 0.1 to 0.5 mg/kg s.c. or i.m. Its i.v. LD_{50} (in mice and rabbits) is 50–100 mg/kg but the i.p. LD_{50} (in mice and guinea pigs) is >1 g/kg. No adverse reactions were seen at adjuvant-active doses s.c. or i.m. in mice, guinea pigs, rabbits, sheep, cats, dogs, horses, and a few humans. Complement activation by inulin had no effect on the clotting cascade in vitro (Cooper, 1993) or in vivo using human volunteers (Nissenson *et al.,* 1979). Particulate inulin containing the gamma form was not antigenic or nephritogenic in rabbits (Verroust *et al.,* 1974).

Dissolved inulin is excreted intact through the kidneys with a short residence time. Particulate inulin is probably digested inside phagocytes (Cooper, 1993; Czop, 1986); γ-IN is apparently metabolized or excreted in vivo and is not cytotoxic or hemolytic in vitro. Dissolved inulin is registered for human i.v. injection and has no pharmacological effect except an osmotic diuresis at very high doses (*British Pharmaceutical Codex,* 1979).

The only effect expected of particulate inulin in vivo is its ACP activation. The effect of acute, massive ACP activation in humans is well documented from studies of human renal dialysis patients (Craddock *et al.,* 1977; Ivanovich *et al.,* 1983; Hakim *et al.,* 1984; Hakim and Schaefer, 1985; Knudsen *et al.,* 1985; Hakim, 1986). These studies provide a good idea of tolerance to identified levels of systemic C3 activation in humans. The rate of such activation by s.c. or i.m. injection of adjuvant-active doses of γ-IN will be far less than those easily tolerated by dialysis patients (Cooper, 1993).

Unlike CFA, even large doses of γ-IN (40 mg/kg) were not encephalitogenic in experimental autoimmune encephalomyelitis (EAE) induced in rats with purified myelin basic protein (BP) plus adjuvant (D. Willenborg and P.D. Cooper, unpublished, reviewed more fully in Cooper, 1993). EAE is thought to be a cell-mediated autoimmune disease similar to multiple sclerosis directed against CNS antigens. However, BP plus γ-IN did produce a primary response for both Ab and cellular reactivity. It is an interesting speculation that autoimmune responses engendered by very strong, pure Th1 adjuvants such as CFA and muramyl peptides may be related to inhibition of $CD8^+$ (Th2-pathway) suppressor T cells, suggested by Bloom *et al.* (1992) as possibly helping to keep autoimmune reactions in check. Thus, an adjuvant such as γ-IN that enhances both Th1 and Th2 pathways may avoid such an imbalance.

8.2. Algammulin

Results of LD_{50} (i.p. or i.v. in mice and rabbits) and pyrogenicity tests in rabbits were identical to those of γ-IN, and so Algammulin is as nonpyrogenic and nontoxic as its components. Both alum and dissolved inulin are registered for human injection.

Local-site reactions to the standard formulation of Algammulin (2- to 3-μm particles) were intermediate between those of alum and γ-IN, but the ultrasonicated fine formulation (~500-nm particles) was quite without reaction at adjuvant-active doses. No adverse reactions to Algammulin were seen in cats, dogs, or sheep at 1–2 mg/kg s.c., or in a few humans at 0.5–1 mg/kg s.c.

9. COMPARISON WITH OTHER VACCINE ADJUVANTS

Evaluation of adjuvanticity studies in the literature is hindered by use of different experimental designs, especially the choice of immunogen. Some modern studies have compared several commercial adjuvants in a single protocol with the extremely potent, toxic, but popular benchmark adjuvant CFA or its component IFA (Kenney *et al.*, 1989; Kensil *et al.*, 1991; Cooper *et al.*, 1991a; Van Nest *et al.*, 1992). The adjuvants followed the principles discussed in Section 2, namely fine particles carrying both the immunogen and an immune modulator. [Surfactants such as QS-21 (Kensil *et al.*, 1991) are likely to present as "particles" in the form of micelles.] They were Algammulin, or monophosphoryl lipid A or lipid-conjugated muramyl peptides with detergent and oil droplets, or purified saponins (Cooper, 1994). All of these preparations when optimally formulated with a compatible Ag gave responses as high as those induced by CFA. Choice of adjuvant may then depend on other factors such as cost and availability, ease of manufacture, side effects, known mode of action, compatibility with target immunogen, and especially the relevance of the type of response to the targeted disease. For this, challenge-protection tests using antigens with commercial potential are probably most decisive.

All adjuvants mentioned enhanced protective Th1 Ig and Th1 cell-mediated immunity responses (Cooper, 1994). Algammulin seemed the most promising for IgA responses, and was one of the few that satisfied the requirement of causing interaction with identified, specific leukocyte receptors and a known mode of action. Algammulin also had the advantage of being able to be adjusted, by varying the alum content, to favor Th2 responses more, or to limit the IgE product of alum-adjuvanted vaccines.

An interesting finding (Cooper, 1994) was that almost all adjuvants tested (including some noncommercial ones; Karagouni and Hadjipetrou-Kourounakis, 1990) behaved as if a leukocyte population(s) (including B cells) was primed in a polyclonal, nonspecific proliferative response for apparently any Ag subsequently presented.

10. SUMMARY AND CONCLUSIONS

Algammulin and γ-IN comprise a novel class of vaccine adjuvant. Their use in vaccines is to exploit the humoral defense known as the alternative pathway of complement. They use a "natural" mechanism and the biochemical basis of their action is well understood in general terms. They are fully researched up to the stage of specific commercial application.

Inulin itself is registered for human use as a solution and is without physiological effect except for ACP activation as γ-IN particles. The ACP comprises a relatively harmless part of the inflammatory response. Gamma inulin is nontoxic in several species including humans and is nonpyrogenic. The amount of systemic C3a produced from adjuvant-active doses of γ-IN is expected to be very much less than that routinely tolerated without effect by human renal dialysis patients. Registration of γ-IN should not be difficult.

Gamma inulin in vivo is either dissolved and excreted unchanged or metabolized to simple foodstuffs. Its primary chemical structure is completely known, and it is inexpensive, readily available, and easy to handle and manufacture. It is completely stable under normal conditions of use and storage. Patent cover is either fully granted or accepted for granting in most developed countries.

Alum is also registered for human use and its combination with γ-IN known as Algammulin is equally nontoxic especially in the fine formulation, and is equally stable. The partial coating with inulin in Algammulin greatly reduces the undesirable effects of alum such as granuloma formation and IgE generation.

Combinations of γ-IN with immunogen carriers other than alum are feasible, either as hybrid particles or as simple mixtures of particles of similar size.

Gamma inulin, and especially Algammulin, are potent enhancers of the Th1 immune response pathway, boosting seroconversion rates and immunological memory in protective Ab classes and enhancing cell-mediated immunity. The responses can equal those of CFA. They are also Th2 pathway enhancers, especially for IgA, and the emphasis on Th2 might be varied by altering the alum-to-inulin ratio in the final formulation. A dual response (balanced Th1 and Th2) may be desirable for several reasons. Their primary targets in vivo are probably lymphocytes rather than macrophages.

Gamma inulin-based adjuvants therefore comprise new, safe, potent, and attractive candidates for enhancing responses to human and veterinary vaccines, especially those requiring cell-mediated defenses.

REFERENCES

Arvieux, J., Yssel, H., and Colomb, M. G., 1988, Antigen-bound C3b and C4b enhance Ag-presenting cell function in activation of T-cell clones, *Immunology* **65**:229–235.

Bitter-Suermann, D., and Burger, R., 1989, C3 deficiencies, *Curr. Top. Microbiol. Immunol.* **153**:223–233.

Bloom, B. R., Salgame, P., and Diamond, B., 1992, Revisiting and revising suppressor T cells, *Immunol. Today* **13**:131–136.

Bokish, V. A., and Müller-Eberhard, H. J., 1970, Anaphylatoxin inactivator of human plasma: Its isolation and characterisation as a carboxypeptidase, *J. Clin. Invest.* **49**:2427–2436.

British Pharmaceutical Codex, 1979, 11th ed., The Pharmaceutical Press, London.

Chevis, R., 1990, Some effects of free radicals in parasite infections, Ph.D. thesis, Australian National University.

Cooper, P. D., 1985, Complement and cancer: Activation of the alternative pathway as a theoretical base for immunotherapy, in: *Advances in Immunology and Cancer Therapy*, Vol. 1 (P. K. Ray, ed.), Springer-Verlag, Berlin, pp. 125–166.

Cooper, P. D., 1993, Solid phase activators of the alternative pathway of complement, in: *Activators and Inhibitors of Complement* (R. B. Sim, ed.), Kluwer Academic Publishers, Dordrecht, pp. 69–106.

Cooper, P. D., 1994, The selective induction of different immune responses by vaccine adjuvants, in: *Vaccination Strategies to Control Infections* (G. L. Ada, ed.), R.G. Landes Co., New York, pp. 125–157.

Cooper, P. D., and Carter, M., 1986a, Anticomplementary action of polymorphic 'solubility forms' of particulate inulin, *Mol. Immunol.* **23**:895–901.

Cooper, P. D., and Carter, M., 1986b, The anti-melanoma activity of inulin in mice, *Mol. Immunol.* **23**:903–908.

Cooper, P. D., and Sim, R. B., 1984, Substances that can trigger activation of the alternative pathway of complement have anti-melanoma activity in mice, *Int. J. Cancer* **33**:686–687.

Cooper, P. D., and Steele, E. J., 1988, The adjuvanticity of gamma inulin, *Immunol. Cell Biol.* **66**:345–352.

Cooper, P. D., and Steele, E. J., 1991, Algammulin: A new vaccine adjuvant comprising gamma inulin particles containing alum, *Vaccine* **9**:351–357.

Cooper, P. D., McComb, C., and Steele, E. J., 1991a, The adjuvanticity of Algammulin, a new vaccine adjuvant, *Vaccine* **9**:408–415.

Cooper, P. D., Turner, R., and McGovern, J., 1991b, Algammulin (gamma inulin/alum hybrid adjuvant) has greater adjuvanticity than alum for hepatitis B surface antigen in mice, *Immunol. Lett.* **27**:131–134.

Cooper, P. D., Steele, E. J., McComb, C., McGovern, J., and Turner, R., 1993, Gamma inulin and Algammulin: Two new vaccine adjuvants, in: *Vaccines 93. Modern Approaches to New Vaccines Including Prevention of AIDS* (H. S. Ginsberg, F. Brown, R. M. Chanock, and R. A. Lerner, eds.), Cold Spring Harbor Laboratory Press, Cold Spring Harbor, NY, pp. 25–30.

Cox, J. C., and Coulter, A. R., 1992, Advances in adjuvant technology and application, in: *Animal Parasite Control Utilizing Biotechnology* (W. K. Yong, ed.), CRC Press, Boca Raton, pp. 49–112.

Craddock, P. R., Fehr, J., Dalmasso, A. P., Brigham, K. L., and Jacob, H. S., 1977, Hemodialysis leukopenia. Pulmonary vascular leukotaxis resulting from complement activation by dialyzer cellophane membranes, *J. Clin. Invest.* **59**:879–888.

Czop, J. K., 1986, Phagocytosis of particulate activators of the alternative complement pathway: Effects of fibronectin, *Adv. Immunol.* **38**:361–398.

Czop, J. K., and Kay, J., 1991, Isolation and characterization of beta-glucan receptors on human mononuclear phagocytes, *J. Exp. Med.* **173**:1511–1520.

Czop, J. K., Fearon, D. T., and Austen, K. F., 1978, Membrane sialic acid on target particles modulates their phagocytosis by a trypsin-sensitive mechanism on human monocytes, *Proc. Natl. Acad. Sci. USA* **75**:3831–3835.

Czop, J. K., Valiant, N. M., and Janusz, M. J., 1989, Phagocytosis of particulate activators of the human alternative complement pathway through beta-glucan receptors, *Prog. Clin. Biol. Res.* **297**:287–296.

Dinarello, C. A., 1987, Interleukins, tumour necrosis factors (cachectin) and interferons as endogenous pyrogens and mediators of fever, in: *Lymphokines*, Vol. 14 (E. Pick, ed.), Academic Press, New York, pp. 1–31.

Erdei, A., Spaeth, E., Alsenz, J., Rüde, E., Schultz, T., Gergely, J., and Dierich, M. P., 1984, Role of C3b receptors in the enhancement of interleukin-2-dependent T-cell proliferation, *Mol. Immunol.* **21**:1215–1221.

Erdei, A., Bajtay, Z., Fabry, Z., Sim, R. B., and Gergely, J., 1988, Appearance of acceptor-bound C3b on HLA-DR positive macrophages and on stimulated U937 cells; inhibition of Fcγ receptors by the covalently fixed C3 fragments, *Mol. Immunol.* **25**:295–303.

Erdei, A., Füst, G., and Gergely, J., 1991, The role of C3 in the immune response, *Immunol. Today* **12**:332–337.

Erdei, A., Köler, V., Schäfer, H., and Burger, R., 1992, Macrophage-bound C3 fragments as adhesion molecules modulate presentation of exogenous antigens, *Immunobiology* **185**:314–326.

Fearon, D. T., and Ahearn, J. M., 1990, Complement receptor type 1 (C3b/C4b receptor: CD35) and complement receptor type 2 (C3d/Epstein–Barr virus receptor: CD21), *Curr. Top. Microbiol. Immunol.* **153**:83–98.

Feingold, D. S., and Avigad, G., 1956, Isolation of sucrose and other related oligosaccharides from partial acid hydrolysate of inulin, *Biochim. Biophys. Acta* **22**:196–197.

Gergeley, J., Erdei, A., and Fabry, Z., 1984, Modulation of Fc receptor mediated functions by split products of C3, *Mol. Immunol.* **21**:1205–1211.

Gilman, A. G., 1987, G proteins, transducers of receptor-generated signals, *Annu. Rev. Biochem.* **56**:615–649.

Götze, O., and Müller-Eberhard, H. J., 1971, The C3 activation system: An alternative pathway of complement activation, *J. Exp. Med.* **134**:90–108.

Gray, D., and Skarvall, H., 1988, B cell memory is short-lived in the absence of antigen, *Nature* **336**:70–72.

Green, S., Dobrjansky, A., Chiasson, M. A., Carswell, E., Schwartz, M. K., and Old, L. J., 1977, *C. parvum* as the priming agent in the production of tumor necrosis factor in the mouse, *J. Natl. Cancer Inst.* **59**:1519–1522.

Greenspan, N. S., and Cooper, L. J. N., 1992, Intermolecular cooperativity: A clue to why mice have IgG3? *Immunol. Today* **13**:164–168.

Griffin, F. M., 1977, Opsonization, in: *Comprehensive Immunology*, Vol. 5 (R. A. Good and S. B. Day, eds.), Plenum Press, New York, pp. 85–113.

Hakim, R. M., 1986, Clinical sequelae of complement activation in hemodialysis, *Clin. Nephrol.* **26**(Suppl. 1):s9–s12.

Hakim, R. M., and Schaefer, A. I., 1985, Hemodialysis-associated platelet activation and thrombocytopenia, *Am. J. Med.* **78**:575–580.

Hakim, R. M., Breillatt, J., Lazarus, J. M., and Port, F. K., 1984, Complement activation and hypersensitivity reactions to dialysis membranes, *N. Engl. J. Med.* **311**:878–882.

Hamilton, T. A., and Adams, D. O., 1987, Molecular mechanisms of signal transduction in macrophages, *Immunol. Today* **8**:151–158.

Hebell, T., Ahearn, J. M., and Fearon, D. T., 1991, Suppression of the immune response by a soluble complement receptor of B lymphocytes, *Science* **254**:102–105.

Heyman, B., Wiersma, E. J., and Kinoshita, T., 1990, In vivo inhibition of the antibody response by a complement receptor-specific monoclonal antibody, *J. Exp. Med.* **172**:665–668.

Ivanovich, P., Chenoweth, D. E., Schmidt, R., Klinkman, H., Boxer, L. A., Jacob, H. S., and Hammerschmidt, D. E., 1983, Symptoms and activation of granulocytes and complement with two dialysis membranes, *Kidney Int.* **24**:758–763.

Johnson, E., Eskeland, T., and Bertheussen, K., 1984, Phagocytosis by human monocytes of particles activating the alternative pathway of complement, *Scand. J. Immunol.* **19**:31–39.

Jones, G. L., Spencer, L., Lord, R., Mollard, R., Pye, D., and Saul, A., 1990, Peptide vaccines derived from a malarial surface antigen: Effects of dose and adjuvants on immunogenicity, *Immunol. Lett.* **24**:253–260.

Karagouni, E. E., and Hadjipetrou-Kourounakis, L., 1990, Regulation of isotype immunoglobulin production by adjuvants in vivo, *Scand. J. Immunol.* **31**:745–754.

Kenney, J. S., Hughes, B. W., Masada, M. P., and Allison, A. C., 1989, Influence of adjuvants on the quantity, affinity, isotype and epitope specificity of murine antibodies, *J. Immunol. Methods* **121**:157–166.

Kensil, C. R., Patel, U., Lennick, M., and Marciani, D., 1991, Separation and characterization of saponins with adjuvant activity from *Quillaja saponaria* Molina cortex, *J. Immunol.* **146**:431–437.

Klaus, G. G. B., and Humphrey, J. H., 1986, A re-evaluation of the role of C3 in B-cell activation, *Immunol. Today* **7**:163–165.

Knudsen, F., Nielsen, A. H., Pedersen, J. O., Grunnet, N., and Jersild, C., 1985, Adult respiratory distress-like syndrome during hemodialysis: Relationship between activation of complement, leukopenia, and release of granulocyte elastase, *Int. J. Artif. Organs* **8**:187–194.

Lachmann, P. J., 1979, Complement, in: *The Antigens*, Vol. 5 (M. Sela, ed.), Academic Press, New York, pp. 283–303.

Lambris, J. D., 1988, The multifunctional role of C3, the third component of complement, *Immunol. Today* **9**:387–393.

Lambris, J. D., Becherer, J. D., Servis, C., and Alsenz, J., 1993, Use of synthetic peptides in exploring and modifying complement reactivities, in: *Activators and Inhibitors of Complement* (R. B. Sim, ed.), Kluwer Academic Publishers, Dordrecht, pp. 201–232.

Lynn, W. A., and Golenbock, D. T., 1992, Lipopolysaccharide antagonists, *Immunol. Today* **13**:271–276.

McAleer, M. A., and Sim, R. B., 1993, The complement system, in: *Activators and Inhibitors of Complement* (R. B. Sim, ed.), Kluwer Academic Publishers, Dordrecht, pp. 1–15.

McDonald, E. J., 1946, The polyfructosans and difructose anhydrides, *Adv. Carbohydr. Chem.* **2**:253–277.

Marchessault, R. H., Bleha, T., Deslandes, Y., and Revol, J. F., 1980, Conformation and crystalline structure of $(2 \rightarrow 1)$-β-D-fructofuranan (inulin), *Can. J. Chem.* **58**:2415–2421.

Melchers, F., Erdei, A., Schultz, T., and Dierich, M. P., 1985, Growth control of activated, synchronized murine B cells by the C3d fragment of human complement, *Nature* **317**:264–267.

Mosmann, T. R., and Coffman, R. L., 1989, Th1 and Th2 cells: Different patterns of lymphokine secretion lead to different functional properties, *Annu. Rev. Immunol.* **7**:145–173.

Müller-Eberhard, H. J., 1981, The human complement protein C3: Its unusual functional and structural versatility in host defense and inflammation, in: *Advances in Immunopathology* (W. O. Weigle, ed.), Symp. Specialists Inc., Miami, pp. 141–160.

Müller-Eberhard, H. J., 1988, Molecular organization and function of the complement system, *Annu. Rev. Biochem.* **57**:321–347.

Müller-Eberhard, H. J., and Schreiber, R. D., 1980, Molecular biology and chemistry of the alternative pathway of complement, *Adv. Immunol.* **29**:1–55.

Nissenson, A. R., Rice, L. E., Potter, E. V., *et al.,* 1979, Variations in serum complement following inulin infusion in man, *Nephron* **23**:218–222.

Palmer, D. G., Cooper, P. D., Carnegie, P. R., Wallace, H., Deol, H. S., Thompson, R. C. A., and Dunsmore, T., 1990, A new polysaccharide adjuvant (Algammulin) useful for the improvement of cell-mediated immune response in sheep. *Aust. Soc. Parasitol. Abstr.,* Fremantle, p. 51.

Phelps, C. F., 1965, The physical properties of inulin solutions, *Biochem. J.* **95**:41–47.

Pollock, C. J., Hall, M. A., and Roberts, D. P., 1979, Structural analysis of fructose polymers by gas–liquid chromatography and gel filtration, *J. Chromatogr.* **171**:411–415.

Romagnani, S., 1992, Induction of Th1 and Th2 responses: A key role for the 'natural' immune response? *Immunol. Today* **13**:379–381.

Rosen, H., and Law, S. K. A., 1990, The leukocyte cell surface receptors for the iC3b product of complement, *Curr. Top. Microbiol. Immunol.* **153**:99–122.

Ross, G. D., and Medof, M. E., 1985, Membrane complement receptors specific for bound fragments of C3, *Adv. Immunol.* **37**:217–267.

Saul, A., Lord, R., Jones, G. L., and Spencer, L., 1992, Protective immunization with invariant peptides of the *Plasmodium falciparum* antigen MSA2, *J. Immunol.* **148**:208–211.

Stewart-Tull, D. E. S., 1989, Recommendations for the assessment of adjuvants (immunopotentiators), in: *Immunological Adjuvants and Vaccines* (G. Gregoriadis, A. C. Allison, and G. Poste, eds.), NATO ASI Series A: Life Sciences, Vol. 179, Plenum Press, New York, pp. 213–226.

Thyphronitis, G., Kinoshita, T., Inoue, K., Schweinle, J. E., Tsokos, G. C., Metcalf, E. S., Finkelman, F. D., and Balow, J. E., 1991, Modulation of mouse complement receptors 1 and 2 suppresses antibody responses in vivo, *J. Immunol.* **147**:224–230.

Van Nest, G. A., Steimer, K. S., Haigwood, N. L., Burke, R. L., and Ott, G., 1992, Advanced adjuvant formulation for use with recombinant subunit vaccines, in: *Vaccines 92. Modern Approaches to New Vaccines Including Prevention of AIDS* (F. Brown, R. M. Chanock, H. S. Ginsberg, and R. A. Lerner, eds.), Cold Spring Harbor Laboratory Press, Cold Spring Harbor, NY, pp. 57–62.

Verroust, P. J., Wilson, C. B., and Dixon, F. J., 1974, Lack of nephritogenicity of systemic activation of the alternative complement pathway, *Kidney Int.* **6**:157–169.

Wiersma, E. J., Kinoshita, T., and Heyman, B., 1991, Inhibition of immunological memory and T-independent humoral responses by monoclonal antibodies specific for murine complement receptors, *Eur. J. Immunol.* **21**:2501–2506.

Chapter 25

A New Approach to Vaccine Adjuvants

Immunopotentiation by Intracellular T-Helper-Like Signals Transmitted by Loxoribine

Michael G. Goodman

1. INTRODUCTION

1.1. Discovery of Loxoribine and Its Analogues

Vaccination with innocuous antigens derived from pathogenic microorganisms is designed to provide protection against the significant morbidity and mortality associated with diseases caused by these pathogens. Vaccination is most important precisely in those patients who are most likely to have difficulty mounting an adequate immune response either to the intact pathogen or to the vaccinating antigen, that is, those patients with acquired permanent or temporary immunodeficiencies. These patients manifest defects in one or more cell lineages that can involve deficient antigen processing, antigen presentation in the context of appropriate major histocompatibility antigen (MHC) molecules, transmembrane signal transduction, signal transmission, cytokine generation, cytokine receptors, and so forth. Among the striking advantages of the compounds discussed in this chapter is the ability to overcome or ameliorate many obstacles to effective immune responses against the epitopes of pathogenic microorganisms. This property appears to be unique to the 7,8-disubstituted guanine nucleosides.

The C8-substituted guanine ribonucleosides were first discovered while studying the role of cyclic GMP (cGMP) in B-cell activation (Goodman and Weigle, 1981, 1982a,b). At the time, there was considerable controversy in the literature concerning the role of cGMP in B-cell activation (Watson *et al.,* 1973; Watson, 1975; Coffey *et al.,* 1977; Diamantstein and Ulmer, 1975; Weinstein *et al.,* 1974, 1975; Wedner *et al.,* 1975; Burleson

Michael G. Goodman • Department of Immunology, The Scripps Research Institute, La Jolla, California 92037.

Vaccine Design: The Subunit and Adjuvant Approach, edited by Michael F. Powell and Mark J. Newman. Plenum Press, New York, 1995.

and Sage, 1976; Weber and Goldberg, 1976). One of the central issues of disagreement was the ability of exogenous cGMP to induce mitogenesis in cultured B cells. However, different investigators used different cGMP analogues, some of which (e.g., dibutyryl cGMP and 8Br-cGMP) were designed to be highly lipophilic to increase the likelihood that the cyclic phosphate would cross the plasma membrane. We discovered that the manner of substitution of various cGMP analogues was relevant to more than the ability of the molecule to cross the plasma membrane. Thus, underivatized cGMP as well as dibutyryl cGMP were not effective B-cell stimulants. However, 8-bromo-cGMP was consistently effective as a B-cell activator. In subsequent experiments the cyclic phosphate nature of the molecule was shown to be irrelevant to its stimulatory capacity, such that 8-bromo-GMP is more active than 8-bromo-cGMP, and more potent by approximately one order of magnitude. 8-Bromoguanosine, lacking the 5′ phosphate group, is more active still. However, 8-bromoguanine, lacking β-D-ribose, was found to be devoid of biological activity. Subsequent structure–activity studies revealed that substitution of the 7-nitrogen with certain aliphatic or aromatic groups enhanced immunological activity even further (Goodman and Hennen, 1986; Chen *et al.*, 1994). The most active of the compounds tested is 7-allyl-8-oxoguanosine (7a8oGuo, loxoribine).

1.2. Overview of Cell Types Activated and Immunobiological Actions Evoked by Loxoribine and Its Analogues

Loxoribine and its analogues augment immunobiological activity of a diverse group of cell types. Perhaps the best studied of these is the B cell. The effects of loxoribine and its analogues on these cells fall into antigen-independent and antigen-dependent categories. Induction of B-cell proliferation (Goodman and Weigle, 1981, 1983d) and antigen-non-specific (polyclonal) immunoglobulin secretion (Goodman and Weigle, 1982b) fall within the former category. Also included in this group of activities is the induction of increased MHC class II molecule expression (Ahmad and Mond, 1986). These properties are best described for the earlier members of the substituted guanosine series such as 8-bro-moguanosine (8BrGuo) and 8-mercaptoguanosine (8MGuo), but are most potently induced by loxoribine. Antigen-dependent effects of loxoribine and its analogues on B cells include antigen-specific enhancement of antibody responses (Goodman and Weigle, 1983b; Scheuer *et al.*, 1985a); T-cell-like signaling to antigen-reactive B cells (Goodman and Weigle, 1983c); inhibition of tolerance induction (Scheuer *et al.*, 1985b); and bypass of tolerant T cells late in the course of experimental tolerance (Scheuer *et al.*, 1985b). Co-stimulus-dependent effects include the augmentation of antigen-induced proliferation of T cells (Goodman, 1991); augmentation of antigen-specific T-cell help (Goodman and Weigle, 1986); enhancement of cytolytic T-cell activity induced by poorly immunogenic stimuli (Feldbush and Ballas, 1985); inhibition of T-cell tolerance induction (Scheuer *et al.*, 1985b); and upregulation of the secretion of certain cytokines (Goodman, 1988a; Pope *et al.*, 1994b).

Effects on macrophages and macrophage-like cell lines have also been studied. Substituted guanine nucleosides induce these cells to secrete monokines such as interleukin (IL)-1β, tumor necrosis factor (TNF)-α, interferon (IFN)-α, and IL-6. Augmentation of macrophage-mediated cytotoxicity toward tumor targets was found to be only partially dependent on IFN (Koo *et al.,* 1988). Recently, Pope and colleagues have described the effects of loxoribine on natural killer cells and lymphokine-activated killer (LAK) cells (Pope *et al.,* 1992a,b, 1993a,b). These effects include augmentation of NK cell-mediated cytolytic activity, augmentation of natural killer-dependent inhibition of metastasis of B-16 melanoma cells to the lungs, and synergy with low-dose IL-2 to enhance LAK cell-mediated cytotoxicity. The mechanism of this latter phenomenon was found to be dependent on the upregulation of IL-2 receptor expression (Pope *et al.,* 1993a).

2. AMPLIFICATION OF ANTIBODY RESPONSES

2.1. Cellular Mechanism of Action

The increased number of antibody-secreting cells observed in plaque assays of B cells stimulated with antigen in the presence of loxoribine could theoretically take its origin from either or both of two sources. The first of these is the clonal expansion, or proliferation, of mature antigen-reactive B cells. This mechanism would be predominantly dependent on the proliferation-inducing properties of loxoribine and its analogues in the presence of antigen. The second possible mechanism is that preexistent quiescent, but potentially antigen-reactive, precursor cells could be recruited to secrete antibody by the conjoint actions of antigen and loxoribine. Kinetic studies indicate that in both the murine and human systems, the action of substituted nucleosides is exerted relatively late in the culture period, well after cycles of B-cell proliferation have been completed (Goodman and Weigle, 1983b, 1985b). Thus, the ability of these compounds to increase the number of cells that secrete antibody in response to antigen appears to be relatively independent of proliferative events.

Several different lines of evidence support this hypothesis. First, using disubstituted nucleosides, we have shown that the dose–response profile for proliferation is dissociable from that for differentiation induced by the same agent. The two dose–response profiles exhibit peaks whose optima differ by one and one-half orders of magnitude (Goodman and Hennen, 1986). Thus, at nucleoside concentrations that induce optimal differentiation to antibody secretion, B cells do not proliferate significantly. Second, the SJL mouse strain has been shown to lack responsiveness to proliferative signals transmitted by 8MGuo, although it exhibits essentially normal responsiveness to the adjuvanticity of this compound (Goodman and Weigle, 1984c, 1985a). Third, as mentioned above, human peripheral blood lymphocytes are entirely unresponsive to the proliferative properties of these molecules while being quite sensitive to their capacity to provoke augmented antibody responses to nominal antigen (Ellis *et al.,* 1990; Goodman, 1991; Goodman and Weigle, 1985b). Fourth, addition of very bulky substituents (e.g., cinnamyl) at the N7 position of the guanine ring enables the resultant compound to induce increased antibody responses in the absence of B-cell proliferation (Goodman, 1991). Finally, these two parameters can be dissociated by exposure to gamma irradiation. At very low doses, B-cell proliferation to 8MGuo is totally eliminated, while approximately 70% of immunoenhancing activity remains intact (Goodman and Weigle, 1984c).

In order to directly assess the contributions of clonal expansion versus recruitment of preexistent lymphocyte reserves, precursor frequency analyses were performed. Results of these studies indicate that for every cell that secretes antibody in the presence of antigen alone, 4.2 additional cells exhibit responsiveness to antigen only in the presence of nucleoside. The contribution of a minor proliferative component in the murine system was indicated by a 50% increase in mean clone size in positive wells containing antigen and nucleoside relative to the size of clones in positive wells with antigen alone. These studies substantiate the existence of a pool of additional precursor cells, responsive to antigen only in the presence of nucleoside, that is recruited into this response (Goodman and Weigle, 1984c; Goodman, 1986a). Whether the recruited cells are totally quiescent, or had previously secreted immunoglobulin at extremely low levels and are upregulated by the nucleoside is at present unresolved.

The observation that these agonists act relatively late in the course of an ongoing immune response is interpreted to reflect the requirement for prior activation by critical signals such as antigens or cytokines (Goodman, 1986b). The recruited cells are likely to be immature B cells or pre-B cells that can be induced to differentiate to a state of antigen reactivity and antibody production by additional signals provided by substituted nucleo- sides. In support of this concept, antigen-unresponsive cells from neonatal mice have been shown to produce adult-level antibody responses in the presence of antigen and 8MGuo (Goodman and Weigle, 1984c). Likewise, polysaccharide-unresponsiveness in human neonatal B cells is overcome by signals from 8MGuo (Rijkers *et al.,* 1988).

The regulatory effects of macrophages and their soluble products on immunopoten- tiation by 8MGuo have also been explored (Goodman, 1986b). Supplementation of macrophage-depleted B-cell cultures with adherent cells enhanced the proliferative re- sponse to anti-immunoglobulin antibodies, but depressed the response to 8MGuo. These changes could be eliminated by adding indomethacin to B-cell cultures containing supple- mental macrophages. Moreover, they could be reproduced by adding exogenous cyclooxy- genase products (e.g., prostaglandins of the E series), but not other macrophage products, to cultured B cells. A number of lipoxygenase products were tested without demonstrable effect on these responses (Goodman and Weigle, 1984a). When addition of prostaglandin was delayed for more than 24 h, the effect on anti-immunoglobulin responses changed from enhancement to inhibition, and the effect on 8MGuo was lost. This suggests that in the course of activation, B cells progress through a series of cell cycle-specific regulatory states. This hypothesis is strengthened by the observation that the mitogenic effects of 8MGuo appear to be selective for large, cycling cells (Goodman, 1986b; Wicker *et al.,* 1987). These data suggest a model for regulation of the B-cell cycle in which prostagland- ins, whose secretion has been elicited by many surface-directed B-cell stimuli, enhance the entry of cells into the cell cycle and subsequently regulate their passage through it.

2.2. T-Helper-Like Signals

Loxoribine and its analogues transmit T-helper-like signals to antigen-activated B cells (Goodman and Weigle, 1983c; Goodman, 1985). Antibody responses to T-dependent antigens are not observed in cultures of T-cell-depleted B cells. Such cultures, however, generate high-level responses when supplemented with a substituted guanosine analogue.

The antigen-specific component of the response far exceeds the nonspecific (polyclonal) component. Similarly, significant antibody responses are observed in the presence of 8MGuo in cultures of spleen cells from congenitally athymic (*nu/nu*) mice, which are unable to respond to T-dependent antigens alone. These compounds can thus be classified as an alternate source of T-cell-like help. This is true in the murine system as well as the human system and has been demonstrated for erythrocyte and viral antigens among others (Goodman and Weigle, 1985b; Callard *et al.*, 1985; Dosch *et al.*, 1988).

However, these observations should not be misconstrued to suggest that T cells play no role in immunoenhancement by derivatized nucleosides. Although substituted nucleosides appear to act directly on B cells in transmitting T-cell-like signals, T cells make an important contribution to the overall response level. The physiological signal produced by normal T cells is distinct from the T-cell-like signal provided by these compounds. This is clear because when populations of purified T cells are added to highly enriched preparations of B cells in the presence of antigen and substituted nucleosides, the overall response level increases by a factor of two- to fourfold (Goodman, 1986a). This response level is much greater than the sum anticipated by adding individual responses of (1) B cells with T cells in the presence of antigen, plus (2) B cells and optimal nucleoside concentrations in the presence of antigen, and accordingly the resulting antibody responses are considered synergistic (Goodman, 1985). This synergistic interaction is not dependent on the presence of intact T cells, as the same effect may be reproduced with supernatants from cultures of activated T cells. Moreover, Braun *et al.* (1986) have generated evidence of synergy between 8MGuo and MRL/lpr culture supernatants in the IgG response of an anti-IgM-activated B-cell line, 670-6. Rollins-Smith and Lawton (1988) demonstrated B-cell differentiative synergy between 8MGuo and anti-μ antibodies, using a different culture system that is soluble factor-dependent.

When cyclosporin A is used to inhibit the activity of T cells, the total response level observed in spleen cell populations can be readily separated into T-dependent and T-independent components. Kinetic studies indicate that 8MGuo may be added late in the culture period with preservation of synergy with T cells. In contrast, optimal synergy requires that T cells and T-cell-derived lymphokines, representing the T-cell-dependent component of the response, be present very early in the culture period. Thus, it appears that a lymphokine(s) of T-cell origin induces sensitivity to substituted nucleosides in a particular subset of B cells (Goodman, 1986a).

A B-cell subset that is dependent on both signals was isolated by purifying B cells from populations of G-10 nonadherent cells from CBA/N mice. This particular group of cells was selected because of the unresponsiveness of B cells from these mice to noncognate interactions and because of the unresponsiveness of G-10 nonadherent B cells to substituted nucleosides (Goodman and Weigle, 1983b). The response of this particular subset, an Lyb 5$^-$ subset, was shown to be entirely dependent on reception of signals both from T-cell-derived lymphokines and from substituted nucleosides (Goodman, 1986a). Limiting dilution analyses of precursor frequency confirmed the existence of this subpopulation among B cells from normal animals. The size of this doubly dependent precursor population is thought to be substantial. The identity of the T-cell-derived cytokine that synergizes with 8MGuo has not been established.

In sum, cellular studies have identified three subpopulations of B cells that contribute to the overall antibody responses observed in spleen cell cultures incubated with antigen and substituted nucleosides. These include the mature antigen-reactive set of B cells that respond to antigen without the need for substituted nucleosides, the nucleoside-dependent subset which becomes antigen-responsive in the presence of signals provided by antigen together with substituted nucleosides, and the sizable subset of B cells requiring antigen and both lymphokine- and nucleoside-mediated signals to become antigen reactive.

2.3. Animal Studies

Initially, the capacity of substituted guanine nucleosides to amplify the magnitude of humoral immune responses was described in studies using sheep erythrocytes as the antigen and 8MGuo as the adjuvant (Goodman and Weigle, 1983b). Further studies in the mouse indicated that this compound amplifies the responses to T-cell-independent as well as T-cell-dependent antigens in vitro and in vivo (Goodman and Weigle, 1983a,b; Scheuer *et al.,* 1985a). Thus, in addition to augmenting the primary and secondary antibody responses to sheep erythrocytes in vitro, and in vivo, the IgG response to the T-dependent protein antigens human gamma globulin (HGG) and trinitrophenyl–keyhole limpet hemocyanin (TNP–KLH) were strikingly increased in vivo (Goodman and Weigle, 1983a; Scheuer *et al.,* 1985a, and unpublished data). Similarly, the responses to so-called T-cell-independent antigens were markedly increased. Responses to TNP–*Brucella abortus* and to TNP–Ficoll fall within this category. The latter antigen is well known for its inability to evoke an immune response in mice of the CBA/N strain, a strain manifesting a defect in a late maturing subset of B cells (Quintans and Kaplan, 1978; Phillips and Campbell, 1982; Stein *et al.,* 1983). However, the response to this antigen can be restored in cultured CBA/N cells as well as in vivo when it is accompanied by 8MGuo (Ahmad and Mond, 1984, 1986; Mond *et al.,* 1989). Nucleoside-augmented responses to TNP–Ficoll and pneumococcal polysaccharide have been shown to involve increased IgG1, IgG2, and IgG3 but not IgM antibodies (Mond *et al.,* 1989).

A number of studies have been conducted to evaluate the capacity of loxoribine and its analogues to enhance antibody responses to recombinant proteins and synthetic peptide antigens. Collaborative studies performed with Altman and co-workers examined the capacity of 7-methyl-8-oxoguanosine (7m8oGuo) to enhance the amplitude of the response to a synthetic peptide, p72, from the hepatitis B surface antigen. This peptide was coupled to tetanus toxoid as a carrier and injected into CAF_1 male mice. A striking and prolonged enhancement of antibody titers resulted from including 7m8oGuo in the incomplete Freund's adjuvant (IFA) used to emulsify the peptide–carrier conjugate. All animals were boosted with immunogen alone at day 110, yet titers remained elevated only in the group that initially received the nucleoside adjuvant (Fig. 1). Dose–response studies had previously indicated that a dose of 40 μg of peptide–carrier conjugate was optimal in this mouse strain. However, with the use of 7m8oGuo, this dose of antigen could be reduced tenfold with retention of maximal immunogenicity.

In other studies done in collaboration with Bittle and colleagues (unpublished), a peptide representing residues 141–160 of the foot-and-mouth disease virus type O_1K VP_1 coupled to tetanus toxoid as a carrier was injected in variable quantities into guinea pigs

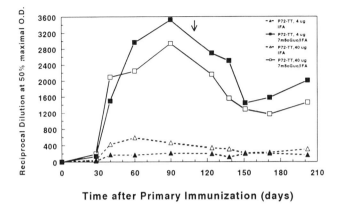

Figure 1. Augmentation of the antibody response to p72-tetanus toxoid by 7m8oGuo. Groups of five mice were immunized with 4 or 40 μg of hepatitis B surface antigen p72 coupled to tetanus toxoid emulsified in IFA, in the presence or absence of 10 mg 7m8oGuo. All animals were boosted with antigen at day 110 (arrow). Results are presented as the arithmetic mean for each group.

together with incremental quantities of 7m8oGuo emulsified in IFA. Serum neutralizing antibody titers were enhanced by one to three orders of magnitude relative to control animals injected with antigen in IFA alone, for the 24-week duration of this study (Fig. 2).

Because of the capacity of loxoribine and its analogues to convert T-cell-dependent antigens into T-cell-independent antigens, and to amplify responses to relatively T-cell-independent antigens such as TNP–Ficoll, collaborative studies were conducted with Dr. Vernon Stevens in an attempt to generate antibody responses to a B-cell-specific epitope in a T-cell-independent fashion. The motivation behind these studies was to avoid the use of T-cell-directed epitopes, with subsequent elimination of potential T-cell-mediated adverse effects such as delayed-type hypersensitivity. Therefore, the B-cell epitope

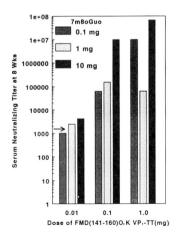

Figure 2. Immunopotentiation of neutralizing titers to FMDV peptide O_1K VP_1 141-160–TT by 7m8oGuo. Groups of four guinea pigs were immunized with incremental doses of FMDV peptide O_1K VP_1 141-160 coupled to tetanus toxoid in IFA with increasing doses of 7m8oGuo, as indicated. Animals were not boosted in these studies. Results are presented as the arithmetic mean for each group. The arrow indicates response level in animals immunized with 0.1 mg antigen in IFA without 7m8oGuo.

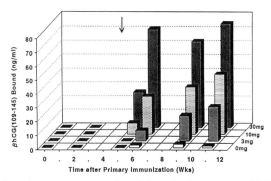

Figure 3. T-cell-independent immunopotentiation of the antibody response to β-hCG–Ficoll. Groups of ten mice were immunized with 200 μg of a B-cell epitope (residues 109–145) of β-hCG coupled to Ficoll either without adjuvant or with incremental doses (3, 10, or 30 mg) of loxoribine as indicated. All animals were boosted at week 4 with the same regimen as was used initially (arrow). Results are presented as the arithmetic mean for each group.

contained in β-hCG peptide residues 109–145 was coupled to Ficoll-70, and 0.2 mg of the conjugate was injected into mice together with 0, 3, 10, or 30 mg of loxoribine. All animals were boosted with immunogen at 4 weeks. Two weeks thereafter, maximal antibody titers were observed in animals receiving the two highest nucleoside doses (Fig. 3). In the absence of loxoribine, the conjugate proved to be a rather poor immunogen.

Further studies were conducted in cynomolgus monkeys. Animals were injected with TNP–KLH together with 0, 1, 10, or 100 mg total dose of 7m8oGuo. Again, IFA was utilized to retard the release of nucleoside. Animals were bled periodically and antibody titers to TNP determined. Although no significant increment in antibody responses was observed at the lowest dose of nucleoside, a dose-dependent increase was noted at doses of 10 and 100 mg 7m8oGuo, the latter eliciting the greatest antibody responses. Significant augmentation of these antibody responses was noted as early as 7 days after immunization. The animals were immunized a second time with either saline or 7m8oGuo identical in amount to that used for the initial immunization. The antibody titers in nucleoside-treated animals remained stable for the duration of the experiment (105 days).

2.4. Immunoprophylaxis

The use of loxoribine pretreatment in anticipation of an immunogenic challenge has also been investigated. Immunodeficient CBA/N (xid) mice were injected with saline, with 8MGuo in IFA subcutaneously (s.c.), or with 8MGuo in a 2% squalene/water emulsion s.c. at day 0. After a 5-day delay, all animals were challenged with an injection of sheep erythrocytes as the immunogen. Five days after this challenge, the capacity of all animals to mount a primary antibody response to antigen was determined. Whereas CBA/N mice that had been preinjected only with saline prior to antigen challenge generated 1100 plaque-forming cells per spleen, animals pretreated with 8MGuo in IFA generated a response of 15,000 PFCs/spleen. Similarly, animals pretreated with 8MGuo in 2% squalene produced an average 22,000 PFCs/spleen. Additional studies, conducted with conventional inbred strains of mice, have demonstrated that administration of 8MGuo in 2% oil may precede immunization by 2 to 3 weeks with retention of full immunopotentiating capacity.

Studies have also been performed to evaluate the potential of these compounds to serve as adjuvants for tumor vaccines. Mice were injected with variable numbers of irradiated (6000 rad) B-16 melanoma cells as a tumor vaccine 21 days and again 14 days prior to intravenous challenge with live B-16 cells (4×10^5). Neither the irradiated B-16 tumor vaccine nor loxoribine alone was capable of stimulating an immune response that protected mice from tumor growth. However, when loxoribine was administered together with the irradiated cell vaccine, dose-related protective immunity was induced, as reflected in up to a 75% diminution in pulmonary metastases. This finding is similar to that made by Sharma *et al.* (1991) who demonstrated that 7-thia-8-oxoguanosine potentiates the efficacy of an L1210 leukemia vaccine.

The immunological mechanism of protection by these compounds is unknown. It is likely that the protective effect is dependent on stimulation of antibodies and/or CTLs against B-16 determinants by weak signals transmitted by the immunogen and amplified by loxoribine. Specific antibodies could exert direct cytotoxic effects on the tumor cells in the presence of complement, or could participate in antibody-dependent cellular cytotoxicity reactions, as shown by others (Jin *et al.*, 1990). CTLs would act directly on the tumor cells. Although it is possible that loxoribine-mediated stimulation of NK cells, LAK cells, cytotoxic macrophages, and/or secretion of cytokines such as TNF-α, IFN, and IL-1 could play a role in this phenomenon, the kinetics of drug turnover together with the transient nature of these latter responses, suggest to us that their participation under these circumstances is unlikely.

2.5. Effects on Human Antibody Responses

In vitro studies have been conducted with normal human peripheral blood lympho-cytes (PBLs). In a culture system that incorporates 10% heat-inactivated autologous plasma, the primary specific antibody response to sheep erythrocytes was found to be dependent on the addition of exogenous IL-2 (Goodman and Weigle, 1985b). In the presence of antigen, but not in its absence, the addition of optimal concentrations of 7m8oGuo augmented the antibody response of PBLs in vitro. Induction of specific antibody responses to antigen in the physical absence of T cells was shown to be nucleoside-dependent.

In separate studies, similar effects of 7m8oGuo were noted in cultures of cells from patients afflicted with common variable immunodeficiency disease (CVID) (Goodman *et al.*, 1991). This disease is attributable to a variety of specific cellular defects, but results in a high incidence of infection in these patients, who are generally dependent on monthly administration of intravenous gamma globulin preparations. In cultured cells from eight of nine patients with CVID, 7m8oGuo restored antigen responses to the mean level of normal donors (without 7m8oGuo) or above. Rijkers *et al.* (1988) examined the effects of 8MGuo on antibody responses of normal human umbilical cord blood B cells to pneumo-coccal polysaccharide antigens. While neonatal cells alone are unresponsive to such antigens, the authors found that responsiveness could be restored with 8MGuo, particularly

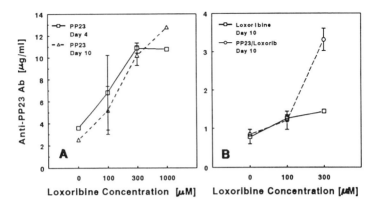

Figure 4. Augmentation of the human PBL response to pneumococcal polysaccharide by loxoribine in vitro. (A) PBLs (10^6/mL) from a normal human donor were cultured with 30 fg/mL pneumococcal polysaccharide antigens either without adjuvant or with incremental concentrations of loxoribine as indicated. Antigen was removed at day 6 and cultures were restimulated with antigen and initial nucleoside dose at day 13. Anti-pneumococcal polysaccharide antibody titers were determined by ELISA 4 or 10 days later. Results are presented as the arithmetic mean of triplicate cultures ± SE. (B) The experimental protocol of panel A was repeated using PBLs from a patient with CVID. Anti-pneumococcal polysaccharide titers were determined 10 days after restimulation.

when added late in the course of culture. This group also found that 8MGuo induces expression of gp350, an Epstein–Barr virus receptor/C3d receptor (CD21) on cultured adult and neonatal B cells (Griffioen *et al.*, 1992).

In studies conducted in our laboratory, normal adult human PBLs were incubated with incremental concentrations of Pneumovax vaccine, a heterogeneous mixture of 23 polysaccharide antigens derived from strains of *Streptococcus pneumoniae*. Although we were unable to induce a primary in vitro antibody response to the pneumococcal polysaccharides, secondary responses were observed when cells were cultured with antigen for 6 days, rested for a week in the absence of antigen, and then restimulated. The secondary responses peaked as early as 4 days after restimulation with the immunogen. Supplementation of cultures with loxoribine in both the primary and secondary stimulatory phases resulted in a striking enhancement of the antibody response (Fig. 4A). As observed for TNP–Ficoll responses in the mouse, very low doses of antigen are required to elicit responses to pneumococcal polysaccharides in cultured human PBLs. When studied in cells from a patient with CVID, loxoribine was observed to induce secondary anti-pneumococcal antibody responses (Fig. 4B). The augmented CVID response appeared to fall within the unaugmented range for normal PBLs.

A double-blind, Phase I, placebo-controlled study of the safety and immunological effectiveness of a single dose of loxoribine was undertaken to evaluate the drug as a potential adjuvant for use in immunization of hemodialysis patients with recombinant hepatitis B vaccine. This recombinant vaccine frequently fails to induce protective antibody titers when administered to chronic renal failure patients in three successive doses according to standard protocol (*Physicians Desk Reference*, 1994). Preliminary evidence from these studies suggests potential efficacy for loxoribine as a vaccine adjuvant in this patient group. Details of this study are presented in Section 7.2.

3. ENHANCEMENT OF T-CELL RESPONSES

3.1. Augmentation of Cytolytic T-Cell Reactivity

Considerably less work has been done examining the adjuvanticity of loxoribine and its analogues for cytolytic T-cell (CTL) responses. The potential of these compounds to augment CTL responses is indicated by the work of Feldbush and Ballas (1985). These investigators found that 8MGuo is a potent immune stimulant for the generation of CTL activity against poorly immunogenic (e.g., heat-inactivated) stimulator cells. In vitro studies showed that these stimulator cells evoked minimal generation of allogeneic CTLs in MLC. However, in the presence of 8MGuo, the response increased to levels comparable to those induced by gamma-irradiated H-2-identical stimulator cells. Similarly, the suboptimal responses that were stimulated by low numbers of fully immunogenic stimulator cells were increased by 8MGuo beyond the levels that were seen in cultures with optimal numbers of irradiated stimulator cells in the absence of 8MGuo. The enhancement of CTL activity was shown to be H-2 restricted, antigen specific, and mediated by nylon wool-nonadherent cells that expressed high-density surface Thy-1 antigen. This differentiative effect of the nucleoside on precursor CTL cells occurs in the absence of T-cell proliferation (Feldbush and Ballas, 1985; Goodman and Weigle, 1983d). Studies are currently in progress to examine the ability of loxoribine and its analogues to augment CTL responses evoked by synthetic influenza peptides bearing CTL epitopes coupled to T-helper epitopes.

3.2. Antigen-Specific T-Cell Proliferation

We have investigated effects of substituted guanine nucleosides on other aspects of T-cell function. Although 8MGuo is not mitogenic for thymocytes, it can alter the mitogenic response of thymocytes cultured with IL-2. The proliferative responses of responding lymphocytes to allogeneic stimulator cells can be similarly augmented by these compounds. 8MGuo was also shown to augment antigen-specific proliferation of lymph node T cells from ovalbumin-primed mice (Goodman, 1991). Thus, these compounds appear to augment proliferation and differentiation of murine T cells only in the presence of other stimulatory signals (Goodman and Weigle, 1986).

The dependence of these phenomena on production of various cytokines from Th1 or Th2 cells is currently unknown. However, there is indirect evidence to suggest that these compounds act on Th1 cells, since cells prestimulated with allogeneic lymphocytes or with mitogenic lectins, such as concanavalin A, produce higher levels of IL-2 when cultured with substituted guanine nucleosides. Resting T cells exhibit no such increase in IL-2 production on nucleoside stimulation (Goodman, 1991). Loxoribine also has been shown to augment IFN-γ secretion in a dose-dependent manner. The origin and phenotype of the secretory cell is presently unknown. Studies with Th1 and Th2 antigen-specific clones are currently in progress to help provide answers to these questions.

4. ROLE OF CYTOKINES

Substituted guanine nucleosides induce the secretion of a number of cytokines, including IFN-α/β, IFN-γ, IL-1β, IL-6, TNF-α, TNF-β, and the p40 chain of IL-12 (Koo *et al.*, 1988; Pope *et al.*, 1994b; Goodman, 1988a, 1991). Increased IL-2 secretion is seen only in the presence of an appropriate co-stimulus. Loxoribine also upregulates the expression of surface receptors for IL-2 (Pope *et al.*, 1993). No increase is seen in mRNA levels of IL-2, IL-3, IL-4, IL-5, IL-7, or GM-CSF.

A dissection of the interrelationships and interdependencies of these cytokines is beyond the scope of this chapter. However, a brief consideration of the effects of these agents on the adjuvanticity of loxoribine and its analogues is of relevance in the present context. We have shown that supplementing cultures of antigen-stimulated murine B cells with exogenous IFN-α or IFN-β together with 8MGuo augments the resultant antigen-specific antibody response in a synergistic manner (Goodman, 1987). However, antibodies against IFN-α or IFN-β at concentrations that abrogate the biological activity of each, fail to diminish the magnitude of antibody responses generated by B cells in the presence of activated T-cell supernatants. This observation suggests that under normal circumstances neither IFN-α nor IFN-β is an important physiological means used by loxoribine to amplify these responses. Similarly, antibodies to IFN-α or IFN-β, added to antigen-stimulated B-cell populations together with substituted nucleosides, fail to diminish the resultant antibody responses (unpublished observations). In contrast to the effects of exogenous IFN-α and IFN-β, the addition of supplemental IFN-γ does not amplify the responses of murine B cells to antigen in the presence of 8MGuo. At concentrations of 5000 units/mL and above, the response is suppressed in dose-dependent fashion. Moreover, when activated T-cell supernatants are treated at pH 2.0 to inactivate IFN-γ, the level of overall responsiveness increases. Thus, IFN-γ plays no demonstrable positive role in the adjuvanticity of these compounds in vitro. It should be noted that cytokines appear to occupy a more critical role in other immunobiological activities evoked by loxoribine. Specifically, anti-IFN-α/β antibodies cause partial but significant inhibition of B-cell proliferative and NK cell responses to loxoribine (Pope *et al.*, 1994a). High doses of rapamycin exhibit similar effects on proliferation (Wicker *et al.*, 1990). Antibodies to the other cytokines mentioned in this section are devoid of significant effects.

Substituted guanine nucleosides induce cultured murine splenic adherent cells as well as the P388D$_1$ macrophage cell line to secrete IL-1 (Goodman, 1988a). Secretion of IL-1-like activity increases in dose-dependent fashion, peaking at nucleoside concentrations that also evoke polyclonal stimulation of B cells (i.e., 0.3–1.0 mM 8BrGuo). Much less IL-1 activity is observed at the lower doses of 8BrGuo, which are optimal for adjuvanticity. When antibodies that neutralize IL-1 bioactivity are added to cultures of antigen-stimulated murine spleen cells in the presence of 8BrGuo, no inhibition of adjuvanticity is observed relative to nonspecific immunoglobulin controls. Thus, IL-1 does not appear to occupy a central position in the events mediating adjuvanticity for these compounds.

The role of TNF-α has been explored with respect to augmentation of humoral immunity. As is observed for IFN-α, and β, exogenous TNF-α appears to be capable of augmenting humoral immune responses generated in cultures of antigen-stimulated murine B lymphocytes in the presence of loxoribine (unpublished observations). However, neutralizing antibodies to TNF-α added to cultures of unseparated murine spleen cells stimulated with antigen and 8MGuo, fail to diminish the level of antigen responsiveness.

The nature of the soluble factor(s) secreted by activated T cells that synergizes with loxoribine and its analogues is undergoing further exploration. IL-2, 3, 4, 5, 6, GM-CSF, and bursin have all been found incapable of further augmenting antibody responses in the presence of substituted nucleosides.

5. BIOCHEMICAL STUDIES

5.1. Transport System

The biochemical mechanism of action of loxoribine and its analogues have been studied in B cells. These compounds are transported across the plasma membrane into B cells by a process of carrier-facilitated diffusion (Goodman and Weigle, 1984b). This process involves a dual-component carrier system comprised of high- and low-affinity components. The Michaelis constant for the high-affinity system is approximately 8 μM, while that for the low-affinity system is 480 μM. These values coincide well with those described in the literature for the uptake of adenosine by murine lymphocytes (Strauss *et al.*, 1976).

Other studies were conducted to determine whether the site of action of these compounds is intracellular or extracellular. 8MGuo, immobilized on Sepharose beads with an interposed spacer arm, was found to be incapable of activating B cells, as was polymerized 8Br-5′GMP (average molecular weight 400,000). Moreover, rigidification of plasma membrane with exogenous cholesterol selectively antagonized stimulation by membrane-directed ligands such as anti-IgM antibodies, while exerting minimal impact on stimulation by 8MGuo. Nucleoside transport antagonists were found to selectively inhibit biological responses to substituted guanine nucleosides at concentrations two to three orders of magnitude lower than those that inhibit activation of cells when stimulated by other agents. These results are consistent with the hypothesis that loxoribine and its analogues act at an intracellular site.

5.2. Loxoribine Binding Proteins: Binding Studies, Autoradiography

Further studies were undertaken to examine the possibility that substituted nucleosides act via a binding interaction with one or more intracellular components. Dose–response studies for immunobiological function had previously suggested that the affinity of any such binding interaction observed would be low enough to make this difficult. Of a number of experimental approaches attempted, only studies performed with whole cell preparations yielded meaningful data. This may be a consequence of secondary stabilizing effects that occur in vivo. Because preceding transport studies had defined a short initial period of unidirectional flux of nucleoside into the cell, followed by bidirectional flux eventuating in the establishment of a state of equilibrium (Goodman and Weigle, 1984b), it appeared likely that the intracellular compartment would contain both free and bound nucleoside pools.

Studies evaluating the kinetics of egress of radiolabeled disubstituted nucleosides demonstrated that indeed a period of rapid nucleoside efflux is followed by a much slower phase (Goodman, 1990). The association kinetics for nucleosides entering the slowly exchangeable pool were complete by approximately 20–30 min of incubation; the half-time for dissociation was 126 min. Nitrogen cavitates prepared from cells from which the rapidly exchangeable (free) pool had been removed, exhibited a peak of radioactivity that did not co-chromatograph with free nucleoside. This activity was found to be much more hydrophobic than free nucleoside on C18 reverse-phase HPLC columns, and eluted from HPLC gel filtration columns at an apparent molecular weight of between 30,000 and 45,000. Cell-associated radioactivity in the slowly exchangeable pool could be released with detergent. Released material co-chromatographed with authentic radiolabeled nucleoside on TLC.

Incubation of murine splenic B cells with incremental amounts of radiolabeled nucleoside demonstrated the existence of two saturable binding interactions. Estimation of the dissociation constants for these interactions by Scatchard analysis yielded an apparent K_d of 4–10 μM for the higher-affinity interaction with about 20,000–40,000 sites/cell, and 700 μM for the lower-affinity interaction (Goodman and Cherry, 1989). In both cases, specific binding was inhibitable by an excess of the identical nucleoside in unlabeled form, as well as by other structural nucleoside analogues, with a hierarchy of inhibition that recapitulated the ordinal relationship for immunobiological activity (i.e., 7a8oGuo > 8BrGuo > 8Br-gua). Binding was not antagonized by irrelevant B-cell antagonists.

Autoradiography was performed on sections of B cells that were first incubated with radiolabeled nucleoside followed by removal of the rapidly exchangeable nucleoside pool. Examination under the electron microscope indicated that the preponderance of radioactivity was associated with the nuclear compartment of B cells (Fig. 5). It is not known whether the origin of the putative nuclear binding component is cytoplasmic or nuclear. If cytoplasmic, this component could be translocated to the nuclear compartment as a complex with nucleoside. If a cytoplasmic binding component serves simply as a shuttle protein, one would anticipate subsequent interaction with a nuclear component in a specific fashion that would directly or indirectly result in initiation of coordinated transcriptional activity.

Alternatively, if the original binding activity is mediated by a nuclear protein, or if it is translocated to the nucleus from the cytosol, it could act directly as a *trans*-acting transcriptional regulatory protein binding to one or more putative regulatory elements near target genes. It is also possible that the nucleoside acts indirectly, binding to a cytosolic nucleoside-binding protein to expose a nuclear localization sequence, or to a nuclear nucleoside-binding protein that might result in configurational alteration that in turn could activate latent protein kinase, phosphatase, or other intrinsic enzymatic activity. These proteins could subsequently activate other nuclear enzymes or regulatory proteins. These possibilities will be addressed in future studies.

5.3. Interaction with Purine Salvage Pathway Enzymes

Inside the cell, loxoribine and its analogues provide a logical substrate for metabolism by purine salvage pathway enzymes. Evaluation of this possibility, how-

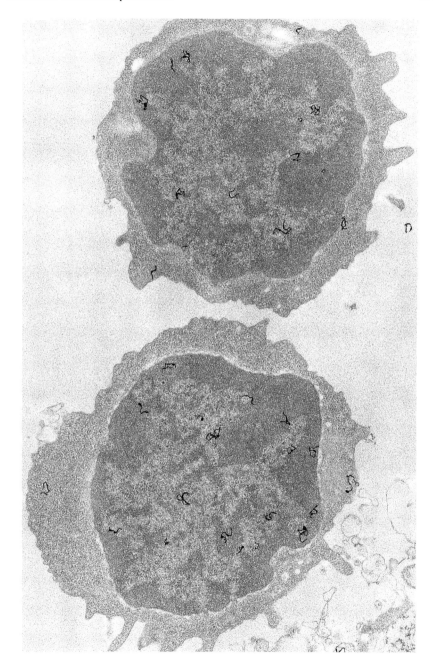

Figure 5. Autoradiographic localization of [^{3}H]7p8oGuo by electron microscopy. CBA/CaJ B cells were cultured with 500 μM [^{3}H]7p8oGuo for 4 h at 37°C. Unbound nucleoside pools were removed and cells were fixed in modified Karnovsky's fixative, and prepared for EM autoradiography as described in Goodman (1990). Photo reproduced with permission of *J. Biol. Chem.*

ever, clearly indicates that the substituted guanine nucleosides are not appropriate sub-strates for this group of enzymes (Goodman and Weigle, 1982a; Goodman, 1988b). Furthermore, it appears unlikely that any substantial degree of phosphorylation of these compounds occurs by direct, kinase-mediated reactions. We have been unable to document any significant degree of incorporation of these compounds into either RNA or DNA (Goodman, 1988b). This lack of incorporation into nucleic acid would be expected on the basis of failure of loxoribine to undergo phosphorylation. Moreover, the fact that this compound is not incorporated into nucleic acid correlates with the lack of mutagenic potential observed to date.

5.4. Protein Kinase C Pathway Independence

Interaction of 7,8-disubstituted guanine nucleosides with specific events in estab-lished signal transduction pathways was evaluated (Goodman *et al.*, 1990). These studies revealed that despite its extensive structural homology with GTP, 7m8oGuo does not inhibit the binding of guanosine 5′-3-O-(thio)triphosphate either to purified G-proteins, or to plasma membrane-associated G-proteins in situ. In contrast to anti-IgM antibodies (Ransom *et al.*, 1988; Bijsterbosch *et al.*, 1985; Grupp *et al.*, 1987; Coggeshall and Cambier, 1984), 7m8oGuo fails to induce elevation of intracellular free calcium ion or of inositol phosphates in B cells (Goodman *et al.*, 1990; Wicker *et al.*, 1990). Moreover, 7m8oGuo does not modify the cellular distribution or activity of protein kinase C (PK-C); nor do inhibitors of PK-C activity diminish stimulation of transcriptional activity induced by 7m8oGuo. Abrogation of B-cell proliferation to anti-IgM antibodies by preincubation with PMA to deplete PK-C, was reversed by supplementation of these cultures with 8MGuo (Mond *et al.*, 1987). PK-C independence has been corroborated for the human antigen-specific response as well, both for cells from normal individuals as well as for those from patients with CVID (Goodman *et al.*, 1991). These data suggest that substituted guanine nucleosides either use a pathway distinct from that mediated by GTP-binding proteins, intracellular free calcium ion, inositol phosphates, and PK-C, or else bypass the early events of this pathway, activating the cell at a point beyond their involvement.

It has been noted that within 1 to 2 h following exposure of B cells to 8MGuo, an increase in the synthesis of a 40-kDa protein of pI 5.0 occurs (Feuerstein and Mond, 1987a). This protein, numatrin, is a nuclear protein that has previously been shown to be associated with induction of B lymphocyte proliferation by a number of mitogens in mice (Feuerstein and Mond, 1987b).

6. PRECLINICAL STUDIES

6.1. Advantageous Features Unique to Loxoribine

1. In addition to its potent activity as an immunobiological adjuvant, loxoribine has a number of unique advantages relative to other immunomodulators. The first of these is that it provides a surrogate source of T-helper-like signal to antigen-reactive B cells, thereby

rendering their antibody responses essentially T cell-independent (Goodman and Weigle, 1983c, 1984c). Thus, it is potentially a very effective adjuvant for patients with functional or absolute T-cell deficiencies, since it can render an otherwise T-cell-dependent vaccine T cell-independent. Examples of this situation include patients with AIDS, patients with CVID with T-helper defects, and patients with congenital T-cell deficiency, such as severe combined immunodeficiency and ataxia-telangiectasia. For vaccines associated with T-cell-mediated adverse effects, such as hypersensitivity reactions, loxoribine should enable vaccine designers to omit T-cell epitope(s) from the immunogen without sacrificing its immunogenicity, as shown in Fig. 3.

2. The ability of loxoribine to augment antibody responses is mediated from an intracellular site, independent of PK-C (Goodman and Weigle, 1984b; Mond *et al.,* 1987; Goodman *et al.,* 1991). Thus, loxoribine strongly enhances antibody responses in cells that are unable to transduce signals from the plasma membrane. Clinical application of this feature would include vaccination of patients with membrane receptor/signal transduction defects, possibly including patients with the immunodeficiencies of senescence and diabetes mellitus. This ability to bypass surface membrane events also enables loxoribine to activate antibody responses in certain defective B cells, such as those from patients with CVID with intrinsic B-cell defects.

3. Loxoribine acts as an adjuvant essentially free of cytokine dependency (Pope *et al.,* 1994b). Therefore, it is anticipated that it will prove valuable for augmenting vaccine-induced immunity in organ transplant patients whose immunity is suppressed by treatment with cyclosporin A and other immunosuppressive agents; it should also induce immune responses to vaccines in patients with specific cytokine defects.

4. Loxoribine has been found to bypass functional immunological immaturity. It is active on B cells from newborn animals as well as on human cord blood lymphocytes (Goodman and Weigle, 1984c; Rijkers *et al.,* 1988). For these reasons, it is anticipated that loxoribine will be useful as an adjuvant for vaccines in infants, whose immune competence remains inadequate against certain pathogens, e.g., *Neisseria meningitidis,* up to the age of 24 months.

6.2. Dose Response, Vehicle, Route of Administration

Extensive preclinical studies have been performed to evaluate the optimal dosage requirements for loxoribine. Antibody responses are observed to increase directly with the dose of nucleoside administered. Working with C8-substituted guanine nucleosides, Mond *et al.* (1989) found that the IgG2 anti-TNP antibody response to TNP–Ficoll in CBA/J mice increased from a titer of 42 in control animals to 81 in animals receiving 10 mg of 8MGuo, to 444 in animals receiving 30 mg, and to 2723 in animals receiving 300 mg of 8MGuo (about a 65-fold increase). Similarly, for N7C8-substituted guanine nucleosides such as loxoribine, response levels continue to increase with escalating dose. Examples of amplified responses to several immunogens are shown in Figs. 1–3. In mice, loxoribine doses of 1 to 4 mg/animal (40–160 mg/kg) are generally effective. The use of these compounds allows for reduction in the dose of immunogen administered by at least one order of magnitude without sacrificing the level of antibody response ultimately achieved. Thus, the dose of p72-tetanus toxoid was reduced from 40 μg to 4 μg per mouse with quantitatively comparable responses (Fig. 1); in the guinea pig, the concentration of foot-and-mouth disease peptide 141–160 type O_1K VP_1 could be decreased from 100 μg to 1 μg/animal without diminution of the neutralizing antibody levels attained so long as each of the latter animals also received a total dose of 0.1 mg 7m8oGuo.

Antibody response levels are controlled significantly by the choice of vehicle for administration of loxoribine. Initial studies were performed using a solution of 8MGuo dissolved in saline or other physiological buffers, but only minimal immunological effects were observed. It was reasoned that the molecule likely had a very short in vivo half-life, and therefore studies were undertaken in which the nucleoside was administered as a suspension in saline, with antigen injected separately. This approach was clearly effective, although the considerable animal-to-animal variation was a consequence of the technically primitive methodology (Goodman and Weigle, 1983a). Subsequently, studies were conducted to compare the virtues of administering 7m8oGuo in a viscous suspension medium such as carboxymethylcellulose versus an oil suspension medium such as sesame oil. In these studies, the antibody responses achieved using nucleosides in carboxymethylcellulose were significantly inferior to those observed with an oil-containing vehicle. A number of different oils were tested, including squalene, sesame oil, oil of anise, bay, cinnamon, and organum. Of these, squalene, sesame oil, and organum were the better vehicles. Direct comparison of carboxymethylcellulose, IFA, 100% sesame oil, and a 2% sesame oil-in-saline emulsion revealed that the latter three appeared optimal, with minimal differences among them (Fig. 6). Sesame oil was chosen as the standard vehicle for further developmental work and for Phase I clinical trials. Other studies indicate essentially equal efficacy for loxoribine dispersed in intralipid, an intravenous medium-chain triglyceride supplement used in hyperalimentation (unpublished observations). Intralipid is much less viscous and accommodates higher concentrations per milliliter of loxoribine.

Differences in the degree of immunobiological activity induced are observed when substituted guanine nucleosides are administered by different routes. At high doses, intravenous administration of loxoribine appears to be of equivalent efficacy to subcutaneous administration. At lower doses, however, subcutaneous administration results in antibody responses of higher magnitude. Direct comparison of the levels of antibody response induced by nucleoside administered by intraperitoneal, subcutaneous, or oral routes revealed that intraperitoneal administration is preferable, being slightly more

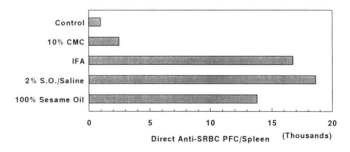

Figure 6. Influence of vehicle on the immunopotentiating activity of loxoribine. Groups of five CBA/CaJ mice were immunized with 2×10^6 SRBCs i.p. either without adjuvant or with 1 mg loxoribine s.c. in a variety of vehicles, as indicated. Results are presented as the arithmetic mean for each group.

effective than the subcutaneous route at moderate and higher doses of nucleoside. At lower doses, intraperitoneal administration is clearly superior to subcutaneous and oral routes. At intermediate to higher doses of nucleoside, oral administration is somewhat inferior to the subcutaneous route. Dose–response profiles indicate that the response to orally administered drug levels off at a time when dose-dependent increases still can be observed under conditions of subcutaneous or intraperitoneal administration. Loxoribine, however, clearly possesses oral activity; certain other analogues have been synthesized that possess a significantly greater degree of oral activity (fivefold) than does loxoribine itself (B. Pope, unpublished observations).

6.3. Effects on Autoimmune-Prone Mice

By its nature as an immunostimulant, loxoribine theoretically might induce undesirable as well as desirable immunological activity, such as exacerbation of autoimmunity. To address this issue, male $(NZB \times W)F_1$ mice were injected subcutaneously with loxoribine in sesame oil, or with sesame oil alone as a control, every other week for a period of 1 year, and subsequently were examined for histopathological changes. Serum IgG, IgM, anti-DNA antibodies, and creatinine levels were also evaluated. No significant increase in autoantibody was noted in loxoribine-treated mice relative to control mice. No evidence of exacerbation of spontaneous systemic lupus erythematosus-like disease was observed on gross or histopathological examination of treated animals. A similar study using 7-allyl-8-thioxoguanosine was conducted with $(NZB \times W)F_1$ male mice, BXSB female mice, MRL +/+ mice as models of chronic autoimmunity. Again, no significant differences between control and experimental animals were noted, indicating that these nucleoside immunostimulants do not induce any consistent trend toward exacerbated autoimmunity in these murine models for human systemic lupus erythematosus.

6.4. Patent Status, Synthesis

Several patents covering the varied potential clinical applications of loxoribine and its predecessors have been filed and have subsequently been issued. A listing of the relevant patents and their dates of issue includes the following:

1. Goodman, M. G., and W. O. Weigle. Modulation of animal cellular responses with compositions containing 8-substituted guanine derivatives. Patent issued September 3, 1985. Patent No. 4,539,205.
2. Goodman, M. G., and W. O. Weigle. Modulation of animal cellular responses with compositions containing 8-substituted guanine derivatives. Patent issued February 17, 1987. Patent No. 4,643,992.
3. Goodman, M.G. Antimicrobial chemotherapeutic potentiation using substituted nucleoside derivatives. Patent issued May 24, 1988. Patent No. 4,746,651.
4. Goodman, M. G., and W. O. Weigle. Modulation of animal cellular responses with compositions containing 8-substituted guanine derivatives. Patent issued July 18, 1989. Patent No. 4,849,411.

5. Goodman, M.G., and E.P. Gamson. Immunostimulating 7-deaza-7-oxa and 7-deaza-7-oxo analogues of 8-substituted-guanine-9-(1'-beta-D-aldoglycosidyl) derivatives and methods of treating test animals. Patent issued November 24, 1992. Patent No. 5,166,141.

6. Goodman, M. G., and W. O. Weigle. Modulation of animal cellular responses with compositions containing 8-substituted guanine derivatives. Patent issued August 14, 1990. Patent No. 4,948,730.

7. Goodman, M. G., W. O. Weigle, S. Bell, R. Chen, R. Robins, and W. J. Hennen. Immunostimulating guanine derivatives, compositions and methods. Patent issued April 30, 1991. Patent No. 5,011,828.

8. Goodman, M. G., and R. Chen. Immunostimulating guanosine derivatives and their pharmaceutical compositions. Patent issued March 3, 1992. Patent No. 5,093,318.

9. Goodman, M. G., and W. O. Weigle. Modulation of animal cellular responses with compositions containing 8-substituted guanine derivatives and interferons. Patent issued September 15, 1992. Patent No. 5,147,636.

10. Goodman, M. G., and W. O. Weigle. Modulation of animal cellular responses with compositions containing 8-substituted guanine derivatives. Patent pending.

11. Goodman, M. G., and L. D. Piro. Cancerous B cell treatment using substituted nucleoside derivatives. Filed November 13, 1992.

Five other patent applications are currently pending.

The synthesis procedure generally utilized for the preparation of loxoribine (7-allyl-8-oxoguanosine) is as follows. In this synthesis, 1-amino-8-oxoguanosine serves as the starting material. It is prepared essentially as described in the method of Rizkalla *et al.* (1969). To a solution of 1-amino-8-oxoguanosine (9.5 g, 30 mmol) in dimethylformamide (DMF) is added sodium methoxide (33 mmol) in 250 mL of DMF. The reaction mixture is stirred at ambient room temperature for 30 min. A DMF solution (10 mL), containing a slight molar excess of the alkylating agent allyl bromide (3-bromopropene), e.g., 33 mmol, is added, and the resulting alkylating reaction mixture is stirred for about 16 h at a temperature of about 20 to 40°C. The solvent is thereafter removed in vacuo and the residue treated with distilled or deionized water (150 mL) and methylene chloride (150 mL). The solid obtained is filtered and recrystallized from an appropriate solvent to yield 1-amino-7-allyl-8-oxoguanosine.

The product of the first stage of synthesis is then dissolved in concentrated HCl (e.g., 4.65 mmol in 15 mL of HCl) to which aqueous sodium nitrite was added (e.g., 4.19 mmol in 5 mL of water) at 0°C. This solution is then stirred for about 1 h. The resulting deaminated product is thereafter obtained by standard crystallization techniques. In this case, 7-allyl-8-oxoguanosine is prepared in about 40% yield from the 1-amino compound as a white powder, mp 230–231°C. NMR (DMSO-d_6): δ 5.6 (d,J=5 Hz 1H); 6.5 (bs, 2H); 10.8 (bs,1H). IR (KBr): 1660, 1590, and 1560 cm^{-1}. The elemental analysis calculated for $C_{13}H_{17}N_3O_6$ is: C, 46.02; H, 5.05; N, 20.64. The observed elemental analysis was found to be: C, 45.63; H, 5.10; N, 20.56

6.5. Safety Profile and Stability

A broad-based pharmacological evaluation has been performed at the R.W.J. Pharmaceutical Research Institute, to assess the physiological activity of loxoribine in a variety of nonimmunological test systems. At 100 mg/kg, subcutaneously administered loxoribine produced weak CNS depression in mice, manifested as a small reduction in open field exploratory activity and bilateral palpebral ptosis. This minor effect lasted for more than 4 h, but was not seen at lower doses (1.0 and 10.0 mg/kg). Loxoribine, administered intravenously at 100 mg/kg, had minimal effects on mean arterial blood pressure and heart rate in conscious instrumented dogs. Two of the three dogs receiving loxoribine experienced emesis which could account for the subsequent slight increase in heart rate and arterial blood pressure. Loxoribine has no significant effect on hemodynamic variables measured 30 and 60 min after intravenous infusion of a single 100 mg/kg dose to anesthetized open-chest dogs. A slight but statistically significant decrease in coronary blood flow was noted during this infusion, but was not present after infusion. Loxoribine, administered as a single 100 mg/kg dose subcutaneously, is devoid of any pro- or anti-inflammatory activity in the established adjuvant arthritic rat model. In a pulmonary function study in anesthetized dogs, intravenous administration of loxoribine at the same dose had no significant effects on dynamic compliance or airway resistance. At $50 \mu g/mL$, loxoribine exhibited no antimicrobial activity against any of the eight microorganisms examined. When administered subcutaneously at 100 mg/kg, loxoribine was found to lack any antigastrolesive activity against ethanol-induced lesions in rats, but did exhibit some marginal antisecretory activity in the pylorus-ligated rat model when tested orally at the same dose level. No contragestational effects were noted when loxoribine was administered subcutaneously at 15 mg/kg for the first 13 days of pregnancy in rats. Finally, loxoribine did not modulate potassium-induced smooth muscle contraction in rabbit aorta or canine trachea, and was devoid of any calcium channel blocking activity at concentrations up to $10 \mu M$.

Stability of loxoribine was also evaluated at the R.W. J. Pharmaceutical Research Institute. Stability of the powdered nucleoside was evaluated at elevated temperatures in an oxygen or nitrogen headspace. After 4 weeks under these conditions, all samples were found to be intact by HPLC assay. In solution, all samples were stable to 4 weeks except that held at 100°C in an atmosphere of oxygen, which exhibited significant degradation. Other stability studies of 8BrGuo and 7m8oGuo emulsified in IFA were conducted by Dr. James Bittle at Scripps. These studies indicated that such preparations retained full biological activity after up to 6 months' storage.

6.6. Activity Relative to Other Immunomodulators

A number of studies have been conducted to evaluate the level of augmentation of antibody responses elicited by loxoribine relative to several other immunomodulatory agents. Most of these studies have been performed in vitro. In the murine system, using sheep erythrocyte antigens, the activity of loxoribine appears to far exceed activity manifested by agents such as muramyl dipeptide (MDP) or levamisole (Fig. 7A); no significant activity has been observed for isoprinosine. In vitro adjuvanticity of bacterial

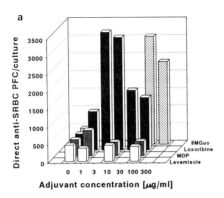
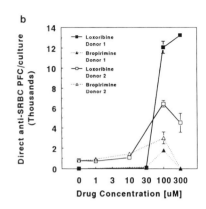

Figure 7. Comparison of the immunopotentiating activity of loxoribine with other adjuvants. (A) CBA/CaJ spleen cells (4×10^6/mL) were cultured with 2×10^6 SRBCs either without adjuvant or with incremental concentrations of levamisole, MDP, loxoribine, or 8MGuo. Direct PFCs to SRBCs were assessed 4 days later. Results are presented as the arithmetic mean of triplicate cultures. (B) The experimental protocol of panel A was repeated using loxoribine or bropirimine in cultures of human PBLs stimulated with SRBCs. Results from two different donors are shown.

lipopolysaccharide is consistently of comparable magnitude to that of loxoribine. The activity of bropirimine is generally comparable to that of loxoribine, but exhibits high-dose cytotoxicity that loxoribine lacks.

When adjuvanticity for human primary antibody responses was evaluated, loxoribine was again found to exhibit activity superior to that of MDP or levamisole. It produced antibody responses that were at least twice the level of those observed with bropirimine. These responses leveled off or continued to increase at high concentrations of loxoribine, whereas at high concentrations, responses to bropirimine fell dramatically to virtually undetectable levels (Fig. 7B).

A number of in vivo studies have also been performed to compare the performance of loxoribine with other immunomodulators. Work done in collaboration with Dr. Vernon Stevens in the murine system indicated that loxoribine is a significantly more effective adjuvant for the secondary antibody responses against synthetic peptide–carrier conjugates than is monophosphoryl lipid A. In an oil vehicle, loxoribine yields responses that are generally comparable to or greater than the magnitude of those produced in mice by antigen in CFA; in dogs, loxoribine appears to be slightly less effective than CFA. Although the ability of loxoribine to enhance antibody responses has not been directly compared to that of bropirimine in vivo, the effects of these two agents have been compared in terms of their abilities to augment NK cell activity. In these assays, conducted by Dr. Barbara Pope, loxoribine was found to be twice as active as bropirimine, and again displayed none of the high-dose toxicity of the latter compound.

7. CLINICAL TRIALS

7.1. Phase I Trial in Advanced Cancer Patients

Loxoribine was initially evaluated in a Phase I safety study conducted in patients with advanced cancer refractory to standard chemotherapy regimens. This study was performed at the University of Pittsburgh Cancer Institute under the direction of Dr. John Kirkwood (Agarwala *et al.*, 1992). Twenty-four patients (14 male, 10 female) were studied in a double-blind crossover trial. Median age of the subjects treated was 60.5 years (range 35–72 years). Patients were divided into three tiers of eight patients each. Within each tier, the patients were divided into two groups of four, one of which received placebo (sesame oil) and the other a single injection of loxoribine in sesame oil. After a 4-week respite, the patients of each group received the opposite treatment. Patients in the first tier received 1 mg/kg loxoribine. After the first tier had been completed and it was deemed safe to proceed, the second tier (at 5 mg/kg) was begun. Similarly, when this tier was completed and the safety of all patients verified, the final tier, at 10 mg/kg, was opened. The malignancies in this group of patients included melanoma (seven; including two ocular), lung (five), colorectal (seven), and one each of breast, larynx, renal, pancreatic, and unknown primary.

Toxicity observed for patients in this study included a flulike syndrome reminiscent of that induced by cytokines such as interferon. In all cases toxicity was less than or equal to grade 1 and included fever, skin rash, nausea/vomiting, and pain at the injection site, with no relation to dosage except for local pain (which was more frequent at 5 mg/kg) and perhaps fever. No maximally tolerated dose (MTD) was achieved. Thus, loxoribine can be given at doses of at least 10 mg/kg without major toxicity. For the most part, constitutional symptoms could be prevented by pretreatment with Tylenol.

In this study, there did not appear to be any changes in clinical laboratory parameters attributable to loxoribine. Autoimmune responses were not induced nor were serum IgE levels increased after loxoribine administration. The most significant effect of loxoribine on cellular immune function in vitro was a transient augmentation of pokeweed mitogen responsiveness of cells taken from loxoribine-treated patients. Maximal effect was noted 24 h after drug administration. Pharmacokinetic data were also gathered in this study. Peak plasma levels of loxoribine were dose-related and occurred 2 h after drug administration. Serum levels remained elevated 24 h after drug administration, particularly for patients in the two higher-dosage tiers. The half-life of loxoribine in these patients was approximately 8 to 12 h. These pharmacokinetic data contrast markedly with those from mice, in which loxoribine is rapidly eliminated from the circulation, with a half-life of approximately 15 min, and is not detectable 6 to 8 h after administration.

7.2. Phase I Trial in Chronic Renal Failure Patients on Hemodialysis

A second clinical trial of loxoribine was subsequently undertaken to evaluate the immunopotentiating capacity of the drug for recombinant hepatitis B vaccine (Recombivax) in patients with chronic renal failure on hemodialysis. This was a Phase I, double-blind placebo-controlled study, conducted jointly at the Mayo Clinic and the Massachusetts General Hospital. The study population is an immunocompromised one; only about 50% of hemodialysis patients given the full course of three injections of hepatitis B surface antigen vaccine attain protective antibody titers (greater than 10 mIU/mL) as compared to more than 90% of normal individuals under age 40 receiving one-quarter the dose administered to hemodialysis patients (*Physicians Desk Reference*, 1994). Moreover, hemodialysis patients attaining protective antibody levels after a full course of vaccination tend to maintain protective antibody levels only transiently. Because of their poor immune responses to vaccination with hepatitis B surface antigen, these patients remain at risk for development of hepatitis B infection.

The study design stipulated that only hemodialysis patients who had failed to establish protective antibody levels against hepatitis B surface antigen after a full course of vaccination were to be enrolled. All patients were to receive Recombivax hepatitis B surface antigen vaccine (40 μg, intramuscularly) as per the manufacturer's instructions. However, rather than three standard injections, only a single injection of the vaccine was to be administered.

A total of nine patients were enrolled. Three were randomized to the sesame oil placebo group and six were randomized to receive 0.75 mg/kg loxoribine [i.e., less than 2% of the dose found effective in mice, on a mg/kg basis (see Section 6.2)]. By 12 weeks after immunization, the three placebo patients showed no increase from baseline in their antibody levels against hepatitis B surface antigen. In contrast, in the low-dose loxorib-ine-treated group, antibody titers against hepatitis B surface antigen increased from baseline through week 12 in three of the six treated patients. Two of these patients had week 12 antibody titers that were elevated beyond the minimum protective level, with a third subject slightly below the protective threshold. The remaining three treated patients showed no significant change from baseline levels. No significant adverse effects were described in any of the patients. Because of preclinical data demonstrating that immunopotentiation increases directly with increasing dose of loxoribine, it is likely that the percent responsiveness as well as the levels of antibody achieved will increase significantly at higher loxoribine doses.

7.3. Future Trials

A third clinical trial has been planned, involving patients with CVID. Because of the small number of these patients available, each patient will serve as his or her own control. Thus, patients will be immunized with a protein vaccine, such as diphtheria or hepatitis vaccine, in the absence of any immunoenhancing agent. All patients will be boosted with antigen alone 1 month after primary immunization. The antibody response will be observed over the ensuing 3-month period. Subsequently, patients will be immunized with a second peptide vaccine (e.g., influenza vaccine) in the presence of 10 mg/kg loxoribine. All patients will be boosted with the immunizing antigen 1 month after primary immunization. Antibody titers will again be followed over the ensuing 3 months, and degree of change compared with that for the first immunogen. Serum immunoglobulins and disease complications will also be monitored regularly.

8. SUMMARY AND CONCLUSIONS

Loxoribine is a potent new immunostimulant with a relatively broad spectrum of immunobiological activities. Both loxoribine and its analogues function as agonists of immune responses in a variety of species, including humans. They upregulate the activity of B cells, T cells, NK cells, macrophages, and LAK cells. Induction of enhanced cytokine secretion has been found to involve IFN-α/β, IFN-γ, TNF-α, TNF-β, IL-1, IL-6, and the 40 kDa chain of IL-12. Evaluation of in vivo activity has been undertaken only for antibody production, NK cell-mediated cytotoxicity, induction of certain cytokines, and LAK cell-mediated cytotoxicity; all four types of activity are markedly upregulated by loxoribine in vivo. Augmentation of antibody production has been observed for protein, recombinant protein, and synthetic peptide antigens, among others. Because loxoribine and its analogues transmit a T-helper-like signal to antibody-producing B cells, it is a highly effective adjuvant even for synthetic peptides that lack T-cell epitopes, effectively replacing the function of T-helper cells in this milieu. It thus provides an alternative, T-cell-independent vaccination strategy if it becomes desirable to avoid untoward T-cell-mediated effects, or in patients with functional or absolute T-cell deficiency.

There are a number of features unique to loxoribine that are highly advantageous under specific circumstances: (1) T cell independence; (2) loxoribine augments antibody responses from an intracellular location (rather than at the surface membrane), independently of protein kinase C involvement; this may be particularly relevant for patients with membrane receptor/signal transduction defects; (3) adjuvanticity of loxoribine is essentially free of cytokine dependency; this may be of particular value for organ transplantation patients whose cytokine-dependent immunity is pharmacologically suppressed; (4) loxoribine bypasses functional immunological immaturity, rendering it particularly useful for vaccines in infants.

In preclinical safety studies, the drug has exhibited a relatively benign profile. Phase I clinical studies to date have produced no toxicity higher than grade 1. The drug appears to be quite stable, and compares very favorably in direct evaluations with a number of other immunostimulators. A number of clinical trials have been planned for the future.

ACKNOWLEDGMENTS

I thank Amnon Altman, Jim Bittle, and Vernon Stevens for their interest in this project and for their permission to reproduce Figs. 1, 2, and 3, respectively. I also thank Alicia Palestini for excellent work in the preparation of the manuscript. This work was supported in part by Grant AI15284 from the National Institutes of Health.

REFERENCES

Agarwala, S., Kirkwood, J. M., Bryant, J., Abels, R., and Troetschel, M., 1992, A double blind, phase I placebo-controlled study of the safety, pharmacokinetics, and immunological effect of single, ascending doses of 7-allyl-8-oxoguanosine in patients with advanced cancer, *Proc. Am. Assoc. Cancer Res.* **33**:263 (abstract 1576).

Ahmad, A., and Mond, J. J., 1984, Restoration of TNP–ficoll induced in vitro immune responsiveness in B cells from xid immune defective mice and in neonatal mice by 8-thioguanosine (8-sGuo), *Fed. Proc.* **43**:1424 (abstract 49).

Ahmad, A., and Mond, J. J., 1986, Restoration of *in vitro* responsiveness of xid B cells to TNP–ficoll by 8-mercaptoguanosine, *J. Immunol.* **136**:1223–1226.

Bijsterbosch, M. K., Meade, C. J., Turner, G. A., and Klaus, G. G. B., 1985, B lymphocyte receptor and polyphosphoinositide degradation, *Cell* **41**:999–1006.

Braun, J., Citri, Y., Baltimore, D., Forouzanpour, F., King, L., Teheranizadeh, K., Bray, M., and Kliewer, S., 1986, B-Lyl cells: Immortal Ly-1$^+$ B lymphocyte cell lines spontaneously arising in murine splenic cultures, *Immunol. Rev.* **93**:5–21.

Burleson, D. G., and Sage, H. J., 1976, Effect of lectins on the level of cAMP and cGMP in guinea pig lymphocytes: early responses of lymph node cells to mitogenic and non-mitogenic lectins. *J. Immunol.* **116**:696–702.

Callard, R. E., Booth, R. J., Brown, M. H., and McCaughan, G. W., 1985, T cell-replacing factor in specific antibody responses to influenza virus by human blood B cells, *Eur. J. Immunol.* **15**:52–59.

Chen, R., Goodman, M. G., Argentieri, D., Bell, S. C., Burr, L. E., Come, J., Goodman, J. H., Klaubert, D. H., Maryanoff, B. E., Pope, B. L., Rampulla, M. S., Schott, M. R., and Reitz, A. B., 1994, Guanosine derivatives as immunostimulants. Discovery of loxoribine, *Nucleosides Nucleotides* **13**:551–562.

Coffey R. G., Hadden E. M., and Hadden, J. W., 1977, Evidence for cyclic GMP and calcium mediation of lymphocyte activation by mitogens, *J. Immunol.* **119**:1387–1394.

Coggeshall, K. M., and Cambier, J. C., 1984, B cell activation. VIII. Membrane immunoglobulins transduce signals via activation of phosphatidylinositol hydrolysis, *J. Immunol.* **133**:3382–3386.

Diamantstein, T., and Ulmer, A., 1975, The antagonistic action of cyclic GMP and cyclic AMP on proliferation of B and T lymphocytes, *Immunology* **28**:113–120.

Dosch, H.-M., Osundwa, V., and Lam, P., 1988, Activation of human B lymphocytes by 8′ substituted guanosine derivatives, *Immunol. Lett.* **17**:125–131.

Ellis, T. M., Fisher, R. I., Bodner, B., and Anderson, D. W., 1990, Enhancement of human lymphokine activated killer cell induction by a guanosine ribonucleoside, *Proc. Am. Assoc. Cancer Res.* **31**:280 (abstract 1661).

Feldbush, T. L., and Ballas, Z. K., 1985, Lymphokine-like activity of 8-mercaptoguanosine: Induction of T and B cell differentiation, *J. Immunol.* **134**:3204–3211.

Feuerstein, N., and Mond, J. J., 1987a, "Numatrin" a nuclear matrix protein associated with induction of proliferation in B cells, *J. Biol. Chem.* **262**: 11389–11397.

Feuerstein, N., and Mond, J. J., 1987b, Identification of a prominent nuclear protein associated with proliferation of normal and malignant B cells, *J. Immunol.* **139**:1818–1822.

Goodman, M. G., 1985, Demonstration of T-cell-dependent and T-cell independent components of 8-mercaptoguanosine-mediated adjuvanticity, *Proc. Soc. Exp. Biol. Med.* **179**:479–486.

Goodman, M. G., 1986a, Mechanism of synergy between T cell signals and C8-substituted guanine nucleosides in humoral immunity: B-lymphotropic cytokines induce responsiveness to 8-mercaptoguanosine, *J. Immunol.* **136**:3335–3340.

Goodman, M. G., 1986b, Regulation of B cell activation by prostaglandins: Cell cycle-specific effects on activation by anti-immunoglobulin and 8-mercaptoguanosine, *J. Immunol.* **137**:3753–3757.

Goodman, M. G., 1987, Interaction between cytokines and 8-mercaptoguanosine in humoral immunity: Synergy with interferon, *J. Immunol.* **139**:142–146.

Goodman, M. G., 1988a, Induction of interleukin 1 activity from macrophages by direct interaction with C8-substituted guanine ribonucleosides, *Int. J. Immunopharmacol.* **10**:579–586.

Goodman, M. G., 1988b, Role of salvage and phosphorylation in the immunostimulatory activity of C8-substituted guanine ribonucleosides, *J. Immunol.* **141**:2394–2399.

Goodman, M. G., 1990, Demonstration of binding components specific for 7,8-disubstituted guanine ribonucleosides in murine B lymphocytes, *J. Biol. Chem.* **265**:22467–22473.

Goodman, M. G., 1991, Cellular and biochemical studies of substituted guanine ribonucleoside immunostimulants, *Immunopharmacology* **21**:51–68.

Goodman, M. G., and Cherry, D. M., 1989, Ligand binding sites for a synthetic B cell growth and differentiation factor, *Cell. Immunol.* **123**:417–426.

Goodman, M. G., and Hennen, W. J., 1986, Distinct effects of dual substitution on inductive and differentiative activities of C8-substituted guanine ribonucleosides, *Cell. Immunol.* **102**:395–402.

Goodman, M. G., and Weigle, W. O., 1981, Activation of lymphocytes by brominated nucleoside and cyclic nucleotide analogues: Implications for the "second messenger" function of cyclic GMP, *Proc. Natl. Acad. Sci. USA* **78**:7604–7608.

Goodman, M. G., and Weigle, W. O., 1982a, Bromination of guanosine and cyclic GMP confers resistance to metabolic processing by B cells, *J. Immunol.* **129**:2715–2717.

Goodman, M. G., and Weigle, W. O., 1982b, Induction of immunoglobulin secretion by a simple nucleoside derivative, *J. Immunol.* **128**:2399–2404.

Goodman, M. G., and Weigle, W. O., 1983a, Manifold amplification of *in vivo* immunity in normal and immunodeficient mice by ribonucleosis derivatized at C8 of guanine, *Proc. Natl. Acad. Sci. USA* **80**:3452–3455.

Goodman, M. G., and Weigle, W. O., 1983b, Derivatized guanine nucleosides: A new class of adjuvant for *in vitro* antibody responses, *J. Immunol.* **130**:2580–2585.

Goodman, M. G., and Weigle, W. O., 1983c, T cell-replacing activity of C8-derivatized guanine ribonucleosides, *J. Immunol.* **130**:2042–2045.

Goodman, M. G., and Weigle, W. O., 1983d, Activation of lymphocytes by a thiol-derivatized nucleoside: Characterization of cellular parameters and responsive subpopulations, *J. Immunol.* **130**:551–557.

Goodman, M. G., and Weigle, W. O., 1984a, Regulation of B lymphocyte proliferative responses by arachidonate metabolites: Effects on membrane-directed versus intracellular activators, *J. Allergy Clin. Immunol.* **74**:418–425.

Goodman, M. G., and Weigle, W. O., 1984b, Intracellular lymphocyte activation and carrier-mediated transport of C8-substituted guanine ribonucleosides, *Proc. Natl. Acad. Sci. USA* **81**:862–866.

Goodman, M. G., and Weigle, W. O., 1984c, Mechanism of 8-mercaptoguanosine mediated adjuvanticity: Roles of clonal expansion and cellular recruitment, *J. Immunol.* **133**:2910–2914.

Goodman, M. G., and Weigle, W. O., 1985a, Dissociation of inductive from differentiative signals transmitted by C8-substituted guanine ribonucleosides to B cells from SJL mice, *J. Immunol.* **134**:91–94.

Goodman, M. G., and Weigle, W. O., 1985b, Enhancement of the human antibody response by C8-substituted guanine ribonucleosides in synergy with interleukin 2, *J. Immunol.* **135**:3284–3288.

Goodman, M. G., and Weigle, W. O., 1986, Enhancement of T cell proliferation and differentiation by 8-mercaptoguanosine, in: *Purine and Pyrimidine Metabolism in Man V* (W. L. Nyhan, L. F. Thompson, and R. W. E. Watts, eds.), Plenum Press, New York, pp. 443–449.

Goodman, M. G., Speizer, L., Bokoch, G. M., Kanter, J., and Brunton, L. L., 1990, Activity of an intracellular lymphocyte stimulator is independent of G-protein interactions, $[Ca^{2+}]_i$ elevation, phosphoinositide hydrolysis, and protein kinase C translocation, *J. Biol. Chem.* **265**:12248–12252.

Goodman, M. G., Gupta, S., Rosenthale, M. E., Capetola, R. J., Bell, S. C., and Weigle, W. O., 1991, C-kinase independent restoration of specific immune responsiveness in common variable immunodeficiency, *Clin. Immunol. Immunopathol.* **59**:26–36.

Greene, D. A., Lattimer, S. A., and Sima, A. A. F., 1987, Sorbitol, phosphoinositides, and sodium-potassium-ATPase in the pathogenesis of diabetic complications, *N. Engl. J. Med.* **316**:599–606.

Griffioen, A. W., Toebes, E. A. H., Zegers, B. J. M., and Rijkers, G. T., 1992, Role of CR2 in the human adult and neonatal *in vitro* antibody response to type 4 pneumococcal polysaccharide, *Cell. Immunol.* **143**:11–22.

Grupp, S. A., Snow, E. C., and Harmony, J. A. K., 1987, The phosphatidylinositol response is an early event in the physiologically relevant activation of antigen-specific B lymphocytes, *Cell. Immunol.* **109**:181–191.

Jin, A., Mhaskar, S., Jolley, W. B., Robins, R. K., and Ojo-Amaize, E. A., 1990, A novel guanosine analogue, 7-thia-8-oxoguanosine, enhances macrophage and lymphocyte antibody-dependent cell mediated cytotoxicity, *Cell. Immunol.* **126**:414–419.

Koo, G. C., Jewell, M. E., Manyak, C. L., Sigal, N. H., and Wicker, L. S., 1988, Activation of murine natural killer cells and macrophages by 8-bromoguanosine, *J. Immunol.* **140**:3249–3252.

Mond, J. J., Feuerstein, N., Finkelman, F. D., Huang, F., Huang, K.-P., and Dennis, G., 1987, B-lymphocyte activation mediated by anti-immunoglobulin antibody in the absence of protein kinase C, *Proc. Natl. Acad. Sci. USA* **84**:8588–8592.

Mond, J. J., Hunter, K., Kenny, J. J., Finkelman, F., and Witherspoon, K., 1989, 8-Mercaptoguanosine-mediated enhancement of *in vivo* IgG1, IgG2 and IgG3 antibody responses to polysaccharide antigens in normal and *xid* mice, *Immunopharmacology* **18**:205–212.

Phillips, N. E., and Campbell, P. A., 1982, IgG subclass distribution of anti-sheep red blood cell plaque-forming cells in mice with the CBA/N defect, *J. Immunol.* **128**:2319–2321.

Physicians Desk Reference, 1994, 48th ed., Medical Economics Data, Montvale, NJ, pp. 1534–1537.

Pope, B. L., Chourmouzis, E., Capetola, R. J., and Lau, C. Y., 1992a, Activation of NK cells by loxoribine, *Int. J. Immunopharmacol.* **14**:1375–1382.

Pope, B. L., Chourmouzis, E., Sigindere, J., and MacIntyre, J. P., 1992b, *In vivo* activation of natural killer cells and priming of IL-2 responsive cytolytic cells by loxoribine (7-allyl-8-oxoguanosine), *Cell. Immunol.* **147**:302–312.

Pope, B. L., Chourmouzis, E., Victorino, L., MacIntyre, J. P., Capetola, R. J., and Lau, C. Y., 1993, Loxoribine (7-allyl-8-oxoguanosine) activates natural killer cells and primes cytolytic precursor cells for activation by IL-2, *J. Immunol.* **151**:3007–3017.

Pope, B. L., Sigindere, J., Chourmouzis, E., MacIntyre, P., and Goodman, M. G., 1994a, 7-Allyl-8-oxoguanosine (loxoribine) inhibits the metastasis of B16 melanoma cells and has adjuvant activity in mice immunized with a B16 tumor vaccine, *Cancer Immunol. Immunother.* **38**:83–91.

Pope, B. L., Chourmouzis, E., MacIntyre, J. P., Lee, S., and Goodman, M. G., 1994b, Murine strain variation in the natural killer cell and proliferative responses to the immunostimulatory compound 7-allyl-8-oxoguanosine: Role of cytokines, *Cell. Immunol.* **159**:194–210.

Quintans, J., and Kaplan, R. B., 1978, Failure of CBA/N mice to respond to thymus-dependent and thymus-independent phosphorylcholine antigens, *Cell. Immunol.* **38**:294–301.

Ransom, J. T., Chen, M., Sandoval, V. M., Pasternak, J. A., Digiusto, D., and Cambier, J. C., 1988, Increased plasma membrane permeability to Ca^{2+} in anti-Ig-stimulated B lymphocytes is dependent on activation of phosphoinositide hydrolysis, *J. Immunol.* **140**:3150–3155.

Rijkers, G. T., Dollekamp, I., and Zegers, B. J. M., 1988, 8-Mercaptoguanosine overcomes unresponsiveness of human neonatal B cells to polysaccharide antigens, *J. Immunol.* **141**:2313–2316.

Rizkalla, B. H., Robins, R. K., and Broom, A. D., 1969, Purine nucleosides. XXVII. The synthesis of 1- and 7-methyl-8-oxoguanosine and related nucleosides, *Biochim. Biophys. Acta* **195**:285–293.

Rollins-Smith, L. A., and Lawton, A. R., 1988, Regulation of B cell differentiation: Anti-μ antibodies have opposite effects on differentiation stimulated by bacterial lipopolysaccharide and 8-mercaptoguanosine, *J. Mol. Cell. Immunol.* **4**:9–19.

Scheuer, W. V., Goodman, M. G., Parks, D. E., and Weigle, W. O., 1985a, Enhancement of the *in vivo* antibody response by an 8-derivatized guanine nucleoside, *Cell. Immunol.* **91**:294–300.

Scheuer, W. V., Goodman, M. G., Parks, D. E., and Weigle, W. O., 1985b, Active transformation of tolerogenic to immunogenic signals in T and B cells by 8-bromoguanosine, *J. Immunol.* **135**:2962–2966.

Sharma, B. S., Balazs, L., Jin, A., Wang, J. C.-J., Jolley, W. B., and Robins, R. K., 1991, Potentiation of the efficacy of murine L1210 leukemia vaccine by a novel immunostimulator 7-thia-8-oxoguanosine. Increased survival after immunization with vaccine plus 7-thia-8-oxoguanosine, *Cancer Immunol. Immunother.* **33**:109–114.

Stein, K. E., Zopf, D. A., Miller, C. B., Johnson, B. M., Mongini, P. K. A., Ahmed, A., and Paul, W. E., 1983, Immune response to a thymus-dependent form of B512 dextran requires the presence of Lyb-5⁻ lymphocytes, *J. Exp. Med.* **157**:657–666.

Strauss, P. R., Sheehan, J. M., and Kashket, E. R., 1976, Membrane transport by murine lymphocytes. I. A rapid sampling technique as applied to the adenosine and thymidine systems, *J. Exp. Med.* **144**:1009–1021.

Watson, J., 1975, Cyclic nucleotides as intracellular mediators of B cell activation, *Transplant Rev.* **23**:223.

Watson, J., Epstein, R., and Cohn, M., 1973, Cyclic nucleotides as intracellular mediators of the expression of antigen-sensitive cells, *Nature* **246**:405–408.

Weber, T. H., and Goldberg, M. L., 1976, Effect of leukoagglutinating phytohemagglutinin on cAMP and cGMP levels in lymphocytes, *Exp. Cell Res.* **97**:432–440.

Wedner, H. J., Dankner, R., and Parker, C. W., 1975, Cyclic GMP and lectin-induced lymphocyte activation, *J. Immunol.* **115**:1682–1688.

Weinstein, Y., Chambers, D. A., Bourne, H. R., and Melmon, K. L., 1974, Cyclic GMP stimulated lymphocyte nucleic acid synthesis, *Nature* **251**:352–355.

Weinstein, Y., Segal, S., and Melmon, K. L., 1975, Specific mitogenic activity of 8-Br-guanosine 3′,5′-monophosphate (Br-cyclic GMP) on B lymphocytes, *J. Immunol.* **115**:112–118.

Wicker, L. S., Boltz, R. C., Jr., Nichols, E. A., Miller, B. J., Sigal, N. H., and Peterson, L. B., 1987, Large, activated B cells are the primary B-cell target of 8-bromoguanosine and 8-mercaptoguanosine, *Cell. Immunol.* **106**:318–329.

Wicker, L. S., Boltz, R. C., Jr., Matt, V., Nichols, E. A., Peterson, L. B., and Sigal, N. H., 1990, Suppression of B cell activation by cyclosporin A, FK506 and rapamycin, *Eur. J. Immunol.* **20**:2277–2283.

Chapter 26

Stearyl Tyrosine

An Organic Equivalent of Aluminum-Based Immunoadjuvants

Christopher Penney

1. INTRODUCTION

In 1966, David Gall reported that although there was a great diversity among the commonly recognized adjuvants, they appeared to possess some common properties. These were the ability to bind proteins, cause local reactions at the site of injection, and interact with cell membranes. Thus, the adjuvants appeared to be surface-active substances as demonstrated by hemolysis of sheep red blood cells. Examples cited included alum precipitates, Freund's adjuvant, saponin, and hexadecylamine. Indeed, he discovered that a number of long-chain alkyl amines were adjuvant active. However, their local toxicity made them unacceptable for use in human vaccines.

Moloney and Wojcik (1981) thought it was possible to retain or improve adjuvanticity but lessen the local toxicity by replacing a long-chain alkyl amine with a long-chain alkyl ester of an amino acid. This would retain a cationic charge and lipophilic tail for binding proteins, but would no longer possess the detergentlike amine or ammonium head group. They reasoned that it was important to retain insolubility and so selected the most insoluble amino acid, tyrosine, for esterification with nontoxic stearyl alcohol. Their early work with stearyl tyrosine describes the improved adjuvanticity and reduced damage at the injection site, relative to aluminum phosphate, when complexed with tetanus toxoid or inactivated polio vaccine. However, this work was preliminary and prompted us to undertake a research program targeted to replace aluminum adjuvant with a more effective, biocompatible biodegradable organic equivalent. This program has spanned approximately one decade.

Christopher Penney • Immunomodulator Research Project, BioChem Therapeutic, Inc., Laval, Quebec H7V 4A7, Canada.

Vaccine Design: The Subunit and Adjuvant Approach, edited by Michael F. Powell and Mark J. Newman. Plenum Press, New York, 1995.

From this work we have discovered a new family of immunoadjuvants headed by the parent compound stearyl tyrosine (ST), or octadecyl tyrosine hydrochloride.

2. WHY REPLACE ALUMINUM?

Insoluble aluminum (phosphate and hydroxide) salts are the only adjuvants used in approved human vaccines in North America. They act primarily by depot formation thereby allowing improved antigen presentation. Other adjuvant mechanisms are operative, such as activation of complement. Billions of doses of aluminum-adjuvanted vaccines have been given to children, and aluminum is considered to be a relatively safe and effective adjuvant. However, aluminum is not totally satisfactory, as illustrated by the recommendation to remove it from DPT vaccine (Gupta and Relyveld, 1991). Aluminum has not been generally approved as an adjuvant by the U.S. FDA, but only as a component in a licensed product. It is not a universal adjuvant, can induce the formation of granuloma on intramuscular (i.m.) injection or cause persistent nodules on subcutaneous (s.c.) injection, and can stimulate the production of IgE antibodies. The latter are responsible for mediating immediate hypersensitive reactions as exemplified by the report of anaphylaxis to adsorbed tetanus toxoid (Ratliff and Burns-Cox, 1984). Aluminum hydroxide gel was recently reported to elicit a vascular permeability increasing effect and toxicity to macrophages (Goto et al., 1993). Aluminum adjuvant is not rapidly biodegradable, cannot be sterilized by filtration, and its preparation is not always reproducible (Landi et al., 1986). Indeed, the importance of the availability of an adjuvant other than aluminum was stressed in a recent letter to the journal Vaccine (Léry, 1994). The majority of experimental adjuvants are organic molecules that function as immunostimulants. However, potent immunostimulation is often accompanied by local and systemic toxic effects. This is complicated further by the susceptibility of certain individuals, especially those of the HLA-B27 haplotype, to develop inflammatory responses and other components of Reiter's syndrome on administration of adjuvants derived from gram-negative bacteria, e.g., muramyl dipeptide, or some other immunomodulators, e.g., levamisole (Allison and Byars, 1991). Thus, despite intensive efforts to replace aluminum with more effective but safe organic immunoadjuvants/immunomodulators, only a few molecules appear to be promising, especially for the purpose of prophylactic immunization of healthy individuals.

3. STEARYL TYROSINE: OVERVIEW

ST, or octadecyl tyrosine hydrochloride, is the octadecyl (18 carbon chain) ester of the amino acid tyrosine (Fig. 1). It is a low molecular-weight synthetic immunoadjuvant. ST has been developed as an organic equivalent of aluminum and, like aluminum adjuvant, is poorly water soluble (<0.01% w/w). It has minimal immunostimulatory properties, but instead adsorbs soluble proteins to form insoluble complexes, thus functioning as an insoluble depot or slow-release vehicle.

An in vitro binding assay was developed to study the interaction of protein antigens with depot (insoluble) adjuvants, and this assay was used to study the interaction of tetanus toxoid with ST and aluminum phosphate (Penney et al., 1985b). A number of trends were

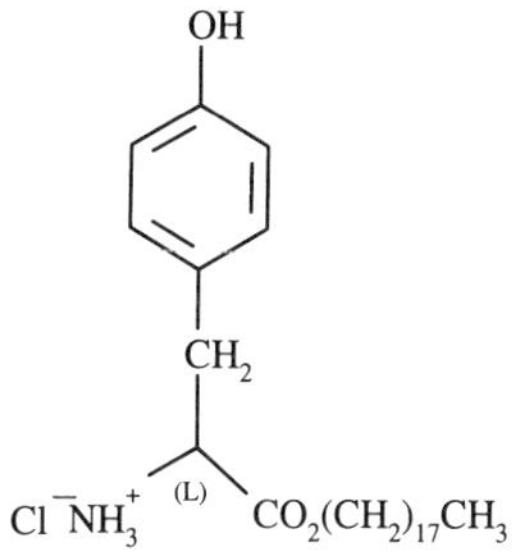

MW = 470.14
MP = 171-173°C

Figure 1. Structure of the immunoadjuvant stearyl tyrosine (octadecyl tyrosine hydrochloride).

observed: (1) agitation of the protein–adjuvant suspension promoted better binding; (2) binding of tetanus toxoid was greater at acidic than at neutral or alkaline pH; and (3) binding of tetanus toxoid was independent of ionic strength.

Phosphate (PBS) was able to desorb tetanus toxoid from aluminum, but not ST. Under the most favorable conditions, ST was able to almost quantitatively bind diphtheria toxoid, insulin, and albumin (Table I). Since ST can effectively extract proteins from solution and confine them to a two-dimensional surface, it was anticipated that ST may induce a number of interesting immunological effects. This would reflect the different affinities each protein antigen would have for the insoluble surface, i.e., the strength of the antigen–adjuvant interaction. Thus, ST was not expected to be a universal adjuvant, but through chemical

Table I
Ability of ST to Bind Vaccine Antigens and Other Proteins[a]

Protein	Agitation	% protein bound[b,c]	
		24 h	7 days
Tetanus toxoid	Stand	24 (32)	47
	Stir	98 (95)	
Diphtheria toxoid	Stand	31 (33)	37
	Stir	84 (91)	
Insulin	Stand	44 (44)	56
	Stir	85 (78)	
Albumin (human)	Stand	31 (25)	44
	Stir	89 (92)	
Albumin (bovine)	Stand	22 (25)	34
	Stir	89 (95)	

[a]1 mg/mL ST, 150 μg/mL protein.
[b]Value in parentheses determined by Bio-Rad Protein Assay.
[c]Penney *et al.* (1985b).

modification of the surface, ST (and analogues) was expected to offer a greater array of adjuvant properties than aluminum adjuvants. First, the surface resulting from the racemic adjuvant due to D,L-tyrosine was expected to differ from the enantiomeric adjuvant (L-tyrosine or D-tyrosine). This was observed in a study with recombinant hepatitis B surface antigen where the racemic adjuvant was less effective than either enantiomer (Nixon-George et al., 1990). Second, tyrosine, because of its phenolic side chain, can participate in a number of important contact interactions (hydrogen bond, charge transfer, hydrophobic) with the protein. Indeed, tyrosine and other aromatic amino acids (phenylalanine, phenylglycine) are found in a number of immunomodulatory substances. These include forphenicinol, bestatin, arphamenine, tyrosyl glycyl glycine, thymopentin, and splenopentin (Penney et al., 1993). Finally, tyrosine can be modified, for example, by introduction of a second long (stearoyl) chain at the phenolic hydroxyl. Alternately, tyrosine can be replaced, for example, with any other amino acid to provide a different surface topography. The ability to provide a diversity of noncovalent interactions with protein antigens as opposed to one strong electrostatic interaction, as is the case with aluminum hydroxide gel, may allow for some lateral two-dimensional movement of antigen and a more compatible interaction with cell membranes. Thus, another mechanism of adjuvanticity may be improved antigen presentation to immune cell subsets.

Another clue regarding the importance of different surface topography, as reflected by the interaction of the adjacent molecules that comprise the insoluble surface, has been recently provided in a study of the rate of polycondensation of stearyl aromatic amino acid monolayers at a water–air interface (Liu et al., 1994). The reaction rate of ST in the stearyl amino acid film was greater than stearyl tryptophan, which was greater than stearyl phenylalanine. It was concluded that these different rates could be ascribed to the distinct packing arrangement between adjacent surface molecules and concomitant steric hindrance caused by the different orientation and size of the aromatic moieties.

3.1. Synthesis

ST may be conveniently synthesized in high yield by the methanesulfonic acid-catalyzed esterification of tyrosine and octadecanol (Penney et al., 1985a). This simple procedure does not require the use of expensive reagents (protected amino acids, coupling reagents) or purification by column chromatography and so is amenable to scaleup. The synthesis consists of three steps: (1) esterification of tyrosine using methanesulfonic acid catalyst in an octadecanol melt to give crude product; (2) conversion of the crude methanesulfonate salt to the free base of ST by stirring the insoluble salt in aqueous bicarbonate; and (3) conversion of the free base to ST hydrochloride by reaction with hydrogen chloride gas. The purified product is obtained in 90% yield. Some variations of the above procedure for the synthesis of ST have been reported in the literature. For example, hydrogen chloride gas has been used as the acid catalyst for the esterification, but the product yield was only 10% (Moloney and Wojcik, 1981). Another procedure employed toluenesulfonic acid as catalyst and refluxing toluene instead of an octadecanol melt, but the product yield was not given (Liu et al., 1994). Tyrosine can be replaced with ethyl tyrosine, but the product yield was 70% (Penney et al., 1985a).

ST hydrochloride possesses well-defined properties which may be characterized by standard chemical methods. These include NMR spectroscopy, elemental analysis, melting point, thin-layer chromatography, and cationic ion exchange HPLC (Penney *et al.*, 1986). Unlike other lipophilic long-chain adjuvants, which tend to be low-melting waxy solids or viscous liquids, ST is a free-flowing, amorphous powder. The white hydrochloride salt of ST is not hygroscopic and the powder can be stored for several years at room temperature or as a refrigerated aqueous suspension. A 1-year stability study of the aqueous suspension of ST showed 0.9, 3.6, and 18.2% degradation to tyrosine at 5, 24, and 37 °C, respectively (Landi *et al.*, 1986). ST possesses another interesting property—it is biocidal. Although a procedure for the dry heat sterilization of ST has been reported (Landi *et al.*, 1986), ST does not require heat sterilization.

3.2. Toxicity

ST is composed of naturally occurring, nontoxic stearyl alcohol and tyrosine, and the esters of these products are also nontoxic. A preliminary acute (mice, guinea pigs) and chronic (rats) toxicity study has been reported (Landi *et al.*, 1986). The LD_{50} in outbred mice was > 2.5 g/kg by intraperitoneal (i.p.) injection. The insolubility of ST precluded an accurate determination of its LD_{50}. However, animals receiving the higher dose gained weight relative to the control. Guinea pigs and rats also received ST by i.p. injection. In these animals, there was no significant difference in the weight gain of the rats, relative to their controls. Gross necropsy of four rats at days 28, 60, and 90 after injection showed that the lungs and kidneys were free of lesions. However, at day 28 all rats had liver and spleen/diaphragm-related peritoneal lesions consistent with the injection of insoluble foreign material into the peritoneal cavity. By day 90, no lesions were observed in the rats. ST was determined to be nonpyrogenic by injection into the ear vein of rabbits (Landi *et al.*, 1986). None of the nine rabbits showed an individual rise in body temperature of more than 0.6°C above normal.

The injection site of ST was examined and compared to aluminum injection sites, using feline rhinotracheitis panleucopenia vaccine (Landi *et al.*, 1986). The cat was selected for this study because it is known to be extremely sensitive to injection of foreign materials. The results demonstrated that ST injected twice at 3 mg/mL did not evoke any local reaction. When the concentration of ST was increased to 9 mg/mL, it induced local indurations in fewer animals than aluminum phosphate at 9 mg/mL, and the indurations were softer and did not persist. In another experiment, it was shown that ST does not induce adjuvant arthritis in rats (Nixon-George *et al.*, 1990). The general lack of toxicity of ST is perhaps best illustrated by the number of studies that have been undertaken with many different animals without any observable toxicity: inbred and outbred mice, rats, guinea pigs, chickens, rabbits, cats, cattle, baboons, and monkeys.

4. ADJUVANTICITY WITH BACTERIAL VACCINES

The first experiments with ST were undertaken with tetanus toxoid vaccine. Aluminum phosphate was used as the standard for comparison since, at the time these studies were initiated, it was the only adjuvant used in human vaccines in Canada. Generally, with regard to antibody response, ST gave higher antibody titers than aluminum phosphate, although the difference was often not significant. More recently, ST has been studied with tetanus and diphtheria toxoids in BALB/c mice (Penney *et al.*, 1993). Animals were immunized on days 0 and 21, and the antibody titer was determined on days 14 and 35. ST was compared with aluminum hydroxide and alum (potassium aluminum sulfate). A small increase in antibody response was observed with both toxoids and the adjuvants 14 days after the primary immunization. On day 35, the antibody response against tetanus toxoid complexed with ST was slightly larger than that observed with alum, but slightly smaller than that observed with aluminum hydroxide. However, neither these differences nor the differences in isotype patterns were significant. On day 35, the antibody response against diphtheria toxoid complexed with ST was slightly larger than that observed with both aluminum adjuvants, but again the differences were not significant. Most recently, a comprehensive study of ST with tetanus toxoid in outbred mice was published (Gupta and Siber, 1994). In this study, toxoid preparations of varying purity were used, and ST was compared with aluminum phosphate and calcium phosphate. The latter is approved for use in DPT vaccine in France. Also, the three toxoid adjuvant complexes were evaluated in guinea pigs according to the U.S. FDA potency test (Gupta and Siber, 1994). All of the adjuvanted toxoids passed the potency test in guinea pigs. ST previously passed the same test in our hands. Mice were immunized on days 0 and 30, and the antibody titers were determined 4 weeks after the primary immunization and 2 weeks after the boosting dose. Interestingly, after the secondary immunization, tetanus toxoids of varying purity and combined with each adjuvant showed similar antibody responses. All of the preparations induced mainly IgG1 antibodies. However, toxoid adjuvanted with ST induced relatively higher titers of IgG2a and IgG2b. In the mouse, the IgG2a and IgG2b antibodies are the most efficient isotype with regard to activation of complement and antibody-dependent cell-mediated cytotoxicity (Kenney *et al.*, 1989). Further, aluminum phosphate induced a significantly higher IgE antibody response than was obtained with ST or calcium phosphate. The increased ratio of IgG2a to IgG1 and the decreased IgE level observed for ST relative to aluminum suggest an improved antigen presentation to specific (Th1) helper cell populations.

In view of the ability of ST to adjuvant toxoids and increase the IgG2a and IgG2b responses, possibly favoring increased protective bactericidal activity, it was expected that ST would be a useful adjuvant for the new generation of polysaccharide–protein conjugate vaccines. The issue of an appropriate adjuvant becomes more important since a number of protein carriers (tetanus toxoid, mutant diphtheria toxin CRM197, and *N. meningitidis* B outer membrane protein) are used in approved pediatric *H. influenzae* b conjugate vaccines. Further, results with aluminum adjuvant have been variable and depend on the type of carrier protein and conjugation technology used to link the polysaccharide with the carrier. For example, an *H. influenzae* b conjugate vaccine prepared with tetanus toxoid carrier and adipic acid dihydrazide linker was less immunogenic in children when adsorbed onto aluminum hydroxide, relative to nonadjuvanted vaccine (Claesson *et al.*, 1988). Another *H. influenzae* b conjugate vaccine which uses an outer membrane protein carrier is adjuvanted with aluminum hydroxide just prior to administration. ST was examined with *N. meningitidis* A, B, and C conjugate vaccines which used tetanus toxoid as the carrier protein (Penney *et al.*, 1993). The meningococcal conjugates were prepared without a linker by reductive amination of toxoid amino groups to terminal aldehyde groups generated on the polysaccharide (Jennings and Lugowski, 1981). Because of the poor immunogenicity of the group B polysaccharide, it was chemically modified whereby sugar *N*-acetyl groups were replaced with *N*-propionyl groups (Jennings *et al.*, 1986). Outbred mice were immunized on days 0, 14, and 28, and the antibody titer was determined on day 39. Aluminum phosphate gave no significant adjuvant effect. Aluminum hydroxide increased the magnitude of the antibody response approximately threefold, relative to saline. ST gave a similar enhancement of the antibody response. However, a significant advantage of ST was the improved stability of the meningococcal A conjugate complexed with ST, relative to aluminum (Penney *et al.*, 1993). The stability of the meningococcal C conjugate was similar with both adjuvants. Also, analysis of the isotype response obtained with ST demonstrated that the increase in IgG2a and IgG2b, relative to IgG1, was greater than that observed without adjuvant. Nonetheless, IgG1 was the most significantly increased antibody, as was noted above for immunization with tetanus toxoid. Interestingly, it was also reported that a dipeptide analogue of ST, stearyl tyrosyl glycine, was able to adjuvant a protective response with the meningococcal B conjugate vaccine when outbred mice were challenged with live *N. meningitidis* B, serotype 2b (Penney *et al.*, 1993). This adjuvant induced an antibody response and isotype pattern similar to that observed with ST. Further, vaccine alone or vaccine adjuvanted with aluminum did not elicit a significantly protective (bactericidal) response.

A preliminary evaluation was undertaken in which ST was compared with aluminum phosphate as adjuvant for an acellular pertussis vaccine (J. Scott, personal communication, Lederle Labs, September, 1988). The two adjuvants induced a similar antibody response to the filamentous hemagglutinin component of the vaccine. However, with regard to pertussis toxin, ST gave a higher response than aluminum phosphate for the pertussis toxin component of the vaccine.

5. ADJUVANTICITY WITH VIRAL VACCINES

The first vaccine to be examined with ST was the formalin-inactivated trivalent poliomyelitis vaccine (IPV) in guinea pigs (Moloney and Wojcik, 1981). The first results were promising and encouraged a long (308 days) study in cynomolgus monkeys (Landi *et al.*, 1986). In this experiment, the monkeys were divided into four groups: IPV; IPV with ST; IPV, diluted 1:4; and IPV, diluted 1:4 with ST. The final concentration of ST in adjuvanted vaccines was 1 mg/mL. The animals were immunized i.m. on days 0, 28, and 168 and the neutralizing antibody titer was determined from bleeds from 15 different days. After the first injection, the antibody titers were low in all groups, and none could be detected in the diluted vaccine without adjuvant. However, following the second injection on day 28, the antibody titers for all vaccines adjuvanted with ST gave, over a period of 140 days, significantly higher titers than the nonadjuvanted vaccines. Also, the diluted adjuvanted vaccine most often gave higher titers than the adjuvanted vaccine. After the third injection on day 168, the antibody titers for the adjuvanted vaccines were higher than those of the nonadjuvanted vaccines over the final 140 days of the study. This experiment demonstrated that the concentration of antigens in commercial IPV could be reduced by at least fourfold without interfering with its immunogenicity, and suggested that it might be possible to reduce the number of injections of vaccine. This is important since IPV is difficult to manufacture and may be eventually formulated as part of a pediatric combination (pertussis, diphtheria, tetanus, *H. influenzae*, hepatitis B, polio) vaccine. More recently, ST has been studied with the same trivalent polio vaccine (IPV) in BALB/c mice (Penney *et al.*, 1993). A significant neutralizing antibody titer was observed after two injections of ST-adjuvanted vaccine, relative to vaccine without adjuvant.

A second primate study was undertaken with an HIV peptide–KLH (keyhole limpet hemocyanin) conjugate vaccine (Nixon *et al.*, 1992) (Fig. 2). This peptide corresponds to amino acid residues 503–535, which represents an immunodominant neutralizing epitope of the HIV envelope protein gp160. In this experiment, six adult baboons were immunized with peptide conjugate vaccine: two were given vaccine alone, two were given vaccine complexed with ST, and two were given vaccine complexed with alum (potassium aluminum sulfate). The animals were hyperimmunized i.m. on days 1, 7, 20, 69, and 178. The antipeptide antibody titer was determined over 8 days. There was no observable antibody titers in the baboons immunized with nonadjuvanted conjugate vaccine. A small specific antibody response was observed in one baboon given peptide conjugate adsorbed onto alum. However, both baboons immunized with peptide conjugate adjuvanted with ST displayed a significant increase in antipeptide antibodies. This response peaked early at day 31 and day 89 in the two animals. Further, the sera from these animals gave a

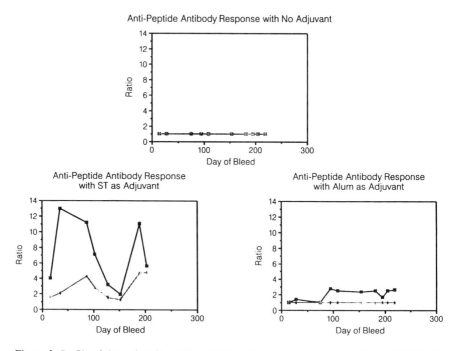

Figure 2. Profile of the antipeptide antibody response in baboons immunized with gp160 (503-535) peptide–KLH conjugate vaccine with no adjuvant, stearyl tyrosine, or alum; ■, baboon 1; ♦, baboon 2.

neutralizing antibody response. No significant neutralizing activity was seen in sera from the other baboons. The observed neutralizing activity was not strong as shown by the fact that 50% of HIV cytotoxicity in a cell killing assay was obtained with a dilution of sera ranging from 1:80 to 1:160. Nonetheless, the results demonstrate that the peptide conjugate vaccine adjuvanted with ST elicited the production of antibodies with neutralizing capacity. A similar neutralizing antibody response was observed when inbred mice were immunized with two injections of the same peptide conjugate vaccine complexed with ST (Nixon *et al.*, 1992).

ST has been extensively evaluated with a recombinant hepatitis B surface antigen derived from transfected human 3T3 cells (Nixon-George *et al.*, 1990; Penney *et al.*, 1993). BALB/c mice were immunized on days 0 and 21, and the antibody titer was determined on days 14, 35, and 42. ST was compared with aluminum hydroxide and alum. Again, the day 14 antibody response was small. However, the secondary antibody response was more than threefold greater with ST when compared with aluminum. Analysis of the isotype of the secondary response revealed that IgG1 antibody was the most significantly increased, but the increase in IgG2a and IgG2b was greater for ST, relative to aluminum. Further, although there was no increase in IgE with ST adjuvant, a significant increase was observed in the secondary response of animals given alum adjuvant. Again, there is a suggestion of improved antigen presentation to specific (Th1) helper cell populations when ST is used as adjuvant. In terms of antigen load in the vaccine, it was shown that 50 ng of hepatitis B vaccine, a subimmunogenic dose, complexed with ST, gave a significantly greater antibody response than 1 μg of vaccine without adjuvant. Finally, the depot effect of ST was illustrated by use of ^{125}I-labeled hepatitis B surface antigen injected into the footpad. The amount of vaccine retained at the site of injection was higher when adsorbed to ST as compared to aluminum (Nixon-George *et al.*, 1990).

Preliminary experiments have been undertaken with ST and other viral vaccines. For example, mice immunized with a recombinant herpes subunit vaccine had more survivors on viral challenge when the vaccine was adjuvanted with ST instead of alum (J. Hilfenhaus, personal communication). Work has also been undertaken with rabies virus, rotavirus, tick-borne encephalitis virus, Newcastle disease virus, and infectious bronchitis virus (Table II).

6. OTHER APPLICATIONS

Based on the ability of tyrosine to adsorb allergen extracts and act as a depot during allergy desensitization therapy, work was undertaken to explore the potential utility of ST and analogues for such an application (Wheeler *et al.*, 1984). It was observed that induction of antibodies to grass pollen extracts was enhanced by increasing chain length of the alkyl ester. Similarly, ST was more effective than tyrosine as an adjuvant in guinea pigs. However, ST increased the irritation at the s.c. injection site compared to controls.

ST has minimal immunostimulatory properties and may be viewed as an inert additive for vaccine formulation. However, it has been reported that adsorption of the influenza glycoproteins neuraminidase (NA) and hemagglutinin (HA) onto ST activated natural killer (NK) cells and macrophages (Arora and Houde, 1988, 1992). The observed NK cell activity was viral antigen specific and both viral glycoproteins stimulated the NK cell

Table II
Summary of Vaccines Using ST as Adjuvant

Vaccine	Test species/comments	Reference
Tetanus toxoid	Outbred mice; increased IgG2a, IgG2b	Gupta and Siber (1994)
	Guinea pigs, passed U.S. FDA potency test	
Diphtheria toxoid	Mice	Penney et al. (1993)
Acellular pertussis (PT, FHA)	Mice; ST better than AlPO₄ with PT	Personal communication
Meningococcal A, B, and C Tetanus conjugates	Outbred mice, rabbits; neutralizing Ab, better than AlPO₄	Penney et al. (1993)
r hepatitis B	Mice; better than Al, no IgE	Nixon-George et al. (1990)
Inactivated polio (Salk)	Mice, rats; neutralizing Ab, Monkeys	Penney et al. (1993) Landi et al. (1986b)
HIV-1 peptide–KLH conjugate	Mice, baboons, neutralizing Ab	Nixon et al. (1992)
r herpes (gD subunit)	Mice, neutralizing Ab	Personal communication
Tick-borne encephalitis virus	Mice, neutralizing Ab	Personal communication
Rabies	Mice, guinea pigs, neutralizing Ab	Personal communication
Other viral vaccines (preliminary: see text)	Mice, Ab	Personal communication

portion of splenocytes of inbred mice. The extent of activation was similar to the standard interferon inducer/NK cell activator polyinosinic acid-polycytidylic acid and was not achieved by ST alone or when ST was replaced by muramyl dipeptide. Macrophages, restimulated with phorbol myristate acetate, exhibited enhanced hydrogen peroxide secretion in the presence of HA or NA and ST. HA alone was ineffective. This work supports the idea noted earlier of improved antigen presentation as a mechanism of adjuvanticity of ST and analogues.

7. ANALOGUES OF STEARYL TYROSINE

The trend observed in animal studies with ST was that this adjuvant displays similar adjuvanticity to alum with bacterial vaccines, but better adjuvanticity with viral vaccines. In view of this adjuvant activity, and the fact that little was reported in the initial publications about the structure–activity relationship of ST, a number of studies have been recently undertaken in an effort to discover the most adjuvant-active compound (Nixon-George et al., 1990; Penney et al., 1993, 1994). As such, over 40 analogues have been made and screened in mice with recombinant hepatitis B surface antigen. These compounds may be broadly classified as follows: (1) stearyl esters of amino acids; (2) stearyl esters of small (di- and tri-) peptides; (3) stearyl amides of amino acids; and (4) ethanolamine O-stearates of amino acids.

The ethanolamine O-stearate represents a novel, long-chain that is not from stearyl alcohol or stearylamine, but instead is derived from stearic acid and ethanolamine (Penney et al., 1994). The stearyl amide of amino acids is identical to the corresponding stearyl ester except that the stearyl chain is connected by an amide bond, instead of an ester linkage. Additionally, tetradecyl tyrosine hydrochloride has been synthesized, and found to be adjuvant active with the hepatitis B vaccine (Penney et al., 1993). However, it gave a more variable response than ST, and was observed to be less active.

Screening of the ST analogues revealed that a number of stearyl amino acids were better adjuvants than aluminum hydroxide or alum with the hepatitis vaccine (Nixon-George et al., 1990; Penney et al., 1993, 1994). Commercial recombinant hepatitis B vaccines use aluminum hydroxide adjuvant. Thus, for example, the amide analogue of ST, tyrosyl stearylamine, displayed approximately the same adjuvanticity as ST. Stearyl glycine and the corresponding amide, glycyl stearylamine, increased the magnitude of the antibody response by approximately 2-fold compared to aluminum. However, except for the dipeptide stearyl glycyl glycine, stearyl peptides were not very effective adjuvants with the hepatitis B antigen. Interestingly, among all of the analogues that were tested, only two compounds were significantly more adjuvant active than ST: stearyl hydroxyphenylglycine and phenylalanylethanolamine O-stearate. Both adjuvants were approximately twice as active as ST, in terms of the magnitude of the secondary antibody response. Relative to saline, this represents an approximately 30-fold increase in antibody response, or an

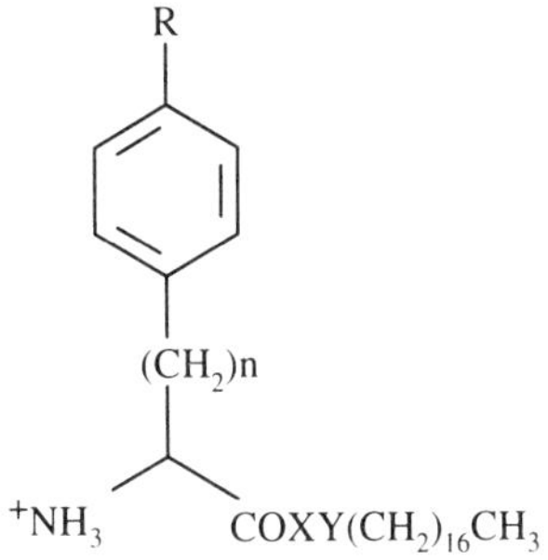

	R	X	Y	n
Stearyl Tyrosine	OH	O	CH_2	1
Stearyl Hydroxyphenylglycine	OH	O	CH_2	0
Tyrosyl Stearylamine	OH	NH	CH_2	1
Stearyl Tyrosyl Glycine	OH	NH	CH_2COOCH_2	1
Phenylalanylethanolamine O-Stearate	H	NH	CH_2CH_2OOC	1

Figure 3. Structure of stearyl tyrosine analogues evaluated with various bacterial and viral vaccines.

approximately 10-fold increase relative to aluminum adjuvant. Further, both adjuvants gave an increased ratio of IgG2a and IgG2b, relative to IgG1, compared to ST.

Based on the results of the hepatitis B antigen-adjuvant screening process, five analogues of ST were selected for further evaluation with a variety of vaccines (Penney *et al.*, 1993, 1994) (Fig. 3). These compounds were stearyl hydroxyphenylglycine, tyrosyl stearylamine, phenylalanylethanolamine *O*-stearate, stearyl glycyl glycine, and stearyl tyrosine glycine. This study showed that in terms of the ability to produce a significant adjuvant effect with a number of bacterial and viral vaccines, no analogue was apparently superior to ST. For example, the next most promising adjuvant appeared to be phenylalanylethanolamine *O*-stearate, and for some vaccines it may be better than ST (Penney *et al.*, 1994). It gave a significantly higher antibody response with hepatitis vaccine, a similar antibody response with tetanus, diphtheria, and HIV peptide vaccines, but it failed to adjuvant an inactivated polio vaccine. It is interesting to note that during the secondary antibody response induced with hepatitis B, tetanus, and diphtheria vaccines, the increase in IgG2a and IgG2b was approximately equal to the increase in IgG1 and this ratio appeared greater than observed with ST. Liposomal (phosphatidylcholine) adjuvants have been reported to increase the ratio of IgG2a and IgG2b to IgG1, relative to aluminum and muramyl dipeptide (Phillips, 1992) and so it is possible that some cationic ethanolamine long-chain compounds offer improved antigen presentation to Th1 helper cell populations.

7. CONCLUSIONS

Stearyl amino acids and peptides represent a new family of immunoadjuvants for vaccines. The parent compound, ST, has been extensively studied and shown to be a potential replacement for aluminum adjuvant in human vaccines. In summary, ST (1) induces a neutralizing antibody response with bacterial and viral vaccines which is similar or superior to aluminum including the magnitude of response and the isotype distribution; (2) possesses defined physical-chemical properties such as free-flowing powder characteristics, high melting point, and precise molecular weight; (3) is amenable to chemical modification resulting in altered modulation of adjuvanticity and the introduction of immunostimulatory signals; (4) is nontoxic and fairly inert showing little damage at the injection site, no adjuvant arthritis, and no pyrogenicity; (5) is biocompatible and biodegradable wherein ST degrades to tyrosine and stearyl alcohol; (6) is inexpensive and easy to prepare; and (7) is biocidal to bacteria and fungi.

ACKNOWLEDGMENTS

I am grateful to Dr. Silvio Landi for numerous useful discussions throughout the course of this project, and for the thorough and thoughtful reading of this manuscript. I appreciate the support given to this writing by BioChem Therapeutic Inc., in particular by Dr. Gervais Dionne. It is a pleasure to acknowledge the skillful typing and additional effort of Ms. Lyne Marcil and the technical editing and final manuscript preparation by Jessica Burdman.

REFERENCES

Allison, A. C., and Byars, N. E., 1991, Immunological adjuvants: desirable properties and side-effects, *Mol. Immunol.* **28**:279–284.

Arora, D. J. S., and Houde, M., 1988, Purified glycoproteins of influenza virus stimulate cell-mediated cytotoxicity *in vivo*, *Nat. Immun. Cell Growth Reg.* **7**:87–94.

Arora, D. J. S., and Houde, M., 1992, Modulation of murine macrophage responses stimulated with influenza glycoproteins, *Can. J. Microbiol.* **38**:188–192.

Claesson, B. A., Trolifors, B., Lagergard, T., Taranger, J., Bryla, D., Otterman, G., Cramton, T., Yang, Y., Reimer, C. B., Robbins, J. B., and Schneerson, R., 1988, Clinical and immunologic responses to the capsular polysaccharide of Haemophilus influenzae type b alone or conjugated to tetanus toxoid in 18- to 23-month-old children, *J. Pediatr.* **112**:695–702.

Gall, D., 1966, The adjuvant activity of aliphatic nitrogenous bases, *Immunology* **11**:369–386.

Goto, N., Kato, H., Maeyama, J., Eto, K., and Yoshihara, S., 1993, Studies on the toxicities of aluminum hydroxide and calcium phosphate as immunological adjuvants for vaccines, *Vaccine* **11**:914–918.

Gupta, R. K., and Relyveld, E. H., 1991, Adverse reactions after injection of adsorbed DPT vaccine are not due only to pertussis organisms or pertussis components in the vaccine, *Vaccine* **9**:699–702.

Gupta, R. K., and Siber, G.R., 1994, Comparison of adjuvant activities of aluminum phosphate, calcium phosphate, and stearyl tyrosine for tetanus toxoid, *Biologicals* **22**:53–63.

Jennings, H. J., and Lugowski, C., 1981, Immunochemistry of groups A, B, and C meningococcal polysaccharide–tetanus toxoid conjugates, *J. Immunol.* **127**:1011–1018.

Jennings, H. J., Roy, R., and Gamian, A., 1986, Induction of meningococcal group B polysaccharide specific IgG antibodies in mice by using N-propionylated B polysaccharide–tetanus toxoid conjugate vaccine, *J. Immunol.* **137**:1708–1713.

Kenney, J. S., Hughes, B. W., Masada, M. P., and Allison, A. C., 1989, Influence of adjuvants on the quantity, affinity, isotype and epitope specificity of murine antibodies, *J. Immunol. Methods* **121**:157–166.

Landi, S., Penney, C. L., Shah, P., Hart, F., Campbell, J. B., and Cucakovich, N., 1986, Adjuvanticity of stearyl tyrosine on inactivated poliovirus vaccine, *Vaccine* **4**:99–104.

Léry, L., 1994, Haemolytic activity of calcium phosphate adjuvant, *Vaccine* **12**:475–480.

Liu, M., Nakahara, H., Shibasaki, Y., and Fukuda, K., 1994, Molecular arrangement and polycondensation of octadecyl esters of aromatic amino acids in Langmuir–Blodgett films, *Thin Solid Films* **237**:244–249.

Moloney, P. J., and Wojcik, G., 1981, Synthetic adjuvants for stimulation of antigenic responses, U.S. Patent No. 4,258,029. Also, 1983, Canadian Patent No. 1,138,773; 1984, European Patent No. 18,189.

Nixon, A., Zaghouani, H., Penney, C. L., Lacroix, M., Dionne, G., Anderson, S. A., Kennedy, R. C., and Bona, C.A., 1992, Adjuvanticity of stearyl tyrosine on the antibody response to peptide 503-535 from HIV gp 160, *Viral Immunol.* **5**:141–152.

Nixon-George, A., Moran, T., Dionne, G., Penney, C. L., Lafleur, D., and Bona, C., 1990, The adjuvant effect of stearyl tyrosine on a recombinant subunit hepatitis B surface antigen, *J. Immunol.* **144**:4798–4802.

Penney, C. L., Shah, P., and Landi, S., 1985a, A simple method for the synthesis of long-chain alkyl esters of amino acids, *J. Org. Chem.* **50**:1457–1459.

Penney, C. L., Shah, P., and Landi, S., 1985b, The interaction of slow-release immunoadjuvants with selected antigens measured *in vitro*, *J. Biol. Stand.* **13**:43–52.

Penney, C. L., Landi, S., Shah, P., Leung, K. H., and Archer, M. C., 1986, Analysis of the immunoadjuvant octadecyl tyrosine hydrochloride, *J. Biol. Stand.* **14**:345–349.

Penney, C. L., Ethier, D., Dionne, G., Nixon-George, A., Zaghouani, H., Michon, F., Jennings, H., and Bona, C. A., 1993, Further studies on the adjuvanticity of stearyl tyrosine and ester analogues, *Vaccine* **11**:1129–1134.

Penney, C. L., Dionne, G., Nixon-George, A., and Bona, C. A., 1994, Further studies on the adjuvanticity of stearyl tyrosine and amide analogues, *Vaccine* **12**:629–632.

Phillips, N. C., 1992, Liposomal carriers for the treatment of acquired immune deficiency syndromes, *Bull. Inst. Pasteur* **90**:205–230.

Ratliff, D. A., and Burns-Cox, C. J., 1984, Anaphylaxis to tetanus toxoid, *Br. Med. J.* **288**:114.

Wheeler, A. W., Whittall, N., Spackman, V., and Moran, D. M., 1984, Adjuvant properties of hydrophobic derivatives prepared from l-tyrosine, *Int. Arch. Allergy Appl. Immunol.* **75**:294–299.

Chapter 27

Cytokines as Vaccine Adjuvants

Current Status and Potential Applications

Penny Dong, Carsten Brunn, and Rodney J.Y. Ho

1. INTRODUCTION

Since Jenner's discovery that cowpox vaccinations protect humans against smallpox, vaccines have been used effectively to protect humans and livestock from contagious and deadly diseases. Most of the marketed vaccines are made from either inactivated or attenuated pathogens (i.e., viruses or bacteria). Although vaccines prepared with inactivated pathogens are often effective, their use may be limited because a small but measurable chance of infection exists, a result of the incomplete inactivation of pathogens in these preparations. The incomplete inactivation of pathogens is particularly a concern for vaccines against viruses that may produce a latent infection (i.e., herpes and retroviruses). Similarly, vaccines constructed with attenuated pathogens may invoke the very disease they are designed to prevent if they are insufficiently attenuated. Therefore, subunit vaccines composed of antigenic components (usually proteins) free of pathogenic components are likely to offer improved safety.

With the advent of recombinant DNA technology, it is possible to manufacture proteins on a large scale for use as subunit vaccines. However, most subunit proteins are weak immunogens compared with inactivated or attenuated vaccines. Therefore, immunogenicity of subunit vaccines must be enhanced with adjuvants to provide antigen-specific protective immunity. Alum (aluminum hydroxide) is the only vaccine adjuvant in products approved by the Food and Drug Administration for human use, despite its weak adjuvanticity. Potent vaccine adjuvants such as Freund's adjuvant, bacillus Calmette–Guérin (BCG), and others are effective in eliciting antigen-specific immune responses; however, their clinical use may be limited because of potential toxicity. In fact, these potent vaccine adjuvants mediate their immune enhancement through nonspecific induction of

---

Penny Dong, Carsten Brunn, and Rodney J.Y. Ho • Department of Pharmaceutics, University of Washington, School of Pharmacy, Seattle, Washington 98195.

Vaccine Design: The Subunit and Adjuvant Approach, edited by Michael F. Powell and Mark J. Newman. Plenum Press, New York, 1995.

several cytokines that regulate immune interactions. Based on this, the selective use of cytokines should effectively and directly improve the immunogenicity of the weak subunit vaccines while minimizing the side effects of nonspecific cytokine inducers, e.g., Freund's adjuvant. Recent advances in our knowledge of cytokine functions and the large availability of recombinant cytokines permit us to systematically test the use of cytokines as adjuvants.

Cytokines are protein factors that produce multiple, pleiotropic effects on many immune cells. In general, they are small (10–50 kDa) proteins that exhibit short biologic half lives and function as autocrines and/or paracrines. The biologic actions of cytokines are often mediated by multiple receptors expressed on the cell surface. The high affinity ($K_a = 10^{10}$ to 10^{12}) and specificity of cytokines for their receptors and their short biologic half-life ensure localized and specific actions on the target cells. It is not a single cytokine but rather the network of cytokines that modulates the immune response. Cytokines generally can be categorized into (1) colony-stimulating factors [e.g., monocyte colony-stimulating factor (M-CSF) and granulocyte CSF (G-CSF)] that are produced primarily in antigen-presenting cells (APCs) and promote the growth of immune progenitor cells and (2) lymphokines such as interleukins that are produced by and stimulate leukocytes and interferons (IFNs).

This chapter focuses on the use of cytokines to enhance the immunogenicity of protein antigens. To systematically develop strategies for using cytokines as vaccine adjuvants, it is essential to understand the roles of cytokines involved in mediating natural immune interactions leading to protective immune responses (i.e., humoral or cellular responses against pathogens). Therefore, we discuss the role of cytokines in antigen presentation and T- and B-cell growth and differentiation. Subsequently, we discuss the application of selected cytokines that have been tested in vivo for vaccine immune enhancement. Finally, we will discuss strategies for optimizing the use of cytokines as vaccine adjuvants.

Because this chapter focuses on the use of cytokines as vaccine adjuvants, the reader should refer to recent reviews on molecular and cellular aspects of cytokine functions for additional details (Kroemer *et al.*, 1993; St. Georgiev and Albright, 1993).

1.1. The Role of Cytokines in Antigen Presentation

When foreign antigen is introduced into the host, the antigen, either in its native form or processed, is presented by APCs at the first step in immune recognition that leads to T- and B-cell responses. The antigen presentation process determines the magnitude and the nature of the immune response. The APCs include monocytes, endothelial cells, fibroblasts, Langerhans cells, dendritic cells, and B cells. With the exception of B cells, antigens taken up by APCs are processed into short peptides either in endosomes or in other proteolytic compartments. The peptide fragments associate with the class II MHC (major histocompatibility complex), or in the cytoplasm with the class I MHC. The efficiency of antigen presentation will depend on the number of surface MHC molecules, the efficiency of antigen uptake, internalization, and processing, and the expression of costimulators for T-cell activation such as IFN and IL-1 (Harding *et al.*, 1988). Cytokines may modulate the antigen presentation process in two ways: (1) increase the number of activated APCs that can present antigen and (2) activate APCs. For example, M-CSF and

G-CSF synthesized by most of the APCs promote differentiation and expansion of mononuclear phagocytes or granulocytes, respectively, while granulocyte–macrophage CSF (GM-CSF) can activate immature progenitor cells and promote the differentiation of both monocytes and granulocytes. IFN-γ, synthesized in T cells or natural killer (NK) cells, activates APCs and induces the synthesis of both class I and class II MHC molecules. Other IFNs, e.g., IFN-α and IFN-β, predominantly produced in monocytes and fibroblasts, can increase expression of class I MHC molecules produced by CD4$^+$ helper T cells. On the other hand, IL-1, synthesized in monocytes and other activated macrophages, may also activate APCs. Transforming growth factor β (TGF-β) secreted from T cells and monocytes, however, acts as an antagonist to the monocyte activation process, impeding the activation of monocytes.

1.2. The Role of Cytokines in T-Cell Growth

Once the antigen is presented to T cells by APCs, a number of cytokines are involved in regulating the clonal expansion of antigen-specific T cells. These antigen-sensitized T cells provide the host with the "proper" cellular immunity against pathogenic diseases. T-cell growth involves the process of immature T-cell activation and differentiation into T-helper cells (Th1 and Th2 cells), cytotoxic T cells (CTLs), and T-cell proliferation. A number of these T-cell growth functions are modulated by cytokines. Immature T cells can be activated by IL-1, TNF (tumor necrosis factor), IL-2, IL-6, and IL-7. Both IL-1 and TNF, secreted by activated monocytes, can activate resting T cells. The activated T cells synthesize IL-2 and express membrane-bound IL-2 receptors (IL-2R). The secretion of IL-2 by activated T cells leads to the growth and expansion of both CD4$^+$ and CD8$^+$ T cells. IL-6, synthesized by APCs in response to IL-1, synergizes with IL-1 in the activation of resting T cells (Lorre *et al.*, 1994; Panzer *et al.*, 1993). IL-7, expressed in a number of thymus cells, has both IL-2-dependent and -independent T-cell activation (Bertagnolli and Herrmann, 1990; Jicha *et al.*, 1992). Differentiation of T cells is regulated by a selective group of cytokines. IL-4 and IL-10 favor Th2 cell development; IFN-γ, IL-2, and IL-12 favor Th1 cell development; IL-2 and IL-7 support CTL growth. In turn, the activated T cells produce cytokines that may affect other immune cells. For example, activated Th1 cells express IL-2, IFN-γ, and TGF-β while activated Th2 cells express primarily IL-4, IL-5, and IL-10. With the complex cytokine network, these growth factors regulate the development of immune responses by modulating the differentiation and expansion of committed T cells.

1.3. The Role of Cytokines in B-Cell Growth

Mature B cells or plasma cells synthesize antibodies against immunogens (or pathogens) in providing the host with humoral immunity. The growth of B cells involves progenitor B-cell proliferation, pre-B-cell activation, and B-cell differentiation to immunoglobulin-producing plasma cells. Similar to the process of T-cell growth, this process is also regulated by a number of cytokines. Stromal cell-derived cytokine IL-7 is characterized as pre- and pro-B-cell growth factor in lymphopoiesis. IL-2, IFN-γ, IL-4, IL-5, and

IL-6 are all activators of B cells. In addition, some of these cytokines are responsible for isotype-switching of antibody-secreting cells: IL- 6, secreted from activated macrophages, stimulates the specialization of IgA-producing B cells (Beagley *et al.*, 1989). IL-4, secreted by $CD4^+$ helper T cells, favors the production of IgE and IgG1 (Coffman *et al.*, 1988; Coffman and Mosmann, 1991). Both IL-5 from T cells and TGF-β from either T cells or phagocytes promote the differentiation of B cells toward the IgA isotype (Ehrhardt *et al.*, 1992). Monokines such as IFN-γ stimulate the synthesis of IgG2a in B cells (Snapper and Paul, 1987). IL-2, on the other hand, enhances antibody production in B cells, but without isotype-switching.

The functional role of individual cytokines, as briefly discussed above, has been studied extensively in recent years as the recombinant forms of protein are now widely available. The results of these studies, mainly performed in vitro, indicate that cytokines may enhance the potency of subunit vaccines through modulation of antigen presentation, and T- and B-cell growth. However, the effect of individual cytokines in vivo cannot be predicted directly from the in vitro data since cytokine functions are mediated through a cellular immune cascade, and the dynamic of biological interactions is much more complicated in vivo than in vitro. Therefore, in the following section, we will describe the role of cytokines in augmenting antigen-specific immune response based on the results of in vivo studies with cytokines. We will also refer to in vitro results where appropriate.

2. APPLICATION OF CYTOKINES IN MODULATING ANTIGEN PRESENTATION

As discussed in Section 1.1, presentation of a given antigen by APCs may be enhanced by increasing the number of APCs competent for antigen presentation and/or activating the existing number of APCs by costimulators. This may be achieved by cytokines themselves or cytokine-inducing chemicals. We will discuss both approaches.

2.1. Cytokines

Cytokines such as CSFs and IFNs have been used to enhance the antigen presentation process. M-CSF, for example, can be used in vivo to activate mononuclear phagocytes and promote their proliferation. For example, Hume *et al.* (1988) have shown that four daily intravenous doses of recombinant human M-CSF increased the number of peripheral blood monocytes, in a dose-dependent fashion, in the liver and peritoneum. These macrophages were larger, indicating their activated state.

Similarly, GM-CSF can be used to enhance the immunogenicity of vaccines. Recently, GM-CSF has been used to overcome the weak immunogenicity of B-cell lymphoma using idiotype antibody (ID)/GM-CSF fusion protein (Tao and Levy, 1993). When free murine GM-CSF (m-GM-CSF) was administered with a murine tumor-derived ID, no change in the mouse survival rate was observed at 120 days after the tumor challenge. In contrast, vaccination with the fusion protein ID/m-GM-CSF provided mice with a 60–70% survival rate at 120 days after tumor challenge. None of the mice survived when treated with ID as antigen alone or with free m-GM-CSF, and only 30% of the mice survived when treated with ID conjugated to keyhole limpet hemocyanin (KLH). In addition, these mice treated with the fusion protein produced a significantly increased anti-ID level, indicating enhanced antigen presentation and, perhaps, B-cell growth. Similarly, irradiated B16 melanoma cells engineered to express m-GM-CSF also stimulate a potent and long-lasting antitumor immunity that includes induction in both CD4$^+$ and CD8$^+$ T cells (Dranoff *et al.*, 1993), suggesting GM-CSF can be useful as an adjuvant to enhance antigen presentation.

Both IFN-γ and IL-1 activate macrophages and enhance antigen presentation. IFN-γ has been used to enhance the immunogenicity of candidate vaccines against malaria, for which the protective immunity may require both humoral and cellular response (Playfair and DeSouza, 1987). When administered concurrently, IFN-γ augments the immune response of an erythrocyte-derived parasite preparation, leading to strong antibody, helper T cell, and delayed-type hypersensitivity (DTH) responses (Playfair and DeSouza, 1987). Comparative studies of IFN-γ, saponin, and IL-1 as adjuvants for a blood stage malaria vaccine indicate that IFN-γ is more effective than IL-1 in suppressing parasite titer counts in CD4$^+$-deficient or low-antibody-responder mice (Heath *et al.*, 1989). In addition to malaria vaccine, IFN-γ has also been shown to delay tumor development in mice immunized with irradiated murine neuroblastoma cells, suggesting its ability to augment the neuroblastoma-associated antigen (Sigal *et al.*, 1990). While IFNs and IL-1 improved the antigenicity of these vaccines, direct enhancement of antigen presentation remains to be verified.

2.2. Cytokine Induction by Other Adjuvants

A number of chemicals are capable of enhancing immune response by elevating cytokine levels. These chemicals, also referred to as cytokine inducers, are often the major active components of laboratory adjuvants that are extremely toxic and potent. Muramyl dipeptide (MDP), for instance, is the minimal active structure of mycobacteria in Freund's adjuvants (Lederer *et al.*, 1975). MDP, and its more lipophilic derivative muramyl tripeptide (MTP), stimulate the synthesis of CSF and IL-1 in monocytes (Maeda *et al.*, 1991). Monophosphoryl lipid A, a nontoxic glycolipid component of endotoxin, also induces IL-1 in activated macrophages (Kiener *et al.*, 1988; Loppnow *et al.*, 1990; Verma *et al.*, 1992). Cholera toxin purified from *Vibrio cholerae* can induce alloantigen Ia expression, as well as IL-1 and IL-6 synthesis in intestinal epithelial cells (Bromander *et al.*, 1993; Lycke *et al.*, 1989).

MDP and MTP have been shown to enhance antigen presentation both in vivo and in vitro (Bahr *et al.*, 1987; Maeda *et al.*, 1991). The increased adjuvanticity provided by MDP and its derivatives is closely correlated to the expression of membrane IL-1 of macrophages (Bahr *et al.*, 1987). Macrophage activation by liposome-encapsulated MTP-phosphatidylethanolamine (MTP-PE) can be observed as their cytotoxic activity against tumor cells increases (Sone *et al.*, 1986) without a significant increase in IFN production (Dietrich *et al.*, 1986). This minimal increase may be advantageous as IFN has the potential to activate nonspecific immune responses, thus producing undesirable side effects in the host. In a vaccination scheme, liposomes containing MTP-PE provide a protective immunity against the weakly immunogenic murine melanoma K1735 cells (Ullrich and Fidler, 1992). In addition, guinea pigs immunized with the herpes simplex virus (HSV) antigen gD in an MTP-PE liposome formulation show enhanced antibody responses, comparable to the same antigen formulated with incomplete (IFA) or complete Freund's adjuvant (CFA) (Sanchez-Pescador *et al.*, 1988). Also, gD formulated in MTP-PE liposomes can effectively suppress virus reactivations in an immunotherapeutic use as vaccine (Ho *et al.*, 1989, 1990). Furthermore, a palmitoylated gD peptide (1-23) formulated in MTP-PE liposomes stimulated a comparable cellular immunity in C3H mice as CFA and a significantly higher level of humoral response (Brynestad *et al.*, 1990). While the protective immunity established using liposome-formulated acylated peptide was still less effective than the HSV infection, it was nonetheless significantly higher than that of other adjuvant formulations. It is possible that acylated peptides may have a lower clearance rate than free peptides, so that a prolonged exposure of peptide to the draining lymph nodes results (Brynestad *et al.*, 1990). The prolonged exposure of peptide and sustained release of MTP-PE could further enhance the time span and intensity of the antigenicity of vaccine alone. Alternatively, liposomes containing MTP-PE can be used as carriers to effectively target antigen to lymphoid cells, thereby further minimizing the potential toxicity of these compounds (Ho *et al.*, 1994). Taken together, liposome-encapsulated MTP-PE may elicit adjuvant effects by increasing the amount of IL-1 synthesized in monocytes, providing a sustained release of MTP that prolongs vaccine exposure to phagocytes and serving as a carrier to preferentially deliver vaccines into APCs. However, the level of cytokine induction by MTP-PE in the above examples is yet to be determined.

Monophosphoryl lipid A (MPL) has also been shown to augment both cellular and humoral immune responses while minimizing hemolysis and other toxicities that are mediated by its parent compound endotoxin. MPL increases the total B-cell number through induction of IFN-γ and IL-1 (Johnson and Tomai, 1990). In particular, MPL enhances the IgM antibody titer against type III pneumococcal polysaccharide in young mice (Baker *et al.*, 1988) with a concurrent increase in nonspecific serum IgG3 and a decrease in serum IgG1 (Hiernaux *et al.*, 1989). The clinical relevance of nonspecific IgG3 production is not clear at present. MPL has been used in various liposome formulations to enhance the induction of antibody against a tetrapeptide-repeat antigen of the circumsporozoite protein of plasmodia (Richards *et al.*, 1989), the capsular polysaccharide components of influenza virus or pneumococcus in polysaccharide–protein conjugates (Schneerson *et al.*, 1991), and a hexapeptide histone H3 antigen (Friede *et al.*, 1993). MPL has also been used to augment the CTL response against ovalbumin (OVA) when liposome-formulated OVA and MPL are given together to mice by intravenous, intraperitoneal, and intramuscular routes (Zhou and Huang, 1993). The fact that injection of liposomal OVA and liposomal MPL at two different sites will not elicit CTL response in the host indicates that both liposomal MPL and OVA must be delivered to the same tissue and perhaps the same cells (Zhou and Huang, 1993). Again, while the level of cytokines such as IFN and IL-1 remains to be determined, it is suggested that MPL elevates the cytokine production based on the observations in vitro.

Cholera toxin (CT), which stimulates IL-1 and IL-6, may enhance antigen presentation, leading to mucosal IgA response. Enhanced antigen presentation provided by CT may be mediated through the cytokines regulated by Th2 cells. Xu-Amano *et al.* (1993) have shown that oral immunization with tetanus toxoid (TT, a protein-based vaccine) and cholera toxin as an adjuvant effectively stimulates the antigen-specific $CD4^+$ T cells both in Peyer's patches and spleen. These helper T cells predominantly secrete IL-4 and IL-5. The elicitation of $CD4^+$ T cells parallels the enhanced secretory IgA and serum IgG production. In this case, CT may enhance the immune response by activating the endothelial cells in Peyer's patches to secrete IL-1 and IL-6.

3. APPLICATION OF CYTOKINES IN MODULATING T-CELL GROWTH TO ENHANCE CELLULAR IMMUNE RESPONSE

Following vaccination and proper antigen presentation, mobilization of antigen-specific T cells is one of the key events triggering the immune responses that lead to immunity against infection. T-cell growth involves the activation of immature thymocytes and differentiation of activated T cells into helper T cells (Th1 and Th2 cells) and CTLs. Th1 and Th2 cells are essential either in DTH reactions or in providing help to B cells, while cytotoxic T cells are essential for controlling infection by eliminating infected cells. Cytokines modulate T-cell growth in at least three aspects: (1) activation of resting T cells, (2) differentiation of activated T cells into T helper cells, and (3) clonal expansion (or growth) of the committed T cells.

A number of laboratories have shown that IL-2 can enhance the growth of both cytotoxic and helper T cells. IL-2 can augment the immune response introduced by MCA-102, a murine sarcoma. Sencer *et al.* (1991) observed that when liposome-formulated IL-2 is administered, mice vaccinated with MCA-102 demonstrated significant delays in tumor growth and in elevated DTH. Ho *et al.* (1992) have shown that four weekly doses of liposome-formulated IL-2 given in conjunction with two doses of gD protein reduce HSV-2 recurrence by 70%, compared with gD administered with soluble IL-2 or the single agent alone. The decreased recurrence rate in HSV-2 is correlated to an elevated antigen-specific T and B cell response. Fusion protein composed of gD and human IL-2 has been genetically constructed to enhance anti-HSV antibody responses; vaccination with this fusion protein in animals provides complete immunity against HSV challenge, while gD formulated in alum did not offer such protection (Hazama *et al.,* 1993). Further characterizations indicated that the effects of IL-2–gD conjugate on immune enhancement are related to the biological effect of IL-2 and not the carrier–hapten effect since no increases in anti-human IL-2 response were detectable. IL-2 and IL-7 produce similar augmentation of CTLs against HSV challenge to naive mice as enhanced immunity was observed; CTLs are primarily responsible for the suppression of viral infection (Ho, unpublished results; Rouse *et al.,* 1985). Another example of IL-2 enhancing the CTL response comes from combination studies with TNF against mouse melanoma. The mean survival time for tumor-bearing mice was greatly prolonged when IL-2 was used in combination with TNF, and 30% of these mice were cured of the tumors. Lymphocytes isolated from spleens of those cured mice exhibit enhanced CTL activity and unchanged lymphokine-activated killer activity against B16 tumors (Urano *et al.,* 1993).

IL-12, primarily secreted by macrophages, is effective in enhancing Th1 response and NK cell activities. Protection against *Leishmania major* requires the cell-mediated immune response established by specific Th1 cells (Scott, 1991). However, when mice are vaccinated with a soluble leishmania antigen (SLA), only the IL-4 level is elevated because of preferential Th2 cell induction. When given together with SLA, IL-12 (0.5 μg) enhances Th1 response and reduces the IL-4 level, leading to augmented immunity against the parasite (Afonso and Scott, 1993). In this case, IL-12 stimulates a significant initial NK cell response; IFN-γ produced in NK cells synergizes IL-12 stimulation of Th1 response. In another study, a poorly immunogenic murine tumor cell line (BL-6) was used as a vaccine in the presence of fibroblasts expressing IL-12. A significantly delayed tumor development was observed after the tumor challenge, compared with controls that did not receive cytokine adjuvant. Histological analysis revealed a peritumoral presence of macrophages and decreased $CD4^+$ cells in the tumor (Tahara *et al.*, 1994).

4. APPLICATION OF CYTOKINES IN MODULATING B-CELL GROWTH TO ENHANCE HUMORAL IMMUNE RESPONSE

The activation of memory B cells by the antigen leads to the growth of B cells, providing humoral immunity to the host. The growth of B cells involves immature B-cell proliferation, B-cell differentiation, and committed B-cell proliferation and function; this process is modulated by a number of cytokines. B-cell growth factors such as IL-7 promote proliferation of immature B cells; other cytokines such as IL-4, IL-5, IL-6, and IFN-γ modulate the differentiation and proliferation of activated B cells. IL-2 enhances overall antibody production. In this section we will discuss the use of cytokines to augment B-cell growth to enhance humoral response.

IFN-γ directly promotes antigen-specific immunoglobulin production. Cao et al. (1992) demonstrated that mice challenged at 10 LD_{50} after intranasal vaccination with inactivated influenza virus and either m-IFN-γ or m-IFN-β as adjuvants displayed a significantly higher survival rate than those in the control group that were immunized with vaccine alone. Further characterization points to a significantly higher IgA and IgG level in bronchoalveolar lavage and serum, which is attributable to the m-IFN-γ adjuvant.

IFN-1 (a mixture of IFN-α and IFN-β) was effective in elevating IgM and IgG production when administered at the time of vaccination against rabies virus (Mifune *et al.*, 1987). It was not, however, very effective in inducing antibody in patients who were undergoing hemodialysis against hepatitis B virus (Grob *et al.*, 1984), indicating that IFN-1 may not be useful in patients with immunodeficiency conditions. IL-2, on the other hand, was effective in inducing anti-hepatitis B antibody synthesis in patients undergoing hemodialysis (Meuer *et al.*, 1989), perhaps through B-cell stimulation.

IL-2 was shown to enhance antibody production with the help of T cells, as discussed previously. Additional examples described by Kawashima and Platt (1989) and Hughes *et al.* (1992) indicate that the adjuvant effects of recombinant IL-2 enhance immunogenicity of a subunit vaccine of porcine pseudorabies virus and glycoprotein IV of bovine herpes virus-1. When IL-2 was given at a 12-h interval in both cases, antibody production was achieved. Williams *et al.* (1992) showed that IL-2 increases specific antibody production against autologous intralymphatic tumor cells. IL-2 secretion from transduced human melanoma cells enhances the response of allogeneic peripheral blood lymphocytes from melanoma patients, suggesting the potential of IL-2 adjuvanticity in treating cancer

(Uchiyama *et al.*, 1993). One interesting result came from the vaccination studies with macaques using vaccinia virus that encodes the envelope gene of HIV-1. The animals vaccinated with vaccinia virus expressing envelope protein and IL-2 produced higher antibody titers and broader cross-reactivity against various strains of virus (Ruby *et al.*, 1990), suggesting the augmented activation of B-cell clones by IL-2.

Both IL-5 and IL-6 favor growth of the IgA isotype B cell. Pockley and Montgomery (1991) showed that daily, 50-unit doses of IL-5 and IL-6 administered concurrently with dinitrophenylated pneumococcus antigen (DNP-Pn) in each eye resulted in enhanced tear IgA secretion against DNP-Pn without changing the total tear IgA. The high level of specific IgA was maintained without the use of other vaccine adjuvants, suggesting the prolonged establishment of IgA immunity against DNP-Pn provided by IL-5 and IL-6 administration. The results suggest that IL-5 and/or IL-6 may support and maintain memory cells secreting IgA.

5. CYTOKINE FRAGMENTS AS VACCINE ADJUVANTS

Because each cytokine is a pleiotropic modulator of the immune system, the cytokine molecule can be divided into several functional domains. Cytokines have at least one binding domain to interact with their receptors, and one or several effector domains that modulate the transcription of the target genes and/or the regulation of certain cellular proteins in different target cells. Since not all of the possible functions of each cytokine are desirable when used as adjuvants, e.g., inducing inflammation, it is helpful to identify individual functional domains. With the availability of advanced techniques in molecular biology and prediction of protein structures, functional domains of cytokines can be produced by peptide synthesis or recombinant technology and then studied in detail.

For instance, IL-1 both activates resting T cells and elicits inflammatory responses. In order to be used as a vaccine adjuvant, the stimulatory effect of IL-1 should be maximized or maintained, while the inflammatory effect should be minimized. There are two IL-1 isomers in humans, IL-1α and IL-1β, both about 17 kDa in size, encoded by two different genes and sharing only 30% homology in the peptide sequence. However, their biological functions are similar, and they bind to the same receptors with similar affinity. The peptide encompassing residues 163–171 of IL-1β was shown to be immunostimulatory but not inflammatory both in vitro (Antoni *et al.*, 1989) and in vivo (Nencioni *et al.*, 1987; Tagliabue and Boraschi, 1993). Unfortunately, 100 mg/kg of the nonapeptide is necessary to achieve an immune stimulation comparable to 20 ng/kg of the parent IL-1β molecule, indicating a drastically decreased affinity between the ligand and the receptor (Nencioni *et al.*, 1987). Subsequent studies indicated that the nonapeptide did not bind to the IL-1 receptor (Boraschi *et al.*, 1992), explaining why an excessive amount of the nonapeptide is necessary to achieve the same level of immunostimulation. If the high dosage requirement of the nonapeptide can eventually be overcome by optimizing the delivery process, these immune stimulatory peptides derived from cytokines may become useful as a vaccine adjuvant with much reduced side effects.

Penny Dong *et al.*

6. LOCAL DELIVERY OF CYTOKINES AND THE SEQUENCE OF ADMINISTRATION

Following antigen exposure, the timing and intra- and extracellular sites of specific cytokine production that mediate antigen-specific cellular and humoral immune development are a highly ordered process. The timing of these immune cascades are highly sequential events elicited by antigens through cytokine mediators. In addition, cytokine effects on immune systems may be localized only at the sites of antigen presentation, lymphocyte expansion, and maturation. Using phosphorylcholine-conjugated OVA as an antigen, Bogen *et al.* (1993) have shown that IFN-γ-producing NK cells appear at the site of immunization by day 3, while T cells producing IL-2, IL-4, and IFN-γ are not detectable at draining lymph nodes until day 7. At that time, antigen-specific B cells can be detected at the site of injection. Not until 2 weeks later do IL-2-producing T cells become detectable at the site of injection. On the other hand, systemically introduced antigen (i.e., by intramuscular or subcutaneous administration) may not produce immune responses at distal mucosal sites, e.g., vaginal or bronchial mucosa. Therefore, the site and timing of antigen and tissue-specific cytokine delivery are important, not only to induce optimum immune responses but also to reduce undesirable effects such as nonspecific lymphoproliferative disorders (Rich *et al.*, 1993), local inflammation, or capillary leak syndrome (at high doses of IL-2). With the rapid progress of our knowledge of natural immune responses, we now can rationally implement strategies to deliver exogenous cytokines and antigens in a scheme that synchronizes with the kinetics of antigen-specific T- and B-cell expansion. Furthermore, we can localize selective cytokines at the sites that support and maintain the development of antigen-specific immune responses in the immunized hosts.

Because of the pleiotropic nature of cytokines, the results of in vitro functional studies may not always predict the broad in vivo activities on multiple cell types, including nonimmune cells, besides their intended use as antigen-specific immune enhancers. In some cases, the pleiotropic effects of cytokines and their numbers on multiple immune cells may be dose dependent (Alderson *et al.*, 1991). At a low dose, most cytokines may exhibit limited specificity and provide vaccine adjuvant activity; at a high dose they may produce undesirable side effects. For example, at 0.1 ng/mL, IL-7 may stimulate T-cell growth, while at high doses (>100 ng/mL), it may also induce the production of IL-1α, IL-1β, IL-6, and TNF-α, cytokines that lead to inflammation (Alderson *et al.*, 1991). In most cases, the high loading dose required to maintain a minimal therapeutic cytokine level may often produce more than three- to fivefold the therapeutic level for a short period of time in the host, possibly leading to induction of nondesirable side effects. The peak cytokine concentration resulting from the initial loading dose may be significantly reduced by using sustained-release approaches. Sustained-release deliveries of IL-7 and IL-2 have been developed to reduce the systemic toxicity of the cytokine while providing enhancement of vaccine immune responses (Bui *et al.*, 1994a,c; Sencer *et al.*, 1991). Specifically, a prolonged and sustained release of cytokines provided by liposome-encapsulated IL-2 has led to a reduction in the frequency of administration and minimized the induction of antibody against these exogenous cytokines. In addition, the reduced frequency of dosing with cytokines has made their application as vaccine adjuvants a viable strategy by lowering cost and potential toxicity. Furthermore, an increased patient compliance rate can be expected with this strategy because considerably fewer injections are necessary. All of these considerations are essential for the practical and eventual development of cytokines as vaccine adjuvants.

The sustained IL-7 release approach has been used to enhance vaccine immune responses of HSV and HIV antigens. In order to elicit T- and B-cell growth in vivo, soluble IL-7 (in its native form) must be administered for 3 to 5 days at least twice daily. In a sustained-release liposome-encapsulated form, IL-7 may be administered on a once-a-week schedule to provide similar T- and B-cell growth as this strategy has increased the mean residence time of IL-7 from 4 h to 7.9 days (Bui *et al.,* 1994b). When liposome-formulated IL-7 is given on day 7 after recombinant HSV or HIV antigen administration in mice and guinea pigs, thus synchronizing antigen-specific T- and B-cell expansion, IL-7 enhances both humoral and CTL responses (Bui *et al.,* 1994a–c). In addition, sustained-release IL-7 has reduced nonspecific NK cell stimulation and platelet counts (Bui *et al.,* 1994b).

Similar effects are seen with sustained delivery of IL-2. In this case, compared with soluble IL-2, a much lower dose of sustained-release IL-2 is needed to provide equivalent or superior enhancement in vaccine immunogenicity. Since the dose of IL-2 used in sustained-release vehicles is far below the level that will induce the NK cell responses and capillary leak syndrome, toxicity is expected to be minimum. In addition, the IL-2 sustained-release approach has made unnecessary the daily doses of IL-2 required to provide vaccine adjuvant effects on HSV immune responses (Ho *et al.,* 1992; Weinberg and Merigan, 1988) and tumor-associated antigens (Sencer *et al.,* 1991).

For cytokine inducers, chemical modification and compound structure may determine their disposition in host organs (i.e., tissue localization, distribution, and elimination). For example, on intravenous administration MTP, a lipophilic derivative of MDP, remains in the host for a longer period of time than MDP. When MTP is conjugated to the amino-terminus (head group of phospholipid) of phosphatidylethanolamine, the resultant MTP-PE (MTP–phospholipid conjugate) can easily be incorporated into bilayer lipid vesicles. Liposome-formulated MTP-PE has further reduced the clearance and toxicity of MTP in vivo. This approach has produced a sustained presence of MTP-PE in lung, liver, spleen, kidneys, and blood of the host well beyond 24 h postinjection (Fogler *et al.,* 1985). Since MTP is capable of stimulating macrophages and enhancing antigen presentation, it is likely that a sustained presence of muramyl peptides (MDP, MTP, MTP-PE) may enhance vaccine immunogenicity. In fact, a number of laboratories including ours have verified the adjuvant effects of muramyl peptides delivered in liposomes or water-in-oil emulsions (i.e., MF59 formulation) that provided sustained presence of antigen and MTP-PE mixture (Sanchez-Pescador *et al.,* 1988; Ho *et al.,* 1988; Bui *et al.,* 1994b,c). Using MTP-PE liposomes and recombinant antigens, we and others have shown that MTP-PE may provide further enhancement of the adjuvant effects of liposomes (Sone *et al.,* 1986; Sanchez-Pescador *et al.,* 1988; Ho *et al.,* 1989, 1990).

In addition to providing a sustained but low level of cytokines, localization of these compounds and antigen at the site of immune interaction is important because the biological functions of cytokines in eliciting antigen-specific responses may be highly localized. Therefore, cytokines must be delivered to tissues of immune interactions, i.e., the specific cell types and the intracellular sites of antigen/cytokine recognition and processing. This can be achieved by choosing a proper route of administration and by use of delivery vehicles that may selectively deliver cytokines and antigen to the sites of actions.

To enhance antigen presentation, it is possible to deliver cytokines to the same site with the antigen, thereby localizing the effect of cytokines within the same cell. With this strategy, one may further reduce the nonspecific immune response to cytokines and their inducers. Taking advantage of preferential liposome accumulation in the spleen, specifically in macrophages, we have demonstrated that HSV recombinant antigen gD encapsulated in liposomes that express MTP-PE can be targeted to spleen macrophages (Fig. 1 and Table I). Of the APCs—macrophages, B cells, and dendritic cells—isolated from animals that were injected with liposome-encapsulated rgD, macrophages, not B cells or dendritic cells, stimulated autologous HSV-sensitized blood T cells (Table I). These data indicate that liposome-mediated preferential localization of antigen, together with MTP-PE, can enhance antigen presentation by spleen macrophages. The enhanced HSV-gD presentation by MTP-PE liposomes has resulted in a significant enhancement in controlling HSV-2 recurrent disease (Ho *et al.*, 1989, 1990).

The site of administration may also control the tissue localization of vaccine antigen. For example, if the MTP formulated in liposomes is given intranasally, the majority of the molecules are delivered to the lung and nasopharynx. If administered intravenously, MTP is found mostly in the lung, liver, spleen, kidney, and blood (Fogler *et al.*, 1985). It is also

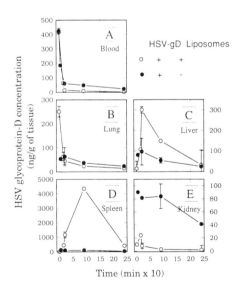

Figure 1. Effects of liposome encapsulation on HSV-gD tissue distribution profile in guinea pigs Liposome-encapsulated (●) or soluble (○) ^{125}I-labled HSV-gD (12 μg in 200 μL) were introduced systemically into guinea pigs weighing 300–350 g. Localization of HSV-gD in each organ was determined at indicated time point based on the radioactivity of HSV-gD. Data were analyzed as nanograms of HSV-gD per gram of tissue, expressed as mean ±SD of four animals. The presented organs were blood (A), lung (B), liver (C), spleen (D), and kidney (E). Adapted from Ho *et al.* (1994). Reprinted from *Vaccine* **12**(3):235–242 (1994), by permission of the publishers Butterworth–Heinemann Ltd. ©

Table I

Differential Localization and Presentation of HSV-gD by Spleen Cells Exposed to
Liposome-Encapsulated HSV-gD in Vivo

Spleen cells	Cell-associated HSV-gD[a] (ng/10[6] cells)	Cell proliferation[b]	
		Spleen T cells[c]	Blood T cells[d]
Total mononuclear cells[e]	18.5 ± 1.2	N.D.[g]	N.D.
Macrophages	17.0 ± 1.8	26,530 ± 3500	23,733 ± 4255
T cells	1.3 ± 0.7	N.D.	N.D.
B cells	0.1 ± 0.2	150 ± 123	255 ± 144
Others	0.6 ± 0.3	N.D.	N.D.
Dendritic cells[f]	0.6 ± 0.4	258 ± 146	330 ± 185

[a]Spleens from guinea pigs, injected with 12 μg liposome-encapsulated HSV-gD, were harvested at 90 min. HSV-gD associated with the indicated spleen cell population are expressed at ng/10[6] cells. Parallel studies with spleens from animals injected with 12 μg soluble HSV-gD produced a nondetectable level of HSV-gD in all spleen cell populations. Data presented as mean ±SD of indicated spleen cells.

[b]The ability of the HSV-gD loaded spleen APCs to stimulate T cells was determined by incubating them with autologous, HSV-2-sensitized T cells for 6 days. Cell proliferation was assessed by [^{3}H]thymidine incorporation into cellular DNA. Data expressed as mean ±SD of four animals.

[c]Spleen T cells were isolated from HSV immune animals at 90 min post HSV-gD administration.

[d]Blood T cells were isolated from HSV immune animals prior to HSV-gD administration.

[e]Total spleen mononuclear cells, isolated on Ficoll–Hypaque gradient, were further separated as adherent macrophages, B, T, and other nonadherent cells.

[f]Dendritic cells were isolated on metrizamide gradient.

[g]N.D., not determined.

possible that organ- or tissue-specific liposomes and other drug carriers can be employed for cytokine transport, which enables cytokines to be released in the desired organ or tissue.

Delivery of cytokines and vaccine antigen to the same cell can also be achieved by physically linking them. Hybrid molecules have been chemically generated by conjugating biotin with IFN-γ (Heath *et al.*, 1989). The biotinylated IFN-γ has been used as an adjuvant/carrier of avidin to elicit immune responses against avidin in mice. The high-affinity binding between biotin and avidin (Diamandis and Christopoulos, 1991) enables biotinylated IFN-γ to target IFN-γ and avidin to the same APCs. Hazama *et al.* (1993) have also chemically conjugated IL-2 with HSV protein gD to enhance immunogenicity of gD in providing immunity against HSV infection. Physical association of antigen and cytokines can also be performed through coexpression as a fusion protein in order to deliver cytokine plus antigen to the same cells. The fusion protein of a tumor-associated antigen and GM-CSF has been constructed and shown to enhance antibody response against tumor-associated antigen (Tao and Levy, 1993). Alternatively, the cytokine gene can be coexpressed with vaccine antigen in a recombinant virus (i.e., vaccinia virus) to enhance vaccine immunogenicity. Ramshaw and his colleagues (Ruby *et al.*, 1990; Karupiah *et al.*, 1992; Ramshaw *et al.*, 1992) demonstrated that IL-2 coexpressed with viral antigens such as the envelope protein gp160 of HIV-1 or the HA protein of the influenza virus in recombinant vaccinia viruses can provide immune enhancement compared to that of vaccinia-expressing antigen alone. However, the uncontrolled expression of cytokines may produce undesirable side effects, so caution in their use is advisable.

Regardless of which cytokines—CSFs, interleukins, monokines, or cytokine inducers—are used to enhance antigen presentation or T- and B-cell development and expansion, a controlled and selective cytokine delivery with proper timing may reduce the toxicity of these pleiotropic compounds while improving their therapeutic and practical value in providing vaccine adjuvant effects.

7. CONCLUSIONS

The purpose of a vaccine adjuvant is to provide the recipient of the vaccine maximum immune protection with minimum toxicity. In some cases, effective protection requires induction of both humoral and cellular immune responses, while others may require only one of the two. With our detailed understanding of cytokine biology and immune cell interactions, we may now systematically develop strategies that may selectively enhance humoral, cellular, or both aspects of immune responses against subunit vaccines.

Thanks to advances in our ability to clone and express the genes of cytokines and immune regulatory factors, we now begin to understand the natural role of cytokines in regulating immune responses. Through these studies, we are beginning to appreciate the complexity of the cytokine network that regulates the overall immune reaction against exogenous antigens, pathogens, or autoimmune antigens. With the development of recombinant technology on an industrial scale, large quantities of pure recombinant cytokines are now available to verify in vivo the putative cytokine functions that are predicted in in vitro studies. Studies with exogenous cytokine administration at therapeutic levels indicate that pleiotropic effects of cytokines may produce not only the intended immune induction, but also undesirable nonspecific responses. In order for cytokines to be used as vaccine adjuvants, a number of criteria must be met: (1) minimum toxicity; (2) ease of administration; (3) reasonable number of injections; and (4) minimal cost.

The broader-acting cytokines may produce more potent adjuvant effects; however, they may also produce higher nonspecific immune responses. The specificity of the broad-acting, less-specific cytokines may be increased by tissue- or cell-selective delivery of cytokines at the sites of immune interactions. By careful consideration of timing, route, and cytokine formulation or carrier, the nonspecific immune responses mediated by pleiotropic cytokines may be minimized. As a result, high doses of cytokines may not be necessary to produce adjuvant effects.

Nonspecific effects of cytokines may also be reduced by functional elucidation of their individual molecular domains. With advances in computing power, and the availability of the protein sequence data base, prediction of the functional domains of cytokines now becomes a practical approach in optimizing cytokine use as adjuvants. Advances in peptide chemistry allowing the synthesis of fairly pure polypeptides now permit studies of cytokine functional domains. This rational peptide design approach may offer a unique way for a further reduction in toxicity and enhanced potency for the application of cytokines as vaccine adjuvants. Overall, a more detailed elucidation of dose-dependent cytokine functions in vivo and development of cytokine targeting strategies will permit us to fine-tune our ability to use cytokines as safe and effective adjuvants for subunit vaccines.

ACKNOWLEDGMENTS

The authors are grateful to C. Shevrin and J. Burdman for their editorial help. The authors' research is supported by National Institutes of Health Grants AI 31854 and 33229.

REFERENCES

Afonso, L. C., and Scott, P., 1993, Immune responses associated with susceptibility of C57BL/10 mice to Leishmania amazonensis, *Infect. Immun.* **61**(7):2952–2959.

Alderson, M. R., Tough, T. W., Ziegler, S. F., and Grabstein, K. H., 1991, Interleukin 7 induces cytokine secretion and tumoricidal activity by human peripheral blood monocytes, *J. Exp. Med.* **173**(4):923–930.

Antoni, G., Presentini, R., Perin, F., Nencioni, L., Villa, L., Censini, S., Ghiara, P., Volpini, G., Bossu, P., Tagliabue, A., and Boraschi, D., 1989, Interleukin 1 and its synthetic peptides as adjuvants for poorly immunogenic vaccines, *Adv. Exp. Med. Biol.* **251**:153–160.

Bahr, G. M., Chedid, L. A., and Behbehani, K., 1987, Induction, in vivo and in vitro, of macrophage membrane interleukin-1 by adjuvant-active synthetic muramyl peptides, *Cell. Immunol.* **107**(2):443–454.

Baker, P. J., Hiernaux, J. R., Fauntleroy, M. B., Stashak, P. W., Prescott, B., Cantrell, J. L., and Rudbach, J. A., 1988, Ability of monophosphoryl lipid A to augment the antibody response of young mice, *Infect. Immun.* **56**(12):3064–3066.

Beagley, K. W., Eldridge, J. H., Lee, F., Kiyono, H., Everson, M. P., Koopman, W. J., Hirano, T., Kishimoto, T., and McGhee, J. R., 1989, Interleukins and IgA synthesis. Human and murine interleukin 6 induce high rate IgA secretion in IgA-committed B cells, *J. Exp. Med.* **169**(6):2133–2148.

Bertagnolli, M., and Herrmann, S., 1990, IL-7 supports the generation of cytotoxic T lymphocytes from thymocytes. Multiple lymphokines required for proliferation and cytotoxicity, *J. Immunol.* **145**(6):1706–1712.

Bogen, S. A., Fogelman, I., and Abbas, A. K., 1993, Analysis of IL-2, IL-4, and IFN-gamma-producing cells in situ during immune responses to protein antigens, *J. Immunol.* **150**(10):4197–4205.

Boraschi, D., Ghiara, P., Scapigliati, G., Villa, L., Sette, A., and Tagliabue, A., 1992, Binding and internalization of the 163-171 fragment of human IL-1 beta, *Cytokine* **4**(3):201–204.

Bromander, A. K., Kjerrulf, M., Holmgren, J., and Lycke, N., 1993, Cholera toxin enhances alloantigen presentation by cultured intestinal epithelial cells, *Scand. J. Immunol.* **37**(4):452–458.

Brynestad, K., Babbit, B., Huang, L., and Rouse, B. T., 1990, Influence of peptide acylation, liposome incorporation, and synthetic immunomodulators on the immunogenicity of a 1-23 peptide of glycoprotein D of herpes simplex virus: Implications for subunit vaccines, *J. Virol.* **64**(2):680–685.

Bui, T., Faltynek, C. R., and Ho, R. J., 1994a, Biologic response of recombinant interleukin-7 on herpes simplex virus infection in guinea pigs, *Vaccine* **12**:646–652.

Bui, T., Faltynek, C., and Ho, R. J., 1994b, Differential disposition of soluble and liposome-formulated human recombinant interleukin-7: Effect on blood lymphocyte population in guinea pigs, *Pharm. Res.* **11**:633–641.

Bui, T., Dykers, T., Hu, S.-L., Faltynek, C. R., and Ho, R. J., 1994c, Effect of MTP-PE liposomes and interleukin-7 on induction of antibody and cell-mediated immune responses to a recombinant HIV-envelope protein, *J. Acquir. Immune Defic. Syndr.* **7**:799–806.

Cao, M., Sasaki, O., Yamada, A., and Imanishi, J., 1992, Enhancement of the protective effect of inactivated influenza virus vaccine by cytokines, *Vaccine* **10**(4):238–242.

Coffman, R. L., and Mosmann, T. R., 1991, CD4$^+$ T-cell subsets: Regulation of differentiation and function, *Res. Immunol.* **142**:7–9.

Coffman, R. L., Seymour, B. W. P., Lebman, D. A., Hiraki, D. D., Christiansen, J. A., Shrader, B., Cherwinski, H. M., Savelkoul, H. F. J., Finkelmann, F. D., Bond, M. W., and Mosmann, T. R., 1988, The role of helper T cell products in mouse B cell differentiation and isotype regulation, *Immunol. Rev.* **102**:5–28.

Diamandis, E. P., and Christopoulos, T. K., 1991, The biotin-(strept)avidin system: Principles and applications in biotechnology, *Clin. Chem.* **37**(5):625–636.

Dietrich, F. M., Hochkeppel, H. K., and Lukas, B., 1986, Enhancement of host resistance against virus infections by MTP-PE, a synthetic lipophilic muramyl peptide. I. Increased survival in mice and guinea pigs after single drug administration prior to infection, and the effect of MTP-PE on interferon levels in sera and lungs, *Int. J. Immunopharmacol.* **8**(8):931–942.

Dranoff, G., Jaffee, E., Lazenby, A., Golumbek, P., Levitsky, H., Brose, K., Jackson, V., Hamada, H., Pardoll, D., and Mulligan, R. C., 1993, Vaccination with irradiated tumor cells engineered to secrete murine granulocyte–macrophage colony-stimulating factor stimulates potent, specific, and long-lasting antitumor immunity, *Proc. Natl. Acad. Sci. USA* **90**(8):3539–3543.

Ehrhardt, R. O., Strober, W., and Harriman, G. R., 1992, Effect of transforming growth factor (TGF)-beta 1 on IgA isotype expression. TGF-beta 1 induces a small increase in sIgA$^+$ B cells regardless of the method of B cell activation, *J. Immunol.* **148**(12):3830–3836.

Fogler, W. E., Wade, R., Brundish, D. E., and Fidler, I. J., 1985, Distribution and fate of free and liposome-encapsulated [^{3}H]nor-muramyl dipeptide and [^{3}H]muramyl tripeptide phosphatidylethanolamine in mice, *J. Immunol.* **135**(2):1372–1377.

Friede, M., Muller, S., Briand, J. P., Van-Regenmortel, M. H., and Schuber, F., 1993, Induction of immune response against a short synthetic peptide antigen coupled to small neutral liposomes containing monophosphoryl lipid A, *Mol. Immunol.* **30**(6):539–547.

Grob, P. J., Joller-Jemelka, H. I., Binswanger, U., Zaruba, K., Descoeudres, C., and Fernex, M., 1984, Interferon as an adjuvant for hepatitis B vaccination in non- and low-responder populations, *Eur. J. Clin. Microbiol.* **3**(3):195–198.

Harding, C. V., Leyva-Cobian, F., and Unanue, E. R., 1988, Mechanisms of antigen processing, *Immunol. Rev.* **106**:77–92.

Hazama, M., Mayumi-Aono, A., Asakawa, N., Kuroda, S., Hinuma, S., and Fujisawa, Y., 1993, Adjuvant-independent enhanced immune responses to recombinant herpes simplex virus type 1 glycoprotein D by fusion with biologically active interleukin-2, *Vaccine* **11**(6):629–636.

Heath, A. W., Devey, M. E., Brown, I. N., Richards, C. E., and Playfair, J. H., 1989, Interferon-gamma as an adjuvant in immunocompromised mice, *Immunology* **67**(4):520–524.

Hiernaux, J. R., Stashak, P. W., Cantrell, J. L., Rudbach, J. A., and Baker, P. J., 1989, Immunomodulatory activity of monophosphoryl lipid A in C3H/HeJ and C3H/HeSnJ mice, *Infect. Immun.* **57**(5):1483–1490.

Ho, R. J., Ting-Beall, H. P., Rouse, B. T., and Huang, L., 1988, Kinetic and ultrastructural studies of interactions of target-sensitive immunoliposomes with herpes simplex virus, *Biochemistry* **27**(1):500–506.

Ho, R. J., Burke, R. L., and Merigan, T. C., 1989, Antigen-presenting liposomes are effective in treatment of recurrent herpes simplex virus genitalis in guinea pigs, *J. Virol.* **63**(7):2951–2958.

Ho, R. J., Burke, R. L., and Merigan, T. C., 1990, Physical and biological characterization of antigen presenting liposome formulations: Relative efficacy for the treatment of recurrent genital HSV-2 in guinea pigs, *Antiviral Res.* **13**(4):187–199.

Ho, R. J., Burke, R. L., and Merigan, T. C., 1992, Liposome-formulated interleukin-2 as an adjuvant of recombinant HSV glycoprotein gD for the treatment of recurrent genital HSV-2 in guinea pigs, *Vaccine* **10**(4):209–213.

Ho, R. J., Burke, R. L., and Merigan, T. C., 1994, Disposition of antigen-presenting liposomes in vivo: Effect on presentation of herpes simplex virus antigen rgD, *Vaccine* **12**(3):235–242.

Hughes, H. P., Campos, M., van Drunen Littel van den Hurk, S., Zamb, T., Sordillo, L. M., Godson, D., and Babiuk, L. A., 1992, Multiple administration with interleukin-2 potentiates antigen-specific responses to subunit vaccination with bovine herpes virus-1 glycoprotein IV, *Vaccine* **10**(4):226–230.

Hume, D. A., Pavli, P., Donahue, R. E., and Fidler, I. J., 1988, The effect of human recombinant macrophage colony-stimulating factor (CSF-1) on the murine mononuclear phagocyte system in vivo, *J. Immunol.* **141**(10):3405–3409.

Jicha, D. L., Schwarz, S., Mule, J. J., and Rosenberg, S. A., 1992, Interleukin-7 mediates the generation and expansion of murine allosensitized and antitumor CTL, *Cell. Immunol.* **141**(1):71–83.

Johnson, A. G., and Tomai, M. A., 1990, A study of the cellular and molecular mediators of the adjuvant action of a nontoxic monophosphoryl lipid A, *Adv. Exp. Med. Biol.* **256**:567–579.

Karupiah, G., Ramsay, A. J., Ramshaw, I. A., and Blanden, R. V., 1992, Recombinant vaccine vector-induced protection of athymic, nude mice from influenza A virus infection. Analysis of protective mechanisms, *Scand. J. Immunol.* **36**(1):99–105.

Kawashima, K., and Platt, K. B., 1989, The effect of human recombinant interleukin-2 on the porcine immune response to a pseudorabies virus subunit vaccine, *Vet. Immunol. Immunopathol.* **22**(4):345–353.

Kiener, P. A., Marek, F., Rodgers, G., Lin, P. F., Warr, G., and Desiderio, J., 1988, Induction of tumor necrosis factor, IFN-gamma, and acute lethality in mice by toxic and non-toxic forms of lipid A, *J. Immunol.* **141**(3):870–874.

Kroemer, G., Moreno de Alboran, I., Gonzalo, J. A., and Martinez, C., 1993, Immunoregulation by cytokines, *Crit. Rev. Immunol.* **13**(2):163–191.

Lederer, E., Adam, A., Ciorbaru, R., Petit, J. F., and Wietzerbin, J., 1975, Cell walls of mycobacteria and related organisms; chemistry and immunostimulant properties, *Mol. Cell. Biochem.* **7**(2):87–104.

Loppnow, H., Durrbaum, I., Brade, H., Dinarello, C. A., Kusumoto, S., Rietschel, E. T., and Flad, H. D., 1990, Lipid A, the immunostimulatory principle of lipopolysaccharides, *Adv. Exp. Med. Biol.* **256**:561–566.

Lorre, K., Kasran, A., Van Vaeck, F., de Boer, M., and Ceuppens, J. L., 1994, Interleukin-1 and B7/CD28 interaction regulate interleukin-6 production by human T cells, *Clin. Immunol. Immunopathol.* **70**(1):81–90.

Lycke, N., Bromander, A. K., Ekman, L., Karlsson, U., and Holmgren, J., 1989, Cellular basis of immunomodulation by cholera toxin in vitro with possible association to the adjuvant function in vivo, *J. Immunol.* **142**(1):20–27.

Maeda, M., Knowles, R. D., and Kleinerman, E. S., 1991, Muramyl tripeptide phosphatidylethanolamine encapsulated in liposomes stimulates monocyte production of tumor necrosis factor and interleukin-1 in vitro, *Cancer Commun.* **3**(10–11):313–321.

Meuer, S. C., Dumann, H., Meyer zum Buschenfelde, K. H., and Kohler, H., 1989, Low-dose interleukin-2 induces systemic immune responses against HBsAg in immunodeficient non-responders to hepatitis B vaccination, *Lancet* **1**(8628):15–18.

Mifune, K., Mannen, K., Cho, S., and Narahara, H., 1987, Enhanced antibody responses in mice by combined administration of interferon with rabies vaccine, *Arch. Virol.* **94**(3–4):287–295.

Nencioni, L., Villa, L., Tagliabue, A., and Boraschi, D., 1987, Adjuvant activity of the 163–171 peptide of human IL-1 beta administered through different routes, *Lymphokine Res.* **6**(4):335–339.

Panzer, S., Madden, M., and Matsuki, K., 1993, Interaction of IL-1 beta, IL-6, and tumor necrosis factor-alpha (TNF-alpha) in human T cells activated by murine antigens, *Clin. Exp. Immunol.* **93**(3):471–478.

Playfair, J. H., and De Souza, J. B., 1987, Recombinant gamma interferon is a potent adjuvant for a malaria vaccine in mice, *Clin. Exp. Immunol.* **67**(1):5–10.

Pockley, A. G., and Montgomery, P. C., 1991, In vivo adjuvant effect of interleukins 5 and 6 on rat tear IgA antibody responses, *Immunology* **73**(1):19–23.

Ramshaw, I., Ruby, J., Ramsay, A., Ada, G., and Karupiah, G., 1992, Expression of cytokines by recombinant vaccinia viruses: A model for studying cytokines in virus infections in vivo, *Immunol. Rev.* **127**:157–182.

Rich, B. E., Campos Torres, J., Tepper, R. I., Moreadith, R. W., and Leder, P., 1993, Cutaneous lymphoproliferation and lymphomas in interleukin 7 transgenic mice, *J. Exp. Med.* **177**(2):305–316.

Richards, R. L., Swartz, G. M., Jr., Schultz, C., Hayre, M. D., Ward, G. S., Ballou, W. R., Chulay, J. D., Hockmeyer, W. T., Berman, S. L., and Alving, C. R., 1989, Immunogenicity of liposomal malaria sporozoite antigen in monkeys: Adjuvant effects of aluminium hydroxide and non-pyrogenic liposomal lipid A, *Vaccine* **7**(6):506–512.

Rouse, B. T., Miller, L. S., Turtinen, L., and Moore, R. N., 1985, Augmentation of immunity to herpes simplex virus by in vivo administration of interleukin 2, *J. Immunol.* **134**(2):926–930.

Ruby, J., Brinkman, C., Jones, S., and Ramshaw, I., 1990, Response of monkeys to vaccination with recombinant vaccinia virus which coexpress HIV gp160 and human interleukin-2, *Immunol. Cell. Biol.* **68**:113–117.

Sanchez-Pescador, L., Burke, R. L., Ott, G., and Van Nest, G., 1988, The effect of adjuvants on the efficacy of a recombinant herpes simplex virus glycoprotein vaccine, *J. Immunol.* **141**(5):1720–1727.

Schneerson, R., Fattom, A., Szu, S. C., Bryla, D., Ulrich, J. T., Rudbach, J. A., Schiffman, G., and Robbins, J. B., 1991, Evaluation of monophosphoryl lipid A (MPL) as an adjuvant. Enhancement of the serum antibody response in mice to polysaccharide–protein conjugates by concurrent injection with MPL, *J. Immunol.* **147**(7):2136–2140.

Scott, P., 1991, IFN-gamma modulates the early development of Th1 and Th2 responses in a murine model of cutaneous leishmaniasis, *J. Immunol.* **147**(9):3149–3155.

Sencer, S. F., Rich, M. L., Katsanis, E., Ochoa, A. C., and Anderson, P. M., 1991, Anti-tumor vaccine adjuvant effects of IL-2 liposomes in mice immunized against MCA-102 sarcoma, *Eur. Cytokine Netw.* **2**(5):311–318.

Sigal, R. K., Lieberman, M. D., Reynolds, J. V., Williams, N., Ziegler, M. M., and Daly, J. M., 1990, Tumor immunization. Improved results after vaccine modified with recombinant interferon gamma, *Arch. Surg.* **125**(3):308–312.

Snapper, C. M., and Paul, W. E., 1987, Interferon-gamma and B cell stimulatory factor-reciprocally regulate Ig isotype production, *Science* **236**:944–947.

Sone, S., Utsugi, T., Tandon, P., and Ogawara, M., 1986, A dried preparation of liposomes containing muramyl tripeptide phosphatidylethanolamine as a potent activator of human blood monocytes to the antitumor state, *Cancer Immunol. Immunother.* **22**(3):191–196.

St. Georgiev, V., and Albright, J. F., 1993, Cytokines and their role as growth factors and in regulation of immune responses, *Ann. N.Y. Acad. Sci.* **685**:584–602.

Tagliabue, A., and Boraschi, D., 1993, Cytokines as vaccine adjuvants: Interleukin 1 and its synthetic peptide 163–171, *Vaccine* **11**(5):594–595.

Tahara, H., Zeh, H. J., Storkus, W. J., Pappo, I., Watkins, S. C., Gubler, U., Wolf, S. F., Robbins, P. D., and Lotze, M. T., 1994, Fibroblasts genetically engineered to secrete interleukin 12 can suppress tumor growth and induce antitumor immunity to a murine melanoma in vivo, *Cancer Res.* **54**(1):182–189.

Tao, M. H., and Levy, R., 1993, Idiotype/granulocyte-macrophage colony-stimulating factor fusion protein as a vaccine for B-cell lymphoma, *Nature* **362**:755–758.

Uchiyama, A., Hoon, D. S., Morisaki, T., Kaneda, Y., Yuzuki, D. H., and Morton, D. L., 1993, Transfection of interleukin 2 gene into human melanoma cells augments cellular immune response, *Cancer Res.* **53**(5):949–952.

Ullrich, S. E., and Fidler, I. J., 1992, Liposomes containing muramyl tripeptide phosphatidylethanolamine (MTP-PE) are excellent adjuvants for induction of an immune response to protein and tumor antigens, *J. Leukocyte Biol.* **52**(5):489–494.

Urano, K., Habu, S., and Nishimura, T., 1993, Potentiation of therapeutic effect of recombinant tumor necrosis factor against B16 mouse melanoma by combination with recombinant interleukin 2, *Cytokine* **5**(3):224–229.

Verma, J. N., Rao, M., Amselem, S., Krzych, U., Alving, C. R., Green, S. J., and Wassef, N. M., 1992, Adjuvant effects of liposomes containing lipid A: Enhancement of liposomal antigen presentation and recruitment of macrophages, *Infect. Immun.* **60**(6):2438–2444.

Weinberg, A., and Merigan, T. C., 1988, Recombinant interleukin 2 as an adjuvant for vaccine-induced protection. Immunization of guinea pigs with herpes simplex virus subunit vaccines, *J. Immunol.* **140**(1):294–299.

Williams, T. W., Yanagimoto, J. M., Mazumder, A., and Wiseman, C. L., 1992, Interleukin-2 increases the antibody response in patients receiving autologous intralymphatic tumor cell vaccine immunotherapy, *Mol. Biother.* **4**(2):66–69.

Xu-Amano, J., Kiyono, H., Jackson, R. J., Staats, H. F., Fujihashi, K., Burrows, P. D., Elson, C. O., Pillai, S., and McGhee, J. R., 1993, Helper T cell subsets for immunoglobulin A responses: Oral immunization with tetanus toxoid and cholera toxin as adjuvant selectively induces Th2 cells in mucosa associated tissues, *J. Exp. Med.* **178**(4):1309–1320.

Zhou, F., and Huang, L., 1993, Monophosphoryl lipid A enhances specific CTL induction by a soluble protein antigen entrapped in liposomes, *Vaccine* **11**(11):1139–1144.

Chapter 28

Cytokines as Immunological Adjuvants

Andrew W. Heath

1. INTRODUCTION

Over the past decade there has been a revolution in the prospects for vaccination against many of the infectious agents that still produce massive mortality and morbidity around the world. The reason for this revolution is the potential of a new technology, molecular biology, applied to the vaccine field, as evidenced by most of the chapters of this volume. However, with very few exceptions this increased potential for vaccination against these diseases has not yet been translated into reality. One of the reasons for this is that the novel recombinant proteins, with all their inherent advantages of safety and defined composition, often also have the disadvantage of lower immunogenicity than whole killed or live vaccines (Allison, 1983). Because of this, there is now a lot of work being done on novel means of enhancing vaccine immunogenicity. This search includes a variety of materials of various origins, including synthetic (Chapters 11 and 20), bacterial (Chapters 12 and 21), and plant (Chapters 22 and 23). This chapter, along with chapters by Lachman *et al.* (Chapter 29) and Dong *et al.* (Chapter 27), focuses on the use of naturally occurring cytokines as immunological adjuvants.

An "adjuvant" might be described as a non-antigen-specific material that enhances antigen-specific immune responses; cytokines might similarly be described as non-anti-gen-specific proteins that can have profound effects on specific immune responses. In light of the above descriptions, attempts at using cytokines as immunological adjuvants were perhaps not too surprising.

The use of cytokines as immunological adjuvants perhaps marks a move away from the more traditional, empirical means of producing possible new adjuvants. This empirical method was used, for instance, when muramyl dipeptide (MDP) was identified as the minimal component from complete Freund's adjuvant. This was done by a process of fractionating mycobacterial cell wall components with assessment of adjuvanticity of successive fractions (Ellouz *et al.,* 1974; Merser *et al.,* 1975) and the actual mode of action

---

Andrew W. Heath • Department of Medical Microbiology, University of Sheffield Medical School, Sheffield S10 2RX, United Kingdom.

Vaccine Design: The Subunit and Adjuvant Approach, edited by Michael F. Powell and Mark J. Newman. Plenum Press, New York, 1995.

of MDP as an adjuvant was the subject of subsequent investigations. The possibility of using cytokines as adjuvants represents an approach to the problem from the opposite direction, that is, by using a knowledge of the workings of the immune system to rationally design vaccine strategies. Of course in the final analysis, everything depends on whether the proposed adjuvant is actually effective in animal studies, and ultimately in clinical trials.

A large number of cytokines (and perhaps all of them!) have been shown to be capable of enhancing various immune responses when administered for prolonged periods during the development of an immune response to a particular antigen. For instance, interleukin-11 (IL-11) enhanced the antibody plaque-forming cell (PFC) response against sheep red blood cells (SRBC) in vivo, but was given twice daily for the 7 days following injection of SRBC, either as a first or second immunization (Yin *et al.*, 1992). IL-6 enhanced primary (about twofold) and secondary (about tenfold) responses against SRBC when given for 6 days following antigen injection (Takatsuki *et al.*, 1988). IL-3 perfusion via osmotic pump for 7 days enhanced the antibody response to human IgG (injected on day 1) about fivefold (Kimoto *et al.*, 1988). For this chapter, however, I have concentrated on cytokines that are effective in a single dose given at or near the time of antigen injection. This is not to imply that cytokines that do not exhibit this property will have no use in vaccination, but for the practical purposes of vaccinating large numbers of people at the lowest possible cost, simultaneous administration of the adjuvant will be necessary. It is likely that developments in slow-release formulations will make feasible other cytokines, such as those above. Although IL-2 in some circumstances needs to be given for prolonged periods, I have included it for several reasons including its occasional effectiveness as a single dose, its potent effect, and the large volume of work reported on this cytokine.

2. PRODUCTION OF CYTOKINES

Cytokines are natural mammalian proteins, but are usually expressed as recombinant proteins for medical purposes. They are not, in general, difficult to manufacture as recombinant proteins. Recombinant cytokines may also be produced in *E. coli* without loss of activity because, although most cytokines are naturally glycosylated, glycosylation is not, in most cases, necessary for cytokine activity. Most cytokines are relatively small (10–25 kDa), and are often monomers, but may occur naturally as homodimers or trimers (IL-12 and lymphotoxin-β are exceptions, both being heterodimers). For further information on expression of cytokines see Clemens *et al.* (1987).

3. PATENT PROTECTION

There are a large number of patents covering the use of various cytokines as immunological adjuvants. The following list, although not comprehensive, illustrates the complexity of cytokines and their use as adjuvants. European patent (EP) 241,725 (Boehringer Ingelheim) covers the use of interferon gamma (IFN-γ) as an immunological adjuvant. The use of IL-2 by multiple injections, and by controlled release, is covered by U.S. patents 5,100,664 and 5,102,872 (Cetus); IL-2 expressed in vaccinia virus is covered by U.S. 7,122,163 (U.S. Department of Health and Human Services). Cytokine–antigen fusion proteins, in particular using IL-2, are covered by EP 406,857 (Takeda Chemical Industry Ltd.). In addition, IL-2 encapsulated within liposomes is the subject of WO 9,004,412 (Minnesota University) and WO 8,905,631 (Institut Pasteur). IL-1 synthetic peptide is covered by EP 8,6830,299 and U.S. 922,066 (Sclavo).

4. A BRIEF SUMMARY OF CYTOKINE ADJUVANTICITY

The first three cytokines shown to be adjuvants were also the three with the greatest potential. These three cytokines are IL-1, IL-2, and IFN-γ. The adjuvant effects of these three cytokines have been covered in some detail in several reviews (Heath and Playfair, 1992, 1993; Hughes and Babiuk, 1992; Tagliabue and Boraschi, 1993) and will only be briefly summarized here.

4.1. Interleukin-1

IL-1 is actually two different proteins, interleukin-1 α and β, which have 25% amino acid homology, but apparently largely overlapping functions. There are some conflicting reports as whether or not both of these forms possess adjuvant activity. This was a question that did not arise in the original work, as the IL-1 used by Staruch and Wood (1983) was purified from LPS-stimulated monocytes rather than recombinant material. An injection of IL-1 was shown to be effective in enhancing the antibody response to BSA about tenfold, but this enhancement was very dose- and time-dependent. There was virtually no enhancement of antibody responses when IL-1 was administered at the same time as the antigen, and the most effective time was 2 h after the antigen. Likewise, the adjuvant effect of 500 units was virtually nonexistent: adjuvanticity was apparent at 1000 and 2000 units, but disappeared by 4000 units. This time dependence of cytokine adjuvanticity has recurred in a number of studies, although it is not absolute, as an inferior effect can be obtained by injecting IL-1 and antigen simultaneously. Nencioni *et al.* (1987) were able to enhance secondary PFC responses to SRBC by threefold using recombinant human IL-1β 1 h after dosing with antigen. This group has done a lot of work on IL-1, in particular using a peptide that apparently has adjuvant effects but no pyrogenicity (Nencioni *et al.,* 1987; Tagliabue and Boraschi, 1993; and Chapter 27). Boraschi *et al.* (1990) found adjuvant effects with IL-1β but not IL-1α, but other data (Heath *et al.,* 1989a; Reed *et al.,* 1989a) indicate that IL-1α is effective in enhancing protection against *P. yoelii* and antibody PFC responses after immunization, and similarly has an improved effect when given after the antigen.

IL-1 presumably acts by enhancing the proliferation of antigen-specific T cells (Reed *et al.,* 1989a), although the finding that IL-1 also enhances antibody responses against the T-independent antigen, pneumococcal polysaccharide (Nencioni *et al.,* 1987), might require another explanation.

Table I
A Summary of Some Effects of the Vaccination Regime on Cytokine Adjuvanticity

Cytokine	Time Given	Effect	Reference
IL-1	2 h after antigen	Antibody ↑ PFC response ↑	Nencioni *et al.* (1987) Reed *et al.* (1989a)
IL-2	With antigen, then daily injections for 5 days or more	Protection against *H.* *pleuropneumoniae*, HSV, rabies Antibody not increased	Nunberg *et al.* (1989) Anderson *et al.* (1987) Weinberg and Merigan (1988)
	Emulsified in oil (with antigen)	Antibody ↑	Kawamura *et al.* (1985) Good *et al.* (1988)
	Encapsulated in liposomes (with antigen)	Antibody ↑	Abraham and Shah (1992) Mbawuike *et al.* (1990)
	Fusion protein with antigen	Antibody ↑ HSV protection ↑	Hazama *et al.* (1993a,b)
IFN-γ	With antigen	Antibody ↑, DTH ↑ Protection against *P. yoelii*, VSV ↑↑	Heath *et al.* (1989a) Playfair and DeSouza (1987) Anderson *et al.* (1989)
	2 days before antigen	DTH ↑, antibody ↓ (Th1 ↑?)	Heath and Playfair (1991)
GM-CSF	Fusion protein with antigen	Antibody ↑ Protection against tumor	Tao and Levy (1993)
IL-12	With antigen	Protection against *Leishmania* ↑ Th1 (DTH)	Alfonso *et al.* (1994)

4.2. Interleukin-2

IL-2 is perhaps the most studied of all cytokines as adjuvants, and has been used as what might loosely be termed an "adjuvant" in three different formats, in which it probably has three different modes of action. In most instances IL-2 has been administered as multiple injections following the antigen, and given by this method it has been very successful in enhancing protection against infectious challenge. The infectious agents immunized against include *Haemophilus pleuropneumoniae* (Anderson *et al.,* 1987), herpes (Weinberg and Merigan, 1988), rabies viruses (Nunberg *et al.,* 1989), and murine malaria (Heath and Playfair, unpublished data). When given in multiple doses, IL-2 presumably acts by helping to expand those T-cell clones that have bound the antigenic peptides. In other instances, IL-2 has been given as a single injection in aqueous solution, where it was useful for enhancing antibody responses to hepatitis B in humans (Meuer *et al.,* 1989; see section on immunodeficiency), or as an emulsion in oil, where it has overcome genetic nonresponsiveness to peptides (Kawamura *et al.,* 1985 ; Good *et al.,* 1988). In overcoming genetic nonresponsiveness, an effect on T-cell expansion was ruled out by the authors, who suggested that a local effect on antigen-specific B cells might be responsible for its action.

4.3. Interferon-γ

IFN-γ is effective at enhancing memory for both cell-mediated immune responses and humoral immunity when given mixed with the antigen in aqueous solution (Playfair and DeSouza, 1987). It appears to be perhaps more practical than IL-1 or IL-2 as an adjuvant, both in terms of timing and dose response, in that the optimal time of administration is at the same time as the antigen, and it is effective across a very wide dose range (Heath and Playfair, 1992). IFN-γ also enhanced the secondary antibody response to, and protection against, vesicular stomatitis virus (VSV) when given mixed with a VSV "G" glycoprotein subunit (Anderson *et al.*, 1989). This cytokine has also been shown to be effective in clinical trials in vaccination against hepatitis B. Inclusion of IFN-γ with the antigen resulted in a more rapid rise in antibody responses in clinical trial (Quiroga *et al.*, 1990). The mode of action of IFN-γ appears to be via enhancement of the efficiency of antigen presentation by increasing MHC class II expression on antigen-presenting cells (APCs) (Heath *et al.*, 1991).

5. MEANS OF IMPROVING ADJUVANT EFFECTS OF CYTOKINES

There are several ways of increasing the adjuvant effects of cytokines. In cases where cytokines exert their adjuvanticity through increasing the efficiency of antigen presentation, an obvious means of increasing adjuvanticity would be to ensure efficient delivery of the cytokine to the APCs that are actually presenting the vaccine antigen. This can be achieved through a physical linkage of cytokine and antigen, and was the premise behind our work in which IFN-γ was biotinylated and then mixed with avidin prior to injection into mice. The adjuvant effect of the interferon–avidin conjugate was clearly superior to that of the controls, which included conjugates lacking cytokine activity, and simple mixtures (Heath and Playfair, 1990). The additional adjuvant effect was manifested mostly as an increased DTH response to avidin, although antibody responses were enhanced slightly. A similar cytokine–antigen association was created more neatly by the manufacture of a fusion protein of granulocyte–monocyte colony-stimulating factor (GM-CSF) and a tumor idiotype (Tao and Levy, 1993). The fusion protein induced enhanced antibody responses against the idiotype, as well as increased protection against the tumor. Again, controls included a cytokine–antigen mixture. Another example of cytokine–antigen fusion proteins was produced by Hazama *et al.* (1993a,b) when they created a fusion of herpes simplex glycoprotein D and IL-2. The glycoprotein–IL-2 fusion protein was used to immunize mice intranasally, and was very efficient at inducing both high serum antibody responses, and protection against challenge with herpes simplex virus (HSV) (Hazama *et al.*, 1993a,b). Another cytokine–antigen fusion molecule was created by making synthetic peptides consisting of the IL-1 adjuvant peptide mentioned above, and an antigenic peptide, which enabled immunization of similar efficiency with 50-fold lower doses of peptide (Rao and Nayak, 1990).

Another means by which cytokine and antigen could be more closely associated would be by the inclusion of both into liposomes. This was done by Abraham and Shah (1992) who incorporated IL-2 into liposomes that also contained bacterial polysaccharides, either levan (from *Aerobacter levanicum*) or a *Pseudomonas aeruginosa* polysaccharide. These liposomes were used to immunize mice intranasally, and inclusion of IL-2 resulted in a significant increase in pulmonary plasma cells producing specific antibody, as well as enhanced protection.

Of course the incorporation of the cytokine into liposomes, even liposomes without antigen, could have effects on cytokine delivery, and IL-2 in liposomes was shown to be effective in enhancing protection against influenza A virus when mixed with the antigen (Mbawuike *et al.,* 1990). IL-2 was also effective in increasing protection against HSV following overlapping injections with glycoprotein D, although in this case protection was against recurrent infection in already infected guinea pigs (Ho *et al.,* 1992; and Chapter 27). Other means of altering cytokine delivery, for instance by lengthening exposure, might involve the use of slow-release vehicles, such as polyethylene glycol–IL-2 (Singh-Hora *et al.,* 1990; Nunberg *et al.,* 1989), or expression in live vectors such as vaccinia virus (Flexner *et al.,* 1987; Ramshaw *et al.,* 1987) or salmonella (Denich *et al.,* 1993; Carrier *et al.,* 1992).

Other means of increasing cytokine adjuvanticity include synergistic or additive combinations of cytokines with conventional adjuvants, or cytokines with other cytokines. There are few publications about combining cytokines and other adjuvants, although we found IFN-γ to be effective in enhancing responses to alum-precipitated *P. yoelii* vaccine (Heath *et al.,* 1989b), combinations of cytokines with liposomes and with avridine have already been mentioned, and the effectiveness of IFN-γ with *C. parvum* is mentioned below. Similarly, combinations of cytokines have not been studied much, although in preliminary experiments we saw some synergy between IFN-γ and tumor necrosis factor α (TNF-α) (Heath and Playfair, unpublished), and an IL-1/IL-2 combination was shown to be effective in enhancing antibody responses to foot-and-mouth disease virus (FMDV) when mixed with the vaccine (McCullough *et al.,* 1991). More work is required in both of these areas, and clearly a knowledge of the modes of action of cytokine adjuvants and conventional adjuvants should enable rational choices of combinations to be made.

6. AREAS OF PARTICULAR POTENTIAL FOR CYTOKINE ADJUVANTS

6.1. Immunodeficiency

The use of cytokines as adjuvants may be particularly useful in some forms of immunodeficiency. As mentioned in the introduction, the modes of action of conventional adjuvants are often not well understood, but are very likely to involve the induction of cytokine release (Odean *et al.,* 1990). Figure 1 is a cartoon in which an adjuvant from a bacterial source induces the release of a cytokine from macrophages, which in turn induces the release of another cytokine from T cells, which acts on B cells and has an enhancing effect on the immune response. In this hypothetical situation, macrophages are unable to produce the first cytokine, and the entire effect of the adjuvant is lost. Artificial substitution of the second cytokine is able to induce normal immune responses, overcoming the deficiency. The point of this example is to illustrate that using a knowledge of the basis of immunodeficiency and the modes of action of cytokines, it may be possible to use cytokines to great advantage in immunization of immunodeficient people. There are a number of examples of the successful use of cytokines as adjuvants in immunization of immunodeficient subjects.

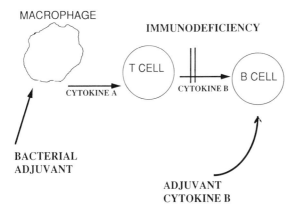

Figure 1. A hypothetical situation in which a cytokine (B) may be particularly effective as an adjuvant in an immunocompromised subject in which conventional adjuvants were ineffective.

IL-1 has been used as an adjuvant in several such situations. For instance, in a model that mimics the situation described in Fig. 1, mice infected with *Trypanosoma cruzi* are deficient in responses to T-dependent antigens, as demonstrated by the inferior PFC response to SRBCs; this defective response is the result of deficient T-cell help. Reed *et al.* (1989b) were able to show a deficiency in IL-1 production from cells of infected mice, and were able to restore immune responses in these mice by the addition of exogenous IL-1. In addition, IL-1 and an IL-1 nonapeptide were effective in enhancing immune responses of mice immunodepressed either through aging or irradiation (Frasca *et al.,* 1989).

IFN-γ has also been effective as an adjuvant in immunocompromised hosts. Since HIV infection results in a lack of T-cell help, we attempted to mimic this situation by depleting mice of CD4$^+$ T cells prior to vaccination. The mice were then immunized with a murine malaria (*P. yoelii*) antigen with saponin (a potent adjuvant for inducing protection in this system). Protection of CD4-depleted mice was markedly lower than that of normal animals (Heath *et al.,* 1989a). In contrast, mice immunized with antigen plus IFN-γ responded similarly whether or not they had been depleted of CD4$^+$ cells. Again, this situation probably mimics somewhat the hypothetical system in Fig. 1, in that CD4$^+$ cells are a major source of IFN-γ. IFN-γ was also markedly effective as an adjuvant in genetically immunocompromised mice, including Biozzi low-antibody-producer animals (Biozzi *et al.,* 1975) and in mice bred to produce antibody of low affinity (Katz and Steward, 1975; Heath *et al.,* 1989a).

As mentioned above, IL-2 has been shown to be effective in immunocompromised humans (Meuer *et al.,* 1989). Hemodialysis patients, who had failed previously to respond to hepatitis B vaccination, were immunized with hepatitis B surface antigen and IL-2, and showed a much higher seroconversion rate. These results also support the mechanism of Fig. 1, in that these immunosuppressed patients had been shown to express abnormally high levels of IL-2 receptor, and so may have been particularly sensitive to the addition of exogenous IL-2. The results also demonstrate the effectiveness of a rational approach to the choice of adjuvant, based on some knowledge of the immunology of the potential vaccinees.

6.2. Direction of the Immune Response

The fact that qualitatively different immune responses could be elicited by different vaccination schedules was noted a long time ago by Parish and Liew (1972) who found that with varying doses of immunogen, animals produced either high antibody responses or strong cellular immunity, as measured by DTH. These responses tended to flip-flop with increasing antigen dose, so that both cellular and humoral immune responses were not maximized. These qualitatively different immune responses were shown to be of practical relevance in animal models, and in particular in *Leishmania major*, in which protection was normally correlated with strong DTH responses, and susceptibility with strong antibody responses. The explanation for these differences in responses did not come until the description of two different types of mouse helper T-cell clones. Mouse T-helper cells can be divided into two groups based on the cytokines produced. Th1 cells are distinguished from Th2 cells by production of IFN-γ, and Th2 cells produce IL-4 and IL-5 (for reviews see Coffman *et al.,* 1988; Mosmann and Coffman, 1989). Th1 cells are potent enhancers of DTH responses, and Th2 cells of antibody; and in the *Leishmania* system, Th1 cells give protection while Th2 cells cause susceptibility (Locksley and Scott, 1991). Much has been written on the subject of Th cell types and their relation to protection against *Leishmania* and other infectious agents. Since the identification of these cells, there has been much interest in the factors controlling which type of response is induced by immunization or natural infection. Factors that might have effects on Th1 versus Th2 differentiation include the type of APC initially presenting antigen, the nature of the antigen itself, and, of course, cytokines, since differential cytokine secretion defined these types of cells. Cytokines have been very clearly shown to play a role in the development of these responses either in vitro, or when administered or removed during the development of an immune response against *Leishmania* in vivo. Thus, in vitro IFN-γ inhibits the growth of Th2 cell clones (Gajewski and Fitch, 1988) whereas IL-4, produced by Th2 cells, acts as an autocrine growth factor for these cells. In vivo, during the development of a *Leishmania* infection, administration of IFN-γ pushes toward a protective, Th1-type response, while IL-4 pushes toward a Th2-type response (Chatelein *et al.,* 1992; Coffman *et al.,* 1991), but these effects require prolonged exposure to the cytokine, and are not equivalent to the adjuvant action of cytokines.

From the earliest studies, there have been various hints that cytokine adjuvants might have differential effects on enhancing the immune responses of these Th subsets, but only recently has a very clear effect been seen.

Initial work using IL-1 as an adjuvant showed enhancing effects on antibody titers and PFC responses (Reed *et al.,* 1989a,b; Nencioni *et al.,* 1987). To date, there have been no reports of IL-1 enhancing cellular immunity, although this may simply not have been assessed in these cases. Thus, it is possible that the use of IL-1 as an adjuvant has a specific enhancing effect on immunization of Th2-like cells. This possibility is supported by the finding that adjuvants that induce good antibody responses tend to also induce IL-1 production, while those that induce good cellular immunity do not (Grun and Maurer, 1989).

Results using IL-2 as an adjuvant, at repeated doses, tend to indicate the opposite, that is, no enhancement of antibody responses (Nunberg *et al.*, 1989; Weinberg and Merigan, 1988). These results suggest that IL-2 given in this manner tends to enhance Th1-like responses and not Th2-like responses, although a formal proof of this is still lacking. In addition, there are exceptions to the findings above in which there has been an enhancement of antibody responses using IL-2. These include an enhancing effect of a single dose of IL-2 given to hemodialysis patients (Meuer *et al.*, 1989), and enhancement of responses to FMDV antigen when IL-2 was mixed with the antigen, and the antigen was used at subimmunogenic levels (McCullough *et al.*, 1991). The effectiveness of IL-2 administered as an emulsion in oil in enhancing antipeptide responses has already been mentioned (Kawamura *et al.*, 1985; Good *et al.*, 1988), and IL-2 (given over $2\frac{1}{2}$ days) was also effective in enhancing antibody responses to bovine herpesvirus glycoprotein emulsified in avridine (Hughes *et al.*, 1992). The relative effects of the use of IL-2 as an adjuvant on the immunization of different T subsets need to be determined more thoroughly, but some enhancement of antibody responses does not necessarily exclude an effect predominantly on Th1 cells; for instance, complete Freund's adjuvant is thought to be a potent Th1 enhancer, but it also enhances antibody responses.

Following initial experiments showing enhancement of protection against *P. yoelii*, and knowing of the effects described above of IFN-γ in enhancing Th1-type responses, we had hoped that the use of IFN-γ as an adjuvant would have a differential effect in enhancing Th1-type immunity. These hopes were not realized, however, as IFN-γ enhanced both DTH and antibody responses (Playfair and DeSouza, 1987) and enhanced IgG1 and IgG2a antibody responses (Heath, unpublished data). There were, however, a few situations in which there did appear to be a preferential effect on this subset.

In assessing the importance of timing in relation to the adjuvanticity of IFN-γ we noticed a very odd effect. The adjuvanticity of the cytokine disappeared as the cytokine injection got temporally further away from the antigen injection. This effect was obvious with only a few hours' difference, and was unusual in that not only did the adjuvant effect disappear, but the protection mediated by the vaccine was actually worse than that of antigen alone, showing a suppressive effect (Heath and Playfair, 1991). Further work, concentrating on cytokine given 2 days before vaccine (day −2), showed that IgG antibody responses (but not IgM) were almost completely abrogated, and that this related to a reduction in T-cell help for IgG. DTH responses were not affected, and the suppression was not affected by depleting CD8 cells in vivo. In addition, IgG1 responses were suppressed whereas IgG2a responses were enhanced. All of these factors point toward a selective suppression of Th2-type responses and an enhancement of Th1 responses, but this has yet to be formally proved.

Another instance in which IFN-γ seemed to have a preferential effect was when it was used conjugated to avidin, a manipulation that caused a further significant enhancement of DTH responses, but not of the antibody response (Heath and Playfair, 1990). A third instance was when Scott *et al.* (1989) used IFN-γ as an adjuvant for vaccination against *Leishmania*. In this case, IFN-γ, along with *Corynebacterium parvum*, when injected with the antigen, protected BALB/c mice that were susceptible to *Leishmania* against infection.

Protection is mediated by the Th1 subset. This protection was not seen using IFN-γ alone; thus, the inclusion of *C. parvum* was necessary for the adjuvant to induce a powerful Th1 response. It appeared that the inclusion of *C. parvum* might be inducing the release of some other factor, possibly from macrophages. This result led toward the most potent effect yet seen of a cytokine adjuvant in influencing the balance of these two Th subsets.

IL-12 is a factor produced by macrophages and other cells that stimulates the production of IFN-γ by NK and T cells (Chan *et al.,* 1991). In an in vitro system involving stimulation of TCR transgenic T cells with antigen and cytokine, the inclusion of IL-12 was able to skew the response to a Th1-like response (Hsieh *et al.,* 1993). IL-12 was also effective as a therapy for *Leishmania* infection when given in multiple doses during the infection, in which case it resulted in resolution of infection with the development of a Th1 response (Sypek *et al.,* 1993; Heinzel *et al.,* 1993). From the above powerful effects of IL-12 on induction of Th1 responses, and the fact that it is produced by macrophages, it would appear likely that this cytokine was the *C. parvum*-induced factor of Scott *et al.* The same group was able to show a potent Th1-inducing adjuvant effect of IL-12 in *Leishmania* vaccination (Afonso *et al.,* 1994). *Leishmania*-susceptible BALB/c mice, when injected in the footpad with soluble leishmanial antigen, are not protected against disease. Draining lymph node cells that are taken 3 days after this injection produced IL-4 but little detectable IFN-γ, whereas cells from C3H/HeN mice, which are disease resistant, produced IFN-γ but little or no IL-4. Injection of IL-12 with the antigen reversed the cytokine profile seen from the BALB/c mice, in that IFN-γ was produced at levels higher than those produced by C3H cells, and IL-4 production was extremely low. The authors postulated that this early IFN-γ may have been produced by NK cells, as NK cytotoxicity was higher in those animals receiving IL-12. When popliteal lymph nodes were taken 10 days after immunization, and restimulated in vitro with leishmanial antigen, similar results were seen; thus, a Th1-like response had been induced by the inclusion of IL-12 along with the leishmanial antigen. The importance of NK cells in the induction of this Th1-like response was confirmed by the finding that mice depleted of NK cells by anti-asialo-GM1 treatment did not show this switch to Th1, even when IL-12 was administered with the antigen. The apparent switch to Th1-type immunity induced by IL-12 was highly functionally significant, in that these mice were very well protected against challenge with *Leishmania.* Footpad swelling was actually as low in these animals as in genetically resistant C3H mice, and the parasite numbers in the lesions were decreased from more than 10^7 parasites to around 1000 parasites. Thus, it would seem that IL-12 has great potential as a Th1-inducing adjuvant, and indeed it is likely that IL-12 production is responsible for the marked effectiveness of many bacterial adjuvants in enhancing cellular immunity. Investigation of the effects of combinations of IL-12 with other cytokines, such as IFN-γ, and clinical trials on the use of IL-12 as an adjuvant should provide much interest in the coming years.

7. CONCLUSIONS

It seems likely that cytokines will find a use in human vaccination in certain circumstances. These are likely to include some types of immunodeficiency states, and probably vaccination against diseases in which a powerful Th1-type response is desired. Cytokine expression by live vaccine vectors is another likely possibility (although not covered in this volume). Continuing rational design of immunological adjuvants will likely lead to the use of other "natural" immunological proteins as immunostimulants. We are not, after all, restricted to using molecules that are *naturally* produced in a soluble form, and many normally membrane-bound proteins involved in cell–cell signaling have already been produced and been shown to have activity in soluble form. The range of soluble molecules with immunological effects is likely to become ever broader.

REFERENCES

Abraham, E., and Shah, S., 1992, Intranasal immunization with liposomes containing IL-2 enhances bacterial polysaccharide antigen-specific pulmonary secretory antibody response, *J. Immunol.* **149**:3719–3726.

Afonso, L. C. C., Scharton, T. M., Viera, L. Q., Wysocka, M., Trinchieri, G., and Scott, P., 1994, The adjuvant effect of interleukin-12 in a vaccine against Leishmania major, *Science* **263**:235–237.

Allison, A. C., 1983, Immunological adjuvants and their mode of action, in: *New Approaches to Vaccine Development* (R. Bell and G. Torrigiani, eds.), WHO, Schwabe & CoAG, Basel, pp. 133–154.

Anderson, G., Urbano, O., Fedorka-Cray, P., Newell, A., Nunberg, J., and Doyle, M., 1987, Interleukin-2 and protective immunity in Haemophilus pleuropneumoniae. Preliminary studies, in: *Vaccines '87*, Cold Spring Harbor Laboratory Press, Cold Spring Harbor, NY, pp. 22–25.

Anderson, K. P., Fennie, E. H., and Yilma, T., 1989, Enhancement of a secondary antibody response to vesicular stomatitis virus "G" protein by IFNg treatment at primary immunization, *J. Immunol.* **140**:3599–3604.

Antoni, G., Presentini, R., Perin, A., Tagliabue, A., Ghiara, P., Censini, S., Volpini, L., Villa, L., and Boraschi, D., 1986, A short synthetic peptide fragment of human IL-1 with immunostimulatory but not inflammatory activity, *J. Immunol.* **137**:3201–3204.

Biozzi, G., Stiffel, C., Mouton, D., and Bouthillier, Y., 1975, Selection of lines of mice with high and low antibody responses to complex immunogens, in: *Immunogenetics and Immunodeficiency* (B. Benacerraf, ed.), MTP Press, Lancaster, p. 179–201.

Boraschi, D., Villa, L., Volpini, G., Bossu, P., Censini, S., Ghiara, P., Scapigliat, G., Nencioni, L., Bartalini, M., Matteucci, G., Cioli, F., Carnasciali, M., Olmastroni, E., Mengozzi, M., Ghezzi, P., and Tagliabue, A., 1990, Differential activity of interleukin-1α and interleukin-1β in the stimulation of immune responses in vivo, *Eur. J. Immunol.* **20**:317–321.

Carrier, M. J., Chatfield, S. N., Dougan, G., Nowicka, U. T. A., O'Callaghan, D., Beesley, J. E., Milano, S., Cillari, E., and Liew, F. Y., 1992, Expression of human IL-1β in Salmonella typhimurium: A model system for the delivery of therapeutic proteins in vivo, *J. Immunol.* **148**:1176–1182.

Chan, S. H., Perussia, B., Gupta, J. W., Kobayashi, M., Pospisil, M., Young, H. A., Wolf, S. F., Young, D., Clark, S. C., and Trinchieri, G., 1991, Induction of IFNg production by natural killer cell stimulatory factor: Characterization of the responder cells and synergy with other inducers, *J. Exp. Med.* **173**:869–879.

Clemens, M. J., Morris, A. G., and Gearing, A. J. H., 1987, *Lymphokines and Interferons: A Practical Approach*, IRL Press, Oxford.

Coffman, R. L., Seymour, B. W. P., Lebman, D. A., Hiraki, D. A., Christiansen, J. A., Shrader, B., Cherwinski, H. M., Savelkoul, H. F. J., Finkelman, F. D., Bond, M. W., and Mosmann, T. R., 1988, The role of helper T cell products in mouse B cell differentiation and isotype regulation, *Immunol. Rev.* **102**:5–26.

Denich, K., Borlin, P., O'Hanley, P., Howard, M. C., and Heath, A. W., 1993, The effects of expression of murine interleukin-4 by Aro A–Salmonella typhimurium: Persistence, immune response and the inhibition of macrophage killing, *Infect. Immun.* **61**:4818–4827.

Ellouz, F., Adam, A., Cirorbaru, R., and Lederer, E., 1974, Minimal structural requirements for adjuvant activity of bacterial peptidoglycan derivatives, *Biochem. Biophys. Res. Commun.* **59**:1317–1325.

Feng, G. S., Gray, P., Shepard, H. M., and Taylor, M. W., 1988, Antiproliferative activity of a hybrid protein between interferon γ and tumor necrosis factor β, *Science* **241**:1501–1503.

Flexner, C., Hugin, A., and Moss, B., 1987, Prevention of vaccinia virus infection in immunodeficient mice by vector-directed IL-2 expression, *Nature* **330**:259–261.

Frasca, D., Boraschi, D., Baschieri, S., Bossu, P., Tagliabue, A., Adorini, L., and Doria, G., 1989, In vivo restoration of T cell functions by human IL-1β or its 163-171 nonapeptide in immunodepressed mice, *J. Immunol.* **141**:2651–2655.

Gajewski, T. F., and Fitch, F. W., 1988, Anti-proliferative effect of interferon gamma in immune regulation. 1. Interferon gamma inhibits the proliferation of Th2 but not Th1 murine helper T lymphocyte clones, *J. Immunol.* **140**:4245–4252.

Gerrard, T. L., Siegel, J. P., Dyer, D. R., and Zoon, K., 1987, Differential effects of interferon alpha and interferon gamma on IL-1 secretion by monocytes, *J. Immunol.* **138**:2535–2540.

Ghiara, P., Boraschi, D., Nencioni, L., Ghezzi, P., and Tagliabue, A., 1987, Enhancement of in vivo immune response by tumor necrosis factor, *J. Immunol.* **139**:3676–3679.

Good, M. F., Pombo, D., Lunde, M. N., Maloy, W. L., Halenbeck, R., Koths, K., Miller, L. H., and Berzofsky, J. A., 1988, Recombinant human IL-2 overcomes genetic nonresponsiveness to malaria sporozoite peptides, *J. Immunol.* **141**:972–977.

Grun, J. L., and Maurer, P. H., 1989, Different T helper subsets elicited in mice utilizing two different adjuvant vehicles; the role of endogenous interleukin in proliferative responses, *Cell Immunol.* **121**:134–145.

Hazama, M., Mayumi-Aono, A., Miyazaki, T., Hinuma, S., and Fujisawa, Y., 1993a, Intranasal immunization against herpes simplex virus infection by using a recombinant glycoprotein D fused with immunomodulating proteins, the B subunit of Escherichia coli heat labile enterotoxin and interleukin-2, *Immunology* **78**:643–649.

Hazama, M., Mayumi-Aono, A., Asakawa, N., Kuroda, S., Hinuma, S., and Fujisawa, Y., 1993b, Adjuvant independent enhanced immune responses to recombinant herpes simplex virus type 1 glycoprotein D by fusion with biologically active interleukin 2, *Vaccine* **11**:629–636.

Heath, A. W., and Playfair, J. H. L., 1990, Conjugation of interferon gamma to antigen enhances its adjuvanticity, *Immunology* **71**:454–456.

Heath, A. W., and Playfair, J. H. L., 1991, Early administration of interferon gamma as an adjuvant; an effect on a T helper subpopulation, in: *Vaccines '91* (R. M. Chanock, H. S. Ginsberg, F. Brown, R. A. and Lerner, eds.), Cold Spring Harbor Laboratory Press, Cold Spring Harbor, NY, pp. 351–354.

Heath, A. W., and Playfair, J. H. L., 1992, Gamma interferon as an adjuvant for vaccines, in: *Anti-infective Applications of Interferon Gamma* (H. S. Jaffe, L. R. Bucalo, and S. A. Sherwin, eds.), Dekker, New York.

Heath, A. W., and Playfair, J. H. L., 1993, Cytokines as immunological adjuvants, *Vaccine* **7**:427–434.

Heath, A. W., Devey, M. E., Brown, I. N., Richards, C. E., and Playfair, J. H. L., 1989a, Interferon gamma as an adjuvant in immunocompromised mice, *Immunology* **67**:520–524.

Heath, A. W., Haque, N. A., DeSouza, J. B., and Playfair, J. H. L., 1989b, Interferon gamma as an effective immunological adjuvant, in: *Vaccines '89,* Cold Spring Harbor Laboratory Press, Cold Spring Harbor, NY, pp. 43–46 .

Heath, A. W., Nyan, O., Richards, C. E., and Playfair, J. H. L., 1991, Effects of interferon gamma and saponin on lymphocyte traffic are inversely related to adjuvanticity and MHC class II expression, *Int. Immunol.* **3**:285–291

Heinzel, F. P., Scoenhaut, D. S., Rerko, R. M., Rosser, L. E., and Gately, M. K., 1993, Recombinant interleukin 12 cures mice infected with Leishmania major, *J. Exp. Med.* **177**:1505–1509.

Ho, R. J. Y., Burke, R. L., and Merigan, T. C., 1992, Liposome formulated interleukin-2 as an adjuvant of recombinant HSV glycoprotein D for the treatment of recurrent genital HSV-2 in guinea-pigs, *Vaccine* **10**:209–213.

Hsieh, C.-S., Macatonia, S. E., Tripp, C. S., Wolf, S. F., O'Garra, A., and Murphy, K. M., 1993, Development of Th1 CD4[+] T cells through IL-12 produced by Listeria-induced macrophages, *Science* **260**:547–549.

Hughes, H. P. A., and Babiuk, L. A., 1992, The adjuvant potential of cytokines, *Biotechnol. Ther.* **3**:101–117.

Hughes, H. P. A., Campos, M., van Drunen Little-van den Hurk, S., Zamb, T., Sordillo, L. M., Godson, D., and Babiuk, L. A., 1992, Multiple administration of interleukin-2 potentiates antigen-specific responses to subunit vaccination with bovine herpesvirus-1 glycoprotein IV, *Vaccine* **10**:226–230.

Katz, D., and Steward, M. W., 1975, The genetic control of antibody affinity in mice, *Immunology* **29**:543.

Kawamura, H., Rosenberg, S., and Berzofsky, J. A., 1985, Immunization with antigen and interleukin-2 in vivo overcomes Ir gene low responsiveness, *J. Exp. Med.* **162**:381–386.

Kimoto, M., Kindler, K., Higaki, M., Ody, C., Izui, S., and Vassail, P., 1988, Recombinant murine IL-3 fails to stimulate T or B lymphopoiesis in vivo, but enhances immune responses to T dependent antigens, *J. Immunol.* **140**:1889–1894.

Locksley, R. M., and Scott, P., 1991, Helper T cell subsets in mouse leishmaniasis: Induction, expansion and effector function, *Immunol. Today* **12**:A58–A61.

McCullough, K. C., Pullen, L., and Parkinson, D., 1991, The immune response against foot-and-mouth disease virus: Influence of the T lymphocyte growth factors IL-1 and IL-2 on the murine humoral response in vivo, *Immunol. Lett.* **31**:41–46.

McCune, C. S., and Marquis, D. M., 1990, Interleukin-1 as an adjuvant for active specific immunotherapy in a murine tumor model, *Cancer Res.* **50**:1212–1215.

Mbawuike, I. N., Wyde, P. R., and Anderson, P. M., 1990, Enhancement of the protective efficacy of inactivated influenza A virus vaccine in aged mice by IL-2-liposomes, *Vaccine* **8**:347–352.

Merser, C., Sinay, P., and Adam, A., 1975, Total synthesis and adjuvant activity of bacterial peptidoglycan derivatives, *Biochem. Biophys. Res. Commun.* **66**:1316–1322.

Meuer, S. C., Dumann, H., Meyer zum Buschenfelde, K. H., and Kohler, H., 1989, Low-dose interleukin-2 induces systemic immune responses against HBsAg in immunodeficient non-responders to hepatitis B vaccination, *Lancet* **1**:15–17.

Mosmann, T. R., and Coffman, R. L., 1989, Different patterns of lymphokine secretion lead to different functional properties, *Annu. Rev. Immunol.* **7**:145–173.

Nakai, S., Kawai, K., Hirai, T., and Tasaka, K., 1990, A mutant protein of human interleukin-1 beta with immunostimulatory but not pyrogenic potency, *Life Sci.* **47**:1707–1714.

Nencioni, L., Villa, L., Tagliabue, A., Antoni, G., Presentini, R., Perin, F., Silvestre, S., and Boraschi, D., 1987, In vivo immunostimulating activity of the 163-171 peptide of human IL-1β, *J. Immunol.* **139**:800–804.

Nunberg, J., Doyle, M. V., York, S. M., and York, C. J., 1989, Interleukin-2 acts as an adjuvant to enhance the potency of inactivated rabies virus vaccine, *Proc. Natl. Acad. Sci. USA* **86**:4240–4243.

Odean, M. J., Frane, C. M., Van der Vieren, M., Tomai, M. A., and Johnson, A. G., 1990, Involvement of gamma interferon in antibody enhancement by adjuvants, *Infect. Immun.* **58**:427–432.

Parish, C. R., and Liew, F. Y., 1972, Immune response to chemically modified flagellin. 3. Enhanced cell-mediated immunity during high and low zone antibody tolerance to flagellin, *J. Exp. Med.* **135**:298–311.

Playfair, J. H. L., and DeSouza, J. B., 1987, Recombinant gamma interferon is a potent adjuvant for a malaria vaccine in mice, *Clin. Exp. Immunol.* **67**:5–10.

Quiroga, J. A., Castillo, I., Porres, J. C., Casado, S., Saez, F., Gracia Martinez, M., Gomez, M., Inglada, L., Sanchez-Sicilia, L., Mora, A., *et al.,* 1990, Recombinant gamma interferon as adjuvant to hepatitis B vaccine in haemodialysis patients, *Hepatology* **12**:661–663.

Ramshaw, I. A., Andrew, M. E., Phillips, S. M. N., Boyle, D. B., and Coupar, B. E. H., 1987, Recovery of immunodeficient mice from a vaccinia virus/IL-2 recombinant infection, *Nature* **329**:545–546.

Rao, K. V. S., and Nayak, A. R., 1990, Enhanced immunogenicity of a sequence derived from hepatitis B virus surface antigen in a composite peptide that includes the immunostimulatory region from human interleukin-1, *Proc. Natl. Acad. Sci. USA* **87**:5519–5522.

Reed, S. G., Pihl, D. K., Conlon, P. J., and Grabstein, K. H., 1989a, IL-1 as adjuvant. Role of T cells in the augmentation of specific antibody production by recombinant human IL-1α, *J. Immunol.* **142**:3129–3133.

Reed, S. G., Pihl, D. K., and Grabstein, K. H., 1989b, Immune deficiency in chronic Trypanosoma cruzi infection. Recombinant IL-1 restores T helper function for antibody production, *J. Immunol.* **142**:2067–2071.

Scott, P., Pearce, E., Cheever, A. W., Coffman, R. L., and Sher, A., 1989, Role of cytokines and CD4[+] T cell subsets in the regulation of parasite immunity and disease, *Immunol. Rev.* **112**:161–182.

Singh-Hora, M., Rana, R. K., Nunberg, J. H., Tice, T. R., Gilley, R. M., and Hudson, M. E., 1990, Controlled release of interleukin-2 from biodegradable microspheres, *Biotechnology* **8**:755–758.

Staruch, M. J., and Wood, D. D., 1983, The adjuvanticity of interleukin-1 in vivo, *J. Immunol.* **130**:2191–2194.

Sypek, J. P., Chung, C. L., Mayor, E. H., Subramanyam, J. M., Goldman, S. J., Sieburth, D. S., Wolf, S. F., and Schaub, R. G., 1993, Resolution of cutaneous leishmaniasis: Interleukin-12 initiates a protective T helper type 1 immune response, *J. Exp. Med.* **177**:1797–1802.

Tagliabue, A., and Boraschi, D., 1993, Cytokines as vaccine adjuvants: Interleukin-1 and its synthetic peptide 163-171, *Vaccine* **11**:594–595.

Takatsuki, F., Okano, A., Suzuki, C., Chieda, R., Takahara, Y., Hirano, T., Kishimoto, T., Hamuro, J., and Akiyama, Y., 1988, Human recombinant IL-6/B cell stimulatory factor 2 augments murine antigen specific antibody responses in vitro and in vivo, *J. Immunol.* **141**:3072–3077.

Talmadge, J. E., Phillips, H., Schneider, M., Rowe, T., Pennington, R., Bowersox, O., and Lenz, B., 1988, Immunomodulatory properties of recombinant murine and human tumor necrosis factor, *Cancer Res.* **48**:544–550.

Tao, M. H., and Levy, R., 1993, Idiotype GMCSF fusion protein as a vaccine for B cell lymphoma, *Nature* **362**:755–758.

Weinberg, A., and Merigan, T. C., 1988, Recombinant interleukin-2 as an adjuvant for vaccine-induced protection. Immunization of guinea pigs with herpes simplex virus subunit vaccines, *J. Immunol.* **140**:294–299.

Weyland, C., Goronzy, J., Fathman, C. G., and O'Hanley, P., 1987, Administration in vivo of recombinant interleukin-2 protects mice against septic death, *J. Clin. Invest.* **79**:1756–1763.

Yin, T. G., Schendel, P., and Yang, Y. C., 1992, Enhancement of in vitro and in vivo antibody responses by interleukin-11, *J. Exp. Med.* **175**:211–216.

Chapter 29

Cytokine-Containing Liposomes as Adjuvants for Subunit Vaccines

Lawrence B. Lachman, Li-Chen N. Shih, Xiao-Mei Rao, Stephen E. Ullrich, and Jeffrey L. Cleland

1. INTRODUCTION

Liposomes provide a carrier function to bring antigen to cells of the immune system and to provide a mechanism for slow release of antigen. Since liposomes are slowly absorbed, they also provide a "depot effect" in which the presence of the antigen may be maintained for a longer period of time compared to soluble antigen (Alving, 1991). In addition to antigen, liposomes may carry other agents that potentiate an immune response. In this chapter we will present our current data concerning the adjuvant effect of a special type of liposomes containing a subunit protein antigen and cytokines.

2. CYTOKINES AS ADJUVANTS

It is now established that adjuvants stimulate the immune response to antigens by activating either Th1 or Th2 $CD4^+$ or $CD8^+$ T lymphocytes to secrete distinct classes of lymphokines (Audibert and Lise, 1993; and see Chapters 27 and 28). Complete Freund's adjuvant (CFA) activates Th1 cells resulting in delayed-type hypersensitivity (DTH) while alum activates Th2 cells, potentiating a humoral response (Audibert and Lise, 1993; Grun and Maurer, 1989). The importance of adjuvants in the induction of DTH has been reinforced by recent findings concerning the gradual loss of cell-mediated immunity (CMI) in HIV-1$^+$ individuals (Salk *et al.*, 1993). Clerici *et al.* (1993a) found that the progression

Lawrence B. Lachman, Li-Chen N. Shih, Xiao-Mei Rao • Department of Cell Biology, University of Texas M.D. Anderson Cancer Center, Houston, Texas 77030. *Stephen E. Ullrich* • Department of Immunology, University of Texas M.D. Anderson Cancer Center, Houston, Texas 77030. *Jeffrey L. Cleland* • Pharmaceutical Research & Development, Genentech, Inc., South San Francisco, California 94080.

Vaccine Design: The Subunit and Adjuvant Approach, edited by Michael F. Powell and Mark J. Newman. Plenum Press, New York, 1995.

of HIV-1 was associated with a switch from a Th1-like cytokine profile (high IL-2, low IL-4 and IL-10) to a Th2-like cytokine profile (low IL-2, high IL-4 and IL-10).

The first cytokine to be used as an adjuvant was IL-1 (Staruch and Wood, 1983). Interestingly, one of the many original names for IL-1 was B-cell activating factor (BAF) since it increased the antibody response to soluble antigen (Wood, 1979a). Subsequent biochemical characterization revealed that BAF was identical to IL-1 (Wood, 1979b). Reed *et al.* (1989) demonstrated that IL-1 increased the immune response to both carrier and hapten and that this effect could not be blocked by an excess of antibody to IL-2. Thus, although IL-1 was known to potentiate T-cell proliferation by increasing the production of IL-2 (Smith *et al.,* 1980), IL-1 increased antibody production by directly stimulating B lymphocytes.

IL-2 also had adjuvant properties and was shown to increase the immune response to hepatitis B antigen in immunodeficient nonresponder patients (Meuer *et al.,* 1989; Piera *et al.,* 1993). The usefulness of IL-2 as an adjuvant is limited by cardiovascular and neuroendocrine toxicity, the need for frequent injection, and timing considerations (Siegel and Puri, 1991). IL-2 is, however, a prime candidate for adjuvant gene therapy and has been transfected into several tumors with promising initial results (Foa *et al.,* 1992).

The ability of IL-6 to stimulate immunoglobulin production (Akira *et al.,* 1990) indicated that IL-6 had significant potential as an adjuvant. In a recent publication, Duits *et al.* (1993) demonstrated that liposomes containing IL-6 were able to enhance the immune response of mice to a weakly immunogenic protein antigen. The recent report of Ramsay *et al.* (1994) has confirmed the importance of IL-6 in the induction of mucosal IgA and highlighted the importance of this cytokine in the induction of mucosal immunity.

Interferon-γ (IFN-γ) is the cytokine most well characterized for its adjuvant properties. A mixture of protein antigen and IFN-γ can activate helper T cells for increased antibody production and DTH (Heath *et al.,* 1989). The adjuvant properties of IFN-γ may be related to its well-established macrophage-activating properties that include increasing IL-1 production and expression of MHC class II molecules (Heath and Playfair, 1992). IFN-γ has been shown to have clinical efficacy as an adjuvant for the immunization of hemodialysis patients to hepatitis B vaccine (Quiroga *et al.,* 1990). Although at significant risk, hemodialysis patients are poor responders to hepatitis vaccine. Vaccinees receiving IFN-γ with the hepatitis vaccine developed greater titers in a shorter interval than control receiving only the vaccine.

The most recent cytokine to demonstrate potential as an adjuvant for HIV-1 and tumor vaccines is IL-12 (Hall, 1994). IL-12 has been demonstrated to dramatically increase CMI and may thus have significant importance as an adjuvant specific for virus infections (Trinchieri, 1993; Gately, 1993). Recently, Clerici *et al.* (1993b) demonstrated that IL-12 could restore the in vitro cell-mediated immune responses of lymphocytes from HIV-1[+] patients and Afonso *et al.* (1994) demonstrated that IL-12 was an effective adjuvant for *Leishmania major.*

3. PRESENTATION OF ANTIGEN BY LIPOSOMES

In 1985, Walden *et al.* demonstrated that planar membranes, phospholipid-covered glass coverslips, containing digested ovalbumin and class II MHC molecules were able to

Table I

Proliferation of an Antigen-Specific T-Cell Hybridoma or
Antigen-Sensitized Spleen Cells to Liposomes[a]

	[³H]-TdR uptake (cpm)	
Liposome	T-cell hybridoma	Spleen cells
Class II + conalbumin + IL-1	125,000	20,000
Class II + conalbumin	77,500	12,000
Class II + IL-1	6,200	5,600
Class II	2,000	1,000

[a]Data from Bakouche and Lachman (1990).

stimulate IL-2 production from an ovalbumin-specific T-cell hybridoma. They also noted that similarly prepared unilamellar vesicles were not able to stimulate the T-cell hybridoma. Watts *et al.* (1984) found that liposomes containing MHC class II molecules and antigen covalently coupled to the phospholipid were able to stimulate antigen-specific cloned T-helper cells and T-cell hybridomas. The major difference between the remarkable finding of Watts *et al.* (1984) and that of Walden *et al.* (1985) was that the protein antigen did not require hydrolysis before attachment to the liposome. The conclusion of Watts *et al.* (1984) was that processing of antigen by APC was not essential for recognition by antigen-specific T cells. After we demonstrated that membrane-associated IL-1 could be extracted from activated monocytes and incorporated on the surface of liposomes (Bakouche *et al.,* 1987), it was a natural extension of the work of Watts *et al.* (1984) to determine if the presence of membrane-associated IL-1 on antigen-containing liposomes would increase the T-cell response. We found these liposomes induced greater proliferation of an antigen-specific hybridoma or antigen-educated splenic T cells than liposomes lacking IL-1 when the whole protein antigen (conalbumin) was presented (Table I). Although IL-1 increased the proliferative response for these conditions, it was not essential to obtain a significant response to the antigen.

If, however, the class II molecule was purified from IFN-γ-activated macrophages that had processed the conalbumin antigen in vitro, the inclusion of IL-1 was also found to augment the proliferative responses (Table II). The proliferation of the T hybridoma and the spleen lymphocytes was enhanced to a much greater extent by including membrane IL-1 on the surface of the liposomes. The purpose of these experiments was to determine if IL-1 could enhance the T-cell response to protein antigen presented on the surface of liposomes. We confirmed the findings of Watts *et al.* (1984) that protein antigens need not be processed if presented on the surface of liposomes and we expanded the findings of Walden *et al.* (1985) by demonstrating that IL-1 enhanced the T-cell response to antigen presented in the context of a class II molecule.

Although it is possible to make liposome-bearing class II molecules for inbred strains of mice, this strategy has limited usefulness for humans. We concluded that a more strategic route leading to a useful adjuvant would be to prepare liposomes containing cytokines on their exterior surface and allow the host's immune cells to take up the liposome and present the antigen. We hypothesized that the cytokine on the surface of the liposome could

Table II
Proliferation of an Antigen-Specific T-Cell Hybridoma or
Antigen-Sensitized Spleen Cells to Liposomes Bearing Processed
Antigen[a]

	[³H]-TdR uptaked (cpm)	
Liposome	T-cell hybridoma	Spleen cells
Class II + conalbumin + IL-1	92,000	39,000
Class II + conalbumin	13,800	4,200
Class II + IL-1	11,500	3,550
Class II	6,650	2,300

[a]Data from Bakouche and Lachman (1990).

potentiate the immune response to the antigen. More specifically, we wanted to address the possibility that liposomes containing Th1-type cytokines could induce DTH and cytotoxic T lymphocytes (CTLs), while liposomes containing Th2-type cytokines could increase humoral immunity through antibody production. This difference in immune response is very important because our current reasoning indicates that effective adjuvants for HIV-1 must induce CTLs (Salk *et al.,* 1993). Also, we hypothesized that T lymphocytes stimulated by cytokines on the surface of liposomes could respond to the antigen in the absence of an immediate source of class II MHC. To investigate these theories, we prepared liposomes that contained cytokines on their exterior surface.

4. DEHYDRATION–REHYDRATION VESICLES (DRVs) CONTAINING CYTOKINES

4.1. Preparation of DRVs

Since our goal was to prepare liposomes that had the maximum amount of cytokine on their exterior surface, we decided to use DRVs as initially described by Gregoriadis *et al.* (1987). The procedure for making DRVs is to prepare traditional liposomes from phospholipids and water and then add the protein(s) of interest to a water suspension of the liposomes, followed by lyophilization of the preparation (dehydration). The dried preparation is then suspended in buffer or medium (rehydration) and extensively vortexed to re-form the liposomes. Tan and Gregoriadis (1989) demonstrated the ability of this type of liposome to increase the adjuvant properties of IL-2.

4.2. Trapping Capacity of DRVs

We prepared DRVs with two lipid combinations, phosphatidylcholine/cholesterol (PC/CH) (1:1) and PC/phosphatidylserine (PC/PS) (7:1). Using preparations of radioiodinated cytokines and the recombinant protein HIV-1 MN rgp120, we determined the

Table III
Trapping Ratio of Radiolabeled Cytokines and HIV-1 MN rgp120 in DRVs

	Trapping ratio (%)[a]	
	PC/PS[b] (7:3)	PC/CH[c] (1:1)
rIL-1α	5.2 ± 1.1	13.5 ± 0.4
rIL-1β	20.2 ± 0.2	24.7 ± 2.6
rTNF-α	17.5 ± 2.1	34.5 ± 3.3
rIL-6	7.2 ± 1.1	24.5 ± 2.8
rIFN-γ	14.5 ± 0.3	22.7 ± 3.8
MN rgp120	16.3 ± 1.6	16.9 ± 0.2
Inulin	12.2 ± 0.6	4.5 ± 0.2

[a]Trapping ratio is the percentage of added radiolabeled cytokine associated with the DRVs following three washes by centrifugation.
[b]Phosphatidylcholine/phosphatidylserine.
[c]Phosphatidylcholine/cholesterol.

percentage of each protein that was trapped by the DRVs. As shown in Table III, the highest trap ratios occurred with PC/CH and the range of trapping was between 13.5 and 34.5%. We determined the liquid volume of the liposomes using inulin (see Chapter 24) as previously described by Nayar *et al.* (1987). It can be estimated that the PC/PS DRVs would be able to trap approximately 12.2% of an added protein if the protein was found exclusively in the liquid phase of the liposomes and PC/CH DRVs would trap approximately 4.5%. These results indicated that the radiolabeled cytokines and HIV-1 MN rgp120 were almost exclusively trapped in the lipid phase of the PC/CH DRVs since the values greatly exceeded the liquid volume.

The mechanism of trapping proteins in DRVs depends on the dehydration step of the DRV preparation (Gregoriadis *et al.*, 1987). In the absence of an aqueous environment, hydrophilic proteins such HIV-1 MN rgp120 and cytokines associate with the charged phospholipids. This association of the cytokines and HIV-1 MN rgp120 with the phospholipids remained quite strong (see Section 4.3) even after the dehydrated liposomes were rehydrated. We selected DRVs, as opposed to classical liposomes, because this type of liposome traps much greater amounts of hydrophilic proteins and has the greatest likelihood to trap proteins on the exterior surface of the liposome (Hume and Nayar, 1989).

4.3. Slow Release of the Trapped Cytokines and HIV-1 MN rgp120 in the DRVs

To determine the stability of the association between the DRVs and the cytokines and HIV-1 MN rgp120, DRVs were prepared with radioiodinated protein components. DRVs prepared in the standard manner using only radiolabeled proteins were washed three times in phosphate-buffered saline (PBS) at room temperature before beginning the experiment shown in Table IV. The DRVs were soaked in RPMI 1640 containing 5% fetal calf serum (FCS) at 37°C in individual tubes and centrifuged at the times shown in Table IV. The amount of radiolabeled protein remaining with the DRV pellet following centrifugation

Table IV
Retention of Radiolabeled Cytokines and HIV-1 MN rgp120 in DRVs Incubated in RPMI
1640 Containing 5% FCS

Time (h)	rIL-1α	rIL-1β	rIL-6	rTNF-α	IFN-γ	HIV-1 MN rgp120
			Retention of radiolabeled protein (%) for PC/PS DRVs			
0	100	100	100	100	100	100
1	93.9	94.7	91.5	94.3	98.6	97.1
2	86.1	99.3	94.4	94.7	97.3	93.2
4	102.7	96.1	97.9	96.6	95.8	96.5
6	93.9	91.6	90.3	93.6	ND	91.6
24	80.9	85.5	84.0	91.0	82.5	73.5
48	81.1	83.8	83.1	90.4	80.2	73.5
72	65.7	84.4	77.3	86.8	ND	74.9
			Retention of radiolabeled protein (%) for PC/CH DRVs			
0	100	100	100	100	100	100
1	99.4	96.7	89.6	102.5	97.3	99.0
2	97.4	98.1	83.9	107.1	90.2	98.0
4	92.1	94.1	80.9	104.0	100.3	92.8
6	101.0	91.2	77.7	107.4	92.6	85.8
24	91.8	93.2	71.4	98.7	86.7	85.5
48	92.3	86.5	69.0	101.0	82.8	81.5
72	88.3	87.4	70.8	94.6	90.1	79.7

was divided by the amount of radiolabeled protein in the time zero sample to calculate the percentages shown. The percentage of radiolabeled cytokine and HIV-1 MN rgp120 remaining with the DRV pellet after soaking was quite high for both DRV formulations. There was a gradual loss of radiolabel from the DRVs in every sample. It should be noted this was an in vitro test to determine if the cytokines could be released from the DRVs by soaking in serum-containing medium. Although this experiment may not be predictive of in vivo events, it clearly indicated that the cytokines and HIV-1 MN rgp120 were associated with the DRVs in a stable manner and gradually released over a 72-h period.

4.4. Localization of Trapped Proteins

To determine if the cytokines associated with the DRVs retained biological activity, DRVs containing IL-1α and IL-6 were prepared and soaked overnight at 37°C in RPMI 1640. The DRVs were washed three times by centrifugation and added to standard biological assays used in our laboratory to measure cytokine levels. Briefly, a 72-h [³H]thymidine proliferation assay was performed for IL-1 and IL-6 using the standard D10 and 7TD1 cell lines, respectively (Bakouche *et al.*, 1987; Krakauer, 1993). As shown in Table V, DRVs containing IL-1α and IL-6 exhibited biological activity with both types of

Table V
Biological Assays for DRVs Containing IL-1α and IL-6

IL-1 biological activity [^{3}H]-TdR incorporation (cpm)

		DRVs	
Dilution	rIL-1α positive control	rIL-1α–PC/PS	rIL-1α–PC/CH
1:5	101,540	59,495	69,412
1:25	114,250	69,580	54,744
1:125	107,205	53,607	11,714
1:625	ND	30,724	3,072

IL-6 biological activity [^{3}H]-TdR incorporation (cpm)

		DRVs	
Dilution	rIL-6 positive control	rIL-6–PC/PS	rIL-6–PC/CH
1:5	32,123	13,529	14,860
1:25	27,175	4,953	5,805
1:125	9,264	3,660	4,347
1:625	3,951	3,527	4,162

phospholipid mixtures. IL-1α and IL-6 may leak from the DRVs and interact with the specific cytokine receptor on the D10 or 7TD1 cells. Another possibility is that the cytokines were able to stimulate the cytokine receptor while remaining attached to the DRVs. Supernatants from DRVs containing IL-1α soaked in RPMI 1640 and 5% FCS for 48 h were also assayed for biological activity. Although the supernatants contained IL-1 activity, the levels were less than observed when DRVs were added directly to the assay, indicating possible interaction of the DRV-bound IL-1α with the cellular receptor.

We have also used thin-section electron microscopy to locate added protein to the surface of the DRVs. DRVs prepared with HIV-1 MN rgp120 were treated in a primary reaction with a rabbit IgG to HIV-1 MN rgp120 and a secondary reaction with goat anti-rabbit IgG conjugated to 30-nm gold particles. As shown in Fig. 1, the DRVs are multilamellar, as expected, and gold particles on the exterior surface of the liposome indicate the presence of HIV-1 MN rgp120. Control preparations lacking the primary antibody were negative for the presence of gold particles.

5. IMMUNIZATION OF MICE WITH DRVs CONTAINING CYTOKINES AND HIV-1 MN rgp120

As shown in Table VI, groups of five mice were immunized twice according to the schedule listed there. The DTH was measured as footpad swelling 24 h after footpad injection of soluble HIV-1 MN rgp120. The p values for Student's two-sample t test are shown comparing the soluble samples with PBS and the DRVs with DRVs containing HIV-1 MN rgp120 but lacking cytokine. The results indicate that HIV-1 MN rgp120 did not significantly increase the footpad swelling when compared to PBS, but did cause an

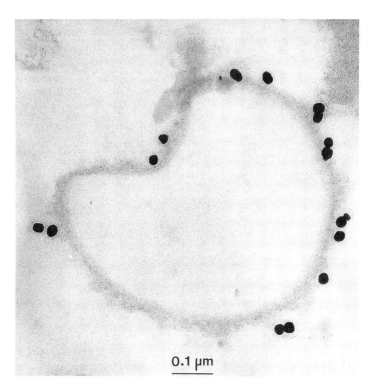

Figure 1. Thin-section electron microscopy of a DRV prepared with MN rgp120 and treated with rabbit IgG to MN rgp120 followed by goat anti-rabbit IgG labeled with gold particles.

increase if used with CFA. Liposomes lacking cytokine also did not significantly increase the DTH response compared to soluble HIV-1 MN rgp120. However, the addition of either 20 units of rIL-6 or 1.0 μg of rIFN-γ per nanomole lipid injection significantly increased the DTH response.

After several repeats of this experiment using a wide range of doses, we concluded that only IL-6 and IFN-γ in DRVs with HIV-1 MN rgp120 were able to stimulate DTH responses. As shown in Table VII, we have expanded the range of doses for these cytokines and titered the serum of individual animals in the groups. With an expanded immunization schedule of three biweekly injections, we found that 20.0 and 30.0 units of IL-6 in DRVs significantly increased both DTH and humoral immune responses. Similarly, 1.0 and 2.0 mg of IFN-γ increased the DTH response. Interestingly, only IL-6 and not IFN-γ increased the antibody responses. When HIV-1 MN rgp120 and IFN-γ (1.0, 2.0, and 5.0 μg) were injected in the soluble form, the DTH response was not significant. There was, however, a significant antibody titer of 8287 $\pm$ 6091 for the dose of 2.0 μg of soluble IFN-γ. This soluble formulation was the only one that induced a significant antibody response.

Soluble HIV-1 MN rgp120 or DRVs containing this protein were not significantly immunogenic, as measured by DTH. If, however, the DRVs contained either murine IFN-γ

Table VI
Immune Response of C3H/HeN Mice to Soluble HIV-1 MN rgp120, to HIV-1 MN rgp120 with Complete Freund's Adjuvant (CFA), and DRVs Containing Cytokines and HIV-1 MN rgp120

Formulation[a]	ΔFootpad ($\times 10^{-2}$ mm)	SD	p[b]
	Soluble		
PBS	6.4	8.7	NB
rgp120	9.4	4.6	0.46
rgp120 + CFA	31.2	9.5	0.0000
	DRVs		
rgp120	12.5	9.7	NB
rgp120–IL-1α (0.03 μg)	9.2	10.9	0.33
rgp120–IL-1β (0.02 μg)	10.3	10.1	0.58
rgp120–IL-6 (20 units)	21.4	11.7	0.056
rgp120–TNF-α (0.02 mg)	15.4	7.4	0.37
rgp120–IFN-γ (0.5 μg)	16.3	11.0	0.37
rgp120–IFN-γ (1.0 μg)	28.8	11.1	0.001
rgp120–IFN-γ (5.0 μg)	15.8	14.6	0.58
Day	Procedure		
1	Subcutaneous injection (15 μg MN rgp120, DRVs or soluble)		
8	Subcutaneous injection (15 μg MN rgp120, DRVs or soluble)		
15	Measure footpad, footpad injection (1 μg soluble MN rgp120)		
16	Measure footpad		

[a]MN rgp120 and murine IFN-γ were provided by Genentech, Inc. Human IL-1α, IL-1β, IL-6 and TNF-α were purchased from Boehringer Mannheim, GMbH, Germany.
[b]p values were determined using Student's two-sample t test for soluble MN rgp120 versus PBS and for DRVs containing MN rgp120 and cytokines versus DRVs containing only MN rgp120.

or human IL-6, a significant DTH response was induced. The humoral immune response, as measured by IgG specific to HIV-1 MN rgp120, was detected only for DRVs containing IL-6 and not the DRVs containing IFN-γ. In the general classification system for cytokines, IL-6 is a Th2 cytokine able to induce humoral immunity, whereas IFN-γ is a Th1 cytokine able to stimulate DTH. Our results indicated that DRVs containing IL-6 and IFN-γ had these respective immunological activities. However, we also found that DRVs containing IL-6 induced DTH. The cytokine classification system is not absolute and contains numerous instances of overlapping activities. We did not, however, observe overlap for induction of humoral immunity by DRVs containing IFN-γ.

6. POSSIBLE MECHANISMS OF ACTION OF DRVs

We have not yet investigated how DRVs are cleared following subcutaneous injection in the abdomen of mice. We know from electron microscopy studies that the DRVs are heterogeneous in size. Fluorescence-activated cell sorting using antibody to gp120 dem-

Table VII

Immune Response of C3H/HeN Mice to Soluble HIV-1 MN rgp120 + Soluble IFNγ, and DRVs Containing Cytokines and HIV-1 MN rgp120

Formulation[a]	ΔFootpad (×10^{-2} mm)	SD	p[b]	Titer[c]	SD	p[b]
		Soluble				
rgp120 + IFN-γ (1.0 μg)	6.5	5.56	0.68	7,213	7,139	0.17
rgp120 + IFN-γ (2.0 μg)	6.9	5.55	0.56	8,287	6,091	0.048
rgp120 + IFN-γ (5.0 μg)	4.4	4.25	0.57	5,847	3,281	0.099
		DRVs				
rgp120	5.5	6.61	NB	3,819	2,040	NB
rgp120–IL-6 (10 U)	6.9	4.96	0.47	5,919	2,698	0.068
rgp120–IL-6 (20 U)	10.5	5.84	0.017	11,193	8,176	0.02
rgp120–IL-6 (30 U)	11.5	6.33	0.028	11,288	7,084	0.0098
rgp120–IFN-γ (0.5 μg)	12.2	8.93	0.056	5,302	5,426	0.42
rgp120–IFN-γ (1.0 μg	17.1	6.79	0.0000	9,125	10,867	0.16
rgp120–IFN-γ (2.0 μg)	14.7	8.01	0.0004	6,088	7,429	0.36
rgp120–IFN-γ (5.0 μg)	8.5	5.08	0.12	4,520	5,054	0.67

Day	Procedure
1	Subcutaneous injection (15 μg MN rgp120, DRVs or soluble)
15	Subcutaneous injection (15 μg MN rgp120, DRVs or soluble)
29	Subcutaneous injection (15 μg MN rgp120, DRVs or soluble)
43	Measure footpad, footpad injection (1 μg soluble MN rgp120)
44	Measure footpad, exsanguinate for ELISA

[a]MN rgp120 and murine IFN-γ were provided by Genentech, Inc. Human IL-1α, IL-1β, IL-6, and TNF-α were purchased from Boehringer Mannheim, GMbH, Germany.

[b]p values were determined using Student's two-sample t Test for soluble MN rgp120 versus PBS and for DRVs containing MN rgp120 and cytokines versus DRVs containing only MN rgp120.

[c]The IgG response to MN gp120 for each mouse was determined by ELISA. The titer equals the reciprocal dilution yielding twice the background response compared to pooled serum from animals immunized with PBS alone. The values shown are the mean and SD determined by averaging the individual titers for the animals in each group.

onstrated that approximately 28% of the DRVs had a mean diameter of 1.66 μm and 53.5% had a mean diameter of 3.99 μm. Most DRVs in this size range could be expected to be taken up by cells of the reticuloendothelial system (Lee *et al.*, 1992; Fan *et al.*, 1990). We have not yet determined if DRVs are transported intact to draining lymph nodes. As discussed in Section 3, DRVs have the ability to present antigen to primed T lymphocytes or antigen-specific hybridomas without prior processing of the antigen. It is possible that DRVs are transported to the lymph nodes and that direct stimulation of T lymphocytes occurs in the node. The effect of cytokines on this type of immune reaction must then be determined. Another mechanism of action for antigen presentation of a heterogeneous population of DRVs could be fusing of the DRVs with the plasma membrane of APCs. Rao *et al.* (1994) recently demonstrated that a repetitive peptide-encapsulated liposome was presented to T lymphocytes by APCs without internalization or intracellular processing. The transfer of the antigen to the plasma membrane of the APC probably represented a fusion of the liposome with the APC, resulting in transfer of the repetitive peptide.

7. FUTURE DIRECTIONS FOR CYTOKINE-CONTAINING DRVs

There are many individual cytokines that could be tested for effectiveness in DRVs and there are an even greater number of combinations of cytokines that might prove effective. For example, even though IL-1α and IL-1β did not appear to be effective in DRVs containing HIV-1 MN rgp120 (Table VI), a combination of IL-1 and a second cytokine could potentially be effective. Rational design of DRVs with multiple cytokines might be possible based on our current knowledge of Th1 and Th2 cells and the cytokines they release (Heath and Playfair, 1992). Our findings with IL-6 indicate that it is possible for a Th2-type cytokine to also induce Th1-type activity when prepared in DRVs. It may be possible to design cytokine-containing DRVs that induce only humoral immunity or only DTH for certain antigens. Our findings to date indicate that DRVs containing IFN-γ induced DTH, but did not induce humoral immunity to HIV-1 MN rgp120. It is possible that DRVs containing distinct cytokine(s) could influence the immune response to subunit proteins leading to a Th1-type DTH response with CTL induction or a Th2-type response primarily expressed as antibody production. It is also possible that the most effective vaccines will induce both types of immunity, regardless of their intended purpose.

In conclusion, DRVs offer novel vehicles for the delivery of protein subunit antigens and cytokines. We are at the initial stages of screening individual and combinations of cytokines for effectiveness in mice. It may be possible to design specific formulations of cytokine-containing DRVs depending on the antigen and the type of immunity desired.

ACKNOWLEDGMENTS

This research was supported by the Department of Health and Human Services, National Institutes of Health, National Institute of Allergy and Infectious Diseases (AI33227). We wish to thank Mr. Kenny Dunner, Jr., and Dr. Corazon Bucana for performing the electron microscopy experiments and Karen Ramirez for the fluorescence-activated cell sorting experiments.

REFERENCES

Afonso, L. C., Scharton, T. M., Vieira, L. Q., Wysocka, M., Trinchieri, G., and Scott, P., 1994, The adjuvant effect of interleukin-12 in a vaccine against Leishmania major, *Science* **263**:235–237.

Akira, S., Hirano, T., Taga, T., and Kishimoto, T., 1990, Biology of multifunctional cytokines: IL-6 and related molecules (IL-1 and TNF), *FASEB J.* **4**:2860–2867.

Alving, C. R., 1991, Liposomes as carriers of antigens and adjuvants, *J. Immunol. Methods* **140**:1–13.

Audibert, F. M., and Lise, L. D., 1993, Adjuvants: Current status, clinical perspectives and future prospects, *Immunol. Today* **14**:281–284.

Bakouche, O., and Lachman, L. B., 1990, Synthetic macrophages: Liposomes bearing antigen, class II MHC and membrane-IL-1, *Lymphokine Res.* **9**:259–281.

Bakouche, O., Brown, D. C., and Lachman, L. B., 1987, Liposomes expressing IL-1 biological activity, *J. Immunol.* **138**:4256–4262.

Clerici, M., Hakim, F. T., Venzon, D. J., Blatt, S., Hendrix, C. W., Wynn, T. A., and Shearer, G. M., 1993a, Changes in interleukin-2 and interleukin-4 production in asymptomatic, human immunodeficiency virus-seropositive individuals, *J. Clin. Invest.* **91**:759–765.

Clerici, M., Lucey, D. R., Berzofsky, J. A., Pinto, L. A., Wynn, T. A., Blatt, S. P., Dolan, M. J., Hendrix, C. W., Wolf, S. F., and Shearer, G. M., 1993b, Restoration of HIV-specific cell-mediated immune responses by interleukin-12 in vitro, *Science* **262**:1721–1724.

Duits, A. J., van Puijenbroek, A., Vermeulen, H., Hofhuis, F. M., van de Winkel, J. G., and Capel, P. J., 1993, Immunoadjuvant activity of a liposomal IL-6 formulation, *Vaccine* **11**:777–781.

Fan, D., Bucana, C. D., O'Brian, C. A., Zwelling, L. A., Seid, C., and Fidler, I. J., 1990, Enhancement of murine tumor cell sensitivity to adriamycin by presentation of the drug in phosphatidylcholine–phosphatidylserine liposomes, *Cancer Res.* **50**:3619–3626.

Foa, R., Guarini, A., and Gansbacher, B., 1992, IL2 treatment for cancer: From biology to gene therapy, *Br. J. Cancer* **66**:992–998.

Gately, M. K., 1993, Interleukin-12: A recently discovered cytokine with potential for enhancing cell-mediated immune responses to tumors, *Cancer Invest.* **11**:500–506.

Gregoriadis, G., Davis, D., and Davies, A., 1987, Liposomes as immunological adjuvants: Antigen incorporation studies, *Vaccine* **5**:145–151.

Grun, J. L., and Maurer, P. H., 1989, Different T helper cell subsets elicited in mice utilizing two different adjuvant vehicles: The role of endogenous interleukin 1 in proliferative responses, *Cell. Immunol.* **121**:134–145.

Hall, S. S., 1994, IL-12 holds promise against cancer, glimmer of AIDS hope, *Science* **263**:1685–1686.

Heath, A. W., and Playfair, J. H., 1992, Cytokines as immunological adjuvants, *Vaccine* **10**:427–434.

Heath, A. W., Devey, M. E., Brown, I. N., Richards, C. E., and Playfair, J. H., 1989, Interferon-gamma as an adjuvant in immunocompromised mice, *Immunology* **67**:520–524.

Hume, D. A., and Nayar, R., 1989, Encapsulation is not involved in the activities of recombinant gamma interferon associated with multilamellar phospholipid liposomes on murine bone marrow-derived macrophages, *Lymphokine Res.* **8**:415–425.

Krakauer, T., 1993, A sensitive, specific immunobioassay for quantitation of human interleukin 6, *J. Immunoassay* **14**:267–277.

Lee, K. D., Hong, K., and Papahadjopoulos, D., 1992, Recognition of liposomes by cells: In vitro binding and endocytosis mediated by specific lipid headgroups and surface charge density, *Biochim. Biophys. Acta* **1103**:185–197.

Meuer, S. C., Dumann, H., Meyer zum Buschenfelde, K. H., and Kohler, H., 1989, Low-dose interleukin-2 induces systemic immune responses against HBsAg in immunodeficient non-responders to hepatitis B vaccination, *Lancet* **1**:15–18.

Nayar, R., Morikawa, K., and Fidler, I. J., 1987, Characterization of liposomes containing the chemotactic peptide N-formyl-methionyl-leucyl-phenylalanine (FMLP) and their interaction with mouse macrophages, *Cancer Drug Deliv.* **4**:233–244.

Piera, M., de Bolos, C., Castro, R., and Real, F. X., 1993, Cytokines as adjuvants: Effect on the immunogenicity of NeuAc alpha 2-6GalNAc alpha-O-Ser/Thr (sialyl-Tn), *Int. J. Cancer* **55**:148–152.

Quiroga, J. A., Castillo, I., Porres, J. C., Casao, S., and Saez, F., 1990, Recombinant gamma-interferon as adjuvant to hepatitis B vaccine in hemodialysis patients, *Hepatology* **12**:661–663.

Ramsay, A. J., Husband, A. J., Ramshaw, I. A., Bao, S., Matthaei, K. I., Koehler, G., and Kopf, M., 1994, The role of interleukin-6 in mucosal IgA antibody responses in vivo, *Science* **264**:561–563.

Rao, M., Wassef, N. M., Alving, C., and Krzych, U., 1995, Processing and presentation of liposome-encapsulated antigens by macrophages, (submitted).

Reed, S. G., Pihl, D. L., Conlon, P. J., and Grabstein, K. H., 1989, IL-1 as adjuvant. Role of T cells in the augmentation of specific antibody production by recombinant human IL-1 alpha, *J. Immunol.* **142**:3129–3133.

Salk, J., Bretscher, P. A., Salk, P. L., Clerici, M., and Shearer, G. M., 1993, A strategy for prophylactic vaccination against HIV, *Science* **260**:1270–1272.

Siegel, J. P., and Puri, R. K., 1991, Interleukin-2 toxicity. *J. Clin. Oncol.* **9**:694–704.

Smith, K. A., Lachman, L. B., Oppenheim, J. J., and Favata, M. F., 1980, The functional relationship of the interleukins, *J. Exp. Med.* **151**:1551–1556.

Staruch, M. J., and Wood, D. D., 1983, The adjuvanticity of interleukin 1 in vivo, *J. Immunol.* **130**:2191–2194.

Tan, L., and Gregoriadis, G., 1989, Effect of interleukin-2 on the immunoadjuvant action of liposomes, *Biochem. Soc. Trans.* **17**:693–694.

Trinchieri, G., 1993, Interleukin-12 and its role in the generation of Th1 cells, *Immunol. Today* **14**:335–338.

Walden, P., Nagy, Z. A., and Klein, J., 1985, Induction of regulatory T-lymphocyte responses by liposomes carrying major histocompatibility complex molecules and foreign antigen, *Nature* **315**:327–329.

Watts, T. H., Brian, A. A., Kappler, J. W., Marrack, P., and McConnell, H. M., 1984, Antigen presentation by supported planar membranes containing affinity-purified I-Ad, *Proc. Natl. Acad. Sci. USA* **81**:7564–7568.

Wood, D. D., 1979a, Mechanism of action of human B cell-activating factor. I. Comparison of the plaque-stimulating activity with thymocyte-stimulating activity, *J. Immunol.* **123**:2400–2407.

Wood, D. D., 1979b, Comparison of the plaque-stimulating and thymocyte-stimulating activities derived from human monocytes, *Ann. NY Acad. Sci.* **332**:491–502.

Chapter 30

Haemophilus influenzae Type b Conjugate Vaccines

Peter J. Kniskern, Stephen Marburg, and Ronald W. Ellis

1. INTRODUCTION

Haemophilus influenzae, a gram-negative rod-shaped bacterium, is a major human pathogen that causes a range of diseases in infants, children, and adults. There are six antigenic types of *H. influenzae*, termed a–f, whose antigenic specificity is provided by the capsular polysaccharide (Ps). There also are nontypeable strains which lack a capsular Ps. *H. influenzae* type b (Hib) is the most pathogenic *H. influenzae* strain for infants and young children and a major cause of invasive bacterial infections. Until the 1990s, Hib caused an estimated 10,000 cases of meningitis per year in children 2 months to 5 years of age in the United States (Vadheim and Ward, 1994). The mortality rate is up to 5% in developed countries, and up to 35% of survivors may develop permanent neurological sequelae. Other invasive Hib infections include cellulitis, empyema, endocarditis, endophthalmitis, epididymitis, epiglottitis, osteomyelitis, pericarditis, pneumonia, septic arthritis, and tracheitis (Kaplan, 1994). While the total incidence of such Hib infections was approximately equal to that of Hib meningitis in the United States, these diseases vary significantly in relative incidence elsewhere in the world. As a result of the development and widespread use of Hib conjugate vaccines in several developed countries, the incidence of invasive Hib diseases has decreased by about 95% in the United States (M.M.W.R., 1994) and 60–80% in other countries (Vadheim and Ward, 1994).

The most significant epidemiological feature of invasive Hib diseases in unvaccinated populations is its age-related incidence, where the risk is generally highest at approximately 6 to 12 months of age. In many areas the risk is lower below 6 months of age because of transplacental acquisition of maternal antibodies. The risk decreases with age above 2

Peter J. Kniskern and Ronald W. Ellis • Virus and Cell Biology, Merck Research Laboratories, West Point, Pennsylvania 19486. *Stephen Marburg* • Synthetic Chemical Research, Merck Research Laboratories, Rahway, New Jersey 07065.

Vaccine Design: The Subunit and Adjuvant Approach, edited by Michael F. Powell and Mark J. Newman. Plenum Press, New York, 1995.

years, presumably as a result of immune maturation as well as exposure to other pathogens serologically cross-reactive with Hib. While the incidence of invasive Hib disease is lower in developed than in developing countries, there are selected populations with significantly higher incidence of disease. For example, Australian aborigines, Eskimos, and native Indian populations of North America have a higher incidence than their respective country averages, perhaps because they live under conditions similar to those in developing areas (Vadheim and Ward, 1994).

A series of classical experiments established the Hib capsular Ps as a candidate vaccine antigen. The basis for antibodies mediating in vitro protection against Hib first was shown in bactericidal assays with normal human sera (Fothergill *et al.*, 1933). Hyperimmune rabbit antisera to Hib then were employed successfully for passive immunotherapy of Hib infections (Alexander *et al.*, 1943); the activity of such sera could be absorbed by purified Hib capsular Ps (Alexander *et al.*, 1944). The Ps was purified and its structure shown to be polyribosylribitol phosphate (PRP) (Crisel *et al.*, 1975). PRP was used to develop a Farr-type radioimmunoassay (RIA) to quantify serum antibodies to PRP (anti-PRP) (Robbins *et al.*, 1973). Levels of such antibodies were shown to correlate with protection from invasive Hib disease (Peltola *et al.*, 1977).

On the basis of these studies, purified PRP was developed into a vaccine. It was shown to be immunogenic in older children and adults, but not in children less than 2 years of age (Robbins *et al.*, 1973; Anderson *et al.*, 1977). When PRP vaccine was tested in a double-blind controlled efficacy trial in 50,000 infants and children in Finland, the rate of efficacy in children 18–71 months old was 90%, but no protection was observed in children less than 18 months old (Peltola *et al.*, 1984). On this basis, the vaccine was licensed in the United States in 1985 for routine use in children at least 2 years old and in children 18–23 months of age at high risk of Hib infection. Long-term protection was shown to correlate with anti-PRP levels ≥ 1.0 μg/mL and short-term protection with levels ≥ 0.15 μg/mL, as quantified by RIA (Käyhty *et al.*, 1983). Nevertheless, since most invasive Hib disease occurs in children less than 18 months old, a second-generation Hib vaccine was needed for optimal disease control.

The strategy for developing a second-generation Hib vaccine can be rationalized from immunological considerations. As is the case for most types of Ps, PRP is a T-independent (TI) antigen, which stimulates B lymphocytes directly to produce anti-PRP without the participation of T lymphocytes such that immunological memory is not established. TI antigens are not immunogenic in infants and young children. On the other hand, T-dependent (TD) antigens, such as proteins, stimulate helper T lymphocytes to interact with B lymphocytes, causing the latter to produce anti-PRP. In the course of the TD immune response, immunological memory is established, antibody class-switching occurs, and antibody affinity increases as a result of somatic mutations in anti-PRP immunoglobulin genes. Since TD antigens are immunogenic in infants and young children, the conversion of PRP from a TI to a TD antigen would be expected to make it immunogenic in infants.

The principle of coupling Ps to protein to increase its immunogenicity had long been established (Goebel and Avery, 1931). Thus, the covalent coupling of PRP to a carrier protein would be expected to convert PRP to a TD antigen that would elicit anti-PRP in infants. This is the immunological basis for Hib conjugate vaccines, the second-generation

Hib vaccines that have been shown to protect infants from invasive Hib diseases as described below.

2. RATIONAL CONJUGATE DESIGN, CHEMISTRY, AND PROCESS CONTROL

2.1. Outline of the Processes

Fundamentally, the processes developed for the four licensed vaccines (Table I) differ from one another in the following attributes: (1) the choice of protein carrier, (2) the size of the starting PRP, (3) the linking or bridging molecule, (4) the architecture of the chemical process steps, i.e., whether the processes flow in a single, sequential stream (PRP-TT and HbOC) or in two parallel derivatization streams which join at the point of chemical conjugation (PRP-OMPC and PRP-DT), and (5) the process steps used to remove unconjugated PRP and other reactants. These differences and other attributes of the four processes are discussed in more detail in the following sections. The quantitative aspects of covalency and removal of unconjugated PRP also are discussed in Sections 2.2 and 2.4, respectively.

2.1.1. PRP-D

This process (Gordon, 1986) begins by hydrolyzing the PRP to reduce its molecular weight, after which it is activated with cyanogen bromide to an electrophilic species (considered to be a cyanate ester). The protein (Pr) carrier for PRP-DT is diphtheria toxoid (DT), which is prepared by formalin treatment of diphtheria toxin secreted by *Corynebacterium diphtheria*. In a second process stream, the carboxyl groups of DT are functionalized with adipic acid dihydrazide, using the water-soluble 1-ethyl-3-(3-dimethylaminopropyl) carbodiimide (EDAC) as the condensing agent, creating a nucleophilic DT derivative. The electrophilic and nucleophilic intermediates then react to form the conjugate product (depicted below and as a schematic model in Fig. 1A) which is purified by ammonium sulfate precipitation:

$$DT–HNNHCO(CH_2)_4CONHNHC(= N)O–PRP$$

Analytical size-exclusion chromatography (SEC) was used to provide indirect proof of covalency (see Section 2.2.1).

2.1.2. PRP-OMPC

This process also proceeds in two streams (Marburg *et al.,* 1986, 1987, 1989). The first, which involves derivatization of native PRP, differs from the equivalent steps used in the other three conjugation processes in that it takes place in a nonaqueous system, eliminating the nucleophilic competition between the hydroxyl groups on PRP and the hydroxyls of water. To accomplish this, PRP is converted from the calcium salt to the dimethylformamide (DMF)-soluble tetrabutyl ammonium salt by titration with tetrabutylammonium hydroxide. This hydrophobic PRP salt is reacted in DMF with carbonyl diimidazole (CDI), which activates some of the PRP hydroxyls to the electrophilic

Table I

Characteristics[a] of the Carrier Proteins and Polysaccharides

Conjugate name[a]	Trade name	Manufacturer	Carrier protein (Pr)	Mass (kDa) of Pr	PRP sizing method	Mass (Da) of PRP[b]
HbOC	HibTITER®[c]	Lederle–Praxis	Mutant diphtheria toxin[d]	58	NaIO$_4$ treatment	3400–11,000
PRP-DT	ProHIBit®	Connaught	Diphtheria toxoid[e]	58	Hydrolysis @ 100°C	2×10^5–2×10^7
PRP-OMPC	PedvaxHIB®	Merck	Outer membrane protein complex[f]	50,000	Oxalic acid treatment[g]	$\sim 8 \times 10^4$
PRP-TT	ActHIB® OmniHIB®[h]	Pasteur–Merieux	Tetanus toxoid[e]	150	None	$\sim 1 \times 10^5$

[a]See Section 2 for relevant reference citations and abbreviations for conjugate names.

[b]Values as reported in the literature or estimated from K_d data reported in the literature.

[c]Also available in combination with DTP as Tetramune®.

[d]Cross-reactive material (CRM$_{197}$).

[e]Characteristics are given for the toxin prior to toxoiding.

[f]Isolated from *Neisseria meningitidis* serogroup B.

[g]This is not a sizing operation *per se*, but rather is the result of a chemical event that occurs during the process.

[h]Distributed by SmithKline Beecham in the United States only.

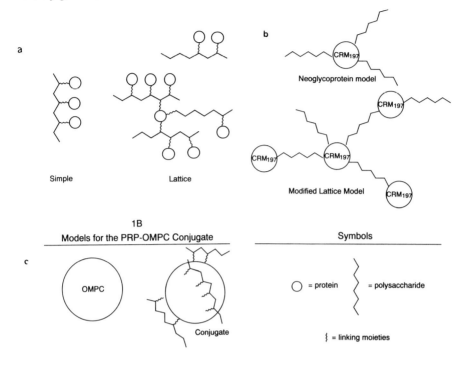

Figure 1. (A) Diagrammatic representation of PRP-DT and PRP-TT. Because of the polyfunctionality of both Pr and Ps, the products are a mixture of geometries which are simple lattice types.

(B) Diagrammatic representation of the PRP-OMPC conjugate. In this case, there are a number of Ps molecules of varying chain length linked through bridging moieties to each large OMPC particle. The term "ladder-type" conjugate seems appropriate in describing the OMPC conjugates. This type of structure differs from the lattice type associated with the PRP-DT and PRP-TT vaccines in that each Ps molecule is linked to only one Pr moiety.

(C) Diagrammatic representation of HbOC. This conjugate can be described as a mixture of a neoglyco-protein model (Dick and Bevrett, 1989) and a lattice (the latter being a modified lattice because the PRP fragment is only bi- and not polyfunctional).

imidazolyl urethane function. The activated PRP then is reacted directly with an aqueous solution of 1,4-butane diamine (BuA_2); the NMR spectrum also indicates that little if any cross-linking has occurred. The final step in the PRP derivatization stream involves the bromoacetylation of the derivatized PRP, which is monitored by NMR for degree of bromoacetylation and derivatization.

The second, parallel process stream functionalizes the Pr carrier which is the outer membrane protein complex (OMPC) from *Neisseria meningitidis* serogroup B. This carrier is a particle (~ 50,000 kDa) that forms a stable colloidal suspension in aqueous systems. This high mass allows OMPC and its conjugates to be ultracentrifuged to a pellet for separation from the soluble nonconjugated PRP. The conjugate also can be retained by ultrafiltration membranes through which unconjugated PRP can permeate. In order to form its thiolated derivative, the OMPC is reacted with *N*-acetylhomocysteine thiolactone; the number of sulfhydryl groups per gram of Pr is determined by Ellman (Ellman, 1959) and Lowry (Lowry *et al.*, 1951) assays.

At this point, the bromoacetylated PRP and thiolated OMPC are reacted to form a thioether bond by bromide displacement from the activated PRP with the thiol functionality on the OMPC. This creates the conjugate, which is shown schematically in Fig. 1B. The thioether (the encircled atoms in the structure depicted below) is the relevant covalent bond:

$$\text{OMPC}-\text{NHCOCHCH}_2\overset{\displaystyle \overset{\text{NHCOCH}_3}{|}}{}\text{CH}_2\text{SCH}_2\text{CONH}\sim\sim\sim\text{PRP}$$

It is unlikely that a significant percentage of Pr is cross-linked, since the final conjugation reaction takes place in the presence of a large excess of activated PRP and light scattering analysis and scanning electron microscopy indicate little change in particle size distribution (J. Hennessey, personal communication).

Excess bromoacetyl groups in the conjugate (those that did not react with the OMPC thiols) next are reacted with *N*-acetylcysteamine to form a "capped" conjugate (~ 50,000 kDa) which then is separated from unconjugated PRP (~ 80 kDa) by diafiltration. The final capped conjugate is characterized as described in Section 3, and an aliquot is hydrolyzed with HCl to cleave all of the peptide bonds in the Pr and the amide bonds. In addition to all of the component amino acids of OMPC, two novel amino acids, *S*-carboxymethylhomo-cysteine (SCMHC) and *S*-carboxymethylcysteamine (SCMC), are released and are detectable in the amino acid analysis spectrum. This approach for defining covalency has been termed the "bigeneric spacer" method (Marburg *et al.*, 1986, 1987, 1989).

2.1.3. PRP-TT

This vaccine (Clemens *et al.*, 1992) is based on the method of Chu *et al.* (1983) and Schneerson *et al.* (1986). In a single process stream, the native PRP is activated with cyanogen bromide and reacted in situ with adipic acid dihydrazide to form a nucleophilic derivative. As discussed further in Section 2.3, the degree of derivatization (the number of adipic hydrazide units per 100 repeat units of PRP) for this intermediate corresponds to about a 2% weight loading, which is approximately 4 adipic hydrazide units per 100 repeat units of PRP. The carrier protein in this case is tetanus toxoid (TT) which is obtained by formalin treatment of tetanus toxin secreted by *Clostridium tetani*. The toxin has a mass of approximately 150 kDa prior to toxoiding (Mangalo *et al.*, 1968). To form the conjugate (depicted below and as a schematic model in Fig. 1A), the carboxyl groups of TT are condensed with the hydrazide group of activated PRP with EDAC:

$$\textit{TT}\text{--CONHNHCO(CH}_2)_4\text{CONHNHC}(=\text{NH})\text{O--}\textit{PRP}$$

Low-mass by-products are removed by SEC. The high-mass material contains the immunogen, which is characterized as described in Section 3.

2.1.4. HbOC

This methodology differs significantly from the other three processes in that the first step in the PRP derivatization process requires generation of aldehyde functionalities in the PRP. This is accomplished by using sodium metaperiodate to cleave the vicinal diols in PRP (Anderson and Eby, 1990), resulting in concomitant size reduction of the PRP polymer to small oligosaccharide fragments. The products of the reaction are fractionated by ultrafiltration. The degree of polymerization, defined as the number of repeat units in a single molecule, is 15–30 and the weight-average is approximately 20.

The Pr carrier used for HbOC is a nontoxic, genetic mutant of diphtheria toxin designated CRM_{197} (58 kDa) (Pappenheimer *et al.,* 1972; Colombatti *et al.,* 1989) which is antigenically equivalent to DT. The use of CRM_{197} offers a potential advantage as carrier over a chemically-created toxoid, because more nucleophilic nitrogens are available to form bonds with electrophilic partners such as aldehyde groups since none of the available lysines in CRM_{197} were reacted with formaldehyde in a toxoiding process.

The bond-forming chemistry used for this process is termed reductive amination and involves the reaction of an amine (from the Pr) with an aldehyde (from the periodate-treated PRP). The resultant Schiff base is reduced in situ by sodium cyanoborohydride, resulting in an alkylated amine. Thus, the activated PRP and CRM_{197} are reacted to form the conjugate:

$$CRM_{197}-NHCH_2CH_2OPO_2-(PRP)_{15-30}-OCH_2CH_2NH-CRM_{197}$$

which also is depicted as a schematic model in Fig. 1C.

The unreacted aldehydes then are reduced with sodium borohydride, and the conjugate is ultrafiltered to remove small reagents and unconjugated PRP. The retentate contains the conjugate, which is characterized as described in Section 3. Since the activated PRP previously was fractionated by ultrafiltration, the copresence of Ps and Pr in the retentate is indirect support for covalency (see Section 2.2 for discussion on direct proof for covalency).

2.2. Process Design and Quantitative Aspects of Covalency

As discussed in Section 1, the immunological basis for the Hib conjugate vaccines is the covalent coupling of PRP to a carrier protein, thereby converting PRP to a TD antigen. If PRP and carrier protein are linked by noncovalent forces, their separation in vivo becomes possible and the efficacy of the conjugate potentially is compromised. Therefore, a covalent bond probably is required, and all of the processes for the licensed Hib conjugates have been designed to use chemical reactions that predictably will achieve covalent linkage. However, the products of these conjugation reactions are of high mass, and the conventional physicochemical analyses of structure are not applicable for demonstrating that covalent bonds have been formed. Therefore, classical approaches to defining the structural nature of the product(s) are not practical for conjugates, and the determination of the covalency of the bond is addressed in two ways.

2.2.1. INDIRECT PROOF OF COVALENCY

This determination relies on separation of products and starting materials on the basis of size or physiochemical property. If Pr and Ps appear, after such a separation, in the same "compartment" (for example, a chromatographic fraction), and such a compartment is different from the "compartments" into which the reactants would separate, it can be concluded that a bond between the two must have been formed. However, these observations do not specify what type of bond (noncovalent versus covalent) exists. All of the conjugates provide methodologies for indirect confirmation of covalency.

2.2.2. DIRECT ASSAYS FOR PROOF AND QUANTITATION OF COVALENCY

Assays that detect a new amino acid that was created during conjugation can provide further proof that a covalent bond has been formed. Since the constituent amino acids of the carrier Pr and the new amino acid formed during conjugation are released by hydrolysis and determined in the same assay, a constituent amino acid can be used as an internal standard. Consequently a ratio can be calculated to define the degree of covalency, a value that is useful as a process control parameter. Because of the fundamental differences among the respective bond-forming chemistries, the optimal degree of covalency must be determined empirically for each conjugate type. Within each vaccine type, such assays, which verify that this ratio is within the specifications, provide another critical process control parameter, along with the Ps/Pr ratio, to verify consistency of manufacture.

As discussed in Section 2.1.2 for PRP-OMPC, SCMHC and SCMC are determined and these values, when referenced internally to a constituent of the conjugate, can be used to calculate the number of covalent bonds formed and the number of unreacted side chains capped after the conjugation reaction. The importance of such analytical control was illustrated clearly when certain postlicensure lots of PRP-OMPC were shown to have less-than-expected immunogenicity in the field. A thorough investigation of this issue by the manufacturer revealed that overderivatization of a subpopulation of PRP molecules with BuA_2 had occurred for some lots. This overderivatized population then preferentially reacted with the thiolated OMPC; this was responsible for the reduced immunogenicity. This phenomenon has been referred to as "hyperconjugation," which has been controlled by a process modification. In addition, levels of SCMHC and SCMC now have been employed to establish release specifications for the ratios of SCMHC/PRP and (SCMHC + SCMC)/PRP, the limits of which provide a check of all lots to ensure that the implemented changes continue to control the process and eliminate possibly hyperconjugated lots.

For HbOC, two types of analysis were developed to provide additional evidence for covalency (Smith *et al.,* 1989; Seid *et al.,* 1989). The first employs demonstration of the coincidence of antigenic reactivity to PRP and to CRM_{197} after SDS-PAGE and immunoblotting. The second approach follows the strategy developed for PRP-OMPC (*vide supra*) and involves the detection of the new amino acid formed when the lysines on the CRM_{197} are reductively aminated with the activated PRP. When the resultant conjugate is hydrolyzed in acid, N_ε-(2-hydroxyethyl)lysine is formed and detected by amino acid analysis.

2.3. Characterization of Starting Materials and Process Intermediates

Heretofore, vaccine materials were natural products, characterized by their isolation processes and the characteristics of the final immunogen. In the case of conjugate vaccines, these natural products are transformed into a series of chemical intermediates that require definition just as do the intermediates in a multistep organic chemical synthesis. This staged analytical system not only provides control of the overall process but also affords an understanding of the final product in structural terms.

The characteristics of the protein carriers (Table I) have been important factors in the development of these vaccines in that they have dictated: (1) the processes used for conjugation and reactant removal; (2) the properties of the final conjugates that bear on vaccine formulation and the immune response to it; and (3) the analytical assays required for characterization of process intermediates and of the final conjugate immunogens. In addition for PRP-TT and PRP-DT, the reaction of the epsilon-amino groups of lysine by formalin treatment in the toxoiding step has implications for subsequent process steps for PRP-DT and PRP-TT. Therefore, this toxoiding step should be consistent for different lots of DT and TT and for any formalin-treated proteins that might be used for other future conjugates.

Numerous publications and patents exist describing the purification and characterization of PRP (Anderson *et al.,* 1976; Kniskern *et al.,* 1981), which has a repeating unit composed of ribose, ribitol, and phosphate in equimolar ratios. Specifications (WHO Technical Report, 1991) require that the PRP preparations must contain > 32% ribose, 6.8–9.0% phosphorus, <1% protein, and <1% nucleic acid content. PRP is a family of polymers that vary in the number of the repeating units (Crisel *et al.,* 1975), hence molecular weight (Table I). In some cases an index of the molecular weight heterogeneity (sometimes termed polydispersity) also is determined (Hennessey *et al.,* 1993). For PRP-DT, PRP-OMPC, and PRP-TT, the size of the PRP that enters the conjugation reaction is only slightly smaller than Ps shed by the Hib bacterium growing in liquid culture. These PRP molecules initially still have several hundred repeating units, but may suffer some size degradation in the process of chemical modification. For the case of HbOC, the chemistry employed results in the partial depolymerization of PRP. By controlling the amount of periodate used for the oxidative depolymerization reaction, oligosaccharide fragments are obtained that are within the range of sizes that result in an immunogenic conjugate (Anderson *et al.,* 1989).

For all of the Hib conjugates, using either oligo- or polysaccharides results in an efficacious vaccine. This indicates that some or all of the protective epitopes are displayed on the final conjugate molecules. It should be noted, however, that some Ps, notably those of *N. meningitidis* B (Lifely *et al.,* 1987), *Streptococcus pneumoniae* type 14 (Wessels and Kasper, 1989) and Group B Streptococcus type III (Jennings *et al.,* 1981), display conformational epitopes that elicit neutralizing antibodies. It is not known whether PRP contains conformational epitopes, but it must be kept in mind that such epitopes may be required for a neutralizing antibody response. Therefore, in the development of new Ps-Pr conjugates, it may be critical that synthesis of a particular conjugate start with Ps of sufficiently high molecular weight to ensure that such size-associated conformers are present in the final conjugate. These data usually are determined immunologically by RIA, ELISA, or nephelose methods which are used to verify that antigenicity has been preserved.

For all of the processes, the derivatized PRP is characterized to ensure consistent functionalization. For the conjugates that proceed in two process streams (PRP-DT and PRP-OMPC), the derivatized Pr carrier also is subject to analytical control. Manufacturers also conduct additional analyses, such as verification of antigenic integrity.

2.4. Separation of Unconjugated Polysaccharide

It is unclear whether rigorous removal of unconjugated Pr from the final products is necessary. However, the effective dosages of the vaccines are based on *conjugated* PRP, and the release assays cannot discriminate between conjugated and unconjugated PRP. Furthermore, there is some evidence from animal immunogenicity studies that the presence of free Ps in a conjugate preparation can reduce the desired immune response (Peeters *et al.,* 1992). Therefore, processes must be employed to reduce the free Ps to appropriate low levels. Processes generally rely on biochemical separations based on the size differences of the conjugates and the free Ps; these size-based separations are most efficient if the starting Ps and Pr have molecular weights that differ by approximately 10-fold (Kniskern and Marburg, 1994). For the licensed vaccines, the specifications for unconjugated PRP (expressed as percent free Ps) are in the range of 10–37% (Table III).

3. CHARACTERIZATION OF BULK CONJUGATES AND FINAL CONTAINER VACCINES

Table II summarizes the assays and methodologies used to release and follow the stability of the Hib conjugate vaccines. Table III provides a compilation of the characteristics of the different immunogens and their corresponding vaccine formulations. Clearly, the inherent differences in the vaccine designs and processes have resulted in as many differences as common features among these products.

The vaccine content of the final container is calculated from the PRP assay. The PRP/Pr ratios vary considerably among the licensed conjugates. However, within a vaccine type, this determination will give an important indication of process consistency. The PRP-OMPC and HbOC conjugates also would be expected to have unique specifications related to the newly synthesized amino acids which relate to degree of conjugation. These parameters, along with the immunochemical and immunobiological assays discussed below, form the basis for releasing consistent and stable vaccine with predictably assured immunogenicity and efficacy in the target population.

The conjugated PRP must maintain its antigenic epitopes which are displayed as structural components on the bacterial capsule in order to elicit antibodies that bind to the bacterium and initiate complement-dependent bacteriolysis and phagocytic destruction of the Hib organism. Chemical assays for PRP do not measure antigenicity, which is determined by binding experiments using antibodies raised to native PRP as displayed on the bacterial capsule (van Dam *et al.,* 1990; Kniskern and Marburg, 1994). Some or all of this antigenicity can be lost during the processing steps. Therefore, such quality control is important not only in the final product but at each phase of a multistep process.

Because antigenicity *a priori* does not predict immunogenicity, the determination of the ability of the final vaccine to elicit functional antibodies in an appropriate animal model is critical. These tests, which will be discussed here only in terms of process control, rejection criteria, and release of vaccine, have been reviewed in detail (Vella and Ellis, 1992). Such in vivo assays, which measure the ability of conjugate vaccines to induce anti-PRP antibodies in experimental animals, have been developed in mice (Chu *et al.,* 1983; Vella *et al.,* 1990) and in infant rabbits (Anderson and Smith, 1977); nonconjugated

Table II
Characterization Assays

Chemical and physical assays	Method[a]	HbOC	PRP-DT	PRP-OMPC	PRP-TT
Assays on Ps and intermediates					
Molecular weight	SEC or UF	Yes	Yes	Yes	Yes
Degree of derivatization or functionalization	NMR	Yes	No	Yes	No
Antigenicity	Nephelose or RIA	Yes	Yes	Yes	Yes
Assays on Pr and intermediates					
Degree of derivatization or functionalization	Ellman	No	No	Yes	No
Assays on conjugate					
Concentration (dosage) Ps	Orcinol	Yes	Yes	Yes	Yes
Concentration Pr	Lowry	Yes	Yes	Yes	Yes
Ps/Pr ratio	Calculation				
Percent unconjugated Ps	SEC or UF	Yes	Yes	Yes	Yes
Direct assay of covalent linkage	AA analysis	Yes	No	Yes	No
Degree of cross-linking	AA analysis	Yes	No	Yes	No
Antigenicity					

(continued)

Table II
(continued)

Chemical and physical assays	Method[a]		Used for conjugate		
		HbOC	PRP-DT	PRP-OMPC	PRP-TT
Preclinical Immunogenicity					
In vivo potency (ED$_{50}$)	Adult mice or rabbits	Yes	Yes	Yes	Yes
T-cell dependency	Athymic (nude) mice	Yes	Yes	Yes	Yes
Infant primate immunogenicity	Infant Rhesus monkeys	No	No	Yes	No
Safety					
Pyrogen	Rabbit thermal induction	Yes	Yes	Yes	Yes
LPS	LAL	Yes	Yes	No	Yes
General safety	Mice and guinea pigs	Yes	Yes	Yes	Yes
Stability-indicating assays					
Antigenicity (in vitro potency)	Nephelose or RIA	Yes	Yes	Yes	Yes
In vivo potency	Adult mice or rabbits	Yes	Yes	Yes	Yes
% unconjugated PRP	SEC or UF or UC	Yes	Yes	Yes	Yes
pH		NS	NS	Yes	NS
Completeness of adsorption[b]	Nephelose or RIA	No	No	Yes	No
Covalency	AA analysis	NS	NS	Yes	NS

[a] Abbreviations: SEC = size-exclusion chromatography; UF = ultrafiltration; NMR = nuclear magnetic resonance; RIA = radioimmunoassay; UC = ultracentrifugation (the size of OMPC allows UC separation for PRP-OMPC); AA = amino acid; LAL = *Limulus* amoebocyte lysate; NS = not specific.

[b] At present, only PRP-OMPC is adsorbed to aluminum as an adjuvant. Other Hib conjugate vaccines in future combination vaccines also will be adsorbed to some extent.

Table III
Characteristics of the Conjugate Vaccines

Vaccine	PRP K_d (CL-4B)[a]	Proof of covalency	Unconjugated PRP removal	% free PRP	PRP dose	Protein dose	PRP/protein ratio	Form	Adjuvant	Preservative	References
HbOC	0.3–0.6[b]	Direct and indirect	Ultrafiltration	<10%	10 μg	ca. 25 μg	ca. 0.4	Liquid	None	Thimerosal[e]	Anderson and Eby (1990), WHO Technical Report (1991), USP DI (1992), *European Pharmacopoeia* (in preparation). *PDR* (1994)
PRP-DT	95% <0.75	Indirect	(NH₄)₂SO₄ precipitation	<37%	25 μg	ca. 18 μg	ca. 1.4[f]	Liquid	None	Thimerosal[e]	Schneerson et al. (1986), Gordon (1986), WHO Technical Report (1991), USP DI (1992) *European Pharmacopoeia* (in preparation), *PDR* (1994)
PRP-OMPC	85% <0.25	Direct and indirect	Ultrafiltration	<15%	15 μg[c]	ca. 250 μg[d]	ca. 0.06	Lyo[h]	Al³⁺	Thimerosal	Marburg et al. (1986, 1987, 1989), WHO Technical Report (1991), USP DI (1992), *European Pharmacopoeia* (in preparation), *PDR* (1994)
PRP-TT	60% <0.20	Indirect	NA[g]	<20%	10 μg	ca. 24 μg	ca. 0.4	Lyo[h]	None	None	Schneerson et al. (1986), WHO Technical Report (1991), *European Pharmacopoeia* (in preparation)

[a] Percentage of starting PRP whose distribution constant (K_d) is below the value specified as analyzed by CL-4B SEC.
[b] K_d (CL-2 B) for the starting PRP before it is reduced to an oligosaccharide by periodate oxidation for conjugation (see text for detailed description of the process).
[c] Developer is in the process of changing dose to 7.5 μg PRP and ca. 125 μg protein based on immunological equivalence.
[d] Reconstituted with diluent supplied by the manufacturer at time of use; manufacturer is in process of developing liquid formulation.
[e] Only in multidose vials.
[f] The release specification is a range from 1.2 to 1.7 (P. H. McVerry, personal communication).
[g] NA = not available.
[h] Manufacturer is developing a liquid formulation.

PRP is not immunogenic in either of these species. It also is possible to verify the functional activity of the induced anti-PRP by examining its ability: (1) to kill Hib organisms in a complement-dependent manner (Musher *et al.,* 1986); (2) to passively protect infant rats from challenge with Hib (Smith *et al.,* 1973); and (3) to enhance the ability of leukocytes to phagocytose and kill Hib (opsonophagocytosis) (Gray, 1990).

The TD nature of the immune response to the conjugates, which provides biological confirmation of covalent linkage, can be determined by comparing the anti-PRP responses of athymic nude mice, which are congenitally devoid of T cells, with those of their heterozygous littermates, which have a normal complement of T-helper cells (Baker, 1975). An infant primate immunogenicity assay also has been developed; this provides a predictor of vaccine immunogenicity in the target human infant population (Vella *et al.,* 1990). The inconsistent seasonal availability of infant Rhesus monkeys makes such an assay impractical for routine testing of every commercial vaccine lot, leaving the mouse and infant rabbit tests as the only practical in vivo release assays.

Table II summarizes the stability-indicating assays that are used to establish vaccine shelf life. Currently all of the licensed vaccines are stable for at least 2 years, which is their recommended shelf life. For the same reasons that it is important as a release specification, the measurement of free Ps also stands out as a critical parameter in determination of vaccine stability. Moreover, the same antigenicity and immunogenicity assays that were used to release the vaccine can be followed over time as an aid in predicting stability of the formulations. Phosphodiester linkages in PRP are susceptible to hydrolysis at elevated temperatures and at extremes of pH. This chemical event causes a pH change; therefore, pH drift is monitored for some of the conjugates as an early indication that such hydrolysis might be occurring. Future combination of the Hib conjugate vaccines with DTP, which is formulated on aluminum-based adjuvants, may necessitate that measurement of Al adsorption be applied to all conjugate vaccines.

The conjugate vaccines are tested for safety in mice and guinea pigs in which they may not cause loss of weight during a specified observation period (*Code of Federal Regulations*, 21CFR 610.11, 1991). Additionally, because PRP is isolated from Hib organisms which contain the pyrogenic lipopolysaccharide (OMPC also contains LPS), the conjugates and the formulated vaccines are tested for pyrogenicity in rabbits (*Code of Federal Regulations*, 21CFR 610.13, 1991). Since these conjugates are produced by reactions involving reactive chemical intermediates, a unique safety concern is raised (WHO Technical Report, 1991), viz., the reactive functional groups that were created for forming the requisite covalent bonds might also modify host Pr and other host macromolecules if they were present in reactive form in the final vaccine preparation. These safety considerations are addressed by incorporating special capping reactions into the processes, as described for PRP-OMPC and HbOC, or by validation of the ability of the process to reduce levels of potential reactive intermediates to insignificant levels. In addition, the question of whether an immune response is elicited to the linker moiety was addressed for PRP-OMPC. In these experiments, no antibody responses to SCMHC were detected in the sera of a group of vaccinated human infants (2 to 16 months of age), even after three doses of vaccine (J. Staub and P. P. Vella, unpublished data). All of the Hib conjugate vaccines have an excellent clinical safety record. Furthermore, Hib conjugate vaccines (and future Ps conjugates for which the PRP conjugates will provide the prototypes) are being developed into combination vaccine formulations with other pediatric vaccine compo-nents. In fact, one such combination of HbOC with DTP (Tetramune™, Lederle–Praxis Biologicals) already has been licensed.

4. IMMUNOGENICITY AND EFFICACY

The four Hib conjugate vaccines elicit anti-PRP in infants and young children but show different immunogenicity profiles. Sufficient studies of the immunogenicity and efficacy of these vaccines in infants were performed in the 1980s to early 1990s such that anti-PRP became accepted as an immunological surrogate for an effective Hib conjugate vaccine, as described below. Evaluations of the immunogenicity of these vaccines in infants typically were performed by immunizations at 2, 4, 6 and 15 months of age to coincide with the ages for administration of diphtheria–tetanus–pertussis (DTP) vaccine in the United States (other ages in other countries) and with regularly scheduled visits to pediatricians. Since there are variations in the quantitation of anti-PRP among different laboratories, the most reliable comparative immunogenicity data have come from head-to-head studies of different vaccines in the same clinical study with all sera assayed in blinded fashion in the same laboratory.

HbOC elicits no detectable anti-PRP post-dose one, low levels (approximately 0.5 μg/mL) post-dose two, but substantial anti-PRP post-dose three (approximately 5 μg/mL). The anti-PRP is of relatively higher avidity than that elicited by PRP-T or PRP-OMPC, is active in bactericidal and opsonophagocytic assays, is predominantly IgG, and primes for a memory response to PRP even after only two doses (Daum and Granoff, 1994). Hence, HbOC shows the properties of a TD antigen. The immune response to HbOC is augmented by carrier priming, in that infants receiving diphtheria toxoid at 1 month of age followed by HbOC (and DTP) at 2 and 4 months of age achieve higher anti-PRP responses than infants not receiving the 1-month dose (Granoff et al., 1993). HbOC was tested in an efficacy trial in north California (Black et al., 1991). Efficacy in 20,800 fully vaccinated children (2, 4, 6 months) compared with unvaccinated controls was 100% post-dose three [95% confidence interval (C.I.) 68–100%], 100% post-dose two (95% C.I. 47–100%), and 26% post-dose one (95% C.I. –166 to +80%). These results mirrored the immunogenicity data in that there was no invasive Hib disease in children receiving two doses of HbOC who are known to be fully primed to a robust post-dose-three or booster response. In a parallel uncontrolled efficacy study in Finland where 55,000 infants were vaccinated at 2, 4, and 14–18 months of age, there were only two cases of invasive Hib disease (Eskola et al., 1990a,b). HbOC was licensed in 1990 in the United States for use in infants at 2, 4, 6, and 15 months of age.

PRP-OMPC is unique among Hib conjugate vaccines in eliciting a significant post-dose-one anti-PRP response (approximately 1–2 μg/mL) which boosts moderately post-dose two (2–5 μg/mL) but does not boost further post-dose three. The anti-PRP is of relatively lower avidity than that elicited by PRP-TT or HbOC, is active in bactericidal and opsonophagocytic assays, is predominantly IgG, and primes for a memory response to PRP (Daum and Granoff, 1994). Thus, PRP-OMPC shows characteristics of both TI antigens (strong post-dose-one response, less efficient boosting) and TD antigens. PRP-OMPC was tested in a double-blind placebo-controlled efficacy study in Navajo Indians in the southwestern United States (Santosham *et al.,* 1991), a population with about ten times the incidence of invasive Hib disease as the general population and an earlier peak incidence of disease. The 5200 infants in the study were randomized to receive either vaccine or placebo at 2, 4, and 15 months of age. Efficacy was 93% post-dose two (95% C.I. 53–98%) and 100% post-dose one (95% C.I. 15–100%). These results were consistent with the immunogenicity data which show a strong post-dose-one anti-PRP response. PRP-OMPC was licensed in 1990 in the United States for use in infants at 2, 4, and 12–15 months of age.

PRP-TT elicits low levels of anti-PRP post-dose one, moderate levels post-dose two (approximately 1 μg/mL), and substantial levels post-dose three (approximately 5 μg/mL). The anti-PRP is of somewhat lower avidity than that elicited by HbOC but higher than that by PRP-OMPC, is active in bactericidal assays, is predominantly IgG, and primes for a memory response to PRP (Daum and Granoff, 1994). The immune response to PRP-TT also is augmented after carrier priming as for HbOC (Granoff *et al.,* 1992). Two double-blind randomized efficacy trials for PRP-TT were begun in the United States (south California and North Carolina) in 1989, but both trials were aborted early because of the licensure of HbOC for infants. While the trials did not proceed long enough for the results to have statistical significance, there were no cases of invasive Hib disease among approximately 6000 vaccinated infants compared to five in controls (Parke *et al.,* 1991; Fritzell and Plotkin, 1992). PRP-TT was used routinely between about 1990 and 1992 to vaccinate Finnish infants at 4 and 6 months of age; there were no cases of invasive Hib disease in 1991 (Peltola *et al.,* 1992). Since it was not possible ethically to conduct another efficacy trial in the United States, the FDA evaluated PRP-TT on the basis of anti-PRP as a surrogate marker of efficacy, where PRP-TT was compared to licensed Hib conjugate vaccines (HbOC, PRP-OMPC) in terms of anti-PRP levels post-dose three and their persistence out to the 15-month booster dose, priming for boost by PRP, bactericidal or opsonophagocytic activity, and class and subclass of anti-PRP. On the basis of this evaluation, PRP-TT was licensed in the United States in 1993 for use in infants at 2, 4, 6, and 15 months of age (Frasch, 1994).

PRP-DT is much less immunogenic in infants than the other Hib conjugate vaccines, eliciting only approximately 0.3 μg anti-PRP/mL post-dose three (Decker *et al.,* 1992). PRP-D was tested in an efficacy trial in Finland from 1985 to 1987 (Frasch, 1994). Efficacy in 58,000 vaccinated children, given doses at 3, 4, 6, and 14–18 months of age, was compared with an equal number of unvaccinated controls and was 90% (95% C.I. 70–96%) post-dose three and 100% post-dose four. PRP-DT also was tested in a double-blind placebo-controlled trial in Native Alaskans from 1984 to 1988 with vaccinations at 2, 4, and 6 months of age (Ward *et al.,* 1990). Efficacy post-dose three was only 43% (95% C.I. –43 to 78%), which was not statistically significant. Since PRP-DT has similar immunogenicity profiles in both efficacy studies, the disparity in outcomes is likely related to differences in epidemiology and study populations. The incidence of disease in Native Alaskans was much higher than in Finnish infants (1700 versus 57/100,000 per year, respectively) and peaks at a much earlier age (6 versus 15 months, respectively). Moreover, Native Alaskan families have a greater average number of children, more crowding, less breast-feeding, far inferior economic conditions, and different racial background compared to Finnish families. Nevertheless, given the difference in outcomes between the trials which have not yet been fully understood coupled with the availability of the more highly immunogenic Hib conjugate vaccines described above, PRP-DT has not been licensed in the United States for use in infants but is available as a booster dose at 15 months of age. In addition, PRP-DT was licensed for infants in both Germany and Iceland on the basis of the Finnish efficacy study, given that these countries have similar epidemiologies of Hib infection as that in Finland.

Thus, three Hib conjugate vaccines are licensed for infants in the United States and in many other developed countries. It is expected that additional Hib conjugate vaccines will be licensed based on immunological comparability to existing vaccines with anti-PRP as a surrogate marker of efficacy.

5. LESSONS FOR THE FUTURE

The vaccines described above are highly immunogenic and efficacious in the at-risk infant population for which they are licensed, and it is unlikely that they will be the subject of further development *per se*. However, they assuredly serve as the prototypes for future Ps conjugate vaccines, and therefore it will be useful to review lessons learned from their development.

5.1. The Implications of Carrier Choice and of Size of Starting Ps

5.1.1. CARRIER CHOICE

The kinetics of response to PRP-OMPC differ from the other three conjugates in that a significant immune response, which usually results in a protective level of antibody, occurs after the primary immunization; there is a moderate boost post-dose two, but no further boost with the third dose. The other three vaccines require a second vaccine administration to achieve similar anti-PRP titers, and this level is boosted by a third immunization. The carrier-specific need for priming with DT and TT is discussed in Section 4, and the processes developed for free Ps removal, which are dictated in part by the physicochemical attributes of the carriers, are discussed in Section 2.4.

5.1.2. SIZE OF STARTING PS

All bacterial capsular Ps are polymers composed of repeating subunits. For PRP, which has a linear structure, this has allowed development of immunogenic conjugates from both oligo- and polysaccharide starting materials. However, for development of other Ps conjugates (such as pneumococcal), the size of the starting Ps may be more constrained, and the immunogenicity of the resultant conjugate will continue to be verified on a case-by-case basis. With this caveat, the size of starting Ps for future conjugates can be chosen to facilitate free Ps removal in the process (see Section 2.4).

5.2. The Importance of Rigorous Process Control and Analytical Testing of the Process Intermediates, Final Products, and Formulated Vaccines

The Hib conjugates are already beginning to serve as models for the development of other Ps conjugate vaccines (see Chapter 31 for a review of the progress for pneumococcal Ps conjugates). To ensure the successful development of such future conjugates, the lessons regarding process control and analytical testing learned during the development of the Hib conjugates will be critical. In this regard, the importance of and proof of covalent conjugation is discussed in Sections 2.2 and 2.3; the importance of process control and analytical qualification for process intermediates is discussed in Section 2.3; the importance of low levels of free Ps is discussed in Section 2.4; and the analytical and immunological release testing of final products and formulated vaccines is discussed in Section 3.

In addition to serving as prototypes for other Ps conjugates, such as those for the Group B Streptococcus, *Staphylococcus aureus* and *N. meningitidis*, as well as for *S. pneumoniae* (as mentioned above), further development of these Hib conjugate vaccines will be necessary as they are incorporated into combined formulations with other licensed vaccines for routine pediatric administration. In addition to Tetramune®, other combinations including DTP with Hib, hepatitis B, and inactivated polio (IPV) vaccines are in advanced stages of development, and incorporation of other Ps conjugates such as those mentioned above (such as pneumococcal) undoubtedly will result in licensing of combinations with perhaps as many as a dozen components. Such combination formulations will make analytical release testing based on physicochemical criteria very challenging, and in vitro and in vivo immunological tests will evolve as the key methods to ensure compatibility and lack of interference among the components.

6. SUMMARY

In summary, all of the Hib conjugate vaccines are highly immunogenic and efficacious in children older than 12–15 months of age, and HbOC, PRP-OMPC, and PRP-T are highly immunogenic and demonstrated to be efficacious in infants as young as 2 months old. HbOC, PRP-OMPC, and PRP-T have been licensed in numerous countries for infants and are recommended for infant immunization. However, perhaps the greatest tribute one can pay to all four Hib vaccines described in this review is to note the dramatic decrease in the incidence of Hib disease that has occurred since their introduction. In fact, according to the *Morbidity and Mortality Weekly Report* (March 4, 1994), the incidence of Hib disease in children less than 5 years old has declined by 95% from 41 cases per 100,000 in 1987 to 2 cases per 100,000 in 1993, timing that coincides with the availability and use of the Hib conjugate vaccines (Anderson, 1994). As universal administration is achieved and the apparent vaccine-induced reduction in carriage of Hib by the population continues, Hib vaccines may follow the lead of past vaccines (such as smallpox, measles, mumps, rubella, and polio) toward eradication of disease or at least a high degree of medical control, thereby virtually eliminating the mortality and insidious morbidity associated with invasive Hib diseases.

REFERENCES

Alexander, H. E., Ellis, C., and Leidy, G., 1943, Treatment of type-specific *Haemophilus influenzae* infections in infancy and childhood, *J. Pediatr.* **20**:673–698.

Alexander, H. E., Heidelberger, M., and Leidy, G., 1944, The protective or curative element in type b *H. influenzae* rabbit serum, *Yale J. Biol. Med.* **16**:425–440.

Anderson, G., 1994, Progress toward elimination of *Haemophilus influenzae* type b diseases among infants and children—1987–1993, *Morbid. Mortal. Weekly Rep.* **48**:144–188.

Anderson, P. W., and Eby, R., 1990, Immunogenic Conjugates, U.S. Patent No. 4,902,506.

Anderson, P. W., and Smith, D. H., 1977, Immunogenicity in weanling rabbits of a polyribophosphate complex from *Haemophilus influenzae* type b, *J. Infect. Dis.* **136** (Suppl.):S63–S70.

Anderson, P. W., Pitt, J., and Smith, D. H., 1976, Synthesis and release of polyribophosphate by *Haemophilus influenzae* type b in vitro, *Infect. Immun.* **13**:581–589.

Anderson, P., Smith, D. H., Ingram, D. L., Wilkins, J., Wehrle, P. F., and Howie, V. M., 1977, Antibody to polyribophosphate of *Haemophilus influenzae* type b in infants and children: Effect of immunization with polyribophosphate, *J. Infect. Dis.* **136** (Suppl):S57–S62.

Anderson, P. W., Pichichero, M. E., Stein, E. C., Porcelli, S., Betts, R. F., Connuck, D. M., Korones, D., Insel, R. A., Zahradnik, J. M., and Eby, R., 1989, Effect of oligosaccharide chain length, exposed terminal group and hapten loading on the antibody response of human adults and infants to vaccines consisting of *Haemophilus influenzae* type b capsular antigen uniterminally coupled to the diphtheria protein CRM$_{197}$, *J. Immunol.* **142**:2464–2468.

Baker, P. J., 1975, Homeostatic control of antibody responses: A model based on recognition of cell-associated antibody by regulatory T cells, *Transplant. Rev.* **26**:3–20.

Black, S. B., Shinefield, H. R., Fireman, B., Hiatt, R., Polen, M., Vittinghoff, E., and the Northern California Kaiser Permanente Study Center Pediatrics Group, 1991, Efficacy in infancy of oligosaccharide conjugate *Haemophilus influenzae* type b (HbOC) vaccine in a United States population of 61,080 children, *Pediatr. Infect. Dis. J.* **10**:97–104.

Chu, C. Y., Schneerson, R., Robbins, J. B., and Rastogi, S. C., 1983, Further studies on the immunogenicity of *Haemophilus influenzae* type b and pneumococcal type 6A polysaccharide–protein conjugates, *Infect. Immun.* **40**:245–256.

Clemens, J. D., Ferreccio, C., Levine, M. M., Horowitz, I., Rao, M. R., Eng, M., Edwards, K. M. and Fritzell, B., 1992, Impact of *Haemophilus influenzae* type b polysaccharide–tetanus protein conjugate vaccine to concurrently administered diphtheria–tetanus–pertussis vaccine, *J. Am. Med. Assoc.* **267**:673–678.

Code of Federal Regulations, 1991, 21CFR 610.13.

Code of Federal Regulations, 1991, 21CFR 610.11.

Colombatti, M., Dell'Arciprete, L., Rappuoli, R., and Tridente, G., 1989, Selective immunotoxins prepared with mutant diphtheria toxins coupled to monoclonal antibodies, *Methods Enzymol.* **178**:404–422.

Crisel, R. M., Baker, R. S., and Dorman, D. E., 1975, Capsular polymer of *Haemophilus influenzae* type b. I. Structural characterization of the capsular polymer of strain Egan, *J. Biol. Chem.* **250**:4926–4930.

Daum, R. S., and Granoff, D. M., 1994, Lessons from the evaluation of immunogenicity, in: *Development and Clinical Use of Haemophilus b Conjugate Vaccines* (R. Ellis and D. M. Granoff, eds.), Dekker, New York, pp. 291–312.

Decker, M. D., Edwards, K. M., Bradley, R., and Palmer, P., 1992, Comparative trial in infants of four conjugate *Haemophilus influenzae* type b vaccines, *J. Pediatr.* **120**:184–189.

Dick, W. E., and Bevrett, M., 1989, Glycoconjucates of bacterial carbohydrate antigens: a survey and consideration of design and preparation factors, *Conjugate Vaccines* (J. M. Cruise and R. E. Lewis, eds.), Karger, Basel, p. 48.

Drug Information for the Health Care Professional, USP DI, Vol. IA, The U.S. Pharmacopeal Convention, Inc. (1992).

Ellman, G. L., 1959, Tissue sulfhydryl groups, *Arch. Biochem. Biophys.* **82**:70–77.

Eskola, J., Käyhty, H., Takala, A. K., Peltola, H., Rönnberg, P.-R., Kela, E., Pekkanen, E., McVerry, P., and Mäkelä, P. H., 1990a, A randomized, prospective field trial of a conjugate vaccine in the protection of infants and young children against invasive *Haemophilus influenzae* type b disease, *N. Engl. J. Med.* **323**:1381–1387.

Eskola, J., Peltola, H., Takala, A., Palmgren, J., and Mäkelä, P. H., 1990b, Protective efficacy of the *Haemophilus influenzae* type b conjugate vaccine HbOC in Finnish infants, *Program and Abstracts of the 30th Interscience Conference on Antimicrobial Agents and Chemotherapy*, Atlanta, October 1990, American Society for Microbiology, Washington, DC (Abstract No. 60).

Fothergill, L. D., Le Roy, D., and Wright, J., 1933, Influenzal meningitis: The relation of age incidence to the bactericidal power of blood against the causal organism, *J. Immunol.* **24**:273–284.

Frasch, C. E., 1994, Regulatory perspectives in vaccine licensure, in: *Development and Clinical Use of Haemophilus b Conjugate Vaccines* (R. Ellis and D. M. Granoff, eds.), Dekker, New York, pp. 435–453.

Fritzell, B., and Plotkin, S., 1992, Efficacy and safety of a *Haemophilus influenzae* type b capsular polysaccharide–tetanus protein conjugate vaccine, *J. Pediatr.* **121**:355–362.

Goebel, W. F., and Avery, O. T., 1931, Chemo-immunological studies on conjugated carbohydrate-protein. V. The immunological specificity of an antigen prepared by combining one capsular polysaccharide of type 3 pneumococcus with foreign protein, *J. Exp. Med.* **54**:431–437.

Gordon, L. K., 1986, Polysaccharide Endotoxoid Conjugate Vaccines, 1986, U.S. Patent No. 4,619,828.

Granoff, D. M., Anderson, E. L., Osterholm, M. T., Holmes, S. J., McHugh, J. E., Belshe, R. B., Medley, F., and Murphy, T. V., 1992, Differences in the immunogenicity of three *Haemophilus influenzae* type b conjugate vaccines in infants, *J. Pediatr.* **121**:187–194.

Granoff, D. M., Holmes, S. J., Belshe, R. B., and Anderson, E. L., 1993, The effect of carrier priming on the anticapsular antibody response to *Haemophilus influenzae* type b conjugate vaccines, *Pediatr. Res.* **33** (No. 4, Part 2):169A.

Gray, B. M., 1990, Opsonophagocidal activity in sera from infants and children immunized with *Haemophilus influenzae* type b conjugate vaccine (meningococcal protein conjugate), *Pediatrics* **85** (Apr. Suppl.):694–697.

Hennessey, J. P., Bednar, B., and Manam, V., 1993, Molecular size analysis of *Haemophilus influenzae* type b capsular polysaccharide, *J. Liquid Chromatogr.* **16**:1715–1729.

Jennings, H. J., Lugowski, C., and Kasper, D. L., 1981, Conformational aspects critical to the immunospecificity of the type 3 group B streptococcal polysaccharide, *Biochemistry* **20**:4511–4518.

Kaplan, S. L., 1994, Pathogenesis and treatment of infants and children, in: *Development and Clinical Use of Haemophilus b Conjugate Vaccines* (R. Ellis and D. M. Granoff, eds.), Dekker, New York, pp. 371–388.

Käyhty, H., Peltola, H., Karanko, V., and Mäkelä, P. H., 1983, The protective level of serum antibodies to the capsular polysaccharide of *Haemophilus influenzae* type b, *J. Infect. Dis.* **147**:1100–1105.

Kniskern, P. J., and Marburg, S., 1994, Conjugation: Design, chemistry and analysis, in: *Development and Clinical Uses of Haemophilus b Conjugate Vaccines* (R. W. Ellis and D. M. Granoff, eds.), Dekker, New York, pp. 37–69.

Kniskern, P. J., Hagopian, A., and Carlo, D. J., 1981, Meningitis Vaccines, U.S. Patent No. 4,307,080.

Lifely, M. R., Moreno, C., and Lindon, J. C., 1987, An integrated molecular and immunological approach towards a meningococcal group B vaccine, *Vaccine* **5**:11–26.

Lowry, O. H., Rosebrough, N. J., Farr, A. L., and Randall, R. J., 1951, Protein measurement with the Folin phenol reagent, *J. Biol. Chem.* **193**:265–275.

Mangalo, R., Bizzini, B., Turpin, A., and Raynaud, M., 1968, The molecular weight of tetanus toxin, *Biochim. Biophys. Acta* **168**:583–584.

Marburg, S., Jorn, D., Tolman, R. L., Arison, B., McCauley, J., Kniskern, P. J., Hagopian, A., and Vella, P. P., 1986, Bimolecular chemistry of macromolecules—Synthesis of bacterial polysaccharide conjugates with *Neisseria meningitidis* membrane protein, *J. Am. Chem. Soc.* **108**:5282–5297.

Marburg, S., Tolman, R. L., and Kniskern, P. J., 1987, Covalently-Modified Polyanionic Bacterial Polysaccharides, Stable Covalent Conjugates of Such Polysaccharides and Immunogenic Protein with Bigeneric Spacers, and Methods of Preparing Such Polysaccharides and Conjugates and of Confirming Covalency, U.S. Patent No. 4,695,624.

Marburg, S., Tolman, R. L., and Kniskern, P. J., 1989, Covalently-Modified Polyanionic Bacterial Polysac-charides, Stable Covalent Conjugates of Such Polysaccharides and Immunogenic Protein with Bigeneric Spacers, and Methods of Preparing Such Polysaccharides and Conjugates and of Confirming Covalency, U.S., Patent No. 4,882,317.

MMWR, 1994, Progress toward elimination of *Haemophilus influenza* type b disease among infants and children, *Morbid. Mortal. Weekly Rep.* **2**(8):144–147.

Musher, D., Gorlee, A., Murphy, T., Chapman, A., Zahradnik, J., Apicella, M., and Baughn, R., 1986, Immunity to *Haemophilus influenzae* type b in young adults: Correlation of bactericidal and opsonizing activity of serum with antibody to polyribosylribitol phosphate and lipooligosaccharide before and after vaccination, *J. Infect. Dis.* **154**:935–943.

Pappenheimer, A. M., Jr., Uchida, T., and Harper, A. A., 1972, An immunological study of the diphtheria toxin molecule, *Immunochemistry* **9**:891–906.

Parke, J. C., Schneerson, R., Reimer, C., Black, C., Welfare, S., Bryla, D., Levi, L., Pavliakova, D., Cramton, T., Schulz, D., Cadoz, M., and Robbins, J. B., 1991, Clinical and immunologic responses to *Haemophilus influenzae* type b–tetanus conjugate vaccine in infants injected at 3, 5, 7, and 18 months of age, *J. Pediatr.* **118**:184–190.

Peeters, C. C. A. M., Tenbergen-Meekes, A.-M. J., Poolman, J. T. M., Zegers, B. J., and Rijkers, G. T., 1992, Immunogenicity of a *Streptococcus pneumoniae* type 4 polysaccharide–protein conjugate is decreased by admixture of high doses of free saccharide, *Vaccine* **10**:833–840.

Peltola, H., Käyhty, H., Sivonen, A., and Mäkelä, P. H., 1977, *Haemophilus influenzae* type b capsular polysaccharide vaccine in children: A double-blind field study of 100,000 vaccinees 3 months to 5 years of age in Finland, *Pediatrics* **60**:730–737.

Peltola, H., Käyhty, H., Virtanen, M., and Mäkelä, P. H., 1984, Prevention of *Haemophilus influenzae* type b bacteremic infections with the capsular polysaccharide vaccine, *N. Engl. J. Med.* **310**:1561–1566.

Peltola, H., Kilpi, T., and Anttila, M., 1992, Rapid disappearance of *Haemophilus influenzae* type b meningitis after routine childhood immunization with conjugate vaccines, *Lancet* **340**:592–594.

Robbins, J. B., Parke, J. C., Jr., Schneerson, R., and Whisnant, J. K., 1973, Quantitative measurement of "natural" and immunization induced *Haemophilus influenzae* type b capsular polysaccharide antibodies, *Pediatr. Res.* **7**:103–110.

Santosham, M., Wolff, M., Reid, R., Hohenboken, M., Bateman, M., Goepp, J., Cortese, M., Sack, D., Hill, J., Newcomer, W., Capriotti, L., Smith, J., Owen, M., Gahagan, S., Hu, D., Kling, R., Lukacs, L., Ellis, R. W., Vella, P. P., Calandra, G., Matthews, H., and Ahonkhai, V., 1991, The efficacy in Navajo infants of a conjugate vaccine consisting of *Haemophilus influenzae* type b polysaccharide and *Neisseria meningitidis* outer-membrane protein complex, *N. Engl. J. Med.* **324**:1767–1772.

Schneerson, R., Robbins, J. B., Parke, J. C., Bell, C., Schlesselman, J. J., Sutton, A., Wang, Z., Schiffman, G., Karpas, A., and Shiloach, J., 1986, Quantitative and qualitative analysis of serum antibodies elicited in adults by *Haemophilus influenzae* type b and pneumococcus type 6A capsular polysaccharide–tetanus toxoid conjugates, *Infect. Immun.* **52**:519–528.

Seid, R. C., Jr., Boykins, R. A., Liu, D.-F., Kimbrough, K. W., Hsieh, C.-L., and Eby, R., 1989, Chemical evidence for covalent linkages of a semisynthetic glycoconjugate vaccine for *Haemophilus influenzae* type b disease, *Glycoconjugate J.* **6**:489–498.

Smith, A. L., Smith, D. H., Averill, D. R., Marino, J., and Moxon, E. R., 1973, Production of *Haemophilus influenzae* b meningitis in infant rats by intraperitoneal inoculation, *Infect. Immun.* **8**:278–290.

Smith, D. H., Madore, D. V., Eby, R. J., Anderson, P. W., Insel, R. A., and Johnson, C. L., 1989, Haemophilus b oligosaccharide–CRM197 and other haemophilus b conjugate vaccines. A status report, in: *Immunobiology of Proteins and Peptides V. Vaccines* (M. Z. Atassi, ed.), Plenum Press, New York, pp. 65–82.

Vadheim, C. M., and Ward, J. I., 1994, Epidemiology in developed countries, in: *Development and Clinical Use of Haemophilus b Conjugate Vaccines* (R. Ellis and D. M. Granoff, eds.), Dekker, New York, pp. 231–245.

van Dam, J. E. G., Fleer, A., and Snippe, H., 1990, Immogenicity of *Streptococcus pneumoniae* capsular polysaccharides, *Antoine van Leevvwenhoek* **58**:1.

Vella, P. P., and Ellis, R. W., 1992, Haemophilus b conjugate vaccines, in: *Vaccines: New Approaches to Immunological Problems* (R. W. Ellis, ed.), Butterworth–Heinemann, London, pp. 1–21.

Vella, P. P., Staub, J. M., Armstrong, J., Dolan, K. T., Rusk, C. M., Szymanski, S., Greer, W. E., Marburg, S., Kniskern, P. J., Schofield, T. L., Tolman, R. L., Hartner, F., Pan, S.-H., Gerety, R. J., and Ellis, R. W., 1990, Immunogenicity of a new *Haemophilus influenzae* type b conjugate vaccine (meningococcal protein conjugate) (PedvaxHIB®), *Pediatrics* **85**(Apr. Suppl.):668–675.

Ward, J., Brenneman, G., Letson, G. W., Heyward, W. L., and the Alaska *H. influenzae* Vaccine Study Group, 1990, Limited efficacy of a *Haemophilus influenzae* type b conjugate vaccine in Alaska native infants, *N. Engl. J. Med.* **323**:1393–1401.

Wessels, R., and Kasper, D. L., 1989, Antibody recognition of the type 14 pneumococcal capsule. Evidence for a conformational epitope in a neutral polysaccharide, *J. Exp. Med.* **169**:2121–2131.

WHO Technical Report, 1991, Requirements for *Haemophilus influenzae* type b Conjugate Vaccines (Requirements for Biological Substances No. 46), No. 814, pp. 15–37.

Chapter 31

Pneumococcal Conjugate Vaccines

Ronald Eby

1. INTRODUCTION

The development of multivalent pneumococcal vaccines for the prevention of both systemic and noninvasive pneumococcal diseases in infants, older adults, and immune-compromised individuals has gained increasing importance over the last decade. The rising cost of medical care has renewed interest in prevention instead of cure for a disease and in many cases cures may not be available with the increase in antibiotic resistance in many bacteria. Capsular polysaccharide vaccines for the prevention of systemic pneumococcal disease in adults and older children have been readily available for over 17 years but use of the vaccine in these age groups has been limited. The recent licensures of Hib–protein conjugate vaccines, 1987 for toddlers, 1990 for infants, have contributed to a dramatic reduction in the incidence of invasive *Haemophilus influenzae* type b disease and have thus demonstrated the tremendous potential of this technology to significantly reduce the incidence of diseases caused by encapsulated bacteria.

This chapter is a review of the published literature on pneumococcal–protein conjugate vaccines. It is not meant to be a review of pneumococcal disease. For more detailed reviews of pneumococcal disease, epidemiology, or the polysaccharide vaccine, the reader is directed to the numerous review articles (MMWR, 1994; Austrian, 1981a, 1989; Becker, 1993; Bruyn *et al.*, 1992; Dick and Beurret, 1989; Fedson, 1988; Gray and Dillon, 1989; Johnston, 1991; Robbins *et al.,* 1983; Schneerson *et al.,* 1982b; Shapiro, 1991; Watson *et al.,* 1993).

1.1. Epidemiology of Pneumococcal Disease

Streptococcus pneumoniae is a capsulated, gram-positive bacterium that is present as normal flora in the human upper respiratory tract and is a major or frequent cause of three systemic diseases: pneumonia, meningitis, and bacteremia and noninvasive bacterial otitis

Ronald Eby • Lederle–Praxis Biologicals, West Henrietta, New York 14586-9728.

Vaccine Design: The Subunit and Adjuvant Approach, edited by Michael F. Powell and Mark J. Newman. Plenum Press, New York, 1995.

media. In the United States, the overall incidence of systemic pneumococcal infections is estimated at 15–19/100,000 per year with rates of 50/100,000 in the geriatric adult and 160/100,000 in children less than 2 years old (MMWR 1989; Austrian, 1981b). The disease incidence are highest at the extremes of age, the infant and geriatric adult, and it is in these two age groups that production of antibodies to capsular polysaccharides are the lowest. Case fatalities can be high (40,000/year), especially in the geriatric population, in spite of the use of antibiotics, as many serotypes of *S. pneumoniae* are developing resistance to the usual antibiotic treatments.

The incidence of otitis media in children approaches 90% by age 5 years and the peak incidence occurs at 6–15 months of age. It was estimated that over 1.2 million cases of otitis media occur annually (Austrian, 1981b). Recent studies in Finland (Eskola *et al.,* 1992) and Israel (Dagan *et al.,* 1992) have shown that the peak incidence of systemic pneumococcal disease occurs around 12 months of age for the infant and that case fatalities from bacteremia, meningitis, and pneumonia are 1.0, 3.9, 1.5% and 2.3, 5, 0.5% (respective countries). Similar studies in northern California (Black *et al.,* 1994) have shown the same incidence of pneumococcal bacteremia and meningitis (Fig. 1) with the peak infection rates occurring around 12–18 months (232/100,000 for bacteremia and 14/100,000 for meningitis) and then dropping after 18 months.

Recent studies on the epidemiology of pneumococcal disease (Dagan *et al.,* 1992; Eskola *et al.,* 1992; Orange and Gray, 1993; Shapiro and Austrian, 1994) have shown that five serotypes (6B, 14, 19F, 23F, and 18C), of the 85 known serotypes, account for 70–80% of pneumococcal disease in infants and that in the United States, types 9V and 4 are ranked sixth and seventh. In Europe and developing countries, types 1 and 5 are more prevalent than types 4 and 9V. Thus, a pneumococcal conjugate vaccine targeted for infants and geriatric adults in the United States should contain at least seven serotypes (4, 6B, 9V, 14, 18C, 19F, and 23F) to achieve a 75–85% coverage. Conjugate vaccine formulations for Europe and elsewhere would include serotypes 1, 5, 6B, 14, 18C, 19F, and 23F. Other serotypes could and probably would be added as needed.

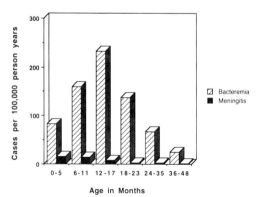

Figure 1. Incidence of systemic pneumococcal disease from 1988 to 1991 in northern California versus age in children less than 5 years of age. The graph was constructed from data provided by Dr. Stephen Black (Black *et al.,* 1994).

1.2. Current Licensed Pneumococcal Vaccines

There are 85 serotypes of *S. pneumoniae*, each having a unique capsular polysaccharide. Antibodies to the capsular polysaccharide have been known since the early 1920s to prevent systemic pneumococcal disease. In the mid-1940s, a hexavalent pneumococcal polysaccharide was licensed for use in the United States. The vaccine was withdrawn shortly after licensure because antibiotic treatment of disease was thought more effective than prevention. A 14-valent polysaccharide vaccine was introduced in 1977 and the valency was increased to 23 in 1983. The 23 pneumococcal serotypes account for 85–90% of all cases of pneumococcal diseases. The current polysaccharide vaccine is licensed for use in adults and children 2 years of age and older. The efficacy of the polysaccharide vaccine has been estimated to be 47–72% in adults and higher (93%) in immunocompromised individuals (Shapiro *et al.*, 1991). The use of the pneumococcal polysaccharide for the prevention of otitis media has been studied (Makela and Karma, 1980, 1989; Makela *et al.*, 1981, 1983a,b; Teele *et al.*, 1981) and the results have been variable. In many studies the incidence of otitis media caused by pneumococcal serotypes included in the vaccine was decreased but the overall incidence of otitis has remained the same. This is a concern since otitis media is caused by many different bacteria and viruses and a vaccine to a single organism—no matter how efficacious—may not lower the overall incidence of disease. The studies showed that older children responded better to the polysaccharide vaccine than did infants but that even in older children protection decreased after 6 months.

1.3. The Need for Pneumococcal Conjugate Vaccines

The efficacy and use of the polysaccharide vaccine in adults and children obviously can be improved primarily because persons at the extremes of age do not respond or respond weakly to T-independent antigens such as polysaccharides. The infant's immune system is not mature enough to respond to most T-independent antigens (polysaccharides). Maturation of the immune response to most capsular polysaccharides in infants occurs around the age of 2 years but the response to some pneumococcal serotypes, such as type 6B, does not mature until almost 5 years of age. The use of saccharide–protein conjugation technology allows for the conversion of T-independent antigens to T-dependent antigens that will induce appropriate immune responses in both infants and older adults.

The increased incidence of antibiotic-resistant *S. pneumoniae* strains is continuing and will continue to increase (Watson *et al.*, 1993). In 1993, over 40 articles and abstracts were presented on the rise in antibiotic-resistant and multiply antibiotic-resistant pneumococci. Vancomycin is the only one of the antibiotics to which *S. pneumoniae* has not developed resistance but this may change shortly. The combination of drug-resistant *S. pneumoniae* with the need to prevent disease in infants, geriatric adults, and immunocompromised persons has led to the development of multivalent saccharide–protein conjugate vaccines. Current U.S. conjugate vaccine in development has seven serotypes (4, 6B, 9V, 14, 18C, 19F, and 23F) (Kennedy and Anderson, 1993) and types 1 and 5 could be added or substituted for European or developing countries. It is ironic that the widespread use of antibiotics caused the first pneumococcal vaccine to be withdrawn from the marketplace and it is the use of antibiotics leading to drug resistance that now demands the development of prevention in the form of vaccines.

2. PNEUMOCOCCAL CONJUGATE VACCINES

2.1. Chemical Structures

Considerable data on the immunogenicity–structure relationships have been amassed for carbohydrate–protein conjugates during the development of the Hib glycoconjugate vaccines (see Chapter 30). It is known that the antibody responses of the carbohydrate-protein conjugates can be affected by the size of the saccharide (such as polysaccharide versus fragments or oligosaccharide), the carrier protein, the nature and number of covalent bonds between the saccharide and protein, and the ratio of saccharide to protein in the final conjugate vaccine, all of which contribute to the three-dimensional structure of the conjugate vaccine (such as neoglycoprotein, lattice or particle). The dose of the carbohydrate, the method of vaccine delivery, and the use of immune stimulants or adjuvants also have an impact on the immune response. The minimum requirements on the synthesis of glycoprotein conjugate vaccines are that the B-cell epitope(s) of the saccharide and the T-cell epitope(s) of the carrier should be functional after covalent attachment. Most of the data accumulated have been on individual vaccines and only a few direct comparisons of glycoconjugates with varied structures have been investigated. One fact that has come out of comparative studies is that the dose of the carbohydrate must be kept constant; if not, the differences in antibody responses seen may be related only to a dose response.

There have been several reviews of carbohydrate–protein conjugate vaccines (Becker, 1993; Dick and Beurret, 1989; Schneerson et al., 1982a, 1982b, 1982c; Stowell and Lee, 1980). One of the more detailed reviews that deals with the concepts of the nature and effect of the chemical structure of glycoconjugates is that of Dick and Beurret (1989) and the reader is directed to that review for a more detailed account of glycoconjugate structure and function. Table I lists most of the pneumococcal saccharide–protein conjugates that have been reported in the literature over the last 60 years, including the first synthetic pneumococcal glycoconjugates (Goebel and Avery, 1931).

2.1.1. NEOGLYCOCONJUGATES

Neoglycoconjugates (Stowell and Lee, 1980) are synthesized by covalently linking a monofunctionalized saccharide moiety to a soluble protein or peptide carrier. Since the saccharide is monofunctional, only one covalent bond between carbohydrate unit and the protein can be formed and the resulting glycoconjugate structure is without cross-linking between protein molecules. Neoglycoconjugates can also be formed between multifunctionalized saccharides and proteins if the conditions are controlled very carefully. Of the glycoconjugates listed in Table I, only a few have truly neoglycoprotein structures. Most of the conjugates were synthesized by coupling either short oligosaccharides activated through the reducing end of the saccharide unit (Arndt and Porro, 1991; Fattom et al., 1988; Goebel, 1938; Lin and Lee, 1982; Paradiso et al., 1993; Porro, 1987; Porro et al., 1985, 1986) or synthetic saccharide repeats that are covalently coupled to a protein or

Table I
Pneumococcal Conjugate Vaccines

Serotype	Saccharide[a]	Protein[b]	Coupling Method[c]	Reference
3	CPS	ESA	Diazobenzylether	Goebel and Avery (1931)
	Cellobiuronic acid	ESA	Diazobenylglucoside	Goebel (1938)
	CPS	BGG	Trichloros-triazine	Paul et al. (1971)
	CPS	DTd,TTd,BSA	Carbodiimide	Beuvery et al. (1982)
	Hexacellobiuronic acid	BSA, KLH, BGG, TTd	Isothiocyanate	Snippe et al. (1983a)
4	CPS or fragment	TTd	Aminocaproic acid	Peeters et al., (1991a)
6A	CPS	TTd	Adipic acid dihydrazide	Chu et al. (1983)
	Fragment	CRM$_{197}$	SIDEA linker	Porro et al. (1986)
8	CPS	S-layers	Reductive amination	Malcolm et al. (1993)
9V	CPS	TTd	Adipic acid dihydrazide	Lu et al. (1991)
12F	CPS	DTd	Thiolation + SPDP	Fattom et al. (1988)
14	CPS	PT	Adipic acid dihydrazide	Schneerson et al. (1992)
	CPS	BSA	Adipic acid dihydrazide	Verheul et al. (1989)
	Fragment	Peptide	SIDEA linker	Paradiso et al. (1993)
17F	Partial synthetic	KLH	Thioether	de Velasco et al. (1993)
19F	CPS	hIgG,BSA	Reductive amination	Lin and Lee (1982)
	CPS	Pneumolysin	Aminocaproic acid	Paton et al. (1991)
6B,14, 19F,23F	Fragments	CRM$_{197}$	SIDEA linker	Arndt and Porro (1991)
	RMwCPS	OMPC	Bigeneric	Vella et al. (1992)
6B,14,18C, 19F,23F	CPS/fragments	DTd	Reductive amination	Anderson and Betts (1989)
6A,6B,18C, 19F,23F	CPS/fragments	CRM$_{197}$	Reductive amination	Eby et al. (1993)

[a]CPS = capsular polysaccharide, RMwCPS = reduced-molecular-weight CPS.
[b]ESA = equine serum albumin, BSA = bovine serum albumin, KLH = keyhole limpet hemocyanin, DTd = diphtheria toxoid, TTd = tetanus toxoid, PT = pertussis toxin, BGG = bovine gamma globulin, CRM$_{197}$ = nontoxic mutant diphtheria toxin, hIgG = human immunoglobulin, OMPC = outer membrane protein complex of *Neisseria meningitidis*.
[c]SIDEA = disuccinimidyl ester of adipic acid, SPDP = *N*-succinimidyl 3-(2-pyridyldithio)propionate.

peptide using a linker group on the reducing end of the molecule (de Velasco et al., 1993; Snippe et al., 1983a). The peptide glycoconjugate reported by Paradiso (Paradiso et al., 1993) is unique in that both the saccharide and the carrier are monofunctional.

The procedure of Porro et al. hydrolyzes the capsular polysaccharide to low-molecular-weight oligosaccharide fragments of three to five repeat units. The oligosaccharides are reacted with either ammonia or diaminoethane at the reducing end to give a free terminal amino group. The amino group is reacted with an excess of the disuccinimidyl ester of adipic acid to introduce an active succinimidyl ester group. The activated oligosaccharide is then reacted with nontoxic mutant of diphtheria toxin (CRM$_{197}$) or any other protein or peptide with free amino group(s) to give a covalent amide bond. The glycoconjugates had up to ten oligosaccharides coupled per protein molecule. The oligosaccharide–peptide conjugate reported by Paradiso (Paradiso *et al.*, 1993) was prepared similarly except that a peptide presenting a T-cell epitope of CRM_{197} was used instead of the native protein.

Lin and Lee (1982) reacted the reducing end of the native 19F pneumococcal polysaccharide directly with the protein through a reductive amination to the lysyl groups by the method of Gray. The resulting conjugate vaccine was not characterized.

The type 3 pneumococcal conjugate of Goebel (Goebel, 1938) was prepared by glycosylating cellobiuronic acid with p-nitrobenzyl alcohol and then converting the nitro group into a diazo function. The monofunctional oligosaccharide was then coupled to albumin to give a pneumococcal conjugate vaccine.

Snippe *et al.* (1983a) prepared a similar type 3 pneumococcal conjugate vaccine by reacting hexacellobiuronic acid with 2-(4-aminophenyl)ethylamine using reductive amination. The terminal arylamino group was converted to a thiocyanate with thiophosgene and then coupled to the free lysyl amino groups of a variety of proteins. The glycoconjugates contained between 6 and 16 hexacellobiuronic acid groups per protein.

De Velasco *et al.* (1993) are exploring the minimum requirements for a pneumococcal type 17F glycoconjugate by synthesizing partial structures of the type 17F repeat unit (di-, tri-, and tetrasaccharides of the heptasaccharide repeat) having a 3-aminopropyl group on the reducing end. The aminopropyl group was converted to a thioacetate function that was then coupled to KLH that had been bromoacetylated to give oligosaccharides coupled by thio ether bonds. Ratio of carbohydrate to protein (w/w) for the conjugates varied between 0.04 (disaccharide) and 0.23 (tetrasaccharide). Type 17F polysaccharide–KLH conjugates were prepared as a control by the adipic acid dihydrazide method (see Section 2.1.2).

All of these glycoconjugates are characterized as soluble conjugates with a molecular weight that is equal to the weight of the protein plus the added weight of the covalently attached saccharide (Arndt and Porro, 1991; Porro, 1987; Porro *et al.*, 1985, 1986). The major advantage of these glycoconjugates is that their structure is easily controlled by the size and structure of the saccharide and the degree of loading on the protein carrier resulting in a fairly uniform composition. This is especially important when trying to relate the vaccine immunogenicity of conjugate vaccines to the structure of the saccharide and the loading on the carrier.

A disadvantage of the neoglycoconjugates can be that their relatively small size, especially when peptide carriers are used, or the use of some native proteins, such as CRM_{197}, can make the vaccines poorly immunogenic because of the short biological half lives of either the carrier or the vaccine unless a depot adjuvant such as alum is used to absorb the vaccine (Arndt and Porro, 1991; Paradiso *et al.*, 1993; Porro, 1987; Porro *et al.*, 1985, 1986). Preclinical and clinical studies by Lederle–Praxis Biologicals have been performed on pneumococcal conjugate vaccines prepared by the method of Arndt and Porro (1991) and the results are reported in Sections 2.2 and 2.3.

2.1.2. LATTICE STRUCTURES

Carbohydrate–protein conjugates that have a lattice or cross-linked structure are usually prepared from capsular polysaccharides or fragments of polysaccharides. The saccharides are randomly activated along the main chain with multiple functional groups that are then covalently coupled to a polyfunctional protein carrier.

The first pneumococcal glycoconjugate reported by Goebel and Avery (1931) involved random etherification of the type 3 polysaccharide with nitrobenzylchloride in base, followed by conversion of the nitrobenzyl group to a diazo functional group and then coupling to albumin. The conjugate formed was insoluble in water presumably because of the extensive cross-linking of the protein with the polysaccharide. This is a common occurrence with lattice-type glycoconjugates. While insolubility is not generally a problem and may be a benefit as far as immunogenicity is concerned, most researchers prefer to work with soluble glycoconjugates for ease of purification, characterization, sterilization, and immunization. Also, aromatic linkers are usually avoided since they are themselves usually highly immunogenic, leading to neoantigens that could cause problems when administered as vaccines in humans.

As shown in Table I, many of the conjugation methods involve randomly reacting the polysaccharide with adipic acid dihydrazide (ADH) and then coupling the activated saccharide to a protein using a carbodiimide (usually EDC) (Chu *et al.*, 1983; Lu *et al.*, 1991; Paton *et al.*, 1991; Verheul *et al.*, 1989). The procedure was developed by Schneerson and Robbins (Schneerson *et al.*, 1980) for preparing Hib glycoconjugates and was later adapted to pneumococcal conjugates (Chu *et al.*, 1983). Again, depending on the reaction conditions, the glycoconjugate synthesized is usually of a large molecular weight with some insoluble material that is usually removed by centrifugation or filtration. In many cases it is the increase in molecular size, especially of the protein carrier, that provides the evidence of a successful conjugation reaction. The large molecular weight of the conjugate usually facilitates the removal of the unreactive protein but it usually interferes with the removal of unreacted saccharide unless low-molecular-weight polysaccharide fragments are used in the coupling.

The ADH method of coupling has been used by Connaught and Pasteur Merieux to prepare their respective Hib glycoconjugate vaccines, ProHIBit® and Act-HIB®. The protein carrier used is diphtheria toxoid and tetanus toxoid for Connaught and Pasteur Merieux, respectively. It has been reported (*Drug Research Reports*, 1993; *FDC Reports*, 1993) that Pasteur Merieux–Connaught are working on pneumococcal conjugate vaccines, but nothing to date has been published on either company's product.

A variation of the ADH coupling method is to use aminocaproic acid as the linker and to couple the acid to the saccharide by the cyanogen bromide method and then couple the activated saccharide to the protein using a carbodiimide (EDC) (Paton *et al.*, 1991).

Another general method is to randomly activate the capsular polysaccharide or fragments of the polysaccharide by reaction with periodate. The reaction leads to a random oxidative cleavage of vicinal hydroxyl groups of the carbohydrates with the formation of reactive aldehyde groups. With most of the pneumococcal serotypes, the reaction with periodate does not cause a reduction in the molecular weight of the polysaccharide or fragment since the oxidation takes place either on branch side chains or on cyclic sugar residues of the main chain. In either case, the main chain is not cleaved and the molecular size remains intact. Coupling to the protein carrier is a direct amination to the lysyl groups of the protein (Anderson and Betts, 1989; Eby *et al.*, 1994; Malcolm *et al.*, 1993) . A spacer group such as aminocaproic acid can be reacted with the aldehydes by reductive amination and then coupled to the protein lysyl groups by EDC coupling (Peeters *et al.,* 1992). The glycoconjugates synthesized are of high molecular weight because of cross-linking of the protein unless very small polysaccharide fragments are used in the coupling reaction. Advantages of the reductive amination procedure are that linker molecules are unnecessary, thus removing a potential neoantigen group, and that a very stable secondary amine or in some cases a tertiary amine linkage is formed between the saccharide and the protein if no linker molecule is used in the reaction.

The direct reductive amination procedure is used by Lederle–Praxis Biologicals to prepare their pneumococcal conjugate vaccines using CRM$_{197}$ as the carrier protein and either polysaccharide or polysaccharide fragments consisting of approximately 20 repeat units, as the saccharide (Eby *et al.,* 1993). Anderson and Betts (1989) and Pichichero and Anderson (1993), working at the University of Rochester Medical Center, are also using direct reductive amination to prepare clinical trial pneumococcal conjugate vaccines.

2.1.3. PARTICLE-BASED VACCINES

Only two of the pneumococcal protein conjugate vaccines listed in Table I use insoluble particles as the protein carrier. These are the Merck vaccines that use outer membrane protein complexes (OMP or OMPC) of *Neisseria meningitidis* (Marburg *et al.,* 1986; Vella *et al.,* 1992) and the S-layer particles of Malcolm (Malcolm *et al.,* 1993).

The Merck pneumococcal conjugate vaccine is prepared using essentially the same procedure as their Hib conjugate vaccine (Marburg *et al.,* 1986). The pneumococcal polysaccharide is first reduced in size (350–600 kDa) by heat or sonication treatment and then derivatized with diaminobutane and carbonyldiimidazole to introduce amino groups into the polysaccharide. The amino groups are then reacted with *p*-nitrophenylbro-moacetate to convert them to bromoacetyl functions. Meanwhile the OMPC is reacted with *N*-acetylhomocysteine thiolactone to introduce thio groups. The conjugation reaction involves the coupling of the thio groups of the derivatized OMPC with the bromoacetyl functions of the polysaccharide resulting in a very stable thioether bond. Unreacted carbohydrate is removed by precipitating the conjugate in water. The supernatant contains the unreacted polysaccharide and other reagents. Unreacted bromoacetyl functions on the polysaccharide are capped with *N*-acetylcysteamine. The coupling method is named by Merck as bigeneric since it involves the use of two linkers that are coupled together. One advantage of the process is that the number of covalent bonds is easily determined by amino acid analysis of the conjugate since each covalent bond between the saccharide and the OMPC results in a new and unique amino acid, *S*-(carboxymethyl)cysteamine. Ratios of carbohydrate to protein range from 0.15 to 0.2 (w/w) (Vella *et al.,* 1992).

The S-layers reported by Malcolm *et al.* (1993) were prepared from *Bacillus alvei* CCM2051. Type 8 pneumococcal oligosaccharides, of one to eight repeat units, were coupled to the S-layers either by reductive amination of the periodate-oxidized oligosac-charide or by carbodiimide-mediated coupling of the uronic acid groups of the oligosac-charide (Davis and Preston, 1981). The physical characteristics of the S-layer conjugate vaccines were not reported.

2.2. Preclinical Analysis

In general, if the pneumococcal protein conjugates have the minimal requirements of a covalent bond between the saccharide and protein carrier, intact B-cell epitopes for the saccharide, and intact T-cell epitopes for the protein, then they will function as T-dependent antigens in animals (Paradiso *et al.*, 1993) and induce an anamnestic response following multiple injections. All of the pneumococcal conjugates shown in Table I have met these minimum requirements and have induced T-dependent responses in either mice, rabbits, or monkeys. The next section will primarily discuss differences seen in pneumococcal conjugates where comparisons have been reported.

2.2.1. IMMUNOLOGICAL ANALYSIS

The first pneumococcal vaccines made by Goebel and Avery (Avery and Goebel, 1931; Goebel, 1938, 1939, 1940a; Goebel and Avery, 1931) demonstrated that rabbits produced type 3-specific antibody responses that were boostable on repeated injections. Similar responses were seen for both the type 3 polysaccharide– and cellobiuronic acid–protein conjugates. Snippe *et al.* (1983b) have shown that mice respond to a hexacellobiuronic acid–protein conjugate producing both IgG and IgM antibodies, but when type 3 polysaccharide was used to immunize mice, only an IgM response was observed. Paul *et al.* (1971) reported that rabbits primed by immunizing with killed type 3 pneumococci could be boosted by a type 3 polysaccharide–bovine gamma globulin (BGG) conjugate but not with the type 3 polysaccharide provided that the rabbits were first immunized with BGG. This group also reported that rabbits would respond to a single injection of type 3 conjugate.

Schneerson and colleagues (Chu *et al.*, 1983; Schneerson *et al.*, 1984) showed that type 6A pneumococcal protein conjugates were immunogenic in mice and in monkeys, both juvenile and infant. The magnitude of type 6A antibody responses in monkeys were much less than those seen for the corresponding Hib conjugate vaccines and the responses of juvenile monkeys were higher than those of infant monkeys. This was one of the first indications that different polysaccharides or different serotype conjugate vaccines can give varied responses in both animals and humans.

Fattom *et al.* (1988, 1990) reported that the magnitude of the type-specific responses in both mice and adult humans injected with type 12F pneumococcal–diphtheria toxoid conjugates appear to be dependent on the size of the saccharide coupled to the protein. Higher-molecular-weight polysaccharide conjugates induce higher antibody responses than the lower-molecular-weight polysaccharide conjugates, although the difference was slightly less than twofold in both mice and humans.

Peeters *et al.* (1991a,b, 1992) have prepared type 4 pneumococcal–tetanus toxoid conjugates using either polysaccharides or oligosaccharides, consisting of 12 repeat units, with and without a six-carbon spacer or linker and variable saccharide-to-protein ratios. Type-specific antibody responses induced in mice were higher for conjugates synthesized with linkers. Antibody responses were also higher for conjugates with higher saccharide-to-protein ratios and polysaccharides were more immunogenic than oligosaccharides. The anti-saccharide isotype antibody response was primarily IgG and IgM; the subclass response was predominantly IgG1 with some IgG3. The effect of free or unreacted saccharide in the pneumococcal conjugate on the type-specific response was also investigated. Low levels of free saccharide had no effect on the immune response, but high levels, 10- to 50-fold over the conjugate dose, did suppress the antibody responses to both the primary and secondary immunizations in both adult and infant mice. Repeated immunizations decreased the saccharide-specific antibody response but not the anti-protein carrier-specific response. They speculated that high doses of conjugates may lead to activation of T-suppressor cells and a subsequent decrease in the saccharide-specific antibody responses.

Lederle–Praxis Biologicals has investigated three pneumococcal vaccine forms: polysaccharide reductively aminated to CRM_{197} (RA-poly), saccharide fragments (20 repeat units) reductively aminated to CRM_{197} (RA-Oligo) (Eby *et al.*, 1994), and short oligosaccharides (3–12 repeat units) coupled to CRM_{197} through a terminal linker group (Linker-Oligo) (Arndt and Porro, 1991). The reductively aminated lattice forms were very immunogenic in mice and rabbits at low doses (less than 2.5 μg) but less immunogenic at higher doses (greater than 10 μg). This held true for either monovalent vaccines or polyvalent vaccines in which the total saccharide dose was greater than 10 μg.

The linker forms, neoglycoproteins, required higher doses (5–30 μg) to induce similar immune responses, especially in mice. The linker form also required absorption to alum (aluminum phosphate or hydroxide) to induce a significant immune response. The size of the oligosaccharide used to synthesize the linker conjugates also was important for immunogenicity. The linker conjugates synthesized with oligosaccharides that were greater than ten repeat units (Dp >10) were poorly immunogenic in both mice and rabbits while linker conjugates synthesized with oligosaccharides of Dp 3–5 were highly immunogenic in both animals (Arndt and Porro, 1991).

Thus, it appears important to formulate these multivalent vaccines so that the total carbohydrate dose is low to avoid suppression and yet high enough for each individual serotype to give a response. Optimal doses in mice ranged between 10 ng and 1 μg per serotype and depended on the specific serotype.

All of the vaccine forms induced low to moderate primary responses and good booster responses as would be expected for T-dependent antigens. The antibodies were mainly of the IgG isotype but IgM antibody levels also increased following the booster dose although this increase was independent of the vaccine form. To date, the animal data obtained using the various vaccine forms are insufficient to allow differentiation of the vaccines prior to testing in humans.

The Merck vaccine (Pnc-OMPC) (types 6B, 14, 19F, and 23F) on aluminum hydroxide has been tested preclinically in mice, chinchillas, and monkeys (Marburg *et al.*, 1986; Giebink *et al.*, 1991, 1993b; Vella *et al.*, 1992). Antisaccharide responses in mice (*nu/+*) were much higher after three i.p. injections (0.5 μg CHO/dose) than the responses in *nu/nu* mice, indicating a T-dependent antigen. The order of the type-specific immune response was 6B>14>19F>>23F. In infant monkeys (Vella *et al.*, 1992), both African green and rhesus, the monovalent vaccines showed an antibody response after one or two injections (either 0.5- or 5-μg doses). There was little difference in the saccharide-specific antibody titers between the two doses in the African green monkeys. Infant rhesus monkeys responded to the 6B-OMPC at doses between 0.02 and 10 μg and again antibody responses were similar. All of the type-specific responses were clearly T-dependent and primarily of the IgG isotype.

The Pnc-OMPC vaccines were tested in chinchillas as monovalent (6B or 23F), bivalent (6B+23F), and tetravalent (6B+14+19F+23F) forms, formulated at doses from 0.5 to 8 μg/kg for the monovalent vaccines and 2.0 μg/kg for the bi- and tetravalent vaccines (Giebink et al., 1991, 1993b). Responses were induced using the monovalent 6B-OMPC after a single injection and a booster response was observed after a second injection. Antibody responses to 6B-OMPC were similar for the different doses. Responses to type 23F were similar after a single injection of the monovalent, bivalent, and tetravalent vaccines at the 2.0 μg/kg dose. Two doses of the tetravalent vaccine induced less antibody to 6B and 23F than a single injection of the monovalent vaccine, whereas type 14 and 19F responses were higher compared to the single injection. IgG and serum IgA but not IgM titers were increased following booster doses.

Another aspect of preclinical studies is the use of adjuvants. Immune responses to most pneumococcal protein conjugates can be improved by absorption to alum, either aluminum phosphate or aluminum hydroxide. All of the companies that have conjugate vaccines in current clinical trials use some type of alum in their formulations. A limited number of experiments of other adjuvants have been conducted (van Dam et al., 1989; van de Wijgert, et al., 1991; Verheul et al., 1989; Zigterman et al., 1988). The nonionic block copolymers, NBPs 1501 and L121, increase the IgG and IgM responses to type 3 pneumococcal conjugates in mice (van Dam et al., 1989; Zigterman et al., 1988). The 1501 stimulated IgG2a and IgG1 responses whereas L121 stimulated IgG2b, IgG3, and IgG1 responses to the same type 3 conjugate (Zigterman et al., 1988). In another study, the responses were about the same for both 1501 and L121 adjuvants, which enhanced IgM and IgG2; avidity also increased over the nonadjuvanted vaccine (van Dam et al., 1989).

Studies using the Quil A saponin adjuvant with type 14–bovine serum albumin pneumococcal conjugates in mice showed increases in the IgG responses but the magnitude of the response depended on both the sex of the mice (females responded much greater than males) and the structure of the conjugate vaccine (soluble forms were more immunogenic than insoluble forms) (van de Wijgert et al., 1991; Verheul et al., 1989).

2.2.2. FUNCTIONAL ANALYSIS

It has been known since the early 1900s that the type-specific antibodies to pneumococcal capsular polysaccharide are protective against systemic S. pneumoniae bacterial disease in animals and humans. The main mode of action of the type-specific antibody is opsonophagocytic. Recent studies have tried to identify which isotype and subclass of antibody is responsible for the protective effects of the antipolysaccharide antibodies (Bruyn et al., 1992; Lortan et al., 1993; Vidarsson et al., 1993). Clearly IgG is protective and subclass analyses have shown that IgG1, IgG2, IgG3, and IgG4 are associated with phagocytosis and protection, but the correlation of phagocytosis or opsonization to the subclass appears to be dependent on the serotype and the source of the antibody (animal, adults, children). One of the characteristics of glycoconjugates is that they convert T-independent antigens to T-dependent antigens and this results in higher IgG responses and usually higher IgG1-to-IgG2 ratios. Preclinical and clinical analyses of antibody responses have demonstrated that pneumococcal conjugate vaccines enhance both the IgG and the IgG1 responses and as a result, one would expect an increase in biological activity.

There are two methods to determine the biological activity of pneumococcal antibodies: in vitro opsonophagocytic assays and in vivo animal protection, either with active or passive immunization. Many of the vaccines listed in Table I have been tested for their ability to induce biologically active antibodies in animals or humans and almost all have been positive. The first pneumococcal conjugate vaccines prepared by Goebel and Avery (1931; Goebel, 1939, 1940a,b) were protective in the mouse challenge model when passively immunized with sera from actively immunized rabbits. The Lederle–Praxis Biologicals vaccines have been tested in animals (McQueen *et al.*, 1991) and human adults (Eby *et al.*, 1994). The antibodies have been shown to be biologically active and there is a direct correlation between the total Ig ELISA titers and the opsonization titers.

The Merck vaccine, Pnc-OMPC, has been shown to induce biologically active antibodies using an opsonophagocidal assay when the vaccines were tested in monkeys. The tetravalent Pnc-OMPC conjugates (6B, 14, 19F, and 23F) have been tested for efficacy in the chinchilla otitis media model (Giebink *et al.*, 1991, 1993b). As stated previously, the antibody responses were primarily IgG and IgM isotypes with little IgA. Protection against types 6B and 19F but not type 14 was observed even though the type 14 antibody response was slightly higher than that of type 6B or 19F. Type 23F was not sufficiently virulent to test for efficacy. These studies provide some promise for the use of pneumococcal conjugate vaccines in humans to prevent otitis media caused by *S. pneumoniae*, but serum antibody responses may not be all that is required to provide protection from otitis media, so additional research is needed.

2.3. Clinical Trial Results

2.3.1. MERCK VACCINES

The Merck pneumococcal conjugate vaccine, Pnc-OMP or Pnc-OMPC, is composed of the pneumococcal polysaccharide covalently linked to an outer membrane protein complex of *Neisseria meningitidis* using a bigeneric linker as described previously. The vaccine has undergone an evolution from a monovalent 6B conjugate in 1991 to currently a heptavalent vaccine composed of serotypes 4, 6B, 9V, 14, 18C, 19F, and 23F. Initial clinical studies of the monovalent 6B conjugate in toddlers and infants investigated the safety, immunogenicity, and dose response (Giebink *et al.*, 1993a; Kennedy *et al.*, 1991; Martin *et al.*, 1992). The studies established that the vaccine was generally safe at doses that ranged from 0.5 to 5 μg CHO/serotype when given in either two or three injections. In both toddlers and infants receiving multiple injections, there were no significant differences in the anti-6B titers based on the dose of the vaccine. Toddlers, 2 to 5 years old, and infants, 2 to 6 months old, given 2 injections two months apart had a tenfold or greater increase in anti-6B titers as a result of the booster injection (Kennedy *et al.*, 1991). Analysis of the isotype response in infants given three injections 2 months apart showed the response to be both IgG and IgM and, in a few of the infants, a low level of IgA was detected (Giebink *et al.*, 1993a).

The next formulation to undergo clinical testing was a tetravalent conjugate vaccine including serotypes 6B, 14, 19F, and 23F formulated at either 0.5 or 1.0 μg carbohydrate/serotype doses. The initial safety studies in adults given a single injection of the 1.0-μg dose

Figure 2. Type-specific antibody responses to pneumococcal polysaccharide
in toddlers receiving two injections of a
four-valent (6B, 14, 19F, 23F) Pnc-OMP
pneumococcal conjugate vaccine (Merck)
(Kayhty *et al.*, 1993b). Toddlers were 24
months of age and the vaccine was injected at 24 and 26 months at a dose of 1
µg carbohydrate per serotype. Antibody
titers were determined by EIA at 24, 25,
and 27 months and are in EIA units of
IgG/mL.

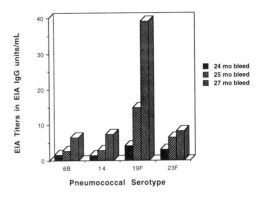

showed the vaccine to be generally safe and immunogenic (Nieminen *et al.*, 1992).
Responses were generally low (less than twofold) for most of the serotypes and for each
of the isotypes (IgA, IgM, and IgG). Mucosal immunity was also investigated but was
found to be poor. The low responses may be related to the single injection of a low dose.
A study of this tetravalent vaccine in Finland using 2-year-old children showed the vaccine
to be generally safe when given as one or two injections at a 1.0-µg dose (Kayhty *et al.*,
1993b). Type-specific antibody responses to the conjugate were higher than a control group
receiving the 23-valent polysaccharide vaccine and the responses could be increased by a
second injection of the conjugate (Fig. 2). About 25% of the toddlers receiving the
pneumococcal conjugate vaccine had measurable IgA titers in their saliva and in some
toddlers with high IgG serum titers, IgG was also found in their saliva.

Three clinical studies in infants receiving two or three injections at 2-month intervals
in both the United States (Keyserling *et al.*, 1993; Yogev *et al.*, 1993) and Finland (Kayhty
et al., 1993a) showed the tetravalent vaccine to have no significant clinical adverse
reactions. The Finnish study investigated the immunogenicity of the vaccine in infants
given two injections at 4 and 6 months of age and in infants given three injections at 2, 4,
and 6 months of age. Type-specific antibody responses were seen for each of the serotypes
and increases in titers occurred after each injection (Fig. 3) indicating a T-dependent

Figure 3. Type-specific antibody responses
to pneumococcal polysaccharide in infants in
Finland receiving three injections of a four-valent (6B, 14, 19F, 23F) Pnc-OMP pneumococcal conjugate vaccine (Merck) (Kayhty *et al.*,
1993a). Infants were 2 months of age and the
vaccine was injected at 2, 4, and 6 months at
a dose of 1 µg carbohydrate per serotype.
Antibody titers were determined by EIA at 0,
4, 6, and 7 months and are in EIA units of
IgG/mL.

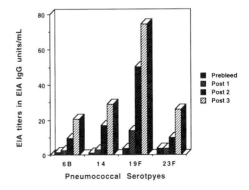

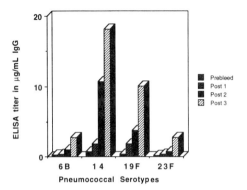

Figure 4. Type-specific antibody responses to pneumococcal polysaccharide in infants in the United States receiving three injections of a four-valent (6B, 14, 19F, 23F) Pnc-OMP pneumococcal conjugate vaccine (Merck) (Keyserling *et al.*, 1993). Infants were 2 months of age and the vaccine was injected at 2, 4, and 6 months at a dose of 1 μg carbohydrate per serotype. Antibody titers were determined by ELISA at 0, 4, 6, and 7 months and are in μg IgG/mL.

response. Responses to three injections ranged from a low of 8-fold for type 23F to a high of 24-fold for type 14 compared to the prevaccination sera.

A similar study in infants in the United States using the tetravalent vaccine at a 1.0-μg dose given at 2, 4, and 6 months showed the same results as the Finnish study (Keyserling *et al.*, 1993). Again, the vaccine was found to be generally safe and the increases in the type-specific antibody responses (Fig. 4) were similar to those seen in Finland. The highest increases were to serotypes 14 and 19F and lower for types 6B and 23F. Over 85% of the infants had greater than 1 μg/mL of antibody specific to each serotype after three injections.

Another study in infants in the United States was conducted using the tetravalent vaccine at a dose of 0.5 μg carbohydrate/serotype given concurrently with DTP, OVP, and Hib vaccines (Yogev *et al.*, 1993). The results again showed the vaccine to be generally safe with only a few significant reactions. The reported serotype-specific antibody responses after two injections were low for types 6B and 23F but higher for types 14 and 19F. The responses after three injections were not reported in this abstract.

Based on the successful results of the clinical studies using the tetravalent pneumococcal conjugate vaccines in toddlers and infants, Merck has formulated a heptavalent vaccine composed of serotypes 4, 6B, 9V, 14, 18C, 19F, and 23F at a dose of 1.0 μg carbohydrate/serotype except for type 6B which is at 2.5 μg reflecting the lower immune response seen in the infants to type 6B. An initial Phase 1 study in adults and children showed the formulation to be generally safe with mild adverse reactions (Kennedy and Anderson, 1993). Adults who received a single injection of the vaccine showed a 1.5- to 2-fold increase in their type-specific responses 1 month after the injection. Children, 2 years old, received two injections 2 months apart and the data reported after the first injection showed a 3- to 10-fold increase in the type-specific responses as compared to the prevaccination sera.

2.3.2. LEDERLE–PRAXIS BIOLOGICALS VACCINES

Lederle–Praxis has tested its three pneumococcal conjugate vaccine models—RA-poly, RA-Oligo, and Linker-Oligo—in Phase 1 clinical trials with adults and toddlers using vaccines formulated as bivalent (types 6A and 23F) vaccines at two dose levels of 2 or 10 μg carbohydrate/serotype. Pnu-Imune® 23 (Lederle–Praxis Biologicals: Pneumococcal

Vaccine Polyvalent; 25 μg each serotype) was used as a control vaccine (Eby *et al.,* 1991, 1994; Steinhoff *et al.,* 1992). Adults ranged in age from 18 to 60 years old and toddlers from 18 to 30 months of age. Each subject, whether adult or toddler, received a single injection of one of the vaccines. All of the conjugate vaccines were found to be generally safe and side effects were mild and transient. None of the vaccines were found to be more reactogenic than the Pnu-Imune® 23 control.

Table II shows the type-specific pneumococcal responses as total Ig determined by ELISA for the adults (Eby *et al.,* 1991, 1994). All of the conjugate models were found to be equally immunogenic at the same dose and it appeared that the 10-μg dose gave slightly but not significantly higher antibody responses than the 2-μg dose. Most adults had at least a fourfold increase in their type-specific responses to the higher dose of conjugate vaccine and the responses were similar to the Pnu-Imune® 23 control vaccine. IgG subclass analysis of the adult responses showed a rise in both the IgG1 and IgG2 antibodies and the ratio of IgG1 to IgG2 showed the response to be mainly IgG1 (Eby *et al.,* 1994). The conjugate vaccines prepared with saccharide fragments coupled either by reductive amination or by linker gave higher IgG1/IgG2 ratios than the polysaccharide-based conjugate vaccine. Analysis of a limited number of adult sera for opsonization activity demonstrated a type-specific biological activity that increased following vaccination and that the increase in opsonization activity correlated with the increase in ELISA titer. The polysaccharide control vaccine induced subclass-specific antibody responses similar to the polysaccharide-based conjugate.

The main purposes of the Phase 1 trials of the bivalent conjugate vaccines in adults and toddlers were to determine safety and immunological differences among the three vaccine models. The same pneumococcal conjugate vaccines tested in toddlers were found to be generally safe with few, mild, and transient side effects. Again, none of the vaccines

Table II

Total Ig Responses in Adults to Bivalent Pneumococcal Conjugate Vaccines

Vaccine[b]	Dose[c]	Anti-6B (μg/mL)[a]				Anti-23F (μg/mL)[a]			
		N[d]	Pre	Post	% 4-fold	N[d]	Pre	Post	% 4-fold
Linker	2 μg	28	3.39	7.16	14%	29	2.37	9.83	38%
	10 μg	27	2.65	11.17	41%	28	1.94	30.19	86%
RA-Oligo	2 μg	28	3.20	8.30	29%	27	2.36	7.74	30%
	10 μg	28	3.00	24.50	61%	27	2.62	16.53	59%
RA-Poly	2 μg	28	2.53	7.60	39%	27	2.26	21.79	56%
	10 μg	27	2.53	10.11	44%	26	2.94	41.01	77%
PS (23v)	25 μg	27	2.53	13.92	56%	28	1.83	13.22	64%

[a]Titers determined by ELISA assay on sera preabsorbed with C-Ps absorbent.

[b]Linker = fragments linked by 6-carbon linker to CRM$_{197}$; RA-Oligo = fragments reductively aminated to CRM$_{197}$; RA-Poly = polysaccharide reductively aminated to CRM$_{197}$; Ps(23v) = 23-valent polysaccharide vaccine (Pnu-Imune® 23).

[c]Micrograms of carbohydrate for each serotype per dose.

[d]Number of subjects.

Table III
IgG Responses in Toddlers to Bivalent Pneumococcal Conjugate Vaccines

Vaccine[b]	Dose[c]	Anti-6B (μg/mL)[a]				Anti-23F (μg/mL)[a]			
		N[d]	Pre	Post	% 4-fold	N[d]	Pre	Post	% 4-fold
Linker	2 μg	15	0.15	0.38	13	17	0.05	0.39	59
	10 μg	15	0.20	0.33[e]	7	17	0.05	0.66	65
RA-Oligo	2 μg	18	0.23	0.50	11	18	0.07	0.34	50
	10 μg	14	0.13	0.27	36	15	0.04	0.46	73
RA-Poly	2 μg	11	0.17	0.40	9	15	0.04	1.22	100[g]
	10 μg	14	0.11	0.57	50	16	0.06	2.84[f]	94[g]
Ps(23v)	25 μg	16	0.42	1.00	25	17	0.11	0.35	53

[a]Titers determined by ELISA assay on sera preabsorbed with C-Ps absorbent.

[b]Linker = fragments linked by 6-carbon linker to CRM_{197}; RA-Oligo = fragments reductively aminated to CRM_{197}; RA-Poly = polysaccharide reductively aminated to CRM_{197}; Ps(23v) = 23-valent polysaccharide vaccine (Pnu-Imune® 23).

[c]Micrograms of carbohydrate for each serotype per dose.

[d]Number of subjects from 18 to 36 months of age.

[e]$p = 0.03$ by ANOVA compared to Ps(23v).

[f]$p = 0.001$ by ANOVA compared to Ps(23v).

[g]$p = 0.002$ by chi square compared to Ps(23v).

were found to be more reactogenic than the Pnu-Imune® 23 control. Table III shows the type-specific pneumococcal responses for the toddlers (Eby *et al.,* 1994). Compared to the adults, the toddlers had lower responses to the 6A conjugates and higher responses to the 23F conjugates. As with the adults, the 10-μg dose induced higher antibody responses than the 2-μg dose and the type 23F polysaccharide conjugate gave the best response (100% of subjects had fourfold or greater increases in titers) compared to either of the oligosaccharide conjugate vaccines. Criteria based on antibody responses demonstrated that none of the vaccines were significantly different and that in general higher responses were observed at higher doses when the vaccines were given as a single injection.

The reductively aminated polysaccharide and oligosaccharide pneumococcal conjugate vaccine forms currently have been formulated as pentavalent vaccines containing serotypes 6B, 14, 18C, 19F, and 23F at doses of 0.5, 2.5, 5, and 10 μg carbohydrate/serotype. Safety studies using the 5-μg dose in a single injection in adults have been completed and the vaccines were found to be generally safe and well tolerated. Type-specific IgG immune responses determined by ELISA for the pentavalent vaccines are shown in Table IV (Eby *et al.,* 1994). Most of the adults responded with a fourfold or greater increase in titers versus their pretiters except for serotypes 6B and 19F, which showed lower responses. There appears to be little difference in the antibody responses to either of the vaccine forms following a single injection in adults. Clinical studies in infants with the three vaccine forms at the four doses following three injections at 2, 4, and 6 months are ongoing.

Table IV
IgG Responses in Adults to Pentavalent Pneumococcal Conjugates

	GMT (IgG μg/mL)[a]							
	RA-Oligo[b]				RA-Poly[b]			
Type	N^c	Pre	Post[d]	%[e]	N^c	Pre	Post[d]	%[e]
6B	14	2.13	13.85	43	12	2.73	7.51	25
14	15	1.28	42.45	73	12	1.75	27.30	67
18C	15	1.58	24.41	73	15	1.90	21.96	87
19F	15	2.91	5.65	20	15	3.27	11.23	40
23F	11	2.92	28.95	82	11	1.29	36.39	100

[a]Titers determined by ELISA assay on sera preabsorbed with C-Ps absorbent.
[b]RA-Oligo = fragments reductively aminated to CRM_{197}; RA-Poly = polysaccharide reductively aminated to CRM_{197}.
  Dose = 5 μg carbohydrate for each serotype per dose.
[c]Number of subjects.
[d]One month after vaccination.
[e]% with $\geq$ fourfold increase over prebleed.

2.3.3. OTHER CONJUGATE VACCINES

Porter Anderson and colleagues at the University of Rochester Medical Center have investigated several pneumococcal vaccines prepared by reductively aminating oxidized polysaccharides or oligosaccharides (types 6A, 6B, 14, 18C, 19F, and 23F) to diphtheria toxoid, tetanus toxoid, or CRM_{197} (Anderson and Betts, 1989; Pichichero and Anderson, 1993; Pichichero et al., 1990).

Initial clinical study in adults used two types of pneumococcal conjugates. Monovalent vaccines were prepared by coupling short oligosaccharides of type 6A having two, three, or four repeat units to diphtheria toxoid. A pentavalent conjugate vaccine was composed of oxidized polysaccharides of types 6A, 14, 18C, 19F, and 23F reductively aminated to diphtheria toxoid individually and mixed together. The carbohydrate dose of 6A in the monovalent vaccines varied between 0.56 and 6.3 μg and the pentavalent vaccine had a different dose for each serotype (6A = 1.3 μg, 14 = 2.6 μg, 18C = 4.2 μg, 19F = 1.3 μg, and 23F = 1.5 μg). The variable saccharide dose was the result of the vaccines having different carbohydrate-to-protein ratios and basing the dose of the vaccines on the protein.

The safety results of the initial study base on three or four subjects per vaccine, indicated that almost all of the subjects experienced minor side effects such as pain and local inflammation at the site of injection. Antibody responses were generally modest for low doses of the 6A monovalent vaccines but higher for the highest dose of the 6A monovalent conjugate vaccine (6.3 μg). Increases in the type-specific response to the polysaccharide conjugates in the pentavalent formulation were seen for all of the serotypes and again the highest responses were seen for the higher doses. Type 23F polysaccharide conjugate in the pentavalent vaccine appeared to induce a very weak response. It is difficult to compare type-specific response to the same serotype in the monovalent and polyvalent vaccines because the doses were different and in general higher doses induce higher antibody responses.

Type 6A pneumococcal conjugates that were produced using oligosaccharide, trimer, or polysaccharide conjugated to diphtheria toxoid by reductive amination were used to immunize 2-year-olds by giving two injections 2 months apart. The resultant immune responses were compared with those induced using the 23-valent polysaccharide vaccine given in one injection (Pichichero *et al.*, 1990). There was little difference in the response to the primary injection but a significant increase, greater than threefold, in the antibody titers to the second injection of the conjugates. Both conjugates appeared to be equal in their antibody response to both the primary and secondary injections. Again, the antibody increases indicate a T-dependent vaccine.

The latest clinical study by Anderson (Pichichero and Anderson, 1993) investigated the effect of vaccine structure on the type-specific antibody responses to a 6A pneumococcal conjugate in 2-year-olds receiving two injections. Conjugate vaccines were prepared by reductively aminating oligosaccharides of type 6A that have 2, 7, or 14 repeat units to tetanus toxoid or type 6A oligosaccharides of 14 repeats to CRM_{197}. The results of the study showed that the conjugate vaccines induce a boostable response and that the magnitude of the response was more dependent on the vaccine carbohydrate dose than on the structure of the conjugates. Also, two doses of the conjugates induced 6A titers that were lower than those to a single dose of the 23-valent polysaccharide vaccine.

Fattom *et al.* (1990) have compared immune responses in adults to pneumococcal type 12F conjugates synthesized by coupling polysaccharides of different sizes to diphtheria toxoid by adipic acid dihydrazide coupling. The conjugate vaccines were give in two injections, 1 month apart at a dose of 25 μg of carbohydrate. The 23-valent polysaccharide vaccine in one injection was used as a control. Adverse effects were mild and transient. Anti-type 12F titers after one injection were increased 3-fold over the pretiters for the polysaccharide, 4.5-fold for the conjugate with the lower-molecular-weight polysaccharide conjugate, and about 9.7-fold for the higher-molecular-weight polysaccharide conjugate. A second injection of either conjugate failed to induce an increase in the type 12F antibody response. A reason for the lack of a booster response is unknown but it was postulated that the response to the first injection was maximal for both the saccharide and the protein carrier.

Schneerson *et al.* (1986) investigated pneumococcal type 6A in adults using polysaccharide conjugated to tetanus toxoid by adipic acid dihydrazide coupling. In adults, the 6A conjugates induced an eightfold rise in anti-6A antibodies after one injection at either a 50- or 100-μg carbohydrate dose. No booster increases in type 6A-specific titers were seen when a second injection of the conjugate was given 3 weeks later. Again it was postulated that the response to the first conjugate injection was maximal. Passive transfer of adult sera to mice after immunization protected the mice from a lethal challenge with type 6 pneumococci. Adverse reactions were seen in most of the adults and were probably related to preexisting tetanus antibodies (Schneerson *et al.*, 1986).

In the children 2 to 5 years of age with sickle-cell disease (Sarnaik *et al.*, 1990), the same 6B conjugate vaccine was injected using a 15-μg dose three times at 2-month intervals. Anti-6B titers increased about 4-fold after the first injection, about 2-fold after the second, and about 1.3-fold after the third. The lack of a significant booster response again may be related to maximal response to either the carrier protein or the carbohydrate.

Anti-6B titers remained elevated for at least 6 months after the third injection. Adverse reactions were mild and resolved within 48 h.

3. CONCLUSIONS

The development of a multivalent pneumococcal protein conjugate vaccine that will prevent systemic and noninvasive diseases will present many challenges to researchers, clinicians, epidemiologists, and manufacturers. Research over the last 60 years has demonstrated conclusively that pneumococcal protein conjugate vaccines can readily convert the normally T-independent capsular polysaccharides into a T-dependent antigen capable of inducing boostable IgG responses in animals and humans. Preclinical research has and will continue to focus on the structure–function relationship of carbohydrate–protein conjugates with the hope of discovering the mechanisms of B and T cell interactions that can lead to vaccines with improved immunogenicity and to the development of new adjuvants and delivery systems.

The current clinical trials of multivalent pneumococcal conjugates look extremely encouraging in both their safety and their ability to induce boostable, type-specific antibody response to all of the serotypes in the vaccines. One of the current vaccines (Merck) has been shown to be immunogenic in the infant. The antibody responses are mainly IgG, which have been shown to be the main protective antibody for the prevention of systemic pneumococcal disease in both animals and humans.

Over the next 2 to 4 years, additional clinical studies will be undertaken to determine optimal pneumococcal conjugate vaccine formulation including dose response, the number of serotypes, the use of adjuvants to enhance or alter antibody responses, and vaccine delivery (systemic or oral). At the same time, questions as to the longevity of the antibody responses and the boostability of these responses by either natural infection or polysaccharide vaccines will be addressed. Phase III studies are expected to begin in 1995. These studies will determine whether the pneumococcal conjugates are effective in reducing the incidence of otitis media caused by *S. pneumoniae*. Standardization of assays for the determination of type-specific pneumococcal antibodies and the development of standard serum will be needed to be able to make comparisons among the various conjugate vaccines and to relate efficacy to antibody titers. Standardization of functional assays, such as mouse protection or opsonization, is also necessary.

The dramatic reduction of systemic *Haemophilus influenzae* type b disease in countries that have licensed and used the Hib–protein conjugate vaccines has been used to demonstrate that saccharide–protein conjugates can prevent systemic bacterial diseases. There is little doubt that the pneumococcal conjugates will be equally efficacious. The prevention of noninvasive diseases such as otitis media by systemic immunization with conjugate vaccines remains to be determined. Will high titers of type-specific systemic antibody be enough to prevent either nasopharyngeal colonization and/or otitis media? Evidence that pneumococcal polysaccharide vaccination can lead to a reduction in the incidence of acute otitis media in infants gives the expectation that the pneumococcal conjugates can induce high antibody titers early in life and that these will have an impact on reducing otitis media disease (Makela and Karma, 1980, 1989; Makela *et al.,* 1981, 1983a,b; Sloyer *et al.,* 1981; Teele *et al.,* 1981).

REFERENCES

Anderson, P., and Betts, R., 1989, Human adult immunogenicity of protein-coupled pneumococcal capsular antigens of serotypes prevalent in otitis media, *Pediatr. Infect. Dis. J.* **8**(Suppl. 1):S50–S53.

Arndt, B., and Porro, M., 1991, Strategies for type-specific glycoconjugate vaccines of *Streptococcus pneumoniae, Adv. Exp. Med. Biol.* **303**:129–148.

Austrian, R., 1981a, Pneumococcus: The first one hundred years, *Rev. Infect. Dis.* **3**:183–189.

Austrian, R., 1981b, Some observations on the pneumococcus and on the current status of pneumococcal disease and its prevention, *Rev. Infect. Dis.* **3**(Suppl.):S1–S17.

Austrian, R., 1989, Pneumococcal polysaccharide vaccines, *Rev. Infect. Dis.* **11**(Suppl. 3):S598–S602.

Avery, O. T., and Goebel, W. F., 1931, Chemo-immunological studies on conjugated carbohydrate-proteins. V. The immunological specificity of an antigen prepared by combining the capsular polysaccharide of type III pneumococcus with foreign protein, *J. Exp. Med.* **54**:437–447.

Becker, R. S., 1993, Conjugate vaccines: Practice and theory, *Springer Semin. Immunopathol.* **15**:217–226.

Beuvery, E. C., van, R. F., and Nagel, J., 1982, Comparison of the induction of immunoglobulin M and G antibodies in mice with purified pneumococcal type 3 and meningococcal group C polysaccharides and their protein conjugates, *Infect. Immun.* **37**:15–22.

Black, S., Shinefield, H., Elvin, L., and Schwalbe, J., 1994, Pneumococcal epidemiology in childhood in a large HMO population, *Pediatr. Res.* **34**(4 Part 2):Abstract 1031.

Bruyn, G. A., Zegers, B. J., and van, F. R., 1992, Mechanisms of host defense against infection with *Streptococcus pneumoniae, Clin. Infect. Dis.* **14**:251–262.

Chu, C., Schneerson, R., Robbins, J. B., and Rastogi, S. C., 1983, Further studies on the immunogenicity of *Haemophilus influenzae* type b and pneumococcal type 6A polysaccharide–protein conjugates, *Infect. Immun.* **40**:245–256.

Dagan, R., Englehard, D., and Piccard, E., 1992, Epidemiology of invasive childhood pneumococcal infections in Israel. The Israeli Pediatric Bacteremia and Meningitis Group, *J. Am. Med. Assoc.* **268**:3328–3332.

Davis, M. T. B., and Preston, J. F., 1981, A simple modified carbodiimide method for conjugation of small-molecular-weight compounds to immunoglobulin G with minimal protein crosslinking, *Anal. Biochem.* **116**:402–407.

de Velasco, E. A., Verheul, A. F. M., Veeneman, G. H., Gomes, L. J. F., van Boom, J. H., Veroef, J., and Snippe, H., 1993, Protein-conjugated synthetic di- and trisaccharides of pneumococcal type 17F exhibit a different immunogenicity and antigenicity than tetrasaccharide, *Vaccine* **11**:1429–1436.

Dick, W. E. J., and Beurret, M., 1989, Glycoconjugates of bacterial carbohydrate antigens, in: *Conjugate Vaccines* Vol. 10 (J. M. Cruse and R. E. J. Lewis, eds.), Karger, Basel, pp. 48–114.

Drug Research Reports, Editorial Board, 1993, Pneumococcal conjugate vaccine may be available within seven years—NIAID's Klein, *Drug. Res. Rep.* **36**(44):6–7.

Eby, R., Koster, M., Arndt, B., Cimino, C., Johnson, C., and Hogerman, D., 1991, Clinical evaluation of a conjugate vaccine for *Streptococcus pneumoniae* type 6A and 23F, Frontiers in Vaccine Research Helsinki, Finland.

Eby, R., Koster, M., Hogerman, D., Malinoski, F., IBS Department, Scale-up and Development Department, 1994, Pneumococcal conjugates, in: *Vaccines 94: Modern Approaches to New Vaccines Including Prevention of AIDS* (E. Norrby, F. Brown, R. M. Chanock, and H. S. Ginsberg, eds.), Cold Spring Harbor Laboratory Press, Cold Spring Harbor, NY, pp. 119–124.

Eskola, J., Takala, A. K., Kela, E., Pekkanen, E., Kalliokoski, R., and Leinonen, M., 1992, Epidemiology of invasive pneumococcal infections in children in Finland, *J. Am. Med. Assoc.* **268**:3323–3327.

Fattom, A., Vann, W. F., Szu, S. C., Sutton, A., Li, X., Bryla, D., Schiffman, G., Robbins, J. B., and Schneerson, R., 1988, Synthesis and physicochemical and immunological characterization of pneumococcus type 12F polysaccharide–diphtheria toxoid conjugates, *Infect. Immun.* **56**:2292–2299.

Fattom, A., Lue, C., Szu, S. C., Mestecky, J., Schiffman, G., Bryla, D., Vann, W. F., Watson, D., Kimzey, L. M., and Robbins, J. B., 1990, Serum antibody response in adult volunteers elicited by injection of

Streptococcus pneumoniae type 12F polysaccharide alone or conjugated to diphtheria toxoid, *Infect. Immun.* **58**:2309–2312.

FDC *Reports*, Editorial Board, 1993, Pneumococcal conjugate vaccines could be seven years from marketing, *FDC Rep.* **55**(44):T&G-6–T&G-7.

Fedson, D. S., 1988, Pneumococcal vaccine, in: *Vaccines* (S. A. Plotkin and E. A. J. Mortimer, eds.), Saunders, Philadelphia, pp. 271–299.

Giebink, G. S., Koskela, M., and Vella, P. P., 1991, Pneumococcal (Pn) capsular polysaccharide (PCP)-group B meningococcal outer membrane protein complex (OMPC) vaccine immunogenicity and efficacy in the chinchilla otitis media (OM) model, *Pediatr. Res.* **29**(4):Abstract 1014.

Giebink, G. S., Alward, C. T., Rzepka, A. A., Daly, K., and Liebeier, C., 1993a, Isotype antibody responses to type 6B pneumococcal polysaccharide (PS) conjugate vaccine in infants, *Pediatr. Res.* **33**(4 Part 2):Abstract 990.

Giebink, G. S., Koskela, M., Vella, P. P., Harris, M., and Le, C. T., 1993b, Pneumococcal capsular polysaccharide–meningococcal outer membrane protein complex conjugate vaccines: Immunogenicity and efficacy in experimental pneumococcal otitis media, *J. Infect. Dis.* **167**:347–355.

Goebel, W. F., 1938, Chemo-immunological properties of an artificial antigen containing cellobiuronic acid, *J. Exp. Med.* **68**:469–484.

Goebel, W. F., 1939, Studies on antibacterial immunity induced by artificial antigens, *J. Exp. Med.* **69**:353–364.

Goebel, W. F., 1940a, Immunity to experimental pneumococcal infection with an artificial antigen containing a saccharide of synthetic origin, *Science* **91**:20–21.

Goebel, W. F., 1940b, Studies on antibacterial immunity induced by artificial antigens. II. Immunity to experimental pneumococcal infections with antigens containing saccharides of synthetic origin, *J. Exp. Med.* **72**:33–48.

Goebel, W. F., and Avery, O. T., 1931, Chemo-immunological studies on conjugated carbohydrate-proteins. IV. The synthesis of the p-aminobenzyl ether of the soluble specific substance of the Type III Pneumococcus and its coupling with protein, *J. Exp. Med.* **54**:431–436.

Gray, B. M., and Dillon, H. J., 1989, Natural history of pneumococcal infections, *Pediatr. Infect. Dis. J.* **8**(Suppl. 1):S23–S25.

Johnston, R. J., 1991, Pathogenesis of pneumococcal pneumonia, *Rev. Infect. Dis.* **13**(Suppl. 6):S509–S517.

Kayhty, H., Ronnberg, P.-R., and Eskola, J., 1993a, Tetravalent pneumococcal (Pnc) capsular polysaccharide (PS)–meningococcal outer membrane protein conjugate vaccine (Pnc-OMP) is immunogenic in early infancy. 33rd Interscience Conference on Antimicrobial Agents and Chemotherapy, New Orleans, Abstract 175.

Kayhty, H., Ronnberg, P.-R., Virolainen, A., and Eskola, J., 1993b, Immunogenicity of tetravalent pneumococcal (Pnc) capsular polysaccharide (PS)–meningococcal outer membrane protein conjugate vaccine (Pnc-OMP) in Finnish 2-year-old children, 33rd Interscience Conference on Antimicrobial Agents and Chemotherapy, New Orleans, Abstract 172.

Kennedy, D. J., and Anderson, E. L., 1993, Safety and immunogenicity of a heptavalent (HV) pneumococcal conjugate vaccine (PCV) in adults (A) and children (C), 33rd Interscience Conference on Antimicrobial Agents and Chemotherapy, New Orleans, Abstract 167.

Kennedy, D. J., Belshe, R. B., and Anderson, E. L., 1991, Safety and immunogenicity of type 6B pneumococcal meningococcal protein conjugate vaccine (6B-OMPC) in children (C) and infants (I), 31st Interscience Conference on Antimicrobial Agents and Chemotherapy, Chicago, Abstract 59.

Keyserling, H. L., Anderson, E. L., and Martin, J. T., 1993, Immunogenicity of a tetravalent (types 6B, 14, 19F, 23F) pneumococcal conjugate vaccine in infants, *Pediatr. Res.* **33**(4 Part 2):Abstract 1016.

Lin, K. T., and Lee, C. J., 1982, Immune response of neonates to pneumococcal polysaccharide–protein conjugate, *Immunology* **46**:333–342.

Lortan, J. E., Kaniuk, A. S., and Monteil, M. A., 1993, Relationship of in vitro phagocytosis of serotype 14 *Streptococcus pneumoniae* to specific class and IgG subclass antibody levels in healthy adults, *Clin. Exp. Immunol.* **91**:54–57.

Lu, C., Kind, P., and Lee, C., 1991, Immune response of neonates to *Streptococcus pneumoniae* type 9V polysaccharide–tetanus toxoid conjugate, 75th Annual Meeting of FASEB, Atlanta, Abstract 5754.

McQueen, K., Phipps, D., Quataert, S., Eby, R., and Pillai, S., 1991, Induction of type-specific, biologically functional antibodies to capsular polysaccharides after immunization with multivalent pneumococcal conjugate vaccines against *Streptococcus pneumoniae, Pediatr. Res.* **31**(4 Part 2):Abstract 1056.

Makela, P. H., and Karma, P., 1980, Can otitis media be prevented with pneumococcal vaccine? *Prog. Clin. Biol. Res.* **47**:95–106.

Makela, P. H., and Karma, P., 1989, Vaccination trials in otitis media: Experiences in Finland since 1977, *Pediatr. Infect. Dis. J.* **8**(Suppl.):S79–S82.

Makela, P. H., Leinonen, M., Pukander, J., and Karma, P., 1981, A study of the pneumococcal vaccine in prevention of clinically acute attacks of recurrent otitis media, *Rev. Infect. Dis.* **3**(Suppl.):S124–S132.

Makela, P. H., Karma, P., and Leinonen, M. K., 1983a, Pneumococcal vaccine and otitis media in infancy, *Bull. Eur. Physiopathol. Respir.* **19**(2):235–238.

Makela, P. H., Karma, P., Sipila, M., Pukander, J., and Leinonen, M., 1983b, Possibilities of preventing otitis media by vaccination, *Scand. J. Infect. Dis. Suppl.* **39**:34–38.

Malcolm, A. J., Best, M. W., Szarka, R. J., Mosleh, Z., Unger, F. M., Messner, P., and Sleytr, U. B., 1993, Surface layers from *Bacillus alveias* a carrier for a *Streptococcus pneumoniae* conjugate vaccine, in: *Advances in Bacterial Paracrystalline Surface Layers* (T. J. Beveridge and S. F. Koval, eds.), Plenum Press, New York, pp. 219–233.

Marburg, S., Jorn, D., Tolman, R. L., Arison, B., McCauley, J., Kniskern, P. J., Hagopian, A., and Vela, P. P., 1986, Bimolecular chemistry of macromolecules: Synthesis of bacterial polysaccharide conjugates with *Neisseria meningitidis* membrane protein, *J. Am. Chem. Soc.* **108**:5282–5287.

Martin, J. T., Kennedy, D. J., Heaney, M. S., and Anderson, E. L., 1992, Evaluation of pneumococcal 6B conjugate vaccine in infants, *Pediatr. Res.* **31**(4 Part 2):Abstract 565.

MMWR, 1989, Pneumococcal polysaccharide vaccine, *Morbid. Mortal. Weekly Rep.* **38**:64–76.

MMWR, 1994, Drug-resistant *Streptococcus pneumoniae*-Kentucky and Tennessee, 1993, *Morbid. Mortal. Weekly Rep.* **43**:23–26, 31.

Nieminen, T., Virolainen, A., Kayhty, H., Leinonen, M., and Eskola, J., 1992, Immune response to tetravalent pneumococcal (PNC) conjugate vaccine (Pn-OMP) in adults, 32nd Interscience Conference on Antimicrobial Agents and Chemotherapy, Anaheim, CA, Abstract 1283.

Orange, M., and Gray, B. M., 1993, Pneumococcal serotypes causing disease in children in Alabama, *Pediatr. Infect. Dis. J.* **12**:244–246.

Paradiso, P. R., Dermody, K., and Pillai, S., 1993, Novel approaches to the development of glycoconjugate vaccines with synthetic peptides as carriers, *Vaccine Res.* **2**:239–248.

Paton, J. C., Lock, R. A., Lee, C. J., Li, J. P., Berry, A. M., Mitchell, T. J., Andrew, P. W., Hansman, D., and Boulnois, G. J., 1991, Purification and immunogenicity of genetically obtained pneumolysin toxoids and their conjugation to Streptococcus pneumoniae type 19F polysaccharide, *Infect. Immun.* **59**:2297–2304.

Paul, W. E., Katz, D. H., and Benacerraf, B., 1971, Augmented anti-S 3 antibody responses to an S 3 –protein conjugate, *J. Immunol.* **107**:685–688.

Peeters, C. C., Tenbergen, M. A., Evenberg, D. E., Poolman, J. T., Zegers, B. J., and Rijkers, G. T., 1991a, A comparative study of the immunogenicity of pneumococcal type 4 polysaccharide and oligosaccharide tetanus toxoid conjugates in adult mice, *J. Immunol.* **146**:4308–4314.

Peeters, C. C., Tenbergen, M. A., Haagmans, B., Evenberg, D., Poolman, J. T., Zegers, B. J., and Rijkers, G. T., 1991b, Pneumococcal conjugate vaccines, *Immunol. Lett.* **30**:267–274.

Peeters, C. C., Tenbergen, M. A., Poolman, J. T., Zegers, B. J., and Rijkers, G. T., 1992, Immunogenicity of a Streptococcus pneumoniae type 4 polysaccharide–protein conjugate vaccine is decreased by admixture of high doses of free saccharide, *Vaccine* **10**:833–840.

Pichichero, M., and Anderson, P., 1993, Boostable pneumococcal type 6A polysaccharide antibody (Pn 6A PS Ab) responses at age 2 Yr to saccharide (sac)–protein conjugates, *Pediatr. Res.* **31**(4 Part 2):Abstract 1054.

Pichichero, M. E., Kochman, L., Porcelli, S. C., and Anderson, P. W., 1990, Memory-type antibody (Ab) responses of two-year-old children to pneumococcal (Pn) type 6A–diphtheria toxoid (D) conjugate vaccines, *Pediatr. Res.* **27**(4 Part 2):Abstract 563.

Porro, M., 1987, Artificial glycoproteins of predetermined multivalent antigenicity as a new generation of candidate vaccines to prevent infections from encapsulated bacteria: Analysis of antigenicity versus immunogenicity, in: *Towards Better Carbohydrate Vaccines* (R. Bell and G. Torrigiani, eds.), Wiley, New York, pp. 279–306.

Porro, M., Costantino, P., Viti, S., Vannozzi, F., Naggi, A., and Torri, G., 1985, Specific antibodies to diphtheria toxin and type 6A pneumococcal capsular polysaccharide induced by a model of semi-synthetic glycoconjugate antigen, *Mol. Immunol.* **22**:907–919.

Porro, M., Costantino, P., Giovannoni, F., Pellegrini, V., Tagliaferri, L., Vannozzi, F., and Viti, S., 1986, A molecular model of artificial glycoprotein with predetermined multiple immunodeterminants for gram-positive and gram-negative encapsulated bacteria, *Mol. Immunol.* **23**:385–391.

Robbins, J. B., Austrian, R., Lee, C. J., Rastogi, S. C., Schiffman, G., Henrichsen, J., Makela, P. H., Broome, C. V., Facklam, R. R., Tiesjema, R. H., and Park, J. C., Jr., 1983, Considerations for formulating the second-generation pneumococcal capsular polysaccharide vaccine with emphasis on the cross-reactive types within groups, *J. Infect. Dis.* **148**:1136–1159.

Sarnaik, S., Kaplan, J., Schiffman, G., Bryla, D., Robbins, J. B., and Schneerson, R., 1990, Studies on Pneumococcus vaccine alone or mixed with DTP and on Pneumococcus type 6B and Haemophilus influenzae type b capsular polysaccharide–tetanus toxoid conjugates in two- to five-year-old children with sickle cell anemia [published erratum appears in *Pediatr. Infect. Dis. J.* 1990, **9** (5): 308], *Pediatr. Infect. Dis. J.* **9**:181–186.

Schneerson, R., Barrera, O., Sutton, A., and Robbins, J. B., 1980, Preparation, characterization and immunogenicity of *Haemophilus influenzae* type b polysaccharide–protein conjugates, *J. Exp. Med.* **152**:361–376.

Schneerson, R., Robbins, J. B., Chu, C. Y., Sutton, A., Schiffman, G., and Vann, W. F., 1982a, Semi-synthetic vaccines composed of capsular polysaccharides of pathogenic bacteria covalently bound to proteins for prevention of invasive disease, *Prog. Allergy* **33**:144–178.

Schneerson, R., Robbins, J. B., Eagan, W., Zon, G., Sutton, A., Vann, W. F., Kaijser, B., Hanson, L. A., and Ahlstedt, S., 1982b, Bacterial capsular polysaccharide conjugates, in: *Seminar in Infectious Diseases: Bacterial Vaccines*, Vol. 4 (L. Weinstein and B. N. Fields, eds.), Thieme Stratton, New York, pp. 311–321.

Schneerson, R., Chu, C. Y., Ahlstedt, S., Soderstrom, T., Sutton, A., Zon, G., and Robbins, J. B., 1982c, Protein–polysaccharide conjugate vaccines, in: *Haemophilus influenzae: Epidemiology, Immunology, and Prevention of Disease* (S. H. Sell and P. F. Wright, eds.), Elsevier, Amsterdam, pp. 265–272.

Schneerson, R., Robbins, J. B., Chu, C., Sutton, A., Vann, W., Vickers, J. C., London, W. T., Curfman, B., Hardegree, M. C., Shiloach, J., and Rastogi, S. C., 1984, Serum antibody responses of juvenile and infant rhesus monkeys injected with *Haemophilus influenzae* type b and pneumococcus type 6A capsular polysaccharide–protein conjugates, *Infect. Immun.* **45**:582–591.

Schneerson, R., Robbins, J. B., Parke, J. J., Bell, C., Schlesselman, J. J., Sutton, A., Wang, Z., Schiffman, G., Karpas, A., and Shiloach, J., 1986, Quantitative and qualitative analyses of serum antibodies elicited in adults by *Haemophilus influenzae* type b and pneumococcus type 6A capsular polysaccharide–tetanus toxoid conjugates, *Infect. Immun.* **52**:519–528.

Schneerson, R., Levi, L., Robbins, J. B., Bryla, D. M., Schiffman, G., and Lagergard, T., 1992, Synthesis of a conjugate vaccine composed of pneumococcus type 14 capsular polysaccharide bound to pertussis toxin, *Infect. Immun.* **60**:3528–3532.

Shapiro, E. D., 1991, Pneumococcal vaccine, in: *Vaccines and Immunotherapy* (S. J. Crys Jr., ed.), Pergamon Press, New York, pp. 127–139.

Shapiro, E. D., and Austrian, R., 1994, Serotypes responsible for invasive *Streptococcus pneumoniae* infections among children in Connecticut, *J. Infect. Dis.* **169**:212–214.

Shapiro, E. D., Berg, A. T., Austrian, R., Schroeder, D., Parcells, V., Margolis, A., Adair, R. K., and Clemens, J. D., 1991, The protective efficacy of polyvalent pneumococcal polysaccharide vaccine, *N. Engl. J. Med.* **325**:1453–1460.

Sloyer, J. J., Ploussard, J. H., and Howie, V. M., 1981, Efficacy of pneumococcal polysaccharide vaccine in preventing acute otitis media in infants in Huntsville, Alabama, *Rev. Infect. Dis.* **3**(Suppl.):S119–S123.

Snippe, H., van, D. J., van, H. A., Willers, J. M., Kamerling, J. P., and Vliegenthart, J. F., 1983a, Preparation of a semisynthetic vaccine to Streptococcus pneumoniae type 3, *Infect. Immun.* **42**:842–844.

Snippe, H., van, H. A., van, D. J., De, R. M., Jansze, M., and Willers, J. M., 1983b, Immunogenic properties in mice of hexasaccharide from the capsular polysaccharide of *Streptococcus pneumoniae* type 3, *Infect. Immun.* **40**:856–861.

Steinhoff, M. C., Edwards, K., Keyserling, H., Johnson, C., Madore, D., and Hogerman, D., 1992, Immunogenicity and safety of 3 bivalent *S. pneumoniae* conjugate vaccines in young children, 32nd Interscience Conference on Antimicrobial Agents and Chemotherapy, Anaheim, CA, Abstract 1284.

Stowell, C. P., and Lee, Y. C., 1980, Neoglycoproteins: The preparations and application of synthetic glycoproteins, *Adv. Carbohydr. Chem. Biochem.* **37**:225–281.

Teele, D. W., Klein, J. O., Bratton, L., Fisch, G. R., Mathieu, O. R., Porter, P. J., Starobin, S. G., Tarlin, L. D., and Younes, R. P., 1981, Use of pneumococcal vaccine for prevention of recurrent acute otitis media in infants in Boston. The Greater Boston Collaborative Otitis Media Study Group, *Rev. Infect. Dis.* **3**(Suppl.):S113–S118.

van Dam, G. J., Verheul, A. F., Zigterman, G. J., De, R. M., and Snippe, H., 1989, Nonionic block polymer surfactants enhance the avidity of antibodies in polyclonal antisera against Streptococcus pneumoniae type 3 in normal and Xid mice, *J. Immunol.* **143**:3049–3053.

van de Wijgert, J. H., Verheul, A. F., Snippe, H., Check, I. J., and Hunter, R. L., 1991, Immunogenicity of Streptococcus pneumoniae type 14 capsular polysaccharide: Influence of carriers and adjuvants on isotype distribution, *Infect. Immun.* **59**:2750–2757.

Vella, P. P., Marburg, S., Staub, J. M., Kniskern, P. J., Miller, W., Hagopian, A., Ip, C., Tolman, R. L., Rusk, C. M., Chupak, L. S., and Ellis, R. W., 1992, Immunogenicity of conjugate vaccines consisting of pneumococcal capsular polysaccharide types 6B, 14, 19F, and 23F and a meningococcal outer membrane protein complex, *Infect. Immun.* **60**:4977–4983.

Verheul, A. F., Versteeg, A. A., De, R. M., Jansze, M., and Snippe, H., 1989, Modulation of the immune response to pneumococcal type 14 capsular polysaccharide–protein conjugates by the adjuvant Quil A depends on the properties of the conjugates, *Infect. Immun.* **57**:1078–1083.

Vidarsson, G., Jonsdottir, I., Jonsson, S. and Valdimarsson, H., 1993, Antibody response to pneumococcal polysaccharides: Relation to opsonic activity, 33rd Interscience Conference on Antimicrobial Agents and Chemotherapy, New Orleans, Abstract 171.

Watson, D. A., Musher, D. M., Jacobson, J. W., and Verhoef, J., 1993, A brief history of the pneumococcus in biomedical research: A panoply of scientific discovery, *Clin. Infect. Dis.* **17**:913–924.

Yogev, R., Gupta, S., Emanuel, B., Williams, K., and Adams, J., 1993, Safety, tolerability and Immunogenicity of tetravalent (6B, 14, 19F, 23F) pneumococcal conjugate vaccine in infants given concurrently with routine immunizations, 33rd Interscience Conference on Antimicrobial Agents and Chemotherapy, New Orleans, Abstract 170.

Zigterman, G. J., Snippe, H., Jansze, M., Ernste, E. B., De, R. M., and Willers, J. M., 1988, Nonionic block polymer surfactants enhance immunogenicity of pneumococcal hexasaccharide-protein vaccines, *Infect. Immun.* **56**:1391–1393.

Chapter 32

Lyme Vaccine Enhancement

N-Terminal Acylation of a Protein Antigen and Inclusion of a Saponin Adjuvant

Richard T. Coughlin, Jianneng Ma, and Daniel E. Cox

1. BACKGROUND

1.1. Lyme Disease, Incidence, Transmission, and Symptoms

Lyme disease is caused by the spirochete *Borrelia burgdorferi* (Burgdorfer *et al*., 1982; Johnson *et al*., 1984) and is the most common tick-borne zoonosis (Steere, 1989). The etiologic spirochete of Lyme disease was first identified by Burgdorfer *et al*. (1982) and subsequently isolated by Barbour *et al*. (1983). If the infection is not treated with antibiotics, the organism can invade the brain, nerves, eyes, joints, and heart and produce morbidity (Steere, 1989). This disease is characterized by early skin lesions termed erythema migrans, and intermittent arthritis, cardiac, and neurologic manifestations. Thus far, at least four genospecies and five seroprotective groups of Lyme disease spirochetes have been proposed on the basis of genetic and molecular determinants (Lovrich *et al*., 1993). To date, all North American isolates of Lyme disease spirochetes are *B. burgdorferi* sensu stricto (Baranton *et al*., 1992). Many European and Asian isolates belong to *B. garinii* sp. nov. and *B. afzelii*, formerly known as the VS461 group (Baranton *et al*., 1992; Canica *et al*., 1993; Park *et al*., 1993). *B. garinii* sp. nov. may be associated with the neurologic and cardiac syndromes and *B. afzelii* with the cutaneous symptoms of erythema migrans or acrodermatitis chronica atrophicans of Lyme disease in Europe (Canica *et al*., 1993; van

Richard T. Coughlin, Jianneng Ma, and Daniel E. Cox • Cambridge Biotech Corporation, Worcester, Massachusetts 01605.

Vaccine Design: The Subunit and Adjuvant Approach, edited by Michael F. Powell and Mark J. Newman. Plenum Press, New York, 1995.

Dam *et al.*, 1993). The fourth genospecies, F63B group of spirochetes, has been identified from ticks in Japan and its etiologic significance is unknown (Postic *et al.*, 1993).

A large number of outer surface proteins (Osp) of Lyme disease spirochetes have been identified (Barbour *et al.*, 1984; Katona *et al.*, 1992; Norris *et al.*, 1992; Preac-Mursic *et al.*, 1992; Reindi *et al.*, 1993; Wilske *et al.*, 1993; Lam *et al.*, 1994). OspA, OspB, and OspC (or pC), the major surface proteins with molecular masses of approximately 31 kDa, 34 kDa, and 22 kDa, respectively, have been extensively characterized genetically (Barbour, 1989; Bergstrom *et al.*, 1989; Fuchs *et al.*, 1992; Marconi *et al.*, 1993). Both OspA and OspB are heterogeneous among the strains and produced by most North American isolates (Barbour and Fish, 1993; Barbour *et al.*, 1984). OspC is commonly seen with European isolates (Wilske *et al.*, 1988) and is also quite heterogeneous.

Shortly after the discovery of *Borrelia* as the etiologic agent of Lyme disease it was shown that hamsters immunized with killed spirochetes are protected against homologous challenge (Johnson *et al.*, 1986a; Schmitz *et al.*, 1991). The feasibility of developing a subunit vaccine has been investigated using OspA, OspB, and OspC as the immunogen in animal models (Fikrig *et al.*, 1990, 1992a,b; Preac-Mursic *et al.*, 1992). The heterogeneity of these proteins makes it challenging to develop a comprehensive vaccine, but worth attempting.

1.2. The Biochemistry of Bacterial Lipoprotein Biosynthesis

A common feature of these targets of protective immunity is that they are lipoproteins. Although lipoproteins are present in all gram-negative, gram-positive, and *Mycoplasma* (Hayashi and Wu, 1990), most research has focused on the murein or Lpp lipoprotein of *E. coli* (Hantke and Braun, 1973). For gram-negative bacteria, the biosynthetic pathway is now well understood and has been reviewed elsewhere (Wu, 1987; Hayashi and Wu, 1990). Since most Lyme vaccine development work has focused on *E. coli*-expressed borrelial proteins, a brief review is appropriate. In *E. coli*, the prolipoprotein is modified by a glyceryl transferase that attaches glycerol to cysteine through a thioether linkage and the ester-linked fatty acids are then attached to the glyceryl moiety by specific phospholipid acyl transferase. In bacteria, two distinct signal peptidases have been identified: SPase I,

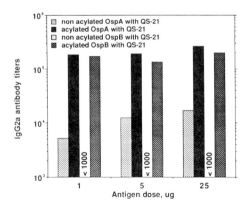

Figure 1. Comparison of acylated and non-acylated forms of OspA and OspB derived from *B. burgdorferi* strain B31 as immunogens. C3H/HeJ mice were immunized twice with either 25, 5, or 1 μg per dose of OspA in sterile PBS with 15 μg of QS-21. IgG2a antibody titers of immunized mice were measured on microtiter plates coated with a whole-cell lysate of *B. burgdorferi* strain B31.

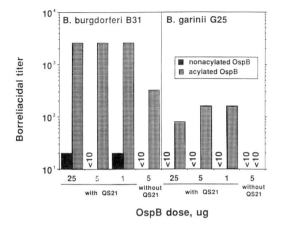

Figure 2. Comparison of borreliacidal titers of C3H/HeJ mice immunized twice with either 25, 5, or 1 μg per dose of acylated OspA derived from *B. burgdorferi* strain B31, in sterile PBS with 15 μg of QS-21. For comparison, another group of C3H/HeJ mice were immunized twice with 5 μg per dose of acylated OspA and no adjuvant. Borreliacidal activity was measured against either the homologous *B. burgdorferi* strain, B31, or the *B. garinii* strain G25.

which removes the signal peptide from the majority of secreted proteins, and SPase II, which cleaves signal peptides from lipoproteins. SPase II is an integral membrane protein that recognizes and cleaves between the sequence -Gly-glycerideCys-. Following cleavage of the glyceride prolipoprotein by SPase II, the third fatty acid is added to the amino-terminus of cysteine. Although subtle differences may exist, this biosynthetic pathway appears to be well conserved among bacteria and allows *E. coli* to be used as an expression system for a wide range of bacterial lipoproteins including *Borrelia* lipoproteins.

1.3. Comparison of Acylated and Nonacylated Forms as Immunogens

Among naturally infected individuals, OspA and OspB are rarely recognized in the early stages of Lyme disease. This is surprising since the mature acylated forms of these proteins expressed in *E. coli* are highly immunogenic. We have compared the acylated and nonacylated forms of OspA and OspB derived from *B. burgdorferi* strain B31 as immunogens (Fig. 1). C3H/HeJ mice were immunized twice with either 25, 5, or 1 μg per dose of OspA in sterile PBS with 15 μg of QS-21 and tested for IgG2a antibody titers on microtiter plates coated with a whole-cell lysate of *B. burgdorferi* strain B31. Acylated OspA produced tenfold higher antibody titers to native antigen than nonacylated OspA. Further, 1 μg of acylated OspA induced tenfold higher antibody titers than 25 μg of nonacylated OspA. The results were even more dramatic for OspB. The nonacylated form of the protein was essentially nonimmunogenic, whereas the acylated form of OspB was just as immunogenic as the acylated form of OspA. Since mouse IgG2a are very efficient components of antibody-dependent complement-mediated killing, it is not surprising that *B. burgdorferi* are readily killed by antisera made against full-length proteins but not truncated proteins even with an adjuvant (Fig. 2).

1.4. Attempts at Synthetic Generation of Lipoproteins

The dramatic difference between the immunogenicity of acylated and nonacylated forms of bacterial lipoproteins has prompted an investigation into the precise structural requirements for immunogenicity and mitogenicity. Chemically synthesized lipopeptide analogues of bacterial lipoproteins have also been shown to be potent adjuvants when combined with or covalently coupled to antigens or haptens. Most of this work has focused on the *E. coli* murein lipoprotein as a prototype and only recently have analogues representing other bacterial lipoproteins been studied. *N*-Palmitoyl-*S*-(2,3-bis(palmitoyloxy)-(2*RS*)-propyl)-(*R*)-cysteine or Pam₃C has been chemically synthesized and tested for a wide range of biological activities (Reitermann *et al.*, 1989).

1.4.1. Pam₃C- DERIVATIVES AS ADJUVANTS

Efforts to develop safe and effective vaccines against viral and bacterial pathogens utilizing recombinant protein technology and synthetic peptides have met with rather limited success. Even if epitopes are known as protective or neutralizing, there have been problems creating long-lasting immunity against the target epitopes. Much of the focus of recombinant vaccines has therefore turned to the use of adjuvants or the other nonantigen components added to stimulate the immune response. Many different compounds have been used in an attempt to control two principal functions of adjuvants, depoting of antigen and direct stimulation of the cells of the immune system. Examples of this approach are described throughout this volume. Depoting adjuvants, such as alum or incomplete Freund's adjuvant, bind to or are emulsified with the antigen to maintain its localization at the injection site resulting in more contact with the immune system. There are many examples of immune-stimulating compounds including components of bacterial cell walls such as lipid A, lipopolysaccharide, or muramyl dipeptide. Other examples of effective adjuvants of nonbacterial origin include nonionic block polymers (Chapter 11), cytokines (Chapters 27–29), and saponins (Audibert and Lise, 1993; Kensil *et al.*, 1993; Chapters 22 and 23). An alternative approach has been to reverse engineer highly immunogenic proteins such as lipoproteins. This has resulted in synthetic lipopeptides based on the N-terminal structure of the outer membrane lipoprotein of *E. coli*. The properties and use of these compounds have recently been reviewed (Bessler and Jung, 1992).

The outer membrane murein lipoprotein of *E. coli* has been shown to be strongly mitogenic and to possess potent immunostimulating activity (Melchers *et al.*, 1975). This activity has been determined to be solely contained within the lipidated amino-terminal pentapeptide of the protein (Bessler *et al.*, 1977). The structure of the lipidated portion of this protein has been known for some time (Hantke and Braun, 1973). The minimum active residue of this sequence is cysteine which is modified with a diacyl diglyceride in thioether linkage (Fig. 3). A third fatty acid is in an amide linkage with the amino group of the cysteine. In the mature murein lipoprotein the majority of the fatty acids are palmitic acid at both the diglyceride and amide position. The lipidated pentapeptide, tripalmitoyl-*S*-glyceryl-cysteinyl-seryl-seryl-asparaginyl-alanine (Pam₃CSSNA), has been chemically synthesized and shown to possess the same mitogenic properties as the intact lipoprotein (Bessler *et al.*, 1985b). There is now an extensive literature in which this synthetic lipopeptide and various modified lipopeptides have been evaluated as adjuvant, primarily

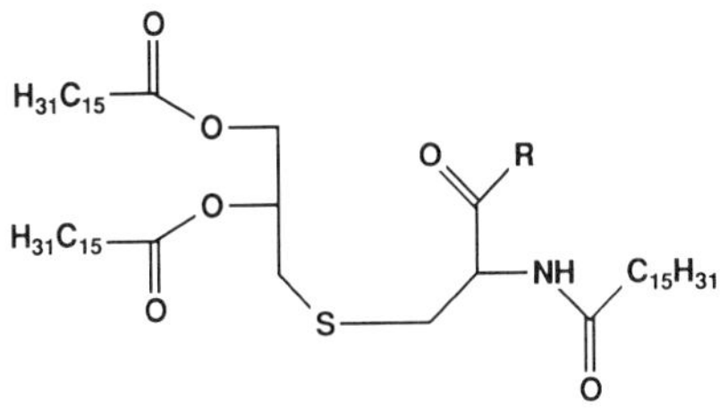

Figure 3. *N*-Palmitoyl-*S*-(2,3-bis(palmitoyloxy)-(2*RS*)-propyl)-(*R*)-cysteine or Pam₃C represents the mature form of the N-terminus of mature bacterial lipoproteins. It has also been chemically synthesized (Reitermann *et al.*, 1989) where *R* can be a hydroxyl group or a small peptide.

for peptide epitopes and conjugated haptens. Through mitogenicity experiments, Bessler *et al.* (1985a) have shown that the minimum structural requirement is tripalmitoyl-*S*-glyceryl-cysteine (Pam₃C) with at least one additional amino acid in a peptide linkage, with the full pentapeptide expressing the highest activity. Pam₃C alone is ineffective. A broad array of substitutions in the amino acid sequence is possible while retaining much of the biological activity (Metzger *et al.*, 1991).

1.4.2. Pam₃C-DERIVATIZED PEPTIDES

The stimulatory activity of the Pam₃C derivatives has been demonstrated by chemically coupling tripalmitoyl-*S*-glyceryl-cysteinyl-serine (Pam₃CS) onto the amino-terminus of poorly immunogenic peptides. One example is the extracytoplasmic domain of epidermal growth factor receptor (Bessler *et al.*, 1985b). A single injection of this conjugate into mice resulted in a strong antibody response to the peptide whereas nonconjugated peptide was virtually nonimmunogenic. The conjugate was also effective in the generation of antibodies during *in vitro* stimulation of cultured spleen cells. In this case the conjugate was approximately 10^4-fold more effective as an immunogen than the peptide alone. Conjugation of the lipopeptide to the peptide was necessary for the full response; simple mixing of the peptide and Pam₃CS was only slightly immunogenic. Monoclonal antibodies generated against this conjugate were able to recognize the native receptor (Muller *et al.*, 1989). Lipopeptides were also shown to be effective adjuvants in the production of antihapten antibodies (Reitermann *et al.*, 1989). In this case, immunization of mice with either the lipopeptide–hapten conjugate or mixing the lipopeptide with a hapten–albumin conjugate both resulted in a strong antihapten response. The lipopeptide tripalmitoyl-*S*-glyceryl-cysteinyl-seryl-lysyl-lysyl-lysyl-lysine (Pam₃CSK₄) albumin conjugate was as effective in stimulating an antibody response as albumin in complete Freund's adjuvant. A similar boost of peptide-specific immune response was observed utilizing lipopeptide-modified peptide epitopes from HIV gp160 (Loleit *et al.*, 1990) and a repetitive epitope of *Plasmodium falciparum* circumsporozoite protein (Wiesmüller *et al.*, 1991). In the latter case, coupling of the minimal structure Pam₃C only to the peptide was as effective as the longer lipopeptide Pam₃SC. This contrasts somewhat with the observed lack of mitogenic activity of Pam₃C alone (Bessler *et al.*, 1985a). Key results in the *Plasmodium* studies are that the relatively simple lipopeptide conjugates were capable of overcoming genetic restriction and inducing a strong antibody response in a low-responder mouse strain. Previously, high antibody titers were only obtained in this strain through the use of complex, high-molecular-weight vaccine mixtures. An additional important humoral antibody effect seen with both the HIV and *Plasmodium* conjugates was isotype switching.

In addition to IgG1, these conjugates induced the production of IgG2a and IgG3 and to a lesser extent IgG2b, indicating the involvement of T cells in the humoral response.

Important aspects of a vaccine candidate are the ability to generate neutralizing antibodies, cell-mediated immunity, and ultimately protection against challenge. Guinea pigs immunized with a T-cell epitope peptide for foot-and-mouth disease virus generated significant neutralizing titers when this peptide was conjugated with Pam₃CSS at the amino-terminus (Wiesmüller *et al.*, 1989). Further, animals that expressed a high neutralizing titer had relatively long-term protection from disease on challenge with live virus. These authors concluded that protection was accomplished via the covalent conjugation of a B-cell mitogen (Pam₃CSS) to the peptide containing the T-cell epitope.

The ability of a vaccine to generate cell-mediated immunity is particularly important in the case of intracellular pathogens. Cytotoxic T lymphocytes (CTLs) kill infected cells by recognizing a complex of MHC class I molecules and peptide fragments of protein synthesized internally. In vivo priming with peptide epitopes is difficult because antigens delivered to antigen-presenting cells are processed in the context of MHC class II molecules and therefore do not stimulate the appropriate T-cell subpopulation. This has been overcome by the use of adjuvants (Chapter 22). Lipopeptide conjugates have been shown to have the capability to induce virus-specific CTLs via an in vivo priming (Deres *et al.*, 1989; Schild *et al.*, 1991). In these experiments, mice were immunized with influenza virus peptides coupled to Pam₃CSS, peptide only, or intact virus. Spleen cells from recipient animals were then isolated and stimulated in culture with either the immunizing peptide or virus. These effector cells were then tested with target cells that were either infected with virus or preincubated with peptide. CTLs were clearly demonstrated to an equivalent degree in animals primed with either virus or lipopeptide conjugate, whereas no CTLs were observed in animals primed with unconjugated peptide. Very similar results were obtained with lipopeptide constructs of HIV envelope glycoprotein epitopes (Martinon *et al.*, 1992). This demonstrates that it is possible to generate CTLs by priming *in vivo* with a totally synthetic molecule, and provides support for the potential utility of this technology for vaccines containing multiple epitopes such as recombinant proteins.

The mechanism of action of lipopeptide adjuvants has not yet been fully explained. It seems clear that the primary effect of the lipidation of immunogens is to direct the interaction of these compounds with the plasma membrane of the cells of the immune system. This effect is evident from the B-cell and macrophage mitogenic activity that many of these lipopeptides are known to possess. A putative lipopeptide receptor or binding protein from B lymphocytes has been described (Biesert *et al.*, 1986), but its relevance to the physiological effects of lipopeptide conjugates remains to be determined. The biochemical sequelae of binding of lipopeptide with immune cells have been studied from many different aspects, including cytokine release and intracellular signaling by various pathways. These results have been recently reviewed (Bessler and Jung, 1992; Wiesmüller *et al.*, 1992). Despite a large body of experimental data, a concrete description of the mechanism of action of lipopeptide adjuvants remains elusive.

An important aspect with regard to the clinical utility of lipopeptide vaccines is their physical effects on animal tissues upon injection. Complete Freund's adjuvant is known to cause severe inflammation and pronounced fibrosis, often leading to abscess formation. This may in part be related to the long-term deposition of this mineral-oil based adjuvant.

Synthetic lipopeptide conjugates, however, cause only a transient inflammation, which rapidly resolves and does not result in fibrous tissue damage (Wiedemann *et al.*, 1991). Thus, lipopeptide adjuvants possess many characteristics that make them ideal candidates as components of effective vaccines.

2. PRODUCT DESCRIPTION OF *BORRELIA BURGDORFERI* LIPOPROTEIN VACCINES

2.1. *E. coli* Expression and Purification

2.1.1. OspA, OspB SIGNAL SEQUENCE

OspA and OspB are tandemly arrayed on a linear plasmid (Howe *et al.*, 1986) and are cotranscribed as one transcriptional unit from an operon situated on an approximately 49-kb double-stranded DNA, linear plasmid of *B. burgdorferi* (Barbour, 1989). Genetic analysis has indicated that both OspA and OspB are lipoproteins with three characteristics typical of prokaryotic signal peptides (Inouye and Halegoua, 1980), including a basic amino-terminus, a hydrophobic central core, and a recognition site for the peptidase (Bergstrom *et al.*, 1989).

The *Borrelia* lipidation and cleavage site differs only slightly from the consensus sequence of 26 other bacterial lipoproteins (Hayashi and Wu, 1990). The consensus motif for positions −4 to +1 is (Leu, Met, Val)-(Leu)-(Ala, Ser)-(Gly, Ala)-(Cys) whereas all reported sequences of the OspA and OspB signal sequence utilize alanine at position −4 and isoleucine at position −2 (Table I). Of 37 known lipoprotein sequences, the bulkier isoleucine substitution at position −2 occurs only in P37 of *Mycoplasma hyorhinis* and Type III PenP of *Bacillus cereus*. Although the isoleucine substitutions are also used in the signal sequence for OspC and OspD, these proteins are unusual in that both have a serine at position −1. Despite these differences, all four of the major borrelial lipoproteins have been expressed and processed into mature acylated proteins when cloned into *E. coli*.

OspA and OspB were confirmed biochemically to be lipoproteins by Brandt *et al.* (1990). As with other lipoproteins, processing of the prolipoproteins to a mature lipoprotein can be altered. Truncating the first 17 codons that represent the signal sequence of the *OspA* gene results in the overproduction of a nonlipidated protein when expressed in *E. coli* (Dunn *et al.*, 1990) which is monomeric after purification. Another construct with an intact *Borrelia* signal sequence was processed correctly and resulted in a lipidated protein, albeit with much lower expression levels. Interestingly, this protein showed a strong tendency for self-association after purification. We have found that expression levels of either OspB or OspA in *E. coli* can reach 11 to 16 mg/g wet cell paste in clones that lack an intact bacterial lipidation recognition site. This compares with 4 to 3.5 mg of OspA or OspB per gram wet cell paste in clones that contain an intact *Borrelia* signal sequence. The disadvantage in protein expression is outweighed by the much greater immunogenicity of the acylated form of the two proteins (Fig. 1).

Table I
Examples of Lipoproteins Found in *Borrelia* and *E. coli*

Lipo-protein	Signal sequence[a]	N-terminus of mature lipoprotein	References
Borrelia OspA			
B31	M KKYLL GIGLI **LALIA**	CKQNV SSLDE KNSVS VDLPG EMKV	this chapter, Eiffert (1992)
N40	M KKYLL GIGLI **LALIA**	CKQNV SSLDE KNSVS VDLPG EMNV	Jonsson *et al.* (1992)
25015	M KKYLL GIGLI **LALIA**	CKQNV SSLDE KNSVS VDLPG EMKV	Fikrig *et al.* (1992c)
GÖ2	M KKYLL GIGLI **LALIA**	CKQNV SSLDE KNSVS VDLPG GMTV	Jonsson *et al.* (1992)
ZS7	M KKYLL GIGLI **LALIA**	CKQNV SSLDE KNSVS VDLPG EMNV	Jonsson *et al.* (1992)
ACAI	M KKYLL GIGLI **LALIA**	CKQNV SSLDE KNSAS VDLPG EMKV	Jonsson *et al.* (1992)
G25	M KKYLL GIGLI **LALIA**	CKQNV SSLDE KNSVS VDLPG GMTV	this chapter
Ip90	M KKYLL GIGLI **LALIA**	CKQNV SSLDE KNSVS VDLPG GMQV	Jonsson *et al.* (1992)
Borrelia OspB			
B31	MRLLI GFALA **LALIG**	CAQKG AESIG SQKEN DLNLE DSSK	this chapter, Eiffert (1992)
GÖ2	MRLLI GFALA **LALIG**	CAQKG AESIG SQKEN DLNLE DSSK	Eiffert (1992)
ACAI	M KQYLL VFALV **LALIA**	CSQKG TEPKS TSQDH NDQEI INSDN	Jonsson *et al.* (1992)
Ip90	M KKYLL GFALV **LALIA**	CGQKG AEPKH NDQDV EDLKK DQKDD	Jonsson *et al.* (1992)
Borrelia OspD			
B31	MKK LIKILL LSLFL **LLSIS**	CVHDK QELSS KSNLN NQKGY LDNEG	Norris *et al.* (1992)
E. coli lipoproteins			
Lpp	MKATK LVLGA VILGS T**LLAG**	CSSNA KIDQL SSDVQ TLNAK VDQLS	Nakamura (1979)

[a]Boldface letters represent the lipidation and cleavage recognition site.

2.1.2. PURIFICATION OF LIPOPROTEINS USING DETERGENT PHASE SEPARATION

Phase partition methods are among the oldest separation techniques for protein purification. One example is the use of membrane-solubilizing nonionic detergents, which can be used to release integral membrane proteins into a monophasic solution. Then, either by raising temperature or increasing ionic strength, a two-phase solution is formed in which hydrophobic proteins intercalate into the predominantly detergent phase while hydrophilic proteins partition into the water phase. This method had been successfully applied to the separation and purification of integral membrane proteins from intracellular or peripheral membrane proteins (Bordier, 1981). More recently, this method has been used to purify membrane proteins of *Treponema pallidum* (Randolf and Norgard, 1988) using Triton X-114. Subsequent analysis of these major *T. pallidum* proteins revealed that they were lipoproteins (Chamberlain *et al.*, 1989). This same approach was successfully used in the extraction of *B. burgdorferi* lipoproteins from *B. burgdorferi* by Brandt *et al.* (1990). Alternately, cloned OspA and OspB that are fully acylated have been purified from *E. coli* using a combination of anion exchange chromatographic techniques (Ma *et al.*, 1994). One disadvantage of this method is that it does not separate acylated from partially or non-acylated protein.

Biophysical studies using fluorescence-quenching of fluorescein-labeled synthetic lipoproteins have revealed that the tripalmitoyl-*S*-glycerylcysteinyl moiety inserts into the hydrophobic lipid bilayer with the protein moiety free to interact with the aqueous phase (Metzger *et al.*, 1991). The lipopeptides also showed a tendency toward self-association and formed membrane patches.

2.2. Vaccine Safety

Two companies, Connaught and SmithKline Beecham, have begun formal efficacy trials of OspA-based vaccines (Rosenthal, 1993; Anon, 1993a) and there has been one report of a Phase I safety and immunogenicity trial (Keller *et al.*, 1994). The Phase I study by Connaught compared a soluble and alum-formulated full-length OspA vaccine in a two- and three-dose schedule. As anticipated, the most common reactions were pain and tenderness at the injection site and reactions did not increase after boosters were given. Although both formulations were well tolerated and immunogenic, there was no statistically significant difference between the immunogenicity of the vaccine with or without alum.

Considering the highly immunogenic nature of borrelial lipoproteins, it may seem odd that an adjuvanted vaccine would be required. Aluminum hydroxide, an adjuvant commonly used for human vaccines, is unable to significantly increase the induction of functional antibody response to OspA (Erdile *et al.*, 1993; Ma *et al.*, 1994), whereas QS-21 can significantly enhance borreliacidal antibody responses to OspA and OspB (Ma *et al.*, 1994; Ma, 1995). Therefore, QS-21 may be an ideal adjuvant candidate for a subunit Lyme disease vaccine. An experimental vaccine containing acylated OspA, OspB, and QS-21 has conferred protection against field-collected, spirochete-infected tick challenge in dogs (Coughlin *et al.*, 1995), and therefore shows promise for the development of an effective vaccine against Lyme disease in humans. QS-21 is also well tolerated and reasonably nontoxic in many animal species including man (Chapter 22).

3. VACCINE EVALUATION

3.1. What Is the Nature of Vaccine-Induced Protection?

Immunization with recombinant OspA and/or OspB formulated with Freund's adjuvant or QS-21 confers protection against homologous challenge either by parenteral injection (Fikrig *et al.*, 1992a; Ma *et al.*, 1994), or by spirochete-infected tick feeding on mice (Fikrig *et al.*, 1992b) and on dogs (Coughlin *et al.*, 1995). Surprisingly, the experimental vaccine can also eliminate *B. burgdorferi* from challenge ticks feeding on the immunized mice (Fikrig *et al.*, 1992b). However, OspA-based vaccine fails to confer protection against heterologous challenge (Fikrig *et al.*, 1992c) and cannot eliminate the infection by postexposure immunization (Fikrig *et al.*, 1993a).

3.1.1. ALTHOUGH IMMUNOGENIC, THESE LIPOPROTEINS ARE NOT NORMALLY RECOGNIZED IN INFECTED ANIMALS

Paradoxically, OspA and OspB as components of vaccines are highly immunogenic targets of immunoprotective antibodies but are only infrequently immunogenic in naturally infected people and animals. Typically, between 5 and 15% of humans who are infected with *B. burgdorferi* and show clinical symptoms have antibodies that react with OspA or OspB by Western blot (Zöller *et al.*, 1991; Ma *et al.*, 1992). Reactivity with OspA or OspB was, however, correlated with the development of late-stage borreliosis (Ma *et al.*, 1992). The low responsiveness to OspA and OspB contrasts with the high responsiveness to any of ten or more other borrelial protein bands including flagellin.

The low OspA and OspB responsiveness can be mimicked when laboratory animals are experimentally infected. Appel *et al.* (1993) observed that needle- or tick-infected dogs differed in Western blot profile. Western blots of needle-inoculated dogs developed OspA and OspB reactivity predominately beginning on day 7, whereas tick-challenged dogs did not develop OspA or OspB reactivity until much later and then only as part of a much broader reactivity with other borrelial proteins. Similarly, hamsters that are infected by needle inoculation developed a potent antibody response to OspA and OspB. In contrast, hamsters infected by tick-transmitted *B. burgdorferi* developed a weak antibody response to OspA and OspB (Roehrig *et al.*, 1992). Roehrig and colleagues proposed that there are low levels of OspA and OspB in the tick inoculum or that the tick or bacteria are able to downregulate the production of OspA and OspB during the initial stages of infection. Reactivity with several other borrelial antigens were uninfluenced by the route of infection.

Changes in the protein profile have also been observed following reintroduction of *B. burgdorferi* strains into *Ixodes* ticks (Hu *et al.*, 1992). In these experiments, low-passage laboratory strains with known protein profiles were fed to ticks through a capillary tube and then reisolated from the tick midgut 1 week later. In several cases, strains that were phenotypically negative for OspA or OspB produced reisolates that expressed either or both of these proteins. Although the mechanism that produced this unusual result is not known, the unique environment of the tick midgut may play a role in the expression level of *B. burgdorferi* outer surface antigens.

3.1.2. PROTECTION IS ANTIBODY MEDIATED

Borrelia are resistant to killing in vitro by nonimmune sera but are readily killed by antibody-dependent complement-mediated killing (Kochi and Johnson, 1988). The mechanism of killing utilizes the classic pathway through the formation of a membrane attack complex and does not involve the alternative complement pathway. In vivo, it has been shown that passive immunization with serum from immunized animals could transfer protection from infection with live *B. burgdorferi* (Johnson *et al.*, 1986b; Schmitz *et al.*, 1990). Thus, humoral immunity appears to be the primary mechanism of protection against infection.

A potential role for phagocytic cells also exists. Georgilis *et al.* (1991) examined the potential of peripheral blood mononuclear cells, monocytes, or polymorphonuclear neutrophils to kill *Borrelia*. They found that 45–67% of high-passage organisms were eliminated whereas only 5–6% of low-passage organisms were eliminated. There was no difference in the ability of the two groups to stimulate oxidative burst. Further, low passage number and resistance to elimination by phagocytic cells was strongly correlated with the ability of *Borrelia* to infect mice.

3.1.3. CELL-MEDIATED IMMUNITY MAY BE NEEDED TO ELIMINATE INTRACELLULAR *BORRELIA*

Although there is a large body of experimental data supporting the ability of antibodies alone to prevent infection by *Borrelia*, there have been reports that *Borrelia* are able to invade human endothelial cells (Comstock and Thomas, 1991; Ma *et al.*, 1991). Whether intracellular *Borrelia* are viable in vivo or are able to reproduce intracellularly is not known. In cell culture, intracellular *Borrelia* are able to evade antibiotics and remain viable, but it is not clear whether host cells are subject to attack by antibody-dependent cell cytotoxicity (ADCC). What is clear is that infected humans are capable of raising Th cells that are able to recognize several epitopes on OspA (Shanafelt *et al.*, 1992). This response usually develops late in disease and is associated with the onset of chronic arthritis and neurologic complications (Steere, 1989). One advantage of vaccination is that resting intracellular *Borrelia* may become targets for ADCC if persistent levels of antibodies can be maintained. If *Borrelia* are capable of reproducing intracellularly, then a vaccine that produces cell-mediated immunity directed against antigens presented at the cell surface in association with MHC class I would be required. An OspA vaccine containing QS-21 (Coughlin *et al.*, 1995; Chapter 22) or the BCG-vectored vaccine described by MedImmune (Anon, 1993b) are likely to produce this kind of cell-mediated immunity.

3.2. Differences in Immunoprotective Antibodies Induced by Acylated versus Nonacylated Outer Surface Proteins

The lipidation of OspA and OspB has been demonstrated to be critical for the enhanced immunogenicity of both antigens including the induction of anti-borrelial antibody (Erdile *et al.*, 1993; Ma and Coughlin, 1993; Ma *et al.*, 1994). Acylated OspA is more immunogenic than non-acylated OspA in mice, as indicated by increased borrelial growth inhibitory activity (Erdile *et al.*, 1993). Recently, a similar observation has been made with both OspA and OspB in dogs (Ma *et al.* 1995).

3.3. Cross Neutralization of Genetically and Geographically Divergent *Borrelia*

Fikrig *et al.* (1992c) observed that a *B. burgdorferi* strain N40 OspA vaccine protected against challenge with strain N40 but not strain 25015 isolated from human cerebrospinal fluid. Conversely, an OspA vaccine based on strain 25015 protected against challenge with strain 25015 but not strain N40. More recently, Jobe *et al.* (1994) have shown that two immunizations of a hamster with a *Borrelia* lysate vaccine induced high borreliacidal titers only to one of four *Borrelia* serogroups. Further, the duration of immunity was short-lived.

Acylated OspA and OspB formulated with adjuvant QS-21 induced significantly higher antibody titers and borreliacidal activity than nonacylated antigens. Of interest is that only the vaccine formulated with OspA, OspB, and QS-21 induced cross-borreliacidal

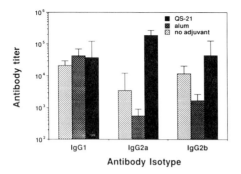

Figure 4. Comparison of antibody titers raised in C3H/HeJ mice immunized twice with 1 μg per dose of acylated OspA in sterile PBS, OspA on 10 μg alum (10:1 alum/protein, w/w), or OspA with 15 μg of QS-21. HRP-conjugated goat anti-mouse IgG1, IgG2a, and IgG2b were used to determine the titer of specific mouse isotypes against recombinant OspA derived from *B. burgdorferi* strain B31.

activity against *B. garinii* strain G25 (Fig. 2). When ten C3H/HeJ mice were immunized twice with acylated OspA from *B. burgdorferi* strain B31 formulated either in sterile PBS, on alum, or with QS-21, very different immune responses were induced (Fig. 4). The OspA specific IgG2a and IgG2b titers were reduced by alum and increased by QS-21 relative to the group receiving OspA and no adjuvant. IgG1 titers were identical for all three vaccine groups.

4. FUTURE DIRECTIONS

4.1. Progress of Clinical Trials in High-Incidence Areas of the United States

Connaught Laboratories has initiated trials of its OspA vaccine on the East Coast (Rosenthal, 1993; Anon, 1993a), eventually enrolling as many as 8000 people. The vaccine would be given in the winter with a booster 30 days later (Anon, 1994). Separate trials are planned by SmithKline Beecham and will be done on Nantucket and Martha's Vineyard, Massachusetts, as well as on Block Island, Rhode Island. Because of the high risk of exposure in these areas, it is likely that results from these trials will be available shortly.

4.2 Social Behavior as a Factor in the Control of Lyme Disease

Although there has been fast progress toward the development of a Lyme disease vaccine, it should be remembered that humans are inadvertent hosts for this spirochete and that even the most successful application of the vaccine will not remove the risk of exposure. It is clear that the etiologic agent of this disease is genetically quite diverse (Marconi and Garon, 1992) and capable of clonal polymorphism in the outer surface proteins in response to selection pressure (Bundoc and Barbour, 1989; Fikrig *et al.*, 1993b). An effective strategy for the control of Lyme disease should include vector surveillance to identify high-risk areas, vector control measures, and eventually vaccination of people at risk of infection (Barbour and Fish, 1993).

ACKNOWLEDGMENTS

We gratefully acknowledge Deborah Davis for sequencing and cloning of *Borrelia* proteins, Barbara Perilli-Palmer for purification of the these proteins, and Patrice Bulger for serologic analysis of immunized animals.

REFERENCES

Anonymous, 1993a, *Biotech Daily* **2**:1–2.

Anonymous, 1993b, *Genetic Tech. News* **13**:2.

Anonymous, 1994, *Vaccine Weekly* p. 7.

Appel, M. J. G., Allan, S., Jacobson, R. H., Lauderdale, T. L., Chang, Y. F., Shin, S. J., Thomford, R. J., Todhunter, R., and Summers, B. A., 1993, Experimental Lyme disease in dogs produces arthritis and persistent infection, *J. Infect. Dis.* **167**:651–664.

Audibert, F. M., and Lise, L. D., 1993, Adjuvants: Current status, clinical perspectives and future prospects, *Trends Pharm. Sci.* **14**:174–178.

Baranton, G., Postic, D., Saint Girons, I., Borlin, P., Piffaretti, J.-C., Assous, M., and Grimont, P. A. D., 1992, Delineation of *Borrelia burgdorferi* sensu stricto, *Borrelia garinii* sp. nov., and group VS461 associated with Lyme borreliosis, *Int. J. Syst. Bacteriol.* **42**:378–383.

Barbour, A. G., 1989, The molecular biology of *Borrelia, Rev. Infect. Dis.* **11**:S1470–S1474.

Barbour, A. G., and Fish, D., 1993, The biological and social phenomenon of Lyme disease, *Science* **260**:1610–1616.

Barbour, A. G., Burgdorfer, W., Hayes, S. F., Peter, O., and Aeschlimann, A., 1983, Isolation of a cultivable spirochete from *Ixodes ricinus* ticks of Switzerland, *Curr. Microbiol.* **8**:123–126.

Barbour, A. G., Tessier, S. L., and Hayes, S. F., 1984, Variation in a major surface protein of Lyme disease spirochetes, *Infect. Immun.* **54**:94–100.

Bergstrom, S., Bundoc, V. G., and Barbour, A. G., 1989, Molecular analysis of linear plasmid-encoded major surface proteins, OspA and OspB, of the Lyme disease spirochete *Borrelia burgdorferi, Mol. Microbiol.* **13**:479–486.

Bessler, W. G., and Jung, G., 1992, Synthetic lipopeptides as novel adjuvants, *Res. Immunol.* **143**:548–553.

Bessler, W. G., Resch, K., Hancock, E., and Hantke, K., 1977, Induction of lymphocyte proliferation and membrane changes by lipopeptide derivatives of the lipoprotein from the outer membrane of *Escherichia coli, Z. Immun-Forsch.* **153**:11–22.

Bessler, W. G., Cox, M., Lex, A., Suhr, B., Wiesmüller, K.-H., and Jung, G., 1985a, Synthetic lipopeptide analogs of bacterial lipoprotein are potent polyclonal activators for murine B lymphocytes, *J. Immunol.* **135**:1900–1905.

Bessler, W. G., Suhr, B., Bühring, H.-J., Muller, C. P., Wiesmüller, K.-H., Becker, G., and Jung, G., 1985b, Specific antibodies elicited by antigen covalently linked to a synthetic adjuvant, *Immunobiology* **170**:239–244.

Biesert, L., Scheuer, W., and Bessler, W. G., 1986, Interaction of mitogenic bacterial lipoprotein and a synthetic analogue with mouse lymphocytes, *Eur. J. Biochem.* **162**:651–657.

Bordier, C., 1981, Phase separation of integral membrane proteins in Triton X-114 solution, *J. Biol. Chem.* **256**:1604–1607.

Brandt, M., Riley, B., Radolf, J., and Norgard, M., 1990, Immunogenic integral membrane proteins of *Borrelia burgdorferi* are lipoproteins, *Infect. Immun.* **58**:983–991.

Bundoc, V. G., and Barbour, A. G., 1989, Clonal polymorphisms of outer membrane protein OspB of *Borrelia burgdorferi, Infect. Immun.* **57**:2733–2741.

Burgdorfer, W., Barbour, A. G., Hayes, S. F., Benach, J. L., Grunwaldt, E., and Davis, J. P., 1982, Lyme disease—a tick borne spirochetosis? *Science* **261**:1317–1319.

Canica, M. M., Nato, F., du Merle, L., Mazie, J. C., Baranton, G., and Postic, D., 1993, Monoclonal antibodies for identification of *Borrelia afzelii* sp. nov. associated with cutaneous manifestations of Lyme borreliosis, *Scand. J. Infect. Dis.* **25**:441–448.

Chamberlain, N. R., Brandt, M. E., Erwin, A. L., Randolf, J. D., and Norgard, M. V., 1989, Major integral membrane protein immunogens of *Treponema pallidum* are proteolipids, *Infect. Immun.* **57**:2872–2877.

Comstock, L. E., and Thomas, D. D., 1991, Characterization of *Borrelia burgdorferi* invasion of cultured endothelial cells, *Microb. Pathog.* **10**:137–148.

Coughlin, R. T., Fish, D., Mather, T. N., Ma, J., Pavia, C., and Bulger, P., 1995, Protection of dogs from Lyme disease with a vaccine containing OspA, OspB, and the saponin adjuvant QS-21, *J. Infect. Dis.* (in press).

Deres, K., Schild, H., Wiesmüller, K.-H., Jung, G., and Rammensee, H.-G., 1989, *In vivo* priming of virus-specific cytotoxic T lymphocytes with synthetic lipopeptide vaccine, *Nature* **342**:561–564.

Dunn, J. J., Lade, B. N., and Barbour, A. G., 1990, Outer surface protein A (OspA) from the Lyme disease spirochete, *Borrelia burgdorferi*: High level expression and purification of a soluble recombinant form of OspA, *Protein Expr. Purif.* **1**:159–168.

Eiffert, H., Ohlenbusch, A., Fehling, W., Lotter, H., and Thomssen, R., 1992, *Infect. Immun.* **60**:1864–1868.

Erdile, L. F., Brandt, M.-A., Warakomski, D. J., Westrack, G. J., Sadziene, A., Barbour, A. G., and Mays, J. P., 1993, Role of attached lipid in immunogenicity of *Borrelia burgdorferi* OspA, *Infect. Immun.* **61**:81–90.

Fikrig, E., Barthold, S. W., Kantor, F. S., and Flavell, R. A., 1990, Protection of mice against the Lyme disease agent by immunizing with recombinant OspA, *Science* **250**:553–556.

Fikrig, E., Barthold, S., Marcantonio, N., Deponte, K., Kantor, F., and Flavell, F., 1992a, Roles of OspA, OspB, and flagellin in protective immunity to Lyme borreliosis in laboratory mice, *Infect. Immun.* **60**:657–661.

Fikrig, E., Telford, S. R., Barthold, S. W., Kantor, F. S., Spielman, A., and Flavell, R. A., 1992b, Elimination of *Borrelia burgdorferi* from vector ticks feeding on OspA-immunized mice, *Proc. Natl. Acad. Sci. USA* **89**:5418–5421.

Fikrig, E., Barthold, S. W., Persing, D. H., Sun, X., Kantor, F. S., and Flavell, R. A., 1992c, *Borrelia burgdorferi* strain 25015: Characterization of outer surface protein A and vaccination against infection, *J. Immunol.* **148**:2256–2260.

Fikrig, E., Barthold, S. W., and Flavell, R. A., 1993a, OspA vaccination of mice with established *Borrelia burgdorferi* infection alters disease but not infection, *Infect. Immun.* **61**:2553–2557.

Fikrig, E., Tao, H., Kantor, F. S., Barthold, S. W., and Flavell, R. A., 1993b, Evasion of protective immunity by *Borrelia burgdorferi* by truncation of outer surface protein B, *Proc. Natl. Acad. Sci. USA* **90**:4092–4096.

Fuchs, R., Jauris, S., Lottspeich, F., Preac-Mursic, V., Wilske, B., and Soutschek, E., 1992, Molecular analysis and expression of a *Borrelia burgdorferi* gene encoding a 22 KDa protein (pC) in *Escherichia coli*, *Mol. Microbiol.* **6**:503–509.

Georgilis, A. K., Steere, A. C., and Klempner, M. S., 1991, Infectivity of *Borrelia burgdorferi* correlates with resistance to elimination by phagocytic cells, *J. Infect. Dis.* **163**:150–155.

Hantke, K., and Braun, V., 1973, Covalent binding of lipid to protein. Diglyceride and amide linked fatty acid at the N-terminal end of the murein lipoprotein of the *Escherichia coli* outer membrane, *Eur. J. Biochem.* **34**:284–296.

Hayashi, S., and Wu, H. C., 1990, Lipoproteins in bacteria, *J. Bioenerg. Biomembr.* **22**:451–471.

Howe, T. R., Laquier, F. R., and Barbour, A. G., 1986, Organization of genes encoding two major outer surface proteins of the Lyme disease agent *Borrelia burgdorferi* within a single transcriptional unit, *Infect. Immun.* **54**:207–212.

Hu, C. M., Gern, L., and Aeschlimann, A., 1992, Changes in the protein profile and antigenicity of different *Borrelia burgdorferi* strains after reintroduction to *Ixodes ricinus* ticks, *Parasite Immun.* **14**:415–427.

Inouye, M., and Halegoua, S., 1980, Secretion and membrane localization of proteins in *Escherichia coli*, *Crit. Rev. Biochem.* **7**:339–371.

Jobe, D. A., Callister, S. M., Lim, L. C., Lovrich, S. D., and Schell, R. F., 1994, Ability of canine Lyme disease vaccine to protect hamsters against infection with several isolates of *Borrelia burgdorferi, J. Clin. Microbiol.* **32**:618–622.

Johnson, R. C., Schmid, G. P., Hyde, F. W., Steigerwalt, A. G., and Brenner, D. J., 1984, *Borrelia burgdorferi* sp. nov.: Etiologic agent of Lyme disease, *Int. J. Syst. Bacteriol.* **34**:496–497.

Johnson, R. C., Kodner, C., and Russell, M., 1986a, Active immunization of hamsters against experimental infection with *Borrelia burgdorferi, Infect. Immun.* **54**:897–898.

Johnson, R. C., Kodner, C., and Russell, M., 1986b, Passive immunization of hamsters against experimental infection with *Borrelia burgdorferi, Infect. Immun.* **53**:713–714.

Jonsson, M., Noppa, L., Barbour, A. G., and Bergström, S., 1992, Heterogeneity of outer membrane proteins in *Borrelia burgdorferi*: Comparison of osp operons of three isolates of different geographic origins, *Infect. Immun.* **60**:1845–1853.

Katona, L. I., Beck, G., and Habicht, G. S., 1992, Purification and immunological characterization of a major low-molecular-weight lipoprotein from *Borrelia burgdorferi, Infect. Immun.* **60**:4995–5003.

Keller, D., Koster, F. T., Marks, D. H., Hosbach, P., Erdile, L. F., and Mays, J. P., 1994, Safety and immunogenicity of a recombinant outer surface protein A Lyme vaccine, *J. Am. Med. Assoc.* **271**:1764–1768.

Kensil, C. R., Newman, M. J., Coughlin, R. T., Soltysik, S., Bedore, D., Recchia, J., Wu, J.-Y., and Marciani, D. J., 1993, The use of Stimulon adjuvant to boost vaccine response, *Vaccine Res.* **2**:273–281.

Kochi, S. K., and Johnson, R. C., 1988, Role of immunoglobulin G in killing *Borrelia burgdorferi* by the classic complement pathway, *Infect. Immun.* **56**:314–321.

Lam, T. T., Nguyen, T.-P. K., Montgomery, R. R., Kantor, F. S., Fikrig, E., and Flavell, R. A., 1994, Outer surface proteins E and F of *Borrelia burgdorferi*, the agent of Lyme disease, *Infect. Immun.* **62**:290–298.

Loleit, M., Tröger, W., Wiesmüller, K.-H., Jung, G., Strecker, M., and Bessler, W. G., 1990, Conjugates of synthetic lymphocyte-activating lipopeptides with segments from HIV proteins induce protein-specific antibody formation, *Biol. Chem. Hoppe-Seyler.* **371**:967–975.

Lovrich, S. D., Callister, S. M., Lim, L. C. L., and Schell, R. F., 1993, Seroprotective groups among isolates of *Borrelia burgdorferi, J. Infect. Dis.* **61**:4367–4374.

Ma, B., Christen, B., Leung, D., and Vigo-Pelfrey, C., 1992, Serodiagnosis of Lyme borreliosis by Western immunoblot: Reactivity of various significant antibodies against *Borrelia burgdorferi, J. Clin. Microbiol.* **30**:370–376.

Ma, J. and Coughlin, R. T., 1993, A simplex colorimetric microtiter assay for borreliacidal activity of antisera, *J. Microbiol. Meth.* **17**:145–153.

Ma, J., Bulger, P., Davis, D. vR., Perilli-Palmer, B., Bedore, D., Kensil, C., Young, E., Hung, C.-H., Seals, J., Pavia, C., and Coughlin, R. T., 1994, Impact of the saponin adjuvant QS-21 and aluminum hydroxide on the immunogenicity of recombinant OspA and OspB of *Borrelia burgdorferi, Vaccine* **12**:925–932.

Ma, J., Bulger, P., Dante, S., Davis, D. vR., Perilli-Palmer, B., and Coughlin, R., 1995, Characterization of canine immune responses to Osp subunit vaccines and natural infection by Lyme disease spirochetes, *J. Infect. Dis.* (in press).

Ma, Y., Sturrock, A., and Weis, J. J., 1991, Intracellular localization of *Borrelia burgdorferi* within human endothelial cells, *Infect. Immun.* **59**:671–678.

Marconi, R. T., and Garon, C. F., 1992, Phylogenetic analysis of the genus *Borrelia*: A comparison of North American and European isolates of *Borrelia burgdorferi, J. Bacteriol.* **174**:241–244.

Marconi, R. T., Samuels, D. S., and Garon, C. F., 1993, Transcriptional analyses and mapping of the ospC gene in Lyme disease spirochetes, *J. Bacteriol.* **175**:926–932.

Martinon, F., Gras-Masse, H., Boutillon, C., Chirat, F., Deprez, B., Guillet, J.-G., Gomard, E., Tartar, A., and Levy, J.-P., 1992, Immunization of mice with lipopeptides bypasses the prerequisite for adjuvant. Immune response of BALB/c mice to Human Immunodeficiency Virus envelope glycoprotein, *J. Immunol.* **149**:3416–3422.

Melchers, F., Braun, V., and Galanos, C., 1975, The lipoprotein of the outer membrane of *Escherichia coli*: A B lymphocyte mitogen, *J. Exp. Med.* **142**:473–482.

Metzger, J., Wiesmüller, K.-H., Schaude, R., Bessler, W. G., and Jung, G., 1991, Synthesis of novel immunologically active tripalmytoyl-S-glyceryl-cysteine lipopeptides as useful intermediates for immunogen preparations, *Int. J. Pept. Protein Res.* **37**:46–57.

Muller, C. P., Bühring, H.-J., Becker, G., Jung, G., Tröger, W., Saalmüller, A., Wiesmüller, K.-H. and Bessler, W. G., 1989, Specific antibody response towards predicted epitopes of the epidermal growth factor receptor induced by a thermostable synthetic peptide adjuvant conjugate, *Clin. Exp. Immunol.* **78**:499–504.

Nakamura, K., Pirtle, R. M., and Inouye, M., 1979, Homology of gene coding for outer membrane lipoprotein with various gram-negative bacteria, *J. Bacteriol.* **137**:595–604.

Norris, S. J., Carter, C. J., Howell, J. K., and Barbour, A. G., 1992, Low-passage-associated proteins of *Borrelia burgdorferi* B31: Characterization and molecular cloning of OspD, a surface-exposed, plasmid-encoded lipoprotein, *Infect. Immun.* **60**:4662–4672.

Park, K.-H., Chang, W.-H., and Schwan, T. G., 1993, Identification and characterization of Lyme disease spirochetes, *Borrelia burgdorferi* sensu lato, isolated in Korea, *J. Clin. Microbiol.* **31**:1831–1837.

Postic, D., Belfaiza, J., Isogai, E., Saint Girons, I., Grimont, P.A.D., and Baranton, G., 1993, A new genomic species in *Borrelia burgdorferi* sensu lato isolated from Japanese ticks, *Res. Microbiol.* **144**:467–473.

Preac-Mursic, V., Wilske, B., Patsuris, E., Jauris, S., Will, G., Soutschek, E., Reinhardt, S., Lehnert, G., Klockmann, U., and Mehraein, P., 1992, Active immunization with pC protein of *Borrelia burgdorferi* protects gerbils against *Borrelia burgdorferi* infection, *Infection* **20**:342–349.

Randolf, J. D., and Norgard, M. V., 1988, Pathogen specificity of *Treponema pallidum* subsp. pallidum integral membrane proteins identified by phase partitioning with Triton X-114, *Infect. Immun.* **56**:1825–1828.

Reindi, M., Redi, B., and Stoffler, G., 1993, Isolation and analysis of a linear plasmid-located gene of *Borrelia burgdorferi* B29 encoding a 27 KDa surface lipoprotein (P27) and its over expression in *Escherichia coli*, *Mol. Microbiol.* **8**:1115–1124.

Reitermann, A., Metzger, J., Wiesmüller, K.-H., Jung, G. and Bessler, W. G., 1989, Lipopeptide derivatives of bacterial lipoprotein constitute potent immune adjuvants combined with or covalently coupled to antigen or hapten, *Biol. Chem. Hoppe-Seyler.* **370**:343–352.

Roehrig, J. T., Piesman, J., Hunt, A. R., Keen, M. G., Happ, C. M., and Johnson, J. B., 1992, The hamster immune response to tick-transmitted *Borrelia burgdorferi* differs from the response to needle-inoculated cultured organisms, *J. Immunol.* **149**:3648–3653.

Rosenthal, E., 1993, *New York Times* **143**:C1–C3.

Schild, H., Deres, K., Wiesmüller, K.-H., Jung, G., and Rammensee, H.-G., 1991, Efficiency of peptides and lipopeptides for *in vivo* priming of virus-specific cytotoxic T cells, *Eur. J. Immunol.* **21**:2649–2654.

Schmitz, J. L., Schell, R. F., Hejka, A. G., and England, D. M., 1990, Passive immunization prevents induction of Lyme arthritis in LSH hamsters, *Infect. Immun.* **58**:144–148.

Schmitz, J. L., Schell, R. F., Lovrich, S. D., Callister, S. M., and Coe, J. E., 1991, Characterization of the protective antibody response to *Borrelia burgdorferi* in experimentally infected LSH hamsters, *Infect. Immun.* **59**:1916–1921.

Shanafelt, M.-C., Anzola, J., Soderberg, C., Yssel, H., Turck, C. W., and Peltz, G., 1992, Epitopes on the outer surface protein A of *Borrelia burgdorferi* recognized by antibodies and T-cells of patients with Lyme disease, *J. Immunol.* **148**:218–224.

Steere, A. C., 1989, Lyme disease, *N. Engl. J. Med.* **321**:586–596.

van Dam, A. P., Kuiper, H., Vos, K., Widjojokusumo, A., de Jongh, B. M., Spanjaard, L., Ramselaar, A. C. P., Kramer, M. D., and Dankert, J., 1993, Different genospecies of *Borrelia burgdorferi* are associated with distinct clinical manifestations of Lyme borreliosis, *Clin. Infect. Dis.* **17**:708–717.

Wiedemann, F., Link, R., Pumpe, K., Jacobshagen, U., Schaeffer, H. E., Wiesmüller, K.-H., Hummel, R.-P., Jung, G., Bessler, W., and Böltz, T., 1991, Histopathological studies on the local reactions induced by complete Freund's adjuvant (CFA), bacterial lipopolysaccharide (LPS) and synthetic lipopeptide (P3C) conjugates, *J. Pathol.* **164**:265–271.

Wiesmüller, K.-H., Jung, G., and Hess, G., 1989, Novel low molecular weight synthetic vaccine against foot and mouth disease containing a potent B-cell and macrophage activator, *Vaccine* **7**:29–33.

Wiesmüller, K.-H., Jung, G., Gillessen, D., Loffl, C., Bessler, W. G., and Böltz, T., 1991, The antibody response in BALB/c mice to the *Plasmodium falciparum* circumsporozoite repetitive epitope covalently coupled to synthetic lipopeptide adjuvant, *Immunology* **72**:109–113.

Wiesmüller, K.-H., Bessler, W. G., and Jung, G., 1992, Solid phase peptide synthesis of lipopeptide vaccines eliciting epitope-specific B-, T-helper and T-killer cell response, *Int. J. Pept. Protein Res.* **40**:255–260.

Wilske, B., Preac-Mursic, V., Schierz, G., Kuhbeck, R., Barbour, A. G., and Kramer, M., 1988, Antigenic variability of *Borrelia burgdorferi*, *Ann. N.Y. Acad. Sci.* **539**:126–143.

Wilske, B., Preac-Mursic, V., Jauris, S., Hofmann, A., Pradel, I., Soutschek, E., Schwab, E., Will, G., and Wanner, G., 1993, Immunological and molecular polymorphisms of OspC, an immunodominant major outer surface protein of *Borrelia burgdorferi*, *Infect Immun.* **61**:2182–2191.

Wu, H. C., 1987, Posttranslational modification and processing of membrane proteins in bacteria, in: *Bacterial Outer Membranes as Model Systems* (M. Inouye, ed.), Wiley, New York, pp. 37–74.

Zöller, L., Burkard, S., and Schäfer, H., 1991, Validity of Western blot band patterns in the serodiagnosis of Lyme borreliosis, *J. Clin. Microbiol.* **29**:174–182.

Chapter 33

Vaccine Research and Development for the Prevention of Filarial Nematode Infections

Robert B. Grieve, Nancy Wisnewski,
Glenn R. Frank, and Cynthia A. Tripp

1. INTRODUCTION

Filarial nematodes constitute a group of pathogens with extraordinary medical and veterinary medical importance. The lymphatic filariae of humans affect almost 90 million people worldwide (Ottesen, 1992). Onchocerciasis is a major cause of infectious blindness, affecting nearly 50 million people in sub-Saharan Africa and the Americas and resulting in blindness in about 1 million people (Taylor, 1985).

Filarial nematodes are complex eukaryotic parasites that have evolved as highly host-adapted parasitic nematodes. The various filarial nematode species universally share several characteristics: (1) they are very host specific, (2) they depend on an arthropod intermediate host for development and host-to-host transmission, and (3) they exhibit lengthy life cycles in the definitive host with attendant long-lasting infection and chronic disease.

The adult forms of these parasites occupy various niches in the definitive host (Table I). Adult worms, depending on the species, are highly variable in size. They are generally small, even threadlike, in diameter and may be from a few centimeters to up to one-half meter in length. The female worms are typically much larger than the male worms with the vast majority of the female's internal volume committed to reproduction.

Through sexual reproduction, adult worms produce an embryonic, prelarval stage called a microfilaria. Depending on the parasite species, these microfilariae preferentially circulate in blood or they can be found in the skin. To perpetuate transmission, microfilariae must be ingested by an appropriate hematophagous arthropod (Table I) where development to a first larval stage (L1), a second larval stage (L2), and a third larval stage (L3) all occur.

Robert B. Grieve, Nancy Wisnewski, Glenn R. Frank, and Cynthia A. Tripp • Paravax, Inc., Fort Collins, Colorado 80525.

Vaccine Design: The Subunit and Adjuvant Approach, edited by Michael F. Powell and Mark J. Newman. Plenum Press, New York, 1995.

Table I

Examples of Principal Filarial Nematode Parasites, Their Intermediate and Definitive Hosts, and Their Sites of Predilection

	Natural definitive host	Intermediate host	Site of predilection
Wuchereria bancrofti	Human	Mosquito	Lymphatics
Brugia malayi	Human	Mosquito	Lymphatics
Brugia pahangi	Cat	Mosquito	Lymphatics
Onchocerca volvulus	Human	Blackfly	Subcutaneous nodules
Loa loa	Human/other primates	Tabanid fly	Subcutaneous tissue, eye
Dirofilaria immitis	Dog	Mosquito	Pulmonary arteries
Acanthocheilonema viteae	Jird	Tick	Subcutaneous tissue
Litomosoides carinii	Cotton rat	Mite	Thoracic cavity

The L3 is adapted to life in both the invertebrate intermediate host as well as the vertebrate definitive host. During, or after, the intermediate host's blood meal, the L3 present in the head and mouthparts of the infected arthropod find their way to the bite wound, thus gaining access to the definitive host. The L3 undergoes yet another morphogenetic change to a fourth larval stage (L4) which, in turn, undergoes the final molt to an immature adult, sometimes termed a fifth stage or L5. The L4 is typically involved with tissue migration and locates the parasite near its preferred site for maturity to the adult worm. Subsequent development to sexual maturity and completion of the life cycle through the generation of microfilariae requires additional time.

The entire developmental cycle within the vertebrate, depending on the parasite species, may require months to over a year. It is noteworthy that in this entire period of larval development in the definitive host, filarial nematodes are extracellular and extravascular. In fact, the L2 is the only stage that dwells intracellularly. Depending on the filarial nematode species, the L2 may be found within the Malpighian tubules, flight muscle, or fat body of the specific arthropod intermediate host.

It is our goal to emphasize the importance of understanding the biology and immunobiology of these unique parasites with the belief that an integrated research approach is necessary for successful vaccine development. Although the various host–filarial parasite systems are unique in many ways, there are conceptual theses that can be transferred from system to system. We have reviewed some of the meaningful literature to underscore those concepts and provided a partial survey of some of the molecules that have been described and molecularly cloned as potential vaccine candidates in these systems. Finally, we derive most of our detailed examples with *Dirofilaria immitis*, a system with which we have had the most experience.

2. EVIDENCE FOR PROTECTIVE IMMUNITY IN FILARIAL NEMATODE INFECTIONS

There are numerous species from at least four related filarial genera (*Wuchereria, Brugia, Onchocerca, Dirofilaria*) that are causative agents of disease in man or animals of veterinary significance. These parasites cause high morbidity related to typically long-lasting, chronic infections in which the life span of the parasite can last for years and repeated exposure is commonplace. The documentation of the existence of naturally acquired protective immunity has focused on epidemiological, immunological, and pathological correlates found within onchocerciasis and lymphatic filariasis endemic populations. These studies are of extreme value, particularly in light of the strict host-specific nature of filariid parasites and the corresponding dearth of suitable animal model systems that would lend themselves to a more systematic, sophisticated study of immune effector mechanisms.

Surrogate definitive host model systems for human filarial parasites that closely mimic the course of disease and pathology of the human infection do not exist. Despite this, initial characterization of host immune responses during experimental manipulation of several nonhuman filarial infections has provided significant information. An extensive body of literature dealing with issues such as the host immune response to single versus repeated infective doses, induction of protection following immunization with crude parasite homogenates, radiation-attenuated parasites, or chemically abbreviated infections, and the putative existence of concomitant immunity has been compiled. The majority of these studies have utilized the following parasite–host interactions: *Dirofilaria immitis*–dog, mouse; *Brugia pahangi*–cat, jird, mouse; *Onchocerca lienalis, O. gutturosa*–jird, mouse; *Acanthocheilonema viteae*–jird, hamster, mouse; and *Litomosoides carinii*–rat, jird, mouse. Several of these infections occur naturally such as *D. immitis* in dogs, *B. pahangi* in cats, and *A. viteae* in jirds, while other interactions, largely in the rodent hosts, constitute surrogate host model systems where the parasite's development is suboptimal.

In the context of vaccine development, it should be remembered that all filarial parasites have complex life cycles in which the definitive host typically is exposed to several distinct developmental stages as the parasite differentiates, such as infective L3, L4, male and female adults, and microfilariae. It is also possible that antigens constitutively present in all stages as well as stage-specific antigens may play a role in immune stimulation. Additionally, it must be remembered that filarial parasites of different genera are heterogeneous in their developmental biology, so various species occupy different habitats within their respective definitive hosts. Correspondingly, different parasitic stages of these various species are known to be the causative agents of what largely has been characterized as immune-mediated pathology associated with clinical disease. This aspect must be considered for each individual filarial species in the development of a suitable vaccine—one that will stimulate immunity and provide protection without inducing or exacerbating pathological sequelae.

2.1. Existence of Naturally Acquired Protective Immunity

2.1.1. HUMAN LYMPHATIC FILARIASIS—THE PUTATIVELY IMMUNE "ENDEMIC NORMAL"

The range of clinical manifestations in lymphatic filariasis is classically referred to as spectral in nature (Ottesen, 1984). In areas endemic for lymphatic filariasis, disease manifestations are categorized into four main clinical types: (1) asymptomatic microfilaremic; (2) microfilaremic with lymphatic pathology, including "filarial fevers" and elephantiasis; (3) amicrofilaremic "occult filariasis" with corresponding tropical pulmonary eosinophilia (TPE) syndrome; and (4) amicrofilaremic, asymptomatic endemic normals. Within the four designated clinical types, certain disease and immunological correlates have been identified. The asymptomatic microfilaremic group is immunologically hyporesponsive, with low levels of antifilarial antibodies (Ottesen *et al.*, 1982) and lymphocytes that do not respond to filarial antigens (Ottesen *et al.*, 1977; Piessens *et al.*, 1980a,b; King *et al.*, 1992). This constitutes a parasite-specific T-cell anergy, Th1 specifically (Ottesen *et al.*, 1977; Piessens *et al.*, 1980b; Nutman *et al.*, 1987; Maizels and Lawrence, 1991; Maizels *et al.*, 1991; King *et al.*, 1993). This group is considered to be immunologically tolerant to adult worms and microfilariae. Symptomatic microfilaremic individuals with lymphatic pathology have measurable cellular and humoral immune responsiveness to filarial antigens (Ottesen *et al.*, 1977, 1982; Piessens *et al.*, 1980a). Amicrofilaremic occult individuals have both humoral, IgG4 and IgE, and cellular, eosinophil and lymphocyte, mediated parasite-specific hyperresponsiveness. This is usually correlated with immune-mediated TPE (Neva and Ottesen, 1978; Ottesen *et al.*, 1979). In essence, the progressively stronger parasite-specific immune responses observed in TPE are associated with both the clearance of microfilariae and onset of severe immune-mediated disease.

Characterization of those individuals without clinical or parasitological evidence of infection has been somewhat ambiguous. It is difficult to differentiate truly immune individuals who are totally free of infection from individuals with single-sex infections, few adult worms, or asymptomatic occult infections (Ottesen, 1984; Day, 1991). Nevertheless, both humoral and cellular-mediated immune responses to parasite antigens are significantly greater in this heterogeneous endemic normal group than in individuals harboring microfilaremic infections, both with and without clinical symptoms (Ottesen *et al.*, 1977, 1982). There is no direct evidence that supports the contention that functional protective immunity is raised in humans. However, the documentation of such subpopulations of putatively immune individuals in areas endemic for *Wuchereria* and *Brugia*, along with the observation that microfilarial rates normally increase until the age of 30 years but remain constant or decrease thereafter (World Health Organization, 1987), provide indirect evidence for naturally acquired protective immunity in humans (Nutman, 1989).

2.1.2. ONCHOCERCIASIS

Direct evidence substantiating the existence of naturally acquired protective immunity against *O. volvulus* infections in humans is similarly absent. Individuals whose infections have been radically cured by chemotherapeutic suramin treatment rapidly become reinfected, indicating that acquired immunity had not developed (Duke, 1968). However, there is increasing circumstantial evidence that a subpopulation of individuals within onchocerciasis-endemic regions, particularly hyper- and meso-endemic regions, may be immune to infection (WHO, 1987; Ward *et al.*, 1988; Elson *et al.*, 1994). These putative endemic normals are exposed to infection, as determined by recombinant antigen-based ELISA and PCR assays, but remain clinically and parasitologically negative. Comparisons of immunological responses using lymphocytes from putatively immune and infected individuals demonstrated a heightened parasite-specific T-cell reactivity, most notably seen as increased interleukin-2 (IL-2) and interleukin-5 (IL-5) production, in the immune group (Ward *et al.*, 1988; Steel and Nutman, 1993). Conversely, putative immune individuals had lower levels of serum onchocerca-specific IgG, IgG subclasses, and IgE than infected subjects (Ward *et al.*, 1988; Boyer *et al.*, 1991; Elson *et al.*, 1994). However, putative immune sera did preferentially recognize several L3-specific antigens by immunoblot (Nutman *et al.*, 1991; Boyer *et al.*, 1991).

Epidemiological data reminiscent of a concomitant-like immunity, showing a decreasing intensity of infection with increasing age (WHO Experts Committee, 1976) and a plateauing of microfilarial concentrations in the skin after 20 to 40 years (Duke and Moore, 1968), also have been reported. In vitro, sera from infected individuals can promote antibody-dependent destruction of microfilariae and infective L3 (Greene *et al.*, 1981, 1985), suggesting that protective antibodies may develop in some portion of the endemic infected population.

It is well documented that immune hyperresponsiveness to microfilarial antigen is associated with localized dermal pathology, termed "sowda," and decreased microfilarial counts, while hyporesponsiveness correlates with generalized infection and high skin microfiladermia (Bartlett *et al.*, 1978; Buttner *et al.*, 1982; Piessens and Mackenzie, 1982). Since clinical dermal and ocular onchocercal disease results from the immune-mediated inflammatory response to damaged or dead microfilariae, there has been a substantial interest in immunity to the microfilarial stage of *Onchocerca*. Animals specifically immunized or spontaneously developing antimicrofilarial antibodies rapidly clear microfilariae without affecting the viability of various adult filarial worms (Wong, 1964; Haque *et al.*, 1978; Weiss and Tanner, 1979; Weil *et al.*, 1982; Kazura and Davis, 1982; Townson and Bianco, 1982; Townson *et al.*, 1984; Carlow and Bianco, 1987; Carlow *et al.*, 1988). However, immunizations against *O. volvulus* microfilariae may intensify the inflammatory response associated with microfilarial death, thereby exacerbating pathology and disease in man. Alternatively, immunity that stimulates inhibition of microfilarial production or release from adult females would be advantageous in preventing pathological manifestations of dermal and ocular onchocerciasis.

2.1.3. NONHUMAN FILARIASIS—*DIROFILARIA IMMITIS, BRUGIA PAHANGI, ACANTHOCHEILONEMA VITEAE*

There are numerous nonhuman filarial species that naturally infect a variety of mammalian hosts. As with human infections, the host immune response to animal filarial infections varies greatly. In addition to infection of their natural host, many animal filarial species can infect surrogate hosts although these infections are typically compromised both qualitatively and quantitatively. These animal model systems exhibit a full range of permissiveness or resistance, again illustrating the host-specific nature of filarial parasites. There are three nonhuman natural host–parasite relationships that have been studied with regard to protective immunity—*Dirofilaria immitis* in the dog, *Brugia pahangi* in the cat, and *Acanthocheilonema viteae* in the Mongolian jird.

There is no definitive evidence of acquired protective immunity in natural infections of dogs harboring *Dirofilaria immitis* infections. Dogs with existing infections can be reinfected repeatedly over their lifetime, and a dog can be reinfected after cure by chemotherapy (Grieve *et al.*, 1983). Probably the best studied natural animal model for human lymphatic filariasis is *Brugia pahangi* in the cat. A range of host immune responses is seen in the *B. pahangi*–cat model system comparable to human filarial infections. Repeated L3 inoculation usually results in patent infections, with microfilariae present in peripheral circulation throughout the lifetime of the adult worms (Denham *et al.*, 1972a). In contrast to the response of the majority of cats, a small percentage of cats never develop a patent microfilaremia, and some microfilaremic cats spontaneously become amicrofilaremic. In an attempt to correlate immune effector mechanisms with amicrofilaremia, antibody recognition of somatic and surface antigens from each infection type was measured (Fletcher *et al.*, 1992). It was found that cats with persistent microfilaremia had the lowest levels of antibody directed against somatic antigens of adults, L3, and microfilariae. Cats that were amicrofilaremic had the highest levels of IgG to each stage, and the microfilaremic cats that spontaneously became amicrofilaremic had somewhat intermediate levels of parasite-specific antibody. No correlation between recognition of specific surface antigen of any stage within any of the three infection phenotypes was found. More recently, a study correlated the presence of parasite-specific IgE in cats where the adult worm populations were killed following repeated larval infections (Baldwin *et al.*, 1993). Parasite-specific IgE was rarely detected in cats in which adult worms survived for years.

Acanthocheilonema viteae, a natural parasite of gerbils, can also be used to experimentally infect the Mongolian jird. Jirds infected with *A. viteae* are resistant to challenge infection during the prepatent period of the primary infection (Tanner and Weiss, 1981a; Abraham *et al.*, 1986b). Through in vivo observations, both parasite-specific and nonspecific cell-mediated and humoral immune responses have been temporally associated with the development of prepatent immunity. Jirds with prepatent infections showed parasite antigen-reactive spleen cells and increasing parasite-specific antibody titers consistent with immune resistance. A nonspecific cellular immunodepression also was seen, potentially related to adherent suppressor cells (Abraham *et al.*, 1986a). Although mechanisms of *A. viteae* larval destruction are unknown, evidence from in vitro experiments supports in vivo studies. Larval *A. viteae* can be killed by immune serum (Tanner and Weiss, 1981b) and cells, including peritoneal exudate cells from normal jirds (Abraham *et al.*, 1986b), and eosinophils and macrophages from normal rats (Haque *et al.*, 1982). Larval development from infective L3 to advanced L3 was essential for in vitro killing, indicating a stage-specific immune response.

Although animal models are useful tools, care must be taken in extrapolating data from one system to another. For example, anti-adult immunity is apparent in several surrogate host model systems. However, the way in which it is manifested varies considerably among different hosts (Wakelin, 1984). In rats, *A. viteae* adults die well before clearance of microfilariae is seen; while in hamsters, *A. viteae* infections become amicrofilaremic, or latent, even though adults remain alive. Latency is related, in part, to the failure of adult females to liberate microfilariae, as latent females resume microfilarial release when transplanted in naive hosts (Haque *et al.*, 1978). Thus, information gained from animal model systems is valuable, but cannot be correlated directly with immunity in human filarial species.

2.2. Evidence of Concomitant Immunity in Filariasis

As discussed above, evidence of protective immunity against lymphatic filariasis originally was based on the existence of a heterogeneous group of amicrofilaremic, asymptomatic endemic normal individuals, presumed to be resistant to infection with L3 (Ward *et al.*, 1988; Freedman *et al.*, 1989). An alternative definition of acquired resistance considers the balance of infection rate and worm mortality, and the corresponding fluctuation of worm burden within any one individual, as a dynamic process. Regulation of this dynamic process may be influenced by host immune responsiveness in the form of concomitant immunity. The development of a protective immune response specifically targeted against a developing larval stage in the face of concurrent homologous infection is referred to as concomitant immunity. Concomitant immunity effectively protects the infected individual from superinfection, as the host gradually develops a resistance to reinfection by infective larvae while the resident fecund adult worms remain functionally intact. This phenomenon is broadly characteristic of many long-lived parasitic helminth infections (Smithers and Terry, 1976).

A variety of experimental studies have shown that *D. immitis* larval stages, along with the larval stages of other filarial species, contain functional antigens that are largely stage-specific (Wong and Guest, 1969; Knight, 1977; Weiss and Tanner, 1981; Maizels *et al.*, 1983; Carlow *et al.*, 1987; Lal and Ottesen, 1988). Such stage-specific antigens may be essential in the development of concomitant immunity. One of the initial demonstrations that concomitant immunity may be functioning in the dynamic host–parasite interplay of filariasis infections came from epidemiological surveys of *D. immitis*-infected dogs. Epidemiological surveys indicated that *D. immitis* populations within individual dogs did not reflect directly the cumulative exposure of the animal to infective larvae. Thus, the suggestion was made that the immune response of infected individuals may have the capacity to somehow regulate parasite populations (Otto, 1969). Further circumstantial evidence in support of possible host regulation was provided in a report documenting that dogs living within endemic areas tended to have a relatively constant mean number of adult worms, regardless of their degree of exposure to infective larval stages (Grieve *et al.*, 1983).

Acquired resistance that could be correlated directly with concomitant immunity was experimentally demonstrated in another natural host–parasite relationship. Cats repeatedly inoculated with *B. pahangi* infective larvae eventually became amicrofilaremic and resistant to reinfection. This resistance was induced by more than 20 "trickle infections," an infection schedule designed to mimic exposure kinetics of natural infections. Immunity was directed primarily against infective L3. After 20 trickle infections, the majority of challenge L3 were destroyed within 24 h of injection, while the existing adult populations remained intact. At a later time point, these cats became amicrofilaremic and the resident adult worms died approximately 1 week later. Animals that had cleared their infection were found to be highly resistant to challenge infection (Denham *et al.*, 1972b, 1983, 1992; Grenfell *et al.*, 1991).

Other trickle infections including *A. viteae*-infected hamsters and jirds (Neilsen, 1976; Barthold and Wenk, 1992), *B. pahangi*-infected jirds (Kowalski and Ash, 1975), and *W. bancrofti*-infected mice (Rajasekariah *et al.*, 1989) demonstrated similar reductions in percent worm recovery. Conversely, most single dose or nontrickle multiple dose infections have not shown such a tendency toward resistance against challenge-infections (Klei *et al.*, 1980). The kinetics of repeated infections with small numbers of larvae over an extended period of time appears to be crucial in the induction of experimentally induced concomitant immunity. Larval migration and host exposure to excretory/secretory (ES) antigens and molting fluids may be vital components in the induction of this specialized stage-specific immune response.

Evidence for concomitant immunity in human filariasis recently has been identified using an immunoepidemiological approach in the *W. bancrofti*-endemic area of Papua New Guinea (Day, 1991; Day *et al.*, 1991a–c). Infection status of the 5 of 92 amicrofilaremic, asymptomatic adults identified in this area of intense, stable transmission was assessed by clinical response to diethylcarbamazine (DEC), as well as by the serological presence of circulating phosphorylcholine-containing antigen (PC-Ag) and filarial-specific IgG4. Both circulating PC-Ag and filarial-specific IgG4 correlate with active lymphatic filarial infection and with microfilarial density (Kwan-Lim *et al.*, 1990; Day *et al.*, 1991a). By these sensitive indicators of infection, all five amicrofilaremic, asymptomatic adults were actually found to harbor active infections, signifying the absence of worm-free endemic normals in this endemic area of intense *W. bancrofti* transmission. Analysis of circulating PC-Ag compared to microfilaremia implied that amicrofilaremic individuals likely have similar worm burdens as individuals with low microfilaremia levels (Day *et al.*, 1991a).

Using PC-Ag as an indirect correlate to adult worm burden in a 12-month longitudinal population dynamics study, it was found that worm burdens seemed to increase rapidly in children and adolescents under age 20, whereas they reached a plateau, and were maintained at constant levels in adults over age 20. Similar results were reported in an epidemiological study of *W. bancrofti* microfilarial infection dynamics in Pondicherry, India. In this report, the rate of gain in infection peaked in the 16–20 age class, while adults over age 20 exhibited a reduced infection rate (Vanamail *et al.*, 1989). These data are consistent with the existence of concomitant immunity—an age-dependent acquisition of resistance to new infections with increasing exposure, presumably directed against the early larval stages and independent of existing worm burden (Day *et al.*, 1991a).

Paralleling this temporal evolution of concomitant immunity, an age-related development of antibodies that were reactive to the surface of *B. malayi* infective L3 was identified in 100% of the immune population, over the age of 20, and only 20% of the under-20 nonimmune population, implicating larval-specific antigen(s) as attractive targets for a protective immune response. This finding suggests that antilarval and antiadult immunity occur independently, and uninfected and infected individuals differing in their antiadult responses both should be capable of engendering an effective anti-L3 immunity. Future analysis of candidate vaccine immunogens and mechanisms of protective immunity in humans should involve age-stratified comparisons between adults who have developed concomitant immunity and preimmune children (Day *et al.*, 1991c; Day, 1991; Maizels and Lawrence, 1991). The concept of concomitant immunity based on the age (exposure)-dependent development of anti-L3 protective immunity is consistent with the existence of immunological tolerance to adult worms and microfilariae, assuming that the T-cell anergy is induced and specific to developing L4, adults, and microfilariae. As such, protective immunity is elicited by L3-specific antigens and occurs independently of both the immune response to other parasite stages and the host's immune-responsiveness, either tolerant or reactive (Maizels and Lawrence, 1991).

Further evidence implicating the L3 stage as the specific target of host concomitant immune responses in the *A. viteae*–jird model system has recently been reported (Eisenbeiss *et al.*, 1994). Repeated low-dose infections of jirds with *A. viteae* appeared to induce concomitant immunity. This was shown in quantitative recovery of parasites from triple-infected jirds, where the challenge larvae were uniformly inactivated at exactly the time of the molt from L3 to L4. Only larvae undergoing the molt, not premolt L3 or postmolt L4, stimulated this concomitant immune response, and only immune jirds, not susceptible jirds, had high serum antibody titers directed against L3 molt-related antigens. Thus, in this system, the protective antigens are, at least temporally, molt-associated. The significant changes seen in the surface composition of developing larvae (Abraham *et al.*, 1988b; Apfel *et al.*, 1992) provide circumstantial evidence that antigens from a specific phase of development, that may not be present in or on other developmental stages, could be crucial to induction of protective immunity.

All available evidence indicates that immune responses to L3 or L4 antigens are nonpathogenic. Uninfected immune individuals presumably kill developing larvae without pathological sequelae, while the infected, older microfilaremic, asymptomatic individuals develop antilarval concomitant immunity preventing superinfection. Thus, vaccination with larval-specific antigen(s) should avoid exacerbation of disease. This should be effective in inducing immunity in naive individuals, in individuals whose infections recently have been cleared by DEC or ivermectin, and in currently infected individuals for protection from new infections (Maizels and Lawrence, 1991; Maizels *et al.*, 1991).

2.3. Experimental Immunization Studies

Immunoepidemiological and experimental investigations documenting the development of acquired protective immunity and concomitant immunity both implicate the infective or early developing filarial larval stages as prime targets for immunological intervention. To this end, numerous investigators have immunized natural and surrogate hosts with some form of worm antigen in an attempt to induce protection against subsequent infective larval challenge infections. Experimental immunogens tested in these studies have taken one of two general forms: (1) crude native antigen or (2) exposure to live larvae, compromised either by irradiation or by chemical treatment.

Experimental infections using different filarial species in a variety of mammalian hosts, with susceptibility ranging from naturally infected permissive hosts to surrogate permissive, semipermissive, and resistant hosts, have provided a unique opportunity to explore mechanisms of acquired immunity. Implantation of challenge larvae within micropore diffusion chambers has facilitated recovery, accurate enumeration, and measurement of surviving larvae. These chambers are typically constructed of inert Lucite rings sealed with porous inert membranes. Larval parasites are contained within the chamber; the porosity of the membrane can be modified to either include or exclude potential effector cells. Thus, both antilarval immune effects can be measured and potential immune effectors can be elucidated. In some instances, experimental immunizations can be correlated with in vitro assays, such as antibody-dependent cell-mediated cytotoxicity, again supplying insight into potential mechanisms of immunity.

2.3.1. IMMUNIZATION STUDIES USING CRUDE PARASITE MATERIAL

Immunization via repeated low-dose infections of *B. pahangi* L3 in cats and jirds and *A. viteae* L3 in hamsters have proven effective in inducing protection against challenge infection (Denham *et al.*, 1972b, 1983; Kowalski and Ash, 1975; Neilson, 1976). Immunizations using crude parasite extracts, consisting of adult and larval stage homogenates and/or excretory–secretory antigens, also have been evaluated in a number of model systems. Early work suggested that dead filarial parasites were not effective in stimulating protective immunity against homologous infection. More recent evidence indicates that resistance to microfilariae and/or infective stage L3 can be induced by immunization with microfilarial or adult worm extracts (Wong, 1964; Bagai and Subrahmanyam, 1970; Kazura and Davis, 1982; Townson and Bianco, 1982; Kazura *et al.*, 1986b; Hayashi *et al.*, 1989), and infective larval extracts (Tanner and Weiss, 1981b; Mehta *et al.*, 1981; Carlow and Philipp, 1987). Most of these studies were done using nonnatural host–parasite systems, and the resistance induced was significantly lower than that induced by live organisms.

In another study using a semipermissive surrogate host, development of protective immunity against challenge *D. immitis* L3 was induced by live infective L3, but not by dead L3 (Abraham *et al.*, 1988a). This immunity was positively correlated with antibody levels to soluble, but not surface, larval antigen. Although it is clear that the stimulation and mechanisms of protective immunity may differ for each host–parasite system, it is generally believed that dead worms or somatic extracts provide modest protection at best (Philipp *et al.*, 1988; Selkirk *et al.*, 1992).

2.3.2. IMMUNIZATION STUDIES USING RADIATION-ATTENUATED LARVAE

Vaccines designed to prevent or substantially reduce canine hookworm and bovine lungworm infection and disease have set a precedent for the use of live, irradiated nematode larvae in commercially available preparations (Jarrett *et al.*, 1960; Miller, 1964). Use of irradiated vaccines is based on the supposition that stimulation of immunity with, and against, the less pathogenic early larval stages should be beneficial in engendering an appropriate protective immune response. Appropriate doses of radiation stunt the growth and retard the development of larvae such that the longevity of the L3 stage is increased. There is also some indication of an enhanced inhibitory effect of irradiation specific to male worms (Devaney *et al.*, 1993). Irradiated filarial larval vaccines have been used to induce high levels of protective immunity in several host–parasite systems normally associated with little naturally acquired resistance. Successful vaccination against L3 challenge has been achieved using live irradiated L3 of *B. malayi* and *B. pahangi* in dogs (Ah *et al.*, 1974), cats (Oothuman *et al.*, 1979), jirds (Storey and Al-Mukhtar, 1982b; Yates and Higashi, 1985; Chusattayanond and Denham, 1986), monkeys (Wong *et al.*, 1969), and mice (Hayashi *et al.*, 1984; Abraham *et al.*, 1989; Bancroft and Devaney, 1993); *A. viteae* in jirds (Tanner and Weiss, 1981a,b; Lucius *et al.*, 1986, 1991); *D. immitis* in dogs (Wong *et al.*, 1974; Mejia and Carlow, 1994); *L. carinii* in rats (Rao *et al.*, 1977); and *O.*

lienalis and *O. volvulus* in mice (Abraham *et al.*, 1992; Lange *et al.*, 1993, 1994; Taylor *et al.*, 1994).

Intensity of radiation has been correlated with extent of developmental inhibition of larvae, therefore allowing experimentally induced protection of varying degrees to be equated with stage-specific developmental inhibition (Oothuman *et al.*, 1978; Yates and Higashi, 1985; Chusattayanond and Denham, 1986). In one such study, dogs were protected by immunization with *D. immitis* L3 irradiated with 20 krad. These irradiated larvae were able to develop into sterile, stunted adults. Higher doses of radiation, which allow less larval development and cause premature larval death, did not confer protection against challenge. These data suggest that development to L4 or immature adult is necessary for effective immunization of dogs against *D. immitis* (Wong *et al.*, 1974).

In a similar study in rats, protection against *L. carinii* infection was induced by immunization with L3 irradiated with greater than 40 krad. This level of radiation prevented molting to L4, suggesting prolonged exposure to L3 is required in this system (Rao *et al.*, 1977). Similarly, *O. lienalis* L3 irradiated with 55–75 krad, which prevented most of the L3 from molting to L4 and killed *O. volvulus* L3, conferred protection against L3 challenge in mice, suggesting that L4 are not essential for induction of protective immunity in this system (Abraham *et al.*, 1992; Lange *et al.*, 1993). Substantiation of this result was provided in a vaccination study with killed *O. volvulus* L4. This approach failed to induce protective immunity against L3 challenge in BALB/c mice (Lange *et al.*, 1993). Conversely, both *B. malayi* L3 and L4 were capable of inducing protective immunity against homologous L3 infection (Carlow and Philipp, 1987). Further evidence of the importance of prolonged or extended L3 development in inducing immunity was reported in an analysis of the immune response of mice to irradiated larval *B. malayi* (Abraham *et al.*, 1989). In this study, irradiated *B. malayi* L3 were used to immunize BALB/c mice three successive times. Following the final immunization, mice were challenged with *B. malayi* L3 in chambers. At 3 weeks postchallenge, evidence of decreased survival in immunized mice, along with stunting and developmental arrest, was seen as 100% of larvae recovered from immunized mice were still L3, while 96% of larvae from control mice were L4. Sera from control mice reacted only with internal, and not with surface, antigens on both L3 and L4. Sera from immunized mice reacted with both internal and external antigens on L3 and L4, suggesting antibodies to surface antigens are important in inducing protective immunity.

Growth retardation or arrested development of parasites in immunized hosts has been reported for several filarial species including *L. carinii* (Weiner *et al.*, 1984), *A. viteae* (Tanner and Weiss, 1981a; Abraham *et al.*, 1986b), and *D. immitis* (Grieve *et al.*, 1988). Generally, live larvae that undergo some degree of limited development and migration induce the highest levels of protective immunity against challenge. Presumably, the longer exposure period of L3 stage-specific antigens stimulates host immune reactivity against subsequent L3 infections. Protective immunity induced by extended exposure to larval antigens is a recurrent theme in both irradiation and trickle infection immunizations.

Immunization studies using irradiated larvae also have provided insight into potential mechanisms of immune-mediated larval killing. Spleen cells from BALB/c mice immunized with irradiated *B. pahangi* L3 produced IL-4, IL-5, and IL-9, but not IFN-γ, after stimulation with parasite antigen or mitogen (Bancroft *et al.*, 1993). Similar results were obtained when BALB/c mice were immunized with irradiated *O. volvulus* L3. In addition to observing a decreased survival rate of challenge larvae contained in diffusion chambers, an influx of eosinophils and IL-5, but not IFN-γ, was found in the chamber microenvironment coincident with the time of parasite killing. The protection induced by immunization with irradiated larvae was substantially reduced in immunized mice treated with monoclonal antibodies that eliminated IL-4 or IL-5 (Lange *et al.*, 1994). Thus, cytokines classically associated with a Th2-like cellular response may play a role in killing of filarial larvae.

In at least one irradiated larval immunization experiment, a higher degree of protection was positively correlated with increased time between challenge and necropsy (Wong *et al.*, 1974). This result indicated a potential multiple stage killing effect, in which vaccination with irradiated L3 stimulated an immune response that is directed not only against L3, but also against developing L4 and immature adult organisms. The fact that antigenic determinants are known to be shared among different stages (Maizels *et al.*, 1983), and that immunization with one stage has been shown to induce protection against challenge of a different stage (Kazura *et al.*, 1986b; Carlow and Philipp, 1987; Hayashi *et al.*, 1989) also support the potential for multiple stage killing.

In addition to the existence of shared determinants between different stages of one species, there is evidence of cross-reacting surface antigens shared among the same stage of several different filarial species. The best known example of this is a surface phosphorylcholine epitope that is highly conserved among filariae (Pery *et al.*, 1974; Maizels *et al.*, 1987). Considerable antigenic similarity also has been demonstrated between *L. carinii* and *W. bancrofti* (Subrahmanyam *et al.*, 1978; Ogilvie *et al.*, 1980), and between *Onchocerca* spp. and *D. immitis* (Grieve *et al.*, unpublished observations).

The potential for cross-reacting antibodies that confer protection against heterologous challenge is also real. Species cross-protection studies, in which irradiated *B. pahangi* L3 conferred protection against *B. malayi* (Carlow and Philipp, 1987) and *B. patei* L3 (Oothuman *et al.*, 1979), and irradiated *O. lienalis* L3 immunization induced protective responses against *O. volvulus* L3 challenge (Lange *et al.*, 1993), provide the experimental evidence. There exists one study in which cross-protection between different filarial genera was induced (Storey and Al-Mukhtar, 1982b). In this investigation, exposure of jirds to radiation-attenuated *L. carinii* L3 conferred resistance against L3 challenge of not only the homologous species *L. carinii* (98%), but also of the heterologous genus *B. pahangi* (71%). Although independent confirmation of cross-protection between filarial genera has not been published by other investigators, the potential for developing zooprophylactic regimes for the control of human filariasis exists in theory.

2.3.3. IMMUNIZATION STUDIES USING CHEMICALLY ABBREVIATED INFECTIONS

Drug treatment of larval infections can induce immune responses that are similar to those raised by vaccination with irradiated larvae. Stimulation of the host's immune system is induced by maximal and repeated exposure to larval stages, without allowing the subsequent normal development of larvae to adult. Protective immune responses against *D. immitis* L3 challenge infections in ferrets (Blair and Campbell, 1981) and dogs (Grieve *et al.*, 1988) have been produced in this manner. These studies utilized the macrolide antiparasitic agent 22,23-dihydroavermectin B1a, ivermectin, active against L3 and L4

(Egerton *et al.*, 1980; Blair and Campbell, 1980) to terminate infections. In the initial study a single dose of ivermectin was given to ferrets 2 months after each of two inoculations of 30 *D. immitis* L3, 5 months apart. High levels of protective immunity were raised, suggesting an immunizing effect of the precardiac developmental stages and demonstrating the capacity to protect ferrets from cardiac invasion and subsequent microfilaremia following experimental reinfection (Blair and Campbell, 1981).

A subsequent investigation of ivermectin-treated *D. immitis* larval infections demonstrated not only immune-mediated protection, but also some insight into the mechanisms involved and parasite developmental stages that were affected (Grieve *et al.*, 1988). Immunization was achieved by three successive administrations of large numbers (150–400) of *D. immitis* L3, followed by ivermectin at 62 days postinfection. Challenge infections consisted of 100 L3 in chambers as well as subcutaneously inoculated L3. Chambers that were recovered 3 weeks after challenge had 63% fewer larvae than controls, and larvae were significantly stunted compared to controls. Assessment of larval growth and development in chambers following drug-treated infections provided clear evidence that larval stages contained the relevant protective antigen(s). Necropsy of dogs 7 months postchallenge also showed a remarkable level of protection, as control dogs had mean of 28.5 adults while immunized dogs had an average of only 0.5 worm (range 0–2). The higher levels of reduction in adult recoveries at 7 months compared to larval recoveries at 3 weeks suggested a multiple stage killing effect occurring in these immune dogs.

Although it was difficult to correlate immunity with antibody reactivity to any of the different larval stages, sera from immune dogs were effective in recognizing larval antigens and passively transferring larval killing and stunting effects (Abraham and Grieve, 1991). Sera from immune dogs were pooled and inoculated into BALB/c mice that were concurrently challenged with *D. immitis* L3 in chambers. At 3 weeks postchallenge, significantly decreased larval survival and larval stunting were observed.

3. CHARACTERISTICS OF THE IDEAL VACCINE

The ideal vaccine would completely prevent transmission to the definitive host. A correlate for vaccines being generated against the sexual stages of the malaria parasite that occur within the vector (Rener *et al.*, 1983) would serve as an example. In that instance the parasite is killed within the vector prior to the development of the stage that is parasitic to vertebrates and that is transmitted with a subsequent bloodmeal. However, very limited research has been conducted in this area with the goal of completely preventing filarial nematode infections.

The next most logical goal for a vaccine is the complete prevention of the development of adult parasites in the definitive host. Parasite destruction would be mediated prior to their access to the site of predilection, thus precluding much of the disease associated with infection and any sequelae following adulticide treatment. A vaccine that induces this type of protective response would target the developing larva while it is still relatively small, accessible in tissue, and prior to the onset of generalized (Grieve *et al.*, 1982) or parasite-specific (Ottesen *et al.*, 1977) immunologic downregulation. Requisite to this research is an appreciation for the many immunobiologic adaptations manifest in the developing larvae. In addition to the L3-to-L4 molt which presents two morphologically different stages, these larval forms have peculiar surface charge characteristics, unique antigenic profiles, and direct complement activation capacities (Abraham *et al.*, 1988b).

Certainly there may be instances where an immunotherapeutic vaccine may be indicated. For example, the adult male nematode of *O. volvulus* may migrate from nodule to nodule inseminating females that remain resident in the nodules. If the adult male worm could be destroyed, or sterilized, sexual reproduction and the generation of disease-causing microfilariae would cease.

One of the most controversial approaches to vaccine development is the targeting of the microfilaria for immunologic destruction. This would preclude transmission of the parasite by eliminating the microfilarial reservoir from exposure to the appropriate arthropod intermediate host. Examples of naturally occurring microfilaria stage-specific immunity abound, and it is relatively easy to experimentally reproduce these phenomena. However, these immunologic effects have proven to be extremely pathogenic to the host. For example, in canine heartworm infections, the stage-specific immunologic destruction of microfilariae accounts for some of the most acute disease states associated with that infection (Knight, 1987). The corollary in human lymphatic filariasis is TPE (Ottesen *et al.*, 1979), an acute disease syndrome. In onchocerciasis, it is theoretically possible that immunization with microfilarial antigens could predispose patients to sowda or more acute ocular disease.

For these various reasons, it would appear that the most logical approach is to target the L3 and L4 larvae. Selection of larval-specific antigens that do not cross-react with microfilariae could be important for generating a protective immune response without the potential for immune pathology. These larval-specific antigens can be discovered with immunologic reagents from immune hosts, or by rational screening approaches searching for novel physiologic and structural targets. As described below, these two screening paths are probably not completely distinct; immune screening can frequently result in the discovery of novel physiologic targets.

A central tenet in the development of an effective vaccine for the prevention of filarial nematode infections is that some form of recombinant antigen vaccine will be necessary. It would be virtually impossible to generate the necessary numbers of larvae to obtain adequate quantities of native antigen(s) for use in a commercial product. With fewer than 10 L3 typically obtained from an intermediate host and the necessity of up to 200 larvae per lane required for an interpretable Western blot, it is clear that a vaccine derived from larval lysates would not be possible for either millions of people or animals. Indeed, the generation of recombinant antigens is necessary even at the level of preliminary immunization experiments in the definitive host.

4. *DIROFILARIA IMMITIS*: A VACCINE IN ANIMALS AND A MODEL FOR HUMAN FILARIASES

D. immitis, the canine heartworm, is a parasite of dogs. It may also complete its life cycle in cats and, interestingly, in sea lions (Grieve *et al.*, 1983). As its common name implies, adult *D. immitis* are typically found in the right ventricle and pulmonary arteries of dogs. The disease associated with this infection is generally chronic and multisystemic, although cardiopulmonary disease certainly provides some of the hallmark symptomatology (Knight, 1987).

Chemoprophylaxis of heartworm infection is readily attainable with chemicals approved for use in dogs by the Food and Drug Administration (FDA). Diethylcarbamazine provided daily, or macrolide antibiotics administered monthly, are highly effective in killing the L3 and early L4 parasites (Knight, 1987; Grieve *et al.*, 1991). There are no FDA approved chemoprophylactic drugs approved for use in host species other than dogs.

While the filarial diseases of humans typically occur in the subtropical and tropical parts of the underdeveloped world, *D. immitis* is widely prevalent in temperate climates of the developed world (Grieve *et al.*, 1983). The infection is of paramount veterinary medical and economic importance in Australia, Japan, and North America. With questions of how to deliver and pay for antifilarial drugs in humans in the underdeveloped world, it is in striking contrast that the annual worldwide market for heartworm chemoprophylactics in dogs is in excess of 150 million U.S. dollars.

Although chemoprophylactics have been demonstrated to be very efficacious, those drugs are not optimal under all conditions. Pet owner compliance with routine medication is a frequent problem; prolonged or frequent treatment lapses can result in treatment failures. Dogs with ongoing microfilaremic infections that receive diethylcarbamazine, for example, may experience severe shocklike reactions (Knight, 1987). Beyond these very real toxicity, or side-effect, concerns are the perceptions of many pet owners that routine chemical treatment over the lifetime of the dog must be dangerous and, consequently, they elect not to use chemoprophylactics.

The concerns over the complete suitability of chemoprophylactic drugs and the size of the market for products that would prevent adult heartworm infection have prompted extensive research into the development of a vaccine. This research has been facilitated by the ready access to both the definitive and intermediate hosts, dogs and mosquitoes. Infected mosquitoes have been available to generate the larval parasites necessary for stage-specific antigens and cDNA libraries, and vaccine candidates can be readily tested in the natural definitive host, the domestic dog.

Research toward the development of a canine heartworm vaccine should benefit similar efforts in the development of vaccines for human filariid infections. The biological similarities among filarial nematodes permit certain conceptual extrapolations from the canine to human host–parasite systems. The data that permitted an insight into the specific *D. immitis* larval stages targeted by immunoprophylaxis should have considerable relevance toward the prevention of human filarial infections. Additionally, based on *D. immitis* gene sequences, homologues of putative vaccine candidates discovered for use in preventing dirofilariasis have been recovered from human filariid cDNA libraries. This should be a particularly powerful approach in light of the relative absence of native parasite antigen, appropriate cDNA libraries, and natural definitive host test systems experienced in all of the human filariases. Finally, because of the cross-reactive potential of various larval-specific antigens among different genera, *D. immitis* antigens may be of direct use in the prevention of human filarial nematode infections.

5. IDENTIFICATION OF CANDIDATE ANTIGENS

One of the most daunting tasks associated with the development of a vaccine against filarial nematode infections is the identification of parasite proteins that can be used as immunogens. Since it is unlikely that a single immunogen will be effective, a pool of immunogens will need to be constructed. Several methods can be used to assemble a list of candidate immunogens. Conceptually, one method, termed rational screening, is to develop schemes to characterize parasite antigens that appeal to the biologist's intuition. These targets include molecules that are necessary for the third and fourth molt, immune evasion, migration, metabolism and growth, and molecules presented on the surface of the parasite. Another method is to use sera from infected individuals or animals immunized with worm lysates to identify immunoreactive proteins. A third method is to utilize antibody reagents derived from immune individuals to specifically identify antigens that are uniquely recognized by the immune system of these individuals and not recognized using similar reagents from infected nonimmune individuals. Although possibly only a part of the effective immune response to filarial infection, antibodies have been shown to mediate or contribute to larval killing and have been used to passively transfer a protective effect. This is the approach we have focused on in this section.

5.1. *Dirofilaria immitis* Antigens Recognized by Antibodies in Immune Dog Sera

Immune dogs were generated by three rounds of experimental infections followed by drug treatment to stop the infections (Grieve *et al.*, 1988). Their sera were passively transferred to mice and shown to kill and stunt *D. immitis* larvae contained in chambers (Abraham and Grieve, 1991). Sera from these immune dogs and their infected nonimmune cohorts were then utilized to identify larval vaccine candidates. Immunoblot analyses of L4 protein preparations allowed for the identification of antigens of 23/24, 39, and 66 kDa that were uniquely recognized by the immune dog sera. Similar analyses using larval ES products collected through the third molt were used to identify antigens of 15, 31, 39, 42, 55, 70, 97, and 207 kDa. Further analysis of the 39-kDa protein demonstrated that it was recognized only by antibodies in sera of four immune dogs, and not two infected cohorts, normal dogs, chronically infected microfilaremic dogs, nor immune-mediated occult infected dogs. The 39-kDa protein was also shown to be stage specific, being found in L3 and L4, but not adults or microfilariae.

Surface labeling of L4 with ^{125}I followed by immunoprecipitation allowed identification of a 33-kDa protein uniquely recognized by antibodies in sera from three of the four immune dogs. Radio-immunoprecipitations performed using the same immune sera and L4 antigens metabolically labeled with [^{35}S]methionine and cysteine were used to identify another antigen of 59 kDa. In a similar experiment (Frank and Grieve, 1991), a doublet of 20/22 kDa was immunoprecipitated from both ^{35}S-labeled ES and L4 lysates. This doublet was probably the same as the 23/24-kDa doublet identified by the immunoblot analyses described above. These protein(s) appeared to be developmentally regulated and were found in L3 and L4, but not microfilariae, L2, or adults, and were released as an ES product coincident with the molt from L3 to L4.

Using this approach, at least 12 antigens have been identified as possible vaccine immunogens. Two of these, the 39-kDa protein and the 20/22-kDa doublet, are larval specific and an association with the L3–L4 molt has been shown with the 20/22-kDa doublet. As such, these molecules fit the criteria for potential vaccine candidates, principally unique recognition by proven immune sera, and larval stage specificity.

5.2. Lymphatic Filariasis

A similar approach for the identification of potential vaccine candidates for *W. bancrofti* has been used with endemic normal sera (Freedman *et al.*, 1989). In this study, putatively immune, infection-free individuals living in a hyperendemic area for subperiodic bancroftian filariasis were identified. The criteria for this classification were based on no prior history of infection or DEC therapy, physical exam, nine negative blood tests for microfilariae, no posttreatment reaction when dosed with DEC, and lack of circulating filarial antigens in their sera. Of 459 individuals screened, 7 met these criteria and were classified as endemic normals and presumed to be immune. Control sera were collected from infected, microfilaremic individuals with no history or evidence of lymphatic obstruction.

Since *W. bancrofti* cannot be maintained in laboratory animals, various stages of the closely related filarial parasite *B. malayi* were used as antigen sources to screen for candidate immunogens. Immunoblot analyses were performed against microfilariae, L3, and adults. Frequency response analyses of the endemic normal and control sera were performed on all of the molecules recognized in these antigen preparations. Although there were trends of differential recognition of three antigens in the adult preparations (15, 86, 88 kDa) and two antigens in the microfilarial preparations (23, 85 kDa), these proved not to be statistically different when frequency response analyses were compared. When L3 antigens were evaluated, all 7 endemic normal sera recognized a 43-kDa protein, subsequently cloned and identified as a chitinase-like antigen (Raghaven *et al.*, 1994), while only 1 of 12 infected patients' sera recognized the same antigen.

Specific immune recognition of *B. malayi* antigens has been studied using the jird model system (Li *et al.*, 1991). Although not the natural host–parasite system, jirds do allow the development of patent infections with *B. malayi*. In this study, serum was collected from immune jirds that had received two infections with irradiated L3, or from control jirds that were infected with normal L3. Immunoblot analyses of L3 antigens were performed. Larval antigens of 97, 60, 55, and 10 kDa were uniquely recognized by antibodies in the immune sera. The 97-kDa molecule was identified to be paramyosin, a muscle protein. Interestingly, immune responses to filarial paramyosin have also been associated with enhanced clearance of transfused *B. malayi* microfilariae in mice (Nanduri and Kazura, 1989). The cloned *B. malayi* paramyosin was subsequently used to immunize jirds (Li *et al.*, 1993), resulting in a 43% reduction in adult worm recoveries and a 10% reduction in adult female length on challenge.

5.3. Onchocerciasis

The endemic normal concept has also been utilized to study potential protective antigens in *O. volvulus* infections. Sera were collected from putatively immune individuals and from microfilaria-positive infected individuals living in a hyperendemic region in Guatemala (Nutman *et al.*, 1991). The criteria for putatively immune individuals were: resident in the area for at least 10 years, three consecutive years of microfilaria-negative skin snips and negative physical examination for nodules, no historical, physical, laboratory, or parasitologic evidence of onchocerciasis at the time of examination; negative ophthalmologic examination, and negative DEC provocative challenge (Mazzotti reaction). IgG and IgE responses were evaluated by immunoblot analyses and by frequency response profiles using antigens recovered from *O. volvulus* adults, and two related species, *O. lienalis* and *B. malayi*. There were no adult *O. volvulus* antigens uniquely recognized by immune IgG and only 8–50% of the immune individuals had unique IgE recognition of four antigens of 92, 70, 25, and 18.5 kDa. There were no larval antigens recognized by all of the putatively immune sera that were not also recognized by at least one infected individual, but there were several significant trends. The *O. lienalis* L3 antigens identified were 50, 47, 45, and 22 kDa. The *B. malayi* L3 antigens were a 151- to 175-kDa triplet, 39 and 35 kDa. Those identified using IgE were 69 and 65 kDa. Thus, there seemed to be not only a larval- and species-specific response, but also a differential recognition by the antibody isotypes.

A similar study performed on individuals from Guatemala was reported the same year (Boyer *et al.*, 1991). Sera were collected from individuals with various clinical and parasitological presentations. Evaluation of immune responses to antigens by immunoblot was performed with adult *O. volvulus* antigens. A glycoprotein of 20 kDa was identified as a potential target in this study in that there appeared to be an IgG3 response to gp20 in immune individuals while infected individuals appeared to have an IgG1 response.

5.4. Microfilaria

Similar methodology was used to identify antigens that may be targets for immune-mediated clearance of microfilariae. Humans living in an endemic *Loa loa* region were divided into two groups, those with and without documented microfilaremic loiasis (Pinder *et al.*, 1988). Individuals with occult loiasis had documented adult *L. loa*, but no microfilaremia. Indirect immunofluorescence analyses using *L. loa* microfilariae demonstrated patchy or no surface fluorescence with microfilaremic sera, while the occult sera all showed positive surface fluorescence. To identify the corresponding surface antigens, microfilariae were surface labeled with ^{125}I and solubilized extracts were immunoprecipitated. A 23-kDa protein was identified by six of seven occult sera, while the microfilaremic sera only marginally precipitated the same molecule. Of note, a 25-kDa protein has been shown to specifically induce enhanced clearance of an intravenous *B. malayi* microfilarial challenge in immunized mice (Kazura *et al.*, 1986a). This protein was identified with immune sera from mice immunized with a crude microfilarial extract.

6. CLONING, CHARACTERIZATION, AND EXPRESSION OF CANDIDATE ANTIGENS

An accumulating body of evidence supporting the role of concomitant immunity in controlling filariid infections points to larval-specific antigens as effective immunogens. This is further supported by the protection engendered by immunization with irradiated larvae or by drug-abbreviated larval infections. However, small quantities of parasite material have limited biochemical and immunological characterization of filariid larval proteins. This is particularly true for larval stage antigens in filarial parasites of humans.

Research efforts consequently have focused on resourceful use of molecular approaches to identify, isolate, and characterize antigens with immunoprophylactic potential. Our goal is to provide selected detailed examples of the discovery and molecular cloning of *D. immitis* genes. A comprehensive review of all filarial genes/proteins that have been described is beyond the scope of this chapter. However, we have provided examples of various molecules in Table II.

To identify immunologically relevant antigens of *D. immitis*, immune sera were generated from dogs receiving chemically abbreviated larval infections. These sera were effective in passive transfer experiments and were subsequently used in immunoblots to uniquely identify larval-specific antigens (Grieve *et al.*, 1992). To molecularly clone the genes encoding these potentially protective antigens, four cDNA expression libraries were prepared from either adult male or female worms, >200,000 in vitro 48 h L3 or >200,000 L4. Differential immunoscreening of these libraries with immune dog sera and sera from naturally infected, nonimmune dogs has identified several vaccine candidate genes from the L3 and L4 cDNA expression libraries (p39, p4, and pDi22) as described in Table II. Clone p39 encodes a novel, larval-specific antigen uniquely recognized by antibodies in immune dog sera and has no significant homology to any sequences published in Genbank data bases. The pDi22 clone is a homologue of the ABA-1 gene product described in *Ascaris* (Spence *et al.*, 1993) which is also referred to as the "ladder protein" because it appears on immunoblots as an ascending ladder of subunits, each larger by 15 kDa. This same gene has been cloned by Poole and colleagues (Poole *et al.*, 1992). The p4 clone contains two nine-amino-acid cysteine-rich Class A motifs described in low-density lipoprotein receptors and epidermal growth factor proteins.

Relevant *D. immitis* genes also have been isolated from larval cDNA libraries by polymerase chain reaction (PCR) amplification or direct screening with degenerate oligonucleotide primers designed from peptide sequence of purified native antigens originally recognized by immune dog sera (DiPLA2). The protein encoded in the DiPLA2 clone is larval specific, uniquely recognized by immune dog sera (Frank and Grieve, 1991), and has homology to phospholipase A2. Using primer sequences designed from the *D. immitis* PLA2 gene, an analogue has been cloned from an *O. volvulus* L3 cDNA library (OvPLA2) (Wisnewski *et al.*, unpublished data). The protein encoded in clone p22U is found in adult and larval stages and shows no significant homology to molecules available in current data bases.

PCR amplification also has been used to target *D. immitis* homologues of specific genes. Degenerate primers designed around highly conserved regions of these genes also have been used in our laboratory to isolate several clones from the *D. immitis* L3 cDNA library (Table II). This approach has been particularly valuable in isolating relevant genes from human filarial parasites where difficulty in obtaining larval material and representative larval cDNA libraries is significant. Small quantities of reverse transcribed RNA were used to generate pools of larval cDNA sequences by PCR (Seeber *et al.*, 1993b). The presence of a highly conserved 22-nucleotide spliced leader (SL) sequence on the 5′ termini of many nematode mature mRNAs enabled the generation of cDNA sequences and minilibraries. This represents a biased compilation of cDNA sequences as not all mature transcripts isolated from filariids have this SL sequence and some transcripts have been

Table II
A Partial Survey and Description of Molecularly Cloned Filarial Nematode Genes[a]

Species	Clone	Homology/similarity	Native Ag (kDa)	Library	References
Bm	Bm-5	paramyosin	97	Bm Ad/mf cDNA	Li et al. (1991)
Di	cDi2	paramyosin	97	Di Ad cDNA	Grandea et al. (1989), Limberger and McReynolds (1990)
Di	p97	paramyosin	—	Di L3/Ad cDNA	Paravax, Inc. (unpublished data)
Ov	OvPmy	paramyosin	—	Ov Ad cDNA	Dahmen et al. (1993)
Ov	Ov1-Ov7	paramyosin	—	Ov Ad cDNA	Limberger and McReynolds (1990)
Ov	2A4/2A5.1	paramyosin-like	92	Ov Ad cDNA	Conraths et al. (1992)
Ov	2A4.1	—	14	Ov Ad cDNA	Conraths et al. (1991)
Ov	Onchag-1	myosin heavy chain	200	Ov Ad cDNA	Donelson et al. (1988), Erondu and Donelson (1990)
Bm	AP18	body wall myosin	—	Bm gDNA	Werner et al. (1989)
Bm	Bm9	myosin	—	Bm Ad cDNA	Dissanayake et al. (1992a)
Ov	Ovmyo-1	myosin	—	Ov Ad cDNA	Werner and Rajan (1992)
Wb	WbN1	myosin-like	—	Wb gDNA	Raghavan et al. (1991, 1992)
Bm	BmColl	collagen	—	Bm gDNA	Caulagi et al. (1991)
Bm, Bp	Bpa22/7	cuticular collagen domains	22	Bp Ad cDNA	Selkirk et al. (1991)
Bm	Ap2	collagen-like	—	Bm gDNA	Werner et al. (1989)
Bm	Bm hs1	HSP70	—	Bm gDNA	Rothstein and Rajan (1991)
Bp	Bpa26/37	HSP70	70	Bp Ad cDNA	Selkirk et al. (1989)
Ov	G15	HSP70	—	Ov Ad cDNA	Rothstein et al. (1989)
Di	Dihsp70	HSP70	70	Di Ad cDNA	Paravax, Inc. (unpublished data)
Ov	Ov7	cystatin	17	Ov Ad cDNA	Lustigman et al. (1991, 1992a)
Ov	Oc 9.3	cystatin	—	Ov Ad cDNA	Chandrashekar et al. (1991)
Di	Di5	ABA-1	multiples of 15	Di Ad cDNA	Poole et al. (1992)
Di	Di22	ABA-1	multiples of 15	Di L4 cDNA	Culpepper et al. (1992)
Bp/Bm	gp15/400	ABA-1	multiples of 15	Bp Ad cDNA	Tweedie et al. (1993)
Di	pD-4	neutrophil chemotactic factor (ABA-1 homolog)	—	Di Ad cDNA	Owhashi et al. (1993)
Ov	Ov33-3	aspartyl protease inhibitor	33	Ov Ad cDNA	Lucius et al. (1988)

Ov	Oc 3.6	aspartyl protease inhibitor	—	Ov Ad cDNA	Chandrashekar et al. (1991)
Bm	Bm33	pepsin inhibitor	—	Bm Ad cDNA	Dissanayake et al. (1993)
Ov	OvB2	aspartyl tRNA synthetase	—	Ov gDNA	Kron et al. (1992)
Bp	gp29	glutathione peroxidase	29	Bp Ad cDNA	Cookson et al. (1992)
Bp, Bm, Wb	gp29	glutathione peroxidase	29	Bp,Bm,Wb (gDNA)	Cookson et al. (1993)
Di	gp29	glutathione peroxidase	29	Di Ad cDNA	Paravax, Inc. (unpublished data)
Ov	OvGST1	glutathione S transferase	31	Ov Ad cDNA	Liebau et al. (1994)
Bp	C-SOD	cytoplasmic CuZn SOD	19	Bp Ad cDNA	Tang et al. (1994)
Bp	EC-SOD	extracellular CuZn SOD	29	Bp Ad cDNA	Tang et al. (1994)
Ov	3B.1.1	extracellular SOD	—	Ov Ad cDNA	James et al. (1994)
Ov	pIEL-12	CuZn SOD	—	Ov Ad cDNA	Henkle et al. (1991)
Bm	MF1	chitinase	70/75	Bm mf cDNA	Fuhrman et al. (1992)
Wb	WbN43	chitinase	43	Wb gDNA	Raghaven et al. (1994), Freedman et al. (1989)
Di	Di PLA2	phospholipase A2	20/22	Di L3 cDNA	Paravax, Inc. (unpublished data)
Ov	Ov PLA2	phospholipase A2	—	Ov L3 cDNA	Paravax, Inc. (unpublished data)
Ov	RAL-1	calreticulin	42	Ov Ad cDNA	Unnasch et al. (1988)
Ov	OvGS1/GS2	major sperm protein	—	Ov gDNA	Scott et al. (1989)
Bm	Bm9	GTP binding protein	22/24	Bm Ad cDNA	Dissanayake et al. (1992b)
Ov	Ov3&20	GTP binding protein	—	Ov Ad cDNA	Dissanayake et al. (1992b)
Ov	OvZf1	zinc finger encoding gene	—	Ov gDNA	Holst and Zipfel (1993)
Ov	EF-1 alpha	trans elong factor 1-a	—	Ov Ad cDNA	Alarcon and Donelson (1991)
Ov	actin 1A/2B	actin	—	Ov Ad cDNA	Zeng and Donelson (1992)
Bm/Bp	Bpa-7	beta-tubulin	50–55	Bp Ad cDNA	Helm et al. (1989)
Bp	beta 1	beta 1 tubulin	—	Bp gDNA	Guenette et al. (1991)
Bp	beta 2	beta 2 tubulin	—	Bp gDNA	Guenette et al. (1992)
Di	p4	LDL receptor motif	—	Di L3 cDNA	Paravax, Inc. (unpublished data)
Di	p39	—	39	Di L3 cDNA	Paravax, Inc. (unpublished data)
Di	p22U	—	22	Di Ad cDNA	Paravax, Inc. (unpublished data)

(continued)

Table II
(continued)

Species	Clone	Homology/similarity	Native Ag (kDa)	Library	References
Di	MPA	astacin metalloprotease	—	Di L3 cDNA	Paravax, Inc. (unpublished data)
Di	CP	cysteine protease	—	Di L3 cDNA	Paravax, Inc. (unpublished data)
Di	cD34	—	34	Di Ad cDNA	Sun et al. (1991)
Bm	SXP-1	—	34/12–14	Bm Ad cDNA	Dissanayake et al. (1992c)
Bm	D1E5.1	—	—	Bm gDNA	Awobuluyi et al. (1991)
Bm	W6	—	63	Bm Ad cDNA	Nilsen et al. (1988)
Bm	Bm19	—	—	Bm gDNA	Arasu et al. (1989)
Ov	pOI5/OI3	—	—	Ov Ad cDNA	Tuan et al. (1991)
Ov	OvL3-1	—	50	Ov Ad cDNA	Seeber et al. (1993a)
Ov	Ov103	—	15	Ov Ad cDNA	Lustigman et al. (1992b)
Ov	Ov39	—	22	Ov Ad cDNA	Braun et al. (1991)
Ov	Ov22/31M	—	~22	Ov Ad cDNA	Bradley et al. (1991)
Ov	Ov20/36M	—	20	Ov Ad cDNA	Bradley et al. (1991)
Ov	RAL-2	—	17	Ov Ad cDNA	Gallin et al. (1989), Bradley et al. (1993)
Ov	M2f.e	—	18	Ov Ad cDNA	Dinman and Scott (1990)
Ov	Ag16	—	26/24	Ov Ad cDNA	Lobos et al. (1990)
Ov	OW-10	—	—	Ov gDNA	Colina et al. (1990)

[a] Abbreviations used: Bm, *Brugia malayi*; Di, *Dirofilaria immitis*; Ov, *Onchocerca volvulus*; Bp, *Brugia pahangi*; Wb, *Wuchereria bancrofti*; L3, third-stage larvae; L4, fourth-stage larvae; Ad, adult; gDNA, genomic DNA library; (gDNA), genomic DNA; cDNA, complementary DNA library; mf, microfilaria; LDL, low-density lipoprotein; SOD, superoxide dismutase; trans elong, translation elongation; CuZn, copper/zinc.

found to contain an internal copy of the SL sequence encoded within the gene (Zeng *et al.*, 1990).

More conventional cloning strategies also have been used to identify potential vaccine immunogens. Genomic and adult cDNA expression libraries from filariid parasites of humans were screened by hybridization with genes of known function to identify a filariid homologue. Because of the lack of larval cDNA expression libraries, adult cDNA expression libraries were differentially screened with a variety of sera to target immunologically relevant proteins. As previously described, these sera have been collected from patients clinically defined as putatively immune. A representative list of certain filarid antigens that have been cloned is presented in Table II.

Vaccine development strategies also have focused on targeting unique filariid proteins with specific biological functions critical to survival. To persist within an immunocompetent host for long periods of time, filariid parasites have developed numerous adaptations to evade the toxic effects of the host leukocyte respiratory burst. To target these potential parasite immune escape mechanisms, parasite-derived antioxidant enzymes such as glutathione peroxidase (gp29), superoxide dismutase, and glutathione S transferase have been cloned from several filariid parasites as potential vaccine targets (see Table II).

7. SUMMARY

The development of vaccines for the prevention of filarial nematode infections is in a state of relative infancy in comparison to vaccines for other parasitic diseases, such as schistosomiasis and malaria. There are many reasons for this slow start. Some of the principal problems are: (1) the lengthy and complex life cycle of these organisms with attendant complex immune responses, (2) the unique characteristics associated with a relatively large number of different pathogens, (3) the lack of suitable model systems for study of medically important infections, (4) the paucity of parasite material for antigen discovery and recombinant library construction, (5) the lack of substantial evidence suggesting the natural occurrence of protective immune responses, and (6) the limited data on mechanisms responsible for protective immunity.

As technical hurdles are considered, it is also critical to focus on the characteristics of a vaccine necessary for its eventual utility. In the case of a vaccine for *D. immitis* a completely successful product will need to approach a 99+% efficacy. This is because of the 99+% efficacy of competitive chemotherapeutic products and the fact that microfilaremia observed on blood examination, resulting from as few as two worms, would present as a vaccine failure. Although very low worm burdens in large dogs could be perceived as success in the context of protection from clinical disease, because of the option of virtually complete chemoprophylactic protection, the typical veterinary practitioner would probably fail to appreciate less than complete vaccine protection.

In contrast, a vaccine that produced a reduction in adult worm burdens without complete protection in either lymphatic filariasis or onchocerciasis would be very important. Highly effective chemoprophylactic agents are not widely available for prevention of the human filariases, and dramatically reduced clinical disease provided by less than a completely effective vaccine could occur as the result of fewer adult worms.

The importance of developing these vaccines has outweighed the obstacles to this research. There has been a great deal of epidemiological and experimental evidence to suggest a vaccine is feasible and antigen discovery has progressed relatively rapidly within just the past few years. Efforts to generate appropriate larval cDNA libraries are beginning to yield dividends and a variety of fascinating vaccine candidates have been cloned.

Additional antigen discovery, research on appropriate modalities for overexpression of genes from these parasites, and the complex tasks associated with vaccinology remain as significant research and development obstacles. There is ample reason for optimism for the integrated immunobiologically centered approach, however, and a certain amount of confidence is warranted in view of the hurdles that have been overcome.

REFERENCES

Abraham, D., and Grieve, R. B., 1991, Passive transfer of protective immunity to larval *Dirofilaria immitis* from dogs to BALB/c mice, *J. Parasitol.* **77**:254–257.

Abraham, D., Weiner, D. J., and Farrell, J. P., 1986a, Cellular and humoral immune responses of jirds resistant to *Dipetalonema viteae* infection, *Infect. Immun.* **52**:742–747.

Abraham, D., Weiner, D. J., and Farrell, J. P., 1986b, Protective immune responses of the jird to larval *Dipetalonema viteae*, *Immunology* **57**:165–169.

Abraham, D., Grieve, R. B., Mika-Grieve, M., and Seibert, M., 1988a, Active and passive immunization of mice against larval *Dirofilaria immitis*, *J. Parasitol.* **74**:275–282.

Abraham, D., Grieve, R. B., and Mika-Grieve, M., 1988b, *Dirofilaria immitis*: Surface properties of third- and fourth-stage larvae, *Exp. Parasitol.* **65**:157–167.

Abraham, D., Grieve, R. B., Holy, J. M., and Christensen, B. M., 1989, Immunity to larval *Brugia malayi* in BALB/c mice: Protective immunity and inhibition of larval development, *Am. J. Trop. Med. Hyg.* **40**:598–604.

Abraham, D., Eberhard, M. L., Lange, A. M., Yutanawiboonchai, W., Perler, F., and Lok, J. B., 1992, Identification of surrogate rodent hosts for larval *Onchocerca lienalis* and induction of protective immunity in a model system, *J. Parasitol.* **78**:447–453.

Ah, H. S., McCall, J. W., and Thompson, P. E., 1974, A simple method for isolation of *Brugia pahangi* and *Brugia malayi* microfilariae, *Int. J. Parasitol.* **4**:677–679.

Alarcon, C. M., and Donelson, J. E., 1991, Translational elongation factor 1alpha (EF-1alpha) of *Onchocerca volvulus*, *Mol. Biochem. Parasitol.* **48**:105–108.

Apfel, H., Eisenbeiss, W. F., and Meyer, T. F., 1992, Changes in the surface composition after transmission of *Acanthocheilonema viteae* third stage larvae into the jird, *Mol. Biochem. Parasitol.* **52**:63–74.

Arasu, P., Nutman, T. B., Steel, C., Mulligan, M., Abraham, D., Tuan, R., and Perler, F. B., 1989, Human T-cell stimulation, molecular characterization and in situ mRNA localization of a *Brugia malayi* recombinant antigen, *Mol. Biochem. Parasitol.* **36**:223–232.

Awobuluyi, M., Maina, C., and Carlow, C., 1991, Cross-linking of a monoclonal antibody–antigen complex enables detection of parasite antigen in immunoblots and in an expression library, *Mol. Biochem. Parasitol.* **44**:149–152.

Bagai, R. C., and Subrahmanyam, D., 1970, Nature of acquired resistance to filarial infection in albino rats, *Nature* **228**:682–683.

Baldwin, C. I., De Medeiros, F., and Denham, D. A., 1993, IgE responses in cats infected with *Brugia pahangi*, *Parasite Immunol.* **15**:291–296.

Bancroft, A. J., and Devaney, E., 1993, The analysis of the humoral response of the BALB/c mouse immunized with radiation attenuated third stage larvae of *Brugia pahangi*, *Parasite Immunol.* **15**:153–162.

Bancroft, A. J., Grencis, R., Else, K., and Devaney, E., 1993, Cytokine production in BALB/c mice immunized with radiation attenuated third stage larvae of the filarial nematode, *Brugia pahangi, J. Immunol.* **150**:1359–1402.

Barthold, E., and Wenk, P., 1992, Dose-dependent recovery of adult *Acanthocheilonema viteae* (Nematoda: Filarioidea) after single and trickle inoculations in jirds, *Parasitol. Res.* **78**:229–234.

Bartlett, A., Turk, J., Ngu, J. L., Mackenzie, C. S., Fuglsang, H., and Anderson, J., 1978, Variation in delayed hypersensitivity in onchocerciasis, *Trans. R. Soc. Trop. Med. Hyg.* **72**:372–377.

Blair, L. S., and Campbell, W. C., 1980, Suppression of maturation of *Dirofilaria immitis* in *Mustela putorius furo* by single dose of ivermectin, *J. Parasitol.* **66**:691–692.

Blair, L. S., and Campbell, W. C., 1981, Immunization of ferrets against *Dirofilaria immitis* by means of chemically abbreviated infections, *Parasite Immunol.* **3**:143–147.

Boyer, A. E., Tsang, V. C. W., Eberhard, M. L., Zea-Flores, G., Hightower, A., Pilcher, J. B., Zea-Flores, R., Zhou, W., and Reimer, C. B., 1991, Guatemalan human onchocerciasis: Evidence for IgG3 involvement in acquired immunity to *Onchocerca volvulus* and identification of possible immune-associated antigens, *J. Immunol.* **146**:4001–4010.

Bradley, J. E., Helm, R., Lahaise, M., and Maizels, R. M., 1991, cDNA clones of *Onchocerca volvulus* low molecular weight antigens provide immunologically specific diagnostic probes, *Mol. Biochem. Parasitol.* **46**:219–228.

Bradley, J., Tuan, R., Shepley, K., Tree, T., Maizels, R., Helm, R., Gregory, W., and Unnasch, T., 1993, *Onchocerca volvulus*: Characterization of an immunodominant hypodermal antigen present in adult and larval parasites, *Exp. Parasitol.* **77**:414–424.

Braun, G., McKechnie, N. M., Connor, V., Gilbert, C. E., Engelbrecht, F., Whitworth, J. A., and Taylor, D. W., 1991, Immunological crossreactivity between a cloned antigen of *Onchocerca volvulus* and a component of the retinal pigment epithelium, *J. Exp. Med.* **174**:169–177.

Buttner, D. W., V. Laer, G., Mannweiler, E., and Buttner, M., 1982, Clinical, parasitological and serological studies on onchocerciasis in the Yemen Arab Republic, *Tropenmed. Parasitol.* **33**:201–212.

Carlow, C. K. S., and Bianco, A. E., 1987, Transfer of immunity to the microfilariae of *Onchocerca lienalis* in mice, *Trop. Med. Parasitol.* **39**:283–286.

Carlow, C. K. S., and Philipp, M., 1987, Protective immunity to *Brugia malayi* larvae in Balb/c mice: Potential of this model for the identification of protective antigens, *Am. J. Trop. Med. Hyg.* **37**:597–604.

Carlow, C. K., Franke, E. D., Lowrie, R. C., Partono, F., and Philipp, M., 1987, Monoclonal antibody to a unique surface epitope of the human filaria *Brugia malayi* identifies infective larvae in mosquito vectors, *Proc. Natl. Acad. Sci. USA* **84**:6914–6918.

Carlow, C. K. S., Dobinson, A. R., and Bianco, A. E., 1988, Parasite-specific immune responses to *Onchocerca lienalis* microfilariae in normal and immunodeficient mice, *Parasite Immunol.* **10**:309–322.

Caulagi, V., Werner, C., and Rajan, T., 1991, Isolation and partial sequence of a collagen gene from the human filarial parasite, *Brugia malayi, Mol. Biochem. Parasitol.* **45**:57–64.

Chandrashekar, R., Masood, K., Alvarez, R. M., Ogunrinade, A. F., Lujan, R., Richards, J., and Weil, G. J., 1991, Molecular cloning and characterization of recombinant parasite antigens for immunodiagnosis of onchocerciasis, *J. Clin. Invest.* **88**:1460–1466.

Chusattayanond, W., and Denham, D. A., 1986, Attempted vaccination of jirds against *Brugia pahangi* with radiation attenuated infective larvae, *J. Helminthol.* **60**:149–155.

Colina, K. F., Perler, F. B., Matsumura, I., Meda, M., and Nutman, T. B., 1990, The identification of an *Onchocerca*-specific recombinant antigen containing a T cell epitope, *J. Immunol.* **145**:1551–1556.

Conraths, F. J., Worms, M. J., Preece, G., Harnett, W., and Parkhouse, R. M. E., 1991, Studies on a 14-kilodalton surface protein of *Onchocerca* microfilariae, *Mol. Biochem. Parasitol.* **46**:103–112.

Conraths, F. J., Harnett, H. W., Worms, M. J., and Parkhouse, R. M. E., 1992, Immunological cross-reaction between an *Onchocerca* paramyosin-like molecule and microfilaria surface antigen, *Trop. Med. Parasitol.* **43**:135–138.

Cookson, E., Blaxter, M. L., and Selkirk, M., 1992, Identification of the major soluble cuticular glycoprotein of lymphatic filarial nematode parasite (gp29) as a secretory homolog of glutathione peroxidase, *Proc. Natl. Acad. Sci. USA* **89**:5837–5841.

Cookson, E., Tang, L., and Selkirk, M. E., 1993, Conservation of primary sequence of gp29, the major soluble cuticular glycoprotein, in three species of lymphatic filariae, *Mol. Biochem. Parasitol.* **58**:155–160.

Culpepper, J., Grieve, R. B., Friedman, L. B., Mika-Grieve, M., Frank, G. R., and Dale, B., 1992, Molecular characterization of a *Dirofilaria immitis* cDNA encoding a highly immunoreactive antigen, *Mol. Biochem. Parasitol.* **54**:51–62.

Dahmen, A., Gallin, M., Schumaucher, M., and Erttmann, K., 1993, Molecular cloning and pre-mRNA maturation of *Onchocerca volvulus* paramyosin, *Mol. Biochem. Parasitol.* **57**:335–338.

Day, K. P., 1991, The endemic normal in lymphatic filariasis: A static concept, *Parasitol. Today* **7**:341–343.

Day, K. P., Gregory, W. F., and Maizels, R. M., 1991a, Age-specific acquisition of immunity to infective larvae in a bancroftian filariasis endemic area of Papua New Guinea, *Parasite Immunol.* **13**:277–290.

Day, K. P., Grenfell, B., Spark, R., Kazura, J. W., and Alpers, M. P., 1991b, Age specific patterns of change in the dynamics of *Wuchereria bancrofti* infection in Papua, New Guinea, *Am. J. Trop. Med. Hyg.* **44**:518–527.

Day, K. P., Spark, R., Garner, P., Raiko, A., Wenger, J. D., Weiss, N., Mitchell, G. F., Alpers, M. P., and Kazura, J. W., 1991c, Serological evaluation of the macrofilaricidal effects of diethylcarbamazine treatment in bancroftian filariasis, *Am. J. Trop. Med. Hyg.* **44**:528–535.

Denham, D. A., Ponnudurai, T., Nelson, G. S., Guy, F., and Rogers, R., 1972a, Studies with *Brugia pahangi*: Parasitological observations on primary infections of cats, *Int. J. Parasitol.* **2**:239–247.

Denham, D. A., Ponnudurai, T., Nelson, G. S., Guy, F., and Rogers, R., 1972b, Studies with *Brugia pahangi*: The effect of repeated infection on parasite levels in cats, *Int. J. Parasitol.* **2**:401–407.

Denham, D. A., McGreevy, P. B., Suswillo, R. R., and Rogers, R., 1983, The resistance to re-infection of cats repeatedly inoculated with infective larvae of *Brugia pahangi*, *Parasitology* **86**:11–18.

Denham, D. A., Medeiros, F., Baldwin, C., Kumar, H., Midwinter, I. C. T., Birch, D. W., and Smail, A., 1992, Repeated infection of cats with *Brugia pahangi*: Parasitological observations, *Parasitology* **104**:415–420.

Devaney, E., Bancroft, A., and Egan, A., 1993, The effect of irradiation on the third stage larvae of *Brugia pahangi*, *Parasite Immunol.* **15**:423–427.

Dinman, J. D., and Scott, A. L., 1990, *Onchocerca volvulus*: Molecular cloning, primary structure, and expression of a microfilarial surface-associated antigen, *Exp. Parasitol.* **71**:176–188.

Dissanayake, S., Xu, M., and Piessens, W., 1992a, Myosin heavy chain is a dominant parasite antigen recognized by antibodies in sera from donors with filarial infections, *Mol. Biochem. Parasitol.* **56**:349–352.

Dissanayake, S., Xu, M., and Piessens, W., 1992b, Filarial parasites contain a *ras* homolog of the TC4/ran/Spi1 family, *Mol. Biochem. Parasitol.* **56**:259–268.

Dissanayake, S., Xu, M., and Piessens, W., 1992c, A cloned antigen for serological diagnosis of *Wuchereria bancrofti* microfilaremia with daytime blood samples, *Mol. Biochem. Parasitol.* **56**:269–278.

Dissanayake, S., Xu, M., Nkenfou, C., and Piessens, W., 1993, Molecular cloning and serological characterization of a *Brugia malayi* pepsin inhibitor homolog, *Mol. Biochem. Parasitol.* **62**:143–146.

Donelson, J. E., Duke, B. O. L., Moser, D., Zeng, W., Erondu, N., Lucius, R., Renz, A., Karam, M., and Flores, G., 1988, Construction of *Onchocerca volvulus* cDNA libraries and partial characterization of the cDNA for a major antigen, *Mol. Biochem. Parasitol.* **31**:241–250.

Duke, B. O. L., 1968, Reinfections with *Onchocerca volvulus* in cured patients exposed to continuing transmission, *Bull. WHO* **39**:307–309.

Duke, B. O. L., and Moore, P. T., 1968, The contribution of different age groups to the transmission of onchocerciasis in a Cameroon forest village, *Trans. R. Soc. Trop. Med. Hyg.* **62**:22–28.

Egerton, J. R., Birnbaum, J., Blair, L. S., Chabala, J. C., Conroy, J., Fisher, M. H., Mrozik, H., Ostlind, D. A., Wilkins, C. A., and Campbell, W. C., 1980, 22,23-dihydroavermectin B1a, a new broad-spectrum antiparasitic agent, *Br. Vet. J.* **136**:88–97.

Eisenbeiss, W. F., Apfel, H., and Meyer, F., 1994, Protective immunity linked with a distinct developmental stage of filarial parasite, *J. Immunol.* **22**:735–742.

Elson, L., Guderian, R., Araujo, E., Bradley, J., Days, A., and Nutman, T., 1994, Immunity to onchocerciasis: Identification of a putatively immune population in a hyperendemic area of Ecuador, *J. Infect. Dis.* **169**:588–594.

Erondu, N. E., and Donelson, J. E., 1990, Characterization of a myosin-like antigen from *Onchocerca volvulus*, *Mol. Biochem. Parasitol.* **40**:213–224.

Fletcher, C., Birch, D. W., and Denham, D. A., 1992, Cats with single *Brugia pahangi* infections: Relationship between parasitological status and humoral responses to somatic and surface parasite antigens, *Parasite Immunol.* **14**:339–350.

Frank, G. R., and Grieve, R. B., 1991, Metabolic labeling of *Dirofilaria immitis* third- and fourth-stage larvae and their excretory–secretory products, *J. Parasitol.* **77**:950–956.

Freedman, D. O., Nutman, T. B., and Ottesen, E. A., 1989, Protective immunity in bancroftian filariasis: Selective recognition of a 43-kD larval stage antigen by infection-free individuals in an endemic area, *J. Clin. Invest.* **83**:14–22.

Fuhrman, J. A., Lane, W. S., Smith, R. F., Piessen, W. F., and Perler, F. B., 1992, Transmission-blocking antibodies recognize microfilarial chitinase in brugian lymphatic filariasis, *Proc. Natl. Acad. Sci. USA* **89**:1548–1552.

Gallin, M. Y., Tan, M., Kron, M. A., Rechnitzer, D., Greene, B. M., Newland, H. S., White, A. T., Taylor, H. R., and Unnasch, T. R., 1989, *Onchocerca volvulus* recombinant antigen: Physical characterization and clinical correlates with serum reactivity, *J. Infect. Dis.* **160**:521–529.

Grandea, A. G., Tuyen, L. K., Asikin, N., Davis, T., Philipp, M., Cohen, C., and McReynolds, L., 1989, A λgt11 cDNA recombinant that encodes *Dirofilaria immitis* paramyosin, *Mol. Biochem. Parasitol.* **35**:31–41.

Greene, B. M., Taylor, H. R., and Aikawa, M., 1981, Cellular killing of microfilariae of *Onchocerca volvulus*: Eosinophil and neutrophil mediated immune serum-dependent destruction, *J. Immunol.* **127**:1611–1618.

Greene, B., Gbakina, A., Albiez, E., and Taylor, H., 1985, Humoral and cellular immune responses to *Onchocerca volvulus* infection in humans, *Rev. Infect. Dis.* **7**:789–795.

Grenfell, B. T., Michael, E., and Denham, D. A., 1991, A model for the dynamics of human lymphatic filariasis, *Parasitol. Today* **7**:318–323.

Grieve, R. B., Brooks, B. O., Babish, J. G., Jacobson, R. H., and Cypess, R. H., 1982, Lymphocyte function in experimental canine dirofilariasis: B-cell responses to heterologous antigen, *J. Parasitol.* **68**:341–343.

Grieve, R. B., Lok, J. B., and Glickman, L. T., 1983, Epidemiology of canine heartworm infection, *Epidemiol. Rev.* **5**:220–246.

Grieve, R. B., Abraham, D., Mika-Grieve, M., and Seibert, B. P., 1988, Induction of protective immunity in dogs to infection with *Dirofilaria immitis* using chemically-abbreviated infections, *Am. J. Trop. Med. Hyg.* **39**:373–379.

Grieve, R. B., Frank, G. R., Stewart, V. A., Parsons, J. C., Belasco, D. L., and Hepler, D. I., 1991, Chemoprophylactic effects of milbemycin oxime against larvae of *Dirofilaria immitis* during prepatent development, *Am. J. Vet. Res.* **52**:2040–2042.

Grieve, R. B., Frank, G. R., Mika-Grieve, M., Culpepper, J. A., and Mok, M., 1992, Identification of *Dirofilaria immitis* larval antigens with immunoprophylactic potential using sera from immune dogs, *J. Immunol.* **148**:2511–2515.

Guenette, S., Prichard, R. K., Klein, R. D., and Matlashewski, G., 1991, Characterization of a *beta*-tubulin gene and *beta*-tubulin gene products of *Brugia pahangi*, *Mol. Biochem. Parasitol.* **44**:153–164.

Guenette, S., Prichard, R. K., and Matlashewski, G., 1992, Identification of a novel *Brugia pahangi beta*-tubulin gene (*B-2*) and a 22-nucleotide spliced leader sequence on *beta*-tubulin mRNA, *Mol. Biochem. Parasitol.* **50**:275–284.

Haque, A., Chassoux, D., Ogilvie, B. M., and Capron, A., 1978, *Dipetalonema viteae* infections in hamsters: Enhancement and suppression of microfilaraemia, *Parasitology* **76**:61–75.

Haque, A., Quaissi, A., Santoro, F., Des Moutis, I., and Capron, A., 1982, Complement-mediated leukocyte adherence to infective larvae of *Dipetalonema viteae* (Filariodea): Requirement for eosinophils or eosinophil products in effecting macrophage adherence, *J. Immunol.* **129**:2219–2225.

Hayashi, Y., Nogami, S., Nakamura, M., Shirasaka, A., and Noda, K., 1984, Passive transfer of protective immunity against *Brugia malayi* in BALB/c mice, *Jpn. J. Exp. Med.* **54**:183–187.

Hayashi, Y., Nakagaki, K., Nogami, S., Hammerberg, B., and Tanaka, H., 1989, Protective immunity against *Brugia malayi* infective larvae in mice: Parameters of active and passive immunity, *Am. J. Trop. Med. Hyg.* **41**:650–656.

Helm, R., Selkirk, M. E., Bradley, J. E., Burns, R. G., Hamilton, A. J., Croft, S., and Maizels, R. M., 1989, Localization and immunogenicity of tubulin in the filarial nematodes *Brugia malayi* and *B. pahangi*, *Parasite Immunol.* **11**:479–502.

Henkle, K. J., Liebau, E., Muller, S., Bergmann, B., and Walter, R. D., 1991, Characterization and molecular cloning of a Cu/Zn superoxide dismutase from the human parasite *Onchocerca volvulus*, *Infect. Immun.* **59**:2063–2069.

Holst, C., and Zipfel, P. F., 1993, Identification of a zinc finger encoding gene in *Onchocerca volvulus*, *Trop. Med. Parasitol.* **44**:147–151.

James, E., McLean, D., and Perler, F., 1994, Molecular cloning of an *Onchocerca volvulus* extracellular Cu-Zn superoxide dismutase, *Infect. Immun.* **62**:713–716.

Jarrett, W., Jennings, F., McIntyre, W., Mulligan, W., Sharp, N., and Urquhart, G., 1960, Immunological studies on *Dictyocaulus viviparus* infection, *Immunology* **3**:145–151.

Kazura, J., and Davis, R. S., 1982, Soluble *Brugia malayi* microfilarial antigens protect mice against challenge by an antibody-dependent mechanism, *J. Immunol.* **128**:1792–1796.

Kazura, J. W., Cicirello, H., and Forsyth, K., 1986a, Differential recognition of a protective filarial antigen by antibodies from humans with bancroftian filariasis, *J. Clin. Invest.* **77**:1985–1992.

Kazura, J. W., Cicirello, H., and McCall, J. W., 1986b, Induction of protection against *Brugia malayi* infection in jirds by microfilarial antigens, *J. Immunol.* **136**:1422–1426.

King, C. L., Kumaraswarmi, V., Poindexter, R. W., Kumria, S., Jayaraman, K., Alling, D. W., Ottesen, E. A., and Nutman, T. B., 1992, Immunologic tolerance in lymphatic filariasis. Diminished parasite-specific T and B lymphocyte precursor frequency in the microfilaremic state, *J. Clin. Invest.* **89**:1403–1410.

King, C. L., Mahanty, S., Kumaraswami, V., Abrahams, J. S., Regunathan, J., Jayaraman, K., Ottesen, E. A., and Nutman, T. B., 1993, Cytokine control of parasite-specific anergy in human lymphatic filariasis. Preferential induction of a regulatory T helper type 2 lymphocyte subset, *J. Clin. Invest.* **92**:1667–1673.

Klei, T. R., McCall, J. W., and Malone, J. B., 1980, Evidence for increased susceptibility of *Brugia pahangi*-infected jirds to subsequent homologous infections, *J. Helminthol.* **54**:161–165.

Knight, D. H., 1977, Heartworm heart disease, *Adv. Vet. Sci. Comp. Med.* **21**:107–149.

Knight, D. H., 1987, Heartworm infection, in: *The Veterinary Clinics of North America*, Vol. 17 (R. B. Grieve, ed.), Saunders, Philadelphia, pp. 1463–1518.

Kowalski, J. C., and Ash, L. R., 1975, Repeated infections in *Brugia pahangi* in the jird, *Meriones unguiculatus, Southeast Asian J. Trop. Med. Public Health* **6**:195–198.

Kron, M., Erttmann, K., Greene, B., and Unnasch, T., 1992, Characterization of a possible tRNA synthetase gene from *Onchocerca volvulus*, *Mol. Biochem. Parasitol.* **52**:289–292.

Kwan-Lim, G., Forsyth, K. P., and Maizels, R. M., 1990, Filarial-specific IgG4 response correlates with active *Wuchereria bancrofti* infection, *J. Immunol.* **145**:4298–4305.

Lal, R. B., and Ottesen, E. A., 1988, Characterization of stage-specific antigens of infective larvae of the filarial parasite *Brugia malayi*, *J. Immunol.* **140**:2032–2038.

Lange, A. M., Yutanawiboochai, W., Lok, J. B., Trpis, M., and Abraham, D., 1993, Induction of protective immunity against larval *Onchocerca volvulus* in a mouse model, *Am. J. Trop. Med. Hyg.* **49**:783–788.

Lange, A. M., Yutanawiboochai, W., Scott, P., and Abraham, D., 1994, IL-4 and IL-5 dependent protective immunity to *Onchocerca volvulus* infective larvae in BALB/cBYJ mice, *J. Immunol.* **153**:205–211.

Li, B., Chandrashekar, R., Alvarez, R. M., Liftis, F., and Weil, G. J., 1991, Identification of paramyosin as a potential protective antigen against *Brugia malayi* infection in jirds, *Mol. Biochem. Parasitol.* **49**:315–324.

Li, B., Ramaswamy, C., and Weil, G., 1993, Vaccination with recombinant filarial paramyosin induces partial immunity to *Brugia malayi* infection in jirds, *J. Immunol.* **150**:1881–1885.

Liebau, E., Walter, R. D., and Henkle-Duhrsen, K., 1994, Isolation, sequence and expression of an *Onchocerca volvulus* glutathione S-transferase cDNA, *Mol. Biochem. Parasitol.* **63**:305–309.

Limberger, R. J., and McReynolds, L. A., 1990, Filarial paramyosin: cDNA sequences from *Dirofilaria immitis* and *Onchocerca volvulus*, *Mol. Biochem. Parasitol.* **38**:271–280.

Lobos, E., Altmann, M., Mengod, G., Weiss, N., Rudin, W., and Karam, M., 1990, Identification of an *Onchocerca volvulus* cDNA encoding a low-molecular-weight antigen uniquely recognized by onchocerciasis patient sera, *Mol. Biochem. Parasitol.* **39**:135–146.

Lucius, R., Ruppel, A., and Diesfeld, H. J., 1986, *Dipetalonema viteae*: Resistance in *Meriones unguiculatus* with multiple infections of stage-3 larvae, *Exp. Parasitol.* **62**:237–246.

Lucius, R., Erondu, N., Kern, A., and Donelson, J. E., 1988, Molecular cloning of an immunodominant antigen of *Onchocerca volvulus*, *J. Exp. Med.* **168**:1199–1204.

Lucius, R., Textor, G., Kern, A., and Kirsten, C., 1991, *Acanthocheilonema viteae*: Vaccination of jirds with irradiation-attenuated stage-3 larvae and with exported larval antigens, *Exp. Parasitol.* **73**:184–196.

Lustigman, S., Brotman, B., Huima, T., and Prince, A. M., 1991, Characterization of an *Onchocerca volvulus* cDNA clone encoding a genus specific antigen present in infective larvae and adult worms, *Mol. Biochem. Parasitol.* **45**:65–76.

Lustigman, S., Brotman, B., Huima, T., Prince, A. M., and McKerrow, J. H., 1992a, Molecular cloning and characterization of onchocystatin, a cysteine proteinase inhibitor of *Onchocerca volvulus*, *J. Biol. Chem.* **267**:17339–17346.

Lustigman, S., Brotman, B., Johnson, E. H., Smith, A. B., Huima, T., and Prince, A. M., 1992b, Identification and characterization of an *Onchocerca volvulus* cDNA clone encoding a microfilarial surface-associated antigen, *Mol. Biochem. Parasitol.* **50**:79–94.

Maizels, R. M., and Lawrence, R. A., 1991, Immunological tolerance: The key feature in human filariasis, *Parasitol. Today* **7**:271–276.

Maizels, R. M., Partono, F., Oemijati, S., Denham, D. A., and Ogilvie, B. M., 1983, Cross-reactive surface antigens on three stages of *Brugia malayi*, *B. pahangi* and *B. timori*, *Parasitology* **87**:249–263.

Maizels, R. M., Burke, J., and Denham, D. A., 1987, Phosphorylcholine-bearing antigens in filarial nematode parasites: Analysis of somatic extracts, in vitro secretions and infection sera from *Brugia malayi* and *B. pahangi*, *Parasite Immunol.* **9**:49–66.

Maizels, R. M., Kurniawan, A., Selkirk, M. E., and Yazdanbakhsh, M., 1991, Immune responses to filarial parasites, *Immunol. Lett.* **30**:249–254.

Mehta, K., Subrahmanyam, D., and Sindhu, R. K., 1981, Immunogenicity of homogenates of the developmental stages of *Litomosoides carinii* in albino rats, *Acta Trop.* **38**:319–324.

Mejia, J. S., and Carlow, C. K., 1994, An analysis of the humoral immune response of dogs following vaccination with irradiated infective larvae of *Dirofilaria immitis*, *Parasite Immunol.* **16**:157–164.

Miller, T. A., 1964, Effect of X-irradiation upon the infective larvae of *Ancylostoma caninum* and the immunogenic effect in dogs of a single infection with 40 kr-irradiated larvae, *J. Immunol.* **50**:735–742.

Nanduri, J., and Kazura, J. W. 1989, Paramyosin-enhanced clearance of *Brugia malayi* microfilaremia in mice, *J. Immunol.* **143**:3359–3363.

Neilsen, J. T. M., 1976, A comparison of the acquired resistance to *Dipetalonema viteae* stimulated in hamsters by trickle versus tertiary infections, *Tropenmed. Parasitol.* **27**:233–237.

Neva, F. A., and Ottesen, E. A., 1978, Tropical (filarial) eosinophilia, *N. Engl. J. Med.* **298**:1129–1131.

Nilsen, T. W., Maroney, P. A., Goodwin, R. G., Perrine, K. G., Denker, J. A., Nanduri, J., and Kazura, J. W., 1988, Cloning and characterization of a potentially protective antigen in lymphatic filariasis, *Proc. Natl. Acad. Sci. USA* **85**:3604–3607.

Nutman, T. B., 1989, Protective immunity in lymphatic filariasis, *Exp. Parasitol.* **68**:248–252.

Nutman, T. B., Kumaraswami, V., and Ottesen, E. A., 1987, Parasite-specific anergy in human filariasis. Insights after analysis of parasite antigen-driven lymphokine production, *J. Clin. Invest.* **79**:1516–1523.

Nutman, T. B., Steel, C., Ward, D. J., Zea-Flores, G., and Ottesen, E. A., 1991, Immunity to onchocerciasis: Recognition of larval antigens by humans putatively immune to *Onchocerca volvulus* infection, *J. Infect. Dis.* **163**:1128–1133.

Ogilvie, B. M., Philipp, M., Jungery, M., Maizels, R. M., and Parkhouse, R. M. E., 1980, The surface of nematodes and the immune response of the host, in: *Host–Invader Interplay* (H. Van Den Bossche, ed.), Elsevier/North-Holland, Amsterdam, pp. 99–104.

Oothuman, P., Denham, D. A., McGreevy, P. B., and Nelson, G. S., 1978, Studies with *Brugia pahangi*. 15. Cobalt 60 irradiation of the worm, *J. Helminthol.* **52**:121–126.

Oothuman, P., Denham, D. A., McGreevy, P. B., Nelson, G. S., and Rogers, R., 1979, Successful vaccination of cats against *Brugia pahangi* with larvae attenuated by irradiation with 10 krad cobalt 60, *Parasite Immunol.* **1**:209–216.

Ottesen, E. A., 1984, Immunological aspects of lymphatic filariasis and onchocerciasis in man, *Trans. R. Soc. Trop. Med. Hyg.* **78**:9–18.

Ottesen, E. A., 1992, Infection and disease in lymphatic filariasis: An immunological perspective, *Parasitology* **104**:871–879.

Ottesen, E. A., Weller, P. F., and Heck, L., 1977, Specific cellular immune unresponsiveness in human filariasis, *Immunology* **33**:413–421.

Ottesen, E. A., Neva, F. A., Paranjape, R. S., Tripathy, S. P., Thiruvengadam, K. V., and Beaven, M. A., 1979, Specific allergic sensitization to filarial antigens in tropical eosinophilia syndrome, *Lancet* 1158–1161.

Ottesen, E. A., Weller, P. F., Lunde, M. N., and Hussain, R., 1982, Endemic filariasis on a Pacific island II. Immunologic aspects: Immunoglobulin, complement, and specific antifilarial IgG, IgM and IgE antibodies, *Am. J. Trop. Med. Hyg.* **31**:953–961.

Otto, G. F., 1969, The immune phenomenon, *J. Am. Vet. Med. Assoc.* **154**:386–387.

Owhashi, M., Futaki, S., Kitagawa, K., Horii, Y., Maruyama, H., Hayashi, H., and Nawa, Y., 1993, Molecular cloning and characterization of a novel neutrophil chemotactic factor from a filarial parasite, *Mol. Immunol.* **30**:1315–1320.

Pery, P., Petit, A., Poulain, J., and Luffan, G., 1974, Phosphorylcholine-bearing components in homogenates of nematodes, *Eur. J. Immunol.* **4**:637–639.

Philipp, M., Davis, T. B., Storey, N., and Carlow, C. K. S., 1988, Immunity in filariasis: Perspectives for vaccine development, *Annu. Rev. Microbiol.* **42**:685–716.

Piessens, W. F., and Mackenzie, C. D., 1982, Lymphatic filariasis and onchocerciasis, in: *Immunology of Parasitic Infections*, Vol. 2 (S. Cohen and K. S. Warren, eds.), Blackwell, Oxford, pp. 622–653.

Piessens, W. F., McGreevy, P. B., Piessens, P. W., McGreevy, M., Koiman, I., Saroso, S., and Dennis, D. T., 1980a, Immune responses in human infections with *Brugia malayi*, *J. Clin. Invest.* **65**:172–179.

Piessens, W. F., McGreevy, P. B., Ratiwayanto, S., McGreevy, M., Piessens, P., Koiman, I., Saroso, J., and Dennis, D. T., 1980b, Immune responses in human infections with *Brugia malayi*: Correlation of cellular and humoral reactions to microfilarial antigens with clinical status, *Am. J. Trop. Med. Hyg.* **29**:563–670.

Pinder, M., Dupont, A., and Egwang, T., 1988, Identification of a surface antigen on *Loa loa* microfilariae the recognition of which correlates with the amicrofilaremic state in man, *J. Immunol.* **141**:2480–2486.

Poole, C. B., Grandea, A. G., Maina, C. V., Jenkins, R. E., Selkirk, M., and McReynolds, L. A., 1992, Cloning of a cuticular antigen that contains multiple tandem repeats from the filarial parasite *Dirofilaria immitis*, *Proc. Natl. Acad. Sci. USA* **89**:5986–5990.

Raghavan, N., McReynolds, L., Maina, C., Feinstone, S., Jayarama, K., Ottesen, E., and Nutman, T., 1991, A recombinant clone of *Wuchereria bancrofti* with DNA specificity for human lymphatic filarial parasites, *Mol. Biochem. Parasitol.* **47**:63–72.

Raghavan, N., Maina, C., Fitzgerald, P., Tuan, R., Slatko, B., Ottesen, E., and Nutman, T., 1992, Characterization of a muscle-associated antigen from *Wuchereria bancrofti*, *Exp. Parasitol.* **75**:379–389.

Raghavan, N., Freedman, D. O., Fitzgerald, P. C., Unnasch, T. R., Ottesen, E. A., and Nutman, T. B., 1994, Cloning and characterization of a potentially protective chitinase-like recombinant antigen from *Wuchereria bancrofti*, *Infect. Immun.* **62**:1901–1908.

Rajasekariah, G. R., Monteiro, Y. M., Nelto, A., Deshpande, L., and Subrahmanyam, D., 1989, Protective immune responses with trickle infections of the third stage filarial larvae, *Wuchereria bancrofti* in mice, *Clin. Exp. Immunol.* **78**:292–298.

Rao, Y. V. B. G., Mehta, K., and Subrahmanyam, D., 1977, *Litomosoides carinii*: Effect of irradiation on the development and immunogenicity of the larval forms, *Exp. Parasitol.* **43**:39–44.

Rener, J., Graves, P. M., Carter, R., Williams, J. L., and Burkot, T. R., 1983, Target antigens of transmission blocking immunity on gametes of *Plasmodium falciparum*, *J. Exp. Med.* **158**:976–981.

Rothstein, N., and Rajan, T. V., 1991, Characterization of an *hsp*70 gene from the human filarial parasite, *Brugia malayi* (Nematoda), *Mol. Biochem. Parasitol.* **49**:229–238.

Rothstein, N. M., Higashi, G., Yates, J., and Rajan, T. V., 1989, *Onchocerca volvulus* heat shock protein 70 is a major immunogen in amicrofilaremic individuals from a filariasis-endemic area, *Mol. Biochem. Parasitol.* **33**:229–236.

Scott, A. L., Dinman, J., Sussman, D., Yenbutr, P., and Ward, S., 1989, Major sperm protein genes from *Onchocerca volvulus*, *Mol. Biochem. Parasitol.* **36**:119–126.

Seeber, F., Brattig, N., Soboslay, P. T., Pogonka, T., Lorz, A., Strote, G., Beck, E., Titanji, V. P. K., and Lucius, R., 1993a, Characterization of a recombinant T cell and B cell reactive polypeptide of *Onchocerca volvulus*, *J. Immunol.* **150**:2931–2944.

Seeber, F., Pogonka, T., and Lucius, R., 1993b, PCR mediated cDNA synthesis from minute amounts of filarial L3 RNA, *Trop. Med. Parasitol.* **44**:57–59.

Selkirk, M. E., Denham, D. A., Partono, F., and Maizels, R. M., 1989, Heat shock cognate 70 is a prominent immunogen in brugian filariasis, *J. Immunol.* **143**:299–308.

Selkirk, M. E., Yazdanbakhsh, M., Freedman, D., Blaxter, M. L., Cookson, E., Jenkins, R. E., and Williams, S. A., 1991, A proline-rich structural protein of the surface sheath of larval *Brugia* filarial nematode parasites, *J. Biol. Chem.* **266**:11002–11008.

Selkirk, M. E., Maizels, R. M., and Yazdanbakhsh, M., 1992, Immunity and the prospects for vaccination against filariasis, *Immunobiology* **184**:263–281.

Smithers, S. R., and Terry, R. J., 1976, The immunology of schistosomiasis, *Adv. Parasitol.* **14**:399–422.

Spence, H., Moore, J., Brass, A., and Kennedy, M., 1993, A cDNA encoding repeating units of the ABA-1 allergen of *Ascaris, Mol. Biochem. Parasitol.* **57**:339–344.

Steel, C., and Nutman, T., 1993, Regulation of IL-5 in onchocerciasis, *J. Immunol.* **150**:5511–5518.

Storey, D. M., and Al-Mukhtar, A. S., 1982a, The development of normal and γ-irradiated *Litomosoides carinii* larvae in cotton rats, *Tropenmed. Parasitol.* **33**:223–226.

Storey, D. M., and Al-Mukhtar, A. S., 1982b, Vaccination of jirds (*Meriones unguiculatus*) against *Litomosoides carinii* and *Brugia pahangi* using irradiated larvae of *L. carinii*, *Tropenmed. Parasitol.* **33**:23–24.

Subrahmanyam, D., Mehta, K., Nelson, D. S., Rao, Y. V., and Rao, C. K., 1978, Immune reactions in human filariasis, *J. Clin. Microbiol.* **8**:228–232.

Sun, S., Matsuura, T., and Sugane, K., 1991, Molecular cloning of the cDNA encoding an immunodominant antigen of *Dirofilaria immitis*, *J. Helminthol.* **65**:149–158.

Tang, L., Ou, X., Henkle-Duhrsen, K., and Selkirk, M., 1994, Extracellular and cytoplasmic CuZn superoxide dismutases from *Brugia* lymphatic filarial nematode parasites, *Infect. Immun.* **62**:961–967.

Tanner, M., and Weiss, N., 1981a, *Dipetalonema viteae* (Filarioidea): Development of the infective larvae in micropore chambers implanted into normal, infected and immunized jirds, *Trans. R. Soc. Trop. Med. Hyg.* **75**:173–174.

Tanner, M., and Weiss, N., 1981b, *Dipetalonema viteae* (Filarioidea): Evidence for a serum-dependent cytotoxicity against developing third and fourth stage larvae in vitro, *Acta Trop.* **38**:325–328.

Taylor, H. R., 1985, Research priorities for immunologic aspects of onchocerciasis, *J. Infect. Dis.* **152**:389–394.

Taylor, M. J., van Es, R. P., Shay, K., Folkard, S., Townson, S., and Bianco, A., 1994, Protective immunity against *Onchocerca volvulus* and *O. lienalis* infective larvae in mice, *Trop. Med. Parasitol.* **45**:17–23.

Townson, S., and Bianco, A. E., 1982, Immunization of calves against the microfilariae of *Onchocerca lienalis*, *J. Helminthol.* **56**:297–303.

Townson, S., Bianco, A. E., Doenhoff, M. J., and Muller, R., 1984, Immunity to *Onchocerca lienalis* microfilariae in mice I. Resistance induced by the homologous parasite, *Tropenmed. Parasitol.* **35**:202–208.

Tuan, R. S., Shepley, K. J., Mulligan, M. M., Abraham, D., and Perler, F. B., 1991, Histochemical localization of gene expression in *Onchocerca volvulus*: In situ DNA histohybridization and immunocytochemistry, *Mol. Biochem. Parasitol.* **49**:191–204.

Tweedie, S., Paxton, W., Ingram, L., Maizels, R., McReynolds, L., and Selkirk, M., 1993, *Brugia pahangi* and *Brugia malayi*: A surface-associated glycoprotein (gp15/400) is composed of multiple tandemly repeated units and processed from a 400-kDa precursor, *Exp. Parasitol.* **76**:156–164.

Unnasch, T. R., Gallin, M. Y., Soboslay, P. T., Erttmann, K. D., and Greene, B. M., 1988, Isolation and characterization of expression cDNA clones encoding antigens of *Onchocerca volvulus* infective larvae, *J. Clin. Invest.* **82**:262–269.

Vanamail, P., Subramanian, S., Das, P. K., Pani, S. P., Rajagopalan, P. K., Bundy, D. A. P., and Grenfell, B. T., 1989, Estimation of age-specific rates of acquisition and loss of *Wuchereria bancrofti* infection, *Trans. R. Soc. Trop. Med. Hyg.* **83**:689–693.

Wakelin, D., 1984, Nematodes which invade tissues: The cuticle as target for effector mechanisms, in: *Immunity to Parasites*, Edward Arnold, London, pp. 117–133.

Ward, D. J., Nutman, T. B., Zea-Flores, G., Portocarrero, C., Lujan, A., and Ottesen, E. A., 1988, Onchocerciasis and immunity in humans: Enhanced T cell responsiveness to parasite antigen in putatively immune individuals, *J. Infect. Dis.* **157**:536–543.

Weil, G. J., Powers, K. G., Parbuoni, B. R., Furrow, R. D., and Ottesen, E. A., 1982, *Dirofilaria immitis*: Antimicrofilarial immunity in experimental filariasis, *Am. J. Trop. Med. Hyg.* **31**:477–483.

Weiner, D. J., Abraham, D., and D'Antonio, R., 1984, *Litomosoides carinii* in jirds (*Meriones unguiculatus*): Ability to retard development of challenge larvae can be transferred with cells and serum, *J. Helminthol.* **58**:129–137.

Weiss, N., and Tanner, M., 1979, Studies on *Dipetalonema viteae* (Filarioidea). 3. Antibody-dependent cell-mediated destruction of microfilariae in vivo, *Tropenmed. Parasitol.* **30**:73–80.

Weiss, N., and Tanner, M., 1981, Immunogenicity of the surface of filarial larvae *Dipetalonema viteae*, *Trans. R. Soc. Trop. Med. Hyg.* **75**:179–181.

Werner, C., and Rajan, T. V., 1992, Comparison of the body wall myosin heavy chain sequences from *Onchocerca volvulus* and *Brugia malayi*, *Mol. Biochem. Parasitol.* **50**:255–260.

Werner, C., Higashi, G. I., Yates, J. A., and Rajan, T. V., 1989, Differential recognition of two cloned *Brugia malayi* antigens by antibody class, *Mol. Biochem. Parasitol.* **35**:209–218.

Wong, M. M., 1964, Studies on microfilaremia in dogs: Levels of microfilaremia in relation to immunologic responses of the host, *Am. J. Trop. Med. Hyg.* **14**:66–77.

Wong, M. M., and Guest, M. F., 1969, Filarial antibodies and eosinophilia in human subjects in an endemic area, *Trans. R. Soc. Trop. Med. Hyg.* **63**:796–799.

Wong, M. M., Fredericks, H. J., and Ramachandran, C. P., 1969, Studies on immunization against *Brugia malayi* infection in the rhesus monkey, *Bull. WHO* **40**:493–501.

Wong, M. M., Guest, M. F., and Lavoipierre, M. J., 1974, *Dirofilaria immitis*: Fate and immunogenicity of irradiated infective stage larvae of beagles, *Exp. Parasitol.* **35**:465–474.

World Health Organization, 1987, Protective immunity and vaccination in onchocerciasis and lymphatic filariasis: Report of the 13th meeting of the scientific working group on filariasis, WHO Document TDR/FIL/SWG (13)/87.3, Geneva.

World Health Organization Experts Committee, 1976, Epidemiology of onchocerciasis, *WHO Tech. Rep. Ser.* **597**:1–94.

Yates, J. A., and Higashi, G. I., 1985, *Brugia malayi*: Vaccination of jirds with [60]cobalt-attenuated infective stage larvae protects against homologous challenge, *Am. J. Trop. Med. Hyg.* **34**:1132–1137.

Zeng, W., and Donelson, J. E., 1992, The actin genes of *Onchocerca volvulus*, *Mol. Biochem. Parasitol.* **55**:207–216.

Zeng, W., Alarcon, C., and Donelson, J., 1990, Many transcribed regions of the *Onchocerca volvulus* genome contain the spliced leader of *Caenorhabditis elegans*, *Mol. Cell. Biol.* **10**:2765–2773.

Chapter 34

Retrovirus and Retrotransposon Particles as Antigen Presentation and Delivery Systems

Sally E. Adams and Alan J. Kingsman

1. INTRODUCTION

The development of technologies to produce recombinant proteins for use as vaccines has made substantial advances during the past decade. In particular, a number of expression systems have been designed to increase the immunogenicity of proteins and peptides by presenting them as polyvalent, particulate structures. Examples of such carrier systems include both the core and surface proteins of hepatitis B virus and poliovirus which have been used to present a variety of immunogens in a particulate form; these include epitopes derived from foot-and-mouth disease virus (Clarke *et al.*, 1987), human immunodeficiency virus (HIV-1) (Michel *et al.*, 1988), and human papillomavirus (Jenkins *et al.*, 1991). In addition, synthetic systems such as immunostimulating complexes (ISCOMs) (Morein *et al.*, 1987; see Chapter 23) and liposomes (Harding *et al.*, 1991; see Chapter 13) have been used to induce both cellular and humoral responses to a range of proteins. Both of these systems result in multiple copies of the protein being presented to the immune system as part of a relatively large particle.

Among the particulate presentation technologies is the manipulation of retroelement particles. The term *retroelement* refers to genetic entities that use reverse transcriptase in their life cycle and includes both retroviruses and retrotransposons. Retroelement particle manipulation started with the yeast retrotransposon Ty. In this system, antigens are genetically fused to the *TYA* gene, which encodes a particle-forming protein that can self-assemble into virus-like particles (VLPs). Fusion at the C-terminus of the *TYA*-encoded protein does not disrupt its ability to form particles, and the *TYA*-fusion proteins therefore

Sally E. Adams • British Bio-technology Ltd., Oxford OX4 5LY, United Kingdom. *Alan J. Kingsman* • British Bio-technology Ltd., Oxford OX4 5LY, and Department of Biochemistry, Oxford University, Oxford OX1 3QU, United Kingdom.

Vaccine Design: The Subunit and Adjuvant Approach, edited by Michael F. Powell and Mark J. Newman. Plenum Press, New York, 1995.

assemble into hybrid VLPs (Adams *et al.*, 1987b). These hybrid particles are able to elicit antibody, T-helper (Th) and cytotoxic T-lymphocyte (CTL) responses.

The similarity of the Ty element to retroviral proviruses has, more recently, led to the extension of these ideas to retroviral systems (Kingsman *et al.*, 1991). The *TYA* gene of Ty is an analogue of the retroviral *gag* gene and this similarity prompted an examination of whether Gag proteins could also be used to carry additional proteins. This has been shown to be the case for the Gag protein from HIV-1 (e.g., Griffiths *et al.*, 1993). An additional advantage of retroviral-based systems is that, unlike Ty-VLPs, virus-derived particles (VDPs) retain their normal ability to bud from cells, acquiring cell surface glycoproteins as they pass through the cell membrane. If the cell can be engineered so that it expresses a heterologous viral envelope glycoprotein in addition to the budding VDP, then it may be possible to produce particulate structures with authentic glycoproteins presented on their surfaces. Such particles would have certain advantages over conventional subunit vaccines, particularly where the conformation of the glycoprotein was critical for retaining immunogenicity.

This chapter describes the basic biology of the Ty-VLP and Gag-derived VDP systems and characterization of the immune responses elicited by a variety of hybrid particulate immunogens.

2. PRESENTATION OF IMMUNOGENS AS HYBRID Ty-VLPs

2.1. The Yeast Ty Element

The term *retrotransposon* refers to a class of eukaryotic transposons that move to new genomic locations via an RNA intermediate and a reverse transcriptase reaction. Detailed analysis of the yeast Ty element has led to a full description of its genetic organization and expression strategies (Kingsman and Kingsman, 1988; Fulton *et al.*, 1990) (Fig. 1). Most Ty elements are 5.9 kb in length and the element can be subdivided into a unique 5.2-kb region and two flanking long terminal repeats or δ regions (Roeder and Fink, 1983; Williamson, 1983). The major 5.7-kb RNA species initiates in the left δ and terminates in the right δ, producing a terminally redundant message that is directly analogous to the full-length, genomic RNA of retroviruses (Elder *et al.*, 1983).

The transcriptional unit of Ty is divided into two overlapping open reading frames, *TYA* and *TYB*, which are analogous to retroviral *gag* and *pol* genes (Mellor *et al.*, 1985a; Fulton *et al.*, 1985; Clare and Farabaugh, 1985). *TYA* encodes a 50-kDa protein, p1, that is subsequently processed by a Ty-encoded protease to generate the cleavage product, p2 (Dobson *et al.*, 1984; Mellor *et al.*, 1985b; Adams *et al.*, 1987a). *TYB* is expressed as a 190-kDa *TYA:TYB* fusion protein, p3, as a result of a specific frameshifting event which avoids the termination codon in *TYA* and shifts translation into the *TYB* reading phase (Mellor *et al.*, 1985a; Wilson *et al.*, 1986). The *TYB*-encoded component of p3 contains protease, reverse transcriptase, and integrase activities (Adams *et al.*, 1987a; Eichinger and Boeke, 1988) (Fig. 1a).

During the transposition cycle of a Ty element, Ty-homologous RNA and a tRNA primer are packaged into VLPs where reverse transcription then generates a double-

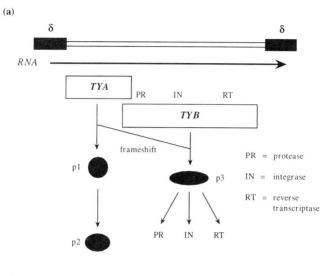

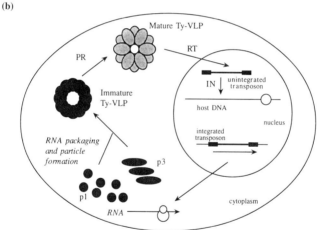

Figure 1. Organization and transposition cycle of the yeast Ty element.

(a) Organization of the yeast Ty element. Black boxes represent δ sequences. Double line denotes internal region. The major 5.7-kb transcript is indicated. Open boxes indicate the *TYA* and *TYB* genes. *TYA* encodes the p1 protein and the p3 protein is expressed from a *TYA:TYB* fusion gene via a specific frameshifting event.

(b) Ty transposition cycle. Ty RNA is transcribed from an integrated Ty element and packaged into an immature particle composed of p1 and p3. The Ty protease cleaves p1 and p3 to form a mature particle. The Ty RNA is reverse transcribed into double-stranded DNA which in turn is integrated into the host chromosome. PR, protease; RT, reverse transcriptase; IN, integrase.

stranded DNA copy (Boeke *et al.*, 1985; Mellor *et al.*, 1985c; Adams *et al.*, 1987a). This double-stranded DNA is then integrated into the chromosome at a new site (Fig. 1b).

2.2. Hybrid Ty-VLPs

When the *TYA* gene alone is expressed in yeast cells, the p1 protein assembles into particles in the absence of any of the *TYB*-encoded proteins (Adams *et al.*, 1987a) (Fig. 2a,b). This observation led directly to the idea that it may be possible to exploit the particle-forming properties of the p1 protein to develop a carrier system where heterologous proteins or peptides could be expressed as hybrid VLPs (Adams *et al.*, 1987b). To produce hybrid particles, genes encoding all or part of the protein of interest are simply inserted at a unique restriction enzyme site at the 3′ end of the *TYA* gene. The resulting fusion genes produce p1-fusion protein which retains the ability to assemble into particulate structures (Fig. 2c,d).

Many VLP constructions that carry a variety of different proteins and peptides have been made. These include HIV-1 structural and regulatory proteins, influenza virus hemagglutinin and nucleoprotein domains, bovine and human papillomavirus proteins, and malaria circumsporozoite peptides (Adams *et al.*, 1987b, 1988; Braddock *et al.*, 1989; Gilmour *et al.*, 1989, 1990; Griffiths *et al.*, 1991, and unpublished data). A remarkable feature of this system is its versatility, in that the assembly of the p1 protein into VLPs seems to be able to accommodate a wide range of material from small peptide-sized fragments through to whole proteins in excess of 40 kDa. This is likely to be related to the unusually flexible assembly process used by p1 (Burns *et al.*, 1990a). Purification of hybrid VLPs is relatively straightforward, and simple procedures have been developed that exploit the physical properties of the particles (Burns *et al.*, 1990b). In brief, the laboratory-scale purification involves a combination of differential centrifugation, rate zonal centrifugation, and size exclusion chromatography. As the sedimentation properties of different hybrid VLPs are similar, this process can be used for any VLP, irrespective of the sequence of the additional protein. The system is therefore extremely flexible, allowing rapid production of a variety of recombinant proteins. Purified VLPs have been stored frozen for periods in excess of 5 years without loss of immunogenicity or structural integrity. VLPs adjuvanted with aluminum hydroxide can be stored for 1 to 2 years at 4°C.

2.3. Immune Responses Elicited by Hybrid VLPs

Each hybrid VLP contains several hundred copies of the fusion protein, and hence several hundred copies of the added immunogen. As a result, a major application of these high-molecular-weight, polyvalent structures is in the development of new vaccines. The immune response required for an effective vaccine may be an antibody response, a CTL response, or both. Underlying these effector mechanisms, there is also a requirement for effective priming of Th cell populations in order to produce cytokines that enhance CTL function, promote differentiation of B lymphocytes into plasma cells, and increase the frequency of memory cells. Studies designed to evaluate and characterize the immune responses induced by hybrid VLPs carrying a variety of heterologous antigens have

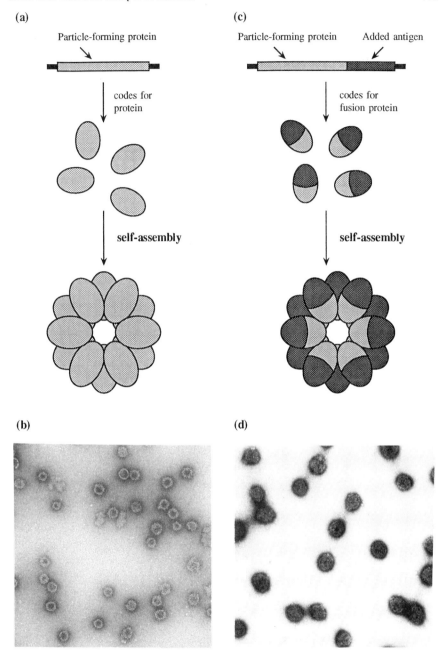

Figure 2. Formation of hybrid particles. (a) Schematic diagram of self-assembly by a particle-forming protein. Examples of particle-forming proteins include the p1 protein of the yeast Ty element and the Gag protein of retroviruses. (b) Electron micrograph of purified p1 VLPs. (c) Schematic diagram of self-assembly by a particle-forming protein fused to an additional antigen. The fusion protein assembles into a hybrid particle. (d) Electron micrograph of purified HIV-1 p24-VLPs.

demonstrated that both humoral and cell-mediated responses are elicited. The induction of antibody, Th cell, and CTL responses are illustrated below, with particular reference to VLPs carrying HIV-1 sequences.

2.3.1. INDUCTION OF HIGH-TITER ANTIBODY RESPONSES BY HYBRID VLps

After infection with HIV-1, an individual mounts an antibody response against the virus, which, broadly speaking, can be divided into antibodies against the core and antibodies against the envelope components of the virus (Kitchen et al., 1984). At the time of AIDS symptoms, antienvelope antibody levels remain high but the level of anticore antibody falls (Lange et al., 1986; Weber et al., 1987). Furthermore, there is evidence that individuals who mount a strong initial immune response against the viral core proteins survive without developing symptoms for longer than those who mount a weak anticore response (Cheingsong-Popov et al., 1991). Although the mechanism remains to be elucidated, these inverse correlations between anticore antibodies and disease progression suggest that inducing and maintaining high levels of anticore antibodies might prevent, or at least delay, the onset of disease.

These observations provide a rationale for the development of VLPs carrying the HIV-1 p24 core protein (p24-VLPs) as a therapeutic vaccine candidate. When used to immunize a variety of animals, including macaques, these hybrid VLPs induced high-titer anticore antibodies (Adams et al., 1988; Mills et al., 1990). More recently, a Phase I study in HIV-1-negative, healthy volunteers demonstrated that the p24-VLPs were well tolerated and immunogenic (Martin et al., 1993). A Phase II double-blind, placebo-controlled trial in 15 asymptomatic infected individuals (CD4 counts >350/mm^3) is underway. This pilot safety study has two dose levels of p24-VLP, with two immunizations being given intramuscularly at 1-month intervals. The study is focusing on safety and tolerance, with measurements for p24 antibody changes and surrogate markers. On the basis of the safety data to date, larger Phase II studies have also been initiated. A multicenter European dose-ranging study has been initiated in HIV-1 positive individuals with CD4 counts greater than 350/mm^3. In this study 72 patients are being randomized to receive one of three doses of p24-VLP or placebo and this will be administered on six occasions at monthly intervals. Additional Phase II studies are also underway in Australia and South Africa, with a parallel track clinical program being followed which focuses on both asymptomatic early stage infection patients and late stage (ARC/AIDS) patients.

The vast majority of antibodies that can neutralize HIV-1 are directed against the envelope proteins, and the V3 sequence within the glycoprotein gp120 is often referred to as the principal neutralizing determinant of the virus (reviewed in Moore and Nara, 1991). There are several lines of evidence suggesting that induction of immunity against the V3 loop may contribute to protection in vivo (Berman et al., 1990; Emini et al., 1992). We therefore constructed VLPs carrying a 40-amino-acid V3 loop sequence from the HIV-1 isolate LAI. Following administration to rabbits, in conjunction with either complete Freund's adjuvant (CFA) or aluminum hydroxide, substantial levels of neutralizing antibodies were elicited. A significant proportion of the antibodies recognized the conserved sequence at the tip of the V3 loop structure and boosting after a 6-month rest period resulted in a rapid recall of the antibody response (Griffiths et al., 1991).

Although high-titer neutralizing antibodies were elicited in the experiments described above, the number of seroconverting animals per group was often variable. In addition, although the LAI-derived particles induced substantial levels of neutralization, the levels induced by particles carrying the V3 sequences from other HIV-1 isolates, such as MN and RF, were modest. In order to overcome these difficulties, new VLP expression vectors were designed in which immunoreactive regions within the p1 protein have been identified and replaced with a V3 sequence derived from isolate MN. The resulting particles appear to be more immunogenic than the original VLPs carrying the MN V3 sequence at the C-terminus of p1 in two important respects. First, high titers of anti-MN neutralizing antibodies are induced, and second, the number of seroconverters per group approaches 100% (unpublished data).

Immunization with a hybrid VLP preparation induces antibodies against the carrier p1 protein in addition to antibodies against the heterologous protein. It could be argued that the presence of a memory response elicited to the Ty component may prevent the development of an antibody response against a second heterologous protein following immunization with a second hybrid VLP construction. However, direct testing of this hypothesis demonstrated that equivalent anti-p24 antibody titers were obtained in rats following immunization with p24-VLPs, irrespective of whether the animals had received previous immunizations with HIV-1 p17-VLPs (unpublished data).

2.3.2. INDUCTION OF Th CELL RESPONSES BY HYBRID VLPs

Studies demonstrating that VLPs could induce Th cell responses have been carried out with both the p24 and V3 constructions. For example, the induction of p24-specific Th cell responses was investigated in macaques immunized with 50-μg doses of p24-VLP. Significant proliferative responses occurred when peripheral blood mononuclear cells were stimulated with p24-VLP. T-cell clones derived from the animals also proliferated in response to p24-VLP. The specificity of the p24 recognition was demonstrated by proliferation of the clones in response to recombinant p24 protein purified from insect cells and to a p24 peptide. Specific p24 responses were also observed in an IL-2-release assay (Mills et al., 1990).

In another series of experiments, mice were immunized with V3-VLPs (HIV-1 isolate LAI). Significant proliferation of lymph node cells was observed following stimulation in vitro with a 40-mer peptide containing the V3 loop sequence from HIV-1 isolate LAI. To assess the efficacy of presenting the V3 loop in this particulate form, we compared the responses induced by using V3-VLPs with those obtained with two nonparticulate immunogens, recombinant gp120 and V3 peptide conjugated to albumin (Fig. 3). V3 responses were reproducibly higher following immunization with V3-VLPs than with either of the other immunogens. This indicates that immunization of mice with the V3 loop as a hybrid VLP results in enhanced proliferative responses (Harris et al., 1992).

2.3.3. INDUCTION OF CTLs BY HYBRID VLPs

The induction of CTLs has been shown to be an important component of protective immunity against viral infections in humans and mice (McMichael et al., 1983; Kast et al., 1986). Although CTL responses are detected during infection, following inoculation

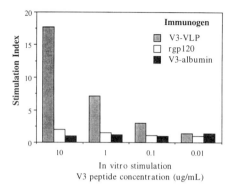

Figure 3. V3-specific proliferative responses in mice immunized with either V3-VLPs, recombinant gp120 (rgp120), or V3 peptide conjugated to albumin. Lymph node cells were removed from the immunized animals and stimulated in vitro with a range of concentrations of V3 peptide. Proliferation was measured as the level of incorporation of [³H]thymidine, converted into stimulation indices by comparison with incorporation of [³H]thymidine by control cells.

with live recombinant vectors (viral or bacterial) (Moss, 1991; Stover *et al.*, 1991) or following direct injection of DNA encoding the protein of interest (Ulmer *et al.*, 1993), the ability to prime CTLs in vivo using protein or peptide immunogens has been a long-sought goal. There has been some progress toward this goal: there are several reports in which peptides have been used to induce CTL responses against influenza, lymphocytic choriomeningitis virus, Sendai, and HIV-1 in mice (Gao *et al.*, 1991; Schultz *et al.*, 1991; Kast *et al.*, 1991; Hart *et al.*, 1991; see Chapter 37). However, in almost every case it has been necessary to present these peptides with adjuvants that are currently unacceptable for use in humans. In the case of whole proteins or large protein fragments there has been less success, although there are a few exceptions where specialized adjuvants (for example, QS-21) (Wu *et al.*, 1992; see Chapter 22) or vehicles such as ISCOMs (Takahashi *et al.*, 1990; see Chapter 23) or liposomes (Reddy *et al.*, 1992; see Chapter 13) have been used. The mechanisms by which these approaches lead to the induction of CTL responses are unknown. However, it has been suggested that the lipid component is the key to accessing the cytoplasmic major histocompatibility complex (MHC) class I molecule processing pathway (required for presentation of the processed peptide to CD8-positive T cells) either by inducing cell membrane fusion with direct release of protein into the cytoplasm or by facilitating escape from the lysosomal processing pathway (Takahashi *et al.*, 1990; Wu *et al.*, 1992; Reddy *et al.*, 1992).

As described above, immunization with V3-VLPs induced both neutralizing antibodies and Th cell responses. The Th cell responses were seen even in the absence of adjuvant. These results prompted us to ask whether the apparent immunogenicity of these particles extended to the induction of CTLs. BALB/c (H-2^d) mice were immunized with V3-VLPs in either CFA, aluminum hydroxide, or saline. The CTL effector activity of splenocytes restimulated in vitro with a synthetic 40-amino-acid V3 peptide was then measured using ^{51}Cr-labeled P815 (H-2^d) target cells pulsed overnight with the same V3 peptide (Fig. 4a). High levels of V3-specific CTLs were induced by V3-VLPs when injected without adjuvant, but CTL activity was barely detectable using effector cells from mice immunized in CFA or aluminum hydroxide (Layton *et al.*, 1993).

When effector cells were preincubated with anti-CD4 or anti-CD8 blocking monoclonal antibodies prior to the addition of target cells, the anti-CD8 antibody inhibited CTL activity, whereas the anti-CD4 antibody had no effect. In addition, CTL activity was not

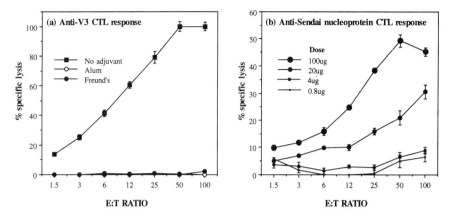

Figure 4. CTL responses induced by hybrid VLPs.

(a) HIV-1 V3-specific CTL responses induced in BALB/c (H-2^d) mice immunized with V3-VLPs in the absence of adjuvant, in the presence of CFA, or as an aluminum hydroxide precipitate (alum). Animals were immunized with a single dose of 20 μg of V3-VLPs. Splenocytes were removed from the immunized animals and stimulated in vitro with V3 peptide for 7 days prior to assessing their ability to lyse ^{51}Cr-labeled, V3 peptide-pulsed P815 (H-2^d) target cells.

(b) Induction of Sendai nucleoprotein (NP)-specific CTLs using Sendai-NP VLPs at four immunization doses. C57BL/6 (H-2^b) mice were immunized and splenocytes stimulated in vitro with Sendai-NP peptide for 7 days. The restimulated splenocytes were then tested for their ability to lyse ^{51}Cr-labeled, Sendai-NP peptide-pulsed EL4 (H-2^b) target cells.

detected using mismatched EL-4 cells (H-2^b) as targets, indicating that the V3-specific CTLs were restricted at the H-2^d locus as previously described (Takahashi et al., 1990). These results demonstrated that the CTL responses were MHC class I molecule-restricted and mediated by CD8-positive cells (Layton et al., 1993).

In order to test whether the ability of hybrid VLPs to induce CTL responses is a general phenomenon, we have selected a number of well-characterized examples for analysis. These include epitopes from the nucleoprotein of influenza, the nucleoprotein of Sendai virus, and the circumsporozoite stage of malaria. All of these epitopes are known to induce a CTL response in particular mouse haplotypes. VLPs that carry each of these sequences have been constructed and their ability to induce CTLs has been examined. To date, all of these hybrid VLPs elicit CTLs (Layton, unpublished data) and an example of the response elicited by VLPs that carry an epitope from Sendai virus nucleoprotein is shown in Fig. 4b. Taken together, the data indicate that VLPs are able to induce a CTL response, in the absence of adjuvant, to a wide range of pathogens.

The CTL priming effect of hybrid VLPs may be related to one or more of several factors. First, it may be the result of optimal stimulation of endocytosis or phagocytosis leading to efficient uptake into specialized antigen-presenting cells (APCs) in the spleen (Rock et al., 1993) or at the site of injection (Rock et al., 1992; Macatonia et al., 1989; Nair et al., 1992). It has been suggested recently that the size of the latex beads conjugated to ovalbumin was a key parameter in determining whether the conjugates induced CTL responses (Kovacsovics-Bankowski et al., 1993), and it may be that the size of the VLP favors uptake by APCs. Second, following uptake into the APC, subsequent leakage of MHC class I molecule-binding V3 peptides may occur from the lysosomal compartment into the cytoplasm. There is evidence that this occurs with acid-sensitive liposome-encapsulated immunogens (Harding et al., 1991). However, it is thought that liposomes gain access via liposome–endosome fusion and as VLPs do not contain any lipid, this does not seem to represent a likely mechanism. Third, hybrid VLPs may access the cytoplasm directly via membrane penetration. This is thought to be a possible mechanism of entry of protein presented either in ISCOMs, with saponins, or as lipopeptides (Deres et al., 1989; Takahashi et al., 1990). However, as already stated, VLPs do not contain lipid nor do they possess any obvious fusion activity like that of the saponins or viral envelope fusion proteins. Studies are now in progress to attempt to define the mechanism of CTL induction by hybrid VLPs.

3. PRESENTATION OF ANTIGENS AS VIRUS-DERIVED PARTICLES

3.1. The Construction of Hybrid Retroviral Cores

As mentioned above, there is a close evolutionary relationship between retro-transposons, such as Ty, and retroviruses. This relationship is reflected in the genetic organization and functional homology between the structural proteins of the two classes of elements (reviewed in Kingsman et al., 1991) (Fig. 5). The fact that the Ty p1 protein can still assemble as a fusion protein, combined with the clear analogy between p1 and retroviral Gag proteins, suggests that it might be possible to produce hybrid retroviral Gag particles.

To test this idea, we chose HIV-1 Gag as the carrier system and the HIV-1 V3 loop as the additional protein. In this case, the Gag component is acting as both vaccine immuno-gen and V3 presentation system. In order to achieve high expression levels, we used a baculovirus expression system as we, and others (Gheyson et al., 1989), had shown previously that expression of HIV-1 Gag alone in insect cells produced high levels of the Gag Pr55 precursor protein. Furthermore, the protein migrates to the cytoplasmic mem-brane and assembles into particles that bud from the cell in much the same way that HIV-1 buds from infected T cells (Fig. 6). The HIV-1 Gag Pr55 protein was fused, close to its C-terminus, to a V3 sequence derived from HIV-1 isolate LAI, and the fusion protein was expressed in insect cells. To determine whether expression resulted in particle formation, the insect cells were examined by electron microscopy. Both Gag alone and Gag:V3 proteins assembled into particles (Fig. 6). However, although some of the Gag:V3 particles budded from the cell surface, approximately half of them were found in the nucleus, presumably because of interference of the normal migration pathway of the Gag Pr55 protein by the V3 sequence (Griffiths et al., 1993).

The ability of Gag:V3 particles to generate anti-Gag and anti-V3 antibodies was then investigated. Following immunization of rats, in conjunction with either CFA or aluminum hydroxide, substantial anti-Gag responses were observed (Fig. 7). Anti-Gag antibodies were also elicited in the absence of adjuvant, albeit with reduced titers. The hybrid Gag:V3

Figure 5. The genetic organization of the yeast Ty element and a simple retrovirus.
(a) Genetic organization of Ty. The *TYA* and *TYB* genes are shown as open boxes below the Ty element. The long terminal repeats or δ sequences are shown as black boxes. *TYA* encodes the p1 protein and the p3 protein is expressed from a *TYA:TYB* fusion gene via a specific frameshifting event. The p3 protein contains protease (PR), integrase (IN), and reverse transcriptase (RT) enzyme activities. The Ty-VLPs contains p1, the p2 cleavage product, and the p3-derived enzyme activities.
(b) Genetic organization of a simple retrovirus. The *gag*, *pol*, and *env* genes are shown as open boxes below the provirus of a simple retrovirus such as avian leukosis virus. The long terminal repeats or LTR sequences are shown as black boxes. The *gag* gene is translated from the full-length RNA to produce a precursor polyprotein, Pr^{gag}. This precursor protein is cleaved to form the viral core proteins by a virally encoded protease. The $\text{Pr}^{\text{gag-pol}}$ precursor protein is expressed from a *gag-pol* fusion gene via a specific frameshifting event. The $\text{Pr}^{\text{gag-pol}}$ protein contains protease (PR), reverse transcriptase (RT), and integrase (IN) enzyme activities. Both the Gag and Pol proteins are incorporated into the core of the virus particle. The *env* gene is expressed by simple translation of a subgenomic spliced RNA containing just the *env* coding sequence. The primary translation product is also a precursor, Pr^{env}, that is cleaved (probably by a cellular protease) to produce a transmembrane protein and a surface protein. Both the transmembrane and surface proteins are usually glycosylated.

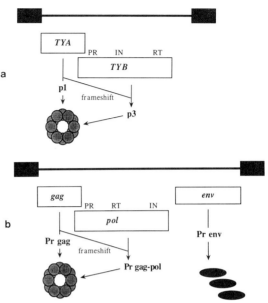

VDPs therefore appear to be potent Gag immunogens. In contrast, the antibody responses to V3 were low, even after multiple injections with adjuvant (Griffiths *et al.*, 1993).

Although the Gag:V3 particles were relatively poor immunogens for generating humoral responses to V3, substantial anti-V3 CTL responses were induced following immunization of mice in the absence of adjuvant (Griffiths *et al.*, 1993) (Fig. 7). No CTLs were induced when CFA or aluminum hydroxide was present in the formulation. Although the mechanism of CTL induction is yet to be elucidated, it is interesting that as with Ty-VLPs, adjuvant-inhibited CTL induction is seen with the Gag VDPs. A feature that is common to particles derived from retroviruses and retrotransposons may therefore facilitate CTL induction.

The production of hybrid Gag:V3 VDPs extends the observation of Weldon *et al.* (1990), who showed that Rous sarcoma virus Gag fused to a yeast isocytochrome *c* was able to form hybrid particles that budded from the cell. Taken together, these data suggest that any retroviral Gag precursor protein could be used to carry additional protein sequences. This may be important for the future use of retroviral systems not only for the development of novel recombinant vaccines, but also for the development of gene delivery

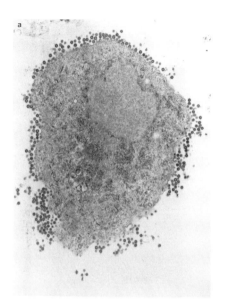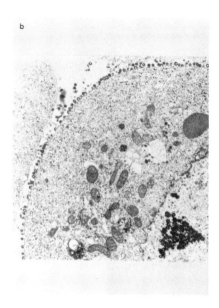

Figure 6. Electron micrographs of insect cells infected with a recombinant baculovirus expressing HIV-1 Gag (a), and a recombinant baculovirus expressing an HIV-1 Gag:V3 fusion protein (b).

systems: hybrid Gag particles could be designed to carry specific RNA or DNA binding domains that would then selectively package a particular nucleic acid molecule.

3.2. Expression of Authentic Glycoproteins Using VDPs

During natural infection, as a retroviral core buds from a cell, it acquires viral envelope glycoproteins as a result of passing through the membrane. These envelope proteins target the virus to a new cell and are therefore a major determinant of retrovirus tropism. It is not clear whether this acquisition process is largely stochastic or a highly organized system that specifically associates the core of the virus with the cytoplasmic domain of the envelope proteins. Whatever the mechanism, if it were possible to replace the viral envelope proteins with a different membrane-bound glycoprotein, then the budding retroviral cores would carry the heterologous protein on their surfaces (Fig. 8). This heterologous protein might be a receptor/ligand molecule that could target the retroviral core to a particular cell type or it might be, for example, a viral glycoprotein antigen derived from a different pathogen.

Implications that incorporation of a heterologous glycoprotein is feasible have come from experiments using a model system. Insect cells were co-infected with two recombinant baculovirus vectors expressing HIV-1 *gag* and influenza virus hemagglutinin (HA). The budding Gag particles carried HA on their surfaces and the HA was functional as determined by its ability to hemagglutinate red blood cells (unpublished data).

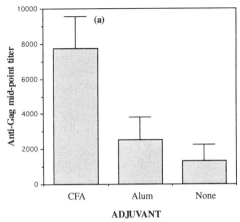

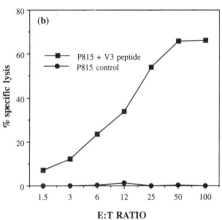

Figure 7. Immune responses induced by Gag:V3 virus-derived particles.

(a) Anti-Gag antibody mid-point titers of rats immunized with 100μg doses of Gag:V3 VDPs in either CFA, as an aluminum hydroxide precipitate (alum) or without adjuvant. Serum samples were taken after a prime and two boost immunizations and tested by enzyme-linked immunosorbent assay (ELISA) against a yeast-derived Gag protein.

(b) Induction of V3-specific CTLs in BALB/c (H-2^d) mice. Mice were immunized with Gag:V3 VDPs and splenocytes restimulated in vitro with V3 peptide for 7 days. The restimulated splenocytes were then tested for their ability to lyse [51] chromium-labelled, V3 peptide-pulsed P815 (H-2^d) target cells or control, non-pulsed P815 cells.

In order to develop this type of technology for general vaccine use, it will be necessary to use a "neutral" retroviral carrier protein, such as the Gag protein from a murine retrovirus rather than the Gag precursor from HIV-1. Incorporation of the glycoproteins from another virus, for example, into the membrane-bound core particle would result in a structure that would closely mimic the native virus. The efficiency of the "pick-up" process remains to be determined and, related to this, there is the possibility that specific recognition sequences that associate Gag and Env are required to maximize incorporation. Candidates for these sequences have been identified in the HIV-1 matrix protein (e.g., Yu *et al.*, 1992). If such sequences exist, they would need to be engineered into the vectors used to express the enveloped particle. Whatever the detailed requirements are, manipulated retrovirus particles may open a new area of vaccine technology by providing the means to present glycoprotein antigens to the immune system in an authentic conformation without the need for replicating recombinant viral vectors or live attenuated viruses.

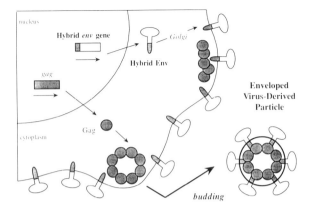

Figure 8. Incorporation of heterologous Env glycoproteins. A retroviral Gag particle is shown budding from the surface of a cell. The cell also contains a gene coding for a hybrid Env glycoprotein. The hybrid Env could contain the surface glycoprotein component of a heterologous virus and is shown anchored in the cell membrane. As the Gag particle buds, it associates with the hybrid Env glycoprotein to form an enveloped, virus-derived particle.

4. CONCLUSIONS

It is clear that it is now possible to construct hybrid retrotransposon and retroviral core structures that carry, potentially, any protein or protein domain. Both hybrid VLPs and VDPs constitute polyvalent, particulate immunogens that induce humoral, Th cell, and CTL responses. In particular, the observation that these particulate antigens induce CTL responses provides a platform for the design of novel nonreplicating vaccines against a variety of viral and parasitic infections or even against cancer cells expressing tumor-specific antigens.

ACKNOWLEDGMENTS

We would like to thank members of the Immunotherapeutics and Biology departments at British Bio-technology for their contributions to the work described in this chapter.

REFERENCES

Adams, S. E., Mellor, J., Gull, K., Sim, R. B., Tuite, M. F., Kingsman, S. M., and Kingsman, A. J., 1987a, The functions and relationships of Ty-VLP proteins in yeast reflect those of mammalian retroviral proteins, *Cell* **49**:111–119.

Adams, S. E., Dawson, K. M., Gull, K., Kingsman, S. M., and Kingsman, A. J., 1987b, The expression of hybrid Ty virus-like particles in yeast, *Nature* **329**:68–70.

Adams, S. E., Senior, J. M., Kingsman, S. M., and Kingsman, A. J., 1988, Induction of HIV antibodies by Ty:HIV hybrid virus-like particles, in: *Technological Advances in Vaccine Development* (L. Lasky, ed.) Liss, New York, pp. 117–126.

Berman, P. W., Gregory, T. J., Riddle, L., Nakamura, G. R., Champe, M. A., Porter, J. P., Worm, F. M., Herschberg, R. D., Cobb, E. K., and Eichberg, J. W., 1990, Protection of chimpanzees from infection with HIV-1 after vaccination with recombinant glycoprotein gp120 but not gp160, *Nature* **345**:622–625.

Boeke, J. D., Garfinkel, D. J., Styles, C. A., and Fink, G. R., 1985, Ty elements transpose through an RNA intermediate, *Cell* **40**:491–500.

Braddock, M., Chambers, A., Wilson, W., Esnouf, M. P., Adams, S. E., Kingsman, A. J., and Kingsman, S. M., 1989, HIV-1 TAT 'activates' presynthesized RNA in the nucleus, *Cell* **58**:269–279.

Burns, N. R., Saibil, H. R., White, N. S., Pardon, J. F., Timmins, P. A., Richardson, S. M. H., Richards, B. M., Adams, S. E., Kingsman, S. M., and Kingsman, A. J., 1990a, Symmetry, flexibility and permeability in the structure of yeast retrotransposon virus-like particles, *EMBO J.* **11**:1155–1164.

Burns, N. R., Gilmour, J. E. M., Kingsman, S. M., Kingsman, A. J., and Adams, S. E., 1990b, Production and purification of hybrid Ty-VLPs, *Methods Mol. Biol.* **8**:277–285.

Cheingsong-Popov, R., Panagiotidi, C., Bowcock, S., Aronstam, A., Wadsworth, J., and Weber, J., 1991, Relation between humoral responses to HIV gag and env proteins at seroconversion and clinical outcome of HIV infection, *Br. Med. J.* **302**:23–26.

Clare, J., and Farabaugh, P., 1985, Nucleotide sequence of a yeast Ty element: Evidence for an unusual mechanism of gene expression, *Proc. Natl. Acad. Sci. USA* **82**:2829–2833.

Clarke, B. E., Newton S. E., Carroll, A. R., Francis, M. J., Appleyard, G., Syred, A. D., Highfield, P. E., Rowlands, D. J., and Brown, F., 1987, Improved immunogenicity of a peptide epitope after fusion to hepatitis B core protein, *Nature* **330**:381–384.

Deres, K., Schild, H., Weismuller, K. H., Jung, G., and Rammensee, H. G., 1989, In vivo priming of virus-specific cytotoxic T lymphocytes with synthetic lipopeptide vaccine, *Nature* **342**:561–564.

Dobson, M. J., Mellor, J., Fulton, A. M., Roberts, N. A., Bowen, B. A., Kingsman, S. M., and Kingsman, A. J., 1984, The identification and high level expression of a protein encoded by the yeast Ty element, *EMBO J.* **3**:1115–1119.

Eichinger, D. J., and Boeke, J. D., 1988, The DNA intermediate in yeast Ty1 transposition copurifies with virus-like particles: Cell-free Ty1 transposition, *Cell* **54**:955–966.

Elder, R. T., Loh, E. Y., and Davis, R. W., 1983, RNA from the yeast transposable element Ty1 has both ends in the direct repeats, a structure similar to retrovirus RNA, *Proc. Natl. Acad. Sci. USA* **80**:2432–2436.

Emini, E. A., Scheif, W. A., Nunberg, J. H., Conley, A. J., Eda, Y., Tokiyoshi, S., Putney, S. D., Matsushita, S., Cobb, K. E., Jett, C. M., Eichberg, J. W., and Murthy, K. K., 1992, Prevention of HIV-1 infection in chimpanzees by gp120 V3 domain-specific monoclonal antibody, *Nature* **355**:728–729.

Fulton, A. M., Mellor, J., Dobson, M. J., Chester, J., Warmington, J. R., Indge, K. J., Oliver, S. G., de la Paz, P., Wilson, W., Kingsman, A. J., and Kingsman, S. M., 1985, Variants within the yeast Ty sequence family encode a class of structurally conserved proteins, *Nucleic Acids Res.* **13**:4097–4112.

Fulton, A. M., Adams, S. E., Rathjen, P. D., Wilson, W., Kingsman, S. M., and Kingsman, A. J., 1990, The biology and exploitation of the yeast retrotransposon Ty, *Adv. Gene Technol.* **1**:1–20.

Gao, X. -M., Zheng, B., Liew, F. Y., Brett, S., and Tite, J., 1991, Priming of influenza virus-specific cytotoxic T lymphocytes in vivo by short synthetic peptides, *J. Immunol.* **147**:3268–3273.

Gheyson, D., Jacobs, E., DeForesta, F., Thiriart, C., Francotte, M., Thines, D., and de Wilde, M., 1989, Assembly and release of HIV-1 precursor Pr55gag virus-like particles from recombinant baculovirus-infected cells, *Cell* **59**:103–112.

Gilmour, J. E. M., Senior, J. M., Burns, N. R., Esnouf, M. P., Gull, K., Kingsman, S. M., Kingsman, A. J., and Adams, S. E., 1989, A novel method for the purification of HIV-1 p24 protein from hybrid Ty-VLPs, *AIDS* **3**:717–723.

Gilmour, J. E. M., Read, S. J., Eglin, R., Ryan, C., Graff, N. R., Stenner, N., Kingsman, S. M., Kingsman, A. J., and Adams, S. E., 1990, Performance characteristics of a novel immunoassay based on hybrid Ty virus-like particles, *AIDS* **4**:967–973.

Griffiths, J. C., Berrie, E. L., Holdsworth, L. N., Moore, J. P., Harris, S. J., Senior, J. M., Kingsman, S. M., Kingsman, A. J., and Adams, S. E., 1991, Induction of high-titer neutralizing antibodies using hybrid human immunodeficiency virus V3-Ty virus-like particles in a clinically relevant adjuvant, *J. Virol.* **65**:450–456.

Griffiths, J. C., Harris, S. J., Layton, G. T., Berrie, E. L., French, T. J., Burns, N. R., Adams, S. E., and Kingsman, A. J., 1993, Hybrid human immunodeficiency virus Gag particles as an antigen carrier system: Induction of cytotoxic T-cell and humoral responses by a Gag:V3 fusion, *J. Virol.* **67**:3191–3198.

Harding, C. V., Collins, D. S., Kanagawa, O., and Unanue, E. R., 1991, Liposome-encapsulated antigens engender lysosomal processing for class II MHC presentation and cytosolic processing for class I presentation, *J. Immunol.* **147**:2860–2863.

Harris, S. J., Gearing, A. J. H., Layton, G. T., Adams, S. E., Kingsman, S. M., and Kingsman, A. J., 1992, Enhanced proliferative cellular responses to V3 peptide and gp120 following immunization with V3:Ty virus-like particles, *Immunology* **77**:315–321.

Hart, M. K., Weinhold, K. J., Scearce, R. M., Washburn, E. M., Clark, C. A., Palker, T. J., and Haynes, B. F., 1991, Priming of anti-human immunodeficiency virus (HIV) CD8+ cytotoxic T cells in vivo by carrier-free HIV synthetic peptides, *Proc. Natl. Acad. Sci. USA* **88**:9448–9452.

Jenkins, O., Cason, J., Burke, K. L., Lunney, D., Gillen, A., Patel, D., McCance, D. J., and Almond, J. W., 1991, An antigen chimera of poliovirus induces antibodies against human papillomavirus type 16, *J. Virol.* **64**:1201–1206.

Kast, W. M., Bronkhorst, A. M., de Waal, L. P., and Melief, C. J. M., 1986, Cooperation between cytotoxic and helper T lymphocytes in protection against lethal Sendai virus infection: Protection by T cells is MHC-restricted, *J. Exp. Med.* **164**:723–738.

Kast, W. M., Roux, L., Curren, J., Blom, H. J. J., Voordouw, A. C., Meloen, R. H., Kolakofsky, D., and Melief, C. J. M., 1991, Protection against lethal Sendai virus infection by in vivo priming of virus-specific cytotoxic T lymphocytes with a free synthetic peptide, *Proc. Natl. Acad. Sci. USA* **88**:2283–2287.

Kingsman, A. J., Adams, S. E., Burns, N. R., and Kingsman, S. M., 1991, Retroelement particles as purification, presentation and targeting vehicles, *Trends Biotechnol.* **9**:303–309.

Kingsman, S. M., and Kingsman, A. J., 1988, Polyvalent recombinant antigens: A new vaccine strategy, *Vaccine* **6**:304–306.

Kitchen, L. W., Barin, F., Sullivan, J. L., McLane, M. F., Brettler, D. B., Levine, P. H., and Essex, M., 1984, Aetiology of AIDS - antibodies to human T-cell leukaemia virus (type III) in haemophiliacs, *Nature* **312**:367–369.

Kovacsovics-Bankowski, M., Clark, K., Benacerraf, B., and Rock, K. L., 1993, Efficient major histocompatibility complex class I presentation of exogenous antigen upon phagocytosis by macrophages, *Proc. Natl. Acad. Sci. USA* **90**:4942–4946.

Lange, J. M. A., Paul, D. A., Huisman, H. G., de Wolf, F., van den Berg, H., Coutinho, R. A., Danner, S. A., vander Noorda, J., and Goudsmit, J., 1986, Persistent HIV antigenaemia and decline of HIV core antibodies associated with transition to AIDS, *Br. Med. J.* **293**:1459–1463.

Layton, G. T., Harris, S. J., Gearing, A. J. H., Hill-Perkins, M., Cole, J. S., Griffiths, J. C., Burns, N. R., Kingsman, A. J., and Adams, S. E., 1993, Induction of HIV-specific cytotoxic T lymphocytes in vivo with hybrid HIV-1 V3:Ty-virus-like-particles, *J. Immunol.* **151**:1097–1107.

Macatonia, S. E., Taylor, P. M., Knight, S. C., and Askonas, B. A., 1989, Primary stimulation by dendritic cells induces antiviral proliferative and cytotoxic T cell responses in vitro, *J. Exp. Med.* **169**:1255–1264.

McMichael, A. J., Gotch, F. M., Noble, G. R., and Beare, P. A. S., 1983, Cytotoxic T cell immunity to influenza, *N. Engl. J. Med.* **309**:13–17.

Martin, S. J., Vyakarnum, A., Cheingsong-Popov, R., Callow, D., Jones, K. L., Senior, J. M., Adams, S. E., Kingsman, A. J., Matear, P., Gotch, F. M., McMichael, A. J., Roitt, I. M., and Weber, J. N., 1993, Immunization of human HIV-seronegative volunteers with recombinant p17/p24:Ty virus-like particles elicits HIV-1 p24-specific cellular and humoral immune responses, *AIDS* **7**:1315–1323.

Mellor, J., Fulton, A. M., Dobson, M. J., Wilson, W., Kingsman, S. M., and Kingsman, A. J., 1985a, A retrovirus-like strategy for expression of a fusion protein encoded by yeast retrotransposon Ty1, *Nature* **313**:243–246.

Mellor, J., Fulton, A. M., Dobson, M. J., Roberts, N. A., Wilson, W., Kingsman, A. J., and Kingsman, S. M., 1985b, The Ty transposon of *Saccharomyces cerevisiae* determines the synthesis of at least three proteins, *Nucleic Acids Res.* **13**:6249–6263.

Mellor, J., Malim, M. H., Gull, K., Tuite, M. F., McCready, S., Dibbayawan, T., Kingsman, S. M., and Kingsman, A. J., 1985c, Reverse transcriptase activity and Ty RNA are associated with virus-like particles in yeast, *Nature* **318**:583–586.

Michel, M. -L., Mancini, M., Sobczack, E., Favier, V., Guetard, D., Bahraqui, E. M., and Tollias, P., 1988, Induction of anti-human immunodeficiency virus (HIV) neutralizing antibodies in rabbits immunized with recombinant HIV–hepatitis B surface antigen particles, *Proc. Natl. Acad. Sci. USA* **85**:7957–7961.

Mills, K. H. G., Kitchin, P. A., Mahon, B. P., Barnard, A. L., Adams, S. E., Kingsman, S. M., and Kingsman, A. J., 1990, HIV p24-specific helper T cell clones from immunized primates recognize highly conserved regions of HIV-1, *J. Immunol.* **144**:1677–1683.

Moore, J. P., and Nara, P. L., 1991, The role of the V3 loop of gp120 in HIV infection, *AIDS* **5**(Suppl. 2):S21–S33.

Morein, J. P., Lovgren, K., Hogland, S., and Sundquist, B., 1987, The ISCOM: An immunostimulating complex, *Immunol. Today* **8**:333–338.

Moss, B., 1991, Vaccinia virus: A tool for research and vaccine development, *Science* **252**:1662–1667.

Nair, S., Zhou, F., Reddy, R., Huang, L., and Rouse, B. T., 1992, Soluble proteins delivered to dendritic cells via pH-sensitive liposomes induce primary cytotoxic T lymphocyte responses in vitro, *J. Exp. Med.* **175**:609–612.

Reddy, R., Zhou, F., Nair, S., Huang, L., and Rouse, B. T., 1992, In vivo cytotoxic T lymphocyte induction with soluble proteins administered in liposomes, *J. Immunol.* **148**:1585–1589.

Rock, K. L., Rothstein, L., Fleischacker, C., and Gamble, S., 1992, Inhibition of class I and class II MHC-restricted antigen presentation by cytotoxic T lymphocytes specific for an exogenous antigen, *J. Immunol.* **148**:3028–3033.

Rock, K. L., Rothstein, L., Gamble, S., and Fleischacker, C., 1993, Characterization of antigen-presenting cells that present exogenous antigens in association with class I MHC molecules, *J. Immunol.* **150**:438–446.

Roeder, S., and Fink, G., 1983, The yeast transposon, Ty, in: *Mobile Genetic Elements* (J. A. Shapiro, ed.), Academic Press, New York, pp. 299–328.

Schultz, M., Zinkernagel, R. M., and Hengartner, H., 1991, Peptide-induced antiviral protection by cytotoxic T cells, *Proc. Natl. Acad. Sci. USA* **88**:991–993.

Stover, C. K., de la Cruz, V. F., Fuerst, T. R., Burlein, J. E., Benson, L. A., Bennett, L. T., Bansal, G. P., Young, J. F., Lee, M. H., Hatfull, G. F., Snapper, S. B., Barletta, R. G., Jacobs, J. R., Jr., and Bloom, B. R., 1991, New use of BCG for recombinant vaccines, *Nature* **351**:456–460.

Takahashi, H., Takeshita, T., Morein, B., Putney, S., Germain, R. N., and Berzofsky, J. A., 1990, Induction of CD8+ cytotoxic T lymphocytes by immunization with purified HIV-1 envelope protein in ISCOMs, *Nature* **344**:873–875.

Ulmer, J. B., Donnelly, J. J., Suezanne, E. P., Rhodes, G. H., Felgner, P. L., Dwarki, V. J., Gromkowski, S. H., Deck, R. R., DeWitt, C. M., Friedman, A., Hawe, L. A., Leander, K. R., Martinez, D., Perry, H. C., Shiver, J. W., Montgomery, D. L., and Liu, M. A., 1993, Heterologous protection against influenza by injection of DNA encoding a viral protein, *Science* **259**:1745–1749.

Weber, J. N., Clapham, P. R., Weiss, R. A., Parker, D., Roberts, C., Duncan, J., Weller, I., Carne, C., Tedder, R. S., Pinching, A. J., and Cheingsong-Popov, R., 1987, Human immunodeficiency virus infection in two cohorts of homosexual men: Neutralizing sera and association of anti-gag antibody with prognosis, *Lancet* **1**:119–122.

Weldon, R. A., Erdie, C. R., Oliver, M. G., and Wills, J. W., 1990, Incorporation of chimeric Gag protein into retroviral particles, *J. Virol.* **64**:4303–4310.

Williamson, V. M., 1983, Transposable elements in yeast, *Int. Rev. Cytol.* **83**:1–25.

Wilson, W., Malim, M. H., Kingsman, A. J., and Kingsman, S. M., 1986, Expression strategies of the yeast retrotransposon Ty: A short sequence directs ribosomal frameshifting, *Nucleic Acids Res.* **14**:7001–7015.

Wu, J. -Y., Gardner, B. H., Murphy, C. I., Seals, J. R., Kensil, C. R., Recchia, J., Beltz, G. A., Newman, G. W., and Newman, M. J., 1992, Saponin adjuvant enhancement of antigen-specific immune responses to an experimental HIV-1 vaccine, *J. Immunol.* **148**:1519–1525.

Yu, X. F., Yuan, X., Matsuda, Z., Lee, T. H., and Essex, M., 1992, The matrix protein of HIV-1 is required for incorporation of viral envelope protein into mature virus, *J. Virol.* **66**:4966–4971.

Chapter 35

Rationale and Approaches to Constructing Preerythrocytic Malaria Vaccines

Stephen L. Hoffman and John B. Sacci, Jr.

1. IRRADIATED SPOROZOITE VACCINATION AS A MODEL FOR MALARIA VACCINE DEVELOPMENT

Parasites belonging to the genus *Plasmodium* are the causative agent for malaria. This disease is primarily found in the tropics and is conservatively estimated to cause 200–300 million new cases each year with approximately 2 million deaths resulting. The parasite has a complex life cycle which is initiated in the host when an anopheline mosquito injects the sporozoite stage as it takes a blood meal. The sporozoites travel through the circulation to the liver where they invade hepatocytes. Once in the hepatocyte the parasite undergoes a cycle of differentiation and division the length of which varies with the species, ultimately producing many thousands of merozoites which reenter the circulation on rupture of the hepatocyte. These liver-stage merozoites invade red blood cells and again multiply. After 48–72 h the red blood cell ruptures, releasing 6–30 merozoites which can then invade other red blood cells. Some parasites differentiate into male and female gametocytes, which when ingested by a mosquito can combine to form a zygote and on further development produce sporozoites that can be inoculated into another host, thereby repeating the cycle.

Vaccine-induced protection, against *Plasmodium* infection, was originally demonstrated by Mulligan *et al.* (1941). They were able to protect chickens by immunizing them with radiation-attenuated *Plasmodium gallinaceum* sporozoites. Nussenzweig *et al.* (1967) subsequently demonstrated that immunization of A/J mice with radiation-attenuated *P.*

The opinions and assertions herein are those of the authors and are not to be construed as official or as reflecting the views of the U.S. Navy or the naval service at large.

Stephen L. Hoffman • Malaria Program, Naval Medical Research Institute, Bethesda, Maryland 20889-5607. *John B. Sacci, Jr.* • Malaria Program, Naval Medical Research Institute, Bethesda, and Department of Microbiology and Immunology, University of Maryland School of Medicine, Baltimore, Maryland 21201.

Vaccine Design: The Subunit and Adjuvant Approach, edited by Michael F. Powell and Mark J. Newman. Plenum Press, New York, 1995.

bergei sporozoites protected mice against challenge with virulent sporozoites. This immunity was stage specific, because mice challenged with infected erythrocytes were not protected. In the early 1970s vaccine-induced protection was demonstrated in humans; vaccination was by the bite of irradiated mosquitoes, carrying *P. falciparum* and in one case *P. vivax* sporozoites in their salivary glands, and the protection was against challenge with live sporozoites (Clyde *et al.*, 1973a,b, 1975; Rieckmann *et al.*, 1974, 1979). This immunity was both stage and species specific since immunization with *P. falciparum* did not protect against *P. vivax*. However, it was not strain specific because immunization with *P. falciparum* sporozoites from Burma protected against challenge with sporozoites from Malaya, Panama, and the Philippines (Clyde *et al.*, 1973a) and immunization with sporozoites from Ethiopia protected against challenge with a strain from Vietnam (Rieckmann *et al.*, 1979). These studies have been repeated recently (Herrington *et al.*, 1991; Egan *et al.*, 1993) and the results were confirmed: irradiated sporozoites are an effective malaria vaccine and can induce protective immunity that lasts for at least 9 months (Edelman *et al.*, 1993).

Radiation-attenuated sporozoites develop only to late trophozoites in the liver. This observation and the finding that irradiated sporozoite-induced immunity does not protect against challenge with infected erythrocytes, indicate that the immunity is directed against the sporozoite in circulation, or parasites developing within hepatocytes. Antibodies may mediate protection by preventing sporozoites from effectively invading hepatoctyes. Either or both antibodies and T cells may recognize parasite antigens expressed by infected hepatocytes once the infection is established and destroy these cells. Unfortunately, irradiated sporozoites have to be delivered alive to be effective as a vaccine. Since mature, infective sporozoites have never been produced in vitro and it is impossible to immunize a large number of individuals by the bite of thousands of sporozoite-infected mosquitoes, this approach is not practical.

The targets and mechanisms of this protective immune response had to be identified so as to construct a synthetic or recombinant vaccine. Initial efforts to develop synthetic preerythrocytic malaria vaccines focused on producing protective antibodies. Currently there is increasing recognition of the requirement to attack the infected hepatocyte, primarily through T-cell-mediated mechanisms.

2. PREVENTING SPOROZOITE INVASION OF HEPATOCYTES

Sera from mice and humans immunized with irradiated sporozoites precipitate the surface coat of live sporozoites; this is called the circumsporozoite (CSP) precipitation reaction (Clyde *et al.*, 1973a,b; Vanderberg *et al.*, 1969). In 1980 Potocnjak *et al.* reported that passive transfer of Fab antibody fragments specific for the 44-kDa *P. berghei* CS protein conferred protection against sporozoite-induced *P. berghei* infections. Passive transfer of monoclonal antibodies against the *P. yoelii* (Charoenvit *et al.*, 1990, 1991b) and *P. vivax* (Charoenvit *et al.*, 1991a) CS proteins have also protected against sporozoite-induced malaria. The mechanism of this action is unknown, but since it can be mediated by Fab fragments of antibodies, is active in mice depleted of complement by injection with cobra venom, and is active in BALB/c *nu/nu* mice (Y. Charoenvit, unpublished), the interaction of sporozoites with antibody appears to be the only critical factor.

The sequences of numerous *Plasmodium* spp. CS proteins have been determined and all have a central region of tandemly repeated amino acids. For example, in *P. falciparum* NANP is repeated 35–40 times (Dame *et al.*, 1984) and in *P. vivax* DRAA/DGQPAG is repeated 19 times (Arnot *et al.*, 1985; McCutchan *et al.*, 1985). There is little resemblance among the tandem repeats of different *Plasmodium* spp. but the flanking sequences contain two highly conserved regions found in CS proteins of all species, simply referred to as region I and region II (Dame *et al.*, 1984).

All of the monoclonal antibodies (Mabs) specific for CS proteins, and capable of protecting animals in passive transfer experiments, recognize the central repeat regions. Furthermore, when polyclonal antibodies were produced in mice against the repeat region and the flanking conserved regions (I and II) of the *P. falciparum* CS protein, only antibodies against the repeat region blocked sporozoite invasion of hepatoma cells in vitro (Ballou *et al.*, 1985). This was not the case when Vergara *et al.* (1985) immunized mice with a synthetic peptide derived from outside the repeat region. They found that these antibodies cross-reacted with *P. berghei* sporozoites and produced some protection in vivo. Recently, though, Pancake *et al.* (1992) and Cerami *et al.* (1992) have demonstrated that sporozoites bind to hepatocytes via sulfated glycoconjugate adhesion motifs in region II of the CS protein. Thus, it is likely that both the repeats and flanking regions may be targets for vaccine-induced antibodies.

Synthetic peptides (Egan *et al.*, 1987; Zavala *et al.*, 1987; Tam *et al.*, 1990) and *E. coli*-produced recombinant CS protein (Egan *et al.*, 1987) have been used in vaccines that induced protective antibody responses in mice against *P. berghei*. Protection ranging from 35% (Egan *et al.*, 1987) to 80% (Tam *et al.*, 1990) has been achieved by immunizing with such vaccines in the *P. berghei* system, demonstrating that vaccine-induced immune responses can protect against sporozoite challenge. Passive transfer of immunoglobulins from vaccinated mice into naive recipient mice protected three of four mice from sporozoite challenge, thus demonstrating the capacity of polyclonal antibodies alone to protect (Egan *et al.*, 1987). Until recently, none of these types of vaccines have induced any protection against the more infectious *P. yoelii* (Charoenvit *et al.*, 1990, 1991b). However, Wang and colleagues (Wang *et al.*, in press) have recently achieved 100% protection against *P. yoelii* sporozoite challenge in outbred mice by immunizing with a vaccine designed to produce antibodies against the repeat region of the PyCSP. This vaccine is a multiple antigenic peptide branched-chain polymer, or MAP (Tam *et al.*, 1990), that utilizes two stretches of amino acids from tetanus toxin for T-cell help, and four copies of the PyCSP repeat sequence, QGPGAP, for B-cell epitopes. It has protected when administered with anionic block copolymers and the combination of liposomes, lipid A, and aluminum hydroxide as delivery systems. A similar *P. falciparum* vaccine is expected to be evaluated in Phase I clinical trials in late 1994, and several similar *P. vivax* vaccines in monkeys in mid-1994. MAP vaccines have also been utilized to assess the immunogenicity of different B- and T-cell epitope combinations derived solely from *P. falciparum* CS (Calvo-Calle *et al.*, 1993). Additionally, significant protection has been achieved, in mice, utilizing a MAP vaccine containing a B-cell epitope and one of two T-cell epitopes from the *P. berghei* CS protein (Migliorini *et al.*, 1993).

Human Vaccine Trials

The gene encoding the *P. falciparum* CS protein was cloned and sequenced in 1984 (Dame *et al.*, 1984) and for the *P. vivax* CS protein in 1985 (McCutchan *et al.*, 1985). Since then, considerable work has been done to develop and test vaccines designed to protect humans by inducing antibodies against the repeat region of these proteins. Most of the work has been in the *P. falciparum* system. In the initial studies an *E. coli*-produced recombinant vaccine called R32tet$_{32}$ or FSV-1 (Ballou *et al.*, 1987) and a synthetic peptide vaccine were tested (Herrington *et al.*, 1987). The R32tet$_{32}$ protein included 32 tetrapeptide repeats from the repeat region of the *P. falciparum* CS protein, (NANP)$_{15}$-NVDP(NANp)$_{15}$NVDP (R32), which were the B-cell epitopes. These were fused to 32 amino acids from the tetracycline resistance region of a plasmid, the T-helper cell epitopes. The immunogen was delivered with aluminum hydroxide as adjuvant or delivery system. The second vaccine included three copies of NANP, the B-cell epitopes, conjugated to tetanus toxoid, the T helper cell epitopes. This product was also given with aluminum hydroxide as an adjuvant. Only a few of the individuals immunized produced the expected levels of antibodies and only one of six individuals challenged in one trial (Ballou *et al.*, 1987), and one of three individuals challenged in the other trial (Herrington *et al.*, 1987) were protected.

In both studies some volunteers with high levels of antibodies had delays in the onset of parasitemia indicating that at least 95% of sporozoites had been rendered noninfectious by the vaccine-induced antibodies. It also appeared that individuals with the highest levels of antibodies were the ones protected. Both R32 and (NANP)$_3$ seemed capable of inducing protective antibodies; therefore, subsequent studies focused on the evaluation of the carrier proteins for providing T-cell help and the adjuvant. These were attempts to improve the interaction of T cells, B cells, and antigen-presenting cells. *Pseudomonas aeruginosa* toxin A (Fries *et al.*, 1992), the nonstructural protein of influenza A (Gordon *et al.*, 1990; Rickman *et al.*, 1991), tetanus toxoid (Herrington *et al.*, 1987), meningococcal outer membrane protein (Sadoff *et al.*, 1987), choleragenoid (Sadoff *et al.*, 1987), hepatitis B virus surface antigen (Vreden *et al.*, 1991), the flanking regions of the CS protein (Herrington *et al.*, 1992), and the carboxy-terminus (D. Gordon, unpublished) of the CS protein have all been tested as carrier proteins. A combination of monophosphoryl lipid A and cell-wall skeleton of mycobacteria (Detox™) (Rickman *et al.*, 1991), liposomes with aluminum hydroxide and monophosphoryl lipid A, hepatitis B surface antigen particles with aluminum hydroxide and monophosphoryl lipid A (D. Gordon, unpublished), and interferon-γ (Sturchler *et al.*, 1989) have all been tested as adjuvants. A number of these have proved promising with 18% (Hoffman *et al.*, 1994) to 25% (D. Gordon, unpublished) of volunteers completely protected against malaria, and equivalent percentages showing a significant delay in the onset of parasitemia indicating that greater than 95% of sporozoites have been inactivated. Antibodies derived from vaccination could be protective, while naturally acquired antibodies to the repeat region were not associated with protection from reinfection (Hoffman *et al.*, 1987) suggesting a qualitative difference in the antibodies elicited.

Thus, in 1994, 15–25% of volunteers can consistently be protected against malaria by vaccines designed to produce protective antibodies against the repeat region of the *P. falciparum* CS protein. Attempts to improve this level of protection by varying B- and T-cell epitopes and delivery systems are ongoing. Ultimately vaccines will require extensive field testing to determine if natural infection will boost the antibody responses to the vaccines. Although the ultimate vaccine formulation has yet to be produced, a multicomponent vaccine inducing both humoral and cellular responses will almost certainly utilize the repeat region of the CS protein.

3. ATTACKING THE INFECTED HEPATOCYTE

3.1. CD8+ T-Cell-Dependent Irradiated Sporozoite Vaccine-Induced Protective Immunity

There is now a strong body of evidence indicating that the immunity induced by the irradiated sporozoite vaccine is mediated by T cells that recognize malaria peptides presented in the context of MHC class I molecules on infected hepatocytes. The potential role of T cells in this immunity was first recognized by Chen *et al.* (1977) who showed that 64% of mu-suppressed mice (anti-IgM treated) that were immunized with irradiated sporozoites were protected, indicating that antibodies were not required for this protection. It was subsequently shown that adoptive transfer of immune T cells, from vaccinated donors, into naive mice protected them from malaria in the absence of antibodies (Egan *et al.*, 1987). Schofield *et al.* (1987b) and Weiss *et al.* (1990) working in the A/J–*P. berghei* and BALB/c–*P. yoelii* systems demonstrated that protective immunity induced by immunization with irradiated sporozoites was abrogated by in vivo depletion of CD8+ T cells. Depletion of CD4+ T cells had no effect on protection. These data demonstrated that antibodies induced by immunization with irradiated sporozoites were not adequate to protect against sporozoite-induced malaria by themselves and that CD8+ T cells were required.

Our interpretation of these data is that this immunity was mediated by CD8+ cytotoxic T lymphocytes (CTLs) that recognized malaria antigens presented on infected hepatocytes. Hoffman *et al.* (1989) reported that when mice immunized with irradiated *P. berghei* sporozoites were challenged with large numbers of live sporozoites, they developed parasite-specific CD8+ T-cell-dependent inflammatory infiltrates in the livers. However, the majority of liver-stage schizonts in naive animals developed normally with no evidence of inflammatory cells (Hoffman *et al.*, 1989). They also used an in vitro system to show that spleen cells from mice immunized with irradiated sporozoites eliminated infected hepatoctyes from culture in an MHC-restricted and species-specific manner (Hoffman *et al.*, 1989). This strongly suggested that immune T cells were recognizing *Plasmodium* sp. antigens presented on infected hepatocytes. Since this activity was not reversed by anti-IFN-γ and not duplicated by culture supernatants, it was thought to be mediated by direct T cell–hepatocyte interaction specifically by CTLs. Although this clearly defined an important mechanism of protective immunity generated by immunization with irradiated sporozoites, it did not identify the specific parasite targets.

3.2. Adoptive Transfer of CD8[+] CTLs against the CS Protein Are Protective

In the late 1980s the only target available for study was the CS protein. Romero *et al.* (1989) working in the *P. berghei* system and Weiss *et al.* (1990) working with *P. yoelii* reported that there was only a single region of these rodent malaria CS proteins that included a CTL epitope in the BALB/c model. CTLs against the *P. yoelii* epitope eliminated infected hepatocytes in vitro in an antigen-specific, MHC-restricted manner and a CTL clone against the analogous region of the *P. berghei* CS protein adoptively transferred complete protection against challenge with *P. berghei* sporozoites (Romero *et al.*, 1989) It was subsequently shown that transfer of a similar CD8[+] CTL clone against the *P. yoelii* CS protein transferred protection (Rodrigues *et al.*, 1991; Weiss *et al.*, 1992) and that if this CD8[+] CTL clone was transferred 3 h after sporozoite inoculation, it still provided protection. Experimentally inoculated sporozoites are not accessible to antibodies within 5 min of inoculation, and are thought to enter hepatocytes within 5–60 minutes of inoculation; this experiment suggested that the CTL clones were recognizing CS protein expressed in infected hepatocytes and either destroying the infected hepatocyte or rendering the parasite nonfunctional. This concept was further supported by data demonstrating that radiolabeled protective, but not nonprotective CTL clones could be found in apposition to infected hepatocytes after adoptive transfer in vivo (Rodrigues *et al.*, 1992). The mechanism whereby these CD8[+] T cells prevent further development of the parasites is unknown. They may act through the release of pore-forming proteins, cytokines, or, as discussed later, the induction of nitric oxide synthase by γ-interferon. There is also evidence that they may require specific adhesion molecules like CD44 on their surfaces to optimally interact with infected hepatocytes (Rodrigues *et al.*, 1992).

3.3. Immunization with CS Protein Vaccines Induces CD8[+] T-Cell-Dependent Partial Protection in Rodent Malaria Model Systems

A substantial effort has been made to generate vaccines that actively induce CTLs against the CS protein. Oral immunization of mice with a recombinant *Salmonella typhimurium* expressing the *P. berghei* CS protein induced CTLs against the *P. berghei* CS protein (Aggarwal *et al.*, 1991) and protected 50–75% of mice against challenge with *P. berghei* sporozoites (Sadoff *et al.*, 1988; Aggarwal *et al.*, 1991). This immunity was abrogated by in vivo depletion of CD8[+] T cells (Aggarwal *et al.*, 1991). Mice immunized with a recombinant vaccinia virus expressing the *P. berghei* CS protein produced CTLs against the *P. berghei* CS protein but were not protected (Satchidanandam *et al.*, 1991). Similarly, mice immunized with recombinant vaccinia, *S. typhimurium*, or pseudorabies virus expressing the *P. yoelii* CS protein produced substantial cellular immune responses, but also were not protected when challenged (Sedegah *et al.*, 1988, 1990, 1992a). However, when BALB/c mice were immunized with irradiated P815 mastocytoma cells transfected with the gene encoding the *P. yoelii* CS protein. CTLs against the CS protein were induced and 50–85% were protected against challenge (Khusmith *et al.*,1991). This protective immunity was eliminated by in vivo depletion of CD8$^+$ T cells and was therefore similar to immunity generated by immunization with irradiated sporozoites (Khusmith *et al.*, 1991).

Transfected tumor cells cannot be given to humans and so work has continued to try to induce protective CD8$^+$ CTLs against the PyCSP using other more acceptable approaches. Immunization of BALB/c mice with a recombinant influenza virus expressing the PyCSP CTL epitope followed by boosting with a vaccinia expressing the PyCSP induces partial, CD8$^+$ T-cell-dependent protection against sporozoite challenge (Li *et al.*, 1993). Most recently, Sedegah *et al.* (1994a) have shown that immunization of BALB/c mice with PyCSP plasmid DNA produces high levels of antibodies and CTL responses that protect up to 83% of the mice against challenge and that this protective immunity is eliminated by treatment of the mice with anti-CD8$^+$ antibodies.

3.4. Induction of CTLs against the *P. falciparum* CS Protein in Humans

The body of data from the rodent malaria system has laid a groundwork for vaccine designers trying to produce vaccines that induce CTLs against the *P. falciparum* CS protein for use in humans. The identification of CTL epitopes on the *P. falciparum* CS protein was first done by Kumar *et al.* (1988). They demonstrated CD8$^+$ T-cell-dependent cytolytic activity against a 23-amino-acid region on the *P. falciparum* CS protein, Pf 7G8 CS 368-390, in B10.BR mice. Malik *et al.* (1991) were able to demonstrate that peripheral blood mononuclear cells from volunteers immunized with irradiated *P. falciparum* sporozoites contained CD8$^+$ T cells with cytolytic activity against the same region, Pf 7G8 CS 368-390 (Kumar *et al.*, 1988). Kenyans with long-term natural exposure to malaria also had CD8$^+$ CTLs against the same region, and Australians who had lived in malarious areas had circulating CTLs of undefined phenotype (Sedegah *et al.*, 1992b; Doolan *et al.*, 1991).

With the establishment of an assay for identifying *Plasmodium*-specific CTLs in humans, a number of groups are studying the capacity of soluble recombinant proteins and recombinant live vectors such as *Salmonella typhi*, vaccinia, and BCG expressing the CS protein to induce antigen-specific CTLs. In a Phase I clinical study one volunteer immunized by oral administration of an attenuated *S. typhi* expressing the PfCSP produced measurable cytolytic activity against PfCSP (Gonzalez *et al.*, 1994). In the next few years there should be abundant information regarding induction of CD8$^+$ CTLs against the CS protein in humans. In parallel there will be considerable work required to consistently protect mice using vaccine constructs and delivery systems that can be applied in humans. Several modifications of vaccine construction and delivery systems are currently being evaluated.

3.5. Identification of Sporozoite Surface Protein 2 as a Target of Vaccine-Induced CD8⁺ Protective CTLs

As we stated previously, immunization with irradiated sporozoites completely protects against malaria, but none of the subunit *P. berghei* or *P. yoelii* CS protein vaccines have induced comparable protection. Furthermore, in the human studies the presence of CTLs against the *P. falciparum* CS protein did not guarantee that the individual would be protected, and likewise, one individual who was not shown to have CTLs was protected against challenge (Malik *et al.*, 1991; Egan *et al.*, 1993). Considering the complexity of sporozoites it was not logical to assume that all protection induced by the whole organism vaccine was mediated by CTLs against a single short stretch of amino acids on a single protein. This has led to the identification of additional antigens that may be responsible for the protection induced by irradiated sporozoite vaccination.

Charoenvit *et al.* (1987) immunized mice with irradiated *P. yoelii* sporozoites and produced a monoclonal antibody directed against a 140-kDa sporozoite protein. The gene encoding this protein was cloned and sequenced (Hedstrom *et al.*, 1990; Rodgers *et al.*, 1992b) and the protein named sporozoite surface protein 2 (SSP2). To determine if immunization with irradiated sporozoites produced not only antibodies, but also CTLs against SSP2, Khusmith *et al.* (1991) transfected a 1.5-kB fragment of the gene into P815 mouse mastocytoma cells and used these as targets in CTL assays. Using mice immunized with irradiated sporozoites they demonstrated the production of CTLs against SSP2. Additionally, a CD8⁺ CTL clone against SSP2 was obtained and when adoptively transferred, complete protection against *P. yoelii* challenge was induced. This established that CTLs specific for SSP2 could completely protect against this highly virulent parasite (Khusmith *et al.*, 1994). Subsequent studies utilized mice that had been immunized with the P815 cells expressing PySSP2; approximately 50% were protected against challenge and the immunity was CD8⁺ T cell dependent (Khusmith *et al.*, 1991). At this point it had been shown that immunization with the PyCS protein or PySSP2 vaccines gave only partial protection against malaria (50–75%), immunity that was in no way comparable to the complete protective immunity found after immunization with irradiated sporozoites. Khusmith *et al.* (1991) then immunized with transfected P815 cells expressing both PyCSP and PySSP2 and achieved 100% protection.

The gene encoding the *P. falciparum* SSP2 (PfSSP2) has now been identified and characterized (Rogers *et al.*, 1992a) and shown to be the previously described thrombospondin-related anonymous protein (TRAP) (Robson *et al.*, 1988). Wizel *et al.* have identified CTL epitopes on PfSSP2 in C57BL/6 mice (1994) and in humans (unpublished). Work is now in progress to produce human vaccines that will induce protective CTLs and perhaps antibodies against SSP2.

3.6. CD4⁺ CTLs against the CS Protein Mediate Protective Immunity

Until recently it had been shown that irradiated sporozoites induced only protective immune responses dominated by CD8⁺ CTLs. Renia *et al.* (1991) have now demonstrated that CD4⁺ T cells specific for an epitope contained in amino acids 59–79 from the amino-terminus of the *P. yoelii* CS protein can recognize CS protein peptides presented on infected hepatocytes and eliminate these infected cells from culture. These CTLs can be adoptively transferred and mediate protection against malaria. Studies are currently under way to actively induce such protective immunity using the rodent model systems with the goal of identifying analogous regions of the *P. falciparum* and *P. vivax* CS proteins that may be incorporated into vaccines for humans. Recently, Moreno *et al.* (1991) reported that immunization of a human with *P. falciparum* sporozoites induced cytotoxic CD4$^+$ T cells that recognized an epitope in the C-terminal region of the CS protein.

3.7. Other Parasite Antigen Targets in Infected Hepatocytes

Although several additional antigens have been identified as being primarily or exclusively expressed in the liver or exoerythrocytic (EE) stage, to date none have been determined to contribute to the protective immunity elicited by immunization with irradiated sporozoites. Of the antigens identified, one is from *P. falciparum*, liver-stage antigen-1 (LSA-1) (Guerin-Marchand *et al.*, 1987; Zhu and Hollingdale, 1991); two from *P. berghei*, *P. berghei* liver 1 (PbL1) (Suhrbier *et al.*, 1990) and a 230-kDa protein LSA-2 (Hollingdale *et al.*,1990); and one 17-kDa *p. yoelli* protein PyHEP17 (Charoenvit *et al.*, in press). Despite the identification of multiple liver-stage proteins, until recently none had been shown to be involved in protective immune responses. A monoclonal antibody, Navy yoelii liver stage 3 (NYLS3), specific for PyHEP17 can reduce the number of infected hepatocytes in vitro and provide partial protection on passive transfer. Furthermore, a DNA vaccine based upon PyHEP17 has been shown to protect up to 83% of challenged mice (Doolan, personal communication). Future work will clarify the potential importance of LSA-1, PbL1, LSA-2, and PyHEP17 and perhaps one or more of these proteins and possibly other liver-stage proteins will be included in multivalent preerythrocytic-stage vaccines.

3.8. Interferon-γ and Other Cytokines

The mechanisms by which CD4$^+$ and CD8$^+$ T lymphocytes actually eliminate infected hepatocytes from culture and protect in vivo have only recently been examined in detail. Most data indicate that cytokines play a dominant role. Systemic administration of IFN-γ partially protects mice and monkeys against *P. berghei* (Ferreira *et al.*, 1986) and *P. cynomolgi* (Maheshwari *et al.*, 1986), respectively, and in vitro treatment of infected hepatocytes with IFN-γ eliminates *P. falciparum* (Mellouk *et al.*, 1987) from culture. Additionally, protection induced by irradiated *P. berghei* sporozoites in A/J mice was abrogated by in vivo treatment of the mice with anti-IFN-γ (Schofield *et al.*, 1987b). But these results could not be reproduced in *P. berghei* (Hoffman *et al.*, 1989) or *P. yoelii* (Rodrigues *et al.*, 1991) immunized BALB/c mice. Recently it has been shown that adoptive transfer of a CD8$^+$ T-cell clone specific for the *P. yoelii* CS protein that produces large quantities of IFN-γ protects against *P. yoelii*, and this protective immunity is eliminated by in vivo treatment of the mice with anti-IFN-γ (Weiss *et al.*, 1992). It may be that the protective *P. berghei* (Sadoff *et al.*, 1988) and *P. yoelii* (Khusmith *et al.*, 1991) vaccines already tested lead to the local release of IFN-γ and that this cytokine is an essential component for protection.

Analysis of the pattern of cytokine production profiles of certain CD4 T-cell clones suggests that other cytokines could be involved (Del Giudice *et al.*, 1990). The inhibitory effect of IL-1 and IL-6 on the intrahepatic development of human and murine parasites has been reported (Mellouk *et al.*, 1987; Pied *et al.*, 1991). Tumor necrosis factor (TNF) inhibited development of *P. berghei* in vitro in a hepatoma cell line (Schofield *et al.*, 1987a), but TNF was not effective alone in cultures of *P. yoelii*-infected hepatocytes (Mellouk *et al.*, 1991; Nussler *et al.*, 1991b), suggesting differences in the way primary cultures of hepatocytes and hepatoma cells respond to cytokines. However, in co-culture experiments using hepatocytes and nonparenchymal cells, TNF induced parasite inhibition by IL-6 release (Nussler *et al.*, 1991a,b). The mechanism by which cytokines kill infected hepatocytes is not well understood; however, recent reports indicate that IFN-γ and other cytokines induce nitric oxide synthase in infected hepatocytes which produce nitrogen oxides, from L-arginine, which is in turn toxic for the EE-stage parasite (Mellouk *et al.*, 1991; Nussler *et al.*, 1991a). It may be that IL-12 is critical in regulating this process. Systemic administration of recombinant IL-12 completely protects mice against sporozoite challenge (Sedegah *et al.*, 1994b). This protection is entirely dependent on the IL-12 inducing other cells to produce IFN-γ and is partially reversed by inhibition of nitric oxide production. Work is in progress to characterize the role of IL-12 in vaccine-induced protection.

4. THE FUTURE: INDUCING MULTIPLE IMMUNE RESPONSES AGAINST MULTIPLE TARGETS

Immunization of humans with radiation-attenuated *P. falciparum* sporozoites consistently protects against challenge. Vaccines that are designed to mimic the effects of irradiated sporozoite vaccination and induce protective immune responses must completely protect against malaria, or, if used in combination with an erythrocytic-stage vaccine, to substantially reduce the number of inoculated sporozoites that develop to mature liver-stage schizonts and release infective merozoites.

It seems logical that the protective immunity induced by the attenuated "whole organism" vaccine must be directed against multiple targets and mediated by multiple immune mechanisms. We know that monoclonal antibodies against the repeat region of the CS protein expressed on the surface of circulating sporozoites, CD8$^+$ CTLs against a single epitope in the carboxy-terminus of the CS protein, CD4$^+$ CTLs against a single epitope in the amino-terminus of the CS protein, and CD8$^+$ CTLs against a single epitope on the PySSP2, can all completely protect against sporozoite-induced malaria in the absence of other parasite-specific immune responses. Furthermore, antibodies against an antigen first expressed in infected hepatocytes (PyHEP17 in the *P. yoelii* system) eliminate infected hepatocytes from culture, presumably by recognizing this protein expressed in infected hepatocytes (Charoenvit *et al.*, in press) and a DNA vaccine based on this gene can provide protection (Doolan, personal communication). Thus, five discrete targets on the sporozoite and infected hepatocytes and at least three different types of immune responses have been shown to contribute to protective immunity.

It is likely that the irradiated sporozoite vaccine actually induces additional protective immune responses against additional targets, and work is in progress to identify these targets and mechanisms. Nonetheless it seems immediately apparent that a coherent strategy would be to try to produce vaccines for humans that induce these varied responses, and such work is in progress (Hoffman *et al.*, 1991, 1993). By designing a vaccine to induce protective antibody and $CD4^+$ and $CD8^+$ T-lymphocyte responses against the CSP, SSP2, and PyHEP17, one could plan to eliminate a portion of the parasites within an individual with each of the responses, but eliminate all of the parasites by hitting five different epitopes with either antibody or T-cell immune responses. Because of genetic restriction of T-cell responses in vaccinees and variation of B and T epitopes in the parasite, it may not be possible to induce all of these types of protective immune responses in all individuals. If such a multivalent vaccine completely protected 20% of the population with each of the five protective immune responses, then the entire population would be protected by the vaccine.

During the past decade, we have made significant progress toward understanding the mechanisms and targets of irradiated sporozoite-induced protective immunity (Hoffman *et al.*, 1993). There will undoubtedly be numerous problems in future attempts to design and construct human vaccines that induce the required immune responses. Research to develop methods for optimal vaccine construction and delivery so as to maximize required immune responses against multiple targets has only just begun. It is not clear whether synthetic peptide, purified recombinant protein, live recombinant vector, plasmid DNA, or other heretofore undiscovered vaccine constructs will prove to be optimal. Nor is it clear what delivery systems will be best. It may be that combinations of multiple types of immunogens and delivery systems will be required to achieve the solid protective immunity required to control malaria. Once effective vaccines are developed, the question of expense of production and delivery will also have to be addressed if such vaccines are ever to be available to the people who need them most. Nonetheless there is now great hope that we will one day have vaccines that protect against malaria by attacking the parasite at multiple stages in its preerythrocytic cycle, and that such vaccines will be combined with vaccines that attack the asexual and sexual erythrocytic stages of the parasite.

ACKNOWLEDGMENT

Supported by Naval Medical Research and Development Command work units 61102A.S13.00101.BFX.1431, 612787A.870.00101.EFX.1432, and 623002A.810. 00101.HFX.1433.

REFERENCES

Aggarwal, A., Kumar, S., Jaffe, R., Hone, D., Gross, M., and Sadoff, J., 1991, Oral Salmonella: Malaria circumsporozoite recombinants induce specific $CD8^+$ cytotoxic T cells, *J. Exp. Med.* **172**:1083–1090.

Arnot, D. E., Barnwell, J. W., Tam, J. P., Nussenzweig, V., Nussenzweig, R. S., and Enea, V., 1985, Circumsporozoite protein of *Plasmodium vivax*: Gene cloning and characterization of the immunodominant epitope, *Science* **230**:815–818.

Ballou, W. R., Rothbard, J., Wirtz, R. A., Gordon, D. M., Williams, J. S., Gore, R. W., Schneider, I., Hollingdale, M. R., Beaudoin, R. L., Maloy, W. L., Miller, L. H., and Hockmeyer, W. T., 1985,

Immunogenicity of synthetic peptides from circumsporozoite protein of *Plasmodium falciparum*, *Science* **228**:996–999.

Ballou, W. R., Hoffman, S. L., Sherwood, J. A., Hollingdale, M. R., Neva, F. A., Hockmeyer, W. T., Gordon, D. M., Schneider, I., Wirtz, R. A., Young, J. F., Wasserman, G. F., Reeve, P., Diggs, C. L., and Chulay, J. D., 1987, Safety and efficacy of a recombinant DNA *Plasmodium falciparum* sporozoite vaccine, *Lancet* **1**:1277–1281.

Calco-Calle, J. M., de Oliveira, G. A., Clavijo, P., Maracic, M., Tam, J. P., Lu, Y. A., Nardin, E. H., Nussenzweig, R. S., and Cochrane, A. H., 1993, Immunogenicity of multiple peptides containing B and T cell epitopes of the circumsporozoite protein of *Plasmodium falciparum*. *J. Immunol.* **150**: 1403–1412.

Cerami, C., Frevert, U., Sinnis, P., Takacs, B., Clavijo, P., Santos, M., and Nussenzweig, V., 1992, The basolateral domain of the hepatocyte plasma membrane bears receptors for the circumsporozoite protein of *Plasmodium falciparum* sporozoites, *Cell* **70**:1021–1033.

Charoenvit, Y., Leef, M. F., Yuan, L.F., Sedegah, M., and Beaudoin, R. L., 1987, Characterization of *Plasmodium yoelii* monoclonal antibodies directed against stage-specific sporozoite antigens, *Infect. Immun.* **55**:604–608.

Charoenvit, Y., Sedegah, M., Yuan, L. F., Gross, M., Cole, C., Bechara, R., Leef, M. F., Robey, F. A., Lowell, G. H., Beaudoin, R. L., and Hoffman, S. L., 1990, Active and passive immunization against *Plasmodium yoelii* sporozoites, *Bull. WHO* **68** (Suppl.):26–32.

Charoenvit, Y., Collins, W. E., Jones, T. R., Millet, P., Yuan, L., Campbell, G. H., Beaudoin, R. L., Broderson, J. R., and Hoffman, S. L., 1991a, Inability of malaria vaccine to induce antibodies to a protective epitope within its sequence, *Science* **251**:668–671.

Charoenvit, Y., Mellouk, S., Cole, C., Bechara, R., Leef, M. F., Sedegah, M., Yuan, L. F., Robey, F. A., Beaudoin, R. L., and Hoffman, S. L., 1991b, Monoclonal, but not polyclonal antibodies protect against *Plasmodium yoeli* sporozoites, *J. Immunol.* **146**:1020–1025.

Charoenvit, Y., Mellouk, S., Sedegah, M., Toyoshima, T., Leef, M., De la Vega, P., Beaudoin, R. L., Aikawa, M., Fallarme, V., and Hoffman, S. L., Characterization of an inhibitory monoclonal antibody against *Plasmodium yoeli* liver and blood stage parasites, *Exp. Parasitol.* (in press).

Chen, D. H., Tigelaar, R. E., and Weinbaum, F. I., 1977, Immunity to sporozoite-induced malaria infection in mice. I. The effect of immunization of T and B cell-deficient mice, *J. Immunol.* **118**:1322–1327.

Clyde, D. F., McCarthy, V. C., Miller, R. M., and Hornick, R. B., 1973a, Specificity of protection of man immunized against sporozoite-induced falciparum malaria, *Am. J. Med. Sci.* **266**:398–401.

Clyde, D. F., Most, H., McCarthy, V. C., and Vanderberg, J. P., 1973b, Immunization of man against sporozoite-induced falciparum malaria, *Am. J. Med. Sci.* **266**:169–177.

Clyde, D. F., McCarthy, V. C., Miller, R. M., and Woodward, W. E., 1975, Immunization of man against falciparum and vivax malaria by use of attenuated sporozoites, *Am. J. Trop. Med. Hyg.* **24**:397–401.

Dame, J. B., Williams, J. L., McCutchan, T. F., Weber, J. L., Wirtz, R. A., Hockmeyer, W. T., Maloy, W. L., Haynes, J. D., Schneider, I., Roberts, D., Sanders, G. S., Reddy, E. P., Diggs, C. L., and Miller, L. H., 1984, Structure of the gene encoding the immunodominant surface antigen on the sporozoite of the human malaria parasite *Plasmodium falciparum*, *Science* **225**:593–599.

Del Giudice, G., Grillot, D., Renia, L., Muller, I., Corradin, G., Louis, J. A., Mazier, D., and Lambert, P. H., 1990, Peptide-primed CD4^{+} cells and malaria sporozoites, *Immunol. Lett.* **25**:59–64.

Doolan, D. L., Houghten, R. A., and Good, M. F., 1991, Location of human cytotoxic T cell epitopes within a polymorphic domain of the *Plasmodium falciparum* circumsporozoite protein, *Int. Immunol.* **3**:511–516.

Edelman, R., Hoffman, S. L., Davis, J. R., Beier, M., Sztein, M. B., Losonsky, G., Herrington, D. A., Eddy, H. A., Hollingdale, M. R., Gordon, D. M., and Clyde, D.F., 1993, Long-term persistence of sterile immunity in a volunteer immunized with x-irradiated *Plasmodium falciparum* sporozoites, *J. Infect. Dis.* **168**:1066–1070.

Egan, J. E., Weber, J. L., Ballou, W. R., Hollingdale, M. R., Majarian, W. R., Gordon, D. M., Maloy, W. L., Hoffman, S. L., Wirtz, R. A., Schneider, I., Woollett, G. R., Young, J. F., and Hockmeyer, W. T., 1987,

Efficacy of murine malaria sporozoite vaccines: Implications for human vaccine development, *Science* **236**:453–456.

Egan, J. E., Hoffman, S. L., Haynes, J. D., Sadoff, J. C., Schneider, I., Grau, G. E., Hollingdale, M. R., Ballou, W. R., and Gordon, D. M., 1993, Humoral immune response in volunteers immunized with irradiated *Plasmodium falciparum* sporozoites, *Am. J. Trop. Med. Hyg.* **49**:166–173.

Fairley, N. H., 1947, Sidelights on malaria in man obtained by subinoculation experiments, *Trans. R. Soc. Trop. Med. Hyg.* **40**:621–676.

Ferreira, A., Schofield, L., Enea, V., Schellekens, H., van der Meide, P., Collins, W. E., Nussenzweig, R. S., and Nussenzweig, V., 1986, Inhibition of development of exoerythrocytic forms of malaria parasites by gamma-interferon, *Science* **232**:881–884.

Fries, L. F., Gordon, D. M., Schneider, I., Beier, J. C., Long, G. W., Gross, M., Que, J. U., Cryz, S. J., and Sadoff, J. C., 1992, Safety, immunogenicity, and efficacy of a *Plasmodium falciparum* vaccine comprising a circumsporozoite protein repeat region peptide conjugated to *Pseudomonas aeruginosa* toxin A, *Infect. Immun.* **60**:1834–1839.

Gonzalez, C., Hone, D., Noriega, F. R., Tacket, C. O., Davis, J. R., Losonsky, G., Nataro, J. P., Hoffman, S., Malik, A., Nardin, E., Sztein, M. B., Heppner, D. G., Fouts, T. R., Isibasi, A., and Levine, M. M., 1994, Salmonella typhi vaccine strain CVD 908 expressing the circumsporozoite protein of *Plasmodium falciparum*: Strain construction and safety and immunogenicity in humans, *J. Infect. Dis.* **169**:927–931.

Gordon, D. M., Cosgriff, T. M., Schneider, I., Wasserman, G. F., Majarian, W. R., Hollingdale, M. R., and Chulay, J. D., 1990, Safety and immunogenicity of a *Plasmodium vivax* sporozoite vaccine, *Am. J. Trop. Med. Hyg.* **42**:527–531.

Guerin-Marchand, C., Druilhe, P., Galey, B., Londono, A., Patarapotikul, J., Beaudoin, R.L., Dubeaux, C., Tartar, A., Mercereau Puijalon, O., and Langsley, G., 1987, A liver-stage-specific antigen of *Plasmodium falciparum* characterized by gene cloning, *Nature* **329**:164–167.

Hedstrom, R. C., Campbell, J. R., Leef, M. L., Charoenvit, Y., Carter, M., Sedegah, M., Beaudoin, R. L., and Hoffman, S. L., 1990, A malaria sporozoite surface antigen distinct from the circumsporozoite protein, *Bull. WHO* **68**:152–157.

Herrington, D. A., Clyde, D. F., Losonsky, G., Cortesia, M., Murphy, J. R., Davis, J., Baqar, S., Felix, A. M., Heimer, E. P., Gillessen, D., Nardin, E., Nussenzweig, R. S., Nussenzweig, V., Hollingdale, M. R., and Levine, M. M., 1987, Safety and immunogenicity in man of a synthetic peptide malaria vaccine against *Plasmodium falciparum* sporozoites, *Nature* **328**:257–259.

Herrington, D., Davis, J., Nardin, E., Beier, M., Cortese, J., Eddy, H., Losonsky, G., Hollingdale, M., Sztein, M., Levine, M., Nussenzweig, R. S., Clyde, D., and Edelman, R., 1991, Successful immunization of humans with irradiated sporozoites: Humoral and cellular responses of the protected individuals, *Am. J. Trop. Med. Hyg.* **45**:539–547.

Herrington, D. A., Losonsky, G. A., Smith, G., Volvovitz, F., Cochran, M., Jackson, K., Hoffman, S. L., Gordon, D. M., Levine, M. M., and Edelman, R., 1992, Safety and immunogenicity in volunteers of a recombinant *Plasmodium falciparum* circumsporozoite protein malaria vaccine produced in lepidopteran cells, *Vaccine* **10**:841–846.

Hoffman, S. L., Oster, C. N., Plowe, C. V., Woollett, G. R., Beier, J. C., Chulay, J. D., Wirtz, R. A., Hollingdale, M. R., and Mugambi, M., 1987, Naturally acquired antibodies to sporozoites do not prevent malaria: Vaccine development implications, *Science* **237**:639–642.

Hoffman, S. L., Isenbarger, D., Long, G. W., Sedegah, M., Szarfman, A., Waters, L., Hollingdale, M. R., van der Miede, P. H., Finbloom, D. S., and Ballou, W. R., 1989, Sporozoite vaccine induces genetically restricted T cell elimination of malaria from hepatocytes, *Science* **244**:1078–1081.

Hoffman, S. L., Nussenzweig, V., Sadoff, J. C., and Nussenzweig, R. S., 1991, Progress toward malaria preerythrocytic vaccines, *Science* **252**:520–521.

Hoffman, S. L., Franke, E. D., Rogers, W. O., and Mellouk, S., 1993, Preerythrocytic malaria vaccine development, in: *Molecular Immunological Considerations in Malaria Vaccine Development* (M. F. Good and A. J. Saul, eds.), CRC Press, Boca Raton, pp. 149–167.

Hoffman, S. L., Edelman, R., Bryan, J., Schneider, I., Davis, J., Sedegah, M., Gordon, D., Church, P., Gross, M., Silverman, C., Hollingdale, M., Clyde, D., Sztein, M., Losonsky, G., Paparello, S., and Jones, T. R., 1994, Safety, immunogenicity, and efficacy of a malaria sporozoite vaccine administered with monophosphoryl lipid A, cell wall skeleton of mycobacteria and squalane as adjuvant, *Am. J. Trop. Med. Hyg.* **51**:603–612.

Hollingdale, M. R., Aikawa, M., Atkinson, C. T., Ballou, W. R., Chen, G., Li, J., Meis, J. F., Sina, B., Wright, C., and Zhu, J., 1990, Non-CS pre-erythrocytic protective antigens, *Immunol. Lett.* **25**:71–76.

Khusmith, S., Charoenvit, Y., Kumar, S., Sedegah, M., Beaudoin, R. L., and Hoffman, S. L., 1991, Protection against malaria by vaccination with sporozoite surface protein 2 plus CS protein, *Science* **252**:715–718.

Khusmith, S., Sedegah, M., and Hoffman, S. L., 1994, Complete protection against *Plasmodium yoelii* by adoptive transfer of a CD8+ T cell clone recognizing sporozoite surface protein 2, *Infect. Immun.* **62**:2979–2983.

Kumar, S., Miller, L. H., Quakyi, I. A., Keister, D. B., Houghten, R. A., Maloy, W. L., Moss, B., Berzofsky, J. A., and Good, M. F., 1988, Cytotoxic T cells specific for the circumsporozoite protein of *Plasmodium falciparum*, *Nature* **334**:258–260.

Li, S., Rodrigues, M., Rodriguez, D., Rodriguez, J. R., Esteban, M., Palese, P., Nussenzweig, R. S., and Zavala, F., 1993, Priming with recombinant influenza virus followed by administration of recombinant vaccinia virus induces CD8+ T-cell-mediated protective immunity against malaria, *Proc. Natl. Acad. Sci. USA* **90**:5214–5218.

McCutchan, T. F., Lal, A. A., De La Cruz, V. F., Miller, L. H., Maloy, W. L., Charoenvit, Y., Beaudoin, R. L., Guerry, P., Hoffman, S. L., Hockmeyer, W. T., Collins, W. E., and Wirth, D., 1985, Sequence of the immunodominant epitope for the surface protein on sporozoites of *Plasmodium vivax*, *Science* **230**:1381–1383.

Maheshwari, R. K., Czarniecki, C. W., Dutta, G. P., Puri, S. K., Dhawan, B. N., and Friedman, R. M., 1986, Recombinant human gamma interferon inhibits simian malaria, *Infect. Immun.* **53**:628–630.

Malik, A., Egan, J. E., Houghton, R. A., Sadoff, J. C., and Hoffman, S. L., 1991, Human cytotoxic T lymphocytes against *Plasmodium falciparum* circumsporozoite protein, *Proc. Natl. Acad. Sci. USA* **88**:3300–3304.

Mellouk, S., Maheshwari, R. K., Rhodes-Feuillette, A., Beaudoin, R. L., Berbiguier, N., Matile, H., Miltgen, F., Landau, I., Pied, S., Chigot, J. P., Friedman, R. M., and Mazier, D., 1987, Inhibitory activity of interferons and interleukin 1 on the development of *Plasmodium falciparum* in human hepatocyte cultures, *J. Immunol.* **139**:4192–4195.

Mellouk, S., Green, S. J., Nacy, C. A., and Hoffman, S. L., 1991, IFN-γ inhibits development of *Plasmodium berghei* exoerythrocytic stages in hepatocytes by an L-arginine-dependent effector mechanism, *J. Immunol.* **146**:3971–3976.

Migliorini, P., Betschart, B., and Corradin, G., 1993, Malaria vaccine: Immunization of mice with a synthetic T cell helper epitope alone leads to protective immunity, *Eur. J. Immunol.* **23**:582–585.

Moreno, A., Clavijo, P., Edelman, R., Davis, J., Sztein, M., Herrington, D., and Nardin, E., 1991, Cytotoxic CD4+ T cells from a sporozoite-immunized volunteer recognize the *Plasmodium falciparum* CS protein, *Int. Immunol.* **3**:997–1003.

Mulligan, H. W., Russell, P., and Mohan, B. N., 1941, Active immunization of fowls against *Plasmodium gallinaceum* by injections of killed homologous sporozoites, *J. Malar. Inst. India* **4**:25–34.

Nussenzweig, R. S., Vanderberg, J., Most, H., and Orton, C., 1967, Protective immunity produced by the injection of X-irradiated sporozoites of *Plasmodium berghei*, *Nature* **216**:160–162.

Nussler, A., Drapier, J.-C., Renia, L., Pied, S., Miltgen, F., Gentilini, M., and Mazier, D., 1991a, L-Arginine-dependent destruction of intrahepatic malaria parasites in response to tumor necrosis factor and/or interleukin 6 stimulation, *Eur. J. Immunol.* **21**:227–230.

Nussler, A. Pied, S., Goma, J., Renia, L., Miltgen, F., Grau, G. E., and Mazier, D., 1991b, TNF inhibits malaria hepatic stages in vitro via synthesis of IL-6, *Int. J. Immunol.* **3**:317–321.

Pancake, S. J., Holt, G. D., Mellouk, S., and Hoffman, S. L., 1992, Malaria sporozoites and circumsporozoite proteins bind specifically to sulfated glycoconjugates, *J. Cell Biol.* **117**:1351–1367.

Pied, S., Renia, L., Nussler, A., Miltgen, F., and Mazier, D., 1991, Inhibitory activity of IL-6 on malaria hepatic stages, *Parasite Immunol.* **13**:211–217.

Potocnjak, P., Yoshida, N., Nussenzweig, R. S., and Nussenzweig, V., 1980, Monovalent fragments (Fab) of monoclonal antibodies to a sporozoite surface antigen (Pb44) protect mice against malaria infection, *J. Exp. Med.* **151**:1504–1513.

Renia, L., Marussig, M. S., Grillot, D., Pied, S., Corradin, G., Miltgen, F., Del Giudice, G., and Mazier, D., 1991, In vitro activity of CD4$^+$ and CD8$^+$ T lymphocytes from mice immunized with a synthetic malaria peptide, *Proc. Natl. Acad. Sci. USA* **88**:7963–7967.

Rickman, L. S., Gordon, D. M., Wistar, R., Krzych, U., Gross, M., Hollingdale, M. R., Egan, J. E., Chulay, J. D., and Hoffman, S. L., 1991, Use of adjuvant containing mycobacterial cell-wall skeleton, monophosphoryl lipid A, and squalane in malaria circumsporozoite protein vaccine, *Lancet* **337**:998–1001.

Rieckmann, K. H., Carson, P. E., Beaudoin, R. L., Cassells, J. S., and Sell, K. W., 1974, Sporozoite induced immunity in man against an Ethiopian strain of *Plasmodium falciparum*, *Trans. R. Soc. Trop. Med. Hyg.* **68**:258–259.

Rieckmann, K. H., Beaudoin, R. L., Cassells, J. S., and Sell, K. W., 1979, Use of attenuated sporozoites in the immunization of human volunteers against falciparum malaria, *Bull. WHO* **57**:261–265.

Robson, K. J., Hall, J. R., Jennings, M. W., Harris, T. J., Marsh, K., Newbold, C. I., Tate, V. E., and Weatherall, D. J., 1988, A highly conserved amino-acid sequence in thrombospondin, properdin and in proteins from sporozoites and blood stages of a human malaria parasite, *Nature* **335**:79–82.

Rodrigues, M. M., Cordey, A.-S., Arreaza, G., Corradin, G., Romero, P., Maryanski, J. L., Nussenzweig, R. S., and Zavala, F., 1991, CD8$^+$ cytolytic T cell clones derived against the *Plasmodium yoelii* circumsporozoite protein protect against malaria, *Int. Immunol.* **3**:579–585.

Rodrigues, M., Nussenzweig, R. S., Romero, P., and Zavala, F., 1992, The in vivo cytotoxic activity of CD8$^+$ T cell clones correlates with their levels of expression of adhesion molecules, *J. Exp. Med.* **175**:895–905.

Rogers, W. O., Malik, A., Mellouk, S., Nakamura, K., Rogers, M. D., Szarfman, A., Gordon, D. M., Nussler, A. K., Aikawa, M., and Hoffman, S. L., 1992a, Characterization of *Plasmodium falciparum* sporozoite surface protein 2, *Proc. Natl. Acad. Sci. USA* **89**:9176–9180.

Rogers, W. O., Rogers, M. D., Hedstrom, R. C., and Hoffman, S. L., 1992b, Characterization of the gene encoding sporozoite surface protein 2, a protective *Plasmodium yoelii* sporozoite antigen, *Mol. Biochem. Parasitol.* **53**:45–52.

Romero, P., Maryanski, J. L., Corradin, G., Nussenzweig, R. S., Nussenzweig, V., and Zavala, F., 1989, Cloned cytotoxic T cells recognize an epitope in the circumsporozoite protein and protect against malaria, *Nature* **341**:323–325.

Sadoff, J. C., Cryz, S., Zollinger, W. D., Furer, E., Loomis, L. D., Hockmeyer, W. T., Chulay, J. D., and Ballou, W. R., 1987, Human immunization with covalent conjugate *Plasmodium falciparum* sporozoite vaccines, *3rd International Congress on Malaria and Babesiosis* p. 269 (Abstract).

Sadoff, J. C., Ballou, W. R., Baron, L. S., Majarian, W. R., Brey, R. N., Hockmeyer, W. T., Young, J. F., Cryz, S. J., Ou, J., Lowell, G. H., and Chulay, J. D., 1988, Oral *Salmonella typhimurium* vaccine expressing circumsporozoite protein protects against malaria, *Science* **240**:336–338.

Satchidanandam, V., Zavala, F., and Moss, B., 1991, Studies using a recombinant vaccinia virus expressing the circumsporozoite protein of *Plasmodium berghei*, *Mol. Biochem. Parasitol.* **48**:89–100.

Schofield, L., Ferreira, A., Nussenzweig, V., and Nussenzweig, R., 1987a, Antimalarial activity of alpha tumor necrosis factor and gamma interferon, *Fed. Proc.* **46**:760.

Schofield, L., Villaquiran, J., Ferreira, A., Schellekens, H., Nussenzweig, R. S., and Nussenzweig, V., 1987b, Gamma-interferon, CD8$^+$ T cells and antibodies required for immunity to malaria sporozoites, *Nature* **330**:664–666.

Sedegah, M., Beaudoin, R. L., De la Vega, P., Leef, M. F., Ozcel, M. A., Jones, E., Charoenvit, Y., Yuan, L. F., Gross, M., Majarian, W. R., Robey, F. A., Weiss, W., and Hoffman, S. L., 1988, Use of a vaccinia construct expressing the circumsporozoite protein in the analysis of protective immunity to *Plasmo-*

dium yoelii, in: Technological Advances in Vaccine Development (L. Lasky, ed.), Liss, New York, pp. 295–309.

Sedegah, M., Beaudoin, R. L., Majarian, W. R., Cochran, M. D., Chiang, C. H., Sadoff, J., Aggarwal, A., Charoenvit, Y., and Hoffman, S. L., 1990, Evaluation of vaccines designed to induce protective cellular immunity against the *Plasmodium yoelii* circumsporozoite protein: Vaccinia, pseudorabies, and salmonella transformed with circumsporozoite gene, *Bull. WHO* **68**(Suppl.):109–114.

Sedegah, M., Chiang, C. H., Weiss, W. R., Mellouk, S., Cochran, M. D., Houghton, R. A., Beaudoin, R. L., Smith, D., and Hoffman, S. L., 1992a, Recombinant pseudorabies virus carrying a plasmodium gene: Herpesvirus as a new live viral vector for inducing T- and B-cell immunity, *Vaccine* **10**:578–584.

Sedegah, M., Sim, B. K. L., Mason, C., Nutman, T., Malik, A., Roberts, C., Johnson, A., Ochola, J., Koech, D., Were, B., and Hoffman, S. L., 1992b, Naturally acquired CD8[+] cytotoxic T lymphocytes against the *Plasmodium falciparum* circumsporozoite protein, *J. Immunol.* **149**:966–971.

Sedegah, M., Hedstrom, R. C., and Hoffman, S. L., 1994a, Protection against malaria by immunization with circumsporozoite protein plasmid DNA, *Clin. Res.* **42**:282A.

Sedegah, M., Finkelman, F., and Hoffman, S. L., 1994b, Interleukin 12 induction of interferon γ-dependent protection against malaria, *Proc. Natl. Acad. Sci.* **91**:10700–10702.

Sturchler, D., Berger, R., Etlinger, H., Fernex, M., Matile, H., Pink, R., Schlumbom, V., and Just, M., 1989, Effects of interferons on immune response to a synthetic peptide malaria sporozoite vaccine in non-immune adults, *Vaccine* **7**:457–461.

Suhrbier, A., Winger, L., O'Dowd, C., Hodivala, K., and Sinden, R. E., 1990, An antigen specific to the liver stage of rodent malaria recognized by a monoclonal antibody, *Parasite Immunol.* **12**:473–481.

Tam, J. P., Clavijo, P., Lu, Y., Nussenzweig, V., Nussenzweig, R., and Zavala, F., 1990, Incorporation of T and B epitopes of the circumsporozoite protein in a chemically defined synthetic vaccine against malaria, *J. Exp. Med.* **171**:299–306.

Vanderberg, J., Nussenzweig, R., and Most, H., 1969, Protective immunity produced by the injection of X-irradiated sporozoites of *Plasmodium berghei*. V. In vitro effects of immune serum on sporozoites, *Mil. Med.* **134**:1183–1190.

Vergara, U., Ruiz, A., Ferreira, A., Nussenzweig, R. S., and Nussenzwieg, V., 1985, Conserved group-specific epitopes of the circumsporozoite proteins revealed by antibodies to synthetic peptides, *J. Immunol.* **134**:3445–3448.

Vreden, S. G., Verhave, J. P., Oettinger, T., Sauerwein, R. W., and Meuwissen, J. H., 1991, Phase I clinical trial of a recombinant malaria vaccine consisting of the circumsporozoite repeat region of *Plasmodium falciparum* coupled to hepatitis B surface antigen, *Am. J. Trop. Med. Hyg.* **45**:533–538.

Wang, R., Charoenvit, Y., Corradin, G. P., Porrozzi, R., Hunter, R. L., Glen, G., Alving, C. R., Church, P., and Hoffman, S. L., Complete protection of outbred mice against *Plasmodium yoelii* by immunization with a circumsporozoite protein multiple antigen peptide vaccine, *J. Immunol.* (in press).

Weiss, W. R., Mellouk, S., Houghten, R. A., Sedegah, M., Kumar, S., Good, M. F., Berzofsky, J. A., Miller, L. H., and Hoffman, S. L., 1990, Cytotoxic T cells recognize a peptide from the circumsporozoite protein on malaria-infected hepatocytes, *J. Exp. Med.* **171**:763–773.

Weiss, W. R., Berzovsky, J. A., Houghten, R., Sedegah, M., Hollingdale, M., and Hoffman, S. L., 1992, A T cell clone directed at the circumsporozoite protein which protects mice against both *P. yoelii* and *P. berghei*, *J. Immunol.* **149**:2103–2109.

Wizel, B., Rodgers, W. O., Houghten, R. A., Lanar, D. E., Tine, J. A., and Hoffman, S. L., 1994, Induction of murine cytotoxic T lymphocytes against Plasmodium falciparum sporozoite surface protein 2, *Eur. J. Immunol.* **24**:1487–1495.

Zavala, F., Tam, J. P., Barr, P. J., Romero, P. J., Ley, V., Nussenzweig, R. S., and Nussenzweig, V., 1987, Synthetic peptide vaccine confers protection against murine malaria, *J. Exp. Med.* **166**:1591–1596.

Zhu, J., and Hollingdale, M. R., 1991, Structure of *Plasmodium falciparum* liver stage antigen-1, *Mol. Biochem. Parasitol.* **48**:223–226.

Chapter 36

The MAP System

A Flexible and Unambiguous Vaccine Design of Branched Peptides

Bernardetta Nardelli and James P. Tam

1. INTRODUCTION

Conventional vaccines consisting of either killed or attenuated infectious agents are limited in their potential by several factors. These include hazards associated with the production, storage that requires a cold chain, presence of contaminating materials, risk of infection in immunocompromised people, and unwanted side effects in the case of incomplete attenuation of the pathogen.

Peptide-based vaccines have advantages, compared to the traditional approaches, of being selective, chemically defined, and safe (Brown, 1990). Short stretches of amino acid sequences, containing epitopes able to elicit a protective immune response, can be selected from a protein. This allows for the elimination of other epitopes, which may be responsible for inducing nonspecific or undesirable stimulation of the immune system (Adorini *et al.*, 1979; Robinson *et al.*, 1990; Robinson and Kehoe, 1992). Peptides can be synthesized to include antigenic determinants that are nonimmunogenic when the whole protein is used (Green *et al.*, 1982). Large quantities of chemically purified peptide vaccines can be prepared with automated methods. Furthermore, peptide-based immunogens are more likely to be resistant to denaturation, and they can be easily stored and transported without refrigeration.

The multiple antigen peptide (MAP) system was created by Tam (Tam, 1988; Posnett *et al.*, 1988) to overcome the requirement for the conjugation of synthetic peptides to carrier proteins. Chemical cross-linking of a peptide to itself or to a carrier has been shown to

Bernardetta Nardelli • Medicine Department, Infectious Diseases Division, New York University Medical Center, New York, New York 10016. *James P. Tam* • Microbiology and Immunology Department, Vanderbilt University, Nashville, Tennessee 37232.

Vaccine Design: The Subunit and Adjuvant Approach, edited by Michael F. Powell and Mark J. Newman. Plenum Press, New York, 1995.

result in modified antigenic determinants (Briand *et al.*, 1985; Flexner, 1990), and undesirable immune responses to the carrier protein have been described (Schutze *et al.*, 1985; Herzenberg and Tokuhisa, 1983). Therefore, the aim of obtaining specific antibodies against predetermined antigenic epitopes may be hindered by the conjugation of the peptides to the carriers.

In this chapter, we summarize the antigenicity, capacity to interact with immune receptors, and immunogenicity, capacity to elicit lymphocyte activation and proliferation, of MAP-based synthetic vaccine models for several infectious diseases. We also describe a new MAP model containing a built-in adjuvant that is effective in inducing humoral and cellular responses following either parenteral or oral administration of the immunogens.

2. MAP DESIGN AND SYNTHESIS

The key feature of the MAP system is the amplification of a peptide antigen in a chemically defined manner. Unlike random polymerization, which usually leads to linear arrays of a wide range distribution of polymers, the MAP system produces branched peptides with an unambiguous structure in a controlled manner. This is achieved by utilizing a core matrix that consists of several sequential levels of trifunctional amino acids as a scaffold (Tam, 1988). Lysine is used because it has two functional ends available for the branching reactions, the α- and ε-amino groups. The first level of coupling produces two reactive amino ends to give a bivalent MAP (Fig. 1). Further sequential propagation of lysines produces MAPs containing tetravalent or octavalent reactive amino ends, which are highly immunogenic. The peptide antigens as well as the core matrix are synthesized in a continuous sequence by the stepwise solid-phase using Boc-benzyl chemistry or Fmoc-tert-butyl chemistry; the synthesis is similar to that used to produce a linear peptide. A conventional method of coupling mediated by dicyclohexylcarbodiimide/1-hydroxy-benzotriazole in dimethylformamide is then used to produce the MAP structure. The MAP resins are treated with deprotecting reagents and the peptides are cleaved from the resins

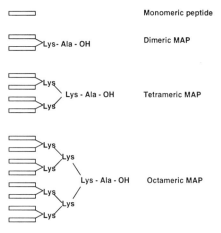

Figure 1.   Schematic representation of MAP constructs.

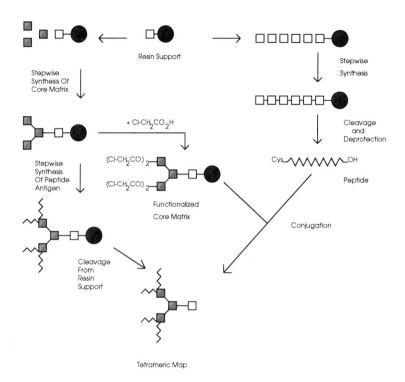

Figure 2. Direct and indirect synthesis methods of MAP constructs.

with low/high hydrogen fluoride (Boc chemistry) or with 95% trifluoroacetic acid (Fmoc chemistry) to yield crude MAPs. The MAPs are then extracted with urea and dialyzed with suitable buffer, and, after lyophilization, characterized by high-performance gel chromatography and amino acid analysis. The resulting molecules contain multiple antigenic determinants surrounding the small branching lysine cores in high-density clusters.

In general, the orientation of a peptide immunogen is important for the generation of antibodies (Dyrberg and Oldstone, 1986). In a MAP construct, the presence of the lysine core at the carboxyl-end creates a polarity preference. If the selected epitope is a carboxyl fragment of a protein, an indirect modular method (Fig. 2) can be used instead of the direct stepwise approach for synthesis. The indirect method consists of the syntheses of a functionalized core matrix and peptide antigens separately, followed by the conjugation of these two components (Lu *et al.*, 1991). There are many methods suitable for conjugating peptide antigens to the core matrix; all of these methods use unprotected peptides. A popular approach is the use of the thiol-alkylation reaction where the peptide is made with a cysteine residue at either the NH_2- or COOH-terminus. This cysteine can be attached to the branching lysine core, which contains a chloroacetyl group (Fig. 2). Other methods developed in our laboratory utilize weak base–aldehyde chemistry. Weak bases, such as cysteine, phenylhydrazine, hydrazide, and amino(oxyl)acetyl groups, can react with aldehydes to form a stable linkage at acidic pH. Unlike the conventional protein carrier conjugation, the immunogen prepared by the indirect method retains the main advantages inherent to the MAP system, namely, small nonimmunogenic core matrix and chemical unambiguity.

Because the backbone of MAPs is made up of amide bonds, most MAPs are remarkably stable in solution between pH 2 and 9. Thus, storage of MAPs should not constitute a significant problem. The design of MAPs using short dendritic peptides makes them resistant to denaturation; therefore, MAPs can be easily stored or shipped as lyophilized powder. These advantages are significant when compared with recombinant proteins or whole pathogen vaccine preparations, which require a cold chain of storage to retain reactivity.

A patent covering the usage of MAPs in vaccines and diagnostics was issued by the U.S. Patent Office (Tam, 1993). Two other related patents on MAPs, including those containing lipidated moieties as built-in adjuvants, were also filed and are in the process of approval. The rights of these patents belong to the Rockefeller University. Others, notably United Biochemical Inc. (Wang, 1989), have also filed patents on aspects of MAPs mainly focusing on specific antigens for AIDS vaccines.

3. MAP ANTIGENICITY

MAP constructs represent a valuable approach for increasing the sensitivity of solid-phase immunoassays that utilize synthetic peptides as antigens (Tam and Zavala, 1989; Marguerite *et al.*, 1992; Briand *et al.*, 1992). MAPs bind to plastic surfaces better than do the corresponding monomers; thus, they can be used at concentrations much lower than the monomeric peptide to detect specific antibodies. This is particularly true when short linear peptides lacking hydrophobic side chains are used (Tam and Zavala, 1989). Tam and Zavala (1989) related the sensitivity of detection to the number of the branching chains in four MAP models. While the dimer was the least reactive, the octameric MAP produced the maximal reactivity. A possible explanation could be that in the MAPs the multimeric arrangement of the branched peptides allows some side chains to bind the surface of the plastic while others are available to interact with the antibody. This is consistent with the study by Marguerite *et al.* (1992) showing that an octameric MAP was a more effective antigen in a solid-phase immunoassay than a tandem repeat, a copolymer composed of glutaraldehyde-cross-linked monomeric peptides, and the peptide alone. MAPs were also suitable to use for the detection of very low levels of serum antibodies (Habluetzel *et al.*, 1991; Marsden *et al.*, 1992). Solid-phase immunoassays based on MAPs are, therefore, a promising tool for serodiagnosis in naturally immunized or infected individuals.

4. MAP IMMUNOGENICITY

In addition to the physical and chemical properties mentioned in Section 1, several points regarding the immunogenic properties of the MAPs should be emphasized.

4.1. Production of a High-Titered Antibody Response

A linear peptide ineffective in raising antibodies can become immunogenic if given in a MAP format (Del Giudice *et al.*, 1990; Kamo *et al.*, 1992). Moreover, antibody titers induced by MAP peptides were found to be superior to those obtained by the corresponding linear form of the peptide conjugated to a carrier protein. For example, an 11-residue MAP construct representing an internal sequence from the tyrosine kinase protein p60[src] elicited higher-titered primary and secondary responses than the same linear peptide conjugated to keyhole limpet hemocyanin (Tam, 1988). An explanation for these observed results is that a MAP attains a polymeric and macromolecular structure when compared to a linear peptide, which in turn may be cleared from the body at a faster rate than a MAP.

It should be pointed out that, in comparison to a carrier-conjugated peptide, the MAP macromolecule has the molecular weight of a small protein in which the antigen peptide represents more than 80% of the total structure. No immune response to the lysine residues has been detected (Posnett *et al.*, 1988; Del Giudice *et al.*, 1990).

4.2. Reactivity of the Elicited Antisera against the Cognate Proteins

Since the initial experiments with MAP constructs, it was evident that the immunization with this polymeric structure resulted in the production of antisera capable of recognizing the cognate sequence of the native protein (Tam, 1988). To demonstrate this, six octameric MAP models were synthesized from sequences of unrelated proteins and injected in mice and rabbits. All MAPs elicited a strong antibody response against the immunizing peptide, and five of them induced antibodies that reacted with the native proteins. Among other reports, we can mention the results obtained by Wolowczuk *et al.* (1991) with a MAP construct consisting of eight copies of the sequence 115–131 derived from the Sm-28-GST antigen of *Schistosoma mansoni*. The immunization with this construct elicited protein-specific antibodies that were able to mediate antibody-dependent cytotoxicity toward the parasite in vitro. Moreover, immunized rats were partially protected against the challenge of infectious *S. mansoni* cercariae. A study was performed to compare the immunogenicity of the octameric MAP and several constructs of the 115–131 peptide, including a single copy peptide, a polymer and a tandem repeat both containing three copies of the peptide (Marguerite *et al.*, 1992). The octameric MAP was found to induce the highest humoral and cellular responses to the Sm-28-GST protein.

In some cases, significant differences have been observed using MAPs and peptide–protein conjugates as immunogens. Immune sera generated by the administration of MAP peptides have been found to react with the cognate protein, whereas antisera generated by the corresponding linear peptide conjugated to a protein carrier induced high antibody titers only against the immunizing peptide (Troalen *et al.*, 1990; Kamo *et al.*, 1992). The MAP format, furthermore, allowed the investigators to overcome the immunodominance of the linker and the carrier used in making the conjugated peptide, and to produce a monoclonal antibody directed against a highly conserved and very poorly immunogenic sequence (Kamo *et al.*, 1992).

4.3. Correlation MAP Structure and Immunogenicity

A frequently asked question relates to the optimal number of branches needed for the MAP construct. This question was partially answered in a comparative study on the major immunogenic epitope of foot-and-mouth disease virus (FMDV) serotype O, which can be defined by the amino acid sequence 141–160 of the protein VP1. This peptide was found to be immunogenic in the absence of protein carrier when polymerized, thus indicating the presence, in the same sequence, of residues recognized by antibody-producing and T-helper cells (Francis *et al.*, 1987). This peptide was, therefore, used as a model to evaluate the effect that varying the number of the branching chains had on MAP immunogenicity (Francis *et al.*, 1991). Guinea pigs were immunized with monomeric, dimeric, tetrameric, and octameric FMDV VP1 emulsified in IFA. Primary and secondary responses elicited by the tetrameric construct were similar to those obtained with the octamer, and significantly superior to that obtained with the dimer. The administration of the monomeric peptide did not generate an antibody response. The antisera were then tested against sets of peptides within the 141–160 linear sequence to map their reactivity sites. It was found that the antibodies elicited by the octameric construct, in comparison to the others, were less specific for the N-terminal residues of the sequence, which are believed to be involved in the neutralization of the virus. It appears, therefore, that in the FMDV system the presentation of an antigenic peptide in a tetrameric structure is sufficient for an optimal response.

4.4. Enhanced Immunogenicity of MAPs Containing B- and T-Cell Epitopes, and Protection Mediated by the Immune Sera

The generation of an optimal antibody response requires the recognition of the antigenic peptide fragments by T-helper cells which in turn promote the engagement of antigen-specific B cells. An effective synthetic immunogen should, therefore, contain sequences known to activate both T and B lymphocytes.

An important characteristic of the MAP system is the ability to incorporate multiple epitopes in the same construct (Fig. 3). The incorporation of both T and B epitopes from the same pathogen into the immunogen might be particularly useful to enhance a specific immune response when infection occurs. These types of MAP constructs have been extensively studied in the malaria vaccine model. An immunodominant B-cell epitope (aa 93–108) in the circumsporozoite protein of the rodent malaria parasite *Plasmodium berghei*, consisting of a repeat of a 16-amino-acid sequence, has been identified. A T-helper cell epitope (aa 265–276) recognized by several mouse strains and mapped in the same protein has also been identified. Ten MAP constructs were synthesized based on these T- and B-cell epitopes. The different constructs were designed to evaluate the relevance of numbers of copies, stoichiometry, and orientation of T- and B-cell sequences in a diepitope model (Tam *et al.*, 1990). This included tetrameric and octameric MAPs containing only the T- and the B-cell epitopes, or containing both epitopes linked in tandem. High antibody titers were induced by the immunization with MAPs containing equimolar amounts of the T- and B-cell epitopes, while monoepitope MAPs and the BT monomer were not immunogenic in the A/J mice used in these experiments. In general, the results indicated that

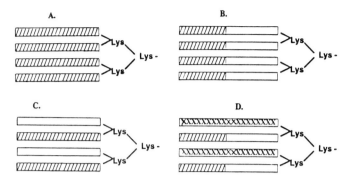

Figure 3. Arrangements of four types of MAP configurations containing one, two, and three antigens connected in tandem or alternating forms to the lysine core (a) mono-antigen, (b) di-antigen (tandem), (c) di-antigen (alternating), (d) tri-antigen.

there was no real advantage to using an octameric over a tetrameric diepitope. The BT construct, in which the T epitope was next to the polylysine core, appeared to be the most efficient immunogen. Most importantly, the antibody responses elicited by the MAP peptides were found to be protective against the intravenous challenge of the immunized mice with 2000 *P. berghei* sporozoites (Tam *et al.*, 1990). The degree of protection correlated with the antibody levels obtained by the immunization protocol (Table I). Administration of the tetrameric BT construct in alum did raise strong humoral response (Chai *et al.*, 1992). However, the antibody titers were lower than those obtained by the same antigen in CFA emulsion.

Table I
Protective Efficacy of Different MAP Models in Mice
Challenged with 2000 *P. berghei* Sporozoites[a]

Immunogen	Antisporozoite (IFA titer $\times 10^{-3}$)[b]	Number protected/challenged[c]	Protection (%)
BT-(4)	128	4/5	80
TB-(4)	32	3/5	60
TB-(8)	32	3/5	60
BT-(8)	8	2/4	50
T-(4)	<0.2	0/4	0
B-(4)	<0.2	0/5	0
B-(8)	<0.2	0/5	0
BT monomer	<0.2	0/5	0
No immunogen	—	0/5	0

[a]Reproduced from Tam *et al.*, 1990, *J. Exp. Med.* **171:**299–306, by copyright permission of the Rockefeller University Press.
[b]A/J mice were injected with 50 μg i.p. of the immunogens emulsified in CFA on day 0, and boosted with 50 μg of the same antigen in IFA on day 21. Sera were collected 34 days later and antibody titers were determined by IFA (immunofluorescence assay) using glutaraldehyde-fixed sporozoites.
[c]Mice were challenged by intravenous inoculations of 2000 sporozoites 35 days after the last booster injection. Pheripheral blood smears were examined daily for parasitized erythrocytes. Protection is defined as absence of parasites from day 3 to 12 after challenge.

Diepitope MAPs were synthesized in the design of a synthetic vaccine model for hepatitis B using a different chemical approach (Tam and Lu, 1989). A B-cell epitope (aa 139–147 of the S protein) and a T-cell epitope (aa 12–26 of the pre-S protein) were used in mono- and diepitope configurations. In the latter, the two peptides were connected in alternating forms on the lysine core, instead of being connected in tandem as in the malaria model. The B-cell determinant was found to be immunogenic in rabbits only when presented in a MAP construct containing the pre-S peptide.

The effectiveness of mono- and diepitope MAP configurations was further analyzed in a synthetic vaccine model for the human immunodeficiency virus type 1 (HIV-1) (Nardelli *et al.*, 1992a). In this paradigm, the monoepitope MAPs consisted of four copies of the major neutralizing determinant of HIV-1, which is localized in the third hypervariable region (V3) of the envelope protein gp120. Different MAPs were synthesized for three HIV-1 isolates (IIIB, RF, and MN). The diepitope MAPs contained a known T-helper cell sequence at the carboxyl-terminus of the various B-cell epitopes (aa 429–443 from gp120). The monoepitopes appeared to elicit a species-dependent antibody response, since mice were partial responders to the IIIB sequences (which contains a murine T-helper determinant), and nonresponders to the monoepitope MAPs of RF and MN isolates (in which no T-helper epitopes have been identified). However, the diepitopes were found to be immunogenic in all of the animal species tested. The antisera generated in rabbits by the diepitope MAPs had higher titers and neutralizing activity against homologous virus than those obtained by immunization with only the B-cell epitope. Moreover, a study by Levi *et al.* (1993) supported the use of MAPs in vaccination protocols based on combination of immunogens. The boosting of gp160-immunized rabbits with a MAP construct, consisting of B- and T-cell epitopes from the HIV-1 envelope protein, induced higher antibody neutralization titers and improved cellular immune responses than the boosting with the recombinant gp160 protein.

These cumulative findings in various experimental systems demonstrate that MAP constructs including appropriate T- and B-cell epitopes can overcome the poor immunogenicity of a monomeric peptide and can give rise to a very effective lymphocyte activation.

4.5. Generation of Long-Term Antibody Responses

An example of induction of a long-lasting humoral response by MAPs can be found in the study of Wang *et al.* (1991). Guinea pigs were immunized with a long linear peptide overlapping the V3 loop of gp120 (aa 297–329) conjugated with bovine serum albumin (BSA) or synthesized in an octameric MAP format. Antibody titers and neutralizing activity of the antisera produced by the BSA-conjugated peptide peaked 4 months after the beginning of the immunization protocol. At the same time point, the antibody titers induced by the MAPs were approximately in the same range. However, the neutralizing activity of the antisera induced by the MAP construct improved strikingly over time, reaching 30 to 50 times that of the BSA-conjugated peptide after 3 years. Moreover, with time the octamer-immunized animals produced cross-reacting antibodies capable of neutralizing unrelated HIV-1 isolates. This study illustrates the usefulness of a MAP construct containing nearly pure immunogenic peptides without the burden of a protein carrier.

4.6. Capacity of Overcoming MHC-Associated Nonresponsiveness

Pessi *et al.* (1991) have shown that the immunogenicity of an antigen not only can be improved but can also be significantly changed when presented in a MAP format. It is known that antibody responses to the repetitive sequence Asn-Ala-Asn-Pro in the malaria circumsporozoite protein of *Plasmodium falciparum* are under the control of the murine major histocompatibility complex (MHC), *H-2*. Synthetic peptides encompassing this repeat induce response only in the $H-2^b$ mice. The administration of a MAP Asn-Ala-Asn-Pro resulted in the antibody production by six different *H-2* haplotypes. The ability to correct the nonresponder status of certain mouse strains using an antigen presented as a MAP has not been reported for other circumsporozoite peptides (Munesinghe *et al.*, 1991). Nevertheless, the study by Pessi *et al.* (1991) is consistent with our experience that short peptides in MAP formats elicit antibody response while they are ineffective as monomeric forms. A plausible explanation may be that new helper epitopes are being generated in the MAP format, which are able to overcome MHC-linked nonresponsiveness. This intriguing property of MAPs is currently under study in our laboratories.

5. LIPIDATED MAP VACCINES

Adjuvants are needed for many immunization protocols using subunit vaccines to both enhance and direct immune responses. In experimental animal models, CFA, consisting of a water-in-oil emulsion of killed mycobacteria, augments antibody responses but is often associated with severe side effects, such as pyrogenicity. The only substances currently used in licensed human vaccines are aluminum salts, which are less effective than CFA in stimulating antibody response and only weakly activate the cellular immune system. In the search for a compound retaining the stimulant activity of CFA but without its toxicity, lipopeptides were isolated from the outer cell membrane of *Escherichia coli* and synthetic analogues were prepared (Wiesmüller *et al.*, 1983). The tripalmitoyl-*S*-glyceryl cysteine (P3C) was found to be particularly promising in the potentiation of antibody responses (Reitermann *et al.*, 1989) and capable of inducing a strong cellular response in vivo when coupled to cytotoxic T-lymphocyte (CTL) epitopes (Deres *et al.*, 1989). Because of these properties, we covalently linked P3C to antigenic MAP peptides to evaluate the possibility of generating a completely synthetic peptide-based vaccine immunogen without the need for a carrier and adjuvant (Defoort *et al.*, 1992). One of the peptides used was a V3 sequence from the gp120 envelope protein of HIV-1, IIIB isolate (aa 308–331), which contains a neutralizing B-cell epitope (Rusche *et al.*, 1988; Goudsmit *et al.*, 1988; Palker *et al.*, 1988; Kenealy *et al.*, 1989), a T-helper cell epitope (Palker *et al.*, 1989), and residues recognized by murine CTLs of the H-2^d phenotype (Takahashi *et al.*, 1988). This peptide was synthesized in a tetrabranched MAP configuration, called B1M, and coupled to the P3C moiety through a Ser-Ser linker (Fig. 4). Mice and guinea pigs were injected with the immunogen, B1M–P3C, free or further amplified by the presentation on liposomes (Table II). The total antibody titers of the immunized animals were lower than those obtained in previous experiments following the immunization with B1M in CFA. However, the neutralization titers of the guinea pig antisera generated by the

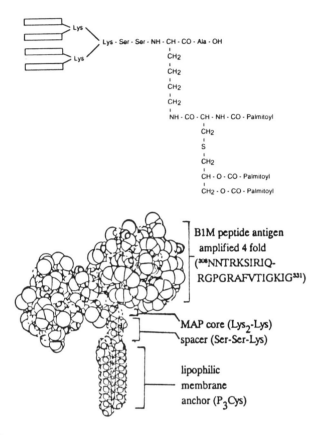

Figure 4. Schematic representation and computer-simulated model of B1M–P3C.

Table II
Antibody Response to B1M–P3C[a]

Immunogen	Antibody titer (×10⁻³)		Inhibition titer	
	Peptide	gp120	Syncytia	RT activity
No immunogen	<0.01	<0.01	0	0
B1M,P3C,liposomes	6.8	1.2	0	0
B1M–P3C/liposomes	6.5	3.2	20	8
B1M–P3C	8.2	3.3	10	8

[a]Dunkin–Hartley guinea pigs were immunized s.c. with 100 μg of the immunogens on days 0 and 14 and with 50 μg on days 30 and 45. Sera were collected 2 weeks after the last boost. The immunogens were: B1M mixed with P3C and liposomes (B1M,P3C,liposomes); B1M covalently linked to P3C and inserted in liposomes (B1M–P3C/liposomes); B1M covalently linked to P3C (B1M–P3C). Antibody titers represent the reciprocal of the end-point dilutions, sera dilutions at which OD were 0.2 unit, as measured in ELISA. Inhibition titers are calculated as fusion inhibition titers (inverse of the dilutions reducing by 90% the number of syncytia formed by CEMT4 cells infected with a recombinant vaccinia virus expressing gp160) and neutralization titers (inverse of the dilutions reducing by 87% the reverse transcriptase activity in HIV-1-infected H9 cells).

Table III
Induction of Peptide-Specific CTL Memory by B2M–P3C
Intraperitoneal or Intravenous Injection[a]

	Days after priming			
	3	7	30	200
i.p. immunization		% lysis		
20:1[b]	56(8)	94(6)	95(2)	58(2)
10:1	41(2)	92(5)	81(1)	45(0)
5:1	27(1)	85(3)	62(1)	30(0)
i.v. immunization				
20:1[b]	94(9)	92(4)	75(3)	ND[c]
10:1	86(6)	85(2)	52(2)	
5:1	71(3)	75(1)	33(2)	

[a]From Nardelli and Tam (1993).
[b]BALB/c mice were injected once i.p. or i.v. with 100 μg of B2M–P3C. The spleen cells were restimulated in vitro with B2M peptide (0.4 μM) at different times after the priming. CTL activity was determined on P815 target cells preincubated with B2M peptide using the effector-to-target cell ratios, E:T, indicated. In parentheses are reported the values obtained on untreated P815 cells.
[c]ND, not determined.

administration of B1M in CFA or B1M–P3C were similar (Nardelli et al., 1992a; Defoort et al., 1992).

B1M–P3C induced a strong T-cell response, as measured by IL-2 production and cytolytic activity of the splenocytes of the immunized mice (Defoort et al., 1992). In particular, the cytotoxic response was induced by the lipopeptide just after one immunization and was superior to the response induced by a full cycle of immunizations (four injections) of B1M in Freund's adjuvant (Nardelli, personal communication). We have

Table IV
CTL Activity Induced by Priming with a Single Peptide or with a Mixture [a,b]

		% specific lysis of peptide-pulsed targets (E:T)			
		P815 + IIIB peptide		P815 + MN peptide	
In vivo priming	HIV-1 isolates	20:1	10:1	20:1	10:1
B2M–P3C	IIIB	84	60	30	18
B8M–P3C	MN	10	5	62	38
B2M–P3C + B8M–P3C	IIIB+MN	90	84	57	38

[a]From Nardelli and Tam (1993).
[b]BALB/c mice were immunized once i.p. with B2M–P3C (20 μg) and B8M–P3C (80 μg) alone or B2M–P3C plus B8M–P3C (20+80 μg). After 5 days' culture, the cytotoxic activity of the IIIB- and MN-specific CTLs was tested against ^{51}Cr-labeled P815 targets pulsed with either 1 μM B2M or 4 μM B8M at the effector:target cell ratios (E:T) indicated.

Table V
Efficacy of B1M–P3C in Inducing Antibody and Cellular Responses following Different
Routes of Administration[a]

	Antibody titers	Cytotoxicity
Intraperitoneal	4300	95%
Subcutaneous	1300	53%
Intragastric	1020	88%
Intravenous	ND[b]	98%

[a]BALB/c mice were immunized with 100 μg of B1M–P3C in phosphate-buffered saline for four times. Sera were collected 10–15 days after the last boost. Antibody titers are expressed as the inverse of the last serum dilution that gave an optical density twofold above the values obtained with preimmune sera in ELISA using the MAP peptide as antigen. Splenic lymphocytes were restimulated in vitro with the relevant peptide for 5 days. Cytotoxicity is expressed as the percentage of specific lysis of radiolabeled syngeneic target cells pulsed with the B1 peptide and incubated for 4 h with splenocytes obtained from the immunized mice at the effector-to-target cell ratio of 20:1.
[b]ND, not determined.

demonstrated that the response was mediated by CD8[+] T lymphocytes, MHC class I molecule-restricted and antigen-specific (Nardelli and Tam, 1993). P815 cells expressing the HIV-1 glycoprotein gp160, following infection with a recombinant vaccinia virus, or pulsed with the relevant peptide aa 308–331 were efficiently killed by the syngeneic effector cells. No cytotoxic activity was generated against P815 cells infected with wild-type vaccinia virus or pulsed with peptides encompassing other sequences of gp120. The reactivity was long-lasting since it was still detectable 7 months after a single antigen injection (Table III). Moreover, the co-injection of MAP–P3C peptides (B2M–P3C, containing a sequence from the V3 region of the IIIB isolate, and B8M–P3C, containing the homologous V3 sequence from the MN isolate) generated CTLs capable of killing syngeneic target cells preincubated with either of the two sequences (Table IV). These results indicate the feasibility of using mixtures of lipidated MAP peptides as multivalent vaccines against infectious agents characterized by antigenic variation, such as HIV-1.

B1M–P3C was found to induce systemic antibody and cellular responses following several routes of immunization, including intraperitoneal, intravenous, subcutaneous, and intragastric (Nardelli et al., 1992b, 1994) (Table V). Moreover, after oral immunization, specific IgA were detected in the mouse saliva. The ability of MAP–P3C constructs to induce mucosal antibody response via oral administration may lead to their use as vaccines for the protection from pathogens that target mucosal surfaces.

6. CONCLUDING REMARKS

The structural and molecular bases for the effectiveness of MAP constructs to generate an improved antibody response in comparison to linear peptides have not yet been fully characterized. Peptides in the MAP format may have in vivo half lives that are longer than those of unconjugated linear peptides. Also the difference of conformation in solution between linear and MAP peptides likely contributes to the observed difference in immunogenicity. The proximity of the multiple copies of the peptide may create new interactions between peptide chains or facilitate the folding of the individual chains, leading to a

Table VI
Advantages of MAPs for Vaccine Design

Physical

No need for conjugation to carrier proteins, avoiding the potential consequences of epitopic suppression related to the carrier or antigenic inactivation of the immunogen resulting from the chemical coupling

Safety; nonreplicating, chemically defined molecules

Flexibility of incorporating multiple epitopes

Feasibility to produce antibody response against conformational determinants present on the native protein

Low cost, lyophilizable chemical product, stable without refrigeration

Immunological

Immunization against predetermined antigenic protein sequences, avoiding the stimulation of immune responses against suppressor or nonprotective immunodominant sequences present in the same protein

Cross-reaction with the parental protein; neutralizing activity against the pathogen infectivity in vitro; protection in vivo (murine malaria model)

Enhancement of specific B- and T-cell responses by presenting more than one immunogenic epitope. Feasibility to overcome genetic unresponsiveness by the incorporation of universal T-helper cell determinants

Generation of a long-lasting antibody response

Following coupling with the lipophilic moiety P3C, stimulation of a strong T-cell immune response; ability to be delivered by oral administration and to elicit IgA response

Feasibility to overcome MHC-associated nonresponsiveness

---

molecular structure of the immunogen similar to that of the native protein. The intracellular processing of a MAP peptide may also be different. The MAP configuration may avoid excessive proteolysis of the peptide and/or cause the formation of products with higher binding affinity to the class II MHC molecules. MAP immunogens do not appear to elicit a T-cell-independent antibody response, based on the observation that athymic *nu/nu* mice were nonresponders to a MAP construct (Del Giudice *et al.*, 1990).

While the answers to these questions await further experimentation, it is evident from the studies reported in this chapter that the MAP design offers several important advantages over other vaccine approaches (summarized in Table VI). It has the potential of being a more efficient vaccine format than those made with whole pathogens or recombinant proteins derived from the infectious agents. Selected linear determinants, known to stimulate protective immunity, can be chemically synthesized in a MAP format, thus avoiding the incorporation of other epitopes that would interfere with the desired response.

MAPs have been shown in several vaccine models to elicit an improved immune response compared to synthetic monomeric peptides covalently linked to carrier proteins. The MAP system represents both the hapten and the carrier, and induces the production of antibodies commonly reacting with the cognate protein. Moreover, there is evidence of qualitative differences between antibodies produced by MAP immunogens and antibodies induced by linear peptides conjugated to a carrier such as BSA (Wang *et al.*, 1991). In general, peptide antigens generate antibodies that bind to the native protein only when the linear sequences from which they are derived are accessible. In contrast, Kelker *et al.* (1994) have shown that two MAP constructs containing sequences of the HIV-1 envelope protein were capable of inducing antibodies reactive against conformational determinants of gp120 and capable of recognizing the virus on the surface of infected cells.

MAPs can be synthesized to include determinants from different proteins or from different regions of the same protein, as has been shown by the constructs containing B- and T-cell epitopes. This property is particularly important since it should make it possible to develop MAP immunogens recognized by a large proportion of the relevant human populations. The immunogenicity of an antigen is regulated by the binding of appropriate fragments to class II MHC molecules on the antigen-presenting cells and by receptors on the T cells which recognize the class II–peptide complex (Schwartz, 1985; Harding and Unanue, 1990). One problem associated with synthetic peptide vaccines is that a given peptide is usually capable of binding only to a minority of the HLA types represented in the population (Schrier *et al.*, 1989; Callahan *et al.*, 1990). Thus, peptides have the potential to be immunogenic in only a small number of individuals. Vaccines consisting of proteins or whole pathogens contain an array of potentially antigenic determinants. Several "universal" T-cell epitopes, i.e., recognized in association with different class II molecules, have been identified in proteins of various pathogens, such as circumsporozoite and a merozoite surface protein of the malaria parasite, tetanus toxoid, influenza hemagglutinin, and envelope glycoprotein of HIV-1 (Sinigaglia *et al.*, 1988; Panina-Bordignon *et al.*, 1989; Roche and Cresswell, 1990; Berzofsky *et al.*, 1991; Kumar *et al.*, 1992). The flexibility of the MAP system to incorporate more than one epitope allows for the use of such universal sequences and consequently may induce antibody responses in the majority of the population, irrespective of the genetic background.

Finally, an effective viral vaccine should induce neutralizing antibodies and trigger cellular immune responses. The latter effect is easily achieved by the MAP conjugation to the lipid tail P3C. At the same time, the immunostimulatory activity of the lipid moiety results in the production of a completely synthetic MAP immunogen with a built-in adjuvant.

REFERENCES

Adorini, L., Harvey, M. A., Miller, A., and Sercarz, E. E., 1979, Fine specificity of regulatory T cells. II. Suppressor and helper T cells are induced by different regions of hen egg-white lysozyme in a genetically non-responder mouse strain, *J. Exp. Med.* **150**:293–306.

Berzofsky, J. A., Pendleton, C. D., Clerici, M., Ahlers, J., Lucey, D. R., Putney, S. D., and Shearer, G. M., 1991, Construction of peptides encompassing multideterminant clusters of HIV envelope to induce in vitro T-cell responses in mice and humans of multiple MHC types, *J. Clin. Invest.* **88**:876–884.

Briand, J. -P., Muller, S., and Van Regenmortel, M. H. V., 1985, Synthetic peptides as antigens: Pitfalls of conjugation methods, *J. Immunol. Methods* **78**:59–69.

Briand, J. -P., Andre, C., Tuaillon, N., Herve, L., Neimark, J., and Muller, S., 1992, Multiple autoepitope presentation for specific detection of antibodies in primary biliary cirrhosis, *Hepatology* **6**:1395–1403.

Brown, F. J., 1990, The potential of peptides as vaccines, *Semin. Virol.* **1**:67–74.

Callahan, K. M., Fort, M. M., Obah, E. A., Reinherz, E. L., and Siliciano, R. F., 1990, Genetic variability in HIV-1 gp120 affects interactions with HLA molecules and T cell receptor, *J. Immunol.* **144**:3341–3346.

Chai, S. K., Clavijo, P., Tam, J. P., and Zavala, F., 1992, Immunogenic properties of multiple antigen peptide systems containing defined T and B epitopes, *J. Immunol.* **149**:2385–2390.

Defoort, J. -P., Nardelli, B., Huang, W., Ho, D. D., and Tam, J. P., 1992, Macromolecular assemblage in the design of a synthetic AIDS vaccine, *Proc. Natl. Acad. Sci. USA* **89**:3879–3883.

Del Giudice, G., Tougne, C., Louis, J. A., Lambert, P. -H., Bianchi, E., Bonelli, F., Chiappinelli, L., and Pessi, A., 1990, A multiple antigen peptide from the repetitive sequence of the Plasmodium malarie circumsporozoite protein induces a specific antibody response in mice of various H-2 haplotypes, *Eur. J. Immunol.* **20**:1619–1622.

Deres, K., Schild, H., Wiesmüller, K. -H., Jung, G., and Rammensee, H. G., 1989, In vivo priming of virus-specific cytotoxic T lymphocytes with synthetic lipopeptide vaccine, *Nature* **342**:561–564.

Dyrberg, T., and Oldstone, M. B., 1986, Peptides as antigens: Importance of orientation, *J. Exp. Med.* **164**:1344–1349.

Flexner, C., 1990, New approaches to vaccination, *Adv. Pharmacol.* **21**:51–99.

Francis, M. J., Fry, C. M., Rowlands, D. J., Bittle, J. L., Houghten, R. A., Lerner, R. A., and Brown, F., 1987, Immune response to uncoupled peptides of foot-and-mouth disease virus, *Immunology* **61**:1–6.

Francis, M. J., Hastings, G. Z., Brown, F., McDermed, J., Lu, Y. -A., and Tam, J. P., 1991, Immunological evaluation of the multiple antigen peptide (MAP) system using the major immunogenic site of foot-and-mouth disease virus, *Immunology* **73**:249–254.

Goudsmit, J., Debouck, C., Meloen, R. H., Smit, L., Bakker, M., Asher, D. M., Wolff, A. V., Gibbs, C. J., Jr., and Gajdusek, D. C., 1988, Human immunodeficiency virus type 1 neutralization epitope with conserved architecture elicits early type-specific antibodies in experimentally infected chimpanzees, *Proc. Natl. Acad. Sci. USA* **85**:4478–4482.

Green, N., Alexander, H., Olson, A., Alexander, S., Shinnick, T. M., Sutcliffe, J. G., and Lerner, R. A., 1982, Immunogenic structure of the influenza hemagglutinin, *Cell* **28**:477–487.

Habluetzel, A., Pessi, A., Bianchi, E., Rotigliano, G., and Esposito, F., 1991, Multiple antigen peptides for specific detection of antibodies to a malaria antigen in human sera, *Immunol. Lett.* **30**:75–80.

Harding, C.V., and Unanue, E. R., 1990, Cellular mechanisms of antigen processing and the function of class I and II major histocompatibility complex molecules, *Cell. Regul.* **1**:499–509.

Herzenberg, L. A., and Tokuhisa, T., 1983, Epitope-specific regulation. I. Carrier-specific induction of suppression for IgG anti-hapten antibody responses, *J. Exp. Med.* **155**:1730–1740.

Kamo, K., Jordan, R., Hsu, H. -T., and Hudson, D., 1992, Development of a monoclonal antibody to a conserved region of p34 ^{cdc2} protein kinase, *J. Immunol. Methods* **156**:163–170.

Kelker, H. C., Schlesinger, D., and Valentine, F. T., 1994, Immunogenic and antigenic properties of an HIV-1 gp120-derived multiple chain peptide, *J. Immunol.* **152**:4139–4148.

Kenealy, W. R., Matthews, T. J., Ganfield, M. -C., Langlois, A. J., Waselefsky, D. M., and Petteway, S. R., Jr., 1989, Antibodies from human immunodeficiency virus-infected individuals bind to a short amino acid sequence that elicits neutralizing antibodies in animals, *AIDS Res. Hum. Retroviruses* **5**:173–182.

Kumar, A., Arora, R., Kaur, P., Chauhan, V. S., and Sharma, P., 1992, "Universal" T helper cell determinants enhance immunogenicity of a Plasmodium falciparum merozoite surface antigen peptide, *J. Immunol.* **148**:1499–1505.

Levi, M., Ruden, U., Birx, D., Loomis, L., Redfield, R., Lovgren, K., Akerblom, L., Sandstrom, E., and Wahren, B., 1993, Effects of adjuvants and multiple antigen peptides on humoral and cellular responses to gp160 of HIV-1, *J. Acquir. Immune Defic. Syndr.* **6**:855–864.

Lu, Y. -A., Clavijo, P., Galantino, M., Shen, Z. -Y., and Tam, J. P., 1991, Chemically unambiguous peptide immunogen: Preparation, orientation and antigenicity of purified peptide conjugated to the multiple peptide system, *Mol. Immunol.* **28**:623–630.

Marguerite, M., Bossus, M., Mazingue, C., Wolowczuk, I., Grass-Masse, H., Tartar, A., Capron, A., and Auriault, C., 1992, Analysis of antigenicity and immunogenicity of five different chemically defined constructs of a peptide, *Mol. Immunol.* **29**:793–800.

Marsden, H. S., Owsianka, A. M., Graham, S., McLean, G. W., Robertson, C. A., and Subak-Sharpe, J. H., 1992, Advantages of branched peptides in serodiagnosis. Detection of HIV-specific antibodies and use of glycine spacers to increase sensitivity, *J. Immunol. Methods* **147**:65–72.

Munesinghe, D. Y., Clavijo, P., Calvo Calle, M., Nussenzweig, R. S., and Nardin, E., 1991, Immunogenicity of multiple antigen peptides (MAP) containing T and B cell epitopes of the repeat region of the P. falciparum circumsporozoite protein, *Eur. J. Immunol.* **21**:3015–3020.

Nardelli, B., and Tam, J. P., 1993, Cellular immune responses induced by in vivo priming with a lipid-conjugated multimeric antigen peptide, *Immunology* **79**:355–361.

Nardelli, B., Lu, Y. -A., Shiu, D. R., Delpierre-Defoort, C., Profy, A. T., and Tam, J. P., 1992a, A chemically defined synthetic vaccine model for HIV-1, *J. Immunol.* **148**:914–920.

Nardelli, B., Defoort, J. -P., Huang, W., and Tam, J. P., 1992b, Design of a complete synthetic peptide-based AIDS vaccine with a built-in adjuvant, *AIDS Res. Hum. Retroviruses* **8**:1405–1407.

Nardelli, B., Haser, P. B., and Tam, J. P., 1994, Oral administration of an antigenic synthetic lipopeptide (MAP-P3C) evokes salivary antibodies and systemic humoral and cellular responses, *Vaccine* **12**:1335–1339.

Palker, T. J., Clark, M. E., Langlois, A. J., Matthews, T. J., Weinhold, K. J., Randall, R. R., Bolognesi, D. P., and Haynes, B. F., 1988, Type-specific neutralization of the human immunodeficiency virus with antibodies to env-encoded synthetic peptides, *Proc. Natl. Acad. Sci. USA* **85**:1932–1936.

Palker, T. J., Matthews, T. J., Langlois, A., Tanner, M. E., Martin, M. E., Scearce, R. M., Kim, J. E., Berzofsky, J. A., Bolognesi, D. P., and Haynes, B. F., 1989, Polyvalent human immunodeficiency virus synthetic immunogen comprised of envelope gp120 T helper cell sites and B cell neutralization epitopes, *J. Immunol.* **142**:3612–3619.

Panina-Bordignon, P., Tan, A., Termijtelen, A., Demotz, S., Corradin, G., and Lanzavecchia, A., 1989, Universal immunogenic T cell epitopes: Promiscuous binding to human MHC class II and promiscuous recognition by T cells, *Eur. J. Immunol.* **19**:2237–2242.

Pessi, A., Valmori, D., Migliorini, P., Tougne, C., Bianchi, E., Lambert, P. -H., Corradin, G., and Del Giudice, G., 1991, Lack of H-2 restriction of the Plasmodium falciparum (NANP) sequence as multiple antigen peptide, *Eur. J. Immunol.* **21**:2273–2276.

Posnett, D. N., McGrath, H., and Tam, J. P., 1988, A novel method for producing anti-peptide antibodies, *J. Biol. Chem.* **263**:1719–1725.

Reitermann, A., Metzger, J., Wiesmüller, K. -H., Jung, G., and Bessler, W. G., 1989, Lipopeptide derivatives of bacterial lipoprotein constitute potent immune adjuvant combined or covalently coupled to antigen or hapten, *Biol. Chem. Hoppe-Seyler* **370**:343–352.

Robinson, J. H., and Kehoe, M. A., 1992, Group A streptococcal M proteins: Virulence factors and protective antigens, *Immunol. Today* **13**:362–366.

Robinson, W. E., Jr., Kawamura, T., Gorny, M. K., Lake, D., Xu, J. -Y., Matsumoto, Y., Sugano, T., Masuho, Y., Mitchell, W. M., Hersh, E., and Zolla-Pazner, S., 1990, Human monoclonal antibodies to the human immunodeficiency virus type 1 (HIV-1) transmembrane glycoprotein gp41 enhance HIV-1 infection in vitro, *Proc. Natl. Acad. Sci. USA* **87**:3185–3189.

Roche, P. A., and Cresswell, P., 1990, High-affinity binding of an influenza hemagglutinin-derived peptide to purified HLA-DR, *J. Immunol.* **144**:1849–1856.

Rusche, J. R., Javaherian, K., McDanal, C., Petro, J., Lynn, D. L., Grimaila, R., Langlois, A., Gallo, R. C., Arthur, L. O., Fischinger, P. J., Bolognesi, D. P., Putney, S. D., and Matthews, T. J., 1988, Antibodies that inhibit fusion of human immunodeficiency virus-infected cells bind a 24-amino acid sequence of the viral envelope, gp120, *Proc. Natl. Acad. Sci. USA* **85**:3198–3202.

Schrier, R. D., Gnann, J. W., Jr., Landes, R., Lockshin, C., Richman, D., McCutchan, A., Kennedy, C., Oldstone, M. B. A., and Nelson, J. A., 1989, T cell recognition of HIV synthetic peptides in a natural infection, *J. Immunol.* **142**:1166–1176.

Schutze, M. -P., Leclerc, C., Jolivet, M., Audibert, F., and Chedid, L., 1985, Carrier-induced epitopic suppression, a major issue for future synthetic vaccines, *J. Immunol.* **135**:2319–2322.

Schwartz, R. H., 1985, T-lymphocyte recognition of antigen in association with gene products of the major histocompatibility complex, *Annu. Rev. Immunol.* **3**:237–261.

Sinigaglia, F., Guttinger, M., Kilgus, J., Doran, D. M., Matilde, H., Etlinger, H., Trzeciak, A., Gillesen, D., and Pink, J. R. L., 1988, A malaria T-cell epitope recognized in association with most mouse and human MHC class II molecules, *Nature* **336**:778–780.

The MAP System 819

Takahashi, H., Cohen, J., Hosmalin, A., Cease, K. B., Houghten, R., Cornette, J. L., DeLisi, C., Moss, B., Germain, R. N., and Berzofsky, J. A., 1988, An immunodominant epitope of the human immunodeficiency virus envelope glycoprotein gp160 recognized by class I major histocompatibility complex molecule-restricted murine cytotoxic T lymphocytes, *Proc. Natl. Acad. Sci. USA* **85**:3105–3109.

Tam, J. P., 1988, Synthetic peptide vaccine design: Synthesis and properties of a high-density multiple antigenic peptide system, *Proc. Natl. Acad. Sci. USA* **85**:5409–5413.

Tam, J. P., 1993, U.S. Patent 5,229,490, Multiple Antigen Peptide System.

Tam, J. P., and Lu, Y. -A., 1989, Vaccine engineering: Enhancement of immunogenicity of synthetic peptide vaccines related to hepatitis in chemically defined models consisting of T- and B-cell epitopes, *Proc. Natl. Acad. Sci. USA* **86**:9084–9088.

Tam, J. P., and Zavala, F., 1989, Multiple antigen peptide. A novel approach to increase detection sensitivity of synthetic peptides in solid-phase immunoassays, *J. Immunol. Methods* **124**:53–61.

Tam, J. P., Clavijo, P., Lu, Y. -A., Nussenzweig, V., Nussenzweig, R., and Zavala, F., 1990, Incorporation of T and B epitopes of the circumsporozoite protein in a chemically defined synthetic vaccine against malaria, *J. Exp. Med.* **171**:299–306.

Troalen, F., Razafindratsita, A., Puisieux, A., Voeltzel, T., Bohuon, C., Bellet, D., and Bidart, J. -M., 1990, Structural probing of human lutropin using antibodies against synthetic peptides constructed by classical and multiple antigen peptide system approach, *Mol. Immunol.* **27**:363–368.

Wang, C. Y., 1989, European Patent Application 89,301,288.0.

Wang, C. Y., Looney, D. J., Li, M. L., Walfield, A. M., Ye, J., Hosein, B., Tam, J. P., and Wong-Staal, F., 1991, Long-term high-titer neutralizing activity induced by octameric synthetic HIV-1 antigen, *Science* **254**:285–288.

Wiesmüller, K. -H., Bessler, W. G., and Jung, G., 1983, Synthesis of the mitogenic S-[2,3-bis(palmitoyloxy)propyl]-N-palmitoyl pentapeptide from the Escherichia coli lipoprotein, *Hoppe Seyler's Z. Physiol. Chem.* **364**:593–606.

Wolowczuk, I., Auriault, C., Bossus, M., Boulanger, D., Gras-Masse, H., Mazingue, C., Pierce, R. J., Grezel, D., Reid, G. D., Tartar, A., and Capron, A., 1991, Antigenicity and immunogenicity of a multiple peptidic construction of the Schistosoma mansoni Sm-28 GST antigen in rat, mouse, and monkey. 1. Partial protection of Fisher rat after active immunization, *J. Immunol.* **146**:1987–1995.

Chapter 37

Design of Experimental Synthetic Peptide Immunogens for Prevention of HIV-1 and HTLV-I Retroviral Infections

Mary Kate Hart, Thomas J. Palker, and Barton F. Haynes

1. INTRODUCTION

The potential for using synthetic peptides to serve as components of protective vaccines or as immunotherapeutics (see Chapter 38) is being explored for a variety of viral or bacterial pathogens. Peptide immunogens that elicit some level of protection in animal models or in clinical trials have been described for foot-and-mouth disease virus (Bittle *et al.*, 1982), murine mammary tumor virus (Dion *et al.*, 1990), Venezuelan equine encephalitis virus (Hunt *et al.*, 1990), respiratory syncytial virus (Trudel *et al.*, 1991), Semliki Forest virus (Snijders *et al.*, 1992), Sendai virus (Kast *et al.*, 1991), lymphocytic choriomeningitis virus (M. Schulz *et al.*, 1991), group A streptococci (Bessen and Fischetti, 1990), and *Plasmodium falciparum* (Rodriguez *et al.*, 1990; Etlinger *et al.*, 1991).

The issues involved in successfully developing a synthetic peptide vaccine have been reviewed (Berzofsky, 1991; Ada, 1991; Milich, 1990; Cease, 1990; Riveau and Audibert, 1990) and will not be discussed in detail here. In this chapter we have dealt specifically with progress toward the development of prototypic immunogens for human immunodeficiency virus (HIV-1) and human T-cell leukemia/lymphotropic virus (HTLV-I) infections using synthetic peptides derived from retroviral proteins.

Using synthetic peptides as immunogens for a preventive HIV vaccine has a number of advantages, including ease of synthesis, the nontoxic nature of the immunogen, the ability to include sequences from a number of HIV isolates, and the absence of the risk of

Mary Kate Hart • Division of Virology, U.S. Army Medical Research Institute for Infectious Diseases, Fort Detrick, Frederick, Maryland 21702. *Thomas J. Palker and Barton F. Haynes* • Department of Rheumatology and Immunology and the Duke Center for AIDS Research, Duke University Medical Center, Durham, North Carolina 27710.

Vaccine Design: The Subunit and Adjuvant Approach, edited by Michael F. Powell and Mark J. Newman. Plenum Press, New York, 1995.

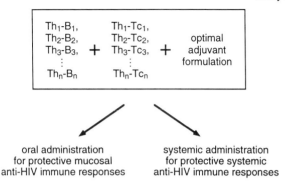

Figure 1. Outline for use of polyvalent peptide immunogens as a preventive vaccine for HIV-1. A practical synthetic peptide vaccine for HIV-1 will require incorporating sufficient Th and CTL epitopes for MHC class I and class II molecules represented in the populations to be immunized, and should include sequences of immunogenic epitopes reflective of HIV-1 isolates in a particular geographic region. Peptides may have to be formulated in an adjuvant that allows maximum immunogenicity for both oral and systemic immune responses. Mucosal immunization may well be needed for induction of protective mucosal, anti-HIV-1 immune responses as well as systemic immune responses.

infection and transmission inherent to live vaccine approaches. The disadvantages of synthetic peptide immunogens are poor immunogenicity, lack of native protein conformation, and the reported inability of soluble proteins and peptides to induce major histocompatibility complex (MHC) class I molecule-restricted cytotoxic T lymphocyte (CTL) responses (Townsend *et al.*, 1986; Takahashi *et al.*, 1990). Moreover, use of the synthetic peptide approach for vaccine design necessitates a strategy for including sufficient T-helper (Th) and CTL epitopes for recognition by diverse MHC antigens in a random-bred population.

In this chapter we have reviewed progress made toward the identification of immunogenic regions of HIV-1 and HTLV-I proteins and the design of peptide immunogens that induce neutralizing antibodies and MHC class I-restricted CTLs. Our strategy for the construction of a synthetic peptide-based polyvalent immunogen for HIV is also presented (Palker *et al.*, 1989; Haynes *et al.*, 1993c) (Fig. 1).

2. SYNTHETIC PEPTIDE APPROACH FOR HIV-1

The correlates of protective immunity for HIV have not been identified, but both neutralizing antibodies (Robert-Guroff *et al.*, 1985; Weiss *et al.*, 1985) and cytotoxic T cells (Walker *et al.*, 1987; Plata *et al.*, 1987; reviewed in Autran *et al.*, 1991) have been detected in HIV-infected patients. Our current hypothesis is that an HIV vaccine candidate should be capable of inducing high levels of virus-neutralizing antibodies as well as anti-HIV CTL responses to lyse infected cells (Haynes *et al.*, 1993c) since both types of responses may be needed for protection from HIV-1 (Berman *et al.*, 1990; Girard *et al.*, 1991; Haynes, 1992; Yasutomi *et al.*, 1993).

2.1. Peptide Synthesis and Purification

The peptides that we used in the studies reviewed herein were synthesized on an Applied Biosystems 431A peptide synthesizer using either *tert*-butoxycarbonyl (t-Boc) or 9-fluorenylmethyloxycarbonyl (Fmoc) chemistry as described elsewhere (Palker *et al.*, 1988b, 1989; Hart *et al.*, 1991). Amino acid analysis, HPLC analysis, N-terminal sequencing, and, more recently, mass spectrometry analysis were performed to verify the identity and purity of the synthesized peptides (Hart *et al.*, 1991; Haynes *et al.*, 1993a,b). Peptide sequences are shown in Table I and Fig. 4.

Unless noted otherwise, for studies using goats and mice, peptides were emulsified in complete Freund's adjuvant (CFA) for the first immunization, and in incomplete Freund's adjuvant (IFA) for all subsequent booster immunizations. Only IFA was used in nonhuman primate models except where noted for the rhesus adjuvant comparison studies.

2.2. Design of HIV-1 Th-B Hybrid Synthetic Peptides

The envelope gene encoding the HIV-1 gp120 molecule contains regions of highly conserved sequences as well as regions that exhibit a high degree of sequence variability among HIV-1 isolates (Starcich *et al.*, 1986; Matthews *et al.*, 1986; Cease *et al.*, 1987; Cheng-Mayer *et al.*, 1988; Takahashi *et al.*, 1988). At the time that our studies were first undertaken, the sequences of HIV-1-neutralizing epitopes had not been identified. Putney *et al.* (1986) observed that type-specific neutralizing antibody reactivity was directed to a 180-amino-acid region in the central portion of HIV-1 env gp120. Palker *et al.* (1988a,b) and three other groups (Rusche *et al.*, 1988; Goudsmit *et al.*, 1988; Kenealy *et al.*, 1989) mapped the binding of anti-HIV-1 neutralizing antibodies to the region now referred to as the principal neutralizing domain of the third variable (V3) loop of HIV-1 gp120.

For the studies described in this chapter, neutralization of HIV-1 was measured using two assays. In the reverse transcriptase (RT) assay (Matthews *et al.*, 1986) 1000 infectious doses of virus were incubated at 37°C for 30 min with diluted test serum in a final volume of 0.2 mL growth medium. H9 cells (1×10^5) were then added to each well and the plates incubated for 10 days, with fresh medium added to the wells daily. Supernatants were then collected from the wells and assayed for RT activity (Poiesz *et al.*, 1980) to determine the ability of the test serum to inhibit viral infectivity. The neutralizing titer was calculated as the reciprocal of the dilution of serum required to inhibit RT activity by 50% relative to controls.

The syncytium inhibition assay (Putney *et al.*, 1986) measured the ability of test sera to inhibit the formation of giant multinucleated cells that occurs in the presence of HIV-1 in vitro. In this assay, $CD4^+$ CEM cells and HIV-1-infected cells fused to form syncytia that can be counted under a microscope within 24 h. Neutralizing titers were calculated as the reciprocal dilution of test serum that yielded a 95% reduction of the number of syncytia formed in control wells.

In the studies of Palker *et al.* (1988b), synthetic peptides designated SP10, containing a neutralizing epitope from the HIV-1 V3 loop, were conjugated to tetanus toxoid (TT) as a carrier molecule, and used to immunize goats after emulsification in CFA/IFA. The sera that were obtained were found to contain antibodies that neutralized either HIV-1$_{\text{IIIB}}$ or

824   Mary Kate Hart *et al.*

Table I
Sequences of HIV and SIV Synthetic Peptides Discussed in This Chapter[a]

Peptide	F	Th	B	CTL	Isolate
			Sequence of region		
F-Th-B-CTL (IIIB)	AVGIGALFLGFL	KQIINMWQEVGKAMYA	CTRPNNNTRKSIRIQRGPG	RAFVTI	HIV-1$_{IIIB}$
F-Th-B-CTL (MN)	AVGIGALFLGFL	KQIINMWQEVGKAMYA	CTRPNYNKRKRIHIGPGRA	FYTTK	HIV-1$_{MN}$
Th-B-CTL (IIIB)		KQIINMWQEVGKAMYA	CTRPNNNTRKSIRIQRGPG	RAFVTI	HIV-1$_{IIIB}$
Th-B-CTL (MN)		KQIINMWQEVGKAMYA	CTRPNYNKRKRIHIGPGRA	FYTTK	HIV-1$_{MN}$
Th-B (RF)		KQIINMWQEVGKAMYA	(C)RKSITKGPGRVIY		HIV-1$_{RF}$
p11C (CTL)				EGCTPYDINQML	SIV
ST1-p11C (Th-CTL)	RQIINTWHKVGKNVYL	....		EGCTPYDINQML	SIV

[a] Amino acids are represented by a single-letter code that is the first letter of its name, except for aspartic acid (D), glutamic acid (E), phenylalanine (F), lysine (K), asparagine (N), arginine (R), glutamine (Q), tryptophan (W), and tyrosine (Y). F (fusogenic) region is amino acids 519–530 from HIV-1$_{IIIB}$. Th (T1) sequence is amino acids 428–443 from HIV-1$_{IIIB}$, B (SP10) sequences are amino acids 303–321 from IIIB, 301–319 from MN, and 325–337 from RF, and the CTL sequences are amino acids 322–327 from IIIB and 320–324 from MN. Amino acids in parentheses were added to facilitate coupling of peptides. HIV-1$_{IIIB}$ sequences are from Ratner *et al.* (1985) and the MN sequences are from Myers *et al.* (1988). The CTL regions complete an MHC class I molecule-restricted epitope that begins IRI (IIIB) and IHI (MN), described in Takahashi *et al.* (1989a). SIV peptides are described in Yasutomi *et al.* (1993).

HIV-1$_{RF}$ in a type-specific manner (Palker *et al.*, 1988b) when tested in the RT inhibition assay or the syncytium inhibition assay. However, when SP10 peptides from three different isolates were conjugated to TT and administered to goats, HIV-1 neutralizing antibody responses were suboptimal (Palker *et al.*, 1989). One possible explanation for the low responses against the HIV-1 sequences is that overwhelming responses to the TT carrier molecule were induced when the three TT-conjugated peptides were administered simultaneously.

To address this possibility and to improve the immunogenicity of the V3 loop peptides, a hybrid peptide construct was synthesized using an HIV-1 Th epitope instead of TT. The T1 gp120 sequence (amino acids 428–443) containing a Th epitope (Cease *et al.*, 1987) was synthesized at the N-terminus of the SP10 sequence, to make a Th–B-cell epitope (Th-B) synthetic peptide construct (Palker *et al.*, 1989). For some peptides, the C-terminal region of SP10 was extended six to eight amino acids to complete an MHC class I molecule-restricted CTL epitope (Takahashi *et al.*, 1988). Adding these amino acids also provided an additional neutralization epitope (Rusche *et al.*, 1988). For some hybrid peptides, the highly conserved fusogenic (F) domain of the HIV-1 transmembrane protein (gp41) was added, in an attempt to produce antibodies against a conserved env region and to facilitate peptide entry into antigen-presenting cells (APCs). Thus, in this chapter, the hybrid peptides will be referred to by the types of epitopes they contain, i.e., Th for helper T cell, B for neutralizing B-cell epitope, CTL for cytotoxic T cell, F for gp41 fusogenic domain, and the HIV-1 isolate designation from which those sequences were derived.

2.3. Induction of Neutralizing Antibody Responses by Th-B Peptide Immunogens

The Th-B hybrid peptides were emulsified in CFA for the initial immunization and in IFA for subsequent boosts. High-titered, type-specific neutralizing antibody responses were measured in sera from goats immunized with the Th-B peptides (Palker *et al.*, 1988b, 1989). More importantly, a trivalent mixture of Th-B peptides from three different HIV-1 isolates also induced high-titered neutralizing antibodies against each of the isolates in goats when the TT carrier protein was replaced with the T1 sequence (Palker *et al.*, 1989). In addition to finding neutralizing antibody responses, these studies also measured T-cell proliferative responses against the T1 epitope and to a second Th epitope in the C-terminal region of the SP10 peptide sequence (Palker *et al.*, 1989). Thus, unconjugated Th-B peptides were demonstrated to be capable of inducing HIV-1 neutralizing antibody responses and T-cell proliferative responses in goats.

In the Semliki Forest virus system, where protection is mediated by antibody, Th-B synthetic peptide immunogens have been evaluated for the ability to induce protective immunity. Snijders *et al.* (1992) protected mice from lethal viral challenge 4 months after immunization with a Th-B peptide construct in Quil A adjuvant. The choice of Th epitope used in the peptide construct was reported to influence the antibody titers measured in mouse sera and the survival rates of subsequently challenged mice. The observations that (1) a second Th-B construct containing the same Th epitope found in the most protective construct, synthesized with a less effective B-cell epitope, was less efficient at inducing protective immunity and (2) a Th-B construct, containing a Th epitope from influenza virus and the protective B-cell epitope from Semliki Forest virus, protected mice from challenge at 4 weeks but not 4 months after immunization, emphasize the importance of evaluating epitopes to ensure that those that best induce and sustain the desired immune responses are included in a vaccine.

An alternative approach to using unconjugated peptides is to link multiple copies of peptides to a lysine backbone structure. This approach, called the multiple antigenic peptide (MAP) system, is described in Chapter 36.

2.4. Rhesus Monkey Studies

Th-B synthetic peptides from HIV-1$_{IIIB}$ were formulated in different adjuvants and used to immunize rhesus monkeys (Hart *et al.*, 1990). Th-B hybrid synthetic peptides from the HIV-1$_{IIIB}$ isolate induced both high-titered type-specific neutralizing antibody responses and T-cell proliferative responses in the monkeys. The induction of neutralizing antibody responses was dependent on the adjuvant used, in that IFA and threonyl-muramyl dipeptide (threonyl-MDP) were found to be superior to alum or poly A:poly U. No differences in the populations of antibodies induced to the peptides were observed between the different adjuvant groups when the sera were tested for reactivity with T1 and SP10 peptides.

Importantly, Th-B peptides were nontoxic when used in experimental vaccine formulations. Renal and liver functions of the monkeys were monitored without observing any toxic effects from peptide immunization. The total numbers of circulating lymphocytes, monocytes, and polymorphonuclear cells did not change after immunization with these peptides. However, the use of poly A:poly U as an adjuvant was observed to decrease the numbers of circulating CD4$^+$ and CD8$^+$ T cells after the first four immunizations and increases in the number of polymorphonuclear cells were measured in animals receiving IFA or threonyl-MDP adjuvants. Reactions at the injection site were observed in animals receiving alum or IFA adjuvants (Hart *et al.*, 1990).

To determine the duration of anti-HIV-1 type-specific neutralizing antibody responses, serum was drawn at 3 months and again at 17 months after the eighth Th-B booster. Anti-HIV-1 neutralizing antibodies were present in sera from monkeys given the peptides in IFA 3 months after the primary series, but were absent after 17 months, although peptide-specific antibodies could still be detected in enzyme-linked immunosorbent assays (ELISAs). Boosting the animals with peptides in IFA induced an anamnestic neutralizing antibody response in sera from three of four monkeys originally given IFA or T-MDP adjuvants (Table II).

In a second study, rhesus monkeys were immunized with Th-B-CTL peptides from the MN isolate of HIV-1. HIV-1$_{MN}$ neutralizing sera obtained from five monkeys were tested for the ability to cross-neutralize HIV-1 isolates with disparate V3-loop sequences. Serum from one monkey was found to cross-neutralize the HIV-1$_{IIIB}$ isolate, the HIV-1$_{RF}$ isolate, and HIV primary isolates CC and Du6587–5, grown in T-cell lines (Haynes *et al.*, 1993a). The HIV-1$_{IIIB}$ cross-neutralizing activity was absorbed by peptides containing the IGPGRAF sequence, found at the tip of the V3 loop. This serum did not neutralize all isolates that contained the IGPGRA sequence, suggesting that flanking or distal amino acids affected the ability of antibodies to bind or neutralize HIV-1 (Haynes *et al.*, 1993a).

Table II
Duration of HIVIIIB-Neutralizing Antibody Responses in Rhesus Monkeys Immunized with
Th-B (IIIB) Synthetic Peptide Immunogens[a]

Neutralization assay	Time of bleed	% inhibition observed in sera			
		T-MDP/IFA		IFA/IFA	
		Rhesus monkey No.			
		17371	*17563*	*19600*	*22214*
Syncytium inhibition	1° series[a]	92	68	100	100
	3 mo rest	0	0	83	53
	17 mo rest	0	0	33	31
	6 wk postboost[b]	93	18	86	50
		RT inhibition observed			
Reverse transcriptase	1° series[a]	+	+	+	+
	3 mo rest	+	+	+	+
	17 mo rest	–	–	–	–
	6 wk postboost[b]	+	–	+	+

[a]Sera from rhesus monkeys immunized with Th-B constructs in T-MDP or IFA adjuvant (Hart *et al.*, 1990) were tested for the presence of antibodies that inhibit HIV-1_{IIIB} in syncytium formation or reverse transcriptase inhibition assays after the completion of the primary series, and again after 3 or 17 months' rest.
[b]Sera were obtained 6 weeks after an additional peptide boost in IFA was administered to each monkey.

Recent data suggest that antibodies raised against recombinant gp120 may be less effective in neutralizing HIV primary isolates grown in peripheral blood mononuclear cells (PBMCs) than in neutralizing laboratory HIV strains or primary isolates grown in T-cell lines (T. Matthews, personal communication). Thus, a key area of research in HIV vaccine development is the study of neutralizing determinants, both conformational and linear, that are expressed on the surface of HIV primary isolates grown in PBMCs, and the design of immunogens that mimic these determinants.

Synthetic peptides derived from the V3 loops of HIV-1 isolates have also been used by White-Scharf *et al.* (1993) as immunogens to elicit broadly neutralizing murine monoclonal antibodies. Overlapping synthetic peptides from other HIV-1 env regions have also been used by others as immunogens to elicit cross-neutralizing antibodies in monkeys (Vahlne *et al.*, 1991; Girard *et al.*, 1991; Ronco *et al.*, 1992).

The observation that only one of the random-bred monkeys tested in our study made a cross-neutralizing antibody response also indicated a need to better define the Th epitope(s) and class II molecule-restriction of these responses, and subsequently to find ways of inducing anti-GPGRAF broadly-reactive antibody responses in human populations expressing disparate MHC class II types (Haynes *et al.*, 1993a).

The issue of defining Th epitopes recognized by different class II molecules has been addressed in a number of studies. The first Th epitopes identified on HIV-1 were described by Cease *et al.* (1987). Peptides of these T-cell epitopes (T1 and T2) induced proliferative responses and interleukin 2 production by T cells of HIV-1-seropositive patients (Clerici *et al.*, 1989). Priming rhesus monkeys with Th peptides induced a proliferative response in half of the monkeys tested (Hosmalin *et al.*, 1991). Following immunization with a suboptimal dose of gp160, increased serum antibody titers to gp160 were measured in those monkeys exhibiting a proliferative response to the Th peptides, as compared to monkeys that were not primed with Th peptides (Hosmalin *et al.*, 1991). Other studies identified clusters of overlapping T-cell epitopes on gp160 that were presented by disparate murine MHC class II molecules (Hale *et al.*, 1989) and by disparate human histocompatibility leukocyte antigen (HLA) types (Berzofsky *et al.*, 1991). These Th epitope clusters were subsequently synthesized N-terminal to a sequence called P18 (HIV-1$_{IIIB}$ sequence RIQRGPGRAFVTIGK, see Table I B/CTL regions) and shown to induce HIV-1 neutralizing antibody responses in mouse strains capable of responding to one of the Th epitopes contained in the cluster (Ahlers *et al.*, 1993). This last study is of particular importance because it provides an approach for overcoming one of the potential limitations of successful synthetic peptide vaccine development, namely the inability to induce immune responses in members of random-bred populations expressing disparate class II molecules.

2.5. Peptide-Induced Anti-HIV-1 Responses in Chimpanzees

The ability of Th-B (IIIB) and Th-B-CTL (IIIB) synthetic peptides to induce neutralizing antibody responses in chimpanzees was also evaluated (Haynes *et al.*, 1993b). Peptides were emulsified in IFA and administered to two chimpanzees at 1-month intervals for a total of seven injections. For the first four injections, 6 mg of Th-B (IIIB) peptide was given and for the last three injections, 30 mg Th-B-CTL (IIIB) was given. The monkeys were then rested for 6 months and given an additional 6-mg dose of Th-B-CTL (IIIB).

No HIVIIIB-neutralizing antibody responses were observed in the syncytium-inhibition assay and no titers > 1:45 were observed in RT inhibition assay using the chimpanzee sera obtained during the initial 6-month phase of the study, although high-titered ELISA antibody responses against Th-B-CTL (IIIB) peptide were observed. The same peptide constructs did induce HIV-1-neutralizing antibody responses when used to immunize goats, however (Haynes *et al.*, 1993b). These data suggested that the chimpanzee sera contained antibodies that reacted with the appropriate V3 loop linear sequence, but that native secondary structures may not have been recognized by the anti-Th-B-CTL (IIIB) chimpanzee antibodies.

In an effort to induce more broadly reactive anti-HIV-1 neutralizing antibodies, another two chimpanzees were immunized with F-Th-B-CTL (IIIB) peptides containing the HIV-1 fusogenic domain of gp41 (F) synthesized N-terminal to the Th-B-CTL HIV-1 env peptide (Haynes *et al.*, 1993b). Whereas the Th-B-CTL peptide was strongly immunogenic and induced antipeptide antibodies, the F-Th-B-CTL peptide was a potent tolerogen for peptide-specific antibody responses (Haynes *et al.*, 1993b).

Following these observations, all four chimpanzees were immunized with three 6-mg doses of Th-B-CTL peptide from the MN isolate. After boosting with Th-B-CTL (MN) peptide, anti-HIV-1 neutralizing antibody responses against both the IIIB and MN isolates were observed in the two chimpanzees that initially received the peptide construct containing the fusogenic region of HIV-1 (F-Th-B-CTL).

As expected, we found no anti-HIV-1 CTLs in peptide-immunized chimpanzees (M. K. Hart, K. Weinhold, and B. F. Haynes, unpublished data), because none of the chimpanzees were the appropriate MHC class I types (A2, A3, B7) for the V3 loop CTL epitopes (Clerici *et al.*, 1991; Safrit *et al.*, 1993; Haynes *et al.*, 1993b).

2.6. Effect of gp41 Fusogenic Domain (F) on Immune Response

Adding both the CTL epitope and the F region to HIV-1 env Th-B peptide constructs could potentially alter the ability of the Th-B peptide construct to induce optimal anti-HIV-1 neutralizing B-cell responses and T-cell proliferative responses. To evaluate this, sera from mice and goats immunized with the different constructs were tested for the presence of neutralizing antibodies. When Th-B or F-Th-B-CTL peptides from HIV-1$_{MN}$ sequences were given to BALB/c or C57BL/6 mice, sera from both strains of mice immunized with either peptide construct inhibited HIV-1$_{MN}$-induced syncytium formation (Table III).

Sera from eight goats given the MN peptide constructs (Th-B, Th-B-CTL, F-Th-B, F-Th-B-CTL) in CFA/IFA inhibited in the RT assay (M. K. Hart, A. J. Langlois, and B. F. Haynes, unpublished data). HIV-1$_{MN}$-induced syncytium formation was inhibited by sera from four goats given Th-B-CTL (MN) or F-Th-B-CTL (MN) after five immunizations (M. K. Hart, T. J. Matthews, and B. F. Haynes, unpublished data), indicating that adding these regions to the construct did not inhibit the ability to induce this type of response. Syncytium-inhibiting antibodies were still present in the sera from one goat given F-Th-B-CTL and one goat given Th-B-CTL 8 months after the fifth immunization (Fig. 2). Administration of a booster 1 month later induced anamnestic antibody responses in both of these goats (Fig. 2), as well as in a second goat given Th-B-CTL, in one goat given F-Th-B, and in one goat given Th-B (MN) peptide (M. K. Hart, T. J. Matthews, and B. F. Haynes, unpublished data).

Although weak anti-F domain antibodies could be detected by ELISA, neutralizing antibodies generated by the hybrid env Th-B and F-Th-B peptides in goats were type-specific, suggesting little or no role for the anti-F antibodies in neutralizing HIV-1 (M. K. Hart, T. J. Matthews, and B. F. Haynes, unpublished data). Indeed, a new panel of anti-F monoclonal

Table III
Ability of Sera from Mice Immunized with Synthetic Peptides to Inhibit HIV-1-Mediated Syncytium Formation[a]

Strain	Peptide	Number of mice with		Total number of mice tested
		>90% inhibition	50–90% inhibition	
BALB/c	Th-B (MN)	1	3	5
BALB/c	F-Th-B-CTL (MN)	2	4	7
C57BL/6	Th-B (MN)	1	3	5
C57BL/6	F-Th-B-CTL (MN)	3	4	7

[a]Sera from BALB/c (H-2^d) or C57BL/6 (H-2^b) mice were tested in syncytium inhibition assays against HIV-1$_{MN}$ after the mice were immunized five times with 10 μg synthetic peptide in CFA/IFA.

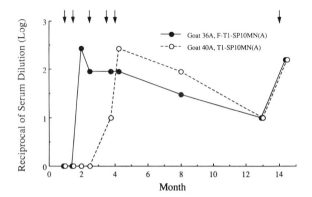

Figure 2. Time course of syncytium-inhibiting antibodies induced in goats by peptide immunogens Tl-SPl0MN(A) (F-Th-B-CTL) or Tl-SPl0MN(A) (Th-B-CTL). The figure represents the level of syncytium-inhibiting antibody against HIV-1$_{MN}$ represented as the log$_{10}$ of the reciprocal of the serum dilution at which 90% inhibition of syncytium formation was observed. Arrows indicate the time of immunizations. Whereas neutralizing antibodies arose later in the goat immunized with the Th-B-CTL peptide, the levels of neutralizing antibodies were similar in the two animals and the duration of neutralizing antibody response was the same. Neutralizing antibodies could be boosted in both animals at month 14.

antibodies that react with HIV-1 gp41 and peptides containing the F sequence did not neutralize HIV-1$_{MN}$ or HIV-1$_{IIIB}$ (K. Casey and B. F. Haynes, unpublished data).

    Peripheral blood T-cell proliferative responses were also measured after immunizing goats with these peptide constructs (Table IV). We observed that the proliferative responses to the peptide constructs containing the F region (i.e., using the peptides containing the F sequence as immunogens in vitro) were, in general, slightly lower than proliferative responses to peptide constructs lacking this region. However, the F-Th-B-CTL peptides were consistently effective when used to stimulate murine CTL responses in vivo, and were also very effective when used to restimulate CTLs in vitro (Hart *et al.*, 1991).

Table IV
Proliferative Responses of Immune Goat PBLs to HIV-1$_{MN}$ Env Peptides after Three Immunizations[a]

		Maximum mean uptake of [^{3}H]thymidine/10^6 cells in culture (cpm)				
Goat	Immunogen	Medium	Th-B	F-Th-B	F-Th-B-CTL	Th-B-CTL
97A	Th-B (MN)	2196	169,308	39,705	30,006	109,998
122A	F-Th-B (MN)	1120	135,766	56,733	119,565	127,808
44A	Th-B-CTL (MN)	1313	278,823	199,051	12,291	178,925
25A	F-Th-B-CTL (MN)	1103	91,588	31,151	10,868	77,880

[a]Cells were incubated with peptides in vitro for 7 days before pulsing with [^{3}H]thymidine for 4 h. Data shown were obtained after three sequential peptide immunizations in CFA/IFA.

It should also be emphasized that even though peptides containing the HIV-1 gp41 fusogenic (F) domain are potent immunogens in mice and goats, such peptides were tolerogens in chimpanzees (Haynes *et al.*, 1993b) and, to a lesser extent, in rhesus monkeys (Haynes *et al.*, 1993a). Since peptides containing the F sequence were tolerogenic in primates, the usefulness of these peptides for developing a preventive vaccine is limited. However, if certain anti-HIV-1 immune responses are clearly determined to be deleterious, then using immunogens containing the F sequence may be a feasible strategy for turning off pathogenic anti-HIV-1 immune responses. Moreover, these data raise the hypothesis that the HIV-1 gp41 F domain might in some way play a role in the failure to generate effective anti-HIV-1 immune responses in humans (Haynes *et al.*, 1993b).

The mechanism by which the F region acts as a tolerogen in nonhuman primates is not understood. Immunization with peptides containing the F sequence was not generally immunosuppressive, as chimpanzee proliferative responses to phytohemaglutinin and Candida were not significantly affected (Haynes *et al.*, 1993b). T-cell lymphopenia was observed in the monkeys receiving peptides with the F region, so we cannot exclude the possibility that these peptides induced more than a state of specific antigen tolerance. The specific tolerance to HIV-1 V3 determinants was transient, however, and was overcome when the monkeys were immunized with Th-B-CTL peptides from a different HIV-1 isolate. It is also interesting that chimpanzees immunized with gp160, containing the F region sequence, did not make strong antibody responses to the V3 loop, whereas immunization with gp120, which did not contain the F sequence, did elicit high V3-specific antibody titers (Berman *et al.*, 1990).

The observation that goats and mice respond to peptides containing the F region, but chimpanzees do not, may indicate that the fusogenic domain of HIV-1 may interact specifically with primate cells. It has been demonstrated that HIV-1 can bind both mouse and human cells although it does not infect mouse cells (Maddon *et al.*, 1986). We have also observed that F-Th-B-CTL peptides have a fivefold increased ability to interact with human cells, as compared to mouse cells (D. Cotsamire and B. F. Haynes, unpublished data). It has been suggested that the inability of HIV-1 to infect mouse cells may be at the level of cell fusion (Maddon *et al.*, 1986), and the lipid composition of target membranes and other factors have been shown to affect F domain-induced fusion (reviewed in White, 1990). It is therefore possible that the biological activity of the fusogenic domain is maintained in peptide form and the induction of tolerance is related to the preferential ability of this sequence to act on primate cells.

2.7. Peptide Induction of MHC Class I Molecule-Restricted Anti-HIV-1 CTLs

The use of synthetic peptides to induce antiviral CTL responses in populations expressing diverse MHC haplotypes has posed some special difficulties. First, it has been generally observed that antiviral MHC class I molecule-restricted CTL responses are induced following viral infection rather than after administration of soluble proteins or synthetic peptides (Townsend *et al.*, 1986; Takahashi *et al.*, 1990). However, there have been reports indicating that appropriate processing and presentation of viral CTL epitopes occurred using derivatized immunogens or synthetic peptides (Staerz *et al.*, 1987; Ishioka *et al.*, 1989; Deres *et al.*, 1989; Carbone and Bevan, 1989; Aichele *et al.*, 1990; M. Schulz *et al.*, 1991; Kast *et al.*, 1991; and see Chapter 38).

A second constraint on the use of synthetic peptides in subunit vaccine formulations for the induction of CTLs in random-bred populations is that a sufficient number of CTL epitopes must be included in the vaccine to induce appropriate responses by cells with disparate MHC haplotypes. This may require that the sequences that serve as T-cell epitopes and the MHC molecules that present those sequences be identified to develop an optimal vaccine. Therefore, synthetic peptide vaccines may have to be a cocktail of peptides containing a variety of epitope sequences designed to elicit the appropriate responses in the majority of recipients (Palker *et al.*, 1989; Haynes *et al.*, 1993c) (Fig. 1). Moreover, given the variability of the HIV-1 genome, the sequences of neutralizing Ab, Th, and CTL epitopes of the HIV-1 variants present in a specific geographic region will have to be taken into consideration and included in a vaccine for a particular region or country (Korber *et al.*, 1993; Haynes *et al.*, 1993c).

Synthetic peptide technology permits the addition or removal of sequences as needed to modify immune responses for a given population. To determine if we could induce anti-HIV-1 MHC class I molecule-restricted CTL responses using synthetic peptide immunogens, we first extended the B sequence of the Th-B peptides to include a previously identified CTL epitope restricted to the H-2D^d molecule in mice (Takahashi *et al.*, 1988, 1989a,b) and HLA A2 and A3 in humans (Clerici *et al.*, 1991). This CTL sequence is shown in Table I. As mentioned, adding the CTL region to the construct (Table I) also completed a second B-cell neutralization epitope in the V3 loop (Rusche *et al.*, 1988). Recently, Safrit *et al.* (1993) described a second MHC class I molecule-restricted CTL epitope, restricted by HLA B7, which is found in the proximal portion of the SP10 peptide.

A second peptide design involved synthesizing Th-B-CTL peptides with a 16-amino-acid sequence from the fusogenic region of HIV-1 gp41 (F, amino acids 519–530) at the peptide N-terminus, making F-Th-B-CTL constructs (Table I). The F region was chosen to make peptides that would potentially insert into the cell membrane of antigen-processing cells to access the MHC class I-associated pathway. Th-B-CTL and F-Th-B-CTL peptides made from sequences from HIV-1$_{\text{IIIB}}$ or HIV-1$_{\text{MN}}$ were used in these studies.

Peptides were used to immunize mice either in CFA/IFA or after being incorporated into liposomes to facilitate entry into the MHC class I-associated processing pathway. We found that HIV-1 env V3 peptides, with either the F-Th or just the Th epitope, induced MHC class I molecule-restricted CTLs in vivo (Hart *et al.*, 1991). We also observed that mice immunized with the peptide constructs containing the CTL epitope produced these responses when the peptide was given in CFA/IFA (Hart *et al.*, 1991) or in liposomes (M. K. Hart and B. F. Haynes, unpublished data). The CTL activity was also observed when the peptides were given in saline, without adjuvant or liposomes (Table V). Peptide-induced anti-HIV-1 CTLs were demonstrated to be type-specific, based on the comparison of the HIV-1$_{\text{IIIB}}$ and HIV-1$_{\text{MN}}$ variants, and were restricted to the D^d class I molecule, as previously shown by Takahashi *et al.* (1988) for the V3 loop distal epitope. H2^d mice given Th-B or F-Th-B peptide constructs lacking the complete CTL epitope failed to generate a CTL response (Hart *et al.*, 1991). Similar findings have been reported by others (Sastry *et al.*, 1992). In studies by Shirai *et al.* (1994), CTL responses were observed when cluster Th epitopes and CTL epitopes (P18) were colinearly synthesized and administered in

Table V
Cytolytic Activity of Immune Spleen Cells from F-Th-B-CTL (MN)-Immunized Mice [a]

			% specific lysis of peptide-coated target cells					
			L5178Y (H-2^d)			EL4 (H-2^b)		
				+ peptide			+ peptide	
Effectors	Adjuvant	E:T	None	(MN)	(IIIB)	None	(MN)	(IIIB)
BALB/c (H2d)	CFA/IFA	50:1	14	52	9	6	1	2
		25:1	8	28	4	1	0	1
BALB/c	None	50:1	5	45	3	0	0	0
		25:1	7	33	3	1	0	0
C57BL/6 (H2b)	None	50:1	8	4	6	0	1	0

[a]Mice were immunized five times with 10 μg F-Th-B-CTL (MN) synthetic peptide in saline or CFA/IFA (CFA used for the first immunization) as indicated. Spleen cells were cultured in vitro with the same peptide as previously described (Hart et al., 1991) and tested for the ability to lyse chromium-labeled L5178Y or EL4 cells coated with Th-B-CTL peptide from the indicated HIV isolate as previously described (Hart et al., 1991). Data are representative of three experiments performed.

QS-21 adjuvant. When Th peptides and P18 peptide were mixed in QS-21, but not colinearly synthesized, only marginal CTL activity was detected.

3. SIMIAN IMMUNODEFICIENCY VIRUS (SIV) ENV SYNTHETIC PEPTIDES INDUCE SIV-SPECIFIC CD8[+] Ctls IN RHESUS MONKEYS

The MHC class I molecule restricting elements for HIV-1-specific CTLs are not known in rhesus monkeys, thus preventing use of the HIV-1-derived Th-B-CTL peptides to determine if synthetic peptides in IFA could prime for MHC class I-restricted antiviral CTLs in primates.

Miller et al. (1991) identified an SIV CTL epitope (p11C) in the SIV core protein p24. They also defined an SIV MHC class I allelic producι called MAMU-A-1 that is a restricting element for MHC class I molecule-restricted cytotoxic T-cell recognition of p11C.

Yasutomi et al. (1993) tested the ability of a p11C peptide and a Th-CTL peptide (ST1-p11C) to induce MHC class I-restricted, anti-SIV CTLs in five MAMU-A-1[+] and four MAMU-A-1[-] rhesus monkeys. ST1 is a peptide from the region of SIV env that is analogous in sequence to HIV-1 T1 (Yasutomi et al., 1993). Either the ST1-p11C or the p11C SIV peptide, formulated in IFA, primed and boosted MHC class I molecule-restricted CTLs in MAMU-A-1[+] but not MAMU-A-1[-] rhesus monkeys. A control HIV-1 Th-CTL peptide did not induce anti-SIV p24 CTLs in two MAMU-A-1[+] monkeys. That the p11C peptide alone induced MHC class I molecule-restricted CTLs suggested either that the p11C peptide contained overlapping Th and CTL epitopes (Yasutomi et al., 1993) or that anti-p11C CTLs could be induced in the absence of CD4[+] T-cell help.

Thus, in both rhesus monkeys and mice, synthetic peptide immunogens formulated in oil-based adjuvants accessed the MHC class I molecule-associated processing pathway and primed MHC class I molecule-restricted CTL responses.

4. HTLV-I

4.1. HTLV-I Pathogenesis and Epidemiology

HTLV-I, the first retrovirus to be linked etiologically to human disease, is the causative agent of adult T-cell leukemia/lymphoma (ATL) (Poiesz *et al.*, 1980, 1981; Haynes *et al.*, 1983) and the chronic progressive neurodegenerative syndrome, tropical spastic paraparesis/HTLV-associated myelopathy (TSP/HAM) (Cruickshank, 1956; Rodgers, 1965; Osame *et al.*, 1986). HTLV-I-associated ATL is a lethal, rapidly progressing malignancy that is refractory to conventional chemotherapy and results in death within 4 to 6 months after diagnosis. While IL-2 receptor-directed, toxin-immunotherapy can occasionally result in clinical remission (Waldmann *et al.*, 1988; Kreitman *et al.*, 1990), attempts to block or ameliorate HTLV-I infection and disease have not been generally successful. HTLV-I infection is also associated with a wide spectrum of secondary disease manifestations, including arthritis (Haynes *et al.*, 1983; Karuyama *et al.*, 1990; Kitajima *et al.*, 1989; Nishioka *et al.*, 1989), infectious dermatitis (La Grenade *et al.*, 1990), immunosuppression (Murai *et al.*, 1990; Taguchi and Miyoshi, 1989), and B-cell chronic lymphocytic leukemia (Mann *et al.*, 1987).

Over 10 million persons are infected with HTLV-I within the endemic regions of southwestern Japan, the Caribbean, Central and South America, Africa, the Middle East, and Melanesia (Mueller, 1991). Within the United States, we and others have identified HTLV-I infection in Japanese immigrants (Haynes *et al.*, 1983), in natives of the southeastern United States with no other risk factors (Gallo *et al.*, 1983; Palker *et al.*, unpublished observation), and in intravenous drug users (Weinberg *et al.*, 1988; Khabbaz *et al.*, 1992). Nationwide, median seroprevalence rates of HTLV-I and II in this cohort range from 0.4 to 17% (Khabbaz *et al.*, 1992; Biggar *et al.*, 1993).

4.2. Feasibility of an HTLV-I Vaccine

The hypothesis that an HTLV-I vaccine is feasible is supported by the existence of natural immunity in humans, successful protection from HTLV-I infection in animals, and the genetic and antigenic relatedness of HTLV-I strains throughout the world (de Thé and Bomford, 1993). MHC-restricted CD8[+] or CD4[+] CTLs against HTLV-I tax, gag, and env as well as neutralizing antibodies to HTLV-I envelope, have been identified in HTLV-I[+] carriers and individuals with ATL and TSP/HAM (Jacobson *et al.*, 1990; Elovaara *et al.*, 1993). Yet, the kinds of immune responses required to limit HTLV-I neuropathology or progression to ATL are poorly understood. Patients with TSP/HAM often have highly elevated CTL precursor frequencies (Elovaara *et al.*, 1993), which might contribute to the autoimmune-like demyelination of long motor neural tracts. Further, elevated maternal antibody titers to a synthetic peptide containing HTLV-I envelope amino acids 190–209 correlated with a threefold increased risk of HTLV-I transmission from mother to child (Wiktor *et al.*, 1993). This region also contains dominant sites recognized by Th cells, CD4$^+$ CTLs, and neutralizing antibodies. Thus, careful selection and presentation of vaccine antigens may well be critical in determining whether immunization protects or enhances HTLV-I infection and disease.

4.3. Envelope Sequence Divergence among HTLV-I Strains

Unlike HIV-1, genetic and antigenic variation does not appear to pose as great a problem for HTLV-I vaccine design, since sequence variation among the env genes of HTLV-I range from 5–7% for Melanesia isolates to 2% among viral isolates from the United States, Canada, Japan, Africa, the Caribbean, and Central and South America (Komurian *et al.*, 1991; Gray *et al.*, 1990; Clapham *et al.*, 1984). There appear to be serological relatedness and cross-neutralization between human immune sera and viral stocks from around the world. However, a mutation in env affecting monoclonal antibody binding has been identified (T. Schulz *et al.*, 1991) and minor envelope sequence changes in MuLV, FeLV, and HIV-1 (Takeuchi *et al.*, 1991) can profoundly alter viral tropism, pathogenicity, and neutralization. We observed that two amino acid changes within the amino-terminal neutralizing region of HTLV-I gp46 (amino acids N_{95} to Q and G_{97} to L) confer HTLV-II-type specificity to this region (Palker *et al.*, 1992). It is therefore conceivable that minor variations of HTLV-I envelope sequences could have a major impact on virus neutralization.

4.4. Vaccine-Induced Protection from HTLV-I Challenge

Protection from experimental challenge with cell-associated HTLV-I has been achieved in animal models. Nakamura *et al.* (1987) protected cynomolgus monkeys against infection by HTLV-I after immunizing with both gp46 external envelope and gp21 transmembrane envelope gene products produced in *E. coli*. After challenge with HTLV-I-producing MT-2 cells, four of six monkeys protected from infection had neutralizing antibody responses to HTLV-I (titers from 1/20 to 1/160) which were absent in the two unprotected monkeys receiving lower levels of inoculum. The authors concluded that neutralizing antibodies to linear determinants of HTLV-I envelope are associated with protection from HTLV-I infection. However, these investigators did not determine whether neutralizing antibodies or antibody-dependent cellular cytotoxicity (ADCC) were components of the protective response; nor did they identify the protective epitopes of HTLV-I envelope. Moreover, achieving protection required five immunizations with a total of 1100 μg over 20 weeks, indicating that further improvements in vaccine design are required to obtain more potent immunogenicity per dose of inoculum.

In rabbits, Shida *et al.* (1987) demonstrated the protective efficacy of recombinant vaccinia constructs expressing HTLV-I envelope glycoproteins. Again, protection from HTLV-I$^+$ T-cell challenge correlated with high levels of anti-HTLV-I envelope antibodies. In this study, investigators did not evaluate the presence of CTLs to HTLV-I envelope or measure neutralizing antibody titers.

As has been demonstrated for HIV, passive administration of immune globulin can prevent HTLV-I infection. Adult rabbits were protected from HTLV-I challenge by the administration of human or rabbit anti-HTLV-I immune sera (Kataoka *et al.*, 1990). Similarly, newborn rabbits were protected from milk-borne transmission of HTLV-I from infected mothers after passive administration of immune globulin (Sawada *et al.*, 1990).

Collectively, these studies convey two vital messages regarding vaccine development: first, the HTLV-I envelope glycoprotein antigen, in either denatured or native form, is protective; and second, circulating antibody contributes to protection, even against cell-associated virus. The observation that linear determinants of HTLV-I gp46 induce protective immunity in animals suggests that synthetic peptides that contain appropriate neutralizing sites of gp46 might prove to be useful as a vaccine. However, further studies are needed to determine the antigenic sequences required for protection, the types of immune responses (ADCC, CTLs) that contribute to protective immunity, and the optimal vaccine designs that potentiate long-lived immunity to HTLV-I.

4.5. Synthetic Peptide Approaches to HTLV-I Vaccine Development

Neutralizing regions of HTLV-I envelope are dispersed throughout both the gp46 external envelope and gp21 transmembrane glycoproteins (Fig. 3). Tanaka *et al.* (1991) reported that rat monoclonal antibodies to gp46 that neutralize HTLV-I bound to sites within amino acids 191–196. This region overlaps a site previously shown to bind the neutralizing human monoclonal antibody 0.5α (Matsushita *et al.*, 1986). Palker and Haynes corroborated the findings of Tanaka *et al.* (1991) and further identified a novel amino-terminal neutralizing site (amino acids 88–98) with a sequence similar to the V3 neutralizing region of HIV-1RF gp120 (Palker *et al.*, 1992). Other neutralizing regions within both HTLV-I gp46 external envelope and gp21 transmembrane glycoproteins have been identified by Inoue *et al.* (1992) and Desgranges *et al.* (1994). Vaccine studies have provided suggestive evidence to indicate that antibody responses to neutralizing sites in either gp46 or gp21 confer protection from HTLV-I challenge infection (Nakamura *et al.*, 1987), although protection induced by immunization with synthetic peptides containing discrete neutralizing sites has not yet been reported.

In addition to a neutralizing site, the central region of gp46 between amino acids 190 and 209 contains dominant sites recognized by Th cells from congenic strains of mice and CD4$^+$ CTLs from HTLV-I-positive individuals with TSP/HAM (Fig. 3). Kurata *et al.* (1989) identified three immunodominant sites for murine Th cells on HTLV-I gp46 (amino acids 190–209, 141–156) and gp21 (amino acids 342–363). Peptides containing these regions could be used to immunize mice to elicit proliferative responses of lymph node cells to native HTLV-I gp46. Jacobson *et al.* (1991) reported that CTL lines generated from two HTLV-I$^+$ patients with HAM/TSP recognized a site within amino acids 196–209. Thus, within a 19-amino-acid sequence of HTLV-I gp46 are found epitopes that bind neutralizing antibodies (amino acids 191–196) and T-cell receptors of both Th cells (191–209) and CTLs (amino acids 196–209). Wiktor *et al.* (1993) found that elevated antibody titers against a peptide SP4al containing envelope amino acids 196–209 correlated significantly with increased mother-to-child transmission of HTLV-I. The proximity of this site to a dominant neutralizing region (amino acids 191–196) suggests the possibility that enhanc-

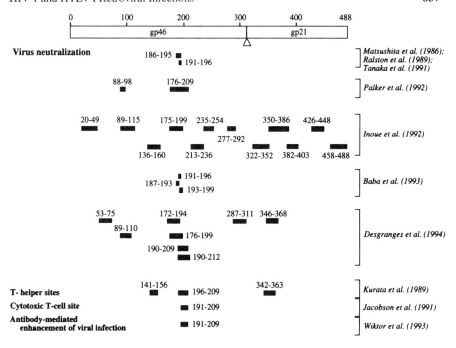

Figure 3. Immunological targets on HTLV-I envelope glycoproteins. Shown are the locations (amino acid numbers) within HTLV-I envelope glycoprotein of sites identified by neutralizing antibodies, Th cells, human CD4[+] CTLs, and antibodies associated with enhanced transmission of HTLV-I from mother to child. Corresponding references are given to the right and in the list of cited literature for this chapter.

ing antibodies that are reactive with amino acids 196–209 could interfere with the binding of neutralizing antibodies to amino acids 191–196. Subunit peptide immunogens that incorporate this region will need to be carefully evaluated for the ability to elicit antibodies that enhance viral infection.

Palker *et al.* (1992) designed a 38-amino-acid chimeric peptide designated DP-91 (Fig. 4) which contains amino-terminal (amino acids 88–98) and central (amino acids 191–196) neutralizing domains of HTLV-I gp46, a dominant Th site, and a site recognized by CD4[+] CTLs. After three subcutaneous immunizations of two goats with DP-91 in CFA (day 0) and IFA (days 14, 21), we measured neutralizing titers to HTLV-I (90% inhibition of syncytium formation) of 1/20 to 1/40 in sera from both animals. While these titers are low compared to neutralizing titers of 1/1280 and greater detected in sera from some HTLV-I[+] patients (T. Palker, personal communication), Nakamura *et al.* (1987) reported similarly low neutralizing titers in vaccinated cynomolgus monkeys that were protected from challenge with HTLV-I-infected cells. Studies are ongoing to evaluate DP-91 and related experimental immunogens as vaccines against HTLV-I infection.

Thus, the presence of circulating antibodies to both native and denatured forms of HTLV-I envelope coincides with protection from HTLV-I challenge. However, to achieve long-lived memory T- and B-cell immunity to HTLV-I, novel constructs and delivery

DP-91 HTLV-I envelope amino acids

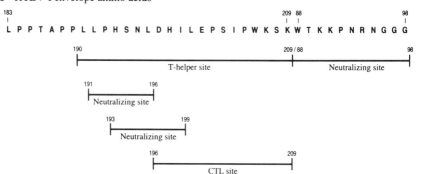

Figure 4. Th-B chimeric HTLV-I envelope peptide DP-91: an HTLV-I immunogen for inducing neutralizing antibodies. Peptide DP-91, containing a dominant Th epitope, three neutralizing antibody epitopes, and a CTL epitope from HTLV-I envelope glycoprotein, induced neutralizing antibodies to HTLV-I (90% inhibition of syncytium formation at 1/20–1/40 dilution) when used with CFA (day 0) and IFA (days 14, 21) to immunize two goats intramuscularly (Palker *et al.*, 1992). Neutralizing antibodies were induced to amino acids 88–98.

systems are needed. Synthetic peptide immunogens offer the advantage that dominant T- and B-cell determinants of HTLV-I can be administered while excluding those sites associated with enhancement of viral infection. With appropriate adjuvants and further delineation of sites of HTLV-I recognized by CTLs, HTLV-I peptide immunogens could conceivably be used to induce multiple effector immune responses, including neutralizing antibodies and priming of Th and MHC class I molecule-restricted, CD8+ CTLs. However, further preclinical studies are warranted to address whether protective immunity, and not enhancement of viral infection, can be achieved with immunization.

5. SUMMARY AND FUTURE DIRECTIONS

Synthetic peptide immunogens can induce high-titered neutralizing antibodies and Th and CTL cellular responses against native human retroviral proteins and virus-infected cells. The usefulness of synthetic peptides as practical immunogens to prevent HIV-1 and HTLV-I infections may be to prime and/or boost certain types of antiretroviral immune responses. Work on retroviral pathogenesis and determination of the correlates of protective immunity to HIV-1 and HTLV-I is moving parallel to work on design of HIV-1 and HTLV-I experimental immunogens. We hope that insights into these parallel avenues of work will be able to guide retroviral vaccine development and speed the development of effective preventive immunogens for human retroviral diseases.

ACKNOWLEDGMENTS

This work was supported by grants P01-CA43447, Centers for AIDS Research Grant AI28662, CA40660, and NCVDG grant AI35351. B. F. H. is a Carter–Wallace Fellow in

Retroviral Research. T. J. P. is a recipient of a Leukemia Society of America Scholar award. The authors thank Thomas J. Matthews, Alphonse J. Langlois, Dani Bolognesi, and Charlene McDanal for performing HIV-1 neutralization assays. Kim R. McClammy provided expert administrative assistance.

REFERENCES

Ada, G., 1991, Strategies for exploiting the immune system in the design of vaccines, *Mol. Immunol.* **28**:225–230.

Ahlers, J. D., Pendleton, C. D., Dunlop, N., Minassian, A., Nara, P. L., and Berzofsky, J. A., 1993, Construction of an HIV-1 peptide vaccine containing a multideterminant helper peptide linked to a V3 loop peptide 18 inducing strong neutralizing antibody responses in mice of multiple MHC haplotypes after two immunizations, *J. Immunol.* **150**:5647–5665.

Aichele, P., Hengartner, H., Zinkernagel, R. M., and Schulz, M., 1990, Anti-viral cytotoxic T cell responses induced by in vivo priming with a free synthetic peptide, *J. Exp. Med.* **171**:1815–1820.

Autran, B., Plata, F., and Debre, P., 1991, MHC-restricted cytotoxicity against HIV, *J. AIDS* **4**:361–367.

Baba, E., Nakamura, M., Tanaka, Y., Kuroki, M., Itoyama, Y., Nakano, S., and Niho, Y., 1993, Multiple neutralizing B-cell epitopes of human T-cell leukemia virus type I (HTLV-I) identified by human monoclonal antibodies, *J. Immunol.* **151**:1013–1024.

Berman, P. W., Gregory, T. J., Riddle, L., Nakamura, G. R., Champe, M. A., Porter, J. P., Wurm, F. M., Hershberg, R. D., Cobb, E. K., and Eichberg, J. W., 1990, Protection of chimpanzees from infection by HIV-1 after vaccination with recombinant glycoprotein gp120 but not gp160, *Nature* **345**:622–625.

Berzofsky, J. A., 1991, Antigenic peptide interaction with MHC molecules: Implications for vaccine development, *Semin. Immunol.* **3**:203–216.

Berzofsky, J. A., Pendleton, C. D., Clerici, M., Ahlers, J., Lucey, D. R., Putney, S. D., and Shearer, G. M., 1991, Construction of peptides encompassing multideterminant clusters of human immunodeficiency virus envelope to induce in vitro T cell responses in mice and humans of multiple MHC types, *J. Clin. Invest.* **88**:876–884.

Bessen, D., and Fischetti, V., 1990, Synthetic peptide vaccine against mucosal colonization by group A streptococci. I. Protection against a heterologous M serotype with shared C repeat region epitopes, *J. Immunol.* **145**:1251–1256.

Biggar, R., Buskell-Boles, Z., Yakshe, P., Caussey, D., Gridley, G., and Seeff, L., 1993, Antibody to human retroviruses among drug abusers in three east coast American cities 1972–1976, *J. Infect. Dis.* **163**:57–63.

Bittle, J. L., Houghten, R. A., Alexander, H., Shinnick, T. M., Sutcliffe, J. G., Lerner, R. A., Rowlands, D. J., and Brown, F., 1982, Protection against FMDV by immunization with a chemically synthesized peptide predicted from the viral nucleotide sequence, *Nature* **298**:30–33.

Carbone, F. R., and Bevan, M. J., 1989, Induction of ovalbumin-specific cytotoxic T cells by *in vivo* peptide immunization, *J. Exp. Med.* **169**:603–612.

Cease, K. B., 1990, Peptide component vaccine engineering: Targeting the AIDS virus, *Int. Rev. Immunol.* **7**:85–107.

Cease, K. B., Margalit, H., Cornette, J. L., Putney, S. D., Robey, W. G., Ouyang, C., Streicher, H. Z., Fischinger, P. J., Gallo, R. C., DeLisi, C., and Berzofsky, J. A., 1987, Helper T cell antigenic site identification in the acquired immunodeficiency syndrome virus gp120 envelope protein and induction of immunity in mice to the native protein using a 16-residue synthetic peptide, *Proc. Natl. Acad. Sci. USA* **84**:4249–4253.

Cheng-Mayer, C., Homsy, J., Evans, L. A., and Levy, J. A., 1988, Identification of human immunodeficiency virus subtypes with distinct patterns of sensitivity to serum neutralization, *Proc. Natl. Acad. Sci. USA* **85**:2815–2819.

Clapham, P., Nagy, K., and Weiss, R., 1984, Pseudotypes of human T-cell leukemia viruses types I and II: Neutralization by patients' sera, *Proc. Natl. Acad. Sci. USA* **81**:2886–2889.

Clerici, M., Stocks, N. I., Zajac, R. A., Boswell, R. N., Bernstein, D. C., Mann, D. L., Shearer, G. M., and Berzofsky, J. A., 1989, Interleukin 2 production used to detect antigenic peptide recognition by T helper lymphocytes from asymptomatic HIV seropositive individuals, *Nature* **339**:383–385.

Clerici, M., Lucey, D. R., Zajac, R. A., Boswell, R. N., Gebel, H. M., Takahashi, H., Berzofsky, J. A., and Shearer, G. M., 1991, Detection of cytotoxic T lymphocytes specific for synthetic peptides of gp160 in HIV-seropositive individuals, *J. Immunol.* **146**:2214–2219.

Cruickshank, E., 1956, A neuropathic syndrome of uncertain origin: Review of 100 cases, *West Indian Med. J.* **5**:147–158.

Deres, K., Schild, H., Weismuller, K. H., Jung, G., and Ramensee, H. G., 1989, In vivo priming of virus-specific cytotoxic T lymphocytes with synthetic lipopeptide vaccine, *Nature* **342**:561–564.

Desgranges, C., Souche, S., Vernant, J.-C., Smadja, D., Vahlne, A., and Horal, P., 1994, Identification of novel neutralization-inducing regions of human T cell lymphotropic virus type I envelope glycoproteins with human HTLV-I seropositive sera, *AIDS Res. Hum. Retroviruses* **10**:163–173.

de Thé, G., and Bomford, R., 1993, An HTLV-I vaccine: Why, how and for whom? *AIDS Res. Hum. Retroviruses* **9**:381–386.

Dion, A. S., Knittel, J. J., and Morneweck, S. T., 1990, Virus envelope-based peptide vaccines against virus-induced mammary tumors, *Virology* **179**:474–477.

Elovaara, I., Koenig, S., Yambasu, A., Brewah, M., Woods, R., Lehky, T., and Jacobson, S., 1993, High human T cell lymphotropic virus type I (HTLV-I)-specific precursor cytotoxic T lymphocyte frequencies in patients with HTLV-I associated neurological disease, *J. Exp. Med.* **177**:1567–1573.

Etlinger, H. M., Renia, L., Matile, H., Manneberg, M., Mazier, D., Trzeciak, A., and Gillessen, D., 1991, Antibody responses to a synthetic peptide-based malaria vaccine candidate: Influence of sequence variants of the peptide, *Eur. J. Immunol.* **21**:1505–1511.

Gallo, R. C., Kalyanaraman, V. S., Sarngadharan, M. G., Sliski, A., Vonderheid, E. C., Maeda, M., Nakao, Y., Yamada, K., Ito, Y., Gutensohn, N., Murphy, S., Bunn, P. A., Catovsky, D., Greaves, M., Blayney, D. W., Haynes, B. F., Jegasothy, B. V., Jaffe, E., Cossman, J., Broder, S., Fisher, R. I., Golde, D. W., and Robert-Guroff, M., 1983, Association of the human type C retrovirus with a subset of adult T-cell cancers, *Cancer Res.* **43**:3892–3899.

Girard, M., Kieny, M. P., Pinter, A., Barre-Sinoussi, F., Nara, P., Kolbe, H., Kusumi, K., Chaput, A., Reinhart, T., Muchmore, E., Ronco, J., Kaczorek, M., Gomard, E., Gluckman, J.-C., and Fultz, P. N., 1991, Immunization of chimpanzees confers protection against challenge with human immunodeficiency virus, *Proc. Natl. Acad. Sci. USA* **88**:542–546.

Goudsmit, J., Boucher, C. A., Meloen, R. H., Epstein, L. G., Smit, L., van der Hoek, L., and Bakker, M., 1988, Human antibody response to a strain-specific HIV-1 gp120 epitope associated with cell fusion inhibition, *AIDS* **2**:157–164.

Gray, G., White, M., Bartman, T., and Marn, D., 1990, Envelope gene sequence of HTLV-I isolate MT-2 and its comparison with other HTLV-I isolates, *Virology* **177**:391–395.

Hale, P. M., Cease, K. B., Houghten, R. A., Ouyang, C., Putney, S., Javaherian, K., Margalit, H., Cornette, J. L., Spouge, J. L., Delisi, C., and Berzofsky, J. A., 1989, T cell multideterminant regions in the human immunodeficiency virus envelope: Toward overcoming the problem of major histocompatability complex restriction, *Int. Immunol.* **1**:409–415.

Hart, M. K., Palker, T. J., Matthews, T. J., Langlois, A. J., Lerche, N. W., Martin, M. E., Scearce, R. M., McDanal, C., Bolognesi, D., and Haynes, B. F., 1990, Synthetic peptides containing T and B cell epitopes from human immunodeficiency virus gp120 induce anti-HIV proliferative responses and high titers of neutralizing antibodies in rhesus monkeys, *J. Immunol.* **145**:2677–2685.

Hart, M. K., Weinhold, K. J., Scearce, R. M., Washburn, E. M., Clark, C. A., Palker, T. J., and Haynes, B. F., 1991, Priming of anti-human immunodeficiency virus (HIV) $CD8^+$ cytotoxic T cells in vivo by carrier-free HIV synthetic peptides, *Proc. Natl. Acad. Sci. USA* **88**:9448–9452.

Haynes, B. F., 1992, Immune responses to HIV infection, in: *AIDS: Etiology, Diagnosis, Treatment, and Prevention*, 3rd ed. (V. DeVita, S. Rosenberg, and A. Fauci, eds.), Lippincott, Philadelphia, pp. 77–86.

Haynes, B., Miller, S., Palker, T., Moore, J., Dunn, P., Bolognesi, D., and Metzgar, R., 1983, Identification of human T-cell leukemia virus in a Japanese patient with adult T-cell leukemia and cutaneous lymphomatous vasculitis, *Proc. Natl. Acad. Sci. USA* **80**:2054–2058.

Haynes, B. F., Torres, J. V., Langlois, A. J., Bolognesi, D. P., Gardner, M. B., Palker, T. J., Scearce, R. M., Jones, D. M., Moody, M. A., McDanal, C., and Matthews, T. J., 1993a, Induction of HIVMN neutralizing antibodies in primates using a prime-boost regimen of hybrid synthetic gp120 envelope peptides, *J. Immunol.* **151**:1646–1653.

Haynes, B. F., Arthur, L. O., Frost, P., Matthews, T. J., Langlois, A. J., Palker, T. J., Hart, M. K., Scearce, R. M., Jones, D. M., McDanal, C., Ottinger, J., Bolognesi, D. P., and Weinhold, K. J., 1993b, Conversion of an immunogenic human immunodeficiency virus (HIV) envelope synthetic peptide to a tolerogen in chimpanzees by the fusogenic domain of HIV gp41 envelope protein, *J. Exp. Med.* **177**:717–727.

Haynes, B. F., Yasutomi, Y., Torres, J. V., Gardner, M. B., Langlois, A. J., Bolognesi, D. P., Matthews, T. J., Scearce, R. M., Jones, D. M., Moody, M. A., McDanal, C., Heinly, C., Bergamo, B., Palker, T. J., and Letvin, N. L., 1993c, Use of synthetic peptides in primates to induce high-titered neutralizing antibodies and MHC class I-restricted cytotoxic T cells against AIDS retroviruses: An HLA-based vaccine strategy, *Trans. Assoc. Am. Physicians* **106**:31–41.

Hosmalin, A., Nara, P. L., Zweig, M., Lerche, N. W., Cease, K. B., Gard, E. A., Markham, P. D., Putney, S. D., Daniel, M. D., Desrosiers, R. C., and Berzofsky, J. A., 1991, Priming with helper T cell epitope peptides enhances the antibody response to the envelope glycoprotein of HIV-1 in primates, *J. Immunol.* **146**:1667–1673.

Hunt, A. R., Johnson, A. J., and Roehrig, J. T., 1990, Synthetic peptides of Venezuelan equine encephalitis virus E2 glycoprotein. I. Immunogenic analysis and identification of a protective peptide, *Virology* **179**:701–711.

Inoue, Y., Kuroda, N., Shiraki, H., Sato, H., and Maeda, Y., 1992, Neutralizing activity of human antibodies against the structural protein of human T-cell lymphotropic virus type I, *Int. J. Cancer* **52**:877–880.

Ishioka, G. Y., Colon, S., Miles, C., Grey, H. M., and Chesnut, R. W., 1989, Induction of class I MHC-restricted, peptide-specific cytolytic T lymphocytes by peptide priming in vivo, *J. Immunol.* **143**:1094–1100.

Jacobson, S., Shida, H., McFarlin, D., Fauci, A., and Koenig, S., 1990, Circulating CD8[+] cytotoxic T lymphocytes specific for HTLV-I pX in patients with HTLV-I associated neurological disease, *Nature* **348**:245–248.

Jacobson, S., Reuben, J., Streilein, R., and Palker, T., 1991, Induction of CD4[+], HTLV-I specific cytotoxic T-lymphocytes from patients with HAM/TSP: Recognition of an immunogenic region of the gp46 envelope glycoprotein of HTLV-I, *J. Immunol.* **146**:1155–1162.

Karuyama, S., Sonoda, A., Yoshida, A., and Osame, M., 1990, Arthritis in a human T-lymphotropic virus type I (HTLV-I) carrier, *Ann. Rheum. Dis.* **49**:718–721.

Kast, W. M., Roux, L., Curren, J., Blom, H. J. J., Voordouw, A. C., Meloen, R. H., Kolakofsky, D., and Melief, C. J. M., 1991, Protection against lethal Sendai virus infection by in vivo priming of virus-specific cytotoxic T lymphocytes with a free synthetic peptide, *Proc. Natl. Acad. Sci. USA* **88**:2283–2287.

Kataoka, R., Takehara, N., Iwahara, Y., Sonoda, T., Ohtsuki, Y., Dawei, Y., Hoshino, H., and Miyoshi, I., 1990, Transmission of HTLV-I by blood transfusion and its prevention by passive immunization in rabbits, *Blood* **76**:1657–1661.

Kenealy, W. R., Matthews, T. J., Ganfield, M. C., Langlois, A. J., Waselefsky, D. M., and Petteway, S. R., Jr., 1989, Antibodies from human immunodeficiency virus-infected individuals bind to a short amino acid sequence that elicits neutralizing antibodies in animals, *AIDS Res. Hum. Retroviruses* **5**:173–182.

Khabbaz, R., Oronato, I., Cannon, R., Hartley, T., Roberts, B., Hosein, B., and Kaplan, J., 1992, Seroprevalence of HTLV-I and HTLV-II among intravenous drug users and persons in clinics for sexually transmitted diseases, *N. Engl. J. Med.* **326**:375–380.

Kitajima, I., Maruyama, I., Maruyama, Y., Ijichi, S., Eiraku, N., Mimura, Y., and Osame, M., 1989, Polyarthritis in human T-lymphotropic virus type I associated myelopathy, *Arthritis Rheum.* **32**:1342–1343.

Komurian, F., Pelloguin, F., and de Thé, G., 1991, *In vivo* genomic variability of HTLV-I depends more upon geography than pathologies, *J. Virology* **65**:3770–3778.

Korber, B. T., Farber, R. M., Wolpert, D. H., and Lapedes, A. S., 1993, Covariation of mutations in the V3 loop of human immunodeficiency virus type 1 envelope protein: An information theoretic analysis, *Proc. Natl. Acad. Sci. USA* **90**:7176–7180.

Kreitman, R., Chaudhury, V., Waldmann, T., Willingham, M., Fitzgerald, D., and Pastan, I., 1990, The recombinant immunotoxin anti-Tac (Fv)-PE40 is cytotoxic toward peripheral blood malignant cells from patients with adult T-cell leukemia, *Proc. Natl. Acad. Sci. USA* **87**:8291–8295.

Kurata, A., Palker, T., Streilein, R., Scearce, R., Haynes, B., and Berzofsky, J., 1989, Immunodominant sites on human T-cell leukemia virus type 1 envelope protein for murine T-cells, *J. Immunol.* **143**:2024–2030.

La Grenade, L., Hanchard, B., Fletcher, V., Cranston, B., and Blattner, W., 1990, Infective dermatitis of Jamaican children: A marker for HTLV-1 infection, *Lancet* **336**:1345–1347.

Maddon, P. J., Dalgleish, A. G., McDougal, J. S., Clapham, P. R., and Axel, R. A., 1986, The T4 gene encodes the AIDS virus receptor and is expressed in the immune system and the brain, *Cell* **47**:333–348.

Mann, D., De Santis, P., Mark, G., Pfeifer, A., Newman, M., Gibbs, N., Popovic, M., Sarngadharan, M., Gallo, R., Clark, J., and Blattner, W., 1987, HTLV-I associated B-cell CLL: Indirect role for retrovirus in leukemogenesis, *Science* **236**:1103–1106.

Matsushita, S., Robert-Guroff, M., Trepel, J., Cossman, H., Mitsuya, H., and Broder, S., 1986, Human monoclonal antibody against an envelope glycoprotein of human T-cell leukemia virus type I, *Proc. Natl. Acad. Sci. USA* **83**:2672–2676.

Matthews, T. J., Langlois, A. J., Robey, W. G., Chang, N. T., Gallo, R. C., Fischinger, P. J., and Bolognesi, D. P., 1986, Restricted neutralization of divergent HTLV-III/LAV isolates by antibodies to the major envelope glycoprotein, *Proc. Natl. Acad. Sci. USA* **83**:9709–9713.

Milich, D. R., 1990, Synthetic peptides: Prospects for vaccine development, *Semin. Immunol.* **2**:307–315.

Miller, M. D., Yamamoto, H., Hughes, A. L., Watkins, D. I., and Letvin, N. L., 1991, Definition of an epitope and MHC class I molecule recognized by gag-specific cytotoxic T lymphocytes in SIVmac-infected rhesus monkeys, *J. Immunol.* **147**:320–329.

Mueller, N., 1991, The epidemiology of HTLV-I infection, *Cancer Causes Control* **2**:37–52.

Murai, K., Tachibana, N., Shiori, S., Shishime, E., Okayama, A., Ishizaki, J., Tsuda, K., and Mueller, N., 1990, Suppression of delayed-type hypersensitivity to PPD and PHA in elderly HTLV-I carriers, *J. AIDS* **3**:1006–1009.

Myers, G., Josephs, S. F., Rabison, A. B., Smith, T. F., and Wong-Staal, F., (eds.), 1988, *Human Retroviruses and AIDS*, Vol. 2, Theoretical Biology and Biophysics Group, Los Alamos National Laboratory, Los Alamos, NM, pp. 68–92.

Nakamura, H., Hayami, M., Ohta, Y., Ishikawa, K., Tsujimoto, H., Kiyokawa, T., Yoshida, M., Sasagawa, A., and Honjo, S., 1987, Protection of cynomolgus monkeys against infection by human T-cell leukemia virus type-I by immunization with viral env gene products in *Escherichia coli*, *Int. J. Cancer* **40**:403–407.

Nishioka, N., Maruyama, I., Sato, K., Kitajima, I., Nakajima, Y., and Osame, M., 1989, Chronic inflammatory arthropathy associated with HTLV-I, *Lancet* **1**:441.

Osame, M., Usuku, K., Izumo, S., Ijichi, N., Amitani, H., Igata, A., Matsumoto, M., and Tara, M., 1986, HTLV-I associated myelopathy, a new clinical entity, *Lancet* **1**:1031–1032.

Palker, T. J., Matthews, T. J., Clark, M. E., Cianciolo, G. J., Randall, R. R., Langlois, A. J., White, G. C., Safai, B., Snyderman, R., Bolognesi, D. P., and Haynes, B. F., 1988a, Mapping of immunogenic and immunodominant epitopes of human immunodeficiency virus gp120 with env-encoded synthetic peptides, in: *Human Retroviruses, Cancer, and AIDS: Approaches to Prevention and Therapy* (D. Bolognesi, ed.), Liss, New York, pp. 161–174.

Palker, T. J., Clark, M. E., Langlois, A. J., Matthews, T. J., Weinhold, K. J., Randall, R. R., Bolognesi, D. P., and Haynes, B. F., 1988b, Type-specific neutralization of the human immunodeficiency virus with antibodies to env-encoded synthetic peptides, *Proc. Natl. Acad. Sci. USA* **85**:1932–1936.

Palker, T. J., Matthews, T. J., Langlois, A. J., Tanner, M. E., Martin, M. E., Scearce, R. M., Kim, J. E., Berzofsky, J. A., Bolognesi, D. P., and Haynes, B. F., 1989, Polyvalent human immunodeficiency virus synthetic immunogen comprised of envelope gp120 T helper cell sites and B cell neutralization epitopes, *J. Immunol.* **142**:3612–3619.

Palker, T., Riggs, E., Spragion, D., Muir, A., Scearce, R., Randall, R., McAdams, M., McKnight, A., Clapham, P., Weiss, R., and Haynes, B., 1992, Mapping of homologous, amino-terminal neutralizing regions of human T-cell lymphotropic virus type I and II gp46 envelope glycoproteins, *J. Virol.* **66**:5879–5889.

Plata, F., Autran, B., Pedroza-Martins, L., Wain-Hobson, S., Raphael, M., Mayaud, C., Denis, M., Guillon, J. M., and Debre, P., 1987, AIDS virus specific cytotoxic T lymphocytes in lung disorders, *Nature* **328**:348–351.

Poiesz, B., Ruscetti, F., Gazdar, A., Bunn, P., Minna, J., and Gallo, R., 1980, Detection and isolation of type-C retrovirus particles from fresh and cultured lymphocytes of a patient with cutaneous T-cell lymphoma, *Proc. Natl. Acad. Sci. USA* **77**:7415–7419.

Poiesz, B., Ruscetti, F., Reitz, M., Kalyanaraman, V., and Gallo, R., 1981, Isolation of a new type-C retrovirus (HTLV) in primary uncultured cells of a patient with Sezary T-cell leukemia, *Nature* **294**:268–271.

Putney, S. D., Matthews, T. J., Robey, W. G., Lynn, D. L., Robert-Guroff, M., Mueller, W. T., Langlois, A. J., Ghrayeb, J., Petteway, S. R., Weinhold, K. J., Fischinger, P. J., Wong-Staal, F., Gallo, R. C., and Bolognesi, D. P., 1986, HTLV-III/LAV neutralizing antibodies to an *E. coli* produced fragment of the virus envelope, *Science* **234**:1392–1395.

Ralston, S., Hoeprich, P., and Akita, R., 1989, Identification and synthesis of the epitope for a human monoclonal antibody which can neutralize human T-cell leukemia/lymphotropic virus type I, *J. Biol. Chem.* **264**:16343–16346.

Ratner, L., Haseltine, W., Patarca, R., Livak, K. J., Starcich, B., Josephs, S. F., Doran, E. R., Rafalski, J. A., Whitehorn, E. A., Baumeister, K., Ivanoff, L., Petteway, S. R., Pearson, M. L., Lautenberger, J. A., Papas, T. S., Ghrayeb, J., Chang, N. T., Gallo, R. C., and Wong-Staal, F., 1985, Complete nucleotide sequence of the AIDS virus, HTLV-III, *Nature* **313**:277–284.

Riveau, G. J., and Audibert, F. M., 1990, Synthetic peptide vaccines against pathogens and biological mediators, *Trends Pharmacol. Sci.* **11**:194–198.

Robert-Guroff, M., Brown, M., and Gallo, R. C., 1985, HTLV-III-neutralizing antibodies in patients with AIDS and AIDS-related complex, *Nature* **316**:72–74.

Rodgers, P., 1965, The clinical features and aetiology of the neuropathic syndrome in Jamaica, *West Indian Med. J.* **14**:36–40.

Rodriguez, R., Moreno, A., Guzman, F., Calvo, M., and Patarroyo, M. E., 1990, Studies in owl monkeys leading to the development of a synthetic vaccine against the asexual blood stages of Plasmodium falciparum, *Am. J. Trop. Med. Hyg.* **43**:339–354.

Ronco, J., DeDieu, J. F., Marie, F. N., Pinter, A., Kaczorek, M., and Girard, M., 1992, High titer HIV-1 neutralizing antibody response of rhesus macaques to gp160 and env peptides, *AIDS Res. Hum. Retroviruses* **8**:1117–1124.

Rusche, J. R., Javaherian, K., McDanal, C., Petro, J., Lynn, D. L., Grimaila, R., Langlois, A., Gallo, R. C., Arthur, L. O., Fischinger, P. J., Bolognesi, D. P., Putney, S. D., and Matthews, T. J., 1988, Antibodies that inhibit fusion of human immunodeficiency virus-infected cells bind a 24-amino acid sequence of the viral envelope gp120, *Proc. Natl. Acad. Sci. USA* **85**:3198–3202.

Safrit, J. T., Lee, A., and Koup, R. A., 1993, Characterization of HLA-B7-restricted cytotoxic T lymphocyte clones specific for the third variable region of HIV gp120, isolated from two patients during acute seroconversion, Abstract presented at *Conferences on Advances in AIDS Vaccine Development, Sixth Annual Meeting of the National Cooperative Vaccine Development Groups for AIDS*, October 30–November 4, 1993.

Sastry, K. J., Nehete, P. N., Venkatnarayanan, S., Morkowski, J., Platsoucas, C. D., and Arlinghaus, R. B., 1992, Rapid *in vivo* induction of HIV-specific CD8[+] cytotoxic T lymphocytes by a 15-amino acid unmodified free peptide from the immunodominant V3-loop of gp120, *Virology* **188**:502–509.

Sawada, T., Tawahara, Y., Ishu, K., Taguchi, H., Hoshino, H., and Miyoshi I., 1990, Immunoglobulin prophylaxis against milkborne transmission of human T-cell leukemia virus in rabbits, *J. Infect. Dis.* **164**:1193–1196.

Schulz, M., Zinkernagel, R. M., and Hengartner, H., 1991, Peptide-induced anti-viral protection by cytotoxic T cells, *Proc. Natl. Acad. Sci. USA* **88**:991–993.

Schulz, T., Calabro, M.-L., Hoad, J., Carrington, C., Matutes, E., Catovsky, D., and Weiss, R., 1991, HTLV-I envelope sequences from Brazil, the Caribbean, and Romania: Clustering of sequences according to geographical origin and variability in an antigenic epitope, *Virology* **184**:483–491.

Shida, H., Tochikura, T., Sato, T., Konno, T., Hirayoshi, K., Seki, M., Ito, Y., Hatanaka, M., Hinuma, Y., Sugimoto, M., Takahashi-Nishimaki, F., Maruyama, T., Miki, K., Suzuki, K., Morita, M., Sashiyama, H., and Hayami, M., 1987, Effect of recombinant vaccinia virus that expresses HTLV-I envelope gene on HTLV-I infection, *EMBO J.* **6**:3379–3384.

Shirai, M., Pendleton, C. D., Ahlers, J., Takeshita, T., Newman, M., and Berzofsky, J. A., 1994, Helper-cytotoxic T lymphocyte (CTL) determinant linkage required for priming of anti-HIV CD8$^+$ CTL in vivo with peptide vaccine constructs, *J. Immunol.* **152**:549–556.

Snijders, A., Benaissa-Trouw, B. J., Snippe, H., and Kraaijeveld, C. A., 1992, Immunogenicity and vaccine efficacy of synthetic peptides containing Semliki Forest virus B and T cell epitopes, *J. Gen. Virol.* **73**:2267–2272.

Staerz, U. D., Karasuyama, H., and Garner, A. M., 1987, Cytotoxic T lymphocytes against a soluble protein, *Nature* **829**:449–451.

Starcich, B. R., Hahn, B. H., Shaw, G. M., McNeely, P. D., Modrow, S., Wolf, H., Parks, E. S., Parks, W. P., Josephs, S. F., Gallo, R. C., and Wong-Staal, F., 1986, Identification and characterization of conserved and variable regions in the envelope gene of HTLV-III/LAV, the retrovirus of AIDS, *Cell* **45**:637–648.

Taguchi, H., and Miyoshi, I., 1989, Immune suppression in HTLV-I carriers: A predictive sign of adult T-cell leukemia, *Acta Med. Okayama* **43**:317–321.

Takahashi, H., Cohen, J., Hosmalin, A., Cease, K. B., Houghten, R., Cornette, J. L., DeLisi, C., Moss, B., Germain, R. N., and Berzofsky, J. A., 1988, An immunodominant epitope of the human immunodeficiency virus envelope glycoprotein gp160 recognized by class I major histocompatibility complex molecule-restricted murine cytotoxic T lymphocytes, *Proc. Natl. Acad. Sci. USA* **85**:3105–3109.

Takahashi, H., Merli, S., Putney, S. D., Houghten, R., Moss, B., Germain, R. N., and Berzofsky, J. A., 1989a, A single amino acid interchange yields reciprocal CTL specificities for HIV-1 gp160, *Science* **246**:118–121.

Takahashi, H., Houghten, R., Putney, S. D., Margulies, D. H., Moss, B., Germain, R. N., and Berzofsky, J. A., 1989b, Structural requirements for class I MHC molecule-mediated antigen presentation and cytotoxic T cell recognition of an immunodominant determinant of the human immunodeficiency virus envelope protein, *J. Exp. Med.* **170**:2023–2035.

Takahashi, H., Takeshita, T., Morein, B., Putney, S., Germain, R. N., and Berzofsky, J. A., 1990, Induction of CD8$^+$ cytotoxic T cells by immunization with purified HIV-1 envelope protein in ISCOMs, *Nature* **344**:873–875.

Takeuchi, Y., Akutsu, M., Murayama, K., Shimuzu, N., and Hoshino, H., 1991, Host range mutant of human immunodeficiency virus type 1: Modification of cell tropism by a single point mutation at the neutralizing epitope in the env gene, *J. Virol.* **65**:1710–1718.

Tanaka, Y., Zeng, L., Shiraki, H., Shida, H., and Toyawa, H., 1991, Identification of a neutralization epitope on the envelope gp46 antigen of human T cell leukemia virus type I and induction of neutralizing antibody by peptide immunization, *J. Immunol.* **147**:354–360.

Townsend, A. R. M., Rothbard, J., Gotch, F. M., Bahadur, G., Wraith, D., and McMichael, A. J., 1986, The epitopes of influenza nucleoprotein recognized by cytotoxic T lymphocytes can be defined with short synthetic peptides, *Cell* **44**:959–968.

Trudel, M., Nadon, F., Seguin, C., and Binz, H., 1991, Protection of BALB/c mice from respiratory syncytial virus infection by immunization with a synthetic peptide derived from the G glycoprotein, *Virology* **185**:749–757.

Vahlne, A., Horal, P., Erikkson, K., Jeansson, S., Rymo, L., Hedstrom, K.-G., Czerkinsky, C., Holmgren, J., and Svennerholm, B., 1991, Immunizations of monkeys with synthetic peptides disclose conserved areas on gp120 of human immunodeficiency virus type 1 associated with cross-neutralizing antibodies and T cell recognition, *Proc. Natl. Acad. Sci. USA* **88**:10744–10748.

Waldmann, T., Goldman, C., Bongiovanni, K., Sharrow, S., Davey, M., Cease, K., Greenberg, S., and Long, D., 1988, Therapy of patients with human T-cell lymphotropic virus-induced adult T-cell leukemia with antiTac, a monoclonal antibody to the receptor for interleukin-2, *Blood* **72**:1805–1816.

Walker, B. D., Chakrabarti, S., Moss, B., Paradis, T. J., Flynn, T., Durno, A. G., Blumberg, R. S., Kaplan, J. C., Hirsh, M. S., and Schooley, R. T., 1987, HIV-specific cytotoxic T lymphocytes in seropositive individuals, *Nature* **328**:345–348.

Weinberg, J., Speigel, R., Blazey, D., Janssen, R., Kaplan, J., Robert-Guroff, M., Popovic, M., Matthews, T., Haynes, B., and Palker T., 1988, Human T-cell lymphotropic virus I and adult T-cell leukemia: Report of a cluster in North Carolina, *Am. J. Med.* **85**:51–58.

Weiss, R. A., Clapham, P. R., Cheingsong-Popov, R., Dalgleish, A. G., Carne, C. A., Weller, I. V. D., and Tedder, R. S., 1985, Neutralization of human T-lymphotropic virus type III by sera of AIDS and AIDS-risk patients, *Nature* **316**:69–72.

White, J. M., 1990, Viral and cellular membrane fusion proteins, *Annu. Rev. Physiol.* **52**:675–697.

White-Scharf, M. E., Potts, B. J., Smith, L. M., Sokolowski, K. A., Rusche, J. R., and Silver, S., 1993, Broadly neutralizing monoclonal antibodies to the V3 region of HIV-1 can be elicited by peptide immunization, *Virology* **192**:197–206.

Wiktor, S., Pate, E., Murphy, E., Palker, T., Champegnie, E., Ramlal, A., Cranston, B., Hanchard, B., and Blattner, W., 1993, Mother-to-child transmission of human T-cell lymphotropic virus type-I (HTLV-I) in Jamaica: Association with antibodies to envelope glycoprotein (gp46) epitopes, *J. AIDS* **6**:1162–1167.

Yasutomi, Y., Palker, T. J., Gardner, M. B., Haynes, B. F., and Letvin, N., 1993, Synthetic peptide in mineral oil adjuvant elicits simian immunodeficiency virus-specific CD8[+] cytotoxic T lymphocytes in rhesus monkeys, *J. Immunol.* **151**:5096–5105.

Chapter 38

Design and Testing of Peptide-Based Cytotoxic T-Cell-Mediated Immunotherapeutics to Treat Infectious Diseases and Cancer

Robert W. Chesnut, Alessandro Sette,
Esteban Celis, Peggy Wentworth, Ralph T. Kubo,
Jeff Alexander, Glenn Ishioka,
Antonella Vitiello, and Howard M. Grey

1. BACKGROUND

1.1. The Role of Cytotoxic T Cells in the Control and Elimination of Infectious Diseases and Cancer

Cytotoxic T lymphocytes (CTLs) have been implicated in the control and elimination of various viral and bacterial infections, tumors, and some parasitic diseases. CTLs that are characterized by the presence of the CD8 antigen generally recognize peptide fragments derived from intracellular processing of various antigens in the form of a complex with MHC class I molecules expressed on the cell surface (Germain and Margulies, 1993). This recognition may result in the lysis of the cell bearing the MHC–peptide antigen complex in an antigen-specific, MHC-restricted manner (Germain and Margulies, 1993). In addition, CTLs also generate a number of different lymphokines including gamma interferon (IFN-γ) and tumor necrosis factor (TNF), which are either directly cytolytic, regulate viral

Robert W. Chesnut, Alessandro Sette, Esteban Celis, Peggy Wentworth, Ralph T. Kubo, Jeff Alexander, Glenn Ishioka, Antonella Vitiello, and Howard M. Grey • Cytel Corporation, San Diego, California 92121.

Vaccine Design: The Subunit and Adjuvant Approach, edited by Michael F. Powell and Mark J. Newman. Plenum Press, New York, 1995.

replication, or function to amplify the ongoing immune response (van der Bruggen and Van den Eynde, 1992; Jassoy *et al.*, 1993; Rosenberg *et al.*, 1988).

The importance of CTLs in recovery from viral infection has been demonstrated both in animal models and in natural infections in humans (Rouse *et al.*, 1988). This type of response is critical for the establishment of protective immunity. Classic adoptive transfer or immunodepletion experiments in murine systems have shown that CTLs are critical for protection against lethal challenges with lymphocytic choriomeningitis virus (LCMV) (Byrne and Oldstone, 1984; Zinkernagel and Doherty, 1979), influenza virus (Yap *et al.*, 1978; Lukacher *et al.*, 1984), herpes simplex virus (HSV) (Sethi *et al.*, 1983), and murine cytomegalovirus (CMV) (Reddehase *et al.*, 1985). Adoptive transfer of CD8$^+$ CTLs into either virus-infected mice or normal mice prior to viral challenge resulted in reversal of disease progression, clearance of the virus, and decreased mortality. In addition, sustained memory was established, resulting in protection from subsequent challenge with virus. Depletion of CD8$^+$ T cells prior to viral challenge generally resulted in increased viremia, acceleration of disease progression, and increased mortality. In humans, the presence of virus-specific CTLs is associated with protective immunity and resolution of infections caused by influenza virus (McMichael *et al.*, 1983) and CMV (Quinnan *et al.*, 1982). Virus-specific, MHC class I-restricted, CD8$^+$ CTL responses have also been demonstrated in natural infection with HIV-1 (Walker *et al.*, 1987, 1988; Johnson *et al.*, 1991, 1992, 1993; Koenig *et al.*, 1988; Nixon *et al.*, 1988), HSV (Yasukawa *et al.*, 1989; Tigges *et al.*, 1993), hepatitis C virus (HCV) (Koziel *et al.*, 1992, 1993), and hepatitis B virus (HBV) (Bertoletti *et al.*, 1991, 1993; Missale *et al.*, 1993; Nayersina *et al.*, 1993).

CTLs have also been implicated in the elimination of tumors and prevention of recurring metastases. Original studies were performed in well-defined murine tumor model systems in which adoptive transfer of tumor-specific CTLs resulted in the eradication of experimentally induced tumors (Melief, 1992; Greenberg, 1991; Urban and Schreiber, 1992). It is now generally accepted that some human tumors express specific tumor-associated antigens (TAAs) which may be recognized by CTLs and may potentially be utilized in vaccination protocols (Urban and Schreiber, 1992). In general, identifying human tumor CTL epitopes is accomplished by analyzing tumor-infiltrating lymphocytes (TILs) or peripheral blood mononuclear cells (PBMCs) that are isolated from cancer patients with tumors (van der Brugen *et al.*, 1991; Jerome *et al.*, 1991; Muul *et al.*, 1987; Anichini *et al.*, 1989; Vose and Bonnard, 1982), by vaccination studies in mice (Skipper and Stauss, 1993; Feltkamp *et al.*, 1993; Chen *et al.*, 1991, 1992), or by examining in vitro induction of CTLs by peptides (Stauss *et al.*, 1992; Houbiers *et al.*, 1993). In humans, few TAAs have been characterized in terms of the presence of CTL epitopes. Potential CTL targets include gene products of oncogenic viruses, mutated oncogenes or suppressor genes, chromosomal translocations, and abnormally expressed or glycosylated self proteins, or overexpressed developmental proteins (Urban and Schreiber, 1992).

Since most tumor cells are weak immunogens, new strategies to enhance the cellular immune response to tumor-specific antigens are being investigated. These strategies include treatment of tumor-bearing hosts with lymphokines such as IL-2, IL-7, IFN-γ, and TNF (Lanzavecchia, 1993). Another strategy to augment tumor immunogenicity is the introduction of costimulatory signals into the tumor cells which may be critical for T-cell activation. Future therapies that may be efficacious in the treatment of a wide variety of tumors may require a combination of different strategies, such as using tumor antigens to generate tumor-specific CTLs in combination with specific lymphokines (Lanzavecchia, 1993).

Depletion and adoptive transfer studies have shown that immunity to parasites is also mediated, in part, by CD8[+] CTLs. Lysis by parasite-specific CTLs is antigen-specific and MHC class I-restricted (Sher and Coffman, 1992). In the malaria system, immunization with various vaccine constructs against antigens that are expressed while the parasite resides in the liver, has resulted in clearance of infection and protection from subsequent infection (Hoffman *et al.*, 1989; Romero *et al.*, 1989, 1990; Khusmith *et al.*, 1991; Widmann *et al.*, 1992). Similar results have also been observed with *Trypanosoma cruzi* and *Toxoplasma gondii* infections (Sher and Coffman, 1992). As in the case of viral infections and tumors, efficacious vaccination strategies for establishing parasite immunity may depend on successfully eliciting antigen-specific CTL responses.

1.2. The Processing and Presentation of Antigen to CD8[+] Cytotoxic T Cells

As mentioned above, CD8[+] CTLs recognize foreign antigen expressed as peptide fragments in association with highly polymorphic MHC class I glycoproteins (Germain and Margulies, 1993; Rammensee *et al.*, 1993). Classic experiments describing the phenomenon of MHC restriction on the one hand (Zinkernagel and Doherty, 1979), and the recognition of antigen in the form of peptide fragments on the other (Townsend *et al.*, 1985) were key to understanding this phenomenon. It was later shown that class I molecules specifically bind peptides derived from proteins synthesized endogenously, such as viral proteins, or from proteins that have been introduced into the class I processing pathway by targeting to the cytosol (Germain and Margulies, 1993; Rammensee *et al.*, 1993). Processing of antigens in the cytoplasm is mediated in part by structures called proteosomes (Goldberg and Rock, 1992) and translocation of peptide fragments to the endoplasmic reticulum (ER) is facilitated by peptide transporter proteins encoded by the TAP-1 and TAP-2 genes (Germain and Margulies, 1993). The function of these transporter proteins was defined by studies of the mutant mammalian cell lines, RMA-S and T2, which are defective in peptide transporter genes and are, therefore, defective in antigen processing and presentation (Attaya *et al.*, 1992; Spies *et al.*, 1992). Once in the ER, peptides associate with the MHC class I heavy chain and the β_2-microglobulin (β_2M) subunit, enabling proper folding of the MHC class I molecule into a trimolecular complex (Germain and Margulies, 1993). The MHC class I/peptide complex is then finally transported to the surface of the cell for recognition by class I-restricted CTLs (Germain and Margulies, 1993).

The interactions between peptides and MHC class I molecules have been more clearly defined by the solution of the three-dimensional structure of several different class I molecules and, importantly, the resolution of the molecular details of the peptide binding groove occupied by single peptide epitopes or by naturally processed peptides (Bjorkman *et al.*, 1987a,b; Garrett *et al.*, 1989; Madden *et al.*, 1991; Saper *et al.*, 1991; Fremont *et al.*, 1992; Matsumura *et al.*, 1992; Zhang *et al.*, 1992; Silver *et al.*, 1992; Young *et al.*, 1994). In addition, significant advances have been made in the isolation and characterization of naturally processed class I binding peptides (Falk *et al.*, 1991; Jardetzky *et al.*, 1991; Rammensee *et al.*, 1993; Rötzschke and Falk, 1991; Falk and Rötzschke, 1991; Van Bleek and Nathenson, 1990; Hunt *et al.*, 1992; Henderson *et al.*, 1992). The majority of the naturally processed peptides that have been characterized by amino acid sequencing either as mixtures or as individual peptides have revealed unique features such as restricted peptide length (generally 9±1 amino acid residues), and the occurrence of key amino acids at defined positions that are referred to as peptide motifs (Falk *et al.*, 1991; Rammensee *et al.*, 1993). In a broad sense, an allele-specific MHC motif can be defined as the set of structural features of peptides that are recognized by a given MHC type, allowing interaction with the MHC molecule and thereby contributing appreciably to the decrease of free energy associated with the formation of the MHC–peptide complex. As will be presented in greater detail in the following sections, our strategy to design peptide-based immunogenic constructs for the induction of specific CTL responses for various infectious diseases and cancers is critically dependent on the successful determination of allele-specific peptide motifs for several frequently expressed HLA-A alleles.

1.3. Summary of Evidence Showing That Synthetic Peptides Can Serve as Immunogens

Given that the technology to analyze naturally processed peptides (Rammensee *et al.*, 1993; Falk *et al.*, 1991; Jardetzky *et al.*, 1991; Van Bleek and Nathenson, 1990; Hunt *et al.*, 1992; Henderson *et al.*, 1992) and to identify CTL epitopes (Rammensee *et al.*, 1993) has been developed, the design of effective peptide-based vaccines can now be realistically contemplated. Formerly, it was thought that in vivo induction of CTLs required immunization with live virus or recombinant viral vectors expressing viral or tumor antigens, since soluble proteins and synthetic peptides were found to be ineffective immunogens. Recently, however, there have been many examples that CTLs are generated in vivo through immunization of animals with free or modified synthetic peptides (Carbone and Bevan, 1989; Kast *et al.*, 1991, 1993; Moore and Fox, 1993; Sastry *et al.*, 1992; Schultz *et al.*, 1991; Gao *et al.*, 1991; Fayolle *et al.*, 1991; Deres *et al.*, 1989; Yasutomi *et al.*, 1993; Zhou *et al.*, 1992). Various techniques have been employed to enhance the immunogenicity of peptides including immunization in the presence of incomplete Freund's adjuvant (IFA), construction of lipopeptides (Deres *et al.*, 1989; Nardelli and Tam, 1993) or fusogenic proteoliposomes (Miller *et al.*, 1992), immunization with hybrid peptides containing a CTL epitope attached to a fusion domain sequence (Hart *et al.*, 1991), use of tetravalent multiple antigenic peptide systems (MAPS) (Nardelli and Tam, 1993, and Chapter 36), immunization with syngeneic, irradiated, peptide-pulsed dendritic cells (Takahashi *et al.*, 1993), or immunization with peptide conjugates that contain CTL and helper T-cell epitopes (Widmann *et al.*, 1992; Yasutomi *et al.*, 1993). Antigen-specific, class I-restricted CTLs in these systems have been generated in both CD4+ T-cell-dependent (Widmann *et al.*, 1992; Fayolle *et al.*, 1991; Yasutomi *et al.*, 1993) and independent manners (Vasilakos and Michael, 1993). It is especially important to note that several of the immunization protocols have resulted in the establishment of protection against viral or tumor challenge (Feltkamp *et al.*, 1993; Kast *et al.*, 1991, 1993). It has also been possible to induce a CTL response in vitro using synthetic peptides (Carbone *et al.*, 1988) and more recently through stimulation with specialized, peptide-pulsed, antigen-presenting cells, such as the RMA-S or T2 cell lines (Stauss *et al.*, 1992; Houbiers *et al.*, 1993; Celis *et al.*, 1994). Finally, several groups, including our own, are investigating the feasibility of using peptide-based vaccines for the treatment of HBV (discussed later), HIV-1 (Gazzard *et al.*, 1992; Kahn *et al.*, 1992), and cancer (discussed later; Ioannides *et al.*, 1993) in humans.

2. SELECTION OF ANTIGENIC PEPTIDES

2.1. Introduction

The identification of the antigenic peptides capable of eliciting specific CTLs that can recognize infected or cancerous cells is crucial to the successful development of therapeutic strategies that target CTL induction (described in detail in the final sections of this chapter). In the following sections, we review the strategy that our group has developed, in order to identify such antigenic peptides from viral proteins and tumor antigens of known amino acid sequence. This strategy is comprised of four major components: (1) definition of MHC-binding peptide motifs; (2) validation of MHC-binding peptide motifs; (3) screening of motif-containing peptides for MHC-binding capacity; (4) testing high-affinity MHC-binding peptides for their capacity to induce CTL responses.

2.2. Definition of MHC-Binding Motifs

We have focused our attention initially on defining the specific MHC motifs for five of the most commonly expressed HLA-A alleles in different ethnic populations: A1, A2.1, A3, A11, and A24. These five alleles allow for coverage of a significant proportion (>90%) of the Caucasian and Asian populations, and for more than 36% of the black population, which is more polymorphic in HLA-A allele type (Imanishi *et al.*, 1992). Given our initial success, we are now expanding our analysis to other HLA-A alleles, as well as several HLA-B and C alleles to increase coverage of the populations that are not adequately covered by the five alleles mentioned. It appears that there may be a limited number of families of motifs that are shared by many different HLA class I alleles. Our research efforts are focused to gain a better understanding of these motif families and to ascertain whether a minimum number of motifs would allow identification of epitopes for many different HLA-A, B, or C alleles. As a consequence, we anticipate that our strategy will result in the ability to cover ≥95% of the population of the major ethnic groups with a reasonable number of peptide epitopes.

As a first step toward defining of the motifs, we have sequenced pooled, naturally occurring MHC–peptide ligands according to the scheme originally described by Rammensee and collaborators (Falk *et al.*, 1991). According to this scheme (Fig. 1), MHC–peptide complexes are purified by affinity chromatography and then treated with acid to dissociate the complexes. The low-molecular-weight peptide fraction is recovered by ultrafiltration and fractionated by HPLC. Pooled peptide fractions are further analyzed by conventional Edman degradation sequencing or by tandem mass spectrometry. Despite the formidable complexity of these peptide fractions, peptides bound to MHC class I display remarkable homogeneity in size, and the amino acid sequence analysis allows the features common to most, if not all, of the peptides bound to a given MHC allele to be discerned.

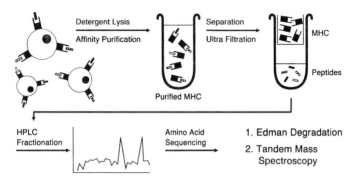

Figure 1. A general scheme for the isolation of naturally processed peptides bound to MHC molecules for amino acid sequencing. A suitable cell source is selected. Homozygous EBV-transformed human B-cell lines are good cell sources which can be readily grown in tissue culture in large quantities ($\sim 10^9-10^{10}$ cells). A cell lysate is prepared by detergent lysis, e.g., using nonionic detergents such as Nonidet P-40 or Triton X-100. The clarified detergent lysate is subjected to affinity purification techniques using the appropriate allele-specific monoclonal antibodies (MAb) or appropriate combinations of pan-reactive antimonomorphic MAbs, e.g., pan-reactive anti-HLA-B, C and pan-reactive anti-HLA-A, B, C. The immune complexes are collected using protein A Sepharose or other suitable matrices by centrifugation. After the thorough washing of the immunoprecipitate, the bound naturally processed peptides are dissociated by treatment of the immunoprecipitate with acid, e.g., 0.1% trifluoroacetic acid or 10% acetic acid, and harvested by ultrafiltration. The low-molecular-weight peptides are further purified by C-18 RP-HPLC. Pooled fractions or individual fractions can be analyzed by direct amino acid sequencing using automated Edman degradation or tandem mass spectrometry (Hunt *et al.*, 1992). For MHC class I peptides, the lengths of the peptides are generally 9 ± 1 amino acids (Falk *et al.*, 1991; Rammensee *et al.*, 1993). Edman degradation analysis of pooled peptide fractions does not yield individual peptide sequences; however, the results of the sequencing reveal the presence of dominant amino acids in some of the positions. Thus, peptide motifs can be derived from the analysis of the peptide sequencing data (Falk *et al.*, 1991; Rammensee *et al.*, 1993).

More specifically, peptides bound to HLA-A molecules are usually remarkably conserved at position 2 and at the C-terminal 9 or 10 position. By definition, amino acids that occupy these positions are referred to as the main anchor residues and form the basis for the allele-specific peptide motif.

By the sequencing of pooled fractions, we have defined the main anchor residues for the five target HLA alleles shown in Table I (Kubo *et al.*, 1994). The HLA-A2.1, A3, and A11 anchor residues defined in our laboratories are in good agreement with those independently defined by other groups (Falk *et al.*, 1991; DiBrino *et al.*, 1993; Zhang *et al.*, 1993). In general, the motifs appeared to be distinct. HLA-A2.1, A3, and A11 all have hydrophobic residues in position 2, but in the case of A3 and A11, a positive charge is present at the C-terminus of the motif, while hydrophobic residues are found at the C-termini of A2.1 bound peptides. A24 appears to utilize mainly aromatic residues at both main anchor positions. Finally, in the case of A1, the C-terminus bears a conserved Y residue, and both positions 2 and 3 are conserved, carrying T or S and D or E residues, respectively.

In order to define the requirements for the interaction between the target MHC types and their peptide ligands, quantitative in vitro binding assays utilizing purified MHC

Table I
HLA-A Allele-Specific Peptide Motifs Identified by Amino Acid Sequencing[a]

	Main anchor residues		
Allele	P-2[b]	P-3	COOH-terminus (P9/10)
A1	T,S	D,E	Y
A2.1	L,M	—[c]	V
A3	V,L,M	—[c]	K
A11	T,V	—[c]	K
A24	Y	—[c]	F,L

[a]Modified from Kubo *et al.* (1994).
[b]Position from the amino-terminus.
[c]No main anchor residues identified.

molecules were established (Sette *et al.,* 1994). These in vitro assays allowed us to define MHC motifs in greater detail. For example, in one set of experiments, the permissiveness of the two main anchor positions was investigated through analyzing the binding of synthetic single amino acid replacement analogues of model MHC-binding peptides as applied to A2.1 molecules (Fig. 2). We found that besides L or M in position 2, analogues carrying I, V, or A could also bind to HLA-A2.1, albeit with 10- to 100-fold lower affinities. Similarly, at position 9, V, I, and L were preferred, but A and M were also tolerated.

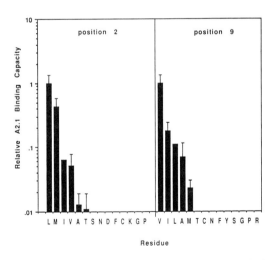

Figure 2. Refining the allele-specific peptide motif for HLA-A2.1 through the binding analysis of polyalanine analogues. Single amino acid substitutions of the parental polyalanine nonamer peptide ALAKAAAAV were tested for binding to purified HLA-A2.1 molecules. The indicated residues were introduced at positions 2 and 9 of the parental peptide. Binding is expressed relative to the parental unsubstituted peptide. From Ruppert *et al.* (1993) with permission from Cell Press.

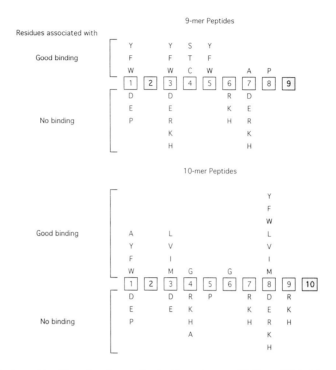

Figure 3. Amino acid residues strongly associated with good or poor binding to HLA-A2.1. Residues are shown that were found to be associated with good binding (ratio >4) or poor binding (ratio <0.25) based on the analysis of polyalanine analogues as described in Fig. 2 for position 2 and in Ruppert *et al.* (1993) for the other positions in nonamer and decamer peptides. Anchor residues in all peptides were L or M in position 2 and V, L, or I at the C-terminus. The amino acids are listed using the single-letter code. From Ruppert *et al.* (1993) with permission from Cell Press.

Following this type of analysis, a more detailed and "expanded" definition of the various MHC motifs was derived (Kubo *et al.,* 1994; Kast *et al.,* 1994). Further experiments in the A2.1 system demonstrated a prominent role for positions other than the two major anchor residues (Ruppert *et al.,* 1993). We found that in many other positions (especially 1, 3, and 7), certain residues were associated with good A2.1 binding, while other residues were associated with little or no A2.1 binding capacity (Fig. 3). These secondary effects appear to be a reflection of steric hindrance effects, as well as critical contributions to the overall binding affinities by secondary anchor residues which engage other pockets in the peptide-binding site of MHC molecules.

In conclusion, specific motifs have been defined for the five major target HLA alleles through the application of the strategy we have outlined above. The specific motifs take into consideration the exact molecular requirements of the major anchor positions, as well as the contributions of other more subtle secondary effects that influence overall binding affinity. These findings underline the highly complex interactions between potential peptide epitopes and MHC molecules. To effectively handle this level of complexity, we have derived computerized algorithms that accept as input the sequences of the proteins considered to be possible antigen targets for CTL induction and automatically calculate, taking into account all of these different factors, the likelihood that a given peptide will bind a given MHC type.

2.3. Validation of the MHC-Binding Motifs

It was of obvious importance to perform further experiments in order to assess the value of the data obtained from the binding assays and to firmly establish the biological relevance of the quantitative measure of MHC binding capacity. Various independent lines of experimentation were undertaken to address these issues.

In a first series of experiments, the relationship between MHC binding capacity and immunogenicity of potential peptide epitopes was investigated. A panel of 20 peptides derived from various viral protein sources, including the core and polymerase antigens of hepatitis B virus (HBV pol) and the E6 and E7 antigens of human papilloma virus (HPV), were selected on the basis of their binding to HLA-A2.1. These peptides spanned several orders of magnitude of A2.1 binding affinity (Sette *et al.*, unpublished data). Mice expressing the human MHC class I allele, HLA-A2.1 as a transgene, were utilized to directly assess the antigenicity of this panel of peptides as a function of A2.1 binding capacity. These transgenic mice have been shown to provide a useful experimental animal model system in which in vivo T-cell responses to potential A2.1 epitopes can be evaluated (Vitiello *et al.*, 1991). The protocol to assess the immunogenicity of selected peptide epitopes involved immunization and assessment of CTL responses of individual transgenic mice that were injected with a high dose of each peptide given with IFA. In order to maximize the chances of detecting positive responses, an equimolar amount of the IA[b]-restricted helper epitope, HBV core 128–140, was also included in the immunizing emulsion. Eleven days later, splenocytes from each individual mouse were recovered and stimulated with the appropriate peptide and, after 6 days of in vitro culture, they were assayed for peptide-specific cytotoxic activity.

It was found that peptides with A2.1 binding affinities of 50 nM or less were uniformly immunogenic. That is, for all five peptides, significant responses were detected in at least two of three mice tested. By contrast, only three of five of the intermediate binders (50 to 500 nM affinity range) were found, by the same criteria, to be immunogenic, and in no instance were low- or negative-binding peptides found to be immunogenic (Sette *et al.*, personal communication). These results indicate that there is a strong correlation between the affinity of binding of peptides to HLA and their ability to be recognized by specific T cells.

Similar results have been obtained by others where the immunogen was not a synthetic peptide but natural epitopes produced during the course of a viral infection (Chisari *et al.*, personal communication). Recall in vitro responses of PBLs derived from A2.1-positive acute hepatitis patients to a panel of 94 different HBV-derived peptides, with affinities in the 5000 to 2 nM range, were measured. Vigorous memory CTL responses were readily obtained from acute hepatitis patients, but not from uninfected individuals. Reproducible CTL responses were detected against nine different peptides. Strikingly, eight of these peptides (89%) were high-affinity binders, and one was an intermediate binder. No reproducible CTL activity was detected in the case of A2.1 low-affinity binders.

Finally, we sought to compare the data obtained following the two experimental approaches described herein with data independently obtained on the affinities of naturally processed peptides eluted from MHC molecules of known HLA-A restriction. In the case of HLA-A naturally processed epitopes, it was previously found that 89% were high-affinity binders, while 6% were intermediate binders and only 5% were low or negative binders (Kubo *et al.*, 1994). Similarly, in the case of known HLA-A-restricted epitopes, it was found that 10/11 (91%) were in a the high-affinity binder category, and 1/11 (9%) was an intermediate binder (Sette *et al.*, personal communication). In no case were low- or negative-binding peptides found.

Thus, the data obtained following four independent experimental approaches are remarkably consistent in indicating an affinity threshold of approximately 500 nM (preferably 50 nM or less) that determines the capacity of a peptide epitope to be recognized by HLA-A-restricted T cells.

We also performed an independent study to assess how effective the MHC motifs (as described in the preceding sections) were in predicting HLA-A binding peptides. A set of 250 peptides comprising all of the possible 9-mer peptides derived from the E6 and E7 proteins of HPV16 were synthesized and tested for binding to various HLA alleles (Kast *et al.*, 1994). Whereas pool sequencing-derived motifs were present in only 27% of high-affinity binders, the more expanded motifs, based on analysis of different amino acid substitutions at the anchor positions, were present in ~90% of high-affinity binders. Furthermore, it was found that the presence of anchor residues in a peptide was, in itself, not sufficient to determine binding to MHC class I molecules, since the majority of motif-containing peptides failed to bind to the relevant MHC. Finally, specific HLA motifs were used to predict peptide binders of 8, 10, and 11 amino acids in length. Several high-affinity binding peptides were identified for each of the various peptide lengths, indicating a significant size heterogeneity in peptides capable of high-affinity binding to HLA-A molecules.

2.4. Screening Vaccine Candidate Peptides for MHC Binding and in Vitro and in Vivo CTL Activation

Having demonstrated that (1) MHC motifs can predict high-affinity binding to MHC class I molecules and (2) there is a strong correlation between immunogenicity and binding, we set out to identify potential vaccine candidate peptides by screening for their capacity to induce a CTL response in vitro and in vivo. We examined the sequences of viral and tumor-associated proteins of interest for the presence of MHC-binding motifs. Synthetic peptides with motif-containing sequences were generated and tested for MHC binding to identify the high (50 nM) and intermediate (50–500 nM) MHC-binding peptides to be screened. This allowed us to reduce the number of potential vaccine candidates from several thousand to a few hundred. These selected peptides were synthesized and screened for the ability to (1) induce primary CTLs in vitro from normal, human PBMCs and (2) induce CTLs in vivo in HLA-A2.1 transgenic mice (see above).

Previously, it was thought that the in vitro generation of CTLs required an in vivo priming event accomplished through either natural infection or vaccination (McMichael *et al.*, 1983; Lamb *et al.*, 1987). However, recent research has shown that primary CTLs may be induced in vitro through stimulation with peptide-loaded mutant cells such as RMA-S (DeBruijn *et al.*, 1991) or T2 (Houbiers *et al.*, 1993). As discussed above, these mutant mouse lymphoma or human lymphoblastoid lines are defective in antigen processing and presentation through the endogenous pathway because of the absence of peptide transporter genes which are responsible for the transfer of peptides from the cytosol to the ER where they bind to MHC class I (Attaya *et al.*, 1992; Spies *et al.*, 1992). These cells, in which the class I molecules are unstable at 37°C, express "empty" class I molecules when cultured at lower temperatures (26–31°C) (Ljunggren *et al.*, 1990). Exogenous peptide, which can be efficiently "loaded" into the peptide binding groove at the reduced temperatures, stabilizes these empty class I molecules. Antigen-specific CTLs have been induced in vitro on stimulation with these peptide-loaded mutant cell lines (Stauss *et al.*, 1992; Houbiers *et al.*, 1993; DeBruijn *et al.*, 1991).

Thus, an APC that can deliver a potent antigen-specific signal in association with appropriate costimulatory signals is one key parameter necessary for the induction of primary CTLs in vitro. However, because of concerns about the safety and utility of the mutant cell lines for adoptive therapy approaches in humans, we have explored other approaches that might allow efficient peptide loading of class I on normal APC sources. We have developed two techniques, using activated human PBMCs instead of mutant cell lines, that facilitate the generation of APCs with a high surface density of peptide/class I complexes. In the first method, PBMCs from normal donors were activated with *Staphylococcus aureus* Cowan-I (Pansorbin, SAC-I cells expressing Protein A), Immunobeads (rabbit anti-human IgM), and human recombinant IL-4. After 4–7 days, the activated PBMCs were preincubated at 26°C overnight to generate empty MHC class I molecules on their surfaces, and then incubated with peptide for 4 h 20°C to effectively load surface class I molecules with relevant peptide (Celis *et al.*, 1994; del Guercio *et al.*, personal communication). These autologous, irradiated, peptide-loaded activated PBMCs were used as the APC population to stimulate responder PBMCs that had been depleted of CD4[+] T cells. Cultures were restimulated on day 12 using autologous, peptide-pulsed, irradiated, adherent cells and tested for cytolytic activity 7 days later against peptide-sensitized targets (homologous HLA-A-expressing EBV-transformed lines). Using this technique, we have successfully identified a nine-amino-acid CTL epitope contained within the tumor-associated MAGE-3 antigen (Celis *et al.*, 1994). As discussed in detail in Section 3.2, this epitope is being considered as the basis of a therapeutic vaccine for the treatment of malignant melanoma.

In the second protocol, SAC-1 activated PBMCs were "stripped" of endogenous peptide associated with surface MHC class I molecules by mild acid treatment (0.13 M citric acid, pH 3.0). This method has been shown to be an effective means of dissociating MHC-bound peptides from class I molecules without affecting the viability of the cells following neutralization (Suguwara *et al.*, 1987; Storkus *et al.*, 1993). The "empty" MHC class I molecules are then loaded with peptide. We have found that when acid-treated cells were neutralized, there was significant stabilization of MHC class I molecules in the presence of exogenous peptides compared to when no exogenous peptide was included in

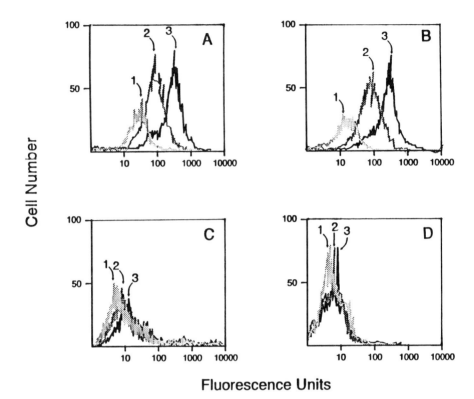

Fluorescence Units

Figure 4. Exogenous loading of peptide to "empty" MHC molecules produced by acid-stripping. Lymphoblasts (induced with PHA) from a normal HLA-A2.1 individual were resuspended for 2 min in ice-cold 0.13 M citric acid, pH 3.0, containing 1% BSA and 10 μg/mL β_2-microglobulin. The cells were neutralized and incubated for 2 h at 20°C with a fivefold volume of 0.15 M phosphate buffer, pH 7.4, containing 1% BSA, 10 μg/mL β_2-microglobulin, and the presence or absence of 20 μg/mL of the HLA-A2.1-binding peptide FLPSDFFPSV from the sequence of hepatitis B virus core protein (residues 18–27). The cells were washed two times with PBS and stained with FITC-labeled pan anti-HLA class I antibody (W6/32) (A), monoclonal antibodies specific for HLA-A2 (B), an antibody specific for HLA-DR molecules (L 243) (C), or normal mouse Ig as a negative control (D). The cells were analyzed by flow microfluorimetry. Peptide-loaded cells (curve 2) were compared with untreated cells (curve 3) and with acid-stripped cells that were neutralized without the addition of peptide (curve 1).

the neutralizing solution (Fig. 4). Presumably, a high number of specific peptide/MHC complexes will result in the former situation, while in the latter case, empty class I molecules degrade following neutralization. This treatment had no significant effect on the expression of HLA-DR class II molecules (Fig. 4). Similar observations have been made by others (Suguwara *et al.,* 1987). We have found that this is an efficient method for loading MHC class I molecules with relevant peptide. These APCs have been used to stimulate normal PBMCs that are depleted of CD4[+] T cells for the induction of primary, antigen-specific CTLs in vitro (Wentworth *et al.,* unpublished observations).

We found that the correlation between immunogenicity and binding observed in the transgenic mice experiments also held with the in vitro peptide screening results. In both systems, a binding threshold was observed in which only high (<50 nM) or intermediate binding (50–500 nM) peptides stimulated the induction of antigen-specific CTLs. Consequently, we routinely screen those peptides with high and intermediate HLA binding affinities for the identification of CTL epitopes that could be used as potential vaccine immunogens. In addition, we have noted that the peptides that induce primary CTL responses in vitro in normal individuals usually induce CTL responses in vivo in transgenic mice. Peptides that are immunogenic in both systems would likely be good candidate epitopes for further development.

Utilizing these techniques, we have screened hundreds of peptides and have successfully identified a number of CTL epitopes in various disease systems such as HBV, cervical cancer, melanoma, HCV, and HIV. This information has prophylactic as well as therapeutic implications for the development of either in vivo injectable immunostimulants or in vitro stimulatory molecules for adoptive cellular therapy.

3. THERAPEUTIC APPLICATIONS

3.1. Background

Once disease-related peptides that are capable of inducing antigen-specific CTLs have been identified, it is still necessary to develop these peptides further into pharmaceutical compositions and/or therapeutic applications that are potentially beneficial for patients. Two types of therapeutic approaches are being developed by Cytel Corp., each with distinct benefits as well as limitations.

One approach is adoptive cellular therapy, in which peripheral blood lymphocytes obtained from patients are activated in vitro to induce disease-specific CTLs. Once induced, the specific CTL population can be expanded and then reinfused into the patient. This therapeutic approach is relatively costly since it must be individualized and because lymphocyte expansion is labor-intensive. However, this may be an effective approach for patients who are immunosuppressed. A second approach involves the injection of patients with therapeutic peptides to directly induce disease-specific CTLs. This application has a number of benefits, including overall low cost. Until recently, however, this approach has been limited by the difficulty of inducing CTL responses in vivo using immunogens other than live viruses. Further, this approach is unlikely to be beneficial in patients who are highly immunosuppressed.

3.2. Adoptive Cellular Therapy

As mentioned in Section 1.1, a large number of experiments in mice have demonstrated that adoptive transfer of antigen-specific CTL lines or clones can treat animals against chronic viral infections, or established tumors. Following this rationale, clinical trials in humans using CTLs that are specific for CMV have been conducted (Riddell *et al.,* 1992; Greenberg *et al.,* 1991). In these trials, immunosuppressed patients who received bone marrow transplants were infused with CTL clones specific for CMV in order to prevent infection with this virus, a common complication associated with immunosuppression. The CTLs utilized in these trials were induced using virus-infected fibroblasts as APCs. Early results showed that these treatments are safe and efficacious in preventing CMV infection, and indicated that the CTLs remain viable and functional for several weeks after the infusion (Riddell *et al.,* 1992; Greenberg *et al.,* 1991).

In a different type of adoptive therapy trial, cancer patients were treated with TILs that were activated and expanded in vitro (Melief, 1992; van der Bruggen and Van den Eynde, 1992; Rosenberg *et al.,* 1988). The TIL population is usually stimulated in culture by autologous tumor cells and IL-2, and as such, the expanded cell population tends to be quite heterogeneous. The proportion of antigen-specific CTLs varies from treatment to treatment, and, in many cases, the total number of specific effector cells is likely to be low. This inconsistency in CTL generation may account for the relatively low success rate of the present adoptive therapy approach.

To overcome these problems, we have developed techniques that enable us to generate in vitro primary, antigen-specific CTL responses. Crucial aspects of our approach include the use of appropriate peptide-loaded stimulatory APCs, depletion of $CD4^+$ T cells, and subsequent enrichment for $CD8^+$ T cells in the responder population to increase precursor frequency, and supplementation of the in vitro cultures with the addition of rIL-7 to enhance the growth and differentiation of the CTL precursors (Kos and Mullbacher, 1992; Alderson *et al.,* 1990). Restimulation of the cultures with autologous, peptide-pulsed adherent cells is also of crucial importance. As discussed above, we have developed protocols to acid-deplete and then load PBMCs with the peptide epitope of choice, thus facilitating the expression of a high density of peptide/class I complex on the cell surface enabling the delivery of a potent antigenic signal to precursor T cells. Second, low CTL precursor frequencies in unprimed individuals may prevent the induction of CTL in numbers sufficiently high for detection and successful expansion. Consequently, we depleted $CD4^+$ T cells from the responder PBMC population, in an effort to enrich the $CD8^+$ precursor T-cell frequency. In addition, depletion of the $CD4^+$ T cells may have prevented the nonspecific expansion of cells that would compete with the antigen-specific CTLs for medium nutrients. Third, since the activation of small, resting T cells for induction of cytolytic activity requires other signals (Azuma *et al.,* 1992; Harding *et al.,* 1992) in addition to an antigen-specific stimulation signal, we also supplemented the cultures with rIL-7. Finally, it is important to successfully expand the antigen-specific CTLs in repetitive restimulation cycles. Thus, we developed and optimized protocols that can be used to expand the cells through one or more restimulation cycles using peptide-pulsed adherent monocytes as APCs.

We recently reported that tumor-specific CTLs could be induced from $CD8^+$ T cells isolated from PBMCs of normal human donors (Celis *et al.,* 1994) that were stimulated with autologous APCs incubated with a peptide derived from a melanoma-associated antigen (MAGE-3). The MAGE-3 protein was described to be expressed in a large proportion of melanoma tumors and to a lesser extent in breast, colon, thyroid, and lung carcinomas, but not in normal tissues except for the testis (van der Bruggen *et al.,* 1991; Zakut *et al.,* 1993). The peptide used in this study was derived from the sequence of the MAGE-3 gene product and it was selected on the basis of having affinity with the HLA-A1

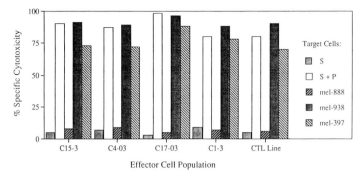

Figure 5. Cytotoxic activity of a MAGE-3-specific CTL line and derived clones. A MAGE-3-specific CTL line derived from a normal individual (Celis *et al.,* 1994), and several CTL clones (C15-3, C4-03, C17-03, and C1-3) selected by limiting dilution from this line, were tested for their capacity to kill various target cell types. A conventional 4-h ^{51}Cr release assay was performed at an effector:target ratio of 15:1. Targets tested were: S, Steinlin cells (a HLA-A1 homozygous EBV-transformed cell line); S + P, Steinlin cells pulsed with the peptide EVDPIGHLY from the MAGE-3 sequence (positions 161–169); mel-888, a MAGE-3-negative HLA-A1 melanoma cell line; mel-938 and mel-397, both MAGE-3-positive and HLA-A1-expressing melanoma tumor cell lines.

binding motif and high binding to purified HLA-A1 molecules (Celis *et al.,* 1994). When PBMCs from a normal volunteer were stimulated in vitro following the protocol described above, peptide-specific HLA-A1-restricted CTL lines were produced. Most importantly, the CTLs lysed melanoma tumor cells that expressed the MAGE-3 protein (Fig. 5). Independently, this same peptide was shown to be the antigen recognized by CTLs isolated from a HLA-A1 patient with melanoma (Gaugler *et al.,* 1994). Thus, it is possible to stimulate and expand specific CTLs in vitro using a motif-selected, class I binding peptide. It will be important to test this approach as well using TILs as the CTL source.

In summary, we have developed a potential strategy for effective adoptive cellular therapy (Fig. 6). According to the strategy, lymphocytes from cancer or chronic virus-infected patients would be obtained from the circulation either from a blood sample or through pheresis. The lymphocytes would be stimulated ex vivo with APCs that have been optimally loaded with the selected antigenic peptide. The addition of cytokines such as IL-1, IL-7, and IL-12 at the early stage of CTL induction should facilitate the stimulation of the antigen-specific CTL precursors. Ten to twelve days after restimulation, with peptide-loaded APCs, the CTLs should be further expanded with use of IL-2. Several cycles of antigen restimulation may be required to obtain the appropriate number of antigen-specific CTLs necessary for the adoptive transfer into the patients.

3.3. In Vivo Injectable Immunotherapeutics

The goal of our efforts toward developing an injectable immunotherapeutic is to produce a drug that, when administered subcutaneously or intramuscularly, would be safe, relatively inexpensive, and able to induce a disease-specific CTL response. Our previous

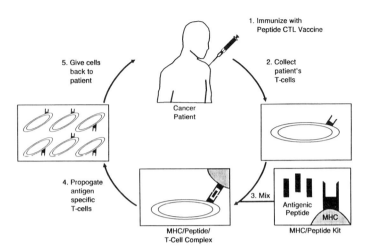

Figure 6. Adoptive immunotherapy strategy using CTLs stimulated (in vitro with synthetic peptides (see text for complete explanation).

experience as well as that of others had demonstrated that some, but not all, optimal length peptides for MHC binding are eight to ten amino acids long and that injection of the optimal length peptide emulsified in Freund's adjuvant into mice gave a CTL response (Aichele *et al.*, 1990; Kast *et al.*, 1991; Gao *et al.*, 1991; Feltkamp *et al.*, 1993; Schultz *et al.*, 1991; Vitiello *et al.*, personal communication). However, there are safety concerns associated with the use of Freund's-like adjuvants in humans for many diseases. Therefore, we undertook to design a novel construct that combined the essential elements that we believed were required to enhance the immunogenicity of the optimal CTL epitope but lacked the safety issues associated with Freund's-like adjuvants.

Initial work was carried out in a murine (BALB/c) model system. A previously identified MHC class I-restricted CTL antigenic peptide from the influenza virus nucleocapsid protein (Flu NP) was selected as the CTL epitope for the study (Flu NP 147–156) (Taylor *et al.*, 1987). In attempting to enhance the immunogenicity of the CTL epitope, we felt that effective adjuvants probably provided at least two important elements. One element is related to the elicitation of a local immune response capable of producing cytokines such as IL-2. The presence of IL-2 and other cytokines at the site of injection or the draining lymph nodes, at the time when CTL precursor cells are expressing IL-2 receptors as a result of recognition of the CTL epitope bound to MHC class I molecules, may be essential for the activation and proliferation of CTL precursor cells (Farrar *et al.*, 1978; Wagner and Rollinghoff, 1978). In order to elicit cytokines, we chose to add a MHC class II-restricted T-helper epitope to the CTL antigenic peptide. The IA^d-restricted ovalbumin (Ova) peptide 323–339 was selected for this purpose. The Ova peptide induces Ova 323–339-specific T-helper cells to secrete cytokines in the same microenvironment where Flu NP 147–156-specific CTL precursor cells were becoming activated and thereby would provide the required "help" for further activation and proliferation.

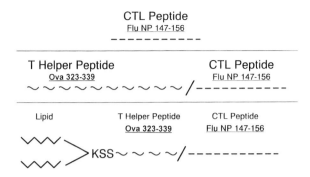

Figure 7. Modifications of the CTL peptide tested for enhancement of in vivo immunogenicity (see text for complete explanation).

The second property of a conventional adjuvant involves a depot effect, that is, localizing the antigen at the site of injection or the draining lymph nodes, and perhaps delivering the antigen to dendritic cells, macrophages, and other "professional" APCs over a sustained period of time. To provide this function, we included two short lipid molecules covalently attached to the lysine residue of a lysine-serine-serine linker (Deres *et al.*, 1989). This lipidated peptide construct is quite insoluble in aqueous solvents and is retained at the site of injection for several days.

In order to test the immunogenicity of the CTL epitope alone, or in combination with the T-helper epitope in the presence or absence of the lipid molecules, an extensive series of in vivo experiments was performed. Although many combinations of peptides alone, as well as lipids plus peptides, were tested for immunogenicity, adding linking of the lipid molecules directly to the T-helper antigenic peptide, which was itself linked to the CTL antigenic peptide, proved to be most effective. The peptide and lipopeptide structures used to define the differences in immunogenicity are shown in Fig. 7. The experimental protocol consisted of immunizing one group of animals with a single subcutaneous injection containing Flu NP 147–156 (10 μg/mouse) formulated in saline alone or in IFA. A second group of mice was injected with a linked peptide in which the Ova 323–339 T-helper epitope was covalently attached to the Flu NP 147–156 CTL epitope. This linked T helper–CTL epitope construct was administered in saline or IFA as described above. The third group of mice was injected with a lipopeptide consisting of two short lipid molecules covalently linked via KSS to the amino-terminus of the Ova 323–339–Flu NP 147–156 linked peptide. This construct, termed the "tripartite immunostimulant," was also administered in saline or IFA as described above.

Representative results are shown in Fig. 8. Immunization of animals with the CTL antigenic peptide (Flu NP 147–156) alone in saline did not induce a detectable CTL response when tested against target cells that were sensitized with the Flu NP 147–156 peptide or infected with influenza virus PR8. CTL activity was detected when mice were immunized with the Flu NP 147–156 emulsified in IFA. However, the level of activity observed was relatively low in that an E:T ratio of 90:1 was required to detect a clear difference from the level of control killing.

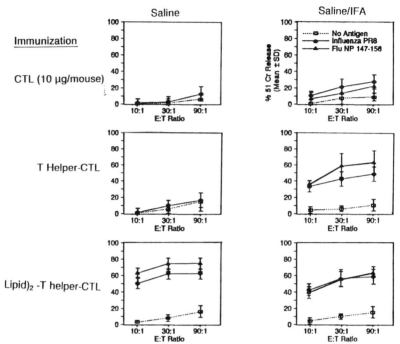

Figure 8. BALB/c mice were injected subcutaneously in the base of the tail with the indicated peptide preparations. Three weeks later the splenocytes were harvested and placed into culture in the presence of Flu NP 147–156 peptide for 1 week. CTL activity was assessed in a conventional 6-h ^{51}Cr release assay using a transformed fibroblast cell line derived from a B10.D2 mouse as target cells. Targets were sensitized with no antigen, the Flu NP 147–156 peptide, or by infection with influenza PR8.

When animals were immunized with a peptide composed of the T-helper epitope linked to the CTL epitope (i.e., Ova 323–339–Flu NP 147–156) in saline, no CTL activity was detected above the control. In contrast, when this linked peptide was administered in IFA, strong CTL activity was detected at an E:T ratio as low as 10:1. These data suggest that the presence of the T-helper peptide did play a role in CTL immunization but that IFA was still required for induction of detectable CTL activity.

Finally, when mice were injected with the lipopeptide containing two lipid molecules attached to the linked T-helper–CTL epitopes in saline, a strong CTL response was detected with lysis of target cells sensitized with the Flu NP 147–156 peptide or by infection with influenza virus PR8. CTL activity was also demonstrated when the lipopeptide was administered to mice in IFA.

Although a number of other combinations of peptides and lipopeptides were tested in a similar manner including lipidated CTL epitope, none induced as potent a CTL response in the absence of IFA as did the lipopeptide described here. Thus, it appeared that the combination of the T-helper epitope and the lipid subserved the function of an adjuvant for induction of a CTL response in vivo.

Although the studies had shown that the tripartite immunostimulant could induce an in vivo response that recognized virus-infected target cells in vitro, it was important to further test the effectiveness of the response in vivo. To accomplish this, another mouse model system utilizing LCMV was employed. Strain 13 LCMV is a virus that can cause chronic infection in adult animals (Ahmed *et al.,* 1984) and, thus, the clearance of strain 13 LCMV from adult animals provides an excellent readout for CTL priming and induction of memory T cells. A tripartite construct was prepared in which a previously defined LCMV CTL epitope was linked to the lipidated Ova 323–339 T-helper antigenic peptide. In collaborative studies carried out by Dr. Rafi Ahmed and co-workers (personal communication), groups of mice were immunized with a single dose of the LCMV-specific tripartite immunogen, with the CTL epitope alone, or the vehicle alone. One month following vaccination, the animals were challenged with strain 13 LCMV. Eight days following challenge, the animals were sacrificed and the level of viremia was quantified. The results showed that while the control group of animals and the group immunized with the CTL epitope alone had high levels of viremia, indicating the establishment of a chronic LCMV infection, the mice vaccinated with the tripartite immunostimulant containing the LCMV CTL antigenic peptide were completely protected against strain 13 LCMV. These results demonstrated two important properties of the tripartite immunogen: (1) it induces memory CTLs since the LCMV challenge was given approximately 1 month after vaccination and (2) the quality of the CTL immunity induced was such that a live viral challenge could be effectively cleared.

Based on this information, we have developed a design for a series of therapeutic peptides for use in humans. The lipid and the T-helper peptide of the construct remain constant whereas the CTL antigenic peptide is specific for the disease indication. A lead compound of this nature has been developed for the treatment of chronic HBV infection. This molecule has been tested in mice expressing the human MHC class I allele, HLA-A2.1, as a transgene (Vitiello *et al.,* 1991). As shown in Fig. 9, animals immunized with a

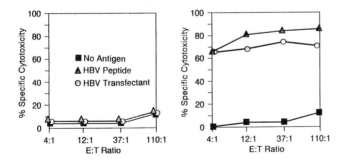

Figure 9. HLA-A2.1 transgenic mice were injected subcutaneously in the base of the tail with either HBc/Ag 18–27 peptide in saline (left panel) or the tripartite immunostimulant containing the HBcAg 18–27 peptide as the CTL epitope (right panel). Three weeks later, splenocytes were harvested and placed into culture in the presence of HBcAg 18–27 peptide for 1 week. CTL activity was determined in a conventional 6-h ^{51}Cr release assay using HLA-A2.1-positive EBV-transformed B cells, JY, as targets. Target cells were sensitized with no antigen, HBcAg 18–27 peptide, or were transfected with the HBV core gene (transfectant provided by Dr. Frank Chisari, The Scripps Research Institute, La Jolla, CA) (Guilhot *et al.,* 1992).

single subcutaneous injection of the CTL epitope, hepatitis B core antigen (HBcAg) 18–27 given in saline generated no detectable CTL response. In contrast, animals similarly injected with the tripartite immunostimulant containing the HBcAg 18–27 peptide generated a strong HBc/Ag-specific CTL response that resulted in the induction of specific CTLs which lysed EBV-transformed B cells sensitized with the HBcAg peptide. In addition, the CTLs were also able to lyse target cells that had been transfected with the HBcAg gene and expressed the HBcAg protein, thus mimicking the endogenous generation of antigenic peptides associated with MHC class I molecules by virus-infected cells.

Thus, the tripartite immunostimulant molecule is able to induce peptide-specific CTL responses in vivo and, therefore, has the potential to play an important role in the immunologic prevention and treatment of a number of different infectious diseases and cancer. Clinical trials are under way to test the safety and efficacy of the molecule in humans. Initial results indicate that the tripartite molecule is safe and is effective at inducing a specific CTL response in man (Vitiello *et al.*, personal communication).

4. SUMMARY AND PERSPECTIVES

It is now well established in animal studies that cytotoxic T cells are capable of affording protection against infectious disease and cancer, as well as in the control or elimination of these diseases once they have become established. The next obvious challenge is to translate these results into prophylactic and therapeutic immunostimulants applicable to human diseases. We believe that the use of selected antigenic peptides to elicit a specific CTL response will play an important role in seeing this challenge met.

The use of antigenic peptides to elicit a CTL response offers several positive features. First, short synthetic peptides can be readily manufactured. Peptide synthesis technology is well established and offers the production of well-defined, cost-effective molecules. Second, peptides are relatively safe molecules. Administration of an eight- to ten-amino-acid fragment derived from a pathogen or tumor cell offers lower safety risks than use of nucleic acids, live vectors, or recombinant proteins, which are more likely to retain inherent biological activities.

The third feature of using antigenic peptides is the capacity to specifically manipulate the immune system. There are only a few potential CTL epitopes within a protein, and the capacity to deliver selected antigenic peptides at relatively high concentrations, in an immunogenic form, is likely to be important in initiating and boosting an immune response where disease already persists. In addition, the use of selected antigenic peptides offers the ability to manipulate the response by choosing "subdominant" antigenic peptides that may shift the immune response to epitopes not normally elicited and, thus, are not subject to "immunologic pressure" to mutate. Selection of this nature is not possible using approaches that involve the whole protein or gene. It is also interesting to note that selection of MHC-bound peptides observed in naturally processed epitopes may also be dependent on the surrounding sequence environment. This phenomenon may reflect sequence preferences of proteolytic enzymes, or even subtle differences in protein structure, leading to differences in antigen processing. The peptide approach may be useful for targeting immune responses to epitopes that are underpresented or nonexistent in the responses normally induced during infection or oncogenesis.

If immunotherapy is going to achieve its rightful role as a tool in the management of human diseases, it will be important to test it in combination with other therapeutic molecules. For instance, in the chronic viral disease setting, it may be important to use antigen-specific immunotherapy along with antiviral drugs that are capable of reducing the viral burden. Similarly, combining forms of immunotherapy may be important in certain disease settings. For example, in late-stage tumor therapy, it may be crucial to prime the patient with the CTL epitope using the tripartite immunogen, then isolate peripheral blood lymphocytes, expand the peptide-specific CTLs ex vivo, deliver these back to the patient, and finally boost the patient periodically with peptide to ensure that a high level of CTL activity is maintained. In addition, the timely administration of cytokines such as the interferons, IL-2, IL-7, and IL-12, are likely to be important for treating disease in at least some patients.

The progress made in recent years in the understanding of T-cell-mediated immunity has opened enormous possibilities in the application of innovative new approaches to stimulate the immune system, the body's natural protective mechanism, to function to its fullest potential. The exciting technologies described in this book attest to the variety of approaches that are being developed. While keeping clearly in mind the fact that T-cell-mediated immunity is capable of doing harm as well as good, these approaches must now be tested in the clinic in order to understand how, when, and where to use antigen-specific immunotherapy to safely, yet more effectively, treat human disease.

ACKNOWLEDGMENTS

This work was supported in part by a grant from the U.S. Public Health Services (AI 18634 to H.M.G.). We wish to thank John Sidney, Scott Southwood, Marie-France del Guercio, Carol Dahlberg, Dung Huynh, and Chu Lee for their excellent technical assistance in the immunochemical studies, particularly in the MHC class I binding assays; Carla Oseroff, Jörg Ruppert, Alessandra Franco, Claire Crimi, Suzette Stitely, Van Tsai, Laura Hale, Peggy Farness, Lunli Yuan, and Renee LaFond for expert technical assistance in the cellular immunology studies; Tom Arrhenius, Ajesh Maewal, Tony Chiem, and Stephanie Shaw for their expert assistance in peptide synthesis and purification. Special thanks to John Fikes for critically reading the manuscript and to Glenna Marshall and Ethel Beltran for their help in preparing the manuscript. We thank Dr. Frank Chisari of The Scripps Research Institute for allowing us to cite some of his preliminary results, and for providing the JY cell line transfected with the HBV core gene.

REFERENCES

Ahmed, R., Solm, A., Butler, L. D., Chiller, J. M., and Oldstone, M. B. A., 1984, Selection of genetic variants of lymphocytic choriomeningitis virus in spleens of persistently infected mice: Role in suppression of cytotoxic T lymphocyte response and viral persistence, *J. Exp. Med.* **160**:521–540.

Aichele, P., Hengartner, H., Zinkernagel, R., and Schultz, M., 1990, Antiviral cytotoxic T cell response induced by in vivo priming with a free synthetic peptide, *J. Exp. Med.* **171**:1815–1820.

Alderson, M., Sassenfeld, H., and Widmer, M., 1990, Interleukin-7 enhances cytolytic T lymphocyte generation and induces lymphokine-activated killer cells from human peripheral blood, *J. Exp. Med.* **172**:577–578.

Anichini, A., Mazzocchi, A., Fossati, G., and Parmiani, G., 1989, Cytotoxic T lymphocyte clones from peripheral blood and from tumor site detect intratumor heterogeneity of melanoma cells: Analysis of specificity and mechanisms of interaction, *J. Immunol.* **142**:3692–3701.

Attaya, M., Jameson, S., Martinez, C. K., Hermel, E., Aldrich, C., Forman, J., Lindahl, K. F., Bevan, M. J., and Monaco, J. J., 1992a, Ham-2 corrects the class I antigen-processing defect in RMA-S cells, *Nature* **355**:647–649.

Azuma, M., Cayabyab, M., Buck, D., Phillips, J. H., and Lanier, L. L., 1992, CD28 interaction with B7 costimulates primary allogeneic proliferative responses and cytotoxicity mediated by small, resting T lymphocytes, *J. Exp. Med.* **175**:353–360.

Bertoletti, A., Ferrari, C., Fiaccadori, F., Penna, A., Margolskee, R., Schlicht, H.-J., Fowler, P., Guilhot, S., and Chisari, F. V., 1991, HLA class I-restricted human cytotoxic T cells recognize endogenously synthesized hepatitis B virus nucleocapsid antigen, *Proc. Natl. Acad. Sci. USA* **88**:10445–10449.

Bertoletti, A., Chisari, F. V., Penna, A., Guilhot, S., Galati, L., Missale, G., Fowler, P., Schlicht, H.-J., Vitiello, A., Chesnut, R. W., Fiaccadori, F., and Ferrari, C., 1993, Definition of a minimal optimal cytotoxic T-cell epitope within the hepatitis B virus nucleocapsid protein, *J. Virol.* **67**:2376–2380.

Bjorkman, P. J., Saper, M. A., Samraoui, B., Bennett, W. S., Strominger, J. L., and Wiley, D. C., 1987a, Structure of the human class I histocompatibility antigen, HLA-A2, *Nature* **329**:506–512.

Bjorkman, P. J., Saper, M. A., Samraoui, B., Bennett, W. S., Strominger, J. L., and Wiley, D. C., 1987b, The foreign antigen binding site and T cell recognition regions of class I histocompatibility antigens, *Nature* **329**:512–518.

Byrne, J.A., and Oldstone, M. B., 1984, Biology of cloned cytotoxic T lymphocytes specific for lymphocytic choriomeningitis virus: Clearance of virus in vivo, *J. Virol.* **51**:682–686.

Carbone, F. R., and Bevan, M. J., 1989, Induction of ovalbumin-specific cytotoxic T cells by in vivo peptide immunization, *J. Exp. Med.* **169**:603–612.

Carbone, F. R., Moore, M. W., Sheil, J. M., and Bevan, M. J., 1988, Induction of cytotoxic T lymphocytes by primary in vitro stimulation with peptides, *J. Exp. Med.* **167**:1767–1779.

Celis, E., Tsai, V., Crimi, C., DeMars, R., Wentworth, P. A., Chesnut, R. W., Grey, H. M., Sette, A., and Serra, H. M., 1994, Induction of anti-tumor cytotoxic T lymphocytes in normal humans using primary cultures and synthetic peptide epitopes, *Proc. Natl. Acad. Sci. USA* **91**:2105–2109.

Chen, L., Thomas, E. K., Hu, S.-L., Hellstrom, I., and Hellstrom, K. E., 1991, Human papillomavirus type 16 nucleoprotein E7 is a tumor rejection antigen, *Proc. Natl. Acad. Sci. USA* **88**:110–114.

Chen, L., Mizuno, M. T., Singhal, M. C., Hu, S.-L., Galloway, D. A., Hellstrom, I., and Hellstrom, K. E., 1992a, Induction of cytotoxic T lymphocytes specific for a syngeneic tumor expressing the E6 oncoprotein of human papillomavirus type 16, *J. Immunol.* **148**:2617–2621.

Chen, L., Ashe, S., Brady, W. A., Hellstrom, I., Hellstrom, K. E., Ledbetter, J. A., McGowan, P., and Linsley, P. S., 1992b, Costimulation of antitumor immunity by the B7 counterreceptor for the T lymphocyte molecules CD28 and CTLA-4, *Cell* **71**:1093–1102.

DeBruijn, M., Schumacher, T., Neiland, J., Ploegh, H., Kast, M., and Melief, C. J. M., 1991, Peptide loading of empty major histocompatibility complex molecules on RMA-S cells allows the induction of primary cytotoxic T lymphocyte responses, *Eur. J. Immunol.* **21**:2963–2970.

Deres, K., Schild, H., Wiesmuller, K.-H., Jung, G., and Rammensee, H.-G., 1989, In vivo priming of virus-specific cytotoxic T lymphocytes with synthetic lipopeptide vaccine, *Nature* **342**:561–564.

DiBrino, M., Parker, K. C., Shiloach, J., Knierman, M., Lukszo, J., Turner, R. V., Biddison, W. E., and Coligan, J. E., 1993, Endogenous peptides bound to HLA-A3 possess a specific combination of anchor residues that permit identification of potential antigenic peptides, *Proc. Natl. Acad. Sci. USA* **90**:1508–1512.

Falk, K., and Rötzschke, O., 1993, Consensus motifs and peptide ligands of MHC class I molecules, *Semin. Immunol.* **5**:81–94.

Falk, K., Rötzschke, O., Stevanovic, S., Jung, G., and Rammensee, H.-G., 1991, Allele-specific motifs revealed by sequencing of self-peptides eluted from MHC molecules, *Nature* **351**:290–296.

Farrar, J. J., Simon, P. L., Koopman, W. J., and Fuller-Bonar, J., 1978, Biochemical relationship of thymocyte mitogenic factor and factors enhancing humoral and cell-mediated immune responses, *J. Immunol.* **124**:1353.

Fayolle, C., Deriaud, E., and Leclerc, C., 1991, In vivo induction of cytotoxic T cell response by a free synthetic peptide requires CD4$^+$ T cell help, *J. Immunol.* **147**:4069–4073.

Feltkamp, M. C. W., Smits, H. L., Vierboom, M. P. M., Minnaar, R. P., de Jongh, B. M., Drijfhout, J. W., ter Schegget, J., Melief, C. J. M., and Kast, W. M., 1993, Vaccination with cytotoxic T lymphocyte epitope-containing peptide protects against a tumor induced by human papillomavirus type 16-transformed cells, *Eur. J. Immunol.* **23**:2242–2249.

Fremont, D. H., Matsumura, M., Stura, E. A., Peterson, P. A., and Wilson, I. A., 1992, Crystal structures of two viral peptides in complex with murine class I H-2K^b, *Science* **257**:919–927.

Gao, X., Zheng, B., Liew, F. Y., Brett, S., and Tite, J., 1991, Priming of influenza virus-specific cytotoxic T lymphocytes in vivo by short synthetic peptides, *J. Immunol.* **147**:3268–3273.

Garrett, T. P., Saper, M. A., Bjorkman, P. J., Strominger, J. L., and Wiley, D. C., 1989, Specificity pockets for the side chains of peptide antigens in HLA-Aw68, *Nature* **342**:692–696.

Gaugler, B., Van den Eynde, B., van der Bruggen, P., Romero P., Gaforio, J. J., DePlaen, E., Lethe, B., Brasseur, F., and Boon, T., 1994, Human gene MAGE-3 codes for an antigen recognized on a melanoma by autologous cytolytic T lymphocytes, *J. Exp. Med.* **179**:921–930.

Gazzard, B., Youle, M., MacDonald, V., O'Toole, C. M., Stambud, D., Rios, A., Achour, A., Zagury, D., Naylor, P. H., Sarin, P. S., and Goldstein, A. L., 1992, Safety and immunogenicity of HGP-30: Evaluation of a synthetic HIV-1 p17 vaccine in healthy HIV-seronegative volunteers, *Vaccine Res.* **1**:129–135.

Germain, R. N., and Margulies, D. H., 1993, The biochemistry and cell biology of antigen processing and presentation, *Annu. Rev. Immunol.* **11**:403–450.

Goldberg, A. L., and Rock, K. L., 1992, Proteolysis, proteasomes and antigen presentation, *Nature* **375**:375–379.

Greenberg, P. D., 1991, Adoptive T cell therapy of tumors: Mechanisms operative in the recognition and elimination of tumor cells, *Adv. Immunol.* **49**:281–355.

Greenberg, P. D., Reuser, P., Goodrich, J. M., and Riddell, S. R., 1991, Development of a treatment regimen for human cytomegalovirus (CMV) infection in bone marrow transplantation recipients by adoptive transfer of donor-derived CMV-specific T cell clones expanded in vitro, *Ann. N.Y. Acad. Sci.* **636**:184–195.

Guilhot, S., Fowler, P., Portillo, G., Morgolskie, R., Ferrari, C., Bartoletti, A., and Chisari, F., 1992, Hepatitis B virus (HBV)-specific cytotoxic T-cell response in humans: Production of target cells by stable expression of HBV-encoded proteins in immortalized human B-cell lines, *J. Virol.* **66**:2670–2678.

Harding, F. A., McArthur, J. G., Gross, J. A., Raulet, D. H., and Allison, J. P., 1992, CD28-mediated signalling co-stimulates murine T cells and prevents induction of anergy in T-cell clones, *Nature* **356**:607–609.

Hart, M. K., Weinhold, K. J., Scearce, R. M., Washburn, E. M., Clark, C. A., Parker, T. J., and Haynes, B. F., 1991, Priming of anti-human immunodeficiency virus (HIV) CD8$^+$ cytotoxic T-cells in vivo by carrier-free HIV synthetic peptides, *Proc. Natl. Acad. Sci. USA* **88**:9448.

Henderson, R. A., Michel, H., Sakaguchi, K., Shabanowitz, J., Appella, E., Hunt, D. F., and Engelhard, V. H., 1992, HLA-A2.1-associated peptides from a mutant cell line: A second pathway of antigen presentation, *Science* **255**:1264.

Hoffman, S. L., Isenbarger, D., Long, G. W., Sedagah, M., Szarfman, A., Waters, L., Hollingdale, M. R., van der Meide, P., Finbloom, D., and Ballou, W. R., 1989, Sporozoite vaccine induces genetically restricted T cell elimination of malaria from hepatocytes, *Science* **244**:1078–1081.

Houbiers, J. G. A., Nijman, H. W., van der Burg, S. H., Drijfhout, J. W., Kenemans, P., van de Velde, C. J. H., Brand, A., Momburg, F., Kast, W. M., and Melief, C. J. M., 1993, In vitro induction of human cytotoxic T lymphocyte responses against peptides of mutant and wild-type p53, *Eur. J. Immunol.* **23**:2072–2077.

Hunt, D. F., Henderson, R. A., Shabanowitz, J., Sakaguchi, K., Michel, H., Sevilier, N., Cox, A. L., Appella, E., and Engelhard, V. H., 1992, Characterization of peptides bound to class I MHC molecule HLA-A2.1 by mass spectrometry, *Science* **255**:1261–1263.

Imanishi, T., Akaza, T., Kimura, A., Tokunaga, K., and Gojobori, T., 1992, Allele and haplotype frequencies for HLA and complement loci in various ethnic groups, in: *HLA 1991, Proc. of the Eleventh International Histocompatibility Workshop and Conference* (K. Tsuji, M. Aizawa, and T. Sasazuki, eds.), Oxford University Press, London, pp. 1066–1077.

Ioannides, C. G., Fisk, B., Jerome, K. R., Irimura, T., Wharton, J. T., and Finn, O. J., 1993, Cytotoxic T cells from ovarian malignant tumors can recognize polymorphic epithelial mucin core peptides, *J. Immunol.* **151**:3693–3703.

Jardetzky, T. S., Lane, W. S., Robinson, R. A., Madden, D.R., and Wiley, D. C., 1991, Identification of self peptides bound to purified HLA-B27, *Nature* **353**:326–329.

Jassoy, C., Harrer, T., Rosenthal, T., Navia, B. A., Worth, J., Johnson, R. P., and Walker, B. D., 1993, Human immunodeficiency virus type-1-specific cytotoxic T lymphocytes release gamma interferon, tumor necrosis factor alpha (TNF-α), and TNF-β when they encounter their target antigens, *J. Virol.* **67**:2844–2852.

Jerome, K. R., Barnd, D. L., Bendt, K. M., Boyer, C. M., Taylor-Papadimitriou, J., McKenzie, I. F., Bast, R. C., Jr., and Finn, O. J., 1991, Cytotoxic T-lymphocytes derived from patients with breast adenocarcinoma recognize an epitope present on the protein core of a mucin molecule preferentially expressed by malignant cells, *Cancer Res.* **51**:2908–2916.

Johnson, R. P., Trocha, A., Yang, L., Marrara, G., Panicali, D., Buchanan, T., and Walder, B. D., 1991, HIV-1 gag-specific cytotoxic T lymphocytes recognize multiple highly conserved epitopes: Fine specificity of the gag-specific response by using unstimulated peripheral blood mononuclear cells and cloned effector cells, *J. Immunol.* **147**:3714–3718.

Johnson, R. P., Trocha, A., Buchanan, T. M., and Walker, B. D., 1992, Identification of overlapping HLA class I-restricted cytotoxic T cell epitopes in a conserved region of the HIV-1 envelope glycoprotein: Definition of minimum epitopes and analysis of the effects of sequence variation, *J. Exp. Med.* **175**:961–971.

Johnson, R. P., Trocha, A., Buchanan, T. M., and Walker, B. D., 1993, Recognition of a highly conserved region of human immunodeficiency virus type 1 gp120 by an HLA-Cw4-restricted cytotoxic T-lymphocyte clone, *J. Virol.* **67**:438–445.

Kahn, J. O., Stites, D. P., Scillian, J., Murcar, N., Stryker, R., Volberding, P. A., Naylor, P. H., Goldstein, A. L., Sarin, P. S., Simmon, V. F., Wang, S.-S., and Heseltine, P., 1992, A phase I study of HPG-30, a 30 amino acid subunit of the human immunodeficiency virus (HIV) p17 synthetic peptide analogue subunit in seronegative subjects, *AIDS Res. Hum. Retroviruses* **8**:1321–1325.

Kast, W. M., Roux, L., Curren, J., Blom, H. J. J., Voordouw, A. C., Meloen, R. H., Kokakofsky, D., and Melief, C. J. M., 1991, Protection against lethal Sendai virus infection by in vivo priming of virus-specific cytotoxic T lymphocytes with a free synthetic peptide, *Proc. Natl. Acad. Sci. USA* **88**:2283–2287.

Kast, W. M., Brandt, R. M. P., and Melief, C. J. M., 1993, Strict peptide length is not required for the induction of cytotoxic T lymphocyte-mediated antiviral protection by peptide vaccination, *Eur. J. Immunol.* **23**:1189–1192.

Kast, W. M., Brandt, R. M. P., Sidney, J., Drijfhout, J.-W., Kubo, R. T., Grey, H. M., Melief, C. J. M., and Sette, A., 1994, The role of HLA-A motifs in identification of potential CTL epitopes in human papillomavirus type 16 E6 and E7 proteins, *J. Immunol.* **152**:3904–3912.

Khusmith, S., Charoenvit, Y., Kumar, S., Sedegah, M., Beaudoin, R. L., and Hoffman, S. L., 1991, Protection against malaria by vaccination with sporozoite surface protein 2 plus CS protein, *Science* **252**:715–718.

Koenig, S., Earl, P., Powell, D., Pantaleo, G., Merli, S., Moss, B., and Fauci, A. S., 1988, Group-specific, MHC class I restricted cytotoxic responses to HIV-1 envelope proteins by cloned peripheral blood T cells from an HIV-1-infected individual, *Proc. Natl. Acad. Sci. USA* **85**:8638–8642.

Kos, F. J., and Mullbacher, A., 1992, Induction of primary anti-viral cytotoxic T cells by in vitro stimulation with short synthetic peptides and interleukin-7, *Eur. J. Immunol.* **22**:3183–3185.

Koziel, M. J., Dudley, D., Wong, J. T., Dienstag, J., Houghton, M., Ralston, R., and Walker, B. D., 1992, Intrahepatic cytotoxic T lymphocytes specific for hepatitis C virus in persons with chronic hepatitis, *J. Immunol.* **149**:3339–3344.

Koziel, M. J., Dudley, D., Afdhal, N., Choo, Q.-L., Houghton, M., Ralston, R., and Walker, B. D., 1993, Hepatitis C virus (HCV)-specific cytotoxic T lymphocytes recognize epitopes in the core and envelope proteins of HCV, *J. Virol.* **67**:7522–7532.

Kubo, R. T., Sette, A., Grey, H. M., Appella, E., Sakaguchi, K., Zhu, N.-Z., Arnott, D., Sherman, N., Shabanowitz, J., Michel, H., Bodnar, W. M., Davis, T. A., and Hunt, D. F., 1994, Definition of specific peptide motifs for four major HLA-A alleles, *J. Immunol.* **152**:3913–3924.

Lamb, J. R., McMichael, A. J., and Rothbard, J. B., 1987, T-cell recognition of influenza viral antigens, *Hum. Immunol.* **19**:79–89.

Lanzavecchia, A., 1993, Identifying strategies for immune intervention, *Science* **260**:937–944.

Ljunggren, H.-G., Stan, N. J., Ohlen, C., Neefjes, J. J., Hoglund, P., Heemels, M.-T., Bastin, J., Schumacher, T. N. M., Townsend, A., Karre, K., and Ploegh, H. L., 1990, Empty MHC class I molecules come out in the cold, *Nature* **346**:476–480.

Lukacher, A. E., Braciale, V. L., and Braciale, T. J., 1984, In vivo effector function of influenza virus, specific cytotoxic T lymphocyte clones is highly specific, *J. Exp. Med.* **160**:814–826.

McMichael, A. J., Gotch, F. M., Noble, G. R., and Beare, P. A. S., 1983, Cytotoxic T-cell immunity to influenza, *N. Engl. J. Med.* **309**:13–17.

Madden, D. R., Gorga, J. C., Strominger, J. L., and Wiley, D. C., 1991, The structure of HLA-B27 reveals nonamer self-peptides bound in an extended conformation, *Nature* **353**:321–325.

Matsumura, M., Fremont, D. H., Peterson, P. A., and Wilson, I. A., 1992, Emerging principles for the recognition of peptide antigens by MHC class I molecules, *Science* **257**:927–934.

Melief, C. J. M., 1992, Tumor eradication by adoptive transfer of cytotoxic T lymphocytes, *Adv. Cancer Res.* **58**:143–175.

Miller, M. D., Gould-Fogerite, S., Shen, L., Woods, R. M., Koenig, S., Mannino, R. J., and Letvin, N. L., 1992, Vaccination of rhesus monkeys with synthetic peptide in a fusogenic proteoliposome elicits simian immunodeficiency virus-specific CD8[+] cytotoxic T lymphocytes, *J. Exp. Med.* **176**:1739–1744.

Missale, G., Redeker, A., Person, J., Fowler, P., Guilhot, S., Schlicht, H.-J., Ferrari, C., and Chisari, F. V., 1993, HLA-A31- and HLA-Aw68-restricted cytotoxic T cell responses to a single hepatitis B virus nucleocapsid epitope during acute viral hepatitis, *J. Exp. Med.* **177**:751–762.

Moore, R. L., and Fox, B. S., 1993, Immunization of mice with human immunodeficiency virus glycoprotein gp160 peptide 315-329 induces both class I- and class II-restricted T cells: Not all T cells can respond to whole molecule stimulation, *AIDS Res. Hum. Retroviruses* **9**:51–59.

Muul, L. M., Spiess, P. J., Director, E. P., and Rosenberg, S. A., 1987, Identification of specific cytolytic immune responses against autologous tumor in humans bearing malignant melanoma, *J. Immunol.* **138**:989–995.

Nardelli, B., and Tam, J. P., 1993, Cellular immune responses induced by in vivo priming with a lipid-conjugated multimeric antigen peptide, *Immunology* **79**:355–361.

Nayersina, R., Fowler, P., Guilhot, S., Missale, G., Cerny, A., Schlicht, H.-J., Vitiello, A., Chesnut, R., Person, J. L., Redeker, A. G., and Chisari, F. V., 1993, HLA-A2-restricted cytotoxic T lymphocyte responses to multiple hepatitic B surface antigen epitopes during hepatitis B virus infection, *J. Immunol.* **150**:4659–4671.

Nixon, D. F., Townsend, A. R. M., Elvin, J. G., Rizza, C. R., Gallwey, J., and McMichael, A. J., 1988, HIV-1 gag-specific cytotoxic T lymphocytes defined with recombinant vaccinia virus and synthetic peptides, *Nature* **336**:484–487.

Quinnan, G. V., Kirmeni, N., Rook, A. H., Manishevitz, J. V., Jackson, L., Moreschi, G., Santos, G. W., Saral, R., and Burns, W. H., 1982, Cytotoxic T cells in cytomegalovirus infection: HLA-restricted T-lymphocyte and non T-lymphocyte cytotoxic response correlate with recovery from cytomegalovirus infection in bone-marrow-transplant recipients, *N. Engl. J. Med.* **307**:6–13.

Rammensee, H.-G., Falk, K., and Rötzschke, O., 1993, Peptides naturally presented by MHC class I molecules, *Annu. Rev. Immunol.* **11**:213–244.

Reddehase, M. J., Weiland, F., Munch, K., Jonjic, S., Luske, A., and Koszinowski, U. H., 1985, Interstitial murine cytomegalovirus pneumonia after irradiation: Characterization of cells that limit viral replication during established infection of the lungs, *J. Virol.* **55**:264–273.

Riddell, S. R., Watanabe, K. S., Goodrich, J. M., Li, C. R., Agha, M. E., and Greenberg, P. D., 1992, Restoration of viral immunity in immunodeficient humans by the adoptive transfer to T cell clones, *Science* **257**:238–241.

Romero, P., Maryanski, J. L., Corradin, G., Nussenzweig, R. S., Nussenzweig, V., and Zavala, F., 1989, Cloned cytotoxic T cells recognize an epitope in the circumsporozoite protein and protect against malaria, *Nature* **341**:323–326.

Romero, P., Maryanski, J. L., Cordey, A.-S., Corradin, G., Nussenzweig, R. S., and Zavala, F. 1990, Isolation and characterization of protective cytolytic T cells in a rodent malaria system, *Immunol. Lett.* **25**:27–32.

Rosenberg, S. A., Packard, B. S., Aebersold, P. M., Solomon, D., Topalian, S. L., Toy, S. T., Simon, P., Lotze, M. T., Yang, J. C., Seipp, C., Simpson, C., Carter, C., Bock, S., Schwartzentruber, D. J., Wei, J. P., and White, D. E., 1988, Use of tumor infiltrating lymphocytes and interleukin 2 in the immunotherapy of patients with metastatic melanoma: A preliminary report, *N. Engl. J. Med.* **319**:1676–1680.

Rötzschke, O., and Falk, K., 1991, Naturally-occurring peptide antigens derived from the MHC class I-restricted processing pathway, *Immunol. Today* **12**:447–455.

Rouse, B. T., Norley, S., and Martin, S., 1988, Antiviral cytotoxic T lymphocyte induction and vaccination, *Rev. Infect. Dis.* **10**:16–33.

Ruppert, J., Sidney, J., Celis, E., Kubo, R. T., Grey, H. M., and Sette, A., 1993, Prominent role of secondary anchor residues in peptide binding to HLA-A2.1 molecules, *Cell* **74**:929–937.

Saper, M. A., Bjorkman, P. J., and Wiley, D. C., 1991, Refined structure of the human histocompatibility antigen HLA-A2 at 2.6Å resolution, *J. Mol. Biol.* **219**:277–319.

Sastry, K. J., Nehete, P. N., Venkatnarayanan, S., Morkowski, J., Platsoucas, C. D., and Arlinghaus, R. B., 1992, Rapid in vivo induction of HIV-specific $CD8^+$ cytotoxic T lymphocytes by a 15-amino acid unmodified free peptide from the immunodominant V3-loop of GP120, *Virology* **188**:502–509.

Schultz, M., Zinkernagel, R. M., and Hengartner, H., 1991, Peptide-induced antiviral protection by cytotoxic T cells, *Proc. Natl. Acad. Sci. USA* **88**:991–993.

Sethi, K. K., Omata, Y., and Schnewer, K. E., 1983, Protection of mice from fatal herpes simplex virus type 1 infection by adoptive transfer of virus-specific and H-2 restricted cytotoxic T lymphocytes, *J. Gen. Virol.* **64**:443–447.

Sette, A., Sidney, J. del Guercio, M.-F., Southwood, S., Ruppert, J., Dahlberg, C., Grey, H. M., and Kubo, R. T., 1994, Peptide binding to the most frequent HLA-A class I alleles measured by quantitative molecular binding assays, *Molec. Immunol.* **31**:813–822.

Sher, A., and Coffman, R. L., 1992, Regulation of immunity to parasites by T cells and T cell-derived cytokines, *Annu. Rev. Immunol.* **10**:385–409.

Silver, M. L., Guo, H., Strominger, J. L., and Wiley, D. C., 1992, Atomic structure of a human MHC molecule presenting an influenza virus peptide, *Nature* **360**:367–369.

Skipper, J., and Stauss, H. J., 1993, Identification of two cytotoxic T lymphocyte-recognized epitopes in the ras protein, *J. Exp. Med.* **177**:1493–1498.

Spies, T., Cerundolo, V., Colonna, M., Cresswell, P., Townsend, A., and DeMars, R., 1992, Presentation of viral antigen by MHC class I molecules is dependent on a putative peptide transporter heterodimer, *Nature* **355**:644–646.

Stauss, H. J., Davies, H., Sadovnikova, E., Chain, B., Horowitz, N., and Sinclair, C., 1992, Induction of cytotoxic T lymphocytes with peptides in vitro: Identification of candidate T-cell epitopes in human papilloma virus, *Proc. Natl. Acad. Sci. USA* **89**:7871–7875.

Storkus, W. J., Zeh, H. J., III, Salter, R. D., and Lotze, M. T., 1993, Identification of T cell epitopes: Rapid elution of class I-presented peptides from viable cells using mild acid elution, *J. Immunother.* **14**:94–103.

Suguwara, S., Abo, T., and Kumagai, K., 1987, A simple method to eliminate the antigenicity of surface class I MHC molecules from the membrane of viable cells by acid treatment at pH 3, *J. Immunol. Methods* **100**:83–90.

Takahashi, H., Nakagawa, Y., Yodomuro, K., and Berzofsky, J. A., 1993, Induction of CD8[+] cytotoxic T lymphocytes by immunization with syngeneic irradiated HIV-1 envelope derived peptide-pulsed dendritic cells, *Int. Immunol.* **5**:849–857.

Taylor, P. M., Davey, J., Howland, K., Rothbard, J., and Askonas, B. A., 1987, Class I MHC molecules rather than other mouse genes dictate influenza epitope recognition by cytotoxic T cells, *Immunogenetics* **26**:267–272.

Tigges, M. A., Koelle, D., Hartog, K., Sekulovich, R. E., Corey, L., and Burke, R. L., 1993, Human CD8[+] herpes simplex virus-specific cytotoxic T-lymphocyte clones recognize diverse virion protein antigens, *J. Virol.* **66**:1622–1634.

Townsend, A. R., Gotch, F. M., and Davey, J., 1985, Cytotoxic T cells recognize fragments of the influenza nucleoprotein, *Cell* **42**:457–467.

Urban, J. L., and Schreiber, H., 1992, Tumor antigens, *Annu. Rev. Immunol.* **10**:617–644.

Van Bleek, G. M., and Nathenson, S. G., 1990, Isolation of an endogenously processed immunodominant viral peptide from the class I H-2K[b] molecule, *Nature* **348**:213–216.

van der Bruggen, P., and Van den Eynde, B., 1992, Molecular definition of tumor antigens recognized by T lymphocytes, *Cur. Opin. Immunol.* **4**:608–612.

van der Bruggen, P., Traversari, C., Chomez, P., Lurquin, C., de Plaen, E., Van den Eynde, B., Knuth, A., and Boon, T., 1991, A gene encoding an antigen recognized by cytolytic T lymphocytes on a human melanoma, *Science* **254**:1643–1647.

Vasilakos, J. P., and Michael, G., 1993, Herpes simplex virus class I-restricted peptide induces cytotoxic T lymphocytes in vivo independent of CD4[+] T cells, *J. Immunol.* **150**:2346–2355.

Vitiello, A., Marchesini, D., Furze, J., Sherman, L. A., and Chesnut, R. W., 1991, Analysis of the HLA-restricted influenza-specific cytotoxic T lymphocyte response in transgenic mice carrying a chimeric human–mouse class I major histocompatibility complex, *J. Exp. Med.* **173**:1007–1015.

Vose, B. M., and Bonnard, G. D., 1982, Human tumor antigens defined by cytotoxic and proliferating responses of cultured lymphoid cells, *Nature* **296**:359–361.

Wagner, H., and Rollinghoff, M., 1978, T–T interactions during in vitro cytotoxic allograft responses. I. Soluble products from activated Ly 1[+] T cells trigger autonomously antigen-primed Ly 23[+] T cells to proliferation and cytolytic activity, *J. Exp. Med.* **148**:1523–1538.

Walker, B. D., Chakrabarti, S., Moss, B., Paradis, T. J., Flynn, T., Durno, A. G., Blumberg, R. S., Kaplan, J. C., Hirsch, M. S., and Schooley, R. T., 1987, HIV-specific cytotoxic T lymphocytes in seropositive individuals, *Nature* **328**:345–348.

Walker, B. D., Flexner, C., Paradis, T. J., Fuller, T. C., Hirsch, M. S., Schooley, R. T., and Moss, B., 1988, HIV-1 reverse transcriptase is a target for cytotoxic T lymphocytes in infected individuals, *Science* **240**:64–66.

Widmann, C., Romero, P., Maryanski, J. L., Corradin, G., and Valmori, D., 1992, T helper epitopes enhance the cytotoxic response of mice immunized with MHC class I-restricted malaria peptides, *J. Immunol. Methods* **155**:95–99.

Yap, K. L., Ada, G. L., and McKenzie, I. F. C., 1978, Transfer of specific cytotoxic T lymphocytes protects mice inoculated with influenza virus, *Nature* **273**:238–239.

Yasukawa, M., Inatsuki, A., and Kobayzashi, Y., 1989, Differential in vitro activation of CD4[+] CD8[−] and CD8[+] CD4[−] herpes simplex virus-specific human cytotoxic T cells, *J. Immunol.* **143**:2051–2057.

Yasutomi, Y., Palker, T. J., Gardner, M. B., Haynes, B. F., and Letvin, N. L., 1993, Synthetic peptide in mineral oil adjuvant elicits simian immunodeficiency virus-specific CD8[+] cytotoxic T lymphocytes in rhesus monkeys, *J. Immunol.* **151**:5096–5105.

Young, A. C. M., Zhang, W., Sacchettini, J. C., and Nathenson, S. G., 1994, The three-dimensional structure of H-2D[b] at 2.4Å resolution: Implications for antigen-determinant selection, *Cell* **76**:39–50.

Zakut, R., Toplian, S. L., Kawakami, Y., Mancini, M., Eliyahu, S., and Rosenberg, S. A., 1993, Differential expression of MAGE-1, -2, and -3 messenger RNA in transformed and normal human cell lines, *Cancer Res.* **53**:5–8.

Zhang, Q., Gavioli, R., Klein, G., and Masucci, M. G., 1993, An HLA-A11-specific motif in nonamer peptides derived from viral and cellular proteins, *Proc. Natl. Acad. Sci. USA* **90**:2217–2221.

Zhang, W., Young, A. C. M., Imarai, M., Nathenson, S. G., and Sacchettini, J. C., 1992, Crystal structure of the major histocompatibility complex class I H-2^b molecule containing a single viral peptide: Implications for peptide binding and T cell receptor recognition, *Proc. Natl. Acad. Sci. USA* **89**:8403–8407.

Zhou, X., Berg, L., Motal, U. M. A., and Jondal, M., 1992, In vivo primary induction of virus-specific CTL by immunization with 9-mer synthetic peptides, *J. Immunol. Methods* **153**:193–200.

Zinkernagel, R. M., and Doherty, P. C., 1979, MHC-restricted cytotoxic T cells: Studies of the biological role of polymorphic major transplantation antigens determining T cell restriction specificity, function, and responsiveness, *Adv. Immunol.* **27**:51–177.

Chapter 39

Development of Active Specific Immunotherapeutic Agents Based on Cancer-Associated Mucins

John Samuel and B. Michael Longenecker

1. INTRODUCTION

The immune system offers the most effective line of defense against infectious organisms. Cancer immunologists are currently attempting to direct the unique defense mechanisms of the immune system to mediate tumor rejection. This approach is based on the assumption that cancer cells express aberrant molecules that have the potential to be recognized by the immune system as "foreign." If such cancer-specific targets can be identified, they may be used as active specific immunotherapeutic (ASI) agents to induce specific immune responses against the cells expressing such structures. Such responses may result in cancer rejection.

Early evidence for the existence of such cancer antigens came from studies reported in the 1950s and 1960s on rodent tumors induced by chemical carcinogens, ultraviolet irradiation, or viruses. Animals preimmunized with such tumor cells were protected against secondary tumor challenge with the same tumor, but not against unrelated cancers (Prehan and Main, 1957; Klein *et al.,* 1960; Khera *et al.,* 1963; Klein and Klein, 1964). However, subsequent studies showed that many naturally arising murine tumors were incapable of inducing such immune-mediated rejection of the tumor (Hewit *et al.,* 1976; Middle and Embleton, 1981). Further, most of the human cancer-associated antigens characterized in the last two decades are also expressed, although to a limited degree, by some normal cells (Hakamori, 1989). Induction of immune responses against such antigens would be difficult, because of self-tolerance of such molecules. Even if such efforts are successful, induction of strong immune responses against self molecules may result in autoimmune disorders.

John Samuel • Faculty of Pharmacy and Pharmaceutical Sciences, University of Alberta, Edmonton, Alberta T6G 2N8, Canada. *B. Michael Longenecker* • Department of Immunology, Faculty of Medicine, University of Alberta, Edmonton, and Biomira Inc., Edmonton, Alberta T6N 1H1, Canada.

Vaccine Design: The Subunit and Adjuvant Approach, edited by Michael F. Powell and Mark J. Newman. Plenum Press, New York, 1995.

Since truly cancer-specific antigens could not be detected in spontaneous human cancers, approaches to develop active specific immunotherapy for common cancers, based on cancer-associated antigens, were viewed with pessimism.

Recent advances in cancer immunology suggest that the development of ASI agents for cancer may be an achievable goal (McMichael and Bodmer, 1992; Pardoll, 1993; Longenecker and MacLean, 1993; Boon, 1993). Although spontaneous human cancers do not express totally "foreign" molecules, there is increasing evidence for subtle cancer-specific alterations of "self" proteins on cancer cells (Urban and Schreiber, 1992). Such changes may result in generation of cancer-specific epitopes recognizable by the immune system. Recent identifications of the single-point mutations of oncogenes and tumor suppressor genes in human carcinomas and the demonstrations that such mutated peptides can be recognized by T cells illustrate this possibility. Although many of these altered cancer-associated molecules are only weakly immunogenic, it may be possible to develop strongly immunogenic ASI formulations that can induce effective immune responses against the epitopes presented on the cancer cells. The results from recent clinical trials using immunogenic formulations of melanoma cell extracts have documented increased survival time and induction of T-cell-mediated immune responses against melanoma-associated epitopes (Mitchell *et al.*, 1993; LeMay *et al.*, 1993; Kan-Mitchell *et al.*, 1993). Thus, efforts to develop ASI agents based on cancer antigens is currently viewed with cautious optimism.

2. IMMUNE RESPONSES RELEVANT TO CANCER REJECTION

The development of effective vaccines and ASI agents requires a clear understanding of the type of immune responses most appropriate for protection against diseases. For the design of vaccines against infectious agents, it is generally recognized that antibody responses are most suited for extracellular pathogens and toxins, whereas protection against intracellular pathogens, such as viruses, requires participation of cell-mediated immune (CMI) responses. In certain infections, inappropriate immune responses may even be harmful (Locksley and Scott, 1991; Clerici and Shearer, 1993). Therefore, the design of effective ASI agents against cancer requires careful consideration of the type of immune responses most effective in cancer rejection.

Humoral immune responses against cancer-associated antigens on autologous tumor cells have been detected in cancer patients (Old, 1981; Furukawa *et al.*, 1989; Ryghetti *et al.*, 1993). Such antibodies may be able to lyse tumor cells by complement-mediated mechanisms or by antibody-dependent cellular cytotoxicity. Induction of antibody responses, epecially IgG responses, to cancer-associated gangliosides in melanoma patients has been correlated with clinical outcome (Livingston *et al.*, 1987). This provides the basis for the development of immunogenic formulations of GM2, GD2, and GD3 as ASI agents for use in melanoma patients (Livingston, 1993).

There is increasing evidence that CMI, particularly cytotoxic T lymphocytes (CTLs) and helper T (Th) cells, may hold even greater potential for initiating cancer rejection. CTLs are predominantly $CD8^+$ lymphocytes that can kill target cells on recognition of peptides in association with MHC class I molecules. Cancer-specific CTLs have been generated in vitro from lymphocytes isolated from patients suffering from a variety of cancers such as melanomas (Anichini *et al.*, 1989; Crowley *et al.*, 1991; Knuth *et al.*, 1992), sarcoma (Solvin *et al.*, 1986), mammary carcinoma (Sato *et al.*, 1986), ovarian carcinoma (Ferrini *et al.*, 1985), B-cell lymphoma (Yssel *et al.*, 1984), and T-cell leukemia (Fisch *et al.*, 1989). These CTLs were able to kill autologous tumor cells in antigen-specific and MHC-restricted fashion. The in vivo relevance of some of these CTL clones has been further demonstrated by their ability to proliferate in the presence of freshly isolated autologous tumor cells (Degiovanni *et al.*, 1990) and/or their ability to kill such target cells (Solvin *et al.*, 1986). CTLs induced by in vivo immunizations or administered by adoptive transfer have effectively eradicated tumors in animal models (Boon *et al.*, 1992; Melief, 1992). Although these studies were done in animals using tumors induced by viruses or carcinogens, which are significantly different from spontaneous human tumors, the results suggest that CTLs elicited against appropriate antigens offer a powerful immunological mechanism for tumor eradication.

Another subpopulation of T cells that are relevant in anticancer immunity are Th cells. The major function of Th cells is the regulation of immune responses. They are predominantly $CD4^+$ T cells that recognize peptides in association with MHC class II molecules on the surface of antigen-presenting cells (APCs), and on activation secrete cytokines that are required for the proliferation and maturation of T and B cells. Two subtypes of Th cells (Th1 and Th2) with distinct cytokine secretion patterns have been recently characterized (Mosmann and Coffman, 1989; Romagnani, 1991; Fitch *et al.*, 1993). Th1 cells that activate mainly the cellular arm of the immune responses, also IgG2a antibodies in mice, secrete interleukin-2 (IL-2), interferon-γ (IFN-γ), and lymphotoxin (LT), but not IL-4, IL-5, IL-6, or IL-10. Th2 cells, which provide help to the humoral immune responses, produce IL-4, IL-5, IL-6, and IL-10, but not IL-2, IFN-γ, or LT. Predominance of one type of Th response over the other has clear consequences in several diseases. For example, in leishmaniasis, activation of the Th1 pathway provides protection, whereas activation of the Th2 pathway exacerbates the disease (Locksley and Scott, 1991). Similarly in human immunodeficiency virus (HIV) infection, progress from asymptomatic infection to development of AIDS is believed to be associated with shift from Th1 to Th2 type of immune responses (Clerici and Shearer, 1993). If cellular immune responses involving cytotoxic T cells and other inflammatory cells, such as natural killer (NK) cells, offer the most potent mechanisms of tumor eradication, then anticancer ASI formulations should be optimized for induction of the dominant Th1 pathway. Th1 cytokines such as IL-2 and IFN-γ have been shown to augment anticancer immunity by potentiating CTLs and other inflammatory cells. A recent report that IL-2 production by tumor cells can bypass the T-helper function in the generation of antitumor responses in an animal model also supports this view (Fearon *et al.*, 1990). Nagarkatti *et al.* (1990) have reported the characterization of tumor-infiltrating $CD4^+$ T cells in a mouse tumor model as Th1 and have shown that these cells can mediate tumor rejection by activating macrophages. Our current efforts are directed toward development of ASI formulations which can potentially activate CTLs and Th1 cells.

3. TARGET ANTIGENS FOR ASI

Since spontaneously arising cancers do not express totally foreign antigens, the search for antigenic targets should be directed to subtle changes in the self proteins. Since T cells recognize processed peptides in association with MHC molecules, peptides derived from intracellular proteins are also important targets for CMI. Further, since antigen processing and presentation are critical steps in T-cell recognition, cancer-associated changes that influence these steps may result in presentation of novel peptide fragments on cancer cells. Tumor-specific single point mutations of oncogenes such as *RAS* and tumor suppressor genes such as *p53* have been reported for a significant proportion of spontaneously arising common cancers such as breast, lung, and colon cancers (Urban and Schrieber, 1992). Although these altered proteins are located intracellularly, the mutated peptide fragments generated from them are presented by MHC molecules and are recognized by T cells (Jung and Schluesener, 1991). The recently characterized cancer rejection gene, *MAGE-1*, expressed by human melanomas, is yet another example of cancer-specific targets for CTLs, generated in cells by point mutations (Boon *et al.*, 1992).

Another subtle, but common change in cancer-associated antigens involves glycosylation (Hakamori, 1989; Singhal and Hakamori, 1990). Can altered glycosylation result in generation of cancer rejection epitopes, especially targets for T-cell recognition? Although aberrant glycosylation is recognized as a common cancer-associated change resulting in humoral immune responses, its consequence to CMI, including MHC presentation of peptide (or glycopeptide) fragments generated from glycoproteins, has not been explored. It is conceivable that glycosylation can affect T-cell recognition of peptides by interfering with proteolytic degradation of proteins into peptides, the binding of peptides to MHC molecules, or by influencing the recognition of peptides by T-cell receptor. There are preliminary reports indicating that glycosylation can influence the generation of peptide epitopes for T-cell recognition (Botarelli *et al.*, 1991; Thomas *et al.*, 1990; Drummer *et al.*, 1993). A category of high-molecular-weight glycoproteins known as mucins are of special interest in relation to aberrant cancer-associated glycosylation and are the focus of our approach to develop ASI agents.

4. CANCER-ASSOCIATED MUCINS AS TARGET ANTIGENS

Mucins are complex large (> 200 kDa) glycoproteins expressed as cell surface molecules and secreted by a variety of normal and malignant epithelial cells (Strous and Dekker, 1992; Devine and McKenzie, 1992). They comprise 50–90% (by weight) oligosaccharide structures that are linked to serines or threonines of core peptides through O-glycosidic bonds. The oligosaccharide structures are made up of linear or branched chains of 1–20 monosaccharides (Hanisch *et al.*, 1989a,b; Capon *et al.*, 1992). The core peptides of several human mucins have been recently characterized by cDNA cloning (Gum *et al.*, 1989, 1990; Gendler *et al.*, 1990; Litenberg *et al.*, 1990; Wreshner *et al.*, 1990; Lan *et al.*, 1990; Porchet *et al.*, 1991; Bobek *et al.*, 1993). The general structural features of mucin core peptides may be illustrated by the amino acid sequence reported for the first and most well characterized mucin, known as MUC1 mucin or polymorphic epithelial mucin (Gendler *et al.*, 1990). The MUC1 core peptide has a large extracellular N-terminal domain, a transmembrane region, and a cytoplasmic C-terminal domain (Fig. 1). The N-terminal domain is largely made of a central region of tandem repeat sequences of 20 amino acids (PPAHGVTSAPDTRPAPGSTA) which is flanked by regions of degenerate tandem repeats. The tandem repeat region is rich in serines and threonines, which are sites

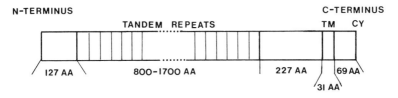

Figure 1. Diagram of MUC1 core peptide, showing a large extracellular domain with a central tandem repeat region (800–1700 AA) flanked by degenerate repeat regions (127 AA at the N-terminus and 227 AA at the C-terminus). The C-terminus also contains the transmembrane (TM) and cytoplasmic (CY) regions. (Adapted from Gendler *et al.*, 1990.)

for *O*-glycosylation. The size of the core peptide varies because of the variability in the number of tandem repeats, a genetic polymorphism. A variable tandem repeat region with multiple *O*-glycosylation sites is a common feature of all mucin core peptides so far characteized.

Cancer cells differ from the normal epithelial cells with respect to expression of mucin molecules (Longenecker and MacLean, 1993). First, the cell surface mucins on the normal epithelial cells are found on the luminal surface and are therefore not exposed to the immune system. This polarized expression of mucins is lost in cancer cells, which express mucins uniformly on their surface, resulting in exposure of mucin molecules to the immune system. Second, the cancer-associated mucins differ from their normal counterparts with respect to glycosylation. They appear to be underglycosylated with truncated carbohydrate chains largely made up of one to six sugar units (Hanisch *et al.*, 1989b; Hull *et al.*, 1989). The normal mucins have extended and branched complex carbohydrate structures (Fig. 2) and the internal sugar units and the core peptide remain hidden by the peripheral carbohydrate structures (Hanisch *et al.*, 1989a). As a result of the truncated carbohydrate structures, the carcinoma mucins have exposed internal sugar units and "naked" peptide sequences that are unexposed in the normal molecule (Burchell *et al.*, 1987; Devine *et al.*, 1990). This can result in generation of three types of cancer-associated epitopes: short carbohydrate, "naked peptide," and possibly glycopeptide structures, all of which are recognizable by the immune system (Longenecker and MacLean, 1993). Such epitopes may be used as the

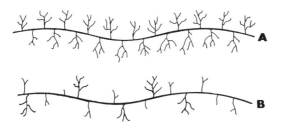

Figure 2. A comparison of normal epithelial mucins (A) with cancer-associated mucins (B). The central thick line represents the core peptide and the thin lines represent the oligosaccharide chains attached to the core peptides. Cancer-associated mucins have fewer and shorter oligosaccharide chains.

basis for the design of ASI agents for stimulating immune rejection of carcinomas expressing mucins.

5. IMMUNE RESPONSES TO CARBOHYDRATE EPITOPES

O-Glycosylation of proteins involves stepwise addition of monosaccharide units to the core peptide (Schachter and Brockhausen, 1989). A simplified presentation of the initial steps in major O-glycosylation pathways for mucins is shown in Fig. 3. The first sugar attached to the core protein is N-acetylgalactosamine (GalNAc). Further elongation of the carbohydrate chain is initiated by formation of one of the four major core structures, core 1 to 4, by β-glycosidic linkages. Addition of a galactose (Gal) or N-acetylglucosamine (GlcNAc) to position 3 of GalNAc gives core structure 1 or 3, respectively. These disaccharide core structures 1 and 3 may be elongated by addition of a GlcNAc to position 6 of GalNAc to give cores 2 and 4, respectively. These core structures are usually further glycosylated by addition of Gal and GlcNAc moieties to produce elongated and branched oligosaccharide structures on mucins. Thus, normal mucins often have many polylactosamine (Galβ1-4GlcNAcβ1-3)$_n$ structures linked to the peptide backbone through one or more of these core structures. The oligosaccharide chains are usully terminated by α-glycosidic linkages of peripheral sugars such as N-acetylneuraminic acid (NeuAc), fucose, Gal, or GalNAc.

As a result of aberrant glycosylation, carcinoma mucins tend to have simpler carbohydrate structures. Two important such structures are the core 1 disaccharide (Galβ→3Gal-

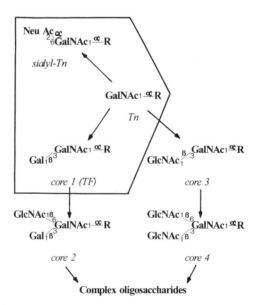

Figure 3. A simplified presentation of the major O-glycosylation pathways for mucins. The epitopes shown in the pentagon are the short cryptic carbohydrate epitopes commonly found on cancer-associated mucins.

NAcα1-R), known as Thomsen–Friedenreich (TF) epitope, and its precursor GalNAcα1-R, known as Tn epitope (Coon *et al.*, 1982; Springer, 1984; Samuel *et al.*, 1990; MacLean and Longenecker, 1991). A third cancer-associated epitope known as sialyl-Tn or STn (Itzkowitz *et al.*, 1989, 1990) is formed by premature sialylation of Tn, which prevents any further glycosylation. These three short carbohydrate epitopes are very commonly found on the cell surface of human cancers and on the mucins secreted by them, but not on normal epithelial cell surfaces or their secreted mucins. Several studies have suggested that TF, Tn, and STn are prognostic markers associated with cancer aggressiveness, invasion, and metastasis (Leathem and Brooks, 1987; Wolf *et al.*, 1988; Itzkowitz *et al.*, 1990; Kobayashi *et al.*, 1992).

The TF epitope served as the first target structure for our initial ASI studies in a mouse model and a subsequent Phase I clinical evaluation in cancer patients (Fung *et al.*, 1990; MacLean *et al.*, 1992). A highly lethal and invasive mouse mammary adenocarcinoma model, TA3-Ha, that secretes and expresses on the cell surface a mucin known as epiglycanin (Van den Eijnden *et al.*, 1979), was used for validation of the concept of ASI using carbohydrate antigens. Epiglycanin contains multiple TF and Tn epitopes. An ASI formulation containing synthetic TF disaccharide, conjugated to the carrier protein keyhole limpet hemocyanin (KLH) and emulsified in Ribi adjuvant, was able to induce both anti-TF antibodies, which bind to both TA3-Ha cells and human tumor cells, and delayed-type hypersensitivity (DTH) to TF determinants on synthetic glycoconjugates and epiglycanin (Fung *et al.*, 1990). The immune response provided a high degree of protection against an otherwise lethal, established, and growing TA3-Ha tumor (Fig. 4). The most effective ASI regimen, with > 90% survival, required pretreatment with a low dose of cyclophosphamide. The use of cyclophosphamide inhibited the formation or activation of cancer-induced suppressor cells. These results demonstrated that a mucin-associated carbohydrate epitope could induce immune responses relevant to the rejection of an already established cancer, even in an aggressive and immune-resistant tumor model. These results have been further supported by Singhal *et al.* (1991), who demonstrated that the Tn epitope can also induce cancer rejection in the same TA3-Ha model.

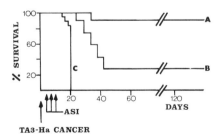

Figure 4. Active specific immunotherapy of TA3-Ha mammary adenocarcinoma tumor-bearing mice. Mice were first given TA3-Ha tumor cells on day 0 and were treated as follows: A: group treated with low-dose cyclophosphamide followed by TF–KLH formulation; B: group treated with TF–KLH formulation only; C: negative control groups such as untreated animals or those treated with irrelevant antigens, adjuvants, or low-dose cyclophosphamide alone. (Adapted from Longenecker and MacLean, 1993.)

Based on these encouraging results, we conducted a Phase I clinical evaluation of an ASI formulation containing TF–KLH and Ribi Detox™ in ten ovarian carcinoma patients with extensive metastatic disease (MacLean *et al.*, 1992). These studies were designed to evaluate the toxicity and immune responses. The results demonstrated that the formulation was nontoxic and effective at inducing TF hapten-specific humoral responses, IgM followed by high-titered IgG antibodies. The IgG antibodies were able to bind to a human cancer-associated mucin containing multiple TF epitopes and to a human cancer cell line in a TF hapten-specific manner. The antibodies were cytotoxic to TF-bearing target cells in a complement-mediated fashion.

We have extended these studies to a second epitope, STn, by evaluation of the immune responses to ASI formulation of STn–KLH in mice and in breast cancer patients in a Phase I clinical trial (MacLean *et al.*, 1993; Longenecker *et al.*, 1993). The antibody response was found to be STn-specific, and was able to induce complement-mediated lysis of STn-bearing tumor targets. In mice, small, but not large, doses of STn–KLH immunogen induced antigen-specific DTH that was inversely proportional to the antibody responses. This suggested that the optimal dose of the ASI formulation for cell-mediated responses would be different from that for humoral responses. Preliminary assessment of the clinical outcome in the 13 breast cancer patients in the STn–KLH study showed that two patients had partial clinical response, six patients had stable disease, and two had mixed response. The three patients who showed progressive disease were those who entered the study with bulky disease. While these early results are encouraging, it is inappropriate to draw any conclusion about the clinical efficacy of the ASI formulation, since this is a small pilot study with patients in an advanced disease stage.

These studies clearly demonstrated that synthetic carbohydrate antigens, designed to mimic the same epitope on cancer-associated mucins, could induce immune responses relevant to the native epitopes on cancer cells in mice and in humans. The immunological mechanisms mediating tumor rejection in mice or the reasons for the apparent clinical responses in few patients are not clear. While these studies have evaluated the humoral responses in mice and patients in detail, the possibility of CMI to the carbohydrate epitopes remains to be explored. However, the observation that the ASI formulation induced DTH reaction, specific for TF and STn epitopes, suggests carbohydrate-specific cell-mediated responses. This is further supported by the results of Singhal *et al.* (1991), who reported T-cell proliferation specific for Tn epitope. Further studies are required to see whether carbohydrate epitopes, possibly presented as glycopeptides, are recognized by T cells in a "classical" MHC-dependent manner.

6. IMMUNE RESPONSES TO MUCIN CORE PEPTIDES

As already discussed, aberrant glycosylation in cancer cells can also result in exposure of cryptic peptide epitopes on the cancer cell surface, providing targets for immune responses. Best evidence for this comes from the studies on cancer-associated MUC1 mucin. This mucin is secreted by and expressed on the surface of several epithelial cells including that of breast, ovary, and pancreas (Zotter *et al.*, 1988). It is also expressed abundantly by breast, pancreatic, and ovarian carcinoma cells. The cancer-associated MUC1 mucin is significantly underglycosylated, with fewer and shorter oligosaccharide chains, when compared to the corresponding normal epithelial mucin. The oligosaccharides isolated from cancer-associated MUC1 mucin tend to be 2 to 6 units in length as compared to the long oligosaccharide chains of up to 20 sugar units isolated from the normal breast epithelial mucin (Hanisch, *et al.*, 1989a; Hull *et al.*, 1989). The peptide sequences exposed on MUC1 mucin as the result of underglycosylation have been characterized by antimucin monoclonal antibodies (MAbs) such as SM-3 and BCP-8 (Burchell *et al.*, 1987; Girling *et al.*, 1989; Xing *et al.*, 1992). The SM-3 and BCP-8 epitopes are mapped within the PDTRP sequence of the 20-amino-acid tandem repeat region. These MAbs bind to this epitope on the MUC1 mucin on human breast cancer cells, but do not bind to the normal epithelial cell MUC1. The relative expression of the SM-3 epitope can be increased by culturing the cells in the presence of inhibitors of O-glycosylation, such as phenyl-N-acetyl-α-galactosaminide. This further demonstrates that the core peptide epitope was generated as a result of underglycosylation (Burchell and Taylor-Papadimitriou, 1993).

The cancer-associated or newly exposed epitopes of MUC1 mucin have the potential to elicit immune responses in cancer patients. Antibody responses to the SM-3 epitope of MUC1 have been demonstrated by using B cells isolated from the draining lymph nodes of an ovarian carcinoma patient (Ryghetti *et al.*, 1993). More importantly, Finn and co-workers have isolated CTL clones specific for cancer-associated MUC1 from pancreatic, breast, and ovarian carcinoma patients (Brand *et al.*, 1989; Jerome *et al.*, 1991, 1993; Ionnides *et al.*, 1993). These were mostly CD8$^+$ clones and were able to kill tumor cells expressing MUC1 in an MHC-unrestricted manner, but not tumor cells not expressing MUC1, nor breast epithelial cells. These data demonstrate the specificity for cancer-expressed mucin epitopes, which were not available for recognition on the normal cells. The CTLs could also kill autologous and allogeneic B cells, transformed with Epstein–Barr virus (EBV) and transfected with cDNA for MUC1. Untransfected B cells were not lysed by these CTLs. The exact mechanism of the apparent MHC-unrestricted antigen recognition by these CTLs is not clear. Finn and co-workers have proposed that the multivalent form of the epitope (repeated 30 to 100 times per molecule) may allow a single mucin molecule to engage many T-cell receptors simultaneously. This may result in cross-linking of the TCR and therefore bypass the need for MHC stabilization of the antigen–receptor complex. However, a recent report on the CTLs isolated from ovarian carcinoma patients indicates that when MUC1-negative cells, pulsed with MUC1 synthetic peptides are used as targets, antigen recognition was MHC restricted (Ionnides *et al.*, 1993). Reddish and co-workers at Biomira Inc. have recently isolated MUC1 peptide fragments by acid elution from affinity-purified HLA class I molecules of several human carcinoma cell lines (unpublished results). It is quite possible that cancer-associated changes including altered glycosylation may result in MHC presentation of MUC1 peptides, which are not presented by normal epithelial cells. Thus, the possibility of classical MHC-restricted CTLs specific for mucin epitopes in carcinoma patients cannot be excluded at this time.

We are currently evaluating the potential of MUC1 peptide epitopes to induce anticancer immune responses with the objective of developing MUC1 peptide ASI formulations for treatment of cancer patients. We have evaluated the immune response of synthetic MUC1 peptide formulations and their ability to induce immune rejection of cancer in a mouse model (Ding *et al.*, 1993; Longenecker and MacLean, 1993). Humoral

Table I
Summary of Immune Responses and Tumor Inhibitory Effects
Induced by MUC1 Peptide Immunogens[a]

Immunogen	Peptide sequence	Antibody response	DTH response	Inhibition of tumor growth
SP1–7-KLH	GVTSAPDTRPAPGSTA	++++	++++	+++
SP1–5	(PDTRPAPGSTAPPAHGVTSA)₄-MAP	NS[b]	++++	++++
SP1–6	(SPDTRPAEKKIAKMEKASSVFNVVNS)₄-MAP	++++	+++	NS

[a]From Ding et al. (1993).
[b]NS, not significant.

and DTH responses against a series of MUC1 peptides with overlapping sequences corresponding to the tandem repeat region of MUC1 were evaluated in CAF1 mice. The anticancer effects of the immune responses were evaluated using a mouse mammary carcinoma model developed by transfection of the human MUC1 gene into the mouse mammary carcinoma cell line, 410.4 (Lalani et al., 1991); the transfected cells are termed E3 cells. Expression of MUC1 mucin on E3 cells was similar to that on human breast cancer cells in that the cryptic peptide epitopes were exposed in a cancer-associated manner.

Immunogenic preparations were made by conjugating the peptides to KLH, by clustering in multiple antigen peptide (MAP) configuration, or by attaching universal T-helper epitopes to MUC1. The immune responses induced by three of the peptide immunogens and their effect on growth of MUC1-bearing tumors are summarized in Table I. While the KLH conjugate of the peptide (SP1-7-KLH) produced strong antibody and DTH responses, the MAP dendritic peptide cluster (SP1-5) induced strong DTH responses, but no detectable antibody responses. Another MAP peptide cluster (SP1-6) incorporating the universal Th epitope (CST-3) of the malarial circumsporozoite protein produced both humoral and DTH responses. The immune responses were shown to be specific for the relevant synthetic peptides and the native human MUC1 mucin expressed on the E3 cells.

The effect of the immunogens on cancer growth was evaluated by tumor size measurements and by survival. This analysis showed that SP1-7-KLH and SP1-5 provided protection, both when used prophylactically as well as therapeutically. No significant effect on tumor growth was induced by SP1-6. The results suggested that cellular immune responses rather than the humoral responses may be the more effective anticancer mechanisms in this model and that antibody responses may sometimes interfere with cancer rejection. These studies demonstrated that MUC1 synthetic peptides can induce immune responses relevant to the peptide sequences exposed on MUC1 mucin on cancer cells and that such responses can mediate rejection of tumor cells expressing such epitopes. Our results are consistent with an independent report from another laboratory, where a recombinant vaccinia virus expressing MUC1 was shown to offer protection to preimmunized rats when challenged with tumor cells expressing MUC1 (Hareuveni et al., 1990).

The major limitation of the above studies is that the tumor antigen expressed is human, and therefore the immune responses against it might be greater than expected from a homologous mouse molecule. Mouse MUC1 has only 34% homology with the human MUC1 in the tandem repeat region (Spicer *et al.,* 1991). A recently developed transgenic mouse model (Peat *et al.,* 1992), expressing human MUC1 in a manner similar to its distribution in normal human tissues, offers a better animal model for further evaluation of the immune responses to the cancer-associated exposed epitopes, since the model would simulate the self-tolerance against the epitopes exposed by the normal cells. This transgenic mouse carrying a syngeneic mouse mammary carcinoma transfected with human MUC1, and expressing it with cancer-associated changes, would provide the most relevant model to simulate the clinical condition of human breast cancer.

7. PHARMACEUTICAL FORMULATION OF ASI AGENTS

Since peptides and glycopeptides by themselves are poor immunogens, ASI formulations based on them should be prepared by their incorporation into immunostimulatory antigen delivery vehicles or by use of adjuvants. Currently there is an increased interest in the development of chemically defined antigen delivery systems suitable for recombinant proteins and synthetic peptides. For the development of anticancer ASI formulations, delivery systems that can induce CTLs in vivo, by antigen delivery to cytoplasm for presentation by MHC class I pathway, are of special interest. Similarly, formulations that can influence the balance of T-helper responses toward a dominant Th1 type would also be of advantage. Antigen delivery systems reported to be effective for targeting antigens for MHC class I presentation such as QS-21 (Newman *et al.,* 1992), tripalmitoyl-*S*-glycerylcysteine (P3C) moiety (Deres *et al.,* 1989), and liposomes containing monophosphoryl lipid A (White *et al.,* 1993) would be expected to be useful for the development of anticancer ASI formulations. However, since the type of immune responses are also influenced by the physicochemical nature of the antigens as much as delivery systems, each formulation should be optimized for the most effective responses.

8. SUMMARY

As a result of aberrant glycosylation, cancer-associated mucins expose to the immune system certain carbohydrate, peptide, and possibly glycopeptide epitopes that are not exposed on the normal mucins. This provides the basis for our development of synthetic carbohydrate, peptide, and glycopeptide-based ASI agents corresponding to the cancer-associated mucin epitopes. Our studies on ASI formulations based on carbohydrate structures such as TF and STn have demonstrated their ability to induce immune response relevant to the native epitopes on the cancer cells in animal models and in cancer patients. Further, such immune responses were able to mediate cancer rejection in an animal model. Similar studies on peptide epitopes of a cancer-associated mucin, MUC1, have also shown the ability of the synthetic antigen to induce anticancer immune responses in an animal model. Ongoing studies on the carbohydrate and peptide epitopes would allow us to define the most important target structures on cancer-associated mucins that can selectively stimulate cancer-specific immune responses. Our long-term goal is to develop multiepitopic gly-copeptide ASI formulations capable of stimulating strong CMI responses against common carcinomas.

REFERENCES

Anichini, A., Fossati, G., and Parmiani, G., 1986, Heterogeneity of clones from human metastatic melanoma detected by autologous cytotoxic T lymphocyte clones, *J. Exp. Med.* **163**:215–220.

Bobek, L. A., Tsai, H., Biesbrock, A. R., and Levine, M. J., 1993, Molecular cloning, sequence, and specificity of expression of the gene encoding the low molecular weight human salivary mucin, *J. Biol. Chem.* **268**:20563–20569.

Boon, T., 1993, Teaching the immune system to fight cancer, *Sci. Am.* **266**:82–89.

Boon, T., De Plaen, E., Larquin, C., Van den Eynde, B., van der Bruggen, P., Traversari, C., Amar-Costesec, A., and Van Pel, A., 1992, Identification of tumour rejection antigens recognized by T lymphocytes, in: *A New Look at Tumor Immunology* (A. J. McMichael and W. F. Bodmer, eds.), Cold Spring Harbor Laboratory Press, Cold Spring Harbor, NY, pp. 23–37.

Botarelli, P., Houlden, B., Haigwood, N., Seevis, C., Montagna, D., and Abrignani, S., 1991, N-Glycosylation of HIV-gp120 may constrain recognition by T lymphocytes, *J. Immunol.* **147**:3128–3132.

Brand, D. L., Lan, M. S., Metzgar, R. S., and Finn, O. J., 1989, Specific, MHC-unrestricted recognition of tumor-associated mucins by human cytotoxic T cells, *Proc. Natl. Acad. Sci. USA* **86**:7159–7164.

Burchell, J., and Taylor-Papadimitriou, J., 1993, Effect of modification of carbohydrate side chains on the reactivity of antibodies with core protein epitopes of the MUC1 gene product, *Epithelial Cell Biol.* **2**:155–162.

Burchell, J., Gendler, S., Taylor-Papadimitriou, J., Girling, A., Lewis, A., Millis, R., and Lamport, D., 1987, Development and characterization of breast cancer reactive monoclonal antibodies directed to the core protein of the human milk mucin, *Cancer Res.* **47**:5476–5482.

Capon, C., Laboisse, C., Wieruszeski, J. M., Maoret, J. J., Augeron, C., and Fournet, B., 1992, Oligosaccharide structures of mucins secreted by human colonic cancer cell line CL. 16E, *J. Biol. Chem.* **267**:19248–19257.

Clerici, M., and Shearer, G. M., 1993, A Th1→Th2 switch is a critical step in the etiology of HIV infection, *Immunol. Today* **14**:107–111.

Coon, J. S., Weinstein, R. S., and Summers, J. L., 1982, Blood group precursor T-antigen expression in human urinary bladder carcinoma, *Am. J. Clin. Pathol.* **77**:692–699.

Crowley, N. J., Darrow T. L., Quinn-Allen, M. A., and Siegler, H. F., 1991, MHC-restricted recognition of autologous melanoma by tumor-specific cytotoxic T lymphocytes: Evidence for recognition by a dominant HLA-A allele, *J. Immunol.* **146**:1692–1699.

Degiovanni, G., Hainaut, P., Lehaye, T., Weynauts, P., and Boon, T., 1990, Antigen recognized on melanoma cell line by autologous cytotoxic T lymphocytes are also expressed on freshly collected tumor cells, *Eur. J. Immunol.* **18**:671–676.

Deres, K., Schild, H., Weismuller, K.-H., Jung, G., and Rammensee, H.-G., 1989, In vivo priming of virus-specific cytotoxic T lymphocytes with synthetic lipopeptide vaccine, *Nature* **342**:561–564.

Devine, P. L., and McKenzie, I. F. C., 1992, Mucins: Structure, function, and associations with malignancy, *BioEssays* **14**:619–625.

Devine, P. L., Warren, J. A., Ward, B. G., McKenzie, I. F. C., and Layton, G. T., 1990, Glycosylation and exposure of tumor-associated epitopes on mucins, *J. Tumor Marker Oncol.* **5**:11–26.

Ding, L., Lalani, E.-N., Reddish, M., Koganty, R., Wong, T., Samuel, J., Yacyshyn, M. B., Taylor-Papadimitriou, J., and Longenecker, B. M., 1993, Immunogenicity of synthetic peptides related to the core-peptide sequence encoded by the human MUC1 mucin gene: Effect of immunization on the growth of murine mammary adenocarcinoma cells tansfected with the human MUC1 gene, *Cancer Immunol. Immunother.* **36**:9–17.

Drummer, H. E., Jackson, D. C., and Brown, L. E., 1993, Modulation of CD4⁺ T-cell recognition of hemagglutination by carbohydrate side chains located outside a T-cell determinant, *Virology* **192**:282–289.

Fearon, E. R., Pardoll, D. M., Itaya, T., Golumber, P., Levitsky, H., Simons, J. W., Karasuyama, H., Vogelstein, B., and Frost, P., 1990, Interleukin-2 production by tumor cells bypass T helper function in the generation of anti-tumor response, *Cell* **60**:397–403.

Fenton, R. G., Taub, D. D., Kwak, L. W., Smith, M. R., and Longo, D. L., 1993, Cytotoxic T cell response and in vivo protection against tumor cells in harboring activated ras proto-oncogenes, *J. Natl. Cancer Inst.* **85**:1294–1302.

Ferrini, S., Biassoni, R., Moretta, A., Bruzzone, M., Nicolin, A., and Moretta, L., 1985, Clonal analysis of T lymphocytes isolated from ovarian carcinoma ascitic fluid: Phenotype and functional characterization of T-cell clones capable of lysing autologous carcinoma cells, *Int. J. Cancer* **36**:337–343.

Fisch, P., Weil-Hilman, G., Uppenskimp, M., Hank, J., Chen, B., Sosman, J., Bridges, A., Colamonici, O., and Sondel, P., 1989, Antigen-specific recognition of autologous leukemia cells and allogenic class-I MHC antigens by IL-2 activated cytotoxic T cells from a patient with acute T-cell leukemia, *Blood* **74**:343–353.

Fitch, F. W., Mckisic, M. D., Lanchi, D. W., and Gajewski, T. F., 1993, Differential regulation of murine T lymphocyte subsets, *Annu. Rev. Immunol.* **11**:29–48.

Fung, P. Y. S., Madej, M., Koganty, R., and Longenecker, B. M., 1990, Active specific immunotherapy of a murine mammary adenocarcinoma using a synthetic tumor-associated glycoconjugate, *Cancer Res.* **50**:4308–4314.

Furukawa, K. S., Furukawa, K., Real, F. X., Old, L. J., and Loyd, K. O., 1989, A unique antigenic epitope of human melanoma is carried on the common melanoma glycoprotein gp95/p97, *J. Exp. Med.* **169**:585–590.

Gendler, S. J., Lancaster, C. A., Taylor-Papadimitriou, J., Duhig, T., Peat, N., Burchell, J., Pemberton, L., Lalani, E.-N., and Wilson, D., 1990, Molecular cloning and expression of human tumor-associated polymorphic epithelial mucin, *J. Biol. Chem.* **265**:15286–15293.

Girling, A., Bartkova, J., Burchell, J., Gendler, S., Gillet, C., and Taylor-Papadimitriou, J., 1989, A core epitope of the polymorphic epithelial mucin detected by the monoclonal antibody SM-3 is selectively exposed in a range of primary carcinomas, *Int. J. Cancer* **43**:1072–1076.

Gum, J. R., Byrd, J. C., Hicks, J. W., Toribara, N. W., Lamport, D. T. A., and Kim, Y. S., 1989, Molecular cloning of human intestinal mucin cDNAs. Sequence analysis and evidence for genetic polymorphism, *J. Biol. Chem.* **264**:6480–6487.

Gum, J. R., Hicks, J. W., Swallow, D. M., Lagase, R. L., Byrd, J. C., Lamport, D. T. A., Siddiki, B., and Kim, Y. S., 1990, Molecular cloning of cDNAs derived from a novel human intestinal mucin gene, *Biochem. Biophys. Res. Commun.* **171**:407–415.

Hakamori, S., 1989, Aberrant glycosylation in tumors and tumor-associated carbohydrate antigens, *Adv. Cancer Res.* **52**:257–331.

Hanisch, F.-G., Uhlenbruck, G., Peter-Katalinic, J., Egge, H., Dabrowski, J., and Dabrowski, U., 1989a, Structure of neutral and O-linked polylactosaminoglycans on human skim milk mucins, *J. Biol. Chem.* **264**:872–883.

Hanisch, F.-G., Uhlenbruck, G., Egge, H., and Peter-Katalinic, J., 1989b, A B72.3 second generation-monoclonal antibody (CC49) defined the mucin-carried carbohydrate epitope Galβ(1-3){NeuAc(2-6)Gal-Nac}, *Biol. Chem. Hoppe Seyler* **370**:21–26.

Hareuveni, M., Gautier, C., Kieny, M. P., Wreschner, D., Chambon, P., and Lathe, R., 1990, Vaccination against tumor cells expressing breast cancer epithelial tumor antigen, *Proc. Natl. Acad. Sci. USA* **87**:9498–9502.

Hewit, H., Blake, E. R., and Walder, A. S., 1976, A critique of the evidence for active host defence against cancer based on personal studies of 27 murine tumors of spontaneous origin, *Br. J. Cancer* **33**:241–259.

Hull, S. R., Bright, A., Carraway, K. L., Abe, M., Hayes, D. F., and Kufe, D. W., 1989, Oligosaccharide differences in DF3 sialomucin antigen from normal human milk and BT-20 human breast carcinoma cell line, *Cancer Commun.* **1**:261–267.

Ionnides, C. G., Fisk, B., Jerome, K. R., Irimura, T., Wharton, J. T., and Finn, O. J., 1993, Cytotoxic T cells from ovarian malignant tumors can recognize polymorphic epithelial mucin core peptides, *J. Immunol.* **151**:3693–3703.

Itzkowitz, S. H., Yuan, M., Montgomery, C. K., Kjelsein, T., Takahashi, H. K., Bigbee, W. L., and Kim, Y. S., 1989, Expression of Tn, sialosyl-Tn, and T antigens in human colon cancer, *Cancer Res.* **49**:197–204.

Itzkowitz, S. H., Bloom, E. J., Kokal, W. A., Modin, G., Hakamori, S.-I., and Kim, Y. S., 1990, Sialosyl-Tn: A novel mucin antigen associated with prognosis in colorectal cancer patients, *Cancer* **66**:1960–1966.

Jerome, K. R., Brand, D. L., Bendt, K. M., Boyer, C. M., Taylor-Papadimitriou, J., McKenzie, I. F. C., Bast, R. C., Jr., and Finn, O.J., 1991, Cytotoxic T lymphocytes derived from patients with breast adenocarcinoma recognize an epitope present on the protein core of a mucin molecule preferentially expressed by malignant cells, *Cancer Res.* **51**:2908–2916.

Jerome, K. R., Domenech, N., and Finn, O. J., 1993, Tumor-specific cytotoxic T cell clones from patients with breast and pancreatic adenocarcinoma recognize EBV-immortalized B cells transfected with polymorphic epithelial mucin complementary DNA, *J. Immunol.* **151**:1654–1662.

Jung, S., and Schluesener, H. J., 1991, Human T lymphocytes recognize a peptide of single point-mutated, oncogenic ras proteins, *J. Exp. Med.* **173**:273–276.

Kan-Mitchell, J., Huang, X.-Q., Steinman, L., Oksenberg, J. R., Harel, W., Parker, J. W., Goedegebuure, P. S., Darrow, T. L., and Mitchell, M. S., 1993, Clonal analysis of in vivo activated CD8$^+$ cytotoxic T lymphocytes from melanoma patient responsive to active specific immunotherapy, *Cancer Immunol. Immunother.* **37**:15–25.

Khera, K. S., Ashkenazi, A., Rapp, F., and Melnick, J. F., 1963, Immunity in hamsters to cells transformed in vitro among the papavo viruses, *J. Immunol.* **91**:604–613.

Klein, G., and Klein, E., 1964, Antigenic properties of lymphomas induced by Moloney agent, *J. Natl. Cancer Inst.* **32**:547–568.

Klein, G., Sjogren, H. O., Klein, E., and Hellstrom, K. E., 1960, Demonstration of resistance against methylcholanthrene-induced sarcomas in primary autochthonous host, *Cancer Res.* **20**:1561–1576.

Knuth, A., Wolfel, T., and Meyer Zum Buschenfelde, K.-H., 1992, T cell responses to human malignant tumors, in: *A New Look at Tumor Immunology* (A. J. McMichael and W. F. Bodmer, eds.), Cold Spring Harbor Laboratory Press, Cold Spring Harbor, NY, pp. 39–52.

Kobayashi, H., Toshihiko, T., and Kawashima, Y., 1992, Serum sialyl Tn as an independent predictor of poor prognosis in patients with epithelial ovarian cancer, *Clin. Oncol.* **10**:95–101.

Lalani, E.-N., Bedichevsky, F., Boshell, M., Shearer, M., Wilson, D., Stauss, H., Gendler, S. J., and Taylor-Papadimitriou, J., 1991, Expression of the gene coding for a human mucin in mouse mammary tumor cell can affect their tumorigenicity, *J. Biol. Chem.* **266**:15420–15426.

Lan, M. S., Hollingsworth, M. A., and Metzgar, R. S., 1990, Polypeptide core of a human pancreatic tumor mucin antigen, *Cancer Res.* **50**:2997–3001.

Leathem, A. J., and Brooks, S. A., 1987, Predictive value of lectin binding on breast cancer recurrence and survival, *Lancet* **1**:1054–1056.

LeMay, L. G., Kan-Mitchell, J., Goedegebuure, P., Harel, W., and Mitchell, M. S., 1993, Detection of melanoma-reactive CD4$^+$ HLA-class I-restricted cytotoxic T cell clones with long-term assay and pretreatment of targets with interferon-γ, *Cancer Immunol. Immunother.* **37**:187–194.

Litenberg, M. J. L., Vos, H. L., Gennisen, A. M. C., and Hilkens, J., 1990, Episialin, a carcinoma-associated mucin, is generated by a polymorphic gene encoding splice variants with alternate amino termini, *J. Biol. Chem.* **265**:5573–5578.

Livingston, P. O., 1993, Approaches to augmenting the IgG antibody response to melanoma ganglioside vaccines, *Ann. N.Y. Acad. Sci.* **690**:204–213.

Livingston, P. O., Natoli, E. J., Jr., Calves, M. J., Stockert, E., Oettgen, H. F., and Old, L. J., 1987, Vaccines containing purified GM2 ganglioside elicit GM2 antibodies in melanoma patients, *Proc. Natl. Acad. Sci. USA* **84**:2911–2915.

Locksley, R. M., and Scott, P., 1991, Helper T cell subsets in leishmaniasis: Induction, expansion and effector functions, *Immunol. Today* **12**:A58–A61.

Longenecker, B. M., and MacLean, G. D., 1993, Prospects for mucin epitopes in cancer vaccines, *Immunologist* **1**:89–93.

Longenecker, B. M., Reddish, M., Koganty, R., and MacLean, G. D., 1993, Immune responses of mice and human breast cancer patients following immunization with synthetic sialyl-Tn conjugated to KLH plus Detox adjuvant, *Ann. N.Y. Acad. Sci.* **690**:276–291.

MacLean, G. D., and Longenecker, B. M., 1991, Clinical significance of the Thomsen–Friedenreich antigen, *Semin. Cancer Biol.* **2**:431–440.

MacLean, G. D., Bowen-Yacyshyn, M. B., Samuel, J., Meikle, A., Stuart, G., Nation, J., Poppema, S., Jerry, M., Koganty, R., Wong, T., and Longenecker, B. M., 1992, Active immunization of breast cancer patients against a common carcinoma (Thomsen–Friedenreich) determinant using a synthetic carbo-hydrate antigen, *J. Immunother.* **11**:292–305.

MacLean, G. D., Reddish, M. A., Koganty, R. R., Wong, T., Gandhi, S., Smolenski, M., Samuel, J., Naholtz, J. M., and Longenecker, B. M., 1993, Immunization of breast cancer patients using a synthetic sialyl-Tn glycoconjugate plus DETOX[TM] adjuvant, *Cancer Immunol. Immunother.* **36**:215–222.

McMichael, A. J., and Bodmer, W. F. (eds.), 1992, *A New Look at Tumor Immunology*, Cold Spring Harbor Laboratory Press, Cold Spring Harbor, NY.

Melief, C. J. M., 1992, Tumor eradication by adoptive transfer of cytotoxic T lymphocytes, *Adv. Cancer Res.* **58**:143–175.

Middle, J., and Embleton, M., 1981, Naturally arising tumors of inbred WAB/Notrat strain II. Immuno-genicity of transplanted tumors, *J. Natl. Cancer Inst.* **67**:637–643.

Mitchell, M. S., Harel, W., Kan-Mitchell, J., LeMay, L. G., Goedegeburre, P., Huang, X. Q., Hofman, F., and Gorshen, S., 1993, Active specific immunotherapy of melanoma with allogeneic cell lysates. Rationale, results, and possible mechanisms of action, *Ann. N.Y. Acad. Sci.* **690**:153–166.

Mosmann, T. R., and Coffman, R. L., 1989, TH1 and TH2 cells: Different pattern of lymphokine secretion lead to different functional properties, *Annu. Rev. Immunol.* **7**:145–173.

Nagarkatti, M., Clary, S. R., and Nagarkatti, P. S., 1990, Characterization of tumor-infiltrating CD4[+] T cells as Th1 cells based on lymphokine secretion and functional properties, *J. Immunol.* **144**:4898–4906.

Newman, M. J., Wu, J.-Y., Gardner, H., Munroe, K. J., Leombruno, D., Recchia, J., Kensil, C. R., and Coughlin, R. T., 1992, Saponin adjuvant induction of ovalbumin-specific CD8[+] cytotoxic T lymphocyte responses, *J. Immunol.* **148**:2357–2362.

Old, L. J., 1981, Cancer immunology: The search for specificity—GHA Clowes Memorial Lecture, *Cancer Res.* **41**:361–375.

Pardoll, D. M., 1993, Cancer vaccines, *Immunol. Today* **14**:310–316.

Peat, N., Gendler, S. J., Lalani, E.-N., Duhig, T., and Taylor-Papadimitriou, J., 1992, Tissue-specific expression of a human polymorphic epithelial mucin (MUC1) in transgenic mice, *Cancer Res.* **52**:1954–1960.

Porchet, N., Nguyen, V. C., Dufosse, J., Audre, J. P., Guyonnet-Duperat, V., Gross, M. S., Denis, C., Degand, P., Bernheim, A., and Aubert, J. P., 1991, Molecular cloning and chromosomal location of tracheo-bron-cheal mucin cDNA containing tandemly repeated sequences of 48 base pairs, *Biochem. Biophys. Res. Commun.* **175**:414–422.

Prehan, R. T., and Main, M. J., 1957, Immunity to methylcholanthrene-induced sarcomas, *J. Natl. Cancer Inst.* **18**:769–778.

Romagnani, S., 1991, Human TH1 and TH2 subsets; doubt no more, *Immunol. Today* **12**:256–257.

Ryghetti, A., Turchi, V., Ghetti, C. A., Scambia, G., Panici, P. B., Roncucci, G., Mancuso, S., Frati, L., and Nuti, M., 1993, Human B cell immune response to the polymorphic epithelial mucin, *Cancer Res.* **53**:2457–2459.

Samuel, J., Noujaim, A. A., MacLean, G. D., Suresh, M. R., and Longenecker, B. M., 1990, Analysis of human tumor-associated Thomsen–Friedenreich antigen, *Cancer Res.* **50**:4801–4808.

Sato, T., Sato, N., Takahashi, S., Koshiba, H., and Kikuchi, K., 1986, Specific cytotoxicity of a long-term cultured T-cell clone on human autologous mammary cancer cells, *Cancer Res.* **46**:4384–4389.

Schachter, H., and Brockhausen, I., 1989, The biosynthesis of branched O-glycans, in: *Mucus and Related Topics* (E. Chantler and N. A. Ratcliff, eds.), The Company of Biologists Ltd., Cambridge, pp. 1–26.

Singhal, A., and Hakamori, S., 1990, Molecular changes in carbohydrate antigens associated with cancer, *BioEssays* **12**:223–230.

Singhal, A., Fohn, M., and Hakamori, S.-I., 1991, Induction of α-N-acetylgalactosamine-O-serine/threonine (Tn) antigen-mediated cellular immune response for active immunotherapy in mice, *Cancer Res.* **51**:1406–1411.

Solvin, S. F., Lackman, R. D., Ferrone, S., Kiely, P. E., and Mastrangelo, M. J., 1986, Cellular immune response to human sarcomas: Cytotoxic T cell clones reactive with autologous sarcomas I. Development, phenotype and specificity, *J. Immunol.* **137**:3042–3048.

Spicer, A. P., Parry, G., Patton, S., and Gendler, S. J., 1991, Molecular cloning and analysis of the mouse homologue of the tumor-associated mucin, MUC1, reveals conservation of potential O-glycosylation sites, transmembrane, and cytoplasmic domains and loss of minisatellite-like polymorphism, *J. Biol. Chem.* **266**:15099–15109.

Springer, G. F., 1984, T and Tn, general carcinoma auto antigens, *Science* **224**:1198–1206.

Strous, G. J., and Dekker, J., 1992, Mucin-type glycoproteins, *Crit. Rev. Biochem. Mol. Biol.* 57–92.

Thomas, D. B., Hodgson, J., Riska, J. F., and Graham, C. M., 1990, The role of endoplasmic reticulum in antigen processing. N-glycosylation of influenza hemagglutinin abrogates CD4[+] cytotoxic T cell recognition of endogenously processed antigen, *J. Immunol.* **144**:2789–2794.

Urban, J. L., and Schreiber, H., 1992, Tumor antigens, *Annu. Rev. Immunol.* **10**:617–644.

Van den Eijnden, D. H., Evans, N. A., Codington, J. F., Reinhold, V., Silber, C., and Jeanloz, R. W., 1979, Chemical structure of epiglycanin, the major glycoprotein of the TA3-Ha ascites cell, *J. Biol. Chem.* **254**:12153–12159.

White, K., Krzych, U., Gordon, G. M., Porter, T. G., Richards, R. L., Alving, C. R., Deal, C. D., Hollingdale, M., Silverman, C., Selvester, D. R., Ballou, W. R., and Gross, M., 1993, Induction of cytolytic and antibody responses using Plasmodium falciparum repeatless circumsporozoite protein encapsulated in liposomes, *Vaccine* **11**:1341–1346.

Wolf, M. F., Ludwig, A., Fritz, P., and Schumacher, K., 1988, Increased expression of Thomsen–Freidenreich (T) antigen during tumor progression in breast cancer patients, *Tumor Biol.* **9**:190–194.

Wreshner, D. H., Haraveuni, M., Tsarfaty, I., Smorodinsky, N., Horev, J., Zaretsky, J., Kotkes, P., Weiss, M., Lathe, R., Dion, A., and Keydar, I., 1990, Human epithelial tumor antigen cDNA sequences , differential splicing may generate multiple protein forms, *Eur. J. Biochem.* **189**:463–473.

Xing, P.-X., Prenzoska, J., Quelch, K., and McKenzie, I. F. C., 1992, Second generation anti-MUC1 peptide monoclonal antibodies, *Cancer Res.* **52**:2310–2317.

Yssel, H., Spits, H., and de Vries, J., 1984, A cloned human T cell line cytotoxic for autologous and allogeneic B lymphoma cells, *J. Exp. Med.* **160**:239–254.

Zotter, S., Hageman, P. C., Lossnitzer, A., Mooi, W. J., and Hilgers, J., 1988, Tissue and tumor distribution of human polymorphic epithelial mucin, *Cancer Rev.* **11**:55–101.

Chapter 40

Synthetic Peptide Vaccines for Schistosomiasis

Donald A. Harn, Sandra R. Reynolds,
Silas Chikunguwo, Steve Furlong, and
Charles Dahl

1. BACKGROUND

Schistosomiasis is a chronic disease that infects an estimated 200 million persons, leading to an estimated 800,000 to 1 million annual deaths. It ranks second only to malaria in terms of morbidity and mortality caused by a parasitic disease. In addition, there is increasing evidence that schistosome infection may have profound effects on growth in children (de Lima e Costa *et al.*, 1988; Corbett *et al.*, 1992; McGarvey *et al.*, 1993). Three species of schistosomes account for the vast majority of human infection: *Schistosoma mansoni*, found in South America, the Caribbean, Africa, and the Middle East; *S. haematobium*, found in Africa and the Middle East; and *S. japonica*, found in Asia and Southeast Asia. In addition, there are other species of schistosomes that infect humans with varying degrees of success such as *S. intercalatum* and *S. mekongi*. Disease is caused by the host immune response to parasite eggs that become trapped in tissues, forming granulomas. Granulomatous responses then lead to the development of fibrotic lesions, which in turn lead to portal hypertension, shunting, and esophageal varices. One or more of these serious disease manifestations are found in *S. japonicum*- and *mansoni*-infected patients who have developed hepatosplenic disease.

Donald A. Harn • Department of Tropical Public Health, Harvard School of Public Health, and Department of Rheumatology and Immunology, Harvard Medical School, Boston, Massachusetts 02115. *Sandra R. Reynolds and Silas Chikunguwo* • Department of Tropical Public Health, Harvard School of Public Health, Boston, Massachusetts 02115. *Steve Furlong* • Department of Rheumatology and Immunology, Harvard Medical School, Boston, Massachusetts 02115. *Charles Dahl* • Department of Biological Chemistry and Molecular Pharmacology, Harvard Medical School, Boston, Massachusetts 02115.

Vaccine Design: The Subunit and Adjuvant Approach, edited by Michael F. Powell and Mark J. Newman. Plenum Press, New York, 1995.

Fortunately, pharmacologic intervention using praziquantel or oxamniquine effectively eliminates egg-laying adult worms. However, reinfection within 1 to 2 years posttreatment occurs in a substantial portion of the population. Therefore, control of morbidity and mortality related to schistosome infection via drug therapy requires continued surveillance of the population to monitor reinfection, and necessitates intermittent drug therapy. Control of schistosomiasis via drug therapy is, therefore, long term (perpetual) and expensive. An inexpensive alternative to drug therapy is the development of an effective and safe vaccine.

The feasibility that a vaccine can be developed to protect against infection with schistosomes has hinged until recently on studies in experimental rodent (mouse and rat) models that demonstrate immune-dependent elimination of challenge organisms in previously vaccinated animals (Doenhoff and Long, 1979; Hsu *et al.*, 1981; Sher *et al.*, 1982; Ford *et al.*, 1984; James, 1987). However, sterilizing immunity in experimental rodent models has not been demonstrated. The highest levels of protective immunity in experimental animal models have been achieved via vaccination with radiation-attenuated infective larval stage (cercariae) (Reynolds and Harn, 1992). When comparing mean numbers of challenge parasites maturing to adult worms among control and vaccinated groups, mice previously vaccinated with radiation-attenuated cercariae have from 40 to 90% fewer adult worms than sham or nonimmunized controls (Reynolds and Harn, 1992); reduction of up to 90% of challenge worm burdens was achieved in mice that were vaccinated four times with irradiated cercariae (Reynolds and Harn, 1992).

In addition to experimental murine schistosomiasis, there is now solid evidence that in endemic sites, there exist resistant and susceptible individuals, and that the development of resistance is age-dependent, occurring predominantly in individuals over 15 years of age (Butterworth *et al.*, 1985). Further, there appear to be a number of immunological correlates associated with the resistant population, specifically the ratios of different immunoglobulin isotypes to peptide or carbohydrate epitopes on parasite antigens (Dessein *et al.*, 1988; Hagan *et al.*, 1991; Rihet *et al.*, 1991, 1992). Thus, it is likely that age-dependent generation of parasiticidal immunological mediators is at least partly responsible for the development of resistance in humans.

2. TARGETS OF IMMUNE RESPONSE

Schistosomes are helminth parasites belonging to the class Trematoda (flukes). Schistosomes have a digenetic life cycle; sexual reproduction occurs in vertebrate hosts and asexual reproduction occurs in invertebrate hosts. The schistosome life cycle is complex in that it presents to the human host five distinct life cycle forms (Fig. 1). Free-swimming infective larvae, cercariae, penetrate mammalian hosts directly, through the skin. The parasite undergoes a dramatic transformation to a schistosomula. This transformation includes many morphological changes such as loss of tail and glycocalyx and generation of a syncytial heptalaminate surface membrane structure. The newly transformed schistosomula migrates via the blood-vascular system to the lungs within 3 to 7 days postinfection, where the larval stage becomes elongated into lung worms. The developing parasites exit the lungs within 10–21 days postinfection via the blood-vascular system and migrate to the liver, where they mature to adult male and female worms. Four

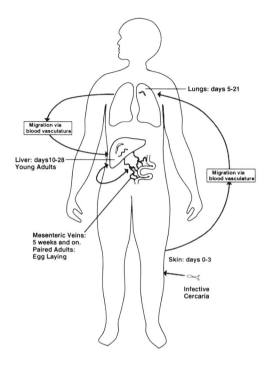

Figure 1. Schistosome life cycle.

to five weeks postinfection, male and female parasites pair, and in the case of *S. mansoni* and *S. japonicum*, move to the mesenteric veins.

Thus, invading parasites are present in the skin, the blood-vascular system of the lungs, the blood-vascular system of the liver, and as adults reside in the blood-vascular system. What stages appear to be most amenable to immune-mediated attack? A number of studies in vivo and in vitro have shown that the skin-, lung-, post-lung-, and pre-liver-stage schistosomula are the targets of immune elimination (Mangold and Dean, 1984). Further, these stages are eliminated in vivo by cellular responses as well as by passive transfer of antibody (Mangold and Dean, 1986; Jwo and LoVerde, 1989; Richter *et al.*, 1993). Mechanisms of resistance in mice vaccinated with irradiated cercariae have been shown to require functional T- and B-cell compartments for the development of resistance (Sher *et al.*, 1982).

3. SELECTION OF CANDIDATE VACCINE ANTIGENS

Several candidate vaccine immunogens have been selected using murine monoclonal antibodies or experimentally infected/vaccinated animal sera as probes (Balloul *et al.*, 1987; Pearce *et al.*, 1988; Harn *et al.*, 1985a,b; Dalton and Strand, 1987; Lanar *et al.*, 1986) (Table I). Two such candidates were initially described by our laboratory (Harn *et al.*, 1985 a,b), the integral membrane protein Sm23 and the glycolytic enzyme triose phosphate

Table I
Candidate Antigens for a Defined Vaccine against Schistosomiasis

Antigen	Mass (kDa)	Stage specificity	Rec/peptide	Adjuvant[a]	Protection (range)[b]
IrV-5	62	Larval/adult	Bacterial recombinant	Proteosomes	32–70%
Sm28	28	"	"	Alum, FA	30–40%
Paramyosin	97	"	"	BCG	30%
TPI	28	All stages	Synthetic peptide	Alum/liposomes	41–82%
Sm23	23	"	"	Alum	36–75%
Sm14	14	Larval	Bacterial recombinant	None	40–65%

[a]Alum, aluminum hydroxide; FA, Freund's adjuvant.
[b]Protection against cercarial challenge in vaccinated mice as compared to adjuvant only or sham-immunized controls. Range equals the mean percent reduction in number of adult worms per group of the vaccinated group compared to control group of mice. In the majority of experiments, $n > 20$.

isomerase (TPI). Both of these proteins have now been expressed in full-length or truncated recombinant forms in bacterial and mammalian expression systems (Shoemaker *et al.*, 1992; Reynolds *et al.*, 1992). In addition, full-length TPI has been expressed in bacillus Calmette–Guérin (BCG) (Reynolds *et al.*, 1995), which is itself a geo-vaccine in addition to being a potent adjuvant.

Our approach for selecting putative protective immunogens was to prepare monoclonal antibodies from mice that had been immunized with a membrane-enriched extract of schistosomula, a larval stage that is a target of the immune response in vitro and in vivo (Harn *et al.*, 1985a,b). Monoclonal antibodies were then screened for binding to the surface membranes of living schistosomula, and those that were positive were then tested for protective efficacy in vivo utilizing passive transfer experiments (Harn *et al.*, 1987, 1992). Two monoclonal antibodies recognizing distinct schistosomula proteins of 23 and 28 kDa were found to bind to the surface membranes of schistosomula and to partially protect against cercarial challenge in vivo (Harn *et al.*, 1985a,b, 1987, 1992).

Sequencing of tryptic peptides obtained from purified native antigens revealed that the 28-kDa antigen was the schistosome homologue of TPI (Harn *et al.*, 1992; Shoemaker *et al.*, 1992), and that the 23-kDa antigen was a structural homologue of a family of mammalian integral membrane proteins including TAPA-1 and Me491 (Reynolds *et al.*, 1992), which was originally cloned for *S. japonicum* by Wright *et al.* (1990). Consensus conserved sequence oligonucleotide probes were constructed and both proteins were produced and expressed as bacterial recombinant proteins (Shoemaker *et al.*, 1992; Reynolds *et al.*, 1992); in addition, full-length Sm23 was also expressed in Cos and CHO cells (Reynolds *et al.*, 1992). The sequences of each recombinant protein were then determined and utilized for construction of synthetic peptides.

3.1. Selection of B- and T-Cell Peptide Epitopes for Sm23 and TPI

Schistosome TPI shares 50% sequence homology with analogous human enzyme, while 25% of the molecule is composed of schistosome-specific residues (Shoemaker *et al.*, 1992). Thus, the potential for generating autoimmunity with this particular immunogen was high if the entire molecule were to be used. Fortunately, the majority of schistosome-specific residues are clustered so that there are considerably long spans with minimal or no homology to the human enzyme (Shoemaker *et al.*, 1992). We therefore decided to produce a synthetic peptide-based vaccine for TPI using exclusively, or largely, schistosome-specific regions of the molecule. We performed identical studies on Sm23 simultaneously with the work on defining immunoreactive portions of TPI (Reynolds *et al.*, 1992). We focused on defining both T- and B- cell epitopes for Sm23 and TPI to maximize immunogenicity of subsequently produced vaccines. Further, to avoid possible problems with the response to individual epitopes being genetically restricted, we mapped the T- and B-cell epitopes using antibodies and lymphocytes from three different mouse strains differing in H-2: C57BL/6J, CBA/J, and BALB/c.

To map B-cell epitopes we utilized sera from chronically infected mice as well as from mice vaccinated with irradiated cercariae (Reynolds *et al.*, 1992, 1994). For both Sm23 and TPI, T-cell epitopes were mapped using lymphocytes from mice vaccinated with irradiated cercariae (Reynolds *et al.*, 1992). For TPI, Th1-type CD4$^+$ T-cell clones from C57BL/6J and CBA/J mice were also used (Reynolds *et al.*, 1994). Initial experiments on mapping immunoreactive portions of TPI utilized tryptic fragments of full-length rec TPI (Reynolds *et al.*, 1994). The immunoreactive fragments were further defined via the construction of synthetic peptide epitopes relevant to these tryptic fragments, and keeping in mind the blocks of schistosome-specific residues (Shoemaker *et al.*, 1992) (Fig. 2). For Sm23, a series of overlapping synthetic peptides were constructed such that the areas of both the large and small hydrophilic domains were covered (Reynolds *et al.*, 1992) (Fig. 2).

For both antibody and T-cell epitopes, we defined synthetic peptide epitopes of Sm23 and TPI that were genetically restricted for one or more of the three mouse strains (Reynolds *et al.*, 1992, 1994). However, there were also consensus peptides that were recognized by antibody and T cells of all three mouse strains and thus represented putative genetically nonrestricted epitopes for Sm23 and TPI (Reynolds *et al.*, 1992, 1994). Based on the observations of Tam *et al.* (1990) who showed that tetrameric MAPs induced optimal responsiveness, the genetically nonrestricted epitopes for TPI were then constructed into three different tetrameric MAPs using Fmoc technology (Fig. 3). The TPI-MAPs were numbered 1, 2, and 4. MAPs 1 and 2 were composed of identical two peptides, P9 and P18 (Fig. 3), differing only in the order of synthesis of the peptides (MAP1 P18-P9, MAP2 P9-P18). P9 was the T-cell epitope defined by CBA/J cells and P18 by C57BL/6J cells. MAPs 1 and 2 were then tested to see if they were immunoreactive with CBA/J and C57BL/6J T-cell clones. CBA/J T clone T9 was stimulated by MAP1 and to a lesser degree MAP2. Surprisingly, and in contrast to T-cell clone T9, the C57BL/6J clone T44 failed to respond to either MAP1 or MAP2. Thus, even though P18 was the most stimulatory peptide for C57BL/6J T-cell clone T44, once it was incorporated into MAP1 or MAP2, T clone T44 failed to respond. This experiment clearly demonstrated that production of MAPs based on linearly synthesized defined T- and B-cell epitopes does not guarantee that the MAP will retain immunoreactivity.

Because of the poor immunoreactivity of MAPs 1 and 2 with cells from C57BL/6J mice we constructed a third tetrameric MAP (MAP4). MAP4 differed from MAP1 and 2

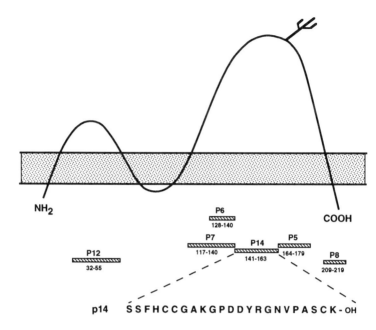

Figure 2. Cartoon of the integral membrane protein Sm23. Sm23 is depicted with four transmembrane domains and two hydrophilic loops. P5–P14 represent synthetic peptides that were produced to map T- and B-cell dominant epitopes. The expanded range of P14 represents the amino acid sequence of this synthetic peptide. The Sm23 tetrameric MAP (M3) is composed entirely of P14.

by replacing synthetic peptide P18 with synthetic peptide P4 (Fig. 4). P4 contains P9, plus an additional eight amino acids on the NH_2 terminus, spanning amino acids 194–210 of TPI (Reynolds *et al.*, 1994) (Fig. 3). Unlike MAPs 1 and 2, MAP4 was highly immunoreactive with T-cell clones from both CBA/J (T9) and C57BL/6J (T44) mice. Therefore, elongation of the P18 synthetic peptide restored immunoreactivity with C57BL/6J T cells, which was lost when P18 was incorporated into the tetrameric MAP. Further, elongation of the P18 T-cell epitope did not significantly alter reactivity of T cells from CBA/J mice (Reynolds *et al.*, 1994). That TPI-MAP4 is a potent immunogen was strengthened by experiments demonstrating that MAP4 could drive expansion of proliferative responses in vivo in CBA/J and C57BL/6J mice that had been previously vaccinated with irradiated cercariae (Reynolds *et al.*, 1994). In the same experiment, MAP4 was shown to drive potent primary responses in naive mice in vivo (Reynolds *et al.*, 1994).

Mapping of B-cell epitopes for Sm23 was more problematic than for TPI because of the previously described conformational nature of the antibody response to Sm23 (Oligino *et al.*, 1987; Reynolds *et al.*, 1992). We observed that reduction of native Sm23 or bacterially expressed Sm23 ablated the majority of antibody binding using rabbit anti-Sm23 sera or sera from chronically infected, or irradiated cercaria-vaccinated CBA/J and C57BL/6J mice. BALB/c and C57BL/6J mice retained minimal Sm23 binding after reduction (Reynolds *et al.*, 1992). Six synthetic peptides spanning the small and large

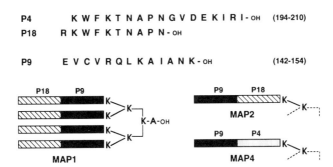

P4   K W F K T N A P N G V D E K I R I - OH   (194-210)
P18   R K W F K T N A P N - OH

P9   E V C V R Q L K A I A N K - OH   (142-154)

Figure 3. Synthetic peptides and MAPs of candidate vaccine antigen TPI. P4, P18, and P9 are synthetic peptides that were found to be immunoreactive with lymphocytes and/or antibodies from naturally infected or mice vaccinated with radiation-attenuated cercariae. Numbers in parentheses indicate corresponding amino acid residues in TPI molecule. MAP1, MAP2, and MAP4 are the tetrameric synthetic peptides that were constructed using P4, P9, or P18.

hydrophilic domains (amino acids 32–55 and 117–179) were tested for antibody binding using BALB/c, C57BL/6J, CBA/J syngeneic mice, and CD-1 outbred mouse sera. Interestingly, the antibody response was limited to two peptides P12 and P14 spanning the small and large hydrophilic domains, respectively (Reynolds *et al.*, 1992) (Fig. 2). P12 and P14 were recognized by antibodies of at least two inbred strains of mice and both peptides were recognized by CD-1 outbred mice. P12 contains one cysteine and P14 contains three; therefore, we tested to determine if either peptide might contain a reduction-sensitive epitope. Mercaptoethanol or dithiothreitol reduction of the peptides resulted in minimal loss of antibody binding for P12, but significant loss of binding for P14, suggesting that P14 contained a reduction-sensitive antibody epitope.

T-cell epitope mapping for Sm23 was simpler in that only one synthetic peptide was recognized by each of the three inbred strains of mice P14 (Reynolds *et al.*, 1992). P6 was recognized by splenocytes from CBA/J and BALB/c mice but not by splenocytes from C57BL/6J mice. Thus, construction of the Sm23 tetrameric MAP was based entirely on P14, which contained the only consensus T-cell epitope as well as a dominant, reduction-sensitive B-cell epitope.

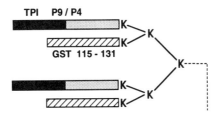

Figure 4. Cartoon of "mixotope" MAP. A combination MAP has been constructed consisting of TPI-MAP (M4) and the protective T-cell peptide from glutathione S-transferase (GST). The "mixotope" is an octapeptide, with four arms each of M4 and GST.

3.2. Vaccination of Mice with TPI and Sm23 MAPs

The goal of our vaccine program was to produce candidate vaccines that could be delivered to developing countries using adjuvant(s) that are simple and stable and a vaccination regimen requiring minimum injections. To mimic this in our animal studies, we initiated our studies in mice using the simple vaccination protocol illustrated in Fig. 5. We utilized two simple adjuvants, aluminum hydroxide (Rehsorptar, Intergen) and liposomes (prepared by S. Furlong, containing equimolar amounts of phosphatidylcholine and cholesterol). Initial vaccine studies were performed using a single TPI MAP, MAP4 and Sm23 MAP3. In the first three studies, mice were immunized with a mixture of 25 μg of MAP in 50 μL and an equal volume of aluminum hydroxide. Mice were challenged with infective-stage cercariae by allowing them to penetrate abdominal skin. Individual experimental groups as well as controls contained from eight to ten mice per group. The numbers of challenge parasites surviving to adult worms were enumerated per mouse 7 to 9 weeks postchallenge, and a mean number of adult worms was then calculated per group. We compared MAP-immunized versus adjuvant control, versus infection control, naive until given challenge infection.

The results of studies I–III using alum are presented in Table II. Data from these studies demonstrate that vaccination of mice with stPI and Sm23 MAPs confer high levels of resistance to challenge infection using alum as adjuvant, and administering the MAPs only

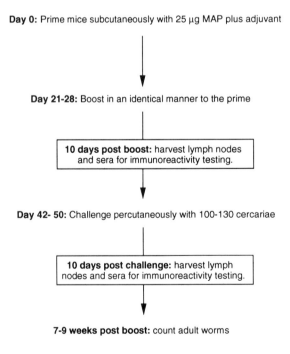

Figure 5. Vaccination protocol and immunoreactivity "flowchart."

Table II
Reduction in Worm Burden after Vaccination with M3 or M4 MAPS and Alum[a]

Expt. No.	Vaccine	% reduction vs. adjuvant	% reduction vs. PBS	p value vs. adjuvant
I	M3/Al	71.5	75.2	<0.05
	M4/Al	46.9	38.9	<0.05
II	M3/Al	69.4	40.6	<0.001
	M4/Al	65.1	82.0	<0.01
III	M3/Al	37.8	36.2	<0.001
	M4/Al	45.3	43.9	<0.001

[a]Mice (eight per group) were primed with 25 μg MAP plus adjuvant by subcutaneous injection. Three weeks later, mice were boosted in an identical manner. Two weeks postboost, mice were challenged with 130 cercariae (Expt. I) or 120 cercariae (Expt. II). Seven weeks postchallenge, mice were killed and adult worm burdens determined by mesenteric vein perfusion in a double-blind fashion. Al, aluminum hydroxide; PBS, phosphate-buffered saline.

two times. Vaccination of mice with TPI-MAP4 reduced mean adult worm burdens from 39 to 82% (average reduction for all three studies of 55%) compared to infection controls. MAP4-vaccinated mouse worm burdens were reduced from 45 to 65% (three-trial average of 52%) compared to adjuvant controls. In study II, three of eight mice vaccinated with MAP4 had absolutely no worms! The levels of protection with MAP3 were comparable to those with MAP4, a range of 36–75% (three-trial average of 51%) versus infection controls, and a range of 38–72% (three-trial range of 60%) versus adjuvant controls. Thus, both MAP3 and MAP4 were highly protective when administered to mice in alum. For each of the study comparisons, the results were highly significant as assessed by ANOVA statistical analysis.

TPI and Sm23 MAPs were also tested for efficacy after incorporation into liposomes. In contrast to the results obtained with alum, only the TPI-MAP4 induced significant resistance to challenge when incorporated into liposomes. The range of protection for MAP4 versus infection control was 42–75% (three-trial average of 60%), and a range of 41–52% (average of 47%) against liposome control. Each of the MAP4-liposome trials was significant assessed by ANOVA analysis. In contrast, MAP3 in liposomes resulted in low and generally nonsignificant protection ranging from 0 to 32% (two-trial average of 16%) against infection control and 25 to 31% (three-trial average of 28%) versus liposome control.

We also performed vaccine studies comparing the efficacy of vaccination with each of the three TPI MAPs to determine if the high levels of protection that we were observing in MAP4-vaccinated mice were related in part to the presence of the P4 epitope. Simultaneously, we compared each of the MAPs at three different concentrations (12.5, 25, and 50 μg/mouse per injection). Using this protocol, we first observed that there was a clear dose dependency for efficacy with MAP4. Using the 50-μg dose we found a mean reduction of adult worms of 86% as compared to adjuvant control mice ($n = 10$ for both groups). MAP1 and MAP2 both have P18 in place of P4 but in different orientations (see Figure 3). Vaccination with MAP1 resulted in marginal and insignificant worm burden reductions at doses of 25 and 50 μg/injection. Vaccination with MAP2 yielded similarly poor efficacy as MAP1 using doses of 50 or 25 μg, respectively. Thus, the additional amino acid residues placed P4 as compared to P18, may be critical for the generation of high levels of protection with MAP4. Alternatively, P4 may be the dominant T-cell epitope for C57BL/6J mice, the strain that was used for all vaccine trials. Therefore, it is likely that vaccination of CBA/J mice with MAP1 or MAP2, which contain the dominant CBA/J T-cell peptide P18, may also result in high levels of protection if T-cell responses are critical for protection.

3.3. Immunobiology of TPI and Sm23 MAP Vaccination

Lymph node cells and sera were taken from all groups 10 days postboost and 10 days postchallenge for analysis of immunoreactivity. The results of several ELISA assays showing that MAP-vaccinated mice produced high levels of antibodies to the relevant peptide and to the homologous recombinant protein are summarized in Table III. There appears to be little or no production of cross-reactive antibodies after vaccination with either MAP3 or MAP4.

Western blot analysis was performed to compare sera obtained from mice vaccinated with the three different TPI-MAPs, as well as to sera from MAP3-vaccinated mice. Interestingly, recombinant TPI was recognized by sera from MAP1- and MAP4-immunized mice but not MAP2-immunized mice. As expected, MAP3-vaccinated mice did not produce antibodies to recombinant TPI (data not shown). The Western blot results are interesting in light of proposing a putative mechanism for the protective immunity induced after vaccination with MAP4 in contrast to the low, insignificant levels of protection obtained after vaccination with MAP1 and MAP2. As indicated by Western blot analysis, MAP1 produces strong antibody responses to full-length recombinant TPI, yet this is not sufficient to achieve high levels of parasite killing in vivo. The Western blot results provide further evidence to suggest that a strong T-cell response is requisite in MAP4-induced protection.

Table III
Antibody Responses[a] of MAP-Vaccinated Mice

Vaccine group[b]	Antigens[c]				
	M3	M4	TP1	VC2	MBP
MAP3/alum					
PB	+++++	–	–	+	–
PC	++++++	–	–	+++	–
MAP4/alum					
PB	–	+	+/–	–	–
PC	–	+++	+	–	–
Alum					
PB	–	–	–	–	–
PC	+/–	+/–	–	+/–	+/–

[a]Antibody responses were assessed by direct binding ELISA of vaccine sera to antigen-coated plates and the results are expressed in terms of optical density of vaccine sera/adjuvant control sera compared to infection control sera which would always be (–) and have an OD range of 0.001–0.15. Thus, +/– would be 0.3–0.5 and ++++++ would be an OD > 2.5.
[b]PB, postboost; PC, postchallenge.
[c]Antigens were plated at 20 μg/mL on Immulon II plates (Dynatech). Abbreviations: M3 and M4 = MAP3 and MAP4, respectively; TPI = triose phosphate isomerase; VC2 = bacterial fusion protein of Sm23; MBP = maltose binding protein.

Table IV
Proliferative Responses of Lymphocytes[a] from MAP-Vaccinated Mice

Vaccine group	Stimulation indices[b]	
	Postboost[c]	Postchallenge[d]
MAP3/alum	–	+++
MAP4/alum	+/–	+++++
Alum	–	++
MAP3/liposomes	–	++
M4P4/liposomes	+/–	++++
Liposomes	–	+/–

[a]Lymphocytes were obtained from axillary lymph nodes of MAP- or sham-vaccinated C57BL/6 mice and pulsed with M3 or M4 for MAP3- and MAP4-immunized mice, respectively.
[b]Stimulation indices equal cpm experimental divided by cpm control (media only).
[c]Axillary lymph nodes were removed 10 days postboost.
[d]Axillary lymph nodes were removed 10–14 days postchallenge.

4. CONCLUSIONS

The development of defined prophylactic vaccines to protect against infection with schistosomes would augment treatment with the available drugs. Unlike other diseases, a sterilizing vaccine, although desirable, is not required in schistosomiasis. As the disease is caused by the host immune response to parasite eggs trapped in tissues, a vaccine that resulted in significant reduction in the numbers of egg-laying adult parasites will likely reduce or eliminate hepatosplenic-related morbidity and mortality. To this end, the Scientific Working Group on schistosomiasis at the World Health Organization Tropical Disease Research Unit has determined that vaccines that lower the adult worm burden by 30–50% will be effective in reducing overall morbidity and mortality.

In addition to the TPI and Sm23 MAPs, there are several other candidate vaccine antigens that have been tested as recombinant antigens or synthetic peptides and shown to be partially protective in mice in vivo (Table I). To compare and contrast these antigens with TPI and Sm23 MAPs, only IrV-5 has shown the same high levels of protection that vaccination with Sm23 or TPI MAPs give. Although IrV-5 appears to require three or four immunizations to achieve this high level of immunity, it can be done in the absence of any adjuvant (Amory Soisson *et al.*, 1992). Sm23 and TPI MAPs require only two immunizations to achieve comparable levels of protection, and it has not been determined if the two MAPs will protect in the absence of alum. The immunization regimen could be critical if compliance with three or four injections is required in developing countries. Additionally, in its present form, IrV-5 has roughly 50% homology with mammalian myosin. Thus, there is great potential risk for the development of autoimmunity. The Sm23 and, more specifically, TPI MAPs were constructed with schistosome-specific residues in an attempt to avoid the induction of autoimmunity. In comparison to GST, it would appear that immunization of mice with TPI or Sm23 MAPs as well as the IrV-5 vaccine induces higher levels of protection. Additionally, GST has been tested in baboons and shown to also possess antifecundity properties (Boulanger *et al.*, 1991), and synthetic peptides have been constructed to map both protective and antifecundity epitopes of GST (Marguerite *et al.*, 1992). Antifecundity has not yet been examined after vaccination with either Sm23 or TPI MAPs. The other major schistosome vaccine candidate, paramyosin, has not given rise to tremendous levels of protection in mice against *S. mansoni* (Pearce *et al.*, 1988). Recently though, Ramirez (1993) has found that the *S. japonicum* homologue of mansoni paramyosin is highly protective against *S. japonicum* infection.

The TDR/World Bank Programme for Research and Training has recently announced that they are preparing to test these candidate vaccine antigens in field sites within the next 1 to 2 years. Barring toxicity reactions, it is probable that the final schistosome vaccine will consist of a "cocktail" of recombinant antigens, or a "mixotope" synthetic peptide such as Spf 66 for falciparum malaria (Pattaroyo *et al.*, 1987). In this regard, a mixotope octameric MAP has now been prepared containing four arms each of the TPI-MAP4 peptide and four arms of the GST peptide (Fig. 5). The TPI-GST octapeptide is currently being tested and the "mixotope–cocktail" approach will likely be expanded in future studies to a number of other combinations.

The ultimate cocktail vaccine will likely include one or more protective (anti-infection epitopes) as well as multiple antipathology epitopes. As the goal of a schistosome vaccine is to reduce parasite egg-associated immunopathology, the inclusion of antifecundity or pathology-modulating epitopes may be equally as important as protective epitopes. In this regard, an antifecundity effect of GST has already been demonstrated in rodents and baboons (Boulanger *et al.*, 1991), and egg antigens identified by granulomatogenic T-cell clones have now been identified and purified (Chikunguwo *et al.*, 1991, 1993).

In order to optimize immunogenicity of these vaccines for use in humans it will be necessary to test the TPI and Sm23 MAPs, as well as each of the other candidate vaccine antigens constructed using murine lymphocytes and antibodies, for immunoreactivity with patient sera and lymphocytes. The possibility that there are small differences in epitope recognition by patient cells or antibodies, requires that we define optimally immunoreactive T- and B-cell epitopes using patient sera and lymphocytes. By comparing lymphoproliferative-, cytokine-, and antibody-binding data with patient HLA class II type, we will also be able to define epitopes that either are not, or have minimal, genetic restriction for use in humans. These studies are in progress for the TPI and Sm23 MAPs using peripheral blood lymphocytes and sera from patients at our field site in Bahia, Brazil. Although these studies are in the early stages, preliminary data suggest that both TPI and Sm23 MAPs are recognized by patient lymphocytes and antibody.

REFERENCES

Amory Soisson, L. M., Masterson, C. P., Tom, T. D., McNally, M. T., Lowell, G. H., and Strand, M., 1992, Induction of protective immunity in mice using a 62-kDa recombinant fragment of a *Schistosoma mansoni* surface antigen, *J. Immunol.* **149**:3612.

Balloul, J. M., Sondermeyer, P., Dreyer, D., Capron, M., Grzych, J. M., Pierce, R. J., Carvalho, D., Lecocq, J. P., and Capron, A., 1987, Molecular cloning of a protective antigen of schistosomes, *Nature* **326**:149.

Boulanger, C., Reid, G. D. F., Sturrock, R. F., Wolowczuk, I., Balloul, J. M., Grezel, D., Pierce, R. J., Otieno, M. F., Guerret, S., Grimaud, J. A., Butterworth, A. E., and Capron, A., 1991, Immunization of mice and baboons with the recombinant Sm28GST affects both worm viability and fecundity after experimental infection with *Schistosoma mansoni*, *Parasite Immunol.* **13**:473.

Butterworth, A.E., Capron, M., Cordingley, J.S., Dalton, P.R., Dunne, D.W., Kariuki, H. C., Kimani, G., Koech, D., Mugambi, M., Ouma, J. H., Prentice, M. A., Richardson, B. A., Arap Siongok, T. K., Sturrock, R. F., and Taylor, D. W., 1985, Immunity after treatment of human *Schistosomiasis mansoni*. II. Identification of resistant individuals, and analysis of their immune responses, *Trans. R. Soc. Trop. Med. Hyg.* **79**:393.

Butterworth, A. E., Dunne, D. W., Fulford, A., Capron, M., Khalife, J., Capron, A., Koech, D., Ouma, J. H., and Sturrock, R., 1988, Immunity in *Schistosomiasis mansoni*: Cross-reactive IgM and IgG2 anti-carbohydrate antibodies block the expression of immunity, *Biochemie* **70**:1053.

Chikunguwo, S. M., Kanazawa, T., Dayal, Y., and Stadecker, M. J., 1991, The cell mediated response to schistosomiasis antigens at the clonal level: In vivo functions of cloned murine egg antigen-specific CD4$^+$ T helper type 1 lymphocytes, *J. Immunol.* **147**:3921.

Chikunguwo, S. M., Quinn, J. J., Harn, D. A., and Stadecker, M. J., 1993, The cell mediated response to schistosomal antigens at the clonal level. III. Identification of soluble egg antigens recognized by cloned specific granulomagenic murine CD4$^+$ Th1-type lymphocytes, *J. Immunol.* **150**:1413.

Corbett, E. L., Butterworth, A. E., Fulford, A. J. C., Ouma, J. H., and Sturrock, R. F., 1992, Nutritional status of children with *Schistosomiasis mansoni* in two different areas of Machakos District, Kenya, *Trans. R. Soc. Trop. Med. Hyg.* **86**:266.

Dalton, J. P., and Strand, M., 1987, *Schistosoma mansoni* polypeptides immunogenic in mice vaccinated with radiation-attenuated cercariae, *J. Immunol.* **139**:2474.

de Lima e Costa, M. M. F., Leite, M. L. C., Rocha, R. S., de Almeida, M. H., Magalhaes, H., and Katz, N., 1988, Anthropometric measures in relation to *Schistosomiasis mansoni* and socioeconomic variables, *Int. J. Epidemiol.* **17**:880.

Dessein, A. J., Begley, M., Demeure, C., Caillol, D., Fueri, J., dos Reis, M. G., Andrade, Z. A., Prata. A., and Bina, J. C., 1988, Human resistance to *Schistosoma mansoni* is associated with IgG reactivity to a 37-kD larval surface antigen, *J. Immunol.* **140**:2727.

Doenhoff, M., and Long, E., 1979, Factors affecting the acquisition of resistance against *Schistosoma mansoni* in the mouse. IV. The inability of T-cell deprived mice to resist re-infection, and other in vivo studies on the mechanism of resistance, *Parasitology* **78**:171.

Ford, M. J., Bickle, Q. D., Taylor, M. G., and Andrews, B. J., 1984, Passive transfer of resistance and the site of immune-dependent elimination of the challenge infection in rats vaccinated with highly irradiated cercariae of *Schistosoma mansoni*, *Parasitology* **89**:461.

Hagan, P., Blumenthal, U. J., Dunne, D., Simpson, A. J. G., and Wilkins, H. A., 1991, Human IgE, IgG4 and resistance to reinfection with *Schistosoma haematobium*, *Nature* **349**:243.

Harn, D. A., Mitsuyama, M., Huguenel, E. D., Oligino, L. D., and David, J. R., 1985a, Identification by monoclonal antibody of a major (28kDa) surface membrane antigen of *Schistosoma mansoni*, *Mol. Biochem. Parasitol.* **16**:345.

Harn, D. A., Mitsuyama, M., Huguenel, E. D., and David, J. R., 1985b, *Schistosoma mansoni*: Detection by monoclonal antibody of a 22,000 dalton surface membrane antigen which may be blocked by host molecules on lung stage parasites, *J. Immunol.* **135**:2115.

Harn, D. A., Quinn, J. J., Oligino, L. D., Percy, A., Ko, A., Pham, K., Gross, A., Gebremichael, A., and Stein, L., 1987, Candidate epitopes for vaccination against *Schistosomiasis mansoni*, in: *Molecular Paradigms for Eradicating Helminthic Parasites* (A. J. MacInnis, ed.), Liss, New York.

Harn, D. A., Gu, W., Oligino, L. D., Mitsuyama, M., Gebremichael, A., and Richter, D., 1992, A protective monoclonal antibody specifically recognizes and alters the catalytic activity of schistosome triosephosphate isomerase, *J. Immunol.* **148**:562.

Hsu, S., Li, Y., Hsu, F., and Burmeister, L.F., 1981, *Schistosoma mansoni*: Vaccination of mice with highly x-irradiated cercariae, *Exp. Parasitol.* **52**:91.

James, S. L., 1987, Induction of protective immunity against *Schistosoma mansoni* by a non-living vaccine. V. Effects of varying the immunization schedule and site, *Parasite Immunol.* **9**:531.

Jwo, J., and LoVerde, P. T., 1989, The ability of fractionated sera from animals vaccinated with irradiated cercariae of *Schistosoma mansoni* to transfer immunity to mice, *J. Parasitol.* **75**:252.

Lanar, D. E., Pearce, E. J., James, S. L., and Sher, A., 1986, Identification of paramyosin as schistosome antigen recognized by intradermally vaccinated mice, *Science* **234**:593.

McGarvey, S. T., Wu, G., Zhang, S., Wang, Y., Peters, P., Olds, G. D., and Wiest, P. M., 1993, Child growth, nutritional status, and *Schistosomiasis japonica* in Jiangxi, Peoples Republic of China, *Am. J. Trop. Med. Hyg.* **48**:547.

Mangold, B. L., and Dean, D. A., 1984, The migration and survival of gamma-irradiated *Schistosoma mansoni* larvae and the duration of host–parasite contact in relation to the induction of resistance in mice, *Parasitology* **88**:249.

Mangold, B. L., and Dean, D. A., 1986, Passive transfer with serum and IgG antibodies of irradiated cercariae-induced resistance against *Schistosoma mansoni* in mice, *J. Immunol.* **136**:2644.

Marguerite, M., Bosus, M., Mazingue, C., Wolowczuk, I., Gras-Masse, H., Tartar, A., Capron, A., and Auriault, C., 1992, Analysis of antigenicity and immunogenicity of five different chemically defined constructs of a peptide, *Mol. Immunol.* **29**:793.

Oligino, L.D., Percy, A.J., and Harn, D.A., 1988, Purification and immunochemical characterization of a 22 kilodalton surface antigen from *Schistosoma mansoni*, *Mol. Biochem. Parasitol.* **28**:95.

Pattaroyo, M.E., Romero, P., Torres, M.L., Clavijo, P., Moreno, A., Martinez, A., Rodriguez, R., Guzman, F., and Cabazas, E., 1987, Induction of protective immunity against experimental infection with malaria using synthetic peptides, *Nature* **328**:629.

Pearce, E. J., James, S. L., Heiny, S., Lanar, D. E., and Sher, A., 1988, Induction of protective immunity against *Schistosoma mansoni* by vaccination with schistosome paramyosin (Sm97), a nonsurface parasite antigen, *Proc. Natl. Acad. Sci. USA* **85**:5678.

Ramirez, B., 1993, TDRU Meeting on Control of Schistosomiasis, November, Manila.

Reynolds, S. R., and Harn, D. A., 1992, Comparison of irradiated-cercariae schistosome vaccine models that use 15- and 50-kilorad doses: The 15-kilorad dose gives greater protection, smaller liver sizes, and higher gamma interferon levels after challenge, *Infect. Immun.* **60**:90.

Reynolds, S. R., Shoemaker, C. B., and Harn, D. A., 1992, T and B cell epitope mapping of SM23, an integral membrane protein of *Schistosoma mansoni*, *J. Immunol.* **149**:3995.

Reynolds, S. R., Dahl, C. E., and Harn, D. A., 1994, T and B epitope determination and analysis of multiple antigenic peptides for the *Schistosoma mansoni* experimental vaccine triose-phosphate isomerase, *J. Immunol.* **152**:193.

Reynolds, S. R., Jacobs, W. R., Cirillo, J. D., Kastens, W. A., Incani, R. N., Edwards, C. S., and Harn, D. A., 1995, Expression of immunologically and enzymatically active *Schistosoma mansoni* triose phosphate isomerase in BCG, (in press).

Richter, D., Incani, R. N., and Harn, D. A., 1993, Isotype responses to candidate vaccine antigens in protective sera obtained from mice vaccinated with irradiated cercariae of *Schistosoma mansoni*, *Infect. Immun.* **61**:3003.

Rihet, P., Demeure, C. E., Bourgois, A., Prata, A., and Dessein, A. J., 1991, Evidence for an association between human resistance to *Schistosoma mansoni* and high anti-larval IgE levels, *Eur. J. Immunol.* **21**:2679.

Rihet, P., Demeure, C. E., Dessein, A. J., and Bourgois, A., 1992, Strong serum inhibition of specific IgE correlated to competing IgG4, revealed by a new methodology in subjects from a *S. mansoni* endemic area, *Eur. J. Immunol.* **22**:2063.

Sher, A., Heiny, S., James, S.L., and Asofsky, R., 1982, Mechanisms of protective immunity against *Schistosoma mansoni* infection in mice vaccinated with irradiated cercariae. II. Analysis of immunity in hosts deficient in T lymphocytes, B lymphocytes, or complement, *J. Immunol.* **128**:1880.

Shoemaker, C., Gross, A., Gebremichael, A., and Harn, D. A., 1992, cDNA cloning and functional expression of the *Schistosoma mansoni* protective antigen triose-phosphate isomerase, *Proc. Natl. Acad. Sci. USA* **89**:1842.

Tam, J. P., Clavijo, P., Lu, Y.-A., Nussenzweig, V., Nussenzweig, R., and Zavala, F.,1990, Incorporation of T and B cell epitopes of the circumsporozoite protein in a chemically defined synthetic vaccine against malaria, *J. Exp. Med.* **171**:299.

Wright, M. D., Henkle, K. J., and Mitchell, G. F., 1990, An immunogenic Mr 23,000 integral membrane protein of *Schistosoma mansoni* worms that closely resembles a human tumor-associated antigen, *J. Immunol.* **144**:3195.

Chapter 41

Synthetic Hormone/Growth Factor Subunit Vaccine with Application to Antifertility and Cancer

Laura L. Snyder, David V. Woo, Pierre L. Triozzi, and Vernon C. Stevens

1. INTRODUCTION

Historically, vaccines were developed to induce immunological memory prior to pathogen exposure so that the immune system could then prevent infection or ameliorate the effects of the ensuing disease. Vaccines of this type were designed for maximum effect because, typically, more was better, and as long as the immune response was directed at the foreign pathogen, the type of response and specific antigenic targets did not cause concern. Today, scientists and physicians wish to direct the immune system against diseases and conditions that have little or no association with foreign pathogens. There is considerable interest in developing active specific vaccines and immunotherapies against self antigens instead of nonself antigens. Success in these efforts depends both on expression on the target tissue of molecules that have the potential to be recognized as "foreign" by the immune system, and on the scientific community's ability to discover safe and effective methods for presenting these molecules to the immune system such that antigenic self-tolerance is broken in a controlled and predictable fashion.

Fertility control and cancer therapy are two areas where vaccination against self antigens holds considerable promise. Because certain embryonic antigens, expressed as oncofetal proteins, are shared by tissues involved in the reproductive process and various malignancies, vaccine development in both areas may benefit from research involving similar immunogenic formulations. In this chapter, we describe the rational design and

Laura L. Snyder and David V. Woo • ImmunoTherapy Corporation, Tustin, California 92680. *Pierre L. Triozzi* • The Ohio State University Comprehensive Cancer Center, The Arthur G. James Cancer Hospital and Research Institute, Columbus, Ohio 43210. *Vernon C. Stevens* • Department of Obstetrics and Gynecology, The Ohio State University, Columbus, Ohio 43210.

Vaccine Design: The Subunit and Adjuvant Approach, edited by Michael F. Powell and Mark J. Newman. Plenum Press, New York, 1995.

development of an antigen-specific vaccine that was originally conceived to provide a safe, effective, and economical means of birth control. This vaccine induces an immune response to human chorionic gonadotropin (hCG) and since hCG is frequently expressed by a variety of cancers, the vaccine is also being developed for cancer immunotherapy. Phase II antifertility trials are ongoing with the vaccine and it is expected to enter Phase II clinical trials for cancer in the near future.

2. SPECIAL CONSIDERATIONS IN VACCINE DEVELOPMENT FOR FERTILITY CONTROL

The current world population is estimated to be 5.6 billion and is expected to reach 8 billion by 2020. Throughout the world, population density is increasing as global population doubling time shortens, causing further encroachment on arable land and greater damage to the environment (Walton, 1993b). Food production during the 1980s lagged behind population growth in two-thirds of all developing countries and in four-fifths of all African nations and is not expected to catch up. As a result, societal economic and health status are adversely affected (Walton, 1993a). More convenient and less costly methods of fertility control are desperately needed to supplement currently available methods, especially in developing countries.

Over 50 years ago, antibodies against pituitary gonadotropins were shown to affect gonadal function (Osterguard, 1942), but efforts to apply this knowledge were frustrated by the phenomena of self-tolerance and species specificity (Glass and Mroueh, 1967; Stevens, 1973). Natural tolerance was first broken using hapten modifications of hormones as vaccine immunogens; antibodies were induced against native luteinizing hormone in baboons (Stevens, 1973) and against native chorionic gonadotropin in women (Stevens and Crystle, 1973).

Development of an antifertility agent designed to regulate human reproduction by immunologic means requires consideration of characteristics specific to that clinical setting. Unlike vaccines developed for prophylaxis in populations at risk for disease or for therapy in populations with conditions that threaten health, virtually no clinical toxicity will be considered tolerable. Keeping the risk-to-benefit ratio unusually low was a priority at every step during development of the prototype antifertility vaccine (AFV), designated hCGβCTP37-DT. An AFV that requires frequent and/or costly monitoring would not be useful for developing nations. The onset and the duration of effective immune response to the AFV must be highly predictable and require minimal effort and compliance on the part of the user. In addition, one can anticipate very specific requirements regarding duration of response: (1) the immune responses to an AFV must be of adequate duration to allow infrequent inoculations, at intervals of no less than 6 months, and (2) immune response durations must be short enough to allow planning of desired births at reasonable intervals. There are also ethical issues to be considered when one seeks to manipulate fertility: (1) it is important that this type of intervention occur early in the reproductive process and (2) since self-control over reproduction is considered a basic human right in most cultures, as much flexibility of use must be designed into the antifertility agent as possible. Obviously, a high level of clinical efficacy, at least 95%, will be required of an AFV and only research approaches with potential to satisfy this requirement were pursued. Some effort should also be devoted to developing a method for reversing the effects of the vaccine as it is almost inevitable that the occasional patient, even though fully informed of the expected effects, will desire a pregnancy before the effects of the vaccine have waned naturally.

Since the antigen targeted will in most cases be a self antigen, a foreign carrier protein or peptide will be needed to provide T-helper cell stimulation. Even a self antigen:carrier conjugate cannot be expected to be strongly immunogenic and the use of immunostimulators, or adjuvants, must also be considered. While designing the hCGβCTP37-DT vaccine, eliciting a cellular immune response was carefully avoided and efforts concentrated on provoking a humoral response capable of preventing pregnancy. It was felt that in circumstances where frequent booster immunizations are anticipated, T-cell activation could result in unacceptable hypersensitivity. Also, cell-mediated immune recognition of the self protein immunogen might be more likely to result in toxicity to normal tissues and possibly permanent sterility. Clearly, an AFV must lend itself well to quality control and economical production so that it can be provided at an affordable cost to its users.

3. IMMUNOLOGICAL FERTILITY CONTROL

Immunological intervention has several potential advantages over nonimmunological approaches to fertility control. Since the active agent in a vaccine can be expected to lack pharmacological activity, direct tissue toxicity is unlikely and monitoring of the patient for levels of vaccine components should not be necessary. Effective prevention of pregnancy with long duration requiring only infrequent treatment or intervention will reduce the incidence of pregnancy resulting from improper use of the method or noncompliance and also facilitates a wide distribution of the vaccine product. Of course, wide distribution can only be supported if the product can be produced on a large scale; some immunologic agents will meet these criteria. Finally, in addition to low cost and ease of use, acceptability of the method is an important consideration and the concept of vaccination is well established and accepted in developing nations.

Production of active specific immunity (ASI) requires that the target immunogen be delivered to a site into which lymphoid cells are then attracted. Antigen-presenting cells (APCs) must then be activated to present the antigen to T cells which must recognize the antigen as "foreign." In the case of fertility regulation, tolerance to a self antigen must be broken to render native reproductive antigens sufficiently immunogenic to induce antibody production. In addition, sustained humoral immunity requires persistent exposure of B cells to antigen, either by frequent booster immunizations, by retention of intact epitope sequences bound to follicular dendritic cells, or by the continuous release of immunogen from depots or microparticles (Stevens, 1993).

The reproductive process from gametogenesis through implantation possesses unique elements that provide potentially immunogenic targets. Strategic development of an immunological contraceptive has involved careful examination of cases of spontaneous infertility with identification of naturally occurring antibodies associated with reproductive failure. Considerable research has been directed toward stimulation of an immune response against sperm, an approach that is supported by clinical evidence that a small proportion of male and female patients attending infertility clinics are found to be infertile as a result of the presence of circulating antibodies against spermatozoa (Boettcher, 1979). This research has progressed slowly and several vaccine formulations have recently entered or are about to enter testing in female nonhuman primates. In a similar approach, a number of antigens have been identified on the zona pellucida, the outer coating of the ovum. Although it has long been known that antibodies raised against the zona pellucida will block fertilization of the mammalian ovum in vivo (Sacco, 1979), attempts to develop a contraceptive vaccine using the most thoroughly researched of these antigens, ZP3, have resulted in permanent loss of ovarian primordial follicles and premature menopause in primates (Paterson *et al.*, 1992).

3.1. Hormones as Target Antigens

Vaccine immunogens should not be expressed by normal tissues or should at least be preferentially expressed by the target tissues. For fertility control, the target immunogen should be (1) pharmacologically inert, (2) specific to reproductive process, and (3) not continuously present. If the antigen is present, it should appear at biologically insignificant levels or should be limited to a site at which a low-grade immune reactivity would not be clinically meaningful.

The hormones that regulate the reproductive system have been considered as potential targets for an immunological contraceptive. Some, like the sex steroids which are necessary for reproductive organ health as well as for activity in other tissues, have not been seriously considered. Others, including follicle-stimulating hormone (FSH), luteinizing hormone (LH), gonadotropin-releasing hormone (GnRH), and chorionic gonadotropin (CG), have received considerable attention and research. Because their continuous presence in the circulation raises safety concerns, FSH and LH are relatively unattractive targets for fertility control. The prospect of persistent formation of circulating immune complexes and the toxicity that may result from deposition of these complexes in tissues, particularly kidney, combined with the possibility of immune reactivity with the pituitary from which these hormones are secreted, have deterred research which might seek to make them targets. Manipulations targeting GnRH would not only invoke the same concerns, by virtue of its role in regulating FSH and LH, but blockade of this hormone would cause gonadal atrophy with loss of secondary sexual characteristics and libido; carefully titrated androgen replacement therapy would become necessary, a level of intensive intervention not practical for a contraceptive vaccine. Of the fertility-regulating hormones, hCG holds the greatest promise as an antifertility target antigen.

3.2. Human Chorionic Gonadotropin

hCG is produced by the trophoblast cells of the human conceptus beginning no later than the blastocyst stage prior to implantation and by the syncytiotrophoblast cells of the placental chorionic villi. It becomes detectable in serum and urine soon after implantation. The physiologic role of hCG in pregnancy includes luteotropic action on the corpus luteum resulting in secretion of progesterone necessary to maintain pregnancy during the first few weeks of gestation.

The hCG molecule is a glycoprotein with a molecular mass of 38 kDa and consists of two noncovalently bound glycoprotein subunits designated α (hCGα) and β (hCGβ) of 14.5 and 23 kDa, respectively (Puett, 1986). The structural genes for the hCG subunits are contained on separate chromosomes; a single gene for hCGα is located on chromosome 6 and multiple genes for hCGβ are located on chromosome 19 (Naylor *et al.*, 1983). The three-dimensional structure of hCG has recently been elucidated in independent investigations using different crystallographic techniques (Lapthorn *et al.*, 1994; Wu *et al.*, 1994). The two subunits have similar topologies, with three disulfide bonds forming a cystine knot on each, making hCG a member of the superfamily of cystine-knot growth factors which also includes nerve growth factor (NGF), transforming growth factor β (TGF-β), and platelet-derived growth factor β (PDGF-β). A segment of the β subunit wraps around the α subunit and is covalently linked like a "seatbelt" by a Cys26–Cys110 disulfide bond; this feature not only stabilizes the heterodimer, but also appears to be important for receptor binding. In its natural state, four simple O-glycosidic oligosaccharides are linked to hCGβ serine residues in positions 121, 127, 132, and 138. Including the N-glycosidic oligosaccharides attached to asparagine residues 52 and 78 of hCGα and 13 and 30 of hCGβ, the total carbohydrate moieties number eight. The α subunit of hCG is chemically identical to the α subunits of human LH, human FSH, and human thyroid-stimulating hormone, but the β subunits differ and provide hormone specificity to target tissue receptors (Hussa, 1980).

Although immunological cross-reactivity exists between the β subunits of these four hormones and hCG antisera cross-react with all four, only human LHβ and hCGβ have significant homology, sharing approximately 80% of their 115 amino-terminal amino acids (Hussa, 1980). Therefore, an immune response stimulated against the entire hCGβ subunit in a vaccine is not specific for hCG and can cross-react with hLH at up to 80% of the reactivity with hCG. But hCGβ is 24 residues longer at the carboxyl-terminal portion of the molecule which is unique by definition (Stevens, 1976).

In the nonpregnant woman, hCG represents a "foreign" molecule, as it is present in physiological quantities in healthy women only following conception. In addition, as a trophoblast hormone, it has the advantage of being expressed at only one anatomical site postfertilization and is in intimate contact with the maternal blood supply. But even at the time hCG is acting to maintain pregnancy, it is present at levels low enough to allow inhibition by a relatively weak immune response and specific hCG neutralization would act silently, without disruption of the endocrine system.

4. DEVELOPMENT OF AN ANTIFERTILITY VACCINE BASED ON HUMAN CHORIONIC GONADOTROPIN

4.1. Peptide Immunogen Selection

Research efforts to identify a highly specific target antigen focused on the unique carboxyl-terminal peptide (CTP) region of hCGβ because of its lack of homology with human LH. Rabbits were immunized with numerous peptides with lengths of 8 to 41 amino acids representing residues within positions 105–145 and all including the carboxyl-terminus. None of the antisera produced reacted with human LH. Peptides with fewer than 20 or more than 40 amino acid residues induced antibodies that were relatively weakly reactive with intact hCG; antisera to peptides with fewer than 35 residues did not consistently neutralize the biological action of hCG in vivo (Stevens, 1976). Peptides containing 35 residues (positions 111–145) and 37 residues (positions 109–145) induced antibody responses that were most highly reactive with hCG and neutralized the biological activity of hCG in vivo. The 37-amino-acid peptide, hCGβ(109–145), was chosen for further development, partly because it contains the cysteine 110 residue, which confers an advantage during conjugation to the carrier. The sequence of the carboxyl-terminal peptide hCGβ(109–145) is Thr-Cys-Asp-Asp-Pro-Arg-Phe-Gln-Asp-Ser-Ser-Ser-Ser-Lys-Ala-Pro- Pro-Pro-Ser-Leu-Pro-Ser-Pro-Ser-Arg-Leu-Pro-Gly-Pro-Ser-Asp-Thr-Pro-Ile-Leu-Pro-Gln-COOH. This peptide will be referred to as hCGβCTP37.

Nine different epitopes have been identified on free hCGβ, seven of which are conserved in assembled hCGβ (Berger *et al.*, 1990). Two of these epitopes are included in hCGβCTP37, one involving amino acid residues 111–118 and the other involving residues 133–145. In a separate study, immunization with short peptides representing the epitopes only, induced antibodies that bound very weakly to hCG and did not neutralize hCG in vivo (Stevens and Jones, 1990; Dirnhofer *et al.*,1993). Additional studies of the structure of carboxyl-terminal peptides using circular dichroism measurements and the Chou–Fasman prediction rules, indicated high likelihood for several β-turns and structural influences of aromatic residues such as phenylalanine within hCGβCTP37, suggesting that the entire peptide fragment would be required to generate significant immunity (Puett *et al.*, 1982).

4.2. Carrier Selection

A series of ten hCGβCTP37:carrier conjugates were prepared using the same conjugation procedures and conditions, and were administered to rabbits in a formulation including complete Freund's adjuvant (CFA). Levels of antibodies produced against hCG and hCGβCTP37 were monitored; the most vigorous immune responses were induced using conjugates incorporating bovine gamma globulin, diphtheria toxoid (DT), or tetanus toxoid (TT) as the carrier (Stevens, 1986). Other carriers evaluated included bacteria and bacterial proteins which provoked moderate levels of antibodies and synthetic polypeptides or carbohydrates which provoked relatively low antibody levels. DT was chosen for the vaccine formulation because of markedly fewer delayed-type hypersensitivity (DTH) reactions compared to TT, and because bovine gamma globulin was considered unsuitable for administration to humans.

4.3. Coupling and Ratio of Peptide to Carrier

In previous experiments, peptide-to-carrier coupling methods resulted in conjugates with highly variable characteristics which do not lend well to adequate production quality control. A method was needed for chemically coupling peptides to carriers covalently and in a predictable fashion, and such a method was developed using 6-maleimido caproic acyl

N-hydroxy succinimide ester (MCS), a bifunctional coupling agent. MCS was first coupled to the carrier amino groups via its active ester and then to the peptide thiol groups via its stable maleimido groups. The hCGβCTP37 peptide contains a cysteine residue at position 110 which was convenient for reactions with its thiol groups. The predictability of the coupling reaction can be attributed to the high degree of reactivity between the quantifiable number of maleimido groups on the MCS-modified conjugate and the thiol groups of the peptide which was present in excess. This method allowed production of conjugate with a highly predictable density of peptide to carrier, which can be expressed in terms of the number of peptides per 100 kDa carrier (Lee *et al.*, 1980).

Additional experiments were designed to determine the optimal peptide:carrier ratios. Rabbits were immunized with conjugates having peptide:carrier densities of 5, 10, 16, 23, 27, and 33 peptides/100 kDa carrier. Densities of 20 to 30 peptides/100 kDa carrier were considered optimal for this immunogen because they induced the highest antibody responses with significantly greater responses developing within 63 days (Stevens *et al.*, 1981a).

4.4. Adjuvant and Vehicle Selection

The hCGβCTP37 peptide, even conjugated to DT, was not expected to be highly immunogenic in women and a variety of compounds were tested for adjuvanticity in rabbits. Conjugates were emulsified in mineral oil with one of several adjuvants. Muramyl dipeptide analogues proved superior to other adjuvants tested and were comparable to CFA in eliciting antibody responses in the rabbits. One of these, nor-muramyl dipeptide (norMDP; N-acetyl-D-glucosamine-3yl-acetyl-L-alanyl-D-isoglutamine sodium salt), was selected for further development (Stevens *et al.*, 1981b).

Likewise a variety of vehicles were tested to replace the mineral oil emulsion, which was not considered acceptable for administration to humans because of concerns regarding potential mutagenic or autoimmune phenomena that might result from continued strong immune stimulation provided by this poorly metabolized compound. A squalene/water emulsion was found to induce the most consistently high antibody response, and was selected for that reason. Preparation of a stable emulsion proved to be of the utmost importance as unstable emulsions resulted in toxicity related to premature release of vaccine components in preliminary studies.

5. PRECLINICAL VACCINE EXPERIENCE IN ANTIFERTILITY

Immunization of nonhuman primates with hCG subunit vaccines prevents or disrupts pregnancy at an early stage; such vaccines have been tested for immunogenicity and efficacy in marmosets, baboons, and bonnet monkeys. Although it is not known whether the resulting antisera would have reacted with marmoset or bonnet monkey CG, they reacted only weakly with baboon CG, at 5–10% of the level of reaction with hCG. Even so, marked antifertility effects were observed in all three species (Stevens, 1975; Hearn, 1976; Talwar *et al.*, 1986; Stevens *et al.*, 1981c). Their effectiveness in fertility regulation

Table I

Comparison of Pregnancy Rates for Female Baboons Immunized with the hCGβCTP37-DT Vaccine Conjugate or Diphtheria Toxoid Alone

Test agent	Mating cycle[a]			Total
	1	2	3	
Diphtheria toxoid				
Number mated	14	4	1	20
Number pregnant	11	3	0	14
Fertility rate (%)	73.3	75.0	0	70.0
hCGß(109–145)-DT				
Number mated	15	15	14	44
Number pregnant	0	1	1	2
Fertility rate (%)	0	6.7	7.1	4.6

[a]Matings commenced during the course of third menstrual cycle after immunization.

in spite of a low level of reactivity with native CG indicates that hCG subunits are potent immunogens for immune system activation.

The hCGβCTP37-DT vaccine was evaluated in baboons for immunogenicity and efficacy. Each of 15 female baboons received three intramuscular inoculations at 1-month intervals; each inoculum contained 1.0 mg of hCGβCTP37-DT conjugate and 1.0 mg of norMDP in a squalene/mannide monooleate/water emulsion. Fifteen female baboons

Table II

Antibody Levels Produced by Female Baboons against CTP-hCGβ, hCG, and Baboon CG (bCG) after Immunization with hCGβCTP37–Diphtheria Toxoid Conjugate

Antibody reactive to	Antibody level during menstrual cycle[a] (mol/L × 10⁻¹⁰)				
	1	2	3	4	5
CTP-hCGβ					
Mean	41.4	186	205.6	252	284.1
SD	28.6	84.1	67.5	118.7	99.7
95% CI[b]	(25.6–57.3)	(139.4–232.5)	(168.3–243.0)	(186.1–317.7)	(226.5–341.7)
hCG					
Mean	31.9	160	172.1	205.5	224.8
SD	23.9	77.7	55	108.2	89.8
95% CI[b]	(18.7–45.2)	(117.0–203.1)	(141.6–202.5)	(145.5–265.4)	(172.9–276.6)
bCG					
Mean	0.7	3.7	5.5	7.7	9
SD	0.6	3.3	3.4	4.8	4.8
95% CI[b]	(0.3–1.0)	(1.9–5.6)	(3.6–7.3)	(5.0–10.4)	(6.3–11.8)
Number of cycles	15	15	15	15	14

[a]Values were determined from serum samples obtained during the early luteal phase of each menstrual cycle.
[b]95% confidence interval.

received control injections (vaccine including unconjugated DT without peptide antigen) on the same schedule. All animals were mated with males of proven fertility until they became pregnant or for a maximum of three matings during three consecutive mating cycles beginning with the third cycle after immunization. Fourteen of twenty matings in the control group resulted in pregnancy (70%) while only 2 of 44 matings in the treated group produced pregnancies (4.6%) as seen in Table I (Stevens and Jones, 1990).

The antibodies produced by the baboons reacted with hCG at 80–90% of its level of reactivity with hCGβCTP37 and with baboon CG at less than 5% of the reactivity with hCG. Antibodies were detected 3 weeks after the first injection and the levels increased after succeeding booster immunizations. Circulating antibody levels to baboon CG were significantly lower in the two treated animals that became pregnant. Mean antibody concentrations reached during the midluteal phase of five menstrual cycles following immunization are shown in Table II. These data suggest that the antigenic sites on hCGβCTP37 are similar to those found on intact hCG and that glycosylation of the terminal peptide of hCGβ does not prevent or inhibit binding of antibodies produced using the peptide immunogen.

6. CLINICAL VACCINE EXPERIENCE IN ANTIFERTILITY

The hCGβCTP37-DT vaccine was demonstrated to be safe and immunogenic in a Phase I trial in Australia and its effectiveness as an antifertility agent is currently the subject of a Swedish Phase II trial; this work is progressing under the auspices of the World Health Organization (WHO). The clinical safety and immunogenicity data were generated by an open-label, controlled trial into which 30 surgically sterilized (tubal ligation) women were enrolled; these data have been reported previously by Jones et al. (1988). The effects of five dose levels with intramuscular inoculations delivering peptide–carrier conjugate doses of 50, 100, 200, 500, and 1000 μg were assessed in groups of six women, four of whom received the complete vaccine. Two control subjects at each dose level received only adjuvant and vehicle. The ratios (w/w) of conjugate to adjuvant and conjugate to vehicle in each inoculum were 2:1 in both cases. Two inoculations were administered to each subject separated by a 6-week interval and subjects were followed for 6 months.

The results of the clinical trial indicated that the vaccine could be safely administered to women aged 26 to 43 and that it was immunogenic. Levels and persistence of anti-hCG antibodies present in serum appeared related to vaccine dose. Calculations based on in vitro anti-hCG binding and knowledge of in vivo hCG levels present during pregnancy as well as the biological neutralizing activity of anti-hCG antibodies indicated that anti-hCG antibodies present in serum at a concentration of 0.52 nmol/L should be sufficient to disrupt pregnancy at the peri-implantation stage. This level of response was induced in all subjects receiving vaccine within 6 weeks after the initial injection and persisted for an average of 3 months. In the subset of women who received inoculations of 500 or 1000 μg conjugate, putatively effective anti-hCG antibody levels persisted for more than 6 months.

The vaccine did not appear to interfere with endocrine function in nonpregnant women. As had been seen in preclinical antifertility studies, no treatment-related interruption or prolongation of menstrual cycle was noted. Likewise, no cross-reactivity was demonstrated between any subject's serum and FSH or LH by radio-binding assay. Two subjects experienced minor reactions local to an inoculation site and one subject developed a functional ovarian cyst which resolved spontaneously. Immediate-type hypersensitivity to DT developed in one subject, reaffirming the need to test for immediate reactivity to DT skin test prior to each vaccine inoculation.

The Phase II clinical trial initiated in Sweden is designed to determine whether the level of immunity elicited by the hCGβCTP37-DT vaccine will provide fertile women with protection against pregnancy. All subjects will receive three vaccine inoculations, the first at study entry, the second 4 weeks later, and the third 6 weeks after the second. Women who respond to the vaccine with anti-hCG antibodies in circulation at levels three times the putatively effective level, will discontinue use of proven birth control methods and rely solely on the vaccine's immunizing effects against hCG for an efficacy evaluation period of up to 6 months. During this period, serum anti-hCG antibody levels will be closely monitored and subjects will be informed when they drop below the arbitrary cutoff. From 125 to 250 women will be enrolled in the trial over the next 2 years in order to achieve a targeted 750 cycles of exposure to pregnancy.

The mechanism of antifertility action is unclear; proposed mechanisms include (1) cytotoxic action mediated by antibodies on the blastocyst after zona pellucida has been shed prior to or shortly after implantation, (2) coating of blastocyst by antibodies which prevent implantation, and (3) blockade of hCG luteotropic effect on ovarian cells preventing excretion of progesterone and therefore maintenance of the pregnancy. Passive administration of antibodies specific for CG to pregnant baboons and marmosets has resulted in miscarriages (Stevens, 1975; Hearn, 1976). Because no extended intervals between menses have been observed in women, preimplantation mechanisms are considered the most likely.

7. APPLICATION TO CANCER: IMMUNOLOGICAL CONTROL OF CANCER

Clearly, there are a great many differences between a human embryo and a human tumor; even so, early human placental development has been termed a "pseudomalignant process" characterized by events also observed in malignant cancer (Ohlsson, 1989). Comparison of these two phenomena reveals similarities relevant to this research: (1) in both, selected genes are activated or reactivated to produce additional factors necessary to sustain rapid cellular proliferation, (2) both enjoy a state of immune privilege, (3) a condition of enhanced growth results, placing the host at risk, and (4) immunologic manipulation of both fertility regulation and cancer will require breaking tolerance to self antigens.

hCG is secreted by cells of the human blastocyst, but not by the fertilized ovum. Similarly, many human cancers can begin to produce and retain or secrete hCG at some point during carcinogenesis. Because of its limited expression in normal tissues, stimulation of the immune system to respond specifically to hCG may be adequate to provide benefit to men and women with cancer while avoiding immune reactivity with normal tissues; it would not be necessary for the immune system to detect subtle malignancy-induced modifications in order to differentiate abnormal from normal antigens.

A number of considerations change when designing ASI vaccines for cancer, perhaps allowing a greater latitude in developing such technologies. A higher level of toxicity will be considered tolerable since available cancer treatments tend to be quite toxic; for example, induction of a treatable autoimmune disorder in exchange for effective treatment of a malignancy may represent an attractive option for the cancer patient. In addition, a vaccine for the treatment of cancer will not be expected to be 95–100% effective in order to be considered promising. A predictable onset of responses will not be as important in a cancer immunotherapy since patients would be closely monitored and nonresponders identified early. Similarly, it will not be necessary to precisely control the duration of the immune response; a longer duration of action will always be considered superior to a shorter one when treating cancer. Convenience of treatment is not as great an issue either, since cancer patients are highly motivated to comply with the requirements of prescribed therapy. Reversibility need not be addressed and the ethical considerations affecting development of products intended to control fertility do not apply to treatments for cancer. Furthermore, activation of cell-mediated immunity (CMI) is an acceptable, even desirable, option in cancer immunotherapy. Activation of cytotoxic T lymphocytes (CTLs) resulting from appropriate immunization appears to contribute to antitumor activity in animal models (Boon *et al.*, 1992; Melief and Kast, 1992). The development of cellular immunity, as demonstrated by DTH to autologous tumor, has correlated with survival in cancer clinical trials (McCune *et al.*, 1990; Berd *et al.*, 1986).

The role of humoral immune responses in antitumor activity remains somewhat controversial. Antibody responses to cancer-associated gangliosides have been correlated with improved clinical outcome (Livingston *et al.*, 1994) and since these gangliosides are unlikely to be recognized by T cells it was suggested that antibodies were mediating the effect. Experiments using nude mice have demonstrated that hCGα-specific antibodies could be passively transferred and induce tumor necrosis of ChaGo cell xenografts (Kumar *et al.*, 1992), thus providing experimental evidence of an in vivo role for antibodies. The potential for passive antibody-mediated immunotherapy for prevention of metastases has been implied by results of monoclonal antibody trials (Riethmuller *et al.*, 1994; Sala *et al.*, 1992), but polyclonal humoral responses generated in vivo appear to be more powerful and longer-lived.

Several mechanisms have been proposed to explain the role of antibodies in immune attack on malignancies; they may elicit antibody-dependent cellular cytotoxicity (ADCC) or complement-dependent cellular cytotoxicity (CDCC), interact directly with growth factor receptors (Murthy *et al.*, 1987), evoke apoptosis (Trauth *et al.*, 1989), or directly mediate cellular lysis (Acevedo *et al.*, 1992b). Antibodies to hCG have been reported to effect complement-mediated cytotoxicity against normal and malignant trophoblasts in vitro and against early human trophoblasts cultured in diffusion chambers in the intraperitoneal cavity of rabbit (Morisada *et al.*, 1972). Numerous animal studies investigating the effect of pretreatment with vaccines incorporating hCGβ (Kellen *et al.*, 1982) or hCGβCTP37 (Acevedo *et al.*, 1987) on the viability of tumor transplants, have established an inverse correlation between levels of circulating antibodies to hCG and tumor growth; it has not been determined whether humoral or cellular immune response was responsible for the antitumor effect seen.

8. APPLICATION TO CANCER: TUMOR EXPRESSION OF CHORIONIC GONADOTROPIN

hCG is produced ectopically by a wide variety of tumor cells of both trophoblastic and nontrophoblastic origin and is considered a biochemical marker of malignancy (Alfthan *et al.*, 1992; Yuen *et al.*, 1977). Intact hCG (hCG-holo), free α subunit (hCGα), free β subunit (hCGβ), and their fragments have been detected in the serum of patients with trophoblastic or nontrophoblastic tumors and in intact biological samples obtained from cancer patients using a variety of methods and antibody reagents (Hussa, 1987a,b; Weintraub and Rosen, 1973; Blackman *et al.*, 1980; Gailani *et al.*, 1976; Rosen and Weintraub, 1974; Borkowski and Muquardt, 1979; Hattori *et al.*, 1978), as presented in Table III.

Immunohistochemical studies of tumor specimens have demonstrated that hCG is generally present more frequently on tumors than in circulation. In a study of 50 colorectal carcinomas, 20 adenomas, 8 ulcerative colitis specimens, and 10 normal mucosa specimens, Campo *et al.* (1987) found hCG-producing cells in 52% of the carcinomas but in none of the normal mucosa or benign lesion specimens. In separate studies, hCG-positive tumor cells were found in 84% of 61 human lung tumors (Wilson *et al.*, 1981) and in 53% of 92 gastric carcinomas examined (Yakeishi *et al.*, 1990). Recent research using a panel of nine monoclonal antibodies that bind to different conformational epitopes on hCG combined with quantitative flow cytometry (Acevedo *et al.*, 1992a), has demonstrated that hCG, its subunits and fragments are highly expressed on the membranes of a large percentage of live cells in all 74 established cancer cell lines examined, including 52 carcinomas, 10 sarcomas, 4 leukemias, 6 lymphomas, and 2 retinoblastomas (Acevedo *et al.*, 1992b), as presented in Table IV. A series of exhaustive studies were performed to differentially quantify independent expression levels of membrane-bound hCG, hCGα, hCGβ, and fragments on these cell lines; antibodies directed at the carboxyl-terminal peptide hCGβCTP37 were more highly reactive with the cancer cells tested, further indicating the abundance of the hCGβ subunit. Likewise, subsequent gene expression studies using specific nucleic acid probes have demonstrated that hCGβ mRNA is present in live cancer cell lines (Krichevsky *et al.*, 1995). Additional flow cytometry studies have extended this effort to live tumor cells obtained directly from surgical biopsy of tumors and demonstrate that many human cancers consistently express the β subunit of hCG preferentially over intact hCG or its α subunit (Acevedo, personal communication, 1993).

Numerous studies monitoring the presence of hCG in patient serum and the secretion of hCG by a great many cultured human tumor cell lines provide convincing evidence that hCG and its subunits, especially hCGβ, may be characteristic phenotypic markers for malignant cancer cells (Tables III and IV). Immunoreactive hCGβ has been demonstrated most commonly in the sera of patients with cancers of the biliary tract (86%), pancreas (72%), testis (67%), bladder (47%), large cell lung (35%), and cervix (30%) (Alfthan *et al.*, 1992; Marcillac *et al.*, 1992). Circulating hCG has been found in approximately 10 to 20% of patients with esophagus, small intestine, breast, and oropharyngeal cancers as well as melanomas and sarcomas (Braunstein, 1990).

Patterns of hCG expression demonstrated by immunocytochemical techniques directed at hCG-holo, hCGα, hCGβ, or fragments suggest that tumors of higher grades and/or

Table III

Ectopic Expression of hCGβ in Patients with Nontrophoblastic Cancers

Cancer	Patients positive/total studied (%)	Determination method	Source	Reference
Lung carcinoma	51/61 (84%)	Immunocytochemical	Fixed tissue[a]	Wilson et al. (1981)
Large cell solid	21/24 (88%)			
Epidermoid	15/17 (88%)			
Adenocarcinoma	12/13 (92%)			
Oat cell	0/3 (0%)			
Small cell anaplastic	2/2 (100%)			
Carcinoid	1/2 (50%)			
Gastric carcinoma	49/92 (53%)	Immunocytochemical	Fixed tissue[a]	Yakeishi et al. (1990)
Well differentiated	10/24 (42%)			
Moderately differentiated	7/16 (44%)			
Poorly differentiated	26/38 (68%)			
Undifferentiated	3/8 (37%)			
Mucinous	3/6 (50%)			
Colorectal carcinoma	26/50 (52%)	Immunocytochemical	Fixed tissue[a]	Campo et al. (1987)
Well differentiated	1/7 (14%)			
Moderately differentiated	10/26 (38%)			
Poorly differentiated	11/12 (92%)			
Mucinous	4/5 (80%)			
Pancreatic carcinoma	21/29 (72%)	Immunofluorometric	Serum	Alfthan et al. (1992)
Biliary cancer	6/7 (86%)			
Pancreatic carcinoma		Immunoradiometric	Serum	Marcillac et al. (1992)
Adenocarcinoma	13/43 (30%)			
Islet cell	2/3 (67%)			
Bladder cancer	18/38 (47%)			
Lung carcinoma				
Adenocarcinoma	3/20 (15%)			
Large cell	8/23 (35%)			
Small cell	1/27 (4%)			
Epidermoid	5/28 (18%)			
Liver carcinoma	6/52 (12%)			
Testicular carcinoma	47/70 (67%)			
Nonseminoma	41/58 (71%)			
Seminoma	6/12 (50%)			
Cervical carcinoma	8/27 (30%)			
Colorectal adenocarcinoma	1/64 (2%)			

[a]Paraffin embedded, formalin or formaldehyde fixed.

Table IV
Expression of Membrane-Bound or Secreted hCG, Its Subunits and Fragments in
Nontrophoblastic Cancer Cell Lines

Cancer	Cell line(s)	Molecules (bound or secreted)	Reference
Squamous cell	LICR-LON-HNn[a]	hCGβ (secreted)	Cowley *et al.* (1985)
Cervix	CaSki	hCGβ (secreted)	Pattillo *et al.* (1977)
	HeLa	hCGα (secreted)	Cox and Rimerman (1988)
	HeLa–fibroblast hybrid	hCGα (secreted)	Stanbridge *et al.* (1982)
Brain (glioblastoma multiforme)	CBT	hCG-holo (secreted) hCGβ (secreted)	Ruddon *et al.* (1980)
Bladder	J82, RT4, SUP, BER, 5637, RT112, DeS2	hCGβ (secreted)	Iles *et al.* (1987)
Lung			
Adenocarcinoma	A-549, A-427, SK-LU1, Calu-3, ERT-17	hCG-holo (bound) hCGα (bound) hCGβ, CTP[b](bound)	Acevedo *et al.* (1992b)
Squamous	RF-8150, Calu-1, SK-MES-1		
Small cell	NCIH69, NCIH128, NCIH146, NCIH526, SHP-77		
Breast	BT-549, MDA-MB-346, MCF7, SK-BR-3, BT-474, MDA-MB-361		
Colorectal	LS180, WiDR, Colo-320DM, Colo-205, SW-620, LoVo, T-84		
Bladder	T24, J82, SCaBER, TCCSUP, 5637, HT1376		
Prostate	DU145, LNCaPFGC, PC-3		
Lymphomas	U937, RPM-I6666, HS445, Daudi, NE-281, Jijoye		

[a]n = 1–9 squamous cell lines (8 of 9 lines positive for hCGβ).

more advanced stages, particularly with metastatic disease, are more likely to show detectable levels of hCG or hCG subunits (Acevedo, personal communication). In patients with gastric cancers, hCG expression may indicate a higher incidence of metastatic disease and a poorer prognosis (Yamaguchi *et al.*, 1989). Similar observations were made in a clinical colorectal cancer trial (Campo *et al.*, 1987) in which 79% of patients with lymph node and/or liver metastases while only 32% of patients without metastases expressed hCG on their tumors ($p < 0.01$). Others have suggested that detection of hCG in nontrophoblastic tumors may indicate the presence of a greater number of proliferative undifferentiated cells representing greater potential tumor aggression (Braunstein *et al.*, 1975; Baylin and Mendelsohn, 1980). Breast cancer patients with high levels of serum hCG have been observed to respond poorly to chemotherapy with remissions of short duration (Tormey *et al.*, 1977). Therefore, the production of hCG by nontrophoblastic tumors appears to be associated with more aggressive tumor behavior.

Derepression of the genes coding for hCG is thought to result in the ectopic production of this hormone in malignancies. While hCG synthesis in normal trophoblasts favors production of hCG-holo, synthesis control of the hCG subunits in malignant cells appears to be decoupled. As a result, some tumor cell lines preferentially secrete hCGβ, such as CaSki (Pattillo *et al.*, 1977), while others such as HeLa predominantly or exclusively produce hCGα in culture (Cox and Rimerman, 1988). Cowley and colleagues demonstrated that the hCGβ secreted by a series of human squamous carcinoma cell lines and detected by radioimmunoassay (RIA) appeared identical to placental hCGβ by high-performance liquid chromatography and in RIA dilution curves (Cowley *et al.*, 1985). However, the hCGα secreted by HeLa cells is not identical to its normal counterpart as determined by SDS-PAGE, Western blot, and tryptic peptide maps. An apparent increase in the molecular weight of the tumor-secreted hCGα compared to urinary hCGα was attributed to more sialic acid groups as a result of increased glycosylation; minor differences in peptide composition were also detected. In addition, the hCGα secreted by HeLa cells did not combine with native hCGβ under normal conditions. These data infer that posttranslational modifications may result in an altered α subunit of hCG which may account for some of the apparent overexpression of hCGβ subunit frequently observed in cancer cells.

The significance of hCG expression and secretion by tumor cells is not known; it has been suggested that hCG plays a functional role in carcinogenesis (Rivera *et al.*, 1989) and that it suppresses T-cell immune function thereby allowing cancer proliferation and local invasion (McManus *et al.*, 1976; Van Rinsum *et al.*, 1986; Strelkauska *et al.*, 1975; Oliver *et al.*, 1989; Schafer *et al.*, 1992). The recent discovery that hCG is a member of the same family of proteins as the growth factors NGF, TGF-β, and PDGF-β provides evidence supporting the suggestion that hCG functions as an autocrine factor in tumor growth (Melmed and Braunstein, 1983). Pattillo *et al.* (1977) reported establishing a cervix carcinoma cell line, CaSki, which was derived from metastatic tumor tissue removed from a woman whose serum contained hCGβ; the CaSki cell line secreted hCG and hCGβ in vitro which inhibited the migration of donor leukocytes obtained from patients with cervix cancer, but not leukocytes from heterologous cancer patients or normal individuals. Although the reasons for hCG expression in tumors and its significance remain unclear, hCG and its subunits represent a promising antigenic epitope for targeting immunotherapeutic agents.

9. APPLICATION TO CANCER: CLINICAL VACCINE EXPERIENCE

In a Phase I dose-escalation safety study, the hCGβCTP37-DT vaccine was demonstrated to be safe and effective in inducing humoral immune responses in patients with various cancers and antitumor responses in patients with advanced colon cancer. Twenty-three patients were enrolled into one of three dose levels and received three intramuscular

Table V
Phase I Clinical Trial: Study Population

Dose Level[a]	Male	Female	Total	Cancer
500/125	5	3	8	6 colon 1 stomach 1 lung
1000/250	6	2	8	5 colon 1 small bowel 2 melanoma
2000/250	5	2	7	1 colon 4 pancreas 1 lung 1 ovary

[a]Represents CTP-DT conjugate (μg)/MDP adjuvant (μg).

vaccine injections at 21-day intervals with single treatments of up to 2000 μg hCGβCPT37-DT conjugate with 250 μg adjuvant. Patients presented with a variety of malignancies and a range of tumor burden; metastatic disease confirmed by surgery and demonstration of intact immune response to one of five common recall antigens were required for study entry. Membrane-bound hCGβCTP37 was detected in 15 of 18 patient tumor specimens, determined by immunohistochemical techniques. Overall, 18 gastrointestinal cancers, 2 lung cancers, 2 melanomas, and 1 ovary cancer were treated (Table V).

The primary measure of efficacy in the study was the generation of an immune response against hCG. Antibody specific for hCG was detected in all patients, generally appearing within 7 weeks of initial vaccine treatment and persisting for more than 10 months. Although there appeared to be a trend toward dose-response, it did not reach statistical significance. Peak antibody levels of more than 30 nmol/L hCG bound were achieved and did not differ according to patient sex; parous women also produced high levels of antibody. Four to ten months after initial treatment, five patients received booster inoculations, four of whom were followed for serum antibody. Anamnestic humoral responses were observed in three of these four patients as presented in Fig. 1; booster immunizations increased serum antibody titers from 6.5- to 10-fold. Other than a shift from IgM to IgG isotype, no evidence of cellular immune involvement was detected.

Measurable tumors were not required for admission into the study, but ten patients had measurable disease prior to vaccine treatment and of these, two (20%) experienced antitumor responses as defined by the study protocol. In both cases, metastatic colon cancer tumors appeared to respond to hCGβCTP37-DT vaccine therapy by 50% or greater reduction of cross-sectional area by CT scan; in one case the lesion disappeared completely and absence of disease was subsequently confirmed by histopathology. Measurement of declining carcinoembryonic antigen (CEA) serum tumor marker after immunization provides some evidence of response in an additional two patients. Interestingly, postvaccination surgical resections of suspicious patient lesions have in several instances yielded tissue samples that were unexpectedly free of disease or largely necrotic.

The vaccine was well tolerated; only one of the 23 patients (4.3%) experienced a mild hypersensitivity reaction to DT and there was no evidence of destructive autoimmunity. It

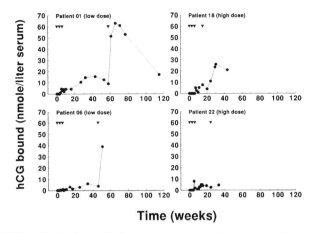

Time (weeks)

Figure 1. Anti-hCG antibody. Serum binding activity in four patients who received hCGβCTP37-DT vaccine at low (500 μg CTP:DT conjugate) or high (2000 μg) doses followed by booster immunizations of 500 μg conjugate. Assay results are reported as nmol hCG bound/L undiluted serum. Arrows indicate timing of immunizations.

may be concluded from the available data that potentially therapeutic doses of hCGβCTP37-DT vaccine are safe and effective in eliciting clinically meaningful humoral immune responses against hCG in patients with various cancers and a range of tumor burden (Triozzi *et al.*, 1993). The clinical responses to date suggest antitumor activity as documented by evidence of tumor regression in patients with advanced disease and reduction in levels of circulating tumor markers. These characteristics make hCGβCTP37-DT vaccine a promising new anticancer agent.

10. THE FUTURE OF THE hCGβCTP37-DT VACCINE

Future efforts to optimize the hCGβCTP37-DT vaccine will, unlike past development, take different directions for antifertility and cancer therapy, according to priorities and considerations unique to the clinical settings. Although both vaccines will benefit from some augmentation of the humoral response, only the cancer therapy can pursue this option without limitation. Likewise, induction of cellular immunity is desirable in the cancer vaccine, but is probably not advisable in immunological fertility regulation.

10.1. Future Development for Antifertility

Although hCGβCTP37-DT vaccine holds considerable promise for fertility regula-tion, effectiveness in preventing human pregnancy has not yet been proved, nor is the duration of its antifertility effect known at this time. Anticipating a probable need to lengthen the duration of protection, a number of design modifications are currently being evaluated. A manipulation that increases antibody presence against hCG will require more persistent presentation of the antigen. Incorporation of the vaccine immunogen into biodegradable microspheres is considered an attractive option. Microspheres are composed of polyglycolic and/or polylactic acids which entrap antigens and release them at the injection site over time (see Chapter 17). Advantages of this system include (1) a decrease in toxicity may result as well as increased immunogenicity and (2) the microspheres lend well to large-scale manufacture. Rabbits that received single immunizations with an hCG peptide immunogen incorporated into microspheres developed high-titered antibody responses that were maintained for more than 1 year (Stevens, 1992). This approach is expected to be widely applied in future vaccine formulations. Liposomes have demonstrated utility as drug carriers and have also been tested as antigen carriers in immunomodulation efforts (Alving, 1993; Allison and Gregoriadis, 1974). They can be prepared simply and can also incorporate adjuvants, markedly improving their capacity to enhance immunity (Fries *et al.*, 1992). These may be an alternative approach.

In order to reduce the incidence of hypersensitivity reactions to DT, alternative methods of inducing T-cell helper activities are being considered. Peptides representing T-cell epitopes of foreign carrier molecules that exhibit minimal levels of MHC restriction, called "promiscuous" T-cell epitopes, such as measles virus protein F, could be incorporated into the vaccine. Similar approaches have worked in rabbits, but it remains to be seen whether they will be effective in overcoming response variability related to human genetic polymorphism (Ho *et al.*, 1990). Alternatively, it may be possible to target the peptide antigen to T-helper cells by linking it to a monoclonal antibody representing a foreign T-cell ligand, and thereby increase the B-cell response while avoiding any threat of a hypersensitivity response (Carayanniotis and Barber, 1987). It has been suggested that this approach may also enhance immunogenicity by stimulating release of cytokines (Palacios, 1985). Antibody production can be induced without T-cell involvement and therefore without risk of hypersensitivity. Achieving B-cell activation without T-cell involvement may also be possible using intracellular B-cell stimulants that mimic the action of cytokines (Golding *et al.*, 1981). Preliminary studies in vivo have demonstrated that an hCG peptide with only B-cell epitopes can induce high levels of antibodies when administered together with one of these B-cell stimulants (Stevens, 1995).

The immunogenicity of the vaccine could be improved if additional epitopes were incorporated into a "cocktail" immunogen; these could be additional hCG epitopes or epitopes derived from sperm, ovum, conceptus, or other reproductive hormones (Stevens *et al.*, 1986). Finally, the induction of generalized mucosal immunity may be possible, limiting the exposure of nonreproductive systems to related toxicity, via oral administration of the vaccine immunogen in a biodegradable polymer antigen delivery system that has shown some promise in rodents (Mestecky, 1987; Eldridge *et al.*, 1989).

10.2. Future Development for Cancer

Results from a preliminary Phase I clinical trial with hCGβCTP37-DT vaccine in patients with metastatic cancer were promising, but continued effort is required to define its mechanism of action and to further augment immune responses, possibly inducing CMI. Although there is evidence that antibodies against hCG may contribute to tumor regression and efforts will be made to augment the humoral response, MHC class I molecule-restricted

CTLs are considered important to effective immunotherapy. CTL induction usually follows processing of antigen through the endogenous pathway in the endoplasmic reticulum before presentation on the cell surface. Since soluble antigens are usually processed through the MHC class II-associated pathway, protein vaccines do not generally induce specific CTL responses. However, several recent studies have indicated that soluble antigens incorporated into various oil- or lipid-based chemical formulations or with adjuvant agents such as QS-21 can promote CTL responses (Raychaudhuri and Morrow, 1993; Newman *et al.,* 1992). Live replicating vectors and nonreplicating DNA plasmids carrying genes encoding vaccine immunogens have been used to induce potent CMI activity (Moss and Flexner, 1987; Fynan *et al.,* 1993; Ulmer *et al.,* 1993; Wang *et al.,* 1993) and similar approaches may prove useful in this system. Although the risks associated with clinical application of these new technologies are unknown, it is known that they can be produced economically.

Recent advances in tumor immunology and vaccine development will allow the development of a new generation of cancer immunotherapeutic vaccines. Our greater understanding of the interplay of immune events involved in active specific immunotherapy will reveal new possibilities toward effective treatment and prevention of cancer. Nevertheless, small steps have been taken in developing strategies that target appropriate self proteins common to fertility regulation and cancer. hCGβCTP37-DT vaccine and similar cancer vaccine approaches can be expected to provide benefit by controlling established cancers, eliminating residual disease postsurgery, and perhaps ultimately preventing cancer metastasis with minimal toxicity and meaningful improvement in patient quality of life.

ACKNOWLEDGMENT

Thanks to C. Van Patten Youngman for editorial assistance.

REFERENCES

Acevedo, H. F., Raikow, R. B., Powell, J. E., and Stevens, V. C., 1987, Effects of immunization against human chorionic gonadotropin on the growth of transplanted Lewis lung carcinoma and spontaneous mammary adenocarcinoma in mice, *Cancer Detect. Prevent. Suppl.* **1**:477–486.

Acevedo, H. F., Krichevsky, A., Campbell-Acevedo, E. A., Galyon, J. C., Buffo, M. J., and Hartsock, R. J., 1992a, Flow cytometry method for the analysis of membrane-associated human chorionic gonadotropin, its subunits, and fragments on human cancer cells, *Cancer* **69**:1818–1828.

Acevedo, H. F., Krichevsky, A., Campbell-Acevedo, E. A., Galyon, J. C., Buffo, M. J., and Hartsock, R. J., 1992b, Expression of membrane-associated human chorionic gonadotropin, its subunits, and fragments by cultured human cancer cells, *Cancer* **69**:1829–1842.

Alfthan, H., Haglund, C., Roberts, P., and Stenman, U., 1992, Elevation of free β subunit of human choriogonadotropin and core β fragment of human choriogonadotropin in the serum and urine of patients with malignant pancreatic and biliary disease, *Cancer Res.* **52**:4628–4633.

Allison, A. C., and Gregoriadis, G., 1974, Liposomes as immunological adjuvants, *Nature* **252**:252–255.

Alving, C. R., 1993, The use of liposomes as vaccine carriers, *J. Immunol. Methods* **140**:1–13.

Baylin, S. B., and Mendelsohn, G., 1980, Ectopic (inappropriate) hormone production by tumors: Mechanisms involved and the biological and clinical implications, *Endocr. Rev.* **1**:45–77.

Berd, D., Maguire, H. C., Jr., and Mastrangelo, M. J., 1986, Induction of cell-mediated immunity to autologous melanoma cells and regression of metastases after treatment with melanoma cell vaccine preceded by cyclophosphamide, *Cancer Res.* **46**:2572–2577.

Berger, P., Klieber, R., Panmoung, W., Madersbacher, S., Wolf, H., and Wick, G., 1990, Monoclonal antibodies against the free subunits of human chorionic gonadotropin, *J. Endocrinol.* **125**:301–309.

Blackman, M. R., Weintraub, B. D., Rosen, S. W., Kourides, I. A., Steinwascher, K., and Gail, M. H., 1980, Human placental and pituitary glycoprotein hormones and their subunits as tumor markers: A quantitative assessment, *J. Natl. Cancer Inst.* **65**:81–93.

Boettcher, B., 1979, Immunity to spermatozoa, *Clin. Obstet. Gynecol.* **6**:385–402.

Boon, T., De Plaen, E., Lurquin, C., Van den Eynde, B., van der Bruggen, P., Traversari, C., Amar-Costesec, A., and Van Pel, A., 1992, Identification of tumour rejection antigens recognized by T lymphocytes, *Cancer Surv.* **13**:23–37.

Borkowski, A., and Muquardt, C., 1979, Human chorionic gonadotropin in the plasma of normal nonpregnant subjects, *N. Engl. J. Med.* **301**:298–302.

Braunstein, G. D., 1990, Placental proteins as tumor markers, in: *Immunodiagnosis of Cancer* (R. B. Herberman and D. W. Mercer, eds.), Dekker, New York, pp. 673–701.

Braunstein, G. D., Rasor, J., and Wade, M. E., 1975, Presence in normal human testes of a chorionic-gonadotropin-like substance distinct from human luteinizing hormone, *N. Engl. J. Med.* **301**:324–326.

Campo, E., Palacin, A., Benasco, C., Quesada, E., and Cardesa, A., 1987, Human chorionic gonadotropin in colorectal carcinoma: An immunohistochemical study, *Cancer* **59**:1611–1616.

Carayanniotis, G., and Barber, B. H., 1987, Adjuvant-free IgG responses induced with antigen coupled to antibodies against class II MHC, *Nature* **327**:59–61.

Cowley, G., Smith, J. A., Ellison, M., and Gusterson, B., 1985, Production of β-human chorionic gonadotrophin by human squamous carcinoma cell lines, *Int. J. Cancer* **35**:575–579.

Cox, G. S., and Rimerman, R. A., 1988, Purification and characterization of the glycoprotein hormone α-subunit-like material secreted by HeLa cells, *Biochemistry* **27**:6474–6487.

Dirnhofer, S., Klieber, R., De Leeuw, R., Bidart, J.-M., Merz, W. E., Wick, G., and Berger, P., 1993, Functional and immunological relevance of the COOH-terminal extension of human chorionic gonadotropin β: Implications for the WHO birth control vaccine, *FASEB J.* **7**:1381–1385.

Eldridge, J. H., Gilley, R. M., Staas, J. K., Moldoveanu, Z., Meulbroek, J. A., and Tice, T. R., 1989, Biodegradable microspheres: Vaccine delivery system for oral immunization, *Curr. Top. Microbiol. Immunol.* **146**:59–66.

Fries, L. F., Gordon, D. M., Richards, R. I., Egan, J. E., Hollingdale, M. R., Gross, M., and Alving, C. R., 1992, Liposomal malaria vaccine in humans: A safe and potent adjuvant strategy, *Proc. Natl. Acad. Sci. USA* **89**:358–362.

Fynan, E. F., Webster, R. G., Fuller, D. H., Haynes, J. R., Santoro, J. C., and Robinson, H. L., 1993, DNA vaccines: Protective immunizations by parenteral, mucosal, and gene-gun inoculations. *Proc. Natl. Acad. Sci. USA* **90**:11478–11482.

Gailani, S., Chu, T. M., Nussbaum, A., Ostrander, M., and Christoff, N., 1976, Human chorionic gonadotrophins (hCG) in nontrophoblastic neoplasms, *Cancer* **38**:1684–1686.

Glass, R. H., and Mroueh, A., 1967, Pregnancy in the rabbit following immunization with human chorionic gonadotropin, *Am. J. Obstet. Gynecol.* **97**:1082–1084.

Golding, B., Chan, S. P., Golding, H., Jones, R. E., Pratt, K. L., Burger, D. R., and Rittenberg, M. B., 1981, Human lymphocytes can generate thymus-independent as well as thymus-dependent anti-hapten plaque-forming cell responses in vitro, *J. Immunol.* **127**:220–224.

Hattori, M., Fukase, M., Yoshimi, H., Matsukura, S., and Imura, H., 1978, Ectopic production of human chorionic gonadotropin in malignant tumors, *Cancer* **42**:2328–2333.

Hearn, J. P., 1976, Immunization against pregnancy, *Proc. R. Soc. London Ser. B* **195**:149–160.

Ho, P. C., Mutch, D. A., Winkel, K. D., Saul, A., Jones, G. L., Doran, T. J., and Rzepczyk, C. M., 1990, Identification of two promiscuous T cell epitopes from tetanus toxin, *Eur. J. Immunol.* **20**:477–483.

Hussa, R. O., 1980, Biosynthesis of human chorionic gonadotropin, *Endocrin. Rev.* **1**:268–294.

Hussa, R. O., 1987a, Clinical applications of hCG tests: Tumors, in: *The Clinical Marker hCG* (R. O. Hussa, ed.), Praeger, New York, pp. 119–136.

Hussa, R. O., 1987b, Subunits of hCG, in: *The Clinical Marker hCG* (R. O. Hussa, ed.), Praeger, New York, pp. 161–178.

Iles, R. K., Oliver, R. T. D., Kitau, M., Walker, C., and Chard, T., 1987, In vitro secretion of human chorionic gonadotropin by bladder tumor cells, *Br. J. Cancer* **55**:623–626.

Jones, W. R., Bradley, J., Judd, S. J., Denholm, E. H., Ing, R. M. Y., Mueller, U. W., Powell, J., Griffin, P. D., and Stevens, V. C., 1988, Phase I clinical trial of a World Health Organization birth control vaccine, *Lancet* **1**:1295–1298.

Kellen, J. A., Kolin, A., Mirakian, A., and Acevedo, H. F., 1982, Effect of antibodies to choriogonadotropin on malignant growth: II Solid transplantable rat tumors, *Cancer Immunol. Immunother.* **13**:2–4.

Krichevsky, A., Campbell-Acevedo, E. A., Tong, J. Y., and Acevedo, H. F., 1995, Immunological detection of membrane-associated human luteinizing hormone correlates with gene expression in cultured human cancer and fetal cells, *Endocrinology* **136**:1034–1039.

Kumar, S., Talwar, G. P., and Biswas, D. K., 1992, Necrosis and inhibition of growth of human lung tumor by anti-α-human chorionic gonadotropin antibody, *J. Natl. Cancer Inst.* **84**:42–47.

Lapthorn, A. J., Harris, D. C., Littlejohn, A., Lustbader, J. W., Canfield, R. E., Machin, K. J., Morgan, F. J., and Isaacs, N. W., 1994, Crystal structure of human chorionic gonadotropin, *Nature* **369**:455–461.

Lee, A. C., Powell, J. E., Tregear, G. W., Niall, H. D., and Stevens, V. C., 1980, A method for preparing β-hCG COOH peptide–carrier conjugates of predictable composition, *Mol. Immunol.* **17**:749–756.

Livingston, P. O., Wong, Y.C., Adluri, S., Tao, Y., Padavan, M., Parente, R., Hanlon, C., Jones-Calves, M., Helling, F., Ritter, G., Oettgen, H. F., and Old, L. J., 1994, Improved survival in stage III melanoma patients with GM2 antibodies: A randomized trial of adjuvant vaccine with GM2 ganglioside, *J. Clin. Oncol.* **12**:1036–1044.

McCune, C. S., O'Donnell, R. W., Mariquis, D. M., and Sahasrabudhe, D. M., 1990, Renal cell carcinoma treated by vaccines for active specific immunotherapy: Correlation of survival with skin testing by autologous tumor cells, *Cancer Immunol. Immunother.* **32**:62–66.

McManus, L. M., Naughton, N. A., and Martinez-Hernandez, A., 1976, Human chorionic gonadotropin in human neoplastic cells, *Cancer Res.* **36**:3476–3481.

Marcillac, I., Troalen, F., Bidart, J. M., Ghillan, P., Ribrag, V., Escudier, B., Malassagne, B., Droz, J. P., Lhommé, C., Rougier, P., Duvillard, P., Prade, M., Lugagne, P. M., Richard, F., Poynard, T., Bohuon, C., Wands, J., and Bellet D., 1992, Free human chorionic gonadotropin β subunit in gonadal and nongonadal neoplasms, *Cancer Res.* **52**:3901–3907.

Melief, C. J., and Kast, W. M., 1992, Lessons from T cell responses to virus induced tumors for cancer eradication in general, *Cancer Surv.* **13**:81–99.

Melmed, S., and Braunstein, G. D., 1983, Human chorionic gonadotropin stimulates proliferation of Nb 2 rat lymphoma cells, *J. Clin. Endocrinol. Metab.* **56**:1068–1070.

Mestecky, J., 1987, The common mucosal immune system and current strategies for induction of immune responses in external secretions, *J. Clin. Immunol.* **7**:265–276.

Morisada, M., Yamaguchi, H., and Iizuka, R., 1972, Toxic action of anti-hCG antibody to human trophoblast, *Int. J. Fertil.* **17**:65–71.

Moss, B., and Flexner, C., 1987, Vaccinia virus expressing vectors, *Annu. Rev. Immunol.* **5**:305–324.

Murthy, U., Basu, A., Rodeck, U., Herlyn, M., Ross, A., and Das, M., 1987, Domain-specificity and antagonistic properties of a new monoclonal antibody to the EGF receptor, *Arch. Biochem. Biophys.* **252**:549–560.

Naylor, S. L., Chin, W. W., Goodman, H. M., Lalley, P. A., Grzeshik, K. H., and Sakaguchi, A. Y., 1983, Chromosomal assignment of genes encoding the α and β subunits of gonadotropin hormones in man and mouse, *Somatic Cell Genet.* **9**:757–770.

Newman, M. J., Wu, J.-Y., Gardner, H., Munroe, K. J., Leombruno, D., Kensil, C. R., and Coughlin, R. T., 1992, Saponin adjuvant induction of ovalbumin-specific CD8[+] cytotoxic T lymphocyte responses, *J. Immunol.* **148**:2357–2362.

Ohlsson, R., 1989, Growth factors, protooncogenes and human placental development, *Cell. Differ. Dev.* **28**:1–16.

Oliver, R. T. D., Nouri, A. M. E., Crosby, D., Iles, R. L., Navarette, C., Martin, J., Bodmer, W., and Festenstein, H., 1989, Biological significance of beta hCG, HLA and other membrane antigen expression on bladder tumors and their relationship to tumour infiltrating lymphocytes (TIL), *J. Immunogenet.* **16**:381–390.

Osterguard, E., 1942, *Antigonadotropic Substances*, Munksgaard, Copenhagen.

Palacios, R., 1985, Monoclonal antibodies against human Ia antigens stimulate monocytes to secrete interleukin 1, *Proc. Natl. Acad. Sci. USA* **82**:6652–6656.

Paterson, M., Koothan, P. T., Morris, K. D., O'Byrne, K. T., Braude, P., Williams, A., and Aitken, R. J., 1992, Analysis of the contraceptive potential of antibodies against native and deglycosylated porcine ZP3 in vivo and in vitro, *Biol. Reprod.* **46**:523–534.

Pattillo, R. O., Hussa, R. O., Story, M. T., Ruckert, A. C. F., Shalaby, M. R., and Mattingly, R. F., 1977, Tumor antigen and human chorionic gonadotropin in CaSki cells: A new epidermoid cervical cancer cell line, *Science* **196**:1456–1458.

Puett, D., 1986, Human choriogonadotropin, *Bioassays* **4**:70–75.

Puett, D., Ryan, R. J., and Stevens, V. C., 1982, Circular dichroic and immunological properties of human choriogonadotropin-carboxyl terminal peptides, *Int. J. Peptide Protein Res.* **19**:506–513.

Raychaudhuri, S., and Morrow, W. J. W., 1993, Can soluble antigen induce CD8$^+$ cytotoxic T cell responses? A paradox revisted, *Immunol. Today* **14**:344–348.

Riethmuller, G., Schneider-Gadicke, E., Schlimok, G., Schmiegel, W., Raab, R., Hoffken, K., Gruber, R., Pichlmaier, H., Hirche, H., Pichlmayr, R., Buggisch, P., Witte, J., and the German Cancer Aid 17-1A Study Group, 1994, Randomised trial of monoclonal antibody for adjuvant therapy of resected Dukes' C colorectal carcinoma, *Lancet* **343**:1177–1183.

Rivera, R. T., Pasion, S. G., Wong, D. T. W., Fei, Y., and Biswas, D. K., 1989, Loss of tumorigenic potential by human lung tumor cells in the presence of antisense RNA specific to the ectopically synthesized alpha subunit of human chorionic gonadotropin, *J. Cell Biol.* **108**:2423–2434.

Rosen, S. W., and Weintraub, B. D., 1974, Ectopic production of the isolated alpha subunit of the glycoprotein hormones: A quantitative marker in certain cases of cancer, *N. Engl. J. Med.* **290**:1441–1447.

Ruddon, R. W., Bryan, A. H., Meade-Cobun, K. S., and Pollack, V. A., 1980, Production of human chorionic gonadotropin and its subunits by human tumor growing in nude mice, *Cancer Res.* **40**:4007–4012.

Sacco, A. G., 1979, Inhibition of fertility in mice by passive immunization with antibodies to isolated zonae pellucidae, *J. Reprod. Fertil.* **56**:533–537.

Sala, A., Gresser, I., Chassoux, D., Maury, C., Santodonato, L., Eid, P., Maunoury, M. T., Barca, S., Cianfrigilia, M., and Belardelli, F., 1992, Inhibition of Freind leukemia cell visceral metastases by a new monoclonal antibody and role of the immune system of the host in its action, *Cancer Res.* **52**:2880–2889.

Schafer, A., Pauli, G., Friedmann, W., and Dudenhausen, J.W., 1992, Human choriogonadotropin (hCG) and placental lactogen (hPL) inhibit interleukin-2 (IL-2) and increase interleukin-1β (IL-1β), -6 (IL-6) and tumor necrosis factor α (TNF-α) expression in monocyte cell cultures, *J. Perinat. Med.* **20**:233–240.

Stanbridge, E. J., Rosen, S. W., and Sussman, H. H., 1982, Expression of the α subunit of human chorionic gonadotropin is specifically correlated with tumorigenic expression in human cell hybrids, *Proc. Natl. Acad. Sci. USA* **79**:6242–6245.

Stevens, V. C., 1973, Immunization of female baboons with hapten-coupled gonadotropins, *Obstet. Gynecol.* **42**:496–506.

Stevens, V. C., 1975, Fertility control through active immunization using placenta proteins, *Acta Endocrinol. Suppl.* **194**:357–375.

Stevens, V. C., 1976, Actions of antisera to hCG-β: In vitro and in vivo assessment, in: *Proceedings of the Fifth International Congress of Endocrinology* (V. H. T. James, ed.), Excerpta Medica, Amsterdam, pp. 379–384.

Stevens, V. C., 1986, Development of a vaccine against human chorionic gonadotropin using a synthetic peptide as the immunogen, in: *Proceedings of the Third International Congress of Reproductive Immunology* (D. A. Clark and B. A. Croy, eds.), Elsevier, Amsterdam, pp. 162–169.

Stevens, V. C., 1992, Future perspectives for vaccine development, *Scand. J. Immunol.* **36** (Suppl. 11):137–143.

Stevens, V. C., 1993, Vaccine delivery systems: Potential methods for use in antifertility vaccines, *Am. J. Reprod. Immunol.* **29**:176–188.

Stevens, V. C., 1995, Prospects for antifertility vaccines, in: *Immunocontraception*, Serono Symposium Series (in press).

Stevens, V. C., and Crystle, C. D., 1973, Effects of immunization with hapten-coupled hCG on the human menstrual cycle, *Obstet. Gynecol.* **42**:485–495.

Stevens, V. C., and Jones, W. R., 1990, Vaccines to prevent pregnancy, in: *New Generation Vaccines* (G. C. Woodrow and M. M. Levine, eds.), Dekker, New York, pp. 879–990.

Stevens, V. C., Cinader, B., Powell, J. E., Lee, A. C., and Koh, S. W., 1981a, Preparation and formulation of a hCG antifertility vaccine: Selection of peptide immunogen, *Am. J. Reprod. Immunol.* **6**:307–314.

Stevens, V. C., Cinader, B., Powell, J. E., Lee, A. C., and Koh, S. W., 1981b, Preparation and formulation of a hCG antifertility vaccine: Selection of adjuvant and vehicle, *Am. J. Reprod. Immunol.* **6**:315–321.

Stevens, V. C., Powell, J. E., Lee, A. C., and Griffin, D., 1981c, Antifertility effects of immunization of female baboons with C-terminal peptides of the β-subunit of human chorionic gonadotropin, *Fertil. Steril.* **36**:98–105.

Stevens, V. C., Chou, W., Powell, J. E., Lee, A. C., and Smoot, J., 1986, The identification of peptide sequences of human chorionic gonadotropin containing a conformational epitope, *Immunol. Lett.* **12**:11–18.

Strelkauska, A. J., Wilson, B. S., Dray, S., and Dodson, M., 1975, Inversion of levels of human T- and B-cells in early pregnancy, *Nature* **258**:331–332.

Talwar, G. P., Singh, O., Singh, V., Rao, D. N., Sharma, N. C., Das, C., and Rao, L. V., 1986, Enhancement of antigonadotropin response to the beta-subunit of ovine luteinizing hormone by carrier conjugation and combination with the beta-subunit of human chorionic gonadotropin, *Fertil. Steril.* **46**:120–126.

Tormey, D. C., Waalkes, T. P., and Simon, R. M., 1977, Biological marker in breast carcinoma: II Clinical correlation with human chorionic gonadotropin, *Cancer* **39**:2391–2396.

Trauth, B. C., Klas, C., Peters, A. M. J., Matzku, S., Moller, P., Falk, W., Debatin, K.-M., and Krammer, P. H., 1989, Monoclonal antibody-mediated tumor regression by induction of apoptosis, *Science* **245**:301–304.

Triozzi, P. T., Martin, E. W., Gochnour, D., and Aldrich, W., 1993, Phase Ib trial of a synthetic β human chorionic gonadotropin vaccine in patients with metastatic cancer, *Ann. N.Y. Acad. Sci.* **690**:358–359.

Ulmer, J. B., Donnelly, J. J., Parker, S. E., Rhodes, G. H., Felgner, P. L., Dwarki, V. J., Stanislaw, H., Gromkowski, R., Deck, R., DeWitt, C. M., Friedman, A., Hawe, L. A., Leander, K. R., Martinez, D., Perry, H. C., Shiver, J. W., Montgomery, D. L., and Liu, M. A., 1993, Heterologous protection against influenza by injection of DNA encoding a viral protein, *Science* **259**:1745–1749.

Van Rinsum, J., Lou, A. S., Van Rooy, H., and Van Den Eunden, D. H., 1986, Specific inhibition of human natural killer cell-mediated cytotoxicity by sialic acid and sialo-oligosaccharides, *Int. J. Cancer* **38**:915–922.

Walton, N. K., 1993a, World hunger: Humanitarian dilemma of the 1990s, *Geo. Global Iss. Q.* **3**(2):16–18.

Walton, N. K., 1993b, Land degradation at odds with earth's growing population, *Geo. Global Iss. Q.* **3**:10–11.

Wang, B., Ugen, K. E., Srikantan, V., Agadjanyan, M., Dang, K., Refaeli, Y., Sato, A. I., Boyer, J., Williams, W. V., and Weiner, D. B., 1993, Gene inoculation induces immune responses against human immunodeficiency virus type I, *Proc. Natl. Acad. Sci. USA* **90**:4156–4160.

Weintraub, B. D., and Rosen, W. S., 1973, Ectopic production of the isolated beta subunit of human chorionic gonadotropin, *J. Clin. Invest.* **52**:3135–3142.

Wilson, T. S., McDowell, E. M., McIntire, R., and Trump, B. F., 1981, Elaboration of human chorionic gonadotropin by lung tumors, *Arch. Pathol. Lab. Med.* **105**:169–173.

Wu, H., Lustbader, J. W., Liu, Y., Canfield, R. E., and Hendrickson, W. A., 1994, Structure of human chorionic gonadotropin at 2.6 angstrom resolution from MAD analysis of the selenomethionyl protein, *Structure* **2**:545–556.

Yakeishi, Y., Masaki, M., and Enjoji, M., 1990, Distribution of β-human chorionic gonadotropin-positive cells in non cancerous gastric mucosa and in malignant gastric tumors, *Cancer* **66**:695–701.

Yamaguchi, A., Ihida, T., Nishimura, G., Kumaki, T., Katch, M., Kosaka, T., Yonemura, Y., and Miyazaki, I., 1989, Human chorionic gonadotropin in colorectal cancer and its relationship to prognosis, *Br. J. Cancer* **60**:382–384.

Yuen, B. H., Cannon, W., Benedet, J. L., and Boyes, D. A., 1977, Plasma β-subunit human chorionic gonadotropin assay in molar pregnancy and choriocarcinoma, *Am. J. Obstet. Gynecol.* **127**:711–712.

Index